DIAGNOSTIC PATHOLOGY

Intraoperative Consultation

SECOND EDITION

LESTER

CASSARINO • CHIRIEAC • CORNELL • COX • DILLON • FOLKERTH
FRISHBERG • HARRISON • JO • KO • KRANE • KRASNOZHEN-RATUSH • LINDBERG • MASON
NOSÉ • QUICK • SNUDERL • SRIVASTAVA • THOMPSON

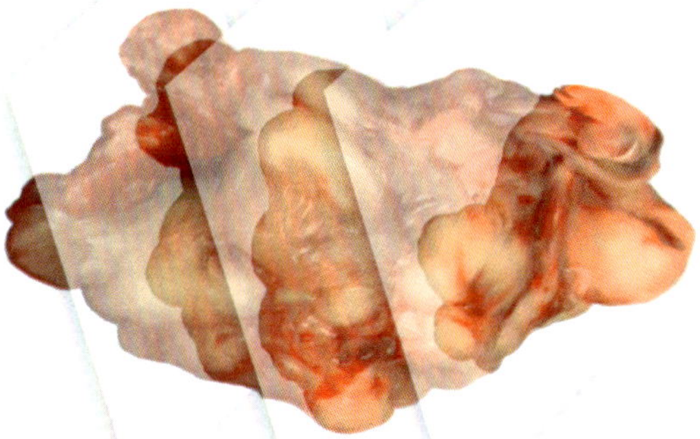

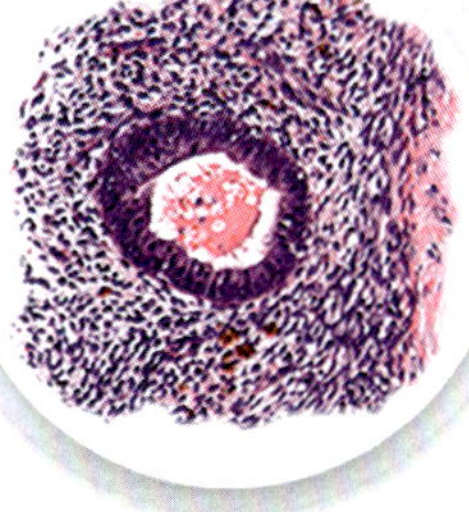

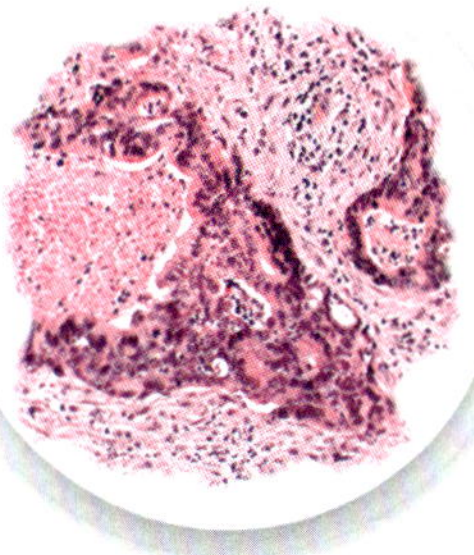

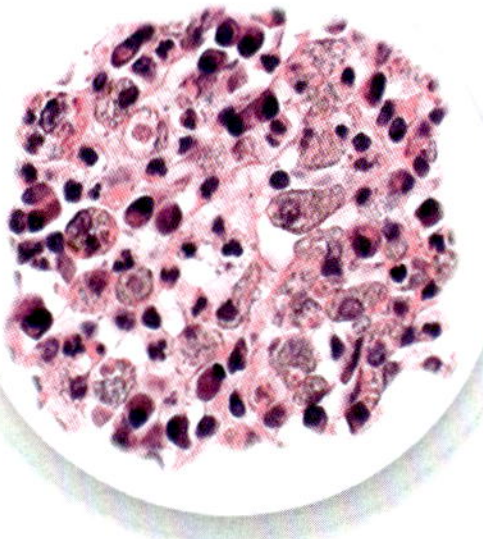

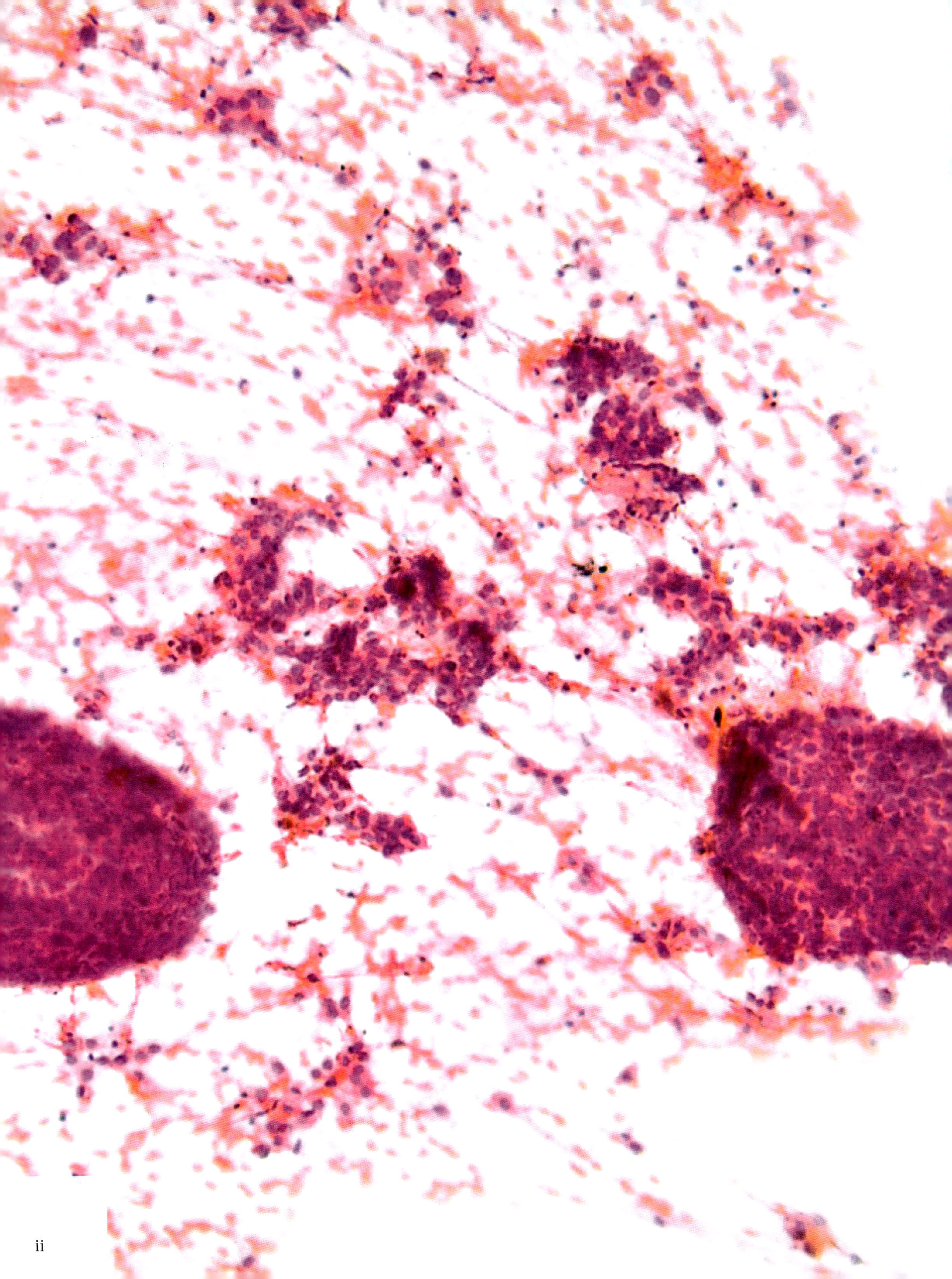

DIAGNOSTIC PATHOLOGY

Intraoperative Consultation

SECOND EDITION

Susan C. Lester, MD, PhD

Chief
Breast Pathology Services
Brigham and Women's Hospital
Assistant Professor
Harvard Medical School
Boston, Massachusetts

ELSEVIER

1600 John F. Kennedy Blvd.
Ste 1800
Philadelphia, PA 19103-2899

DIAGNOSTIC PATHOLOGY: INTRAOPERATIVE CONSULTATION, SECOND EDITION

ISBN: **978-0-323-57019-0**

Notices

Knowledge and best practice in this field are constantly changing. As new research and experience broaden our understanding, changes in research methods, professional practices, or medical treatment may become necessary.

Practitioners and researchers must always rely on their own experience and knowledge in evaluating and using any information, methods, compounds, or experiments described herein. In using such information or methods they should be mindful of their own safety and the safety of others, including parties for whom they have a professional responsibility.

With respect to any drug or pharmaceutical products identified, readers are advised to check the most current information provided (i) on procedures featured or (ii) by the manufacturer of each product to be administered, to verify the recommended dose or formula, the method and duration of administration, and contraindications. It is the responsibility of practitioners, relying on their own experience and knowledge of their patients, to make diagnoses, to determine dosages and the best treatment for each individual patient, and to take all appropriate safety precautions.

To the fullest extent of the law, neither the Publisher nor the authors, contributors, or editors, assume any liability for any injury and/or damage to persons or property as a matter of products liability, negligence or otherwise, or from any use or operation of any methods, products, instructions, or ideas contained in the material herein.

Publisher Cataloging-in-Publication Data

Names: Lester, Susan Carole.
Title: Diagnostic pathology. Intraoperative consultation / [edited by] Susan C. Lester.
Other titles: Intraoperative consultation.
Description: Second edition. | Salt Lake City, UT : Elsevier, Inc., [2018] | Includes bibliographical references and index.
Identifiers: ISBN 978-0-323-57019-0
Subjects: LCSH: Pathology, Surgical--Handbooks, manuals, etc. | Medical consultation--Handbooks, manuals, etc. | MESH: Pathology, Surgial--Atlases. | Cytodiagnosis--methods--Atlases. | Frozen Sections--methods--Atlases. | Intraoperative Period--Atlases.
Classification: LCC RD57.D515 2018 | NLM WO 517 | DDC 617.075--dc23

International Standard Book Number: 978-0-323-57019-0

Cover Designer: Tom M. Olson, BA

Printed in Canada by Friesens, Altona, Manitoba, Canada

Last digit is the print number: 9 8 7 6 5 4 3 2 1

Dedication

This book is dedicated to all the pathologists whose hearts race when alerted by the frozen section pager, to the support staff in the intraoperative consultation room who are always there to assist them, to the surgeons who request essential information to help guide their operations, and most of all, to the patients who have entrusted their care into our hands.

SCL

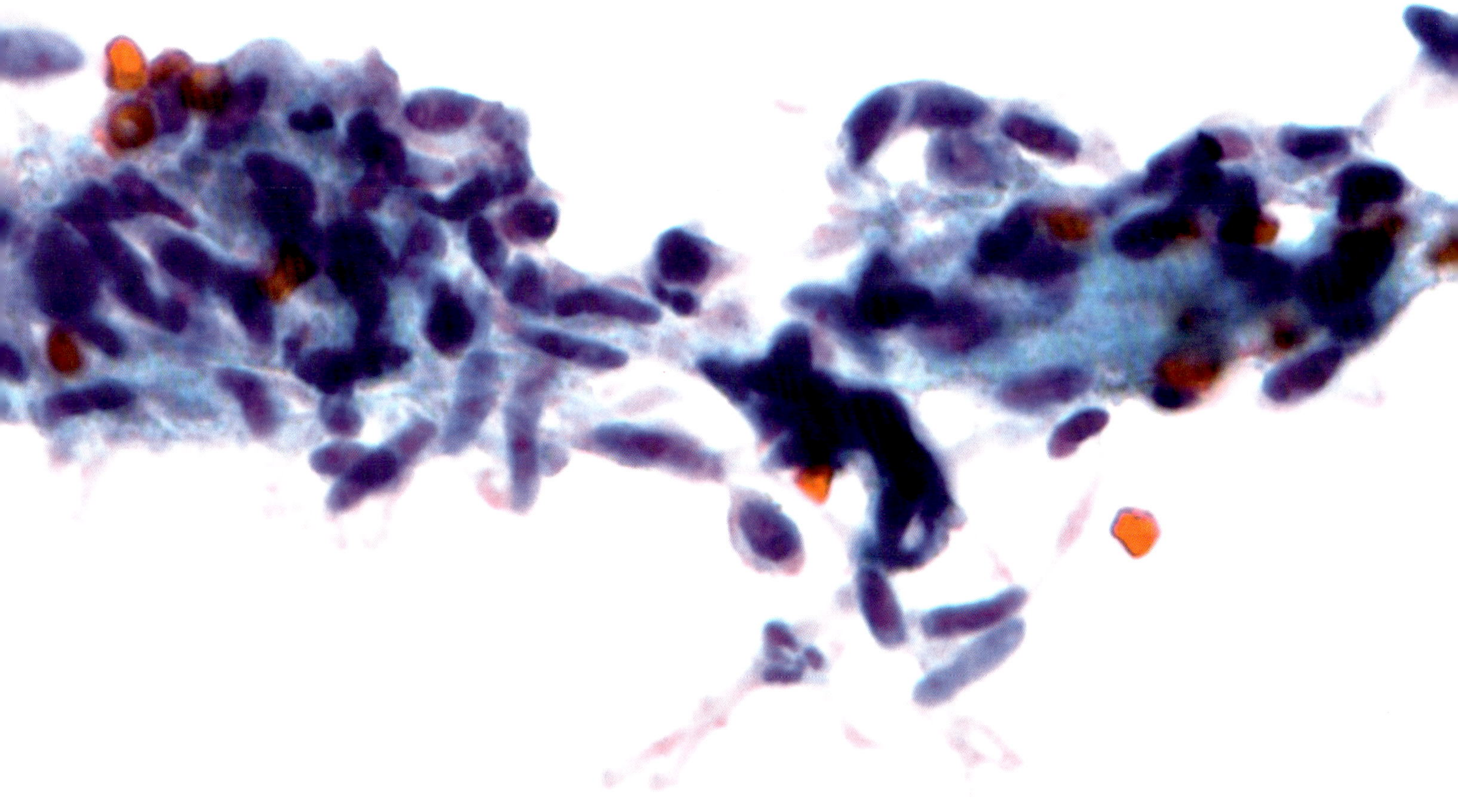

Contributing Authors

David Cassarino, MD, PhD
Consultant Dermatopathologist and Staff Pathologist
Southern California Permanente Medical Group
Los Angeles, California
Clinical Professor
Department of Dermatology
University of California, Irvine
Irvine, California

Lucian R. Chirieac, MD
Associate Pathologist
Brigham and Women's Hospital
Associate Professor of Pathology
Harvard Medical School
Boston, Massachusetts

Lynn D. Cornell, MD
Consultant
Division of Anatomic Pathology
Associate Professor of Laboratory Medicine
and Pathology
Mayo Clinic College of Medicine and Science
Rochester, Minnesota

Roni Michelle Cox, MD
Cleveland Clinic
Cleveland, Ohio

Deborah A. Dillon, MD
Director, Breast Tumor Bank and Clinical
Trials Laboratory
Dana Farber Cancer Institute
Associate Pathologist
Brigham and Women's Hospital
Assistant Professor of Pathology
Harvard Medical School
Boston, Massachusetts

Rebecca D. Folkerth, MD
Department of Forensic Medicine
New York University School of Medicine
New York, New York

David P. Frishberg, MD
Professor of Pathology and Laboratory Medicine
Cedars-Sinai Medical Center
Los Angeles, California
Associate Clinical Professor of Pathology
George Washington University School of
Medicine and Health Sciences
Washington, D.C.

Beth T. Harrison, MD
Associate Pathologist
Brigham and Women's Hospital
Instructor in Pathology
Harvard Medical School
Boston, Massachusetts

Vickie Y. Jo, MD
Pathologist
Brigham and Women's Hospital
Assistant Professor of Pathology
Harvard Medical School
Boston, Massachusetts

Christine J. Ko, MD
Professor of Dermatology and Pathology
Yale University School of Medicine
New Haven, Connecticut

Jeffrey F. Krane, MD, PhD
Associate Director, Cytology Division
Chief, Head and Neck Pathology Service
Brigham and Women's Hospital
Associate Professor of Pathology
Harvard Medical School
Boston, Massachusetts

Olga Krasnozhen-Ratush, MD
Neuropathology Fellow
Department of Pathology
NYU Langone Medical Center
New York, New York

Matthew R. Lindberg, MD
Assistant Professor
Department of Pathology
University of Arkansas for Medical Sciences
Little Rock, Arkansas

Emily F. Mason, MD, PhD
Assistant Professor of Pathology
Vanderbilt University
Nashville, Tennessee

Vania Nosé, MD, PhD
Associate Chief of Pathology
Director of Anatomic and Molecular Pathology
Massachusetts General Hospital
Professor of Pathology
Harvard Medical School
Boston, Massachusetts

Charles Matthew Quick, MD
Associate Professor of Pathology
Director of Gynecologic Pathology
Department of Pathology
University of Arkansas for Medical Sciences
Little Rock, Arkansas

Matija Snuderl, MD
Assistant Professor of Pathology
Director of Molecular Pathology and Diagnostics
NYU Langone Medical Center
New York, New York

Amitabh Srivastava, MD
Associate Professor of Pathology
Harvard Medical School
Associate Director, Surgical Pathology
Director, Surgical Pathology Fellowship Program
Brigham and Women's Hospital
Boston, Massachusetts

Karen S. Thompson, MD
Professor and Interim Chair, Department of Pathology
John A. Burns School of Medicine
University of Hawaii
Pan Pacific Pathologists, Clinical Laboratories of Hawaii
Kapiolani Medical Center for Women and Children
Honolulu, Hawaii

Additional Contributing Authors

Stefan Kraft, MD

Rolf Pfannl, MD

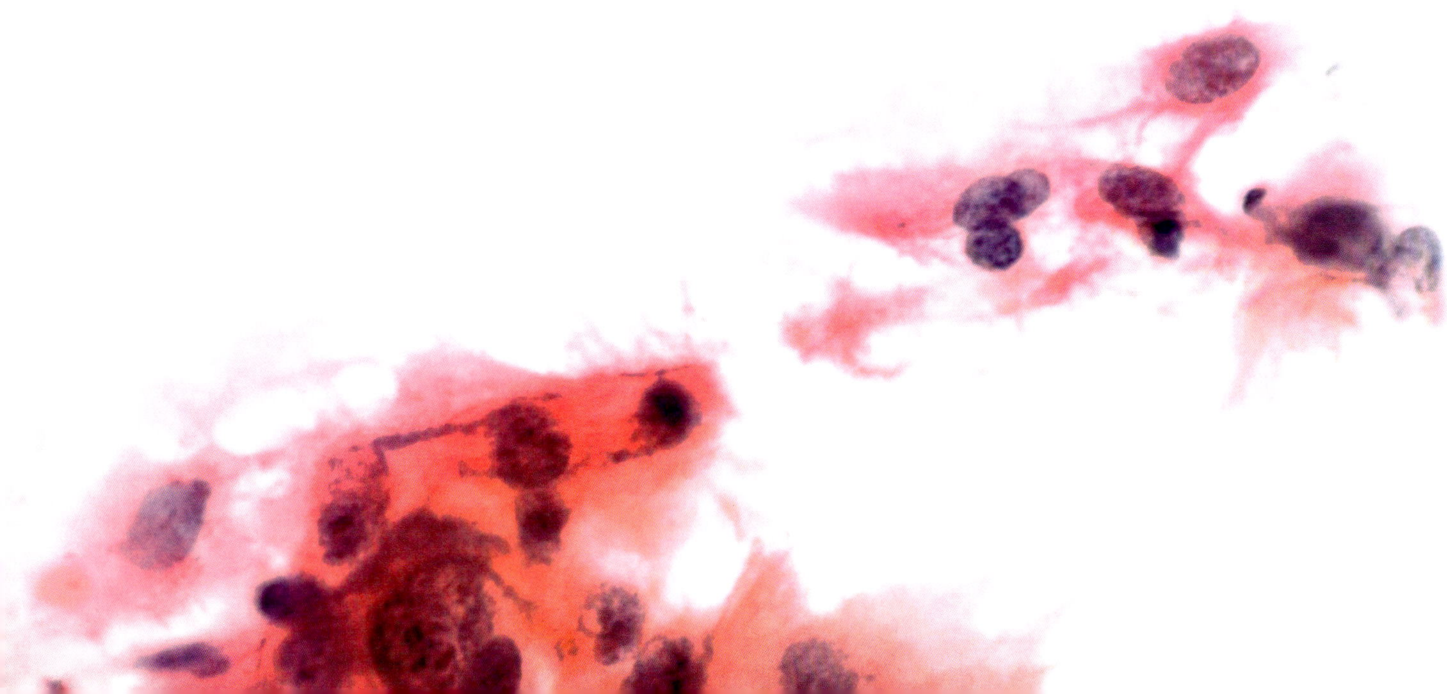

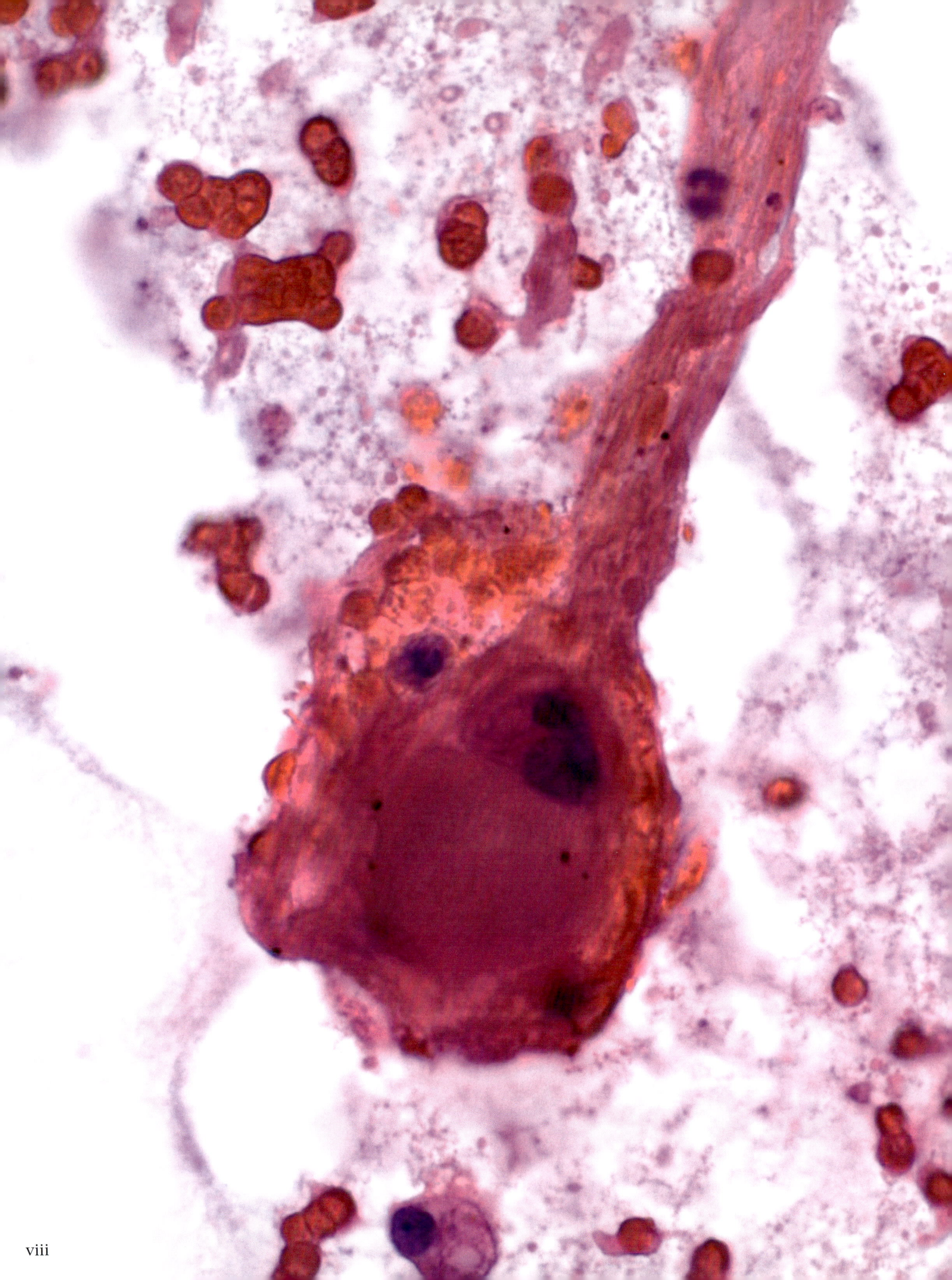

Preface

A very memorable event from my first year in residency was a frozen section. A young woman was under anesthesia being prepared to receive a kidney transplant. The surgeon unexpectedly discovered a firm nodule in the peritoneal cavity. If the diagnosis was cancer, the transplant would not be performed. If benign, she would receive the kidney. I was so impressed by the senior pathologist being able to quickly look at the frozen section and call back the surgeon to tell her the diagnosis was endometriosis and, therefore, the operation that would profoundly change this patient's life could proceed.

Pathology practice has changed in the ensuing years, but the critical importance of intraoperative consultation for patient care has not. In this second edition of *Diagnostic Pathology: Intraoperative Consultation*, the dedicated team of authors has taken the opportunity to extensively update and expand the information essential for pathologists to have available immediately when faced with a question from a surgeon during an operation. The easily accessible format of the first edition has been maintained. There are new chapters on lung wire localization biopsy, nipple margin evaluation, radioactive seed identification, and evaluation of specimens from patients with epilepsy. Essential techniques to rapidly preserve biomolecules for molecular assays are addressed. I am grateful to Dr. Lynette Sholl and Ms. Vivian M. Chan for allowing us to include a new technique recently developed by them to evaluate the staple margins of lung wedge resections. I am also grateful to Dr. Raphael Bueno and Dr. Ritu R. Gill for including the new technique of T-bar localization for lung biopsies.

Preparing a book spanning so many topics requires the assistance of many people. Ms. Kristen K. Gill, Ms. Vivian M. Chan, and the other members of Brigham and Women's Hospital "Team Frozen" are treasured colleagues and collaborators. We also must thank and acknowledge our clinical colleagues, including Dr. Esther Rhei, Dr. Catherine S. Giess, Dr. Rajan Jain, Judyth O'Hara, RN and numerous others. We also thank Dr. Danielle Costigan, Dr. Alexander Christakis, Dr. Inga-Marie Schaefer, Dr. Christine E. Gruessner, Dr. David Hicks, Dr. Richard Owings, Dr. Richard H. Hewlett, Dr. William Welch, Dr. Joseph Corson, Dr. Martina Zink, Dr. Rolf Pfannl, Dr. Stefan Kraft, Ms. Alice Sedlak, Mr. Dennis Poliferno, Ms. Lucy Ross, Ms. Lindsey Cheney, and Ms. Deborah O'Leary.

This book would not have been completed without the outstanding assistance of the Elsevier staff. Our lead editor, Megg Morin, headed the project, kept us all on track, and provided invaluable help and enthusiasm all along the way. Lane Bennion, Rich Coombs, and Laura Wissler created excellent new graphic illustrations. Tom Olson designed a beautiful cover for the book. Lisa Steadman and Jeffrey Marmorstone thoroughly edited each image of every chapter. Rebecca Bluth, Angela Terry, and Emily Fassett saw the book to production. And Arthur Gelsinger, Nina Bennett, Terry Ferrell, Lisa Gervais, and Matt Hoecherl edited the book for months before it came to production.

We hope that, like the first edition, this is the book that every pathologist will want at his or her side the next time a page calls them to an intraoperative consultation.

Susan C. Lester, MD, PhD
Chief
Breast Pathology Services
Brigham and Women's Hospital
Assistant Professor
Harvard Medical School
Boston, Massachusetts

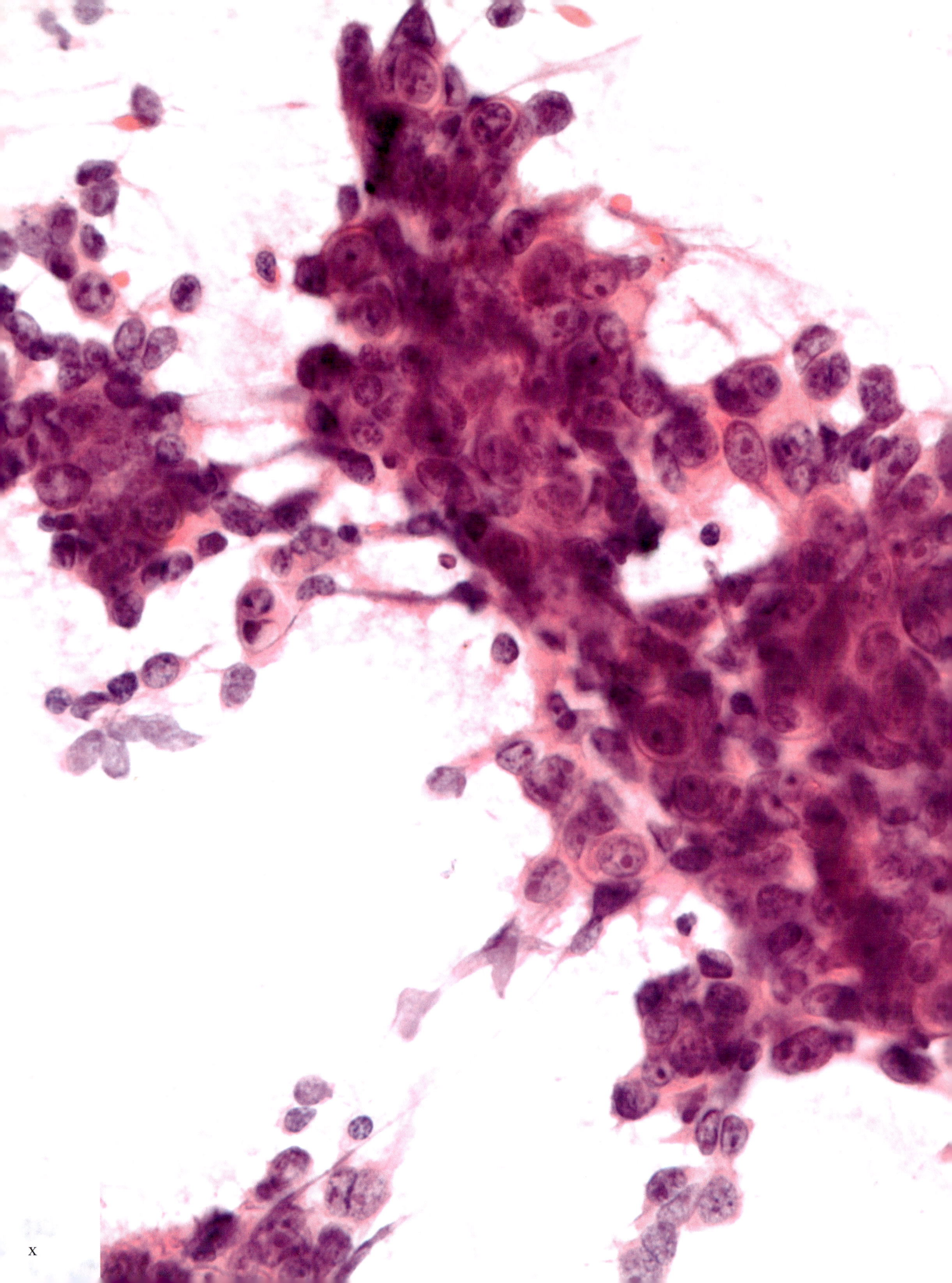

x

Acknowledgments

Lead Editor

Megg Morin, BA

Text Editors

Arthur G. Gelsinger, MA
Rebecca L. Bluth, BA
Nina I. Bennett, BA
Terry W. Ferrell, MS
Lisa A. Gervais, BS
Matt W. Hoecherl, BS

Image Editors

Jeffrey J. Marmorstone, BS
Lisa A. M. Steadman, BS

Illustrations

Richard Coombs, MS
Lane R. Bennion, MS
Laura C. Wissler, MA

Art Direction and Design

Tom M. Olson, BA
Laura C. Wissler, MA

Production Coordinators

Angela M. G. Terry, BA
Emily C. Fassett, BA

ELSEVIER

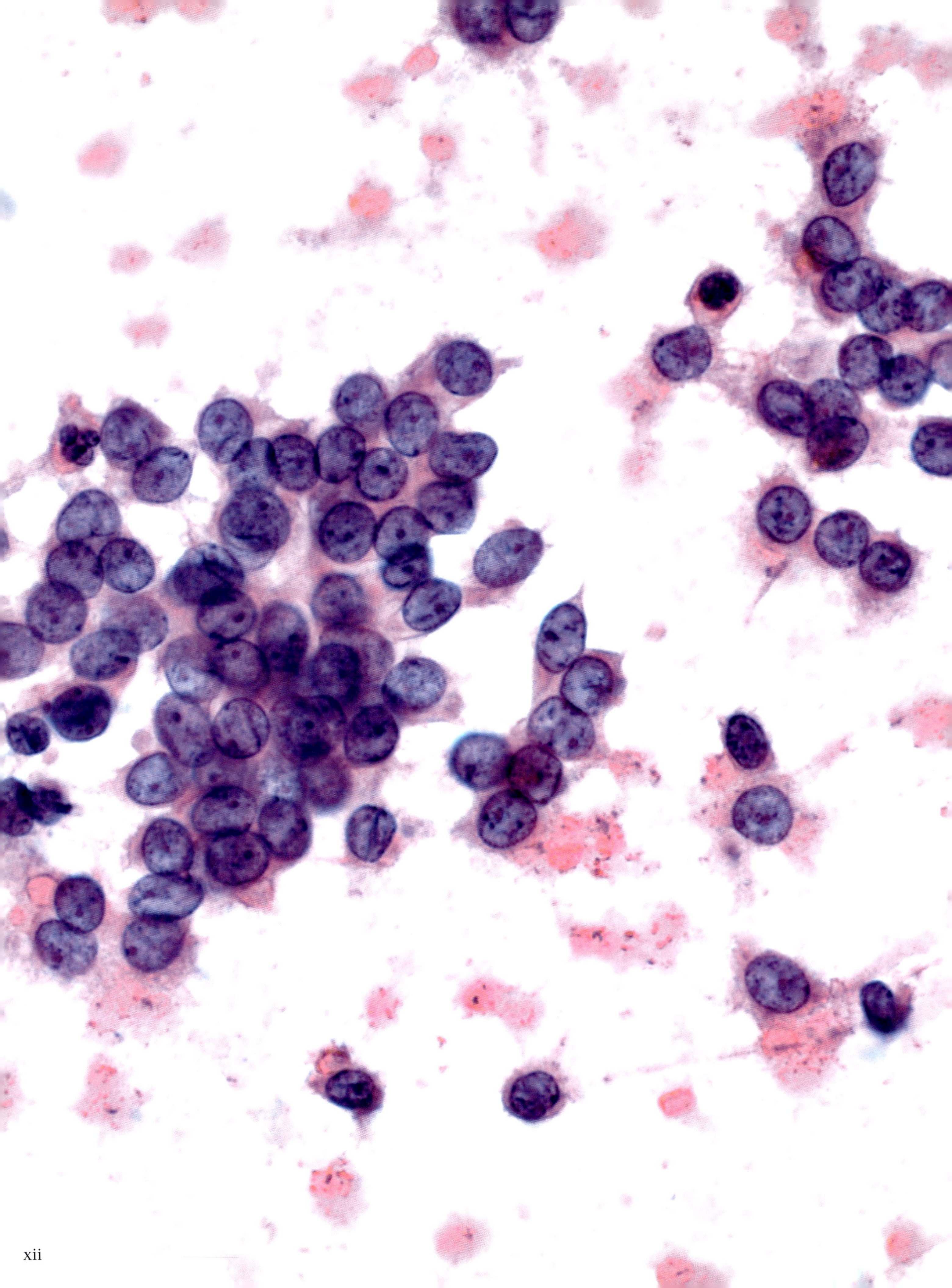

Sections

TABLE OF CONTENTS

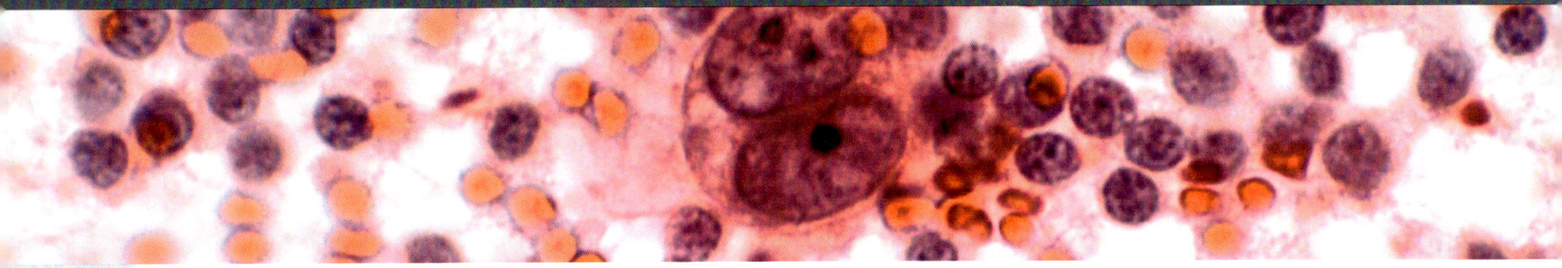

TABLE OF CONTENTS

DIAGNOSTIC PATHOLOGY

Intraoperative Consultation

SECOND EDITION

LESTER

CASSARINO • CHIRIEAC • CORNELL • COX • DILLON • FOLKERTH
FRISHBERG • HARRISON • JO • KO • KRANE • KRASNOZHEN-RATUSH • LINDBERG • MASON
NOSÉ • QUICK • SNUDERL • SRIVASTAVA • THOMPSON

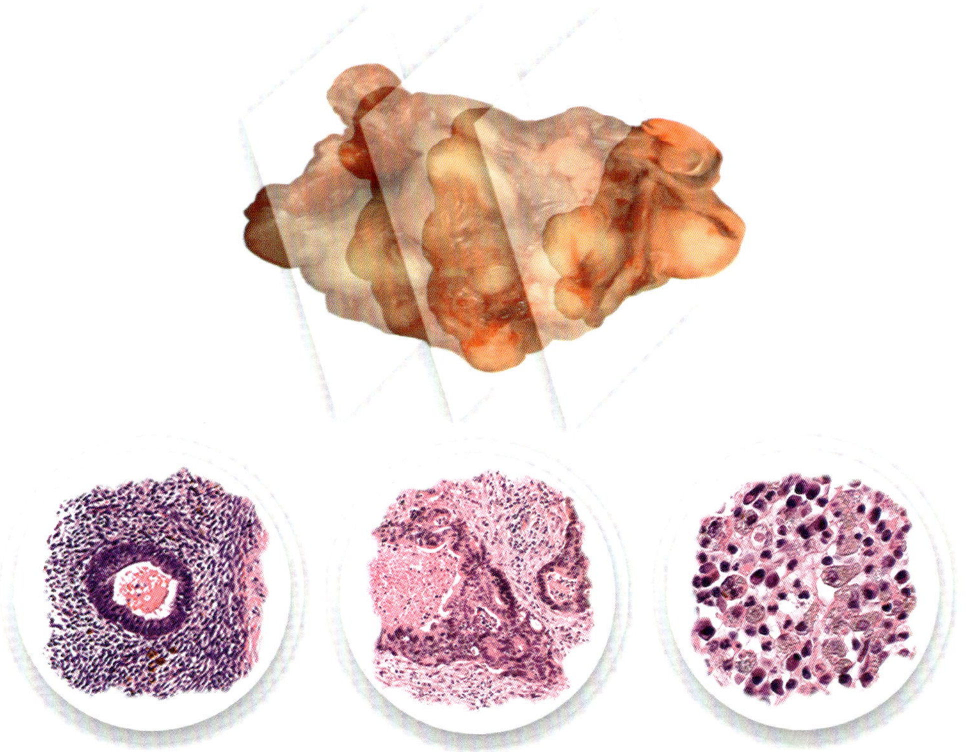

SECTION 1

General

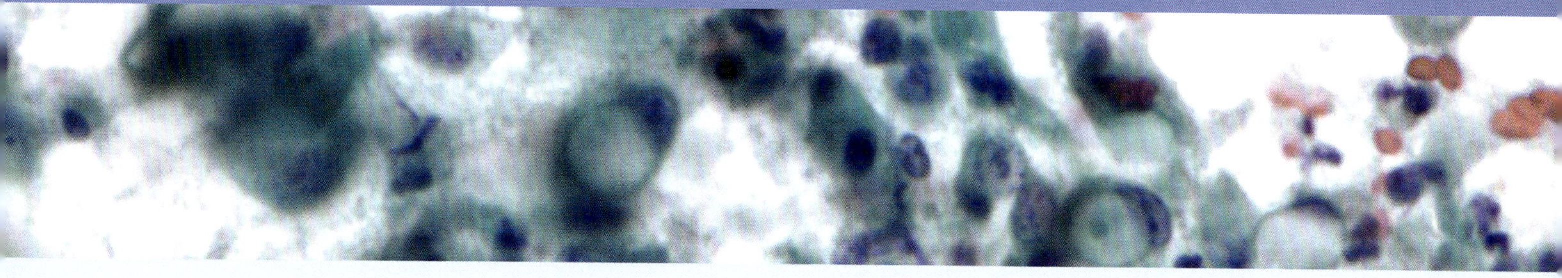

THE ART OF INTRAOPERATIVE CONSULTATION

More Than Pathology at High Speed

- Intraoperative consultation (IOC) has significant differences compared to general pathology practice
  - Major purpose is to answer a specific question required for directing surgery
    - Diagnosis has immediate impact on care of patient
  - Definitive diagnosis generally not necessary or optimal
    - Information should be limited to that essential for immediate management of patient
    - Majority of special studies not available; diagnosis based almost exclusively on H&E slides
    - Only limited sampling of large specimens possible within time limits
  - Judicious interpretation of findings often necessary given limitation of frozen sections
    - Conservative approach, but not too conservative, is appropriate
    - Degrees of uncertainty when a definitive diagnosis is not possible may need to be shared with surgeon
  - Time-limited consultation
    - Ideally, an answer is available to surgeon within 20 minutes
    - Takes precedence over all other activities
    - In most institutions, a pathologist is available on call for consultation at all times
  - Direct interaction between pathologist and surgeon is preferred
    - Precise oral and written communication is essential
  - Often occurs at a site distant from pathology department
    - Pathologists typically prefer using their own microscope in their own workspace
  - Does not occur at predetermined time
    - May be requested at times outside normal working hours (e.g., nights and weekends)
  - Reference material may be limited or difficult to access (e.g., books and journals)
  - Consultation with colleagues often not possible
  - Not subspecialized; pathologists may see specimens outside their areas of expertise
- Pathologist plays important role in advocating for patient during IOC
  - Should only comply with requests for frozen section when they are in best interest of patient
  - Should request additional biopsies when received material is not sufficient for diagnosis
  - Must ensure that tissue is used 1st for diagnosis and clinical care and only 2nd for investigational studies and other uses
- Pearls of knowledge are suggestions and advice
  - Pearls start as grain of sand but gain value over time
  - Knowledge is gained after long years of experience with IOC, many close calls, and a few errors
  - Learning from errors is an excellent method to improve practice (especially when errors are not yours)

Goals of Intraoperative Consultation

- There are 3 principal reasons for immediate microscopic evaluation of specimens
  - **Diagnosis to guide intra- or perioperative patient management**
    - Identification or confirmation of pathologic process
    - Evaluation of margins for known malignancy
  - **Confirm sufficient lesional tissue is present for diagnosis on permanent sections &/or after special studies**
    - Definitive diagnosis is not necessary intraoperative
    - Pathologist confirms to surgeon there is no need to remove additional tissue, resulting in possible additional morbidity
  - **Optimally process tissue for ancillary studies to be used for diagnosis, treatment, or research**
    - Lymphomas
    - Sarcomas
    - Pediatric tumors
    - Other tumors requiring special handling

Intraoperative Consultation: Gross Findings

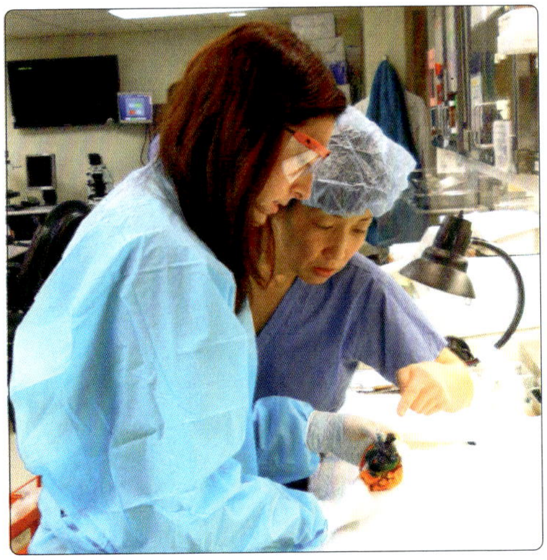

Intraoperative Consultation: Microscopic Findings

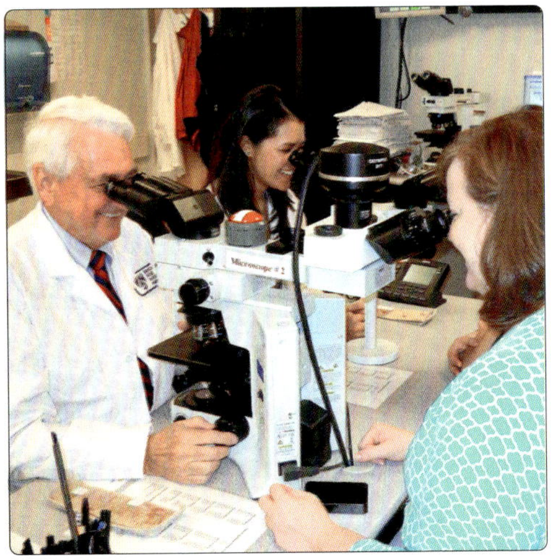

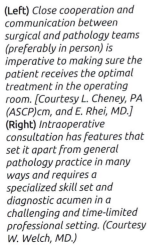

(Left) *Close cooperation and communication between surgical and pathology teams (preferably in person) is imperative to making sure the patient receives the optimal treatment in the operating room. [Courtesy L. Cheney, PA (ASCP)cm, and E. Rhei, MD.]* **(Right)** *Intraoperative consultation has features that set it apart from general pathology practice in many ways and requires a specialized skill set and diagnostic acumen in a challenging and time-limited professional setting. (Courtesy W. Welch, MD.)*

Most Common Diagnostic Questions

- **Diagnosis of primary lesion (~ 20%)**
  - In many cases, preoperative diagnosis is possible using needle or endoscopic biopsies
    - In some cases, prior attempt to diagnose may have been unsuccessful or contraindicated due to location or type of lesion
  - Definitive diagnosis need only be provided when relevant to immediate patient management
    - Often benign vs. malignant is sufficient for intraoperative management
    - Provisional diagnosis can aid in allocation of tissue for ancillary studies
    - In many cases (e.g., lymphomas, small round blue cell tumors, and soft tissue tumors), ancillary studies are often critical; definitive diagnosis at time of IOC is unnecessary
- **Evaluation of margins for known malignant tumor (~ 40%)**
  - Additional tissue may be taken to achieve negative margins in a single procedure
  - Accuracy is generally very high
- **Identification of lymph node metastasis (~ 20%)**
  - Resection with curative intent may be canceled if metastatic disease is identified
    - Additional nodes may not need to be sampled
    - Patients may be treated with systemic therapy prior to definitive resection
  - If a positive sentinel node is identified, additional nodes may be excised
- **Adequacy of tissue for future diagnosis (~ 5%)**
  - Presurgical treatment is becoming more widely used to reduce tumor burden and as a measure of tumor response
  - Tumors must be diagnosed with certainty prior to treatment
    - Fresh tissue may also be desirable for ancillary studies to identify cellular constituents vulnerable to targeted therapy
    - Patients may also consent to have tissue taken for tumor banks
  - Pathologist must request additional tissue when appropriate
- **Evaluation of organ prior to transplant (< 5%)**
  - Scarcity of organs has resulted in donor pool being expanded to include donors with possibly marginally functional organs
  - Intraoperative assessment is important to avoid transplantation of organs with high likelihood of failure

Changes in Intraoperative Consultation Over Time

- Need for IOC changes as treatment of patients changes
- **Consultations becoming more common**
  - Evaluation of lung lesions detected by screening
    - United States Preventative Services Task Force issued recommendations for screening for lung cancer using annual low-dose computed tomography for individuals between the ages of 55-80 with 30-year history of smoking and who currently smoke or have quit smoking within last 15 years
    - Lesions detected by screening are typically small or of low density (ground glass)
    - Lesions can be difficult or impossible for surgeon to palpate
      - □ Special localization techniques may be required
    - More limited surgery may be considered for adenocarcinoma in situ or minimally invasive adenocarcinoma
  - Evaluation of margins of partial nephrectomies
    - Small renal tumors are detected by imaging
    - Increased effort is being made to preserve renal function to avoid need for dialysis
  - Radioactive seed retrieval
    - The use of radioactive seeds rather than wires to mark breast lesions has many advantages for patients and surgeons
    - Retrieval of the seed in the IOC room may be preferred to ensure all seeds are identified, documented, and stored until they can be disposed of safely
  - Nipple margin of mastectomies
    - Nipple- and skin-sparing mastectomies offer cosmetically superior procedure for carefully selected women
    - The base of the nipple may be examined intraoperatively with removal of nipple when carcinoma is detected
  - Evaluation of organs prior to transplant
  - Evaluation of small biopsies for adequacy
- **Consultations currently rarely performed**
  - Identification of parathyroid adenomas
    - Intraoperative measurement of parathyroid hormone level is a useful functional assay that is used to guide surgery
  - Sentinel node evaluation for breast carcinoma
    - Studies have shown good outcomes for carefully selected women with positive sentinel nodes without axillary dissection
    - The need to determine if metastatic carcinoma is in sentinel node intraoperatively has diminished
  - Primary diagnosis of breast lesions
    - Core needle biopsies are highly accurate and allow decisions to be made concerning choice of surgery and systemic therapy (neoadjuvant or adjuvant)
    - Definitive surgery can be planned based on the core needle biopsy diagnosis

Limitations

- Frozen sections are not equivalent to evaluation of specimens on permanent sections
  - Diagnoses on frozen section should be limited to information needed for intraoperative management of patient
- **Sampling**
  - Tissue sections must be small to freeze well and quickly
  - Amount of tissue examined is less than that examined by permanent sections
  - **Pearl of knowledge**: The pathologist evaluating microscopic slides should always perform, or be aware of, the gross findings
    - If macroscopic and microscopic findings are not compatible, pathologist should suspect error

    - A good gross examination is often more accurate than a suboptimal microscopic section
    - Ink can often leak into specimens or smear, making it difficult to identify true margin
- **Ice crystal artifact**
  - Freezing introduces permanent changes in tissues by disrupting cell membranes and other structures
  - Although artifact can be minimized by rapid freezing of small samples, it is usually present
  - Artifacts can make diagnosis difficult or even impossible in extreme cases
    - Nuclei can look larger and more variable in size and shape
    - Holes in tissue can mimic intracellular vacuoles or fat
  - Tissue should only be frozen if benefit to patient outweighs risk of compromising eventual diagnosis
  - **Pearl of knowledge**: Nonpathologists often do not understand that patients can be harmed by inappropriate freezing of tissue due to artifacts permanently introduced
    - This fact can be helpful as part of explanation as to why frozen section should not be performed
- **Technical issues**
  - Some tissues (e.g., adipose tissue) do not freeze well
  - Tissues may be cut thickly
  - Tissue folds can complicate interpretation
- **Absence of special studies**
  - Histochemical and immunohistochemical studies are generally not available
  - Some diagnoses require additional studies

Inappropriate Intraoperative Consultations

- If IOC is requested but the information is not needed for intraoperative or immediate perioperative patient management, the request may be inappropriate
  - Inappropriate IOC can squander valuable resources and time
    - Could delay appropriate IOC for other patients
    - Generates unnecessary medical cost
  - May compromise ultimate diagnosis
- **Unnecessary and potentially harmful to patient**
  - Completely freezing any lesion may preclude ultimate definitive diagnosis
    - Freezing artifact can obscure diagnostic features
    - Tissue loss can occur during sectioning in cryostat
  - Pigmented lesions of skin and small breast lesions should not be entirely frozen
    - These lesions should be diagnosed and features evaluated on optimal permanent sections
    - Freezing artifact and potential loss of tissue can preclude making a definitive diagnosis
  - Pathologist must be advocate for patient
    - Surgeon must be informed as to why freezing entire lesion could be harmful to patient
    - Alternatives can be discussed, such as expedited processing of permanent sections
  - **Pearl of knowledge**: There are rare occasions in which unusual requests for frozen section examination are appropriate
    - Rather than refusing to perform examination, it can be more helpful to ask surgeon how examination will benefit patient
    - Pathologist and surgeon can reach an agreement about best course of action
    - Ultimately, pathologist must act in the best interest of patient
- **Unnecessary but not harmful to patient**
  - There is usually no need for frozen section diagnosis on large tumor that has been completely excised
    - However, performing a frozen section on a small portion of tumor will not interfere with eventual diagnosis
    - Surgeon may request IOC to provide information to the patient or family
  - Request should be discussed with surgeon to determine how intraoperative or immediate postoperative management would be changed by diagnosis
    - If there would be no change, then discuss why frozen section is unnecessary
    - In some cases, there may be clinical indications for diagnosis of which the pathologist is not aware
  - **Pearl of knowledge**: It can be difficult to discuss departmental policy with a surgeon while the patient is under anesthesia
    - If inappropriate requests are recurring problem, departmental and institutional policies should be developed by surgeons and pathologists and discussed in a multidisciplinary setting
- **IOCs known to have low sensitivity or specificity**
  - Value of performing frozen section may be very low in some situations
    - Evaluation of follicular thyroid lesions for capsular invasion
    - Evaluation of margins of large breast excisions
  - Surgeon should be aware of likelihood of a change in diagnosis on permanent sections
  - Departmental and institutional policies should be developed for evaluating these types of specimens

PATIENT HISTORY

Prior to Intraoperative Consultation

- Knowledge about clinical setting helps establish a safety net for patient
  - Substantial number of errors occur because pathologist interprets specimen without adequate information (e.g., not knowing patient has received radiation or chemotherapy)
  - Especially helpful in some situations
    - Biopsies of mediastinal lymph nodes (important to know if for tumor staging or to evaluate lymphadenopathy)
      - Determines if entire specimen should be frozen or only a representative portion
    - Resections after neoadjuvant chemotherapy or radiation therapy
      - Changes in normal cells due to treatment can be mistaken for malignancy
    - Rare tumor types

- Tumors for which imaging appearance is critical for final diagnosis (central nervous system tumors, bone tumors)
  - **Pearl of knowledge**: Reviewing clinical histories prior to IOC leads to faster and more confident diagnoses and considerably less anxiety
    - Some people believe that pathologists should be able to divine all clinical information from surgical specimens as the haruspices in ancient Rome were able to divine information from examining organs—this is not true
- IOC requiring the allocation of tissue for purposes beyond diagnosis must be identified
  - Tissue required for patient treatment should be distinguished from tissue requested for research
    - Patients may require tissue sampling to be eligible for clinical trials
  - Special procedures may be required
    - Sterile tissue is necessary for cell cultures (e.g., vaccine studies)
    - Warm ischemia time (in operating room) and cold ischemia time (until tissue is frozen or placed in fixative should be minimized)
  - Patient care must always take precedence over use of tissue for research that does not directly impact patient
- Obtaining information prior to IOC is preferable, when possible
  - Does not extend the time of the IOC while patient is under anesthesia
  - Allows time to review prior pathology or imaging studies when available
- Well-designed electronic medical records can facilitate obtaining key information prior to the operation

Important Information for Pathologic Interpretation

- Age: Likelihood of diagnosis can be highly dependent on age
- Gender: Some tumors have gender-specific frequencies
- Prior history of malignancy
  - Metastatic disease must always be considered
  - Type of malignancy, stage, and prior treatment are all important factors
  - Treatment-related changes can be mistaken for malignancy
  - Tumors with treatment effect may be difficult to recognize
- Prior history of surgery
  - Surgical changes can be mistaken for malignancy
- Drug use or therapy
  - Drug use can cause changes (e.g., increased mitoses) that can be mistaken for malignancy
- Current pregnancy or lactation
  - Benign breast lesions can have increased mitotic rate &/or necrosis
    - These changes can mimic malignancy
- Known or suspected infection
  - Some diseases may require modifications to protect pathology personnel
    - Special respiratory masks are required to protect from *Mycobacterium tuberculosis*
    - Specimens from patients with suspected Creutzfeldt-Jakob disease should not be examined
  - Specimens should be kept sterile in order to obtain cultures
- Imaging findings
  - In some settings, appearance on imaging is critical
    - Essential to develop differential diagnosis
    - Particularly important for brain lesions, bone tumors, and lung lesions
    - May be necessary to locate lesion in large resections

Information Provided at Time of Intraoperative Consultation

- **Requisition form**
  - Patient identification, surgeon name, operating room number (including phone number) are all essential information
    - Known or suspected infectious diseases should be specified
  - Type of specimen submitted
    - Location
    - Biopsy or complete excision
    - Orientation
  - Purpose of consultation
    - In many cases, will be clear from type of specimen submitted and operative procedure
    - If purpose is not clear, pathologist should discuss with surgeon
    - **Pearl of knowledge**: If the reason for examining specimen is not immediately clear, it is an unusual case and best course of action is to contact surgeon
- **Information obtained during IOC**
  - If information is obtained from surgeon that is helpful for interpretation of frozen section, this will also be helpful for final diagnosis
  - Information should be recorded on requisition form and available to pathologist reviewing case for final sign out
- **Information obtained in operating room**
  - In some institutions, it may be possible for the pathologist to directly observe operative field and to discuss the case face to face with the surgeon

REPORTING RESULTS

Written Report

- Diagnosis is written and signed by attending pathologist
  - Most laboratories have a specific form for this purpose
  - Form should be labeled with patient name, medical record number, and surgical pathology number
  - Specific specimen and subdesignation for frozen section are included
- The diagnosis should directly address the question posed by the surgeon to successfully complete the operation
  - **Pearl of knowledge**: Diagnoses should be brief and include only the information necessary (e.g., "no tumor present" or "metastatic cancer present")
    - Long and wordy reports are difficult to communicate orally and more likely to be misunderstood
  - Avoid using abbreviations
    - An abbreviation saves time for 1 person and aggravates everyone else

History of Intraoperative Consultations

Era	Clinical Setting	Surgery	Pathology
Pre-1800s	Cancer less common as patients often die due to other diseases at early ages	Usually, rapid brutal procedures performed late in course of disease; does not change ultimate outcome	Capacity to evaluate tumors by microscopic examination not available
1800s	Patients come to medical attention late in disease when cancers are locally advanced	Anesthesia and aseptic technique allow earlier surgery and better outcomes; malignant tumors easily identified by gross features; radical surgical procedures performed	Advances in microscopy, microtomes, formalin, and tissue dyes allow identification and classification of tumors
1891	First recorded intraoperative consultation	William S. Halsted requests intraoperative consultation on mastectomy specimen	William H. Welch performs frozen section, but procedure requires an hour and results are not available until after operation has been completed
Early 1900s	Awareness of utility of early diagnosis and new imaging techniques results in patients presenting with smaller tumors	Gross examination not sufficient to identify smaller tumors as benign or malignant; growing impetus for more limited surgery; "When cancer becomes a microscopic disease, there must be tissue diagnosis in the operating room" (Joseph Colt Bloodgood, 1927)	In 1905, Louis B. Wilson publishes frozen section technique that can be performed in a few minutes
Current	Screening and modern imaging modalities detect many cancers at early stage; cancer is truly microscopic disease for many patients	Modern surgery minimizes tissue removed to maintain function and optimize cosmesis	Intraoperative diagnosis plays important role in providing information surgeon needs to ensure tumors have been removed and margins are clear

    - Abbreviations may vary among specialties and may be misunderstood
      - For example, pathologists understand "c/w" to mean "consistent with," whereas radiologists understand "c/w" to mean "compared with"
  - Superfluous information (typically histologic type or grade) is unnecessary and can create potential discrepancies with the final diagnosis
  - **Pearl of knowledge**: It is critical to know the consequences of a diagnosis (e.g. surgery for potential cure terminated or continued) when making diagnostic judgement calls when a definitive diagnosis is not obvious
    - The harm of a false-negative vs. a false-positive diagnosis for a patient is often not equivalent
- Copy of report is made and provided for patient's medical record
- Written reports of IOC may not be available to patient's caregivers for hours to days
  - When possible, documentation of IOC in manner that is available in patient's record is preferable
  - In electronic medical records, this may be possible using hold note

Oral Report

- Final diagnosis is called back to operating room
  - It is preferable to read written report exactly
- When possible, information should be relayed directly to surgeon
  - **Pearl of knowledge**: Complex or unusual diagnoses are best communicated directly between pathologist and surgeon
    - There is high rate of miscommunication when diagnosis is other than "benign" or "malignant"
    - Reports including terms indicating degrees of certainty ("suspicious for," "cannot exclude," "atypical") can be interpreted differently by pathologist and surgeon
    - Similar terms (e.g., "carcinoid" and "carcinoma") must be clearly distinguished
- The person receiving information should write down information and read diagnosis back to pathologist
  - This is requirement of The Joint Commission (TJC), formerly, The Joint Commission on Accreditation of Healthcare Organizations (JCAHO)

SELECTED REFERENCES

1. Norgan AP et al: Implementation of a software application for presurgical case history review of frozen section pathology cases. J Pathol Inform. 8:3, 2017
2. Sams SB et al: Discordance between intraoperative consultation by frozen section and final diagnosis. Int J Surg Pathol. 25(1):41-50, 2017
3. McIntosh ER et al: Frozen section: guiding the hands of surgeons? Ann Diagn Pathol. 19(5):326-9, 2015
4. Roy S et al: Frozen section diagnosis: is there discordance between what pathologists say and what surgeons hear? Am J Clin Pathol. 140(3):363-9, 2013
5. Winther C et al: Accuracy of frozen section diagnosis: a retrospective analysis of 4785 cases. APMIS. 119(4-5):259-62, 2011
6. Taxy JB: Frozen section and the surgical pathologist: a point of view. Arch Pathol Lab Med. 133(7):1135-8, 2009
7. Gal AA et al: The 100-year anniversary of the description of the frozen section procedure. JAMA. 294(24):3135-7, 2005
8. Lechago J: The frozen section: pathology in the trenches. Arch Pathol Lab Med. 129(12):1529-31, 2005
9. Acs G et al: Intraoperative consultation: an historical perspective. Semin Diagn Pathol. 19(4):190-1, 2002
10. Wright JR Jr: The development of the frozen section technique, the evolution of surgical biopsy, and the origins of surgical pathology. Bull Hist Med. 59(3):295-326, 1985

Specimen Delivery to Intraoperative Consultation Room

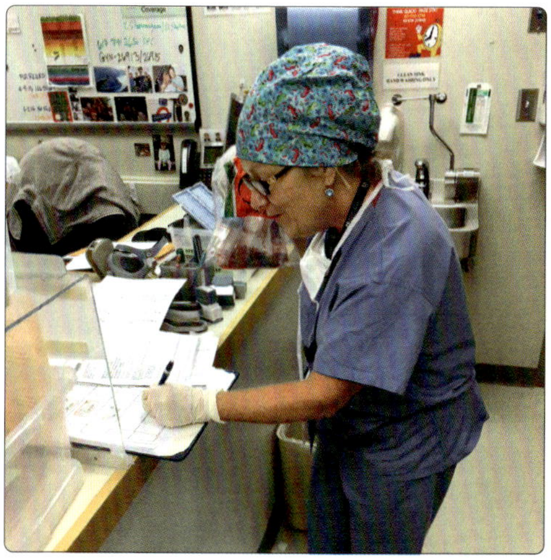

Requisition Form

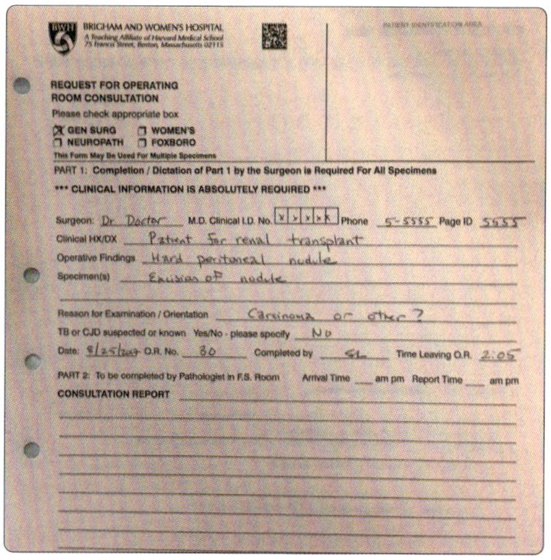

BRIGHAM AND WOMEN'S HOSPITAL
A Teaching Affiliate of Harvard Medical School
75 Francis Street, Boston, Massachusetts 02115

REQUEST FOR OPERATING ROOM CONSULTATION
Please check appropriate box
☒ GEN SURG ☐ WOMEN'S
☐ NEUROPATH ☐ FOXBORO
This Form May Be Used For Multiple Specimens

PART 1: Completion / Dictation of Part 1 by the Surgeon is Required For All Specimens
*** CLINICAL INFORMATION IS ABSOLUTELY REQUIRED ***

Surgeon: Dr Doctor M.D. Clinical I.D. No. x x x x x Phone 5-5555 Page ID 5555
Clinical HX/DX Patient for renal transplant
Operative Findings Hard peritoneal nodule
Specimen(s) Excision of nodule

Reason for Examination / Orientation Carcinoma or other?
TB or CJD suspected or known Yes/No - please specify No
Date: 5/25/2017 O.R. No. 30 Completed by SL Time Leaving O.R. 2:05
PART 2: To be completed by Pathologist in F.S. Room Arrival Time ___ am pm Report Time ___ am pm
CONSULTATION REPORT

(Left) *A consultation begins when a specimen arrives from an operating room and is entered into the log book of the intraoperative consultation room. (Courtesy J. O'Hara, RN.)* **(Right)** *The surgeon must inform the pathologist about the surgical setting and the need for consultation. In this case, the surgeon has palpated an unexpected hard nodule in the peritoneum and needs to know the diagnosis. If malignant, the surgeon will cancel the procedure and not continue with the kidney transplantation.*

Gross Examination

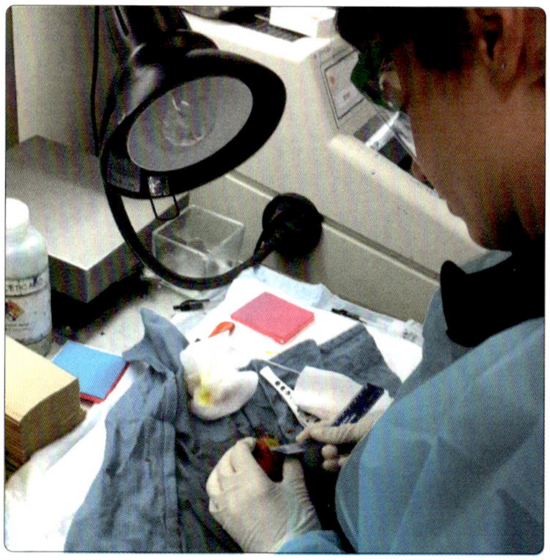

Frozen Section

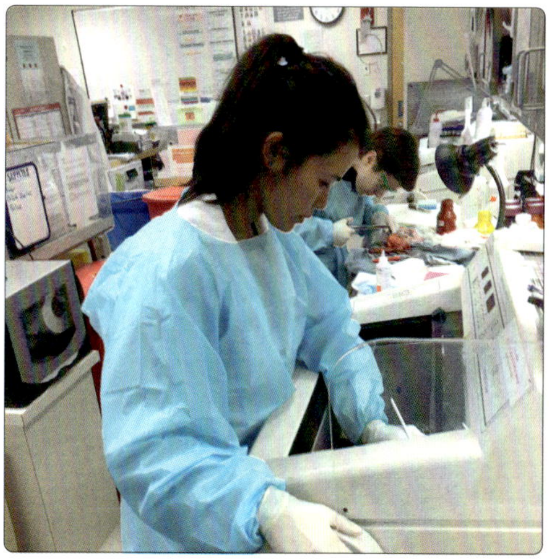

(Left) *Careful gross examination is essential for all consultations to determine the type of tissue present and to select the best area for frozen section. (Courtesy D.C. Costigan, MBBCh.)* **(Right)** *Good frozen section technique is essential to creating high-quality slides that can be used for diagnosis. (Courtesy V. Chan, BS.)*

Microscopic Evaluation

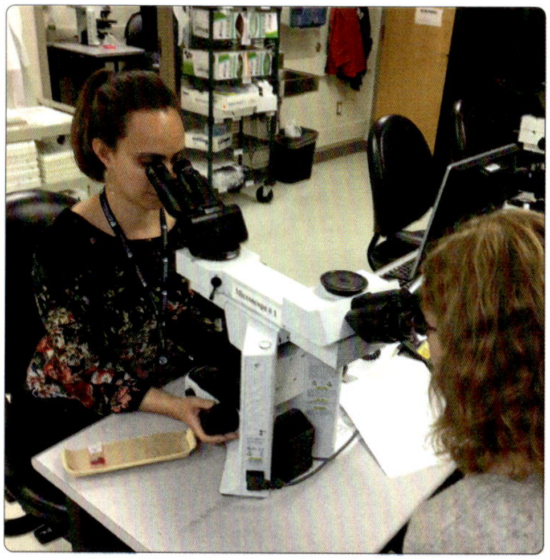

Communication With Surgeon

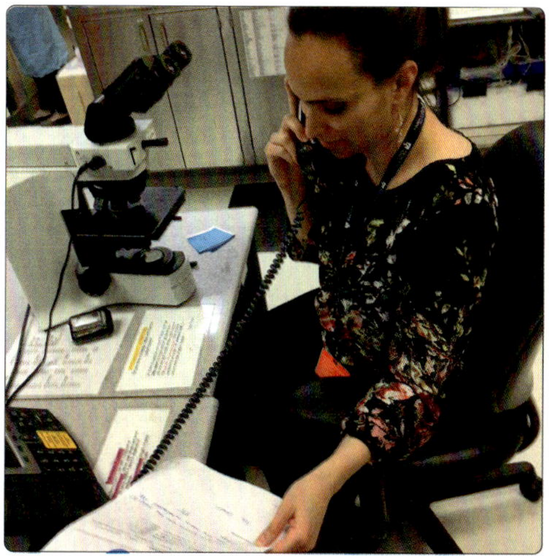

(Left) *A microscopic diagnosis can be provided within minutes due to the ability to harden tissue by freezing to create thin sections. (Courtesy B. T. Harrison, MD.)* **(Right)** *Clear communication with the operating team is essential. Ideally, the pathologist speaks directly with the surgeon by phone or in person. In this case, there is good news. A peritoneal mass discovered during an operation is endometriosis. The surgeon can proceed to completing a kidney transplant. (Courtesy B. T. Harrison, MD.)*

INTRODUCTION

Quality Assessment

- Successful rendering of an intraoperative consultation (IOC) requires a complex series of steps
- Each department needs to develop standards to ensure that best care is provided for each patient, and best practices are utilized for each institution
  - Errors can result in immediate harm or delay optimal care to patients
  - Inappropriate use of IOC generates unnecessary workload and healthcare cost
- Association of Directors of Anatomic and Surgical Pathology (ADASP) and College of American Pathologists (CAP) have issued recommendations for quality assurance (QA) and benchmarks for performance

ELEMENTS OF QUALITY IMPROVEMENT

Quality Improvement Plan

- Mission statement: Clear statement of goals
  - IOCs will prospectively offer patients best care and minimize possibility of error
    - Mechanisms to detect errors are utilized
    - Errors are used as means to educate and to modify system to reduce and prevent future errors
- All elements of test cycle are addressed
  - Preanalytic
  - Analytic
  - Postanalytic
- Sets priorities for targeting resources to best effect
- Complies with regulatory requirements
- Makes appropriate use of internal and external benchmarks
- Uses data tracking to develop strategies for error reduction and prevention

Operational Elements Contributing to High-Quality Service

- Diagnostic capability appropriate to clinical setting
  - Adequate expertise to handle institutional case complexity
    - Peer consultation availability
    - Subspecialist consultation or subspecialty call service if appropriate
  - Sufficient assigned pathologists to handle volume
- Availability of pathologist appropriate to clinical setting
  - May be provided at all times and every day in large hospitals
  - May be by prearranged request for specific types of surgery in small community hospitals or surgicenters
- Physical work environment
  - Adequate space, lighting, and ventilation
  - Tracking log to document receipt of all specimens
  - Well-maintained cryostats and staining stations
  - Well-maintained microscopes
    - Preferably with ability to share images with consultants, trainees, &/or clinicians via multiple heads, telepathology, or digital scanning
  - Proximity of special media, equipment, specimen containers, and requisition slips for ancillary studies
  - Availability of printed and online resources for information related to IOC
  - Telephone, intercoms, or other means to communicate with operating room staff
- Clinical staff
  - Competent, accountable, and expeditious courier service
    - Time spent in transferring specimen for IOC should be minimized
  - Medical/nursing staff provide accurate and sufficient information on requisition slips
    - Inadequate information is detrimental for patient care
      - Increases likelihood of errors in sampling and interpretation
      - May delay diagnosis while additional information is sought

QUALITY ASSURANCE MONITORS AND REPORTING

Volume Statistics

- May be general or subcategorized by specimen type

Possible Block Sampling Error: Small Lesion

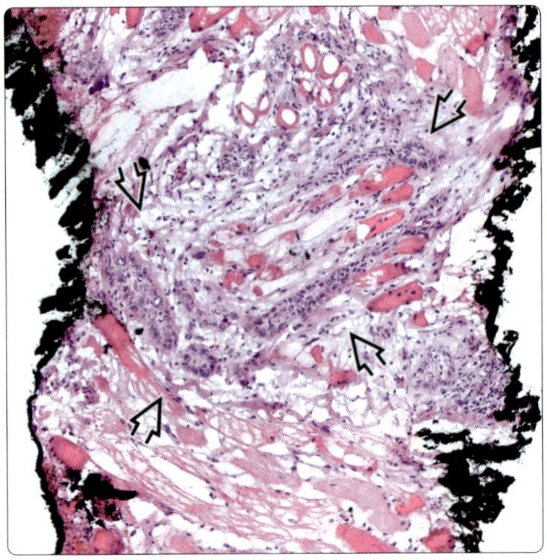

Possible Interpretative Error: Inflammation Obscuring Subtle Findings

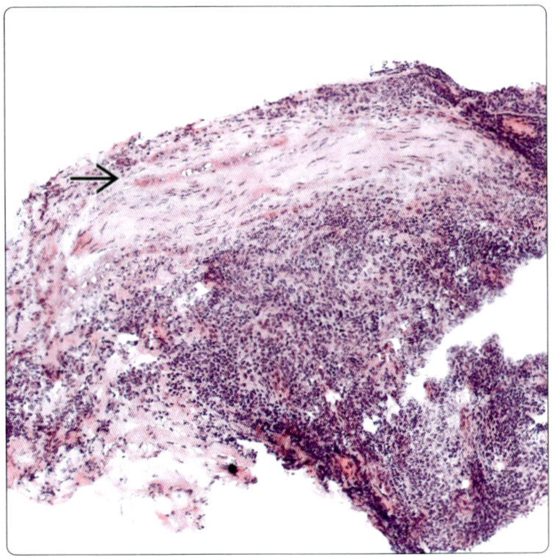

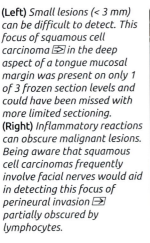

(Left) *Small lesions (< 3 mm) can be difficult to detect. This focus of squamous cell carcinoma* ⇨ *in the deep aspect of a tongue mucosal margin was present on only 1 of 3 frozen section levels and could have been missed with more limited sectioning.* **(Right)** *Inflammatory reactions can obscure malignant lesions. Being aware that squamous cell carcinomas frequently involve facial nerves would aid in detecting this focus of perineural invasion* ⇨ *partially obscured by lymphocytes.*

- Required to determine quality indicators per specimen

Turnaround Time

- Defined as time from delivery of specimen to IOC room to time diagnosis is communicated to surgeon
  - These times should be documented in defined manner (e.g., in specimen tracking log, IOC report, separate QA database)
- Traditionally, expected turnaround time (TAT) is < 20 minutes for routine single-block specimen received by itself with no other concurrent specimens
  - 90% of IOCs can typically be performed during this length of time
  - CAP checklist no longer stipulates threshold for accreditation purposes
- TAT perceived by surgeon is time specimen leaves operating room to time he/she receives diagnosis
  - It may be of value to monitor transit time from operating room to IOC room (preanalytic variable)

Case Review

- IOCs are periodically reviewed
- Errors and deferred cases are detected
- Statistics on performance calculated
- Report should be available &/or presented to department
- Follow-up on issues indicating system problems or need for peer review

ADASP Recommendation

- All IOCs should be reviewed on regular basis and classified into following categories
  - Agreement (no discrepancy between intraoperative and final diagnosis)
  - Disagreement: Minor
  - Disagreement: Major
  - Deferral: Appropriate
  - Deferral: Inappropriate
- Cases in "Disagreement: Major" and "Deferral: Inappropriate" categories should be further classified according to source of problem and according to severity of likely medical consequences

ERRORS

Error Detection and Classification

- All frozen section slides and intraoperative cytology preparations should be reviewed at time of final sign-out of cases with permanent sections
- Any discordant findings should be investigated and reported
  - **Interpretive error**: Findings present on slides used for IOC but not reported
  - **Block sampling error**: Findings not present on slides used for IOC but present in deeper levels on permanent section
    - Errors due to failure to sample lesion the thickness of tissue section (~ > 2-3 mm) because only superficial sections were taken are preventable
      - Representative sections of all tissue fragments should be present on frozen section slides
    - Errors due to failure to detect a lesion smaller than tissue section (~ < 2-3 mm) are not avoidable in all cases
      - Detection of all very small lesions would require exhaustive sectioning and evaluation of numerous levels
      - In general, such extensive sectioning is not feasible or clinically warranted
  - **Gross sampling error**: Findings not present on slides used for IOC or on deeper levels but present in other sections of specimen
- If change in diagnosis will affect patient care, surgeon should be notified immediately, and notification should be documented in final pathology report
  - Such notifications should be addressed by department policy regarding significant and unexpected findings in anatomic pathology

Sources of Error

- Preanalytic
  - Incorrect case or patient identification
  - Incorrect site identification
  - Inadequate clinical information
    - Failure to notify of prior diagnosis of malignancy
    - Failure to provide information about prior chemotherapy (adjuvant or neoadjuvant) or radiation therapy
  - Purpose for IOC unclear or inappropriate
- Analytic
  - Sampling
    - Gross (lesion not selected for frozen section or cytologic preparation)
    - Block (lesion present but not seen on prepared slides)
  - Technical
    - Poor freezing, cutting, or staining technique interferes with interpretation
    - Tissue lost during processing
    - Slides mislabeled
  - Interpretation
    - Change in category (benign vs. malignant)
    - Change within category (type of malignancy)
    - Change in threshold (grade, stage; e.g., atypical ductal hyperplasia vs. ductal carcinoma in situ of breast, atypical adenomatous hyperplasia vs. adenocarcinoma in situ of lung)
    - Change in lymph node status
    - Change in margin status
- Postanalytic
  - Diagnosis not communicated to surgeon
  - Incorrect diagnosis communicated to surgeon
  - Surgeon has understanding of reported diagnosis different from that of pathologist

Classification by Consequences

- ADASP recommends classifying errors according to severity of medical consequences
  - No clinical significance
  - Minor or questionable clinical significance
  - Major or potentially major clinical significance
- Some QA systems classify according to actual rather than potential harm
  - At philosophical discretion of institution but should be defined in quality improvement plan

DEFERRED DIAGNOSES

Definition

- In very broad sense, all IOC diagnoses are deferred to final diagnosis on permanent sections
- For QA purposes, diagnosis is defined as deferred when no diagnosis can be rendered
  - Should be reserved for cases in which information requested cannot be provided using specimen provided
  - Typically, < 5% of IOCs are deferred

Types

- There are 5 major sources of deferred diagnoses
- **Difficult to classify lesions**: Definitive diagnosis (i.e., benign vs. malignant) may not be possible for some specimens submitted for IOC
  - Common examples
    - Pancreatic adenocarcinoma vs. chronic pancreatitis
    - Lepidic pattern adenocarcinoma vs. reactive changes in lung
    - Residual/recurrent squamous cell carcinoma vs. radiation-induced atypia in squamous metaplasia
  - Deferral is appropriate if sufficient diagnostic features are not present
    - Number of appropriately deferred cases is measure of number of very difficult cases encountered in IOC
  - Deferral is inappropriate if, on QA review of frozen section, diagnosis is deemed to be (reasonably) possible
    - Number of inappropriately deferred cases is measure of knowledge base/experience of pathologists
  - Corrective measure: Review diagnostic features with pathologist
    - Provide books and online resources with diagnostic criteria that are readily accessible in IOC room
    - Consider methods to facilitate 2nd opinions for difficult cases (e.g., telepathology)
- **Biopsy induced artifacts**: Extensive crushing &/or cautery can cause tissue damage that precludes interpretation
  - Deferral is appropriate for severely damaged tissue specimens
    - Number of deferred cases is measure of surgical ability to provide high-quality specimens
  - Corrective measure: Explore alternative methods (e.g., cutting needle vs. pinching forceps &/or excision without cautery for diagnostic biopsies submitted for IOC)
    - Some tumors, notably small cell carcinoma, are friable and very difficult to biopsy without significant artifact
- **Artifacts or tissue loss due to pathology processing**: Poor selection of tissue (e.g., freezing large fragments &/or wet tissue), poor cutting technique (e.g., thick, wrinkled sections), poor staining (e.g., contamination of stains with xylene), and loss of tissue in cryostat may preclude interpretation
  - When feasible and appropriate, additional tissue should be frozen or additional biopsy should be requested from surgeon
  - Deferral is not appropriate if better technique would have yielded interpretable slide
    - Number of deferred cases is measure of capacity of pathology personnel to produce high-quality slides
  - Corrective measure: Review appropriate preparation of frozen sections slides with pathology personnel
- **Specimens not amenable to frozen section or cytologic examination**: It may not be possible to evaluate fatty tissue or heavily calcified specimens, such as bone
  - Deferral is appropriate if tissue cannot be examined
    - Number of deferred cases is measure of number of cases that are submitted for IOC that cannot be examined
  - Corrective measure: Surgeons can be informed about types of specimens that cannot be evaluated by IOC
    - Some specimens not amenable to cryostat sectioning can be interpreted using intraoperative cytology preparations
- **Lack of sufficient clinical information for evaluation**: In some cases, clinical information is essential to provide diagnosis
  - Common examples
    - Brain and bone lesion evaluation requires information about imaging findings
    - Information about prior radiation or chemotherapy is necessary to determine if cells with atypia are more likely malignant or due to treatment-induced changes
    - Thyroid follicles associated with lymphocytes and germinal centers could be metastatic carcinoma to lymph node or area of nodular lymphocytic thyroiditis, depending on history of malignancy and location of nodule
  - In majority of cases, further inquiry will yield appropriate information
  - Deferral is appropriate if information cannot or is not provided by surgeon
    - Number of deferred cases is measure of cases without essential clinical information
  - Corrective measure: Surgeons are informed of information needed by pathologist for IOC
    - Review of hospital &/or laboratory information system for patients with scheduled operations likely to generate IOC can be helpful

Cases Not Considered Deferred

- In some situations, definitive diagnosis is not provided but case should not be considered deferred for QA purposes
- **Provisional diagnosis**: In many cases, it is appropriate to provide some diagnostic information on IOC, but final diagnosis is best made after evaluation of permanent sections and possible ancillary studies
  - Common examples
    - Spindle cell neoplasm
    - Lymphoproliferative disorder
    - Encapsulated follicular neoplasm of thyroid
    - Lesional tissue present
  - Not attempting to provide final diagnosis at IOC that is unnecessary for intraoperative management &/or which may reasonably be altered later is good pathology practice
  - Number of such cases should not be used as measure of quality of IOC
- **Canceled diagnosis**: In some cases, IOC may be requested that is considered inappropriate or unnecessary by pathologist
  - Pathologist should discuss case with surgeon to come to decision to cancel request

  - This should be considered canceled request and not deferred diagnosis

BENCHMARKS

Studies of General Accuracy

- Overall accuracy generally in 90-98% range across specimen types in large studies
- False-negatives much more frequent (~ 7x) than false-positives
  - Some specimen types, particularly sentinel lymph nodes, may have high false-negative rate due to sampling error but nevertheless retain high positive and negative predictive values
- Sampling error more common than interpretive error
- Accuracy generally higher for more narrowly defined (e.g., margin assessment of known malignancy) than of general ("what is this mass") questions

ADASP Benchmarks

- Recommendations for maximum acceptable rates
  - Disagreement: Major cases = 3%
  - Deferral: Inappropriate cases = 10%

Variables Affecting Accuracy

- Incidence of target lesion in population
  - If true positives are rare, even studies with low sensitivity may have high negative predictive value
- Reason for IOC
  - Defined question, such as margin positivity of known cancer type, may yield accuracy approaching 100%
  - Accuracy of primary diagnosis of unknown tumor type closer to 80%
- Inclusion or exclusion of lesions difficult to diagnose on frozen section
  - Noninvasive follicular thyroid neoplasm with papillary-like nuclear features
  - Paget disease of vulva
  - Skin margins for melanoma
  - Primary diagnosis of Hirschsprung disease
- Inclusion or exclusion of small lesions difficult or impossible to reliably detect by frozen section
  - Micropapillary carcinoma of thyroid
  - Micrometastases or isolated tumor cells in sentinel nodes for breast cancer
- Inclusion or exclusion of deferred cases
  - Definition of "deferred" diagnosis varies
  - Exclusion of these cases reduces total number of cases and, therefore, increases error rate

Site-Specific Accuracy

- Accuracy varies according to specific case mix
- For specialty hospitals and centers of excellence, it may be appropriate to set specimen-specific benchmarks for reporting
- Positive/negative predictive value of IOC by specimen type may have more clinical utility than sensitivity/specificity/accuracy

STRATEGIES TO PREVENT ERROR

Clinical Information

- Preoperative conferences for complex cases (e.g., orthopedic tumors) are very useful
- Ensure surgeons are aware of information that can alter IOC interpretation
- Utilize medical records, when possible, to obtain essential information prior to IOC
- Request additional information from surgeon if reason for IOC unclear or if unusual findings are encountered

Patient Identification

- Use of 2 identifiers on specimen and slide labels
- Read back of patient identification by operating room team
- Accession case with laboratory ID number as early as possible in handling process
  - All paperwork, slides, and specimen containers must be labeled

Sampling

- Careful gross examination and sectioning of mass lesions is essential
- Additional sampling of gross specimen or block is appropriate when only limited lesion is present for evaluation on slide
- Beware of secondary processes, such as scar, abscess, and granulomata
  - Sampling from edge of malignancy may only reveal reactive changes
- Examples of site-specific strategies to improve sampling
  - Additional gross or microscopic sectioning of lung granulomas and scars
  - Additional sampling of large ovarian/adnexal masses, particularly mucinous tumors
  - If malignancy is not seen on initial sections, staff pathologist should reexamine gross specimen
  - Complete exhaustion of negative tissue margins in skin excisions
  - Submission by surgeon of en face margins distinct from resection specimen for complex anatomic specimens (e.g., pancreatic duct margin, head and neck mucosal excisions)
- If diagnosis is not possible, request additional samples from surgeon if feasible or defer diagnosis if not

Interpretation

- Cases appropriate for IOC should be determined by institution
  - Inappropriate requests can be harmful to patients and may be more prone to error
    - e.g., small primary lesions should not be completely frozen for diagnosis
- Preview of scheduled cases, including review of any available prior slides for comparison, is helpful
- Use cytology preparations as adjunct to conventional frozen sections
- Use of differential diagnosis lists
  - A diagnosis not considered cannot be made
  - Have relevant resources with information about IOC readily available
- Consideration of metastatic disease

- Pathologist should be aware of clinical consequence of diagnosis
  - In some cases, a false-negative diagnosis may cause less patient harm than false-positive diagnosis
  - Communication of degree of certainty of diagnosis may be helpful to surgeon
- False-negative diagnoses are more common than false-positive diagnoses
  - Pathologists tend to be conservative
  - Specific criteria for malignancy can be helpful (e.g., for pancreatic carcinoma)
- Obtain 2nd opinion when possible
  - General "2nd eye"
  - Subspecialist expertise
  - On site or via telepathology
  - May be ad hoc or institutional policy for certain case types

Technical Factors

- Make sure cryostats are working at beginning of day by cutting test slide
- Ensure all personnel using cryostats and stain lines are adequately trained
- Do not hesitate to cut additional sections if tissue folds or holes make interpretation difficult

Communication

- Reporting diagnoses by telephone or intercom should follow recommended procedures
  - Confirm patient identity
  - Identify pathologist rendering diagnosis
  - Identify operating room team member receiving report
  - State findings in clearest terms possible; engage surgeon in discussion or have member of surgical team acknowledge any ambiguous findings
    - Avoid unnecessarily wordy diagnostic text
    - Be aware that qualifiers, such as "favor" or "suspicious," may be misunderstood
    - Uncertain (often deferred) diagnoses are more frequently misunderstood than benign or malignant
    - Similar terms may be confused (especially carcinoma vs. carcinoid)
  - Read back of diagnosis by operating team
    - Pathologist must listen to confirm correct understanding
    - Required by The Joint Commission (TJC) [formerly, Joint Commission on Accreditation of Healthcare Organizations (JCAHO)]
      - Standard DC.01.02.01: "Before taking action on a verbal order or verbal report of a test result, staff uses a record and 'read back' process to verify the information."
- Direct discussion between pathologist and surgeon may be preferable in some cases
  - Nuanced or complex diagnoses
  - Unclear indication for IOC
  - Elicitation of additional significant history
- Recording diagnoses
  - Written record of IOC should be incorporated in final diagnostic report
  - Include pathologist(s) issuing diagnosis
  - Include clinician who was informed of diagnosis
  - Pathology information should include
    - Diagnosis as reported to clinical staff
    - Qualifying comments as reported to clinical staff
    - Description of gross specimen received, particularly if changed by IOC
      - Collapse of cystic structure
      - Documentation of tissue submitted for special diagnostic or research studies or tissue banking
    - Orientation information
    - Ink &/or slide key, as appropriate

TOOLS TO IMPROVE PERSONAL PERFORMANCE

Quality Assurance Dashboard

- Dashboard refers to easily accessible user friendly set of tools and information
  - Analogous to gauges and information available to driver of car
- Can be used to compare individual pathologist performance against departmental or national benchmarks
- Useful for direct feedback to pathologist on overall performance using objective data
- Useful for institutional credentialing and peer review processes

Root Cause Analysis of Errors

- Errors should be discussed with pathologist(s) involved
- Useful for analysis of variables leading to error and feedback about specific case issues
  - Major errors resulting in changes in patient care due to lapses in knowledge may require focused retraining
  - Minor errors not resulting in changes in patient care should also be reviewed to keep pathologist aware of discrepancies

Intraoperative Consultation Conference

- Highly useful for sharing common challenges for complex or problematic cases through vicarious learning
  - All errors are opportunities for learning
  - In some cases, it may be appropriate to not identify pathologist involved
  - In other cases, it may be appropriate to have pathologist present case

Individual Pathologist Case Log

- Used by many pathologists for individual unofficial tracking of problematic or interesting cases
- Very helpful to for self-education and continued learning

SELECTED REFERENCES

1. Sams SB et al: Discordance between intraoperative consultation by frozen section and final diagnosis. Int J Surg Pathol. 25(1):41-50, 2017
2. McIntosh ER et al: Frozen section: guiding the hands of surgeons? Ann Diagn Pathol. 19(5):326-9, 2015
3. Roy S et al: Frozen section diagnosis: is there discordance between what pathologists say and what surgeons hear? Am J Clin Pathol. 140(3):363-9, 2013
4. Winther C et al: Accuracy of frozen section diagnosis: a retrospective analysis of 4785 cases. APMIS. 119(4-5):259-62, 2011

Block Sampling Error: Focal Lesion

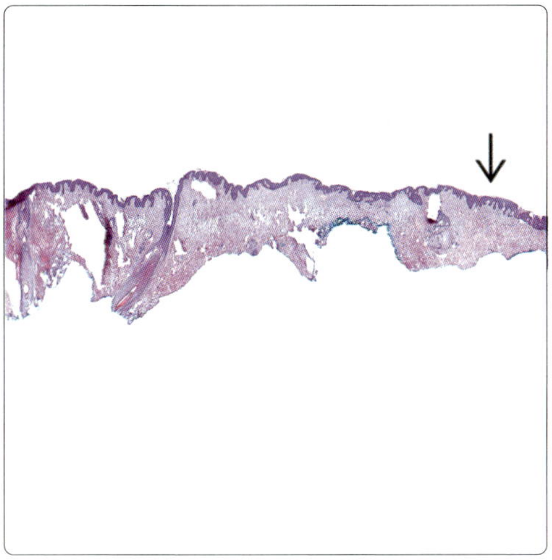

Block Sampling Error: Focal Lesion

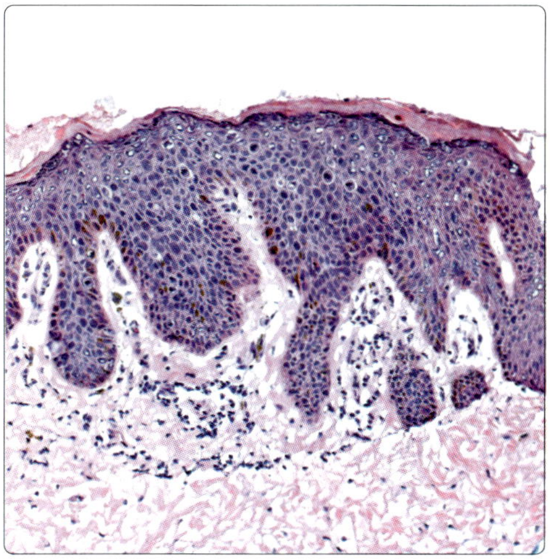

(Left) *Small lesions are easily missed. The margin of this 2.2-cm skin excision was interpreted as negative on frozen section. A < 0.5-mm focus of Bowen disease was seen on permanent section, requiring reexcision.* **(Right)** *Very small focus of penile Bowen disease (squamous cell carcinoma in situ) shows near full-thickness keratinocytic dysplasia, mitotic figures, and apoptosis of lesional cells. The focus involved < 2% of the width of the margin strip and was initially missed on frozen section.*

Possible Interpretive Error: Frozen Section Artifact

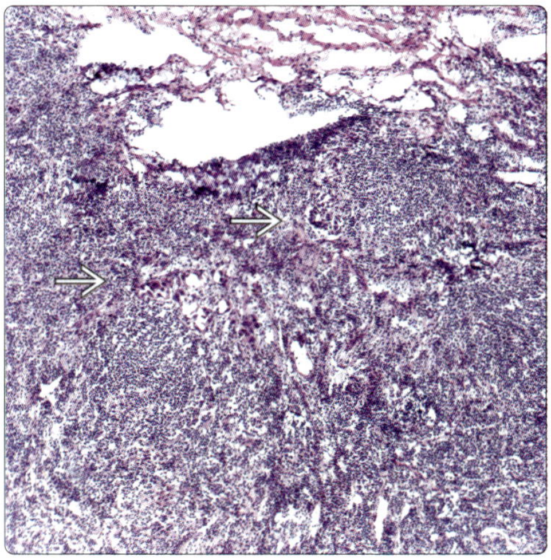

Block Sampling: Lesions Too Small for Routine Detection

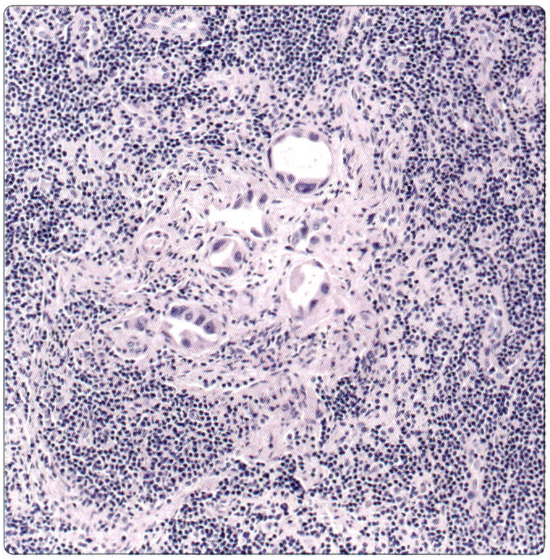

(Left) *Metastases may be difficult to detect or interpret in tissue distorted by frozen section artifact. This lymph node was reported as "atypical cells present, deferred" and proved to be metastatic carcinoma on permanent section.* **(Right)** *Small lymph node metastases (< 2 mm) are not detected in all cases without exhaustive evaluation, which is not clinically warranted. This focus of carcinoma was not present in the frozen sections but was seen in the permanent section. This should not be considered a frozen section error.*

Block Sampling Error: Focal Lesion

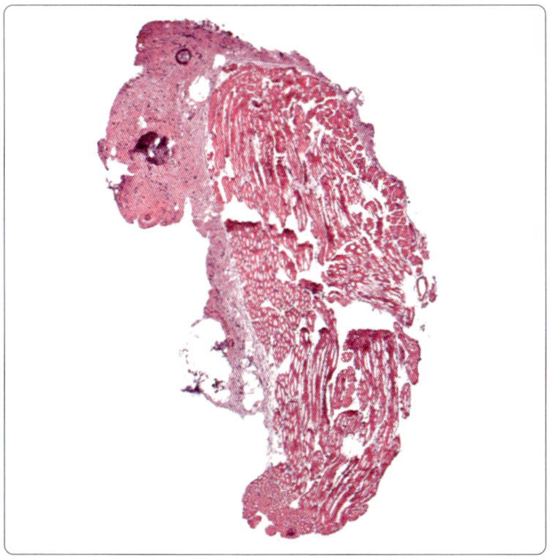

Block Sampling Error: Soft Tissue Margin

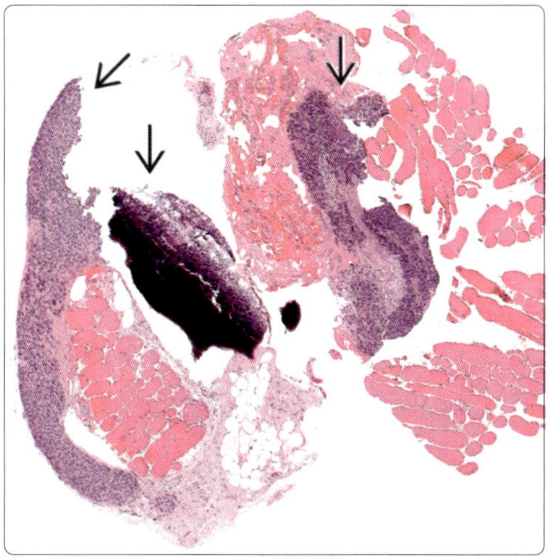

(Left) *This soft tissue margin from a melanoma resection shows no tumor on frozen section. However, tumor was found in the deeper permanent sections prepared from the same tissue block.* **(Right)** *Melanoma was not present in the frozen section slides of this margin. However, multiple foci of tumor are present in the deeper permanent sections. Comparison of the slides revealed that the frozen section only showed a small superficial area of the tissue present in the block, resulting in sampling error.*

Interpretive Error: Section Quality and Crush Artifact

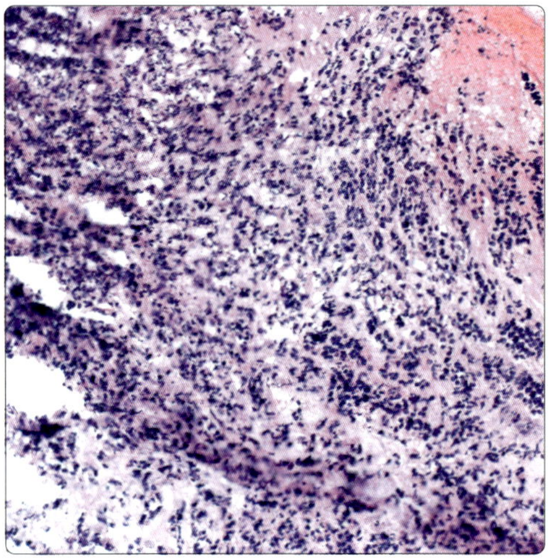

Interpretive Error: Section Quality and Crush Artifact

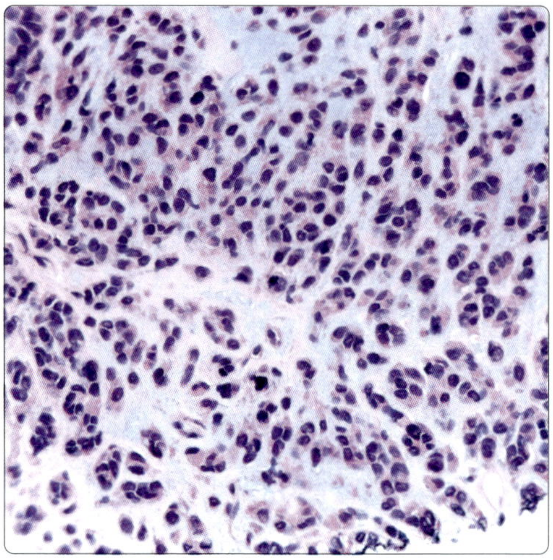

(Left) *This gastric wall biopsy with crush and sectioning artifact was interpreted as "malignancy, carcinoma vs. lymphoma." The final diagnosis was gastrointestinal stromal tumor. Use of differential diagnosis checklists based on morphology, anatomic site, &/or clinical scenario can expand intraoperative diagnostic considerations.* **(Right)** *The frozen sections from this gastrointestinal stromal tumor were virtually uninterpretable, leading to a nonspecific intraoperative diagnosis.*

Gross Sampling Error: Elastotic Scar in Lung Mass

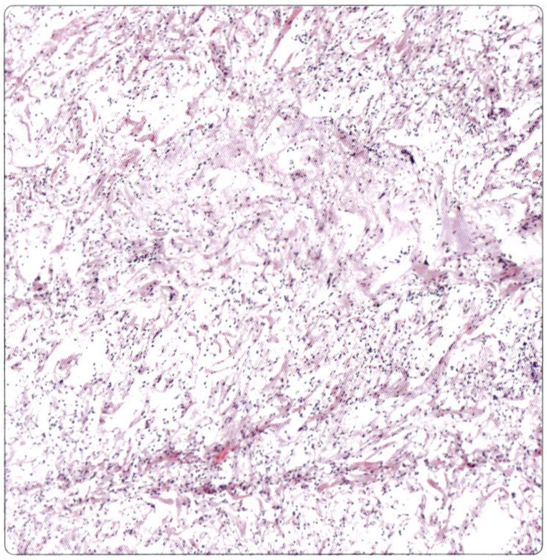

Gross Sampling Error: Elastotic Scar in Lung Mass

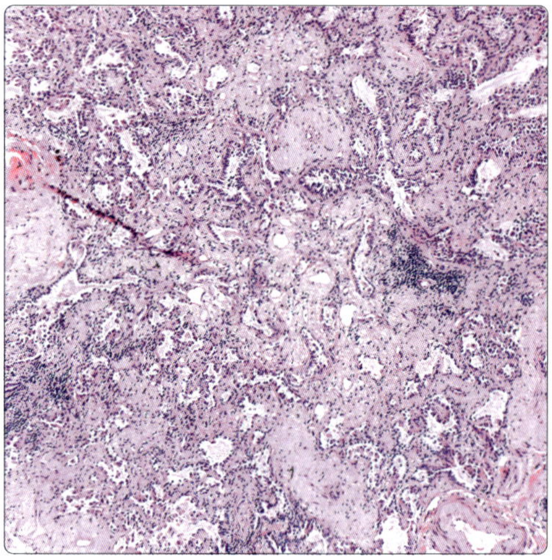

(Left) *This frozen section was correctly interpreted as showing no malignancy. A small focus of adenocarcinoma was found in additional sections. Adenocarcinoma of the lung is often associated with elastotic scar. A negative initial frozen section should prompt consideration of additional block or mass sampling.* **(Right)** *This 3-mm lung adenocarcinoma was present in a 6-mm mass. The frozen sections showed elastotic scar only.*

Gross Sampling Error: Granulomatous Response to Lung Carcinoma

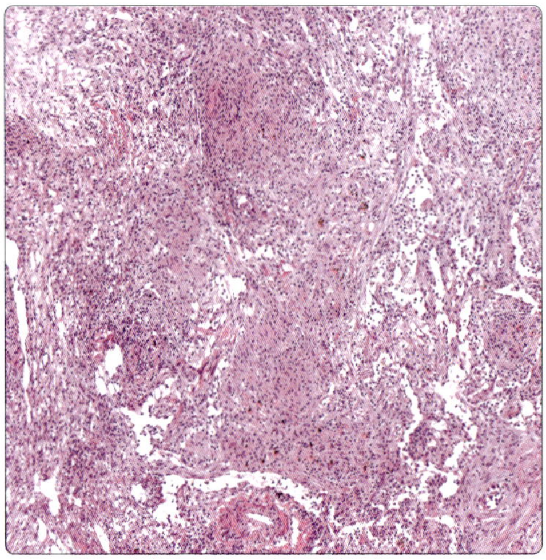

Gross Sampling Error: Granulomatous Response to Lung Carcinoma

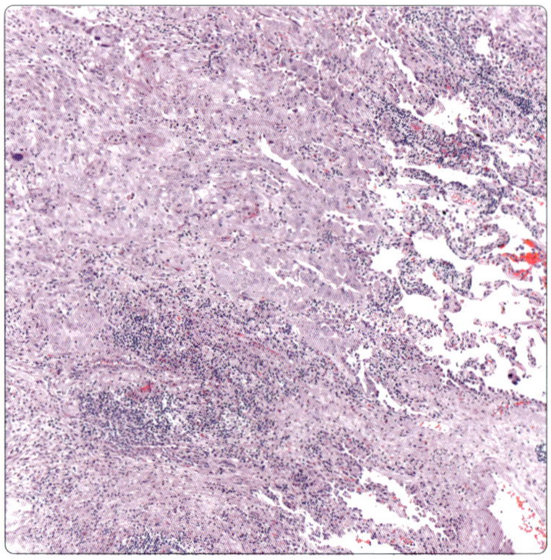

(Left) *On occasion, lung carcinoma may prompt a granulomatous response in nearby nonneoplastic tissue. This frozen section showed only palisading granulomas but was located adjacent to a 3.2-cm adenocarcinoma. Careful gross examination is necessary to select the tissue most likely to show diagnostic findings.* **(Right)** *This permanent section of lung adenocarcinoma shows inflammation and granulomatous response in the adjacent lung tissue. Intraoperative frozen sections showed granulomata only.*

Gross Sampling: Focal Lesion

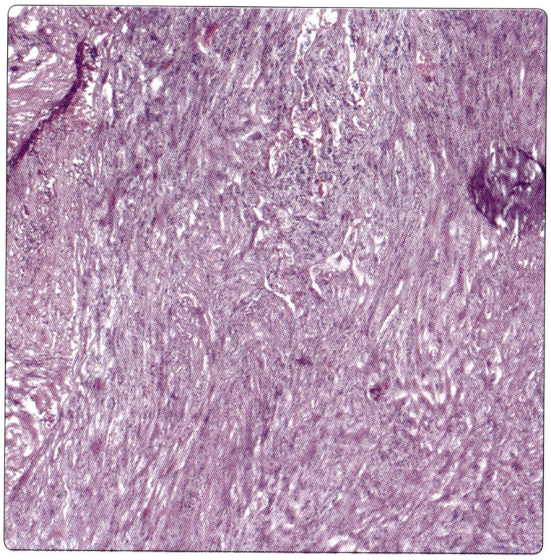

Gross Sampling: Focal Lesion

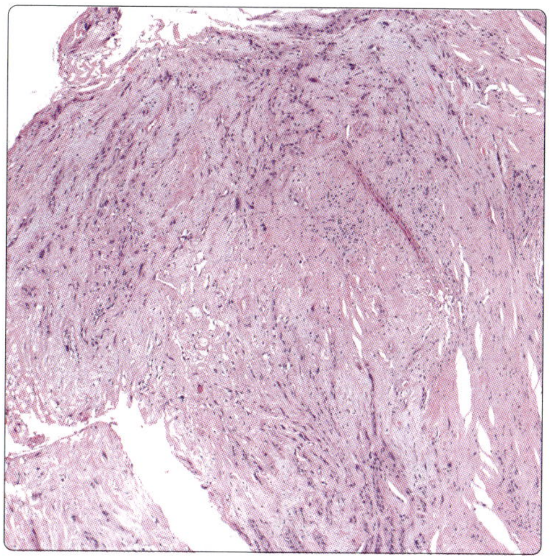

(Left) *Soft tissue biopsy of a previously radiated head and neck squamous cell carcinoma shows extensive fibrosis, reactive atypia of fibroblasts, and ill-defined necrotic cells.* **(Right)** *The frozen sections of this treated squamous cell carcinoma did not reveal malignancy. However, residual viable tumor was evident on permanent sections. Treated tumors are often paucicellular and difficult to detect. Small lesions cannot always be detected by reasonable sampling for frozen section.*

Possible Interpretive Error: Cautery Effect at Specimen Margin

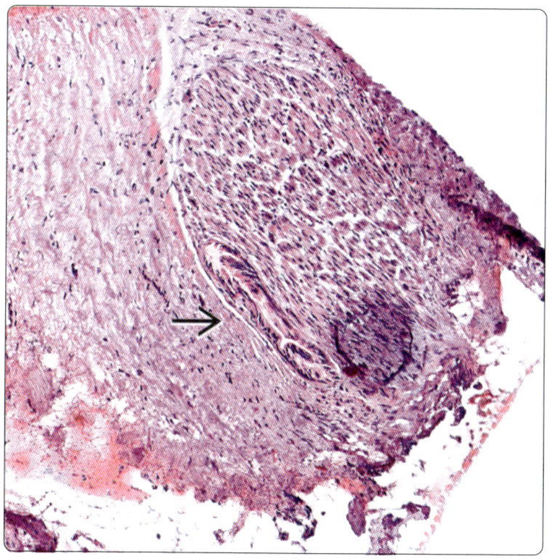

Possible Interpretive Error: Cautery Artifact

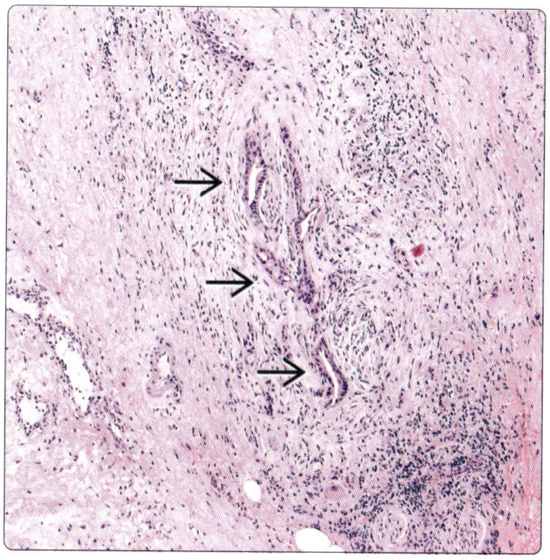

(Left) *This frozen section of a bile duct margin shows a focus of perineural invasion by adenocarcinoma ⇒. Detection is hampered by cautery effect that makes the tumor cells smaller, spindled in morphology, and aligned with nerve fibers. In addition, the focus is located away from the actual duct margin.* **(Right)** *This previously frozen, paraffin-embedded section of nerve shows much more extensive perineural tumor ⇒ and less cautery effect than were present on the original frozen section slides.*

Interpretation Requiring Ancillary Studies: Detection of Organisms

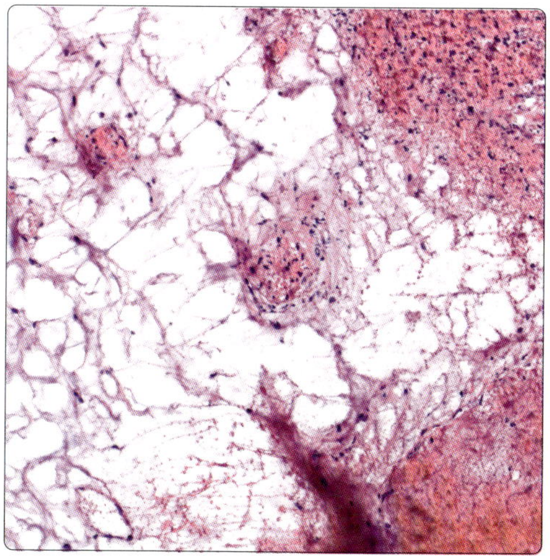

Interpretation Requiring Ancillary Studies: Detection of Organisms

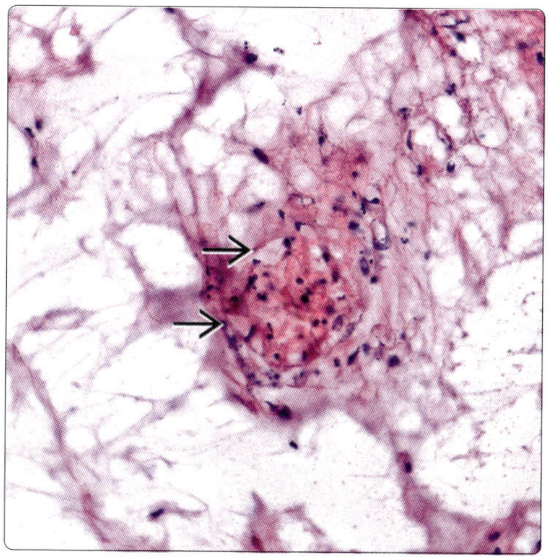

(Left) *Sinus biopsies may be performed to identify invasive fungal infections. This frozen section shows fascicular inflammation, fibrin, and hemorrhage. Although the pattern is suggestive of infection, no organisms are seen. In many cases, special stains are required for identification.* **(Right)** *A frozen section of a sinus biopsy shows refractile structures ⇒ suggestive, but not diagnostic, of fungi. A clinical history of minimal bleeding during biopsy supports a diagnosis of invasive fungi.*

INTRODUCTION

Factors Predisposing to Injury

- Risk to personnel in intraoperative consultation (IOC) room is greater than risk to pathology personnel in general due to multiple factors
  - **Time constraints**
    - Activities (e.g., examining specimens, cutting sections) need to be performed quickly
  - **Multiple people from different departments use IOC room**
    - Pathology personnel, surgeons, operating room nurses, and researchers may be present
    - Not all people may be familiar with best practices for room and specimens
  - **Multiple people may be involved in examining single specimen**
    - Each person must be responsible for appropriate and careful handling and disposal of sharps
  - **Unfamiliarity with room &/or equipment**
    - Some personnel may only use room intermittently
      - Safety equipment may not always be used appropriately
      - Materials may not be replaced or replenished appropriately
    - Room may be used at night and on weekends when personnel familiar with room are not present
  - **Less experienced personnel may perform tasks at irregular intervals**
    - May only use cryostat during IOCs
  - **Patients undergoing surgery may have undiagnosed infectious disease**
    - Pathology personnel who are immunocompromised or with compromised skin (dermatitis, weeping skin lesions, or wounds) may have increased vulnerability
- It is important to have protocols and personnel in place to ensure safety
  - One person should be designated as being in charge of IOC room
    - Ensures room is properly equipped and maintained
    - Provides training to new personnel
    - Supervises daily use of room
  - New pathology personnel should be trained in appropriate procedures during IOC
    - Training should occur annually or when new procedure is introduced

TRAUMATIC INJURIES

Sources

- Razor blades
  - Should have single blade and always be used with protective sheath
- Cryostat blades
  - Blades should never be cleaned with hands
  - Large swab (e.g., gauze wrapped around applicator) is safer method to brush shavings away from blade
  - Injuries from cryostat blades are particularly problematic as exposure to multiple specimens is possible
  - If chuck or block needs to be manipulated, this should be done outside of cryostat
    - Removal of excess embedding material
    - Removal of staples from tissue
- Scalpels
  - Blades must be removed with caution using hemostat or forceps
  - Common source of injuries is during removal of blade when it is contaminated
- Large cutting blades
  - Disposable blades are preferred
    - Can be disposed rather than cleaned
    - Do not require sharpening
- Syringe needles
  - Use of needles is rarely indicated and should be avoided due to risk of penetrating injuries
  - If used, needle should be directly discarded into sharps container and not recapped
  - Needles should not be used to mark site of lesion for later evaluation

Face Protection: Splashes

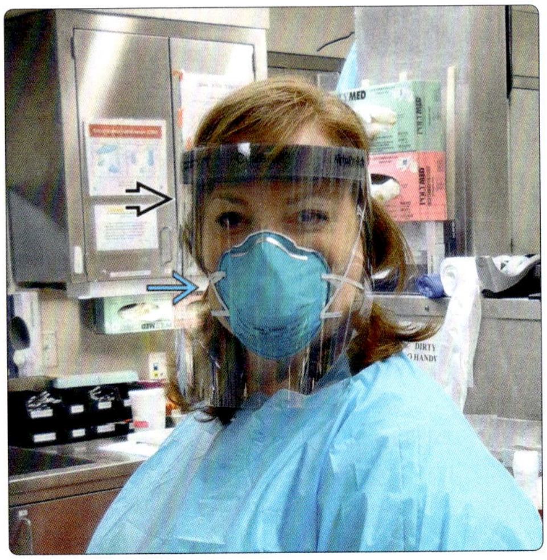

Face Protection: Chemical Exposure

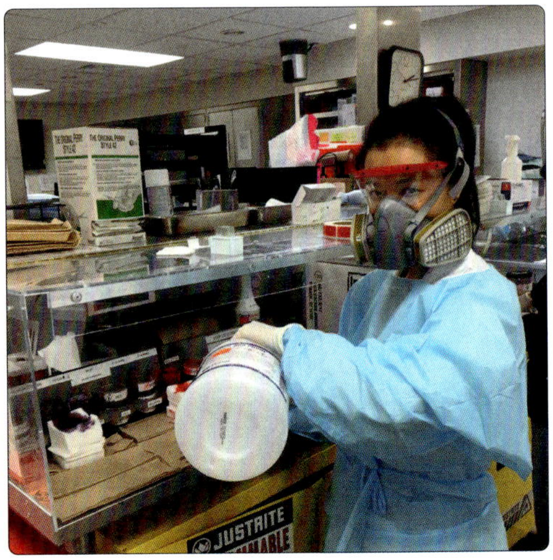

(Left) *When there is a risk of splashing (e.g., opening large cystic masses), a full face shield ⇨ provides the best protection. A face mask ⇨ provides additional protection for the lower face and mouth. (Courtesy K. Gill, PA.)* **(Right)** *Special masks designed to protect against chemical fumes may be worn when performing tasks such as changing solutions on a staining rack. (Courtesy V. Chan, BS.)*

- Large paperclips can be threaded through tissue to mark lesions (e.g., site where radio seed was removed)

Types of Injuries

- Most common type of injury is laceration from blade
- Nondominant hand injuries most common but also occur to dominant hand
- Injuries can potentially convey infectious agents

Prevention

- All blades must be discarded by person using blade
  - Common source of injury is from blades hidden by surgical drapes, paper towels, or tissue
  - Blades should be discarded rather than left on work space after use
- The hand holding the specimen should be well away from the hand holding the blade
  - Hard specimens that require increased force to section are particularly hazardous
  - Specimen can be held with gauze, which provides firmer grip and helps keep nondominant hand away from blade
- Kevlar gloves or metal mesh gloves are available
  - In actual practice, these gloves are unwieldy and difficult to use
- Use of needles and other piercing instruments should be avoided
- Frozen embedding medium should not be removed from chuck using blade
  - Common source of injury
  - Chuck can be kept at room temperature until block is melted or chuck and block can be briefly dipped into formalin container to speed melting
- Cytologic preparations should be used rather than frozen sections when infection is suspected

INHALATION

Sources

- Tissue from patients with infectious disease
- Chemicals (stains, fixatives)
  - Formaldehyde and xylene are of most concern

Mechanism of Injury

- Infection
  - Only reported when aerosolized coolants have been used to freeze blocks with tissue containing *Mycobacterium tuberculosis*
    - Coolants should not be sprayed directly onto tissue
    - If used to cool block, resulting aerosol should be contained within cryostat and not inhaled
    - Better alternative methods for cooling blocks rapidly are available
  - Specimens are unlikely to pose threat under other conditions
- Chemical inhalation
  - Unlikely to occur unless chemicals are not stored properly or unless there is large spill

Prevention

- Infection
  - Masks designed to protect from aerosolized bacteria are available
  - Specific masks for protection from *M. tuberculosis* should be used when specimens from patients with known infections are examined
- Chemical inhalation
  - Appropriate ventilation of IOC room is essential
  - Chemicals must be tightly capped and stored
    - Staining racks should be kept covered when not in use to prevent evaporation as well as air contamination
  - Spill kit and protocol must be available

MUCOCUTANEOUS EXPOSURE

Sources

- Bloody specimens
- Cysts with fluid under pressure

Types of Injuries

- Splash injury into eyes or mouth
- Cutaneous exposure into breaks in skin

Prevention

- Personal protective equipment must always be worn
  - Protective goggles or face masks must be worn when handling specimens that are likely to pose risk of splashing
  - Double gloves should be worn when handling particularly bloody specimens or specimens of known or suspected infectious risk
- Extreme care should be exercised when cutting into hard, intact mass that could be cystic
  - Piercing cyst can result in forceful ejection of fluid several feet
  - Waterproof barrier may be kept over site of incision until it is determined if fluid is present or not
  - Cysts should be opened near sink to aid in disposal of fluid cyst contents
- Eating, drinking, smoking, and application of cosmetics or lip balm are not allowed in IOC room
  - Food cannot be stored in room or refrigerators and must not be discarded in waste containers
- Material that will leave IOC room must be clean to protect personnel outside room from exposures
  - Outer specimen container is kept clean
  - All paperwork is kept clean
    - If contamination occurs, paperwork can be placed inside protective plastic sleeve or information copied onto clean form

INFECTIOUS AGENTS

General Guidelines

- Freezing does not inactivate infectious agents
- Formalin inactivates many infectious agents but may require many hours to do so
  - Prions remain infective after routine fixation
- IOCs should only be performed when absolutely necessary on specimens suspected to harbor infectious agent
- However, majority of infectious agents do not pose risks to immunocompetent individuals

Tuberculosis

- 3 cases of conversion to positive skin tests have been reported during performance of frozen section

- All involved use of aerosolized coolant and inhalation
- Aerosols should be avoided
- Yearly tuberculous (TB) tests are recommended for all hospital personnel

Creutzfeldt-Jakob Disease

- 3 cases have been reported in 2 histotechnologists and 1 pathologist
  - Exposure was to fixed tissues
  - No cases have been reported during performance of IOC
- Special techniques are necessary to inactivate prion proteins
  - Formalin fixation for 24 hours
  - 95% formic acid for 1 hour
  - Formalin fixation for another 24 hours
- Symptoms suggestive of Creutzfeldt-Jakob disease (CJD) include
  - Rapidly progressive dementia
  - Myoclonus
  - Nonspecific neurologic findings
- Tissue handling
  - Specimens from patients with suspected CJD should not be examined by IOC
  - Tissue should be fixed immediately following suggested protocols and stored in secure location
  - Clinical necessity of tissue processing should be considered carefully before placing personnel at risk

HIV

- No cases have been reported during performance of IOC
  - 1 reported case of pathologist infected after scalpel injury to hand during performance of autopsy
- ~ 0.3% risk of infection after penetrating injury
- Postexposure prophylaxis includes 4-week treatment with 2 drugs

Hepatitis B Virus

- No cases have been reported during performance of IOC
- 30% risk of infection after percutaneous penetrating injury
  - Likely also high risk after mucocutaneous exposure
- Infectious hepatitis B virus (HBV) can exist in dried blood for at least 1 week
- Pathology personnel should be vaccinated for hepatitis B
- If nonvaccinated person is exposed, postexposure prophylaxis includes vaccination for HBV
  - Hepatitis B immune globulin can also be used

Hepatitis C Virus

- No cases have been reported during performance of IOC
- ~ 1.8% risk of exposure after penetrating injury
  - Risk after mucocutaneous exposure is likely low
- Hepatitis C virus (HCV) degrades rapidly in environment
- Personnel should be monitored for infection after exposure
  - Postexposure prophylaxis has not been shown to be effective

TUMORS

Risk After Exposure

- Single case report of sarcoma transferred to physician
  - Surgeon suffered injury to hand during excision of sarcoma
  - Sarcoma developed at site of injury
  - Genetic analysis showed that tumor was derived from patient
  - Physician remained well 2 years later
- Rare reports of injected tumor cell lines growing in recipient
- Procedures to avoid exposure to infectious agents also prevent exposure to tumors
  - Risk of transferring tumor to another person is extremely low

RADIATION

Specimens

- Radioactive agents are sometimes used intraoperatively
  - Sentinel lymph node identification
  - Radioactive seeds for localization of breast lesions
  - Octreotide to localize neuroendocrine lesions
- Dose used is generally too low to result in significant exposure to pathology personnel
  - Special procedures are generally not required to limit exposure
    - Standard gloves are adequate for protection
  - Radioactive seeds contain iodine-125 that emits low energy gamma rays of 20-30 keV
    - Titanium capsule surrounds internal core filament containing iodine-125
    - If internal core filament is damaged, area must be treated as radioactive spill
      - Damaging seed should be avoided by not using scissors and very carefully sectioning specimen with scalpel under guidance with gamma probe
- Adequate storage area required for retrieved radioactive material
  - Radioactive seeds can be safely stored in metal container
    - Seed must be stored in closed container listing corresponding surgical pathology number
    - Log book is required to document specific seed, when retrieved from specimen and when released to Radiation Safety Department

Prevention

- If radioactive agents used during surgery, risk to pathology personnel should be considered
- If radioactive materials need to be retrieved (e.g., radioactive seeds), procedures for doing so must be instituted
- Pathologists must have necessary equipment (e.g., Geiger counter, gamma probe) to monitor radioactive material and to detect radioactive medical devices

PERSONAL PROTECTIVE EQUIPMENT

General Guidelines

- Personal protective equipment (PPE) is defined as equipment designed to prevent exposure of skin or clothing to blood or other infectious materials
  - Worn to minimize exposure to hazards that cause serious workplace injuries and illnesses

- Includes chemical, radiological, physical, electrical, mechanical, or other workplace hazards
- Must be provided by institution to employees
- Must be discarded appropriately when contaminated and when leaving IOC room

Hands

- Gloves must always be worn when handling tissues
  - Rings with sharp surfaces should be removed as they can increase likelihood of puncture
- 2 pairs of gloves are recommended if infectious agent suspected
- Latex gloves protect against biohazards but not chemicals
  - Latex is permeable to chemicals and can rapidly degrade when exposed to some types
- Nitrile and neoprene gloves protect against biohazards and exposure to fixatives
  - Personnel with latex allergy may use nitrile gloves
- Metal mesh and Kevlar cloth gloves are available if puncture injuries are possible
  - Latex or nitrile gloves are worn beneath and over gloves
- Soiled gloves should be discarded and replaced when touching other objects in room
  - Gloves should also be changed between specimens to avoid any chance of contamination
- Hands must always be washed after handling specimens and when leaving IOC room
  - Small, inapparent breaks in gloves are common
  - If 2 gloves are worn and blood is present between gloves, gloves should immediately be removed to determine source of blood
    - If hand injury is identified, first aid and evaluation of infection exposure is required

Head and Face

- Eye protection should be worn if splash injuries are possible
  - Safety glasses or goggles
  - Full face mask
  - Face protection should include side shields
- Special respiratory masks protect against aerosolized TB
  - N-95 masks filter at least 95% of particulates that are 3 μm or larger
  - Requires each person to be individually fitted for mask
  - In practice, these masks are uncomfortable and not often used
- Surgical masks
  - Designed to protect patients from exhalations of person wearing mask
  - Inadequate to protect pathology personnel from aerosolized infectious agents
    - Can provide protection of mouth and lower face from splashes

Body

- Scrub suits may be worn when exposure is probable
  - These clothes can be easily exchanged for clean replacements if exposure occurs
- Aprons are used over clothes or scrub suits to protect torso
  - Sleeve protectors or aprons with sleeves are preferable when numerous specimens are handled
- Disposable jumpsuits offer complete coverage of body
- Lab coats should not be used for protection if also worn outside of IOC room

EQUIPMENT AND ROOM

Cryostat

- Ideally, 1 cryostat should be designated for known or possible infectious cases
  - Cases requiring decontamination include known or suspected HIV, HBV, HCV, SARS-related coronavirus, prion disease, myobacterial disease, or systemic fungal disease
  - After cryostat is used for such cases, it must be marked and not used again until after decontamination
- All cryostats must be decontaminated at defined intervals
  - Cryostat is defrosted
  - Tuberculocidal disinfectant is used to clean interior
  - Trimmings and sections of tissues must be removed
- More frequent decontamination is necessary if known infectious cases have been processed

Room

- "Clean" areas should be designated where gloves must not be worn
  - Typically microscopes, telephones, door knobs
    - Most common items used by personnel not directly involved in processing specimens
  - Only clean hands without gloves are allowed to handle material in these areas
  - Avoids possible contamination with biohazardous material that has touched gloves
- All soiled disposable material should be immediately placed in appropriate biohazard containers
- Exposed surfaces are cleaned and disinfected with diluted bleach or other appropriate sterilants

Specimens

- Fix in adequate amount of formalin as soon as possible
- Container must be leakproof and securely sealed
- Specimens that may be infected with CJD must be specifically labeled as biohazard and stored separately
  - These specimens require additional handling to inactivate prions

Chemicals

- Fixatives and stains are associated with health risks if inhaled, ingested, or if exposure to mucous membranes
  - Formalin: Acute effects
    - Strong eye and throat irritation
    - Coughing, wheezing, chest tightness
    - Bronchitis, laryngitis
    - Corneal clouding, loss of vision
  - Xylene: Acute effects
    - Strong irritant of eyes, nose, throat, mucous membranes, skin
    - At high concentrations, can cause headache, dizziness, nausea
  - Aerosol freezing agent: Acute effects
    - Usually use carbon dioxide and propellant
    - Effects are dependent on specific formulation
- Material safety data sheets must be available in room

- Includes information on hazardous ingredients, physical/chemical characteristics, fire and explosion data, reactivity data, information on health hazards, precautions for safe handling and use of chemicals, response to spills, storage and safe disposal methods, and effect on environment
- Flammable chemicals must be kept in metal cabinet
  - Fire extinguisher suitable for chemical fires must be available
- Containers should be kept sealed when not in use and staining racks should be kept covered
- When chemicals are handled, protective gloves must be worn
- Spill kit must be available for small amounts of chemical
  - Absorbent material is poured around spill for containment
  - Absorbent material is then poured over chemical
  - Material can then be swept or brushed into appropriate hazardous waste container
- If large spill cannot be contained, additional help must be requested
  - Room should be evacuated and doors kept closed

Safety Equipment

- Removal of scalpel handles
  - Injuries may occur when removing blade from handle
    - Blades should not be removed using hands
  - Forceps or hemostats can be used
    - Handle is held firmly
    - Blade is pointed away from prosector and other people
    - Blade and blade lock must be facing upward with slanted edge of blade facing toward prosector
    - Base of blade is grasped with forceps or hemostat and pulled outward away from handle until blade lock hole lifts off lock
    - Blade is then carefully moved forward (toward tip) to remove
    - Blade is then placed in sharps container
  - Special devices can also be used to remove handles
- Sharps containers
  - Used to dispose of all blades and needles
    - Must be red &/or marked with biohazard sign
    - Leakproof
  - Should be emptied frequently so that sharps can be dropped into container
    - Sharps should never be pushed into container

Waste Disposal

- Materials contaminated or possibly contaminated with blood or infectious agents
  - All PPE and other materials in contact with specimens and blood must be disposed into specific containers

POST INJURY OR EXPOSURE TREATMENT

Immediate Care

- Administer first aid as necessary
- Wash penetrating injuries with soap and water
  - Allow bleeding injuries to continue to bleed liberally
- Eye and mucous membrane injuries are flushed with water
  - Copious amounts of water should be used and eyelids should be held open
  - There should be access to eyewash fountain
- Record name and other identifiers of patient whose specimen was involved in exposure
  - Occupational Safety and Health Administration (OSHA) requires maintaining logs of occupational exposure and sharps injuries

Subsequent Care

- Consult institutional healthcare team
  - Each institution should have policies for treatment after injury or exposure
  - Incident reports are important to identify repeated problems
  - For some exposures, prophylactic treatment is indicated
    - National Clinicians' Postexposure Prophylaxis Hotline (888) 448-4911

RESOURCES

OSHA

- Refer to OSHA website, Bloodborne pathogens, standard 1910.1030 (see references)
  - Includes regulations for PPE, labeling and disposing of hazardous waste, record keeping (sharps injury log, occupational exposure log, training log) as well as many others
- Refer to OSHA website, Respiratory protection, standard 1910.134 (see references)
  - Primarily issues related to protection from particulates and toxic fumes
- Refer to OSHA website, Personal protective equipment

Clinical and Laboratory Standard Institute (CLSI)

- Protection of laboratory workers from occupationally acquired infection guidelines

College of American Pathologists

- Laboratory Accreditation Program Manual
  - Requirements related to pathology personnel safety include
    - All solutions and stains are properly labeled and changed on defined schedule
    - Cryostats are decontaminated at defined intervals and record is kept of this procedure

SELECTED REFERENCES

1. Fritzsche FR et al: Cut-resistant protective gloves in pathology–effective and cost-effective. Virchows Arch. 452(3):313-8, 2008
2. Jeffries D: Decontamination and CJD: the latest guidance. J Perioper Pract. 16(11):555-60, 2006
3. Kubiczek P et al: Occupational injuries in a pathology residency program. Arch Pathol Lab Med. 130(2):146-7, 2006
4. OSHA. Bloodborne pathogens, standard 1910.1030. https://www.osha.gov/pls/oshaweb/owadisp.show_document?p_id=10051&p_table=STANDARDS. Accessed August 24, 2017
5. OSHA. Respiratory protection, standard 1910.134. https://www.osha.gov/pls/oshaweb/owadisp.show_document?p_table=STANDARDS&p_id=12716. Accessed August 25, 2017
6. OSHA. Personal protective equipment. https://www.osha.gov/SLTC/personalprotectiveequipment/index.html. Accessed August 25, 2017

Types of Gloves

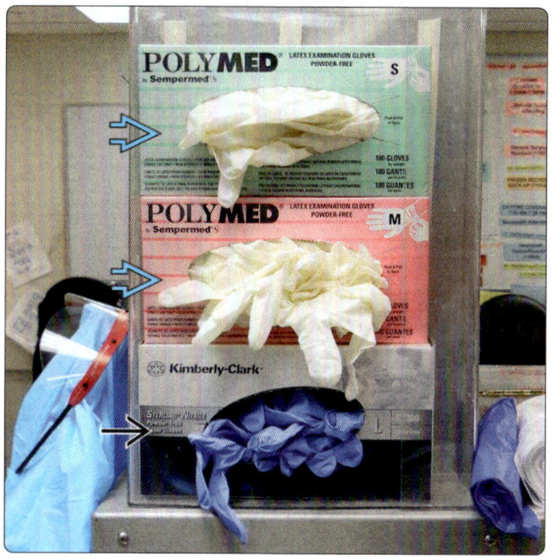

Cut-Resistant Gloves

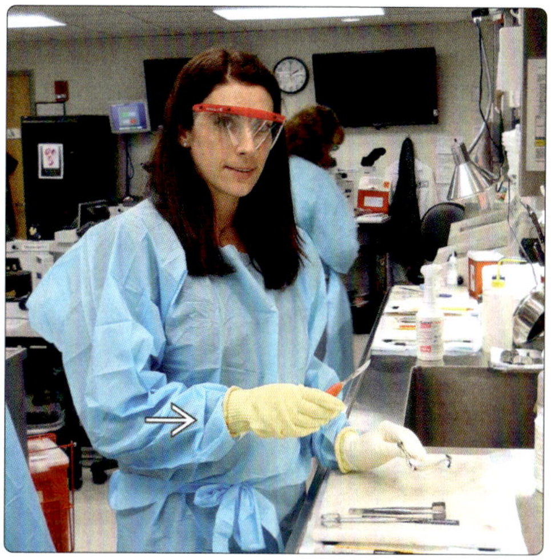

(Left) *Latex gloves* ⇨ *protect against biological materials but are not protective against chemicals. Some people have latex allergies and need to avoid this type of glove. Nitrile gloves* ⇨ *or neoprene gloves protect against both biological materials and chemicals such as formalin.* **(Right)** *Gloves designed with metal mesh or synthetic fibers such as Kevlar* ➡ *can be used in addition to latex gloves when there is a danger of laceration. However, these gloves may reduce dexterity and are not commonly used. (Courtesy L. Cheney, PA.)*

Blades

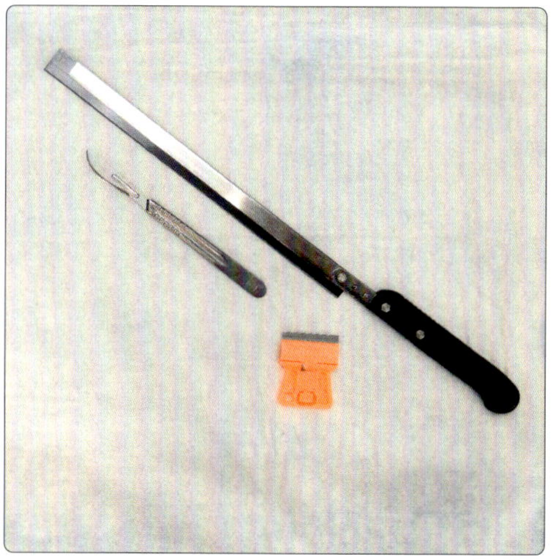

Most Common Hand Injuries

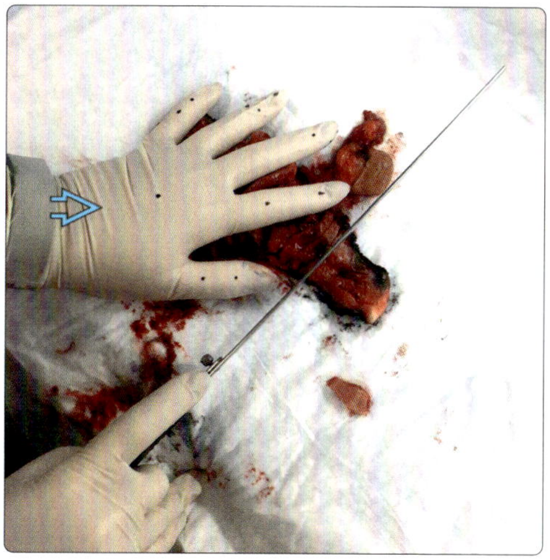

(Left) *The majority of injuries incurred during intraoperative consults are lacerations due to razor blades, scalpels, knives, or cryostat blades. The need for rapid diagnosis must not override safe practices. Blades should be used with the correct handles and discarded appropriately immediately after use.* **(Right)** *The nondominant hand* ⇨ *is more susceptible to injury, as it is often used to hold specimens while sectioning. The dots on the glove indicate the most frequent sites of injury.*

Clearing Cryostat Blade With Brush

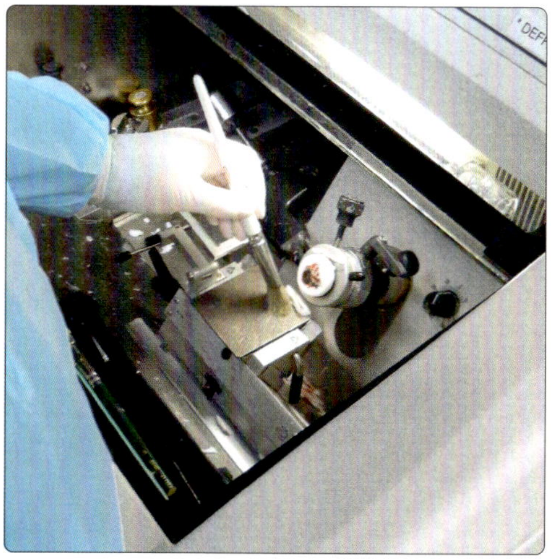

Glove Perforation

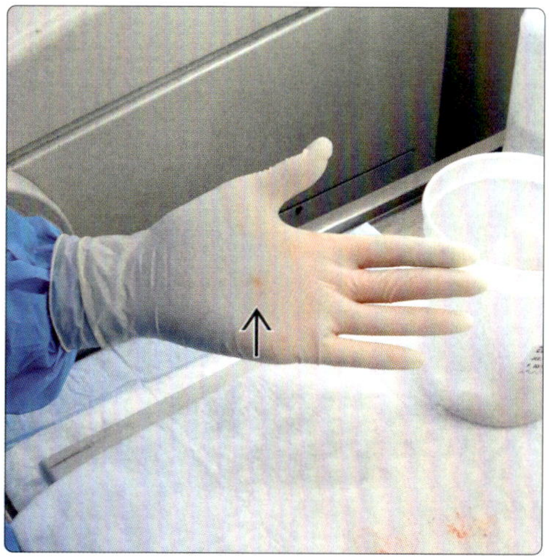

(Left) *The cryostat blade is cleaned of shavings before cutting a new block, or when shavings accumulate when facing a block. A large brush or swab should be used for this purpose. This should never be done with a hand because of the danger of laceration from the cryostat blade.* **(Right)** *If 2 gloves are used and blood is seen between the gloves* ⇨*, there has been a perforation in the outer glove or in both gloves. The gloves should be immediately removed and the hand examined for possible injuries.*

(Left) *The work space must be kept clean and free of clutter. Blades* ⇨ *should be kept at the far side of the area (with the blade pointed away from the prosector) when not in use.* **(Right)** *Cluttered work spaces greatly increase the likelihood of injury and errors. Blades* ⇨ *may not be seen if left intermingled in paper towels and discarded gloves. A common source of injury is a laceration due to a hidden blade when cleaning a workspace. Blood* ⇨ *and tissue contamination also should be avoided.*

Clean Work Space

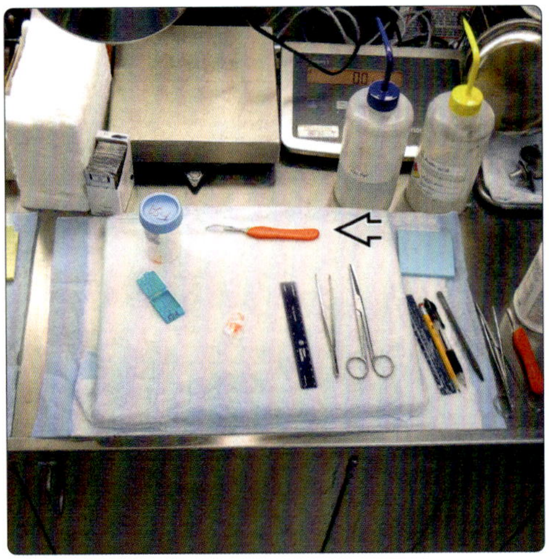

Cluttered Work Space

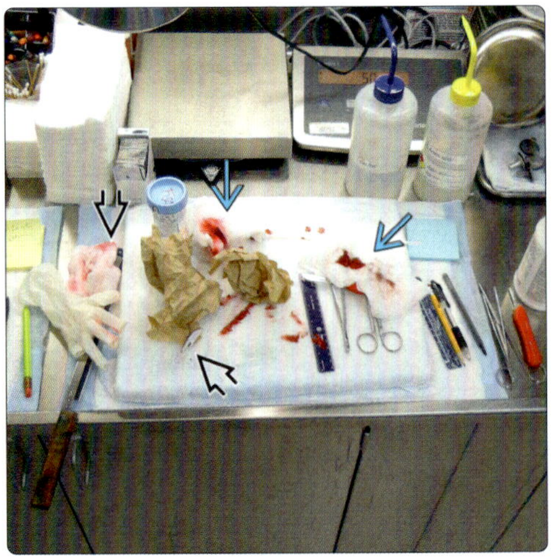

(Left) *A frozen block must be removed from the chuck to process the tissue. This should never be done with a blade, as the force required can result in deep injuries to the hand. The block can be allowed to partially melt at room temperature or will melt more quickly if dipped into formalin. A softened block is easily removed with a finger.* **(Right)** *After a block is slightly softened, it can be removed safely from the chuck with a finger or a ruler. The remnant is wrapped in lens paper and placed in formalin.*

Removing Block From Chuck

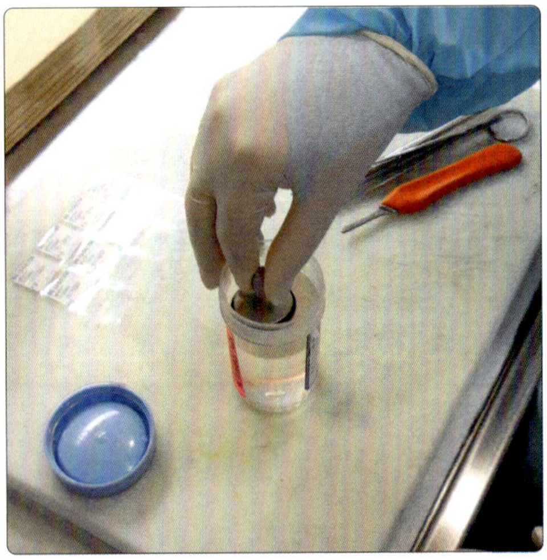

Removing Block From Chuck

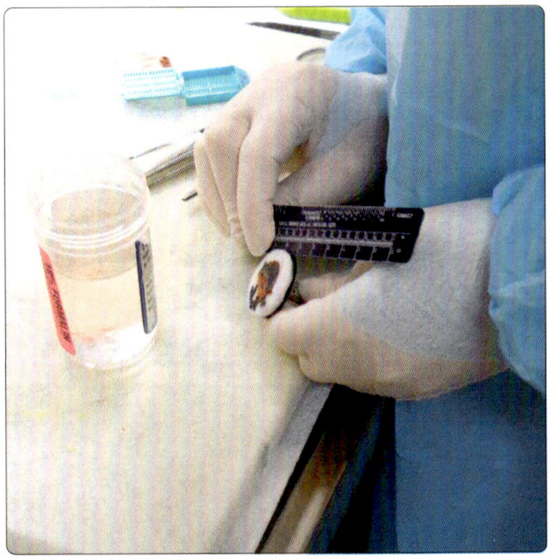

(Left) *Materials, such as paperwork, that are transferred to other locations cannot be contaminated* ⇨*. Paperwork will be handled by transcriptionists and other personnel who do not use personal protective equipment. If contamination occurs, protective sleeves can be used for soiled paperwork.* **(Right)** *All blades, needles, and unused glass slides must be disposed into appropriate containers designed for safe disposal. This container is not safe because sharp objects* ⇨ *are protruding from the top and pose a hazard.*

Soiled Paperwork

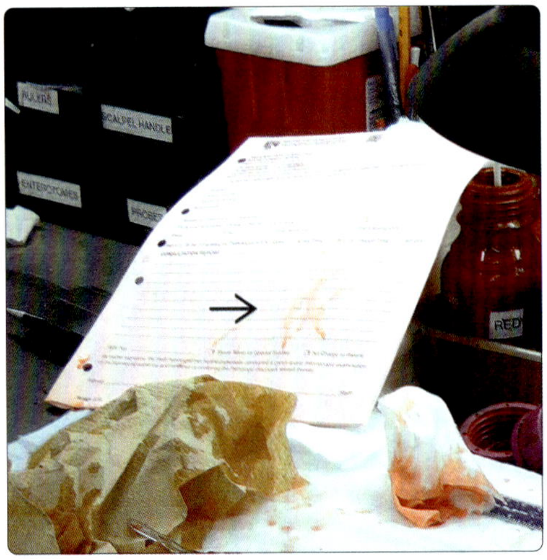

Unsafe Sharps Container

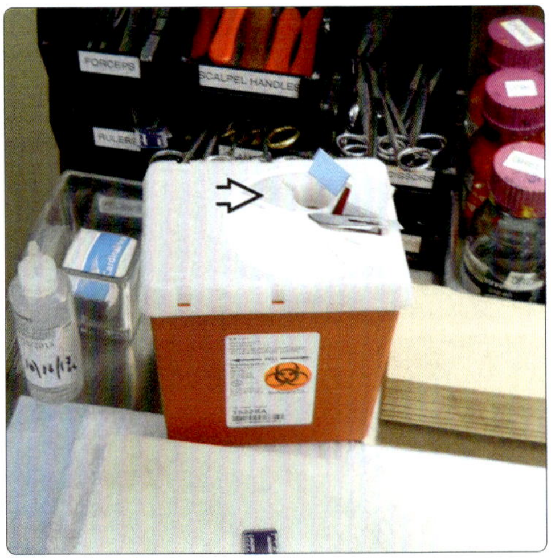

N-95 Mask

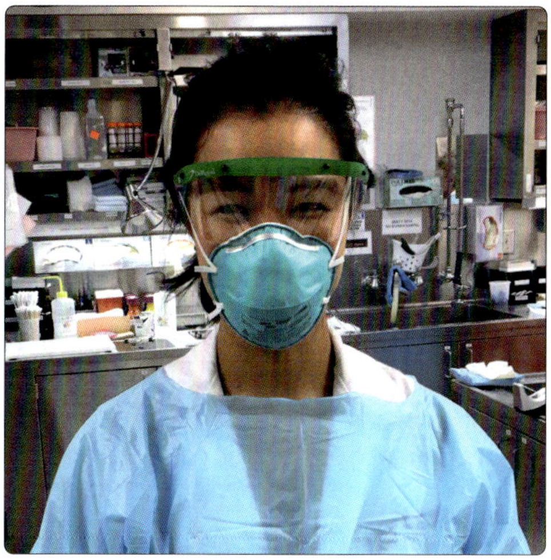

Radiation Sensors

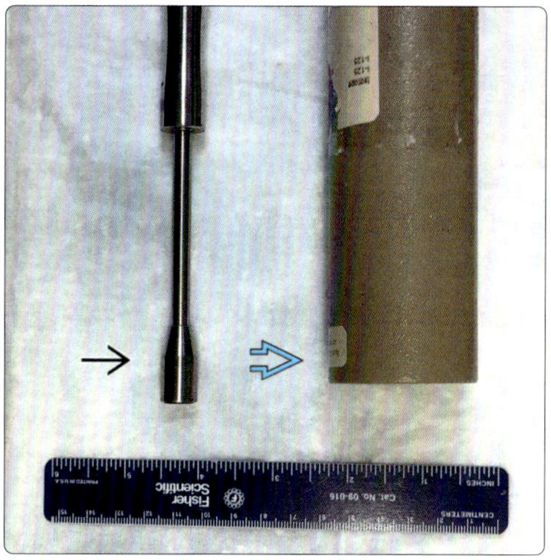

(Left) *Specially designed masks are required to protect against infectious agents such as M. tuberculosis. This is an N-95 mask. It is important that the correct size be used for maximum protection. (Courtesy V. Chan, BS.)* **(Right)** *Geiger counters have a broad sensor ⇨ and are helpful for detecting a variety of types of radiation that can be encountered in medicine. Gamma detectors are used to identify radioactive seeds used to mark breast lesions. A narrower tip → is necessary to localize the small seed in the specimen.*

Radioactive Material: Storage

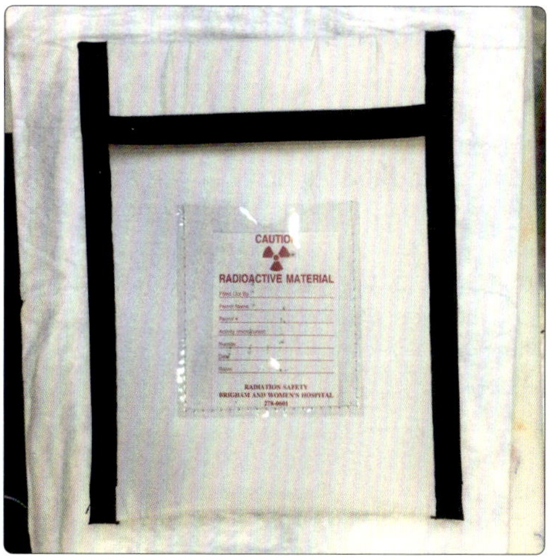

Locked Storage

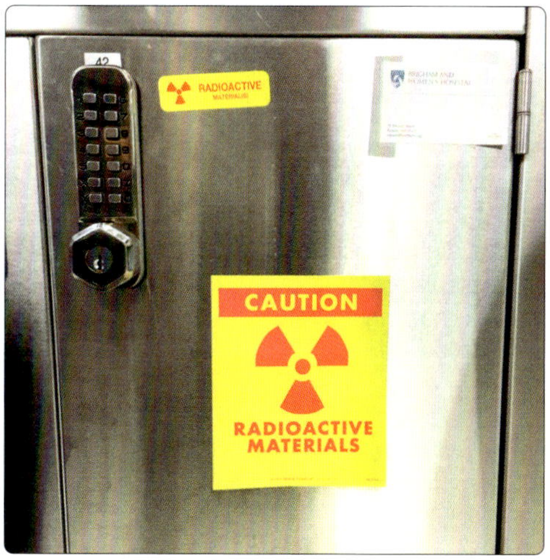

(Left) *After radioactive material is retrieved, a shielded container is required to store the material until it can be safely discarded. This is an envelope lined with lead.* **(Right)** *A locked storage area must be available for storage of radioactive materials. The area must be marked with appropriate signage.*

Chemical Cabinet

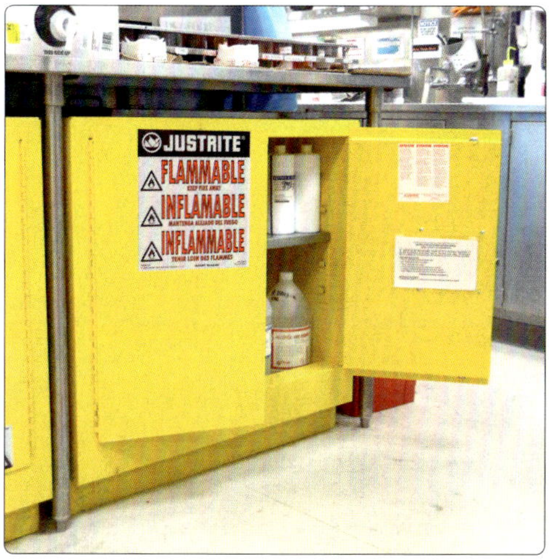

Spill Kit

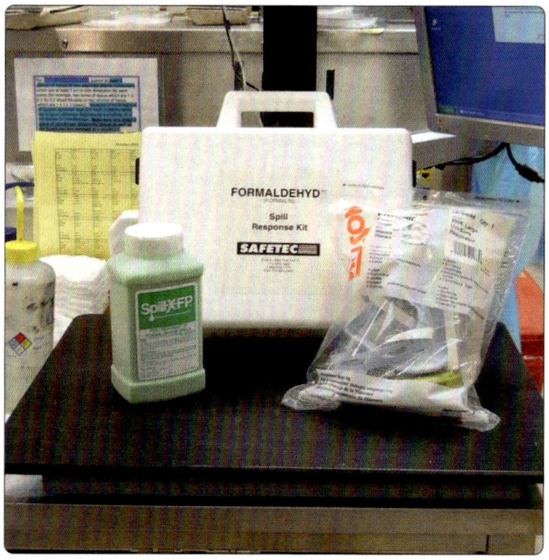

(Left) *Each intraoperative consultation room must have a fireproof cabinet to store the flammable chemicals used for fixation of tissue and staining tissue sections.* **(Right)** *A spill kit contains the materials required to absorb chemicals for disposal and protective wear to keep personnel safe (e.g., face masks). If the spill is too large to be safely contained by such a kit, the room should be evacuated and closed, and the institutional hazardous waste team should be called.*

INTRODUCTION

Definition

- College of American Pathologists (CAP) definition: "The practice of pathology in which digitized or analog video or still images are viewed and the interpretation is part of a formal diagnostic report or the patient record"

Uses/Indications for Telepathology for Intraoperative Consultation

- Diagnosis at a distance
  - Pathologists can provide consultations from locations remote from intraoperative consultation (IOC) room
    - May be used for 1st-line diagnosis or consultation
    - Available outside working hours
    - Applicable to underserved locations (regions or countries with few pathologists)
    - Applicable to remote locations (Antarctica, space stations)
- Access to multiple opinions
  - Some cases are very difficult and benefit from multiple reviewers
    - Unusual tumors
    - Evaluation of margins, particularly in cases in which there is extensive cautery or crush artifact
    - Subtle judgments of invasion
    - Tumors post neoadjuvant therapy
- Access to subspecialty expertise
  - Pathology practice is increasingly subspecialized
    - Maintaining subspecialist availability 24 hours/day, 7 days/week for IOC is logistical challenge for all pathology groups, including large academic departments
    - In some healthcare systems, hospitals with specialized clinical centers of excellence may require more intense subspecialty pathology support than can be provided on site
  - Consultation with subspecialists on-site or at distant sites can be facilitated
- Efficiency in staffing
  - In large networks or multihospital systems, telepathology (for both IOC and permanent section consultation) allows for more efficient use of pathologist resources
  - Mismatch of case volume and need for on-site presence can be alleviated through case flow not limited by proximity to slide production
  - Mix of general and subspecialty expertise can be more flexibly accommodated
  - Creates opportunities for smaller pathology groups to work cooperatively for IOC or expertise sharing
- Access to prior pathology
  - In institutions with digital archives, images of patients' prior pathology specimens may be accessible for real-time comparison to frozen section findings
    - Review of prior tumor histology can be critical for interpretation of intraoperative findings, especially after neoadjuvant treatment
    - Availability of images to IOC team not limited by time needed to retrieve archived glass slides
- Easy archiving of digital images
  - Images readily accessible
    - Quality assurance studies
    - Conferences and teaching
    - Medicolegal purposes
  - Focal findings on a specific intraoperatively prepared slide can be annotated and saved
    - Easier correlation with final permanent section evaluation
    - Annotation does not permanently obscure finding
- Computer-aided interpretation
  - Image analysis to assist in interpretation of slides may become an option in future
    - Computer-assisted diagnosis
    - Identification of focal findings, such as small metastases
    - Quantification of findings important for assessment (e.g., counting neutrophils in cases of suspected joint infection)
    - Eye tracking to ensure entire slide has been observed

Telepathology: Integrated System

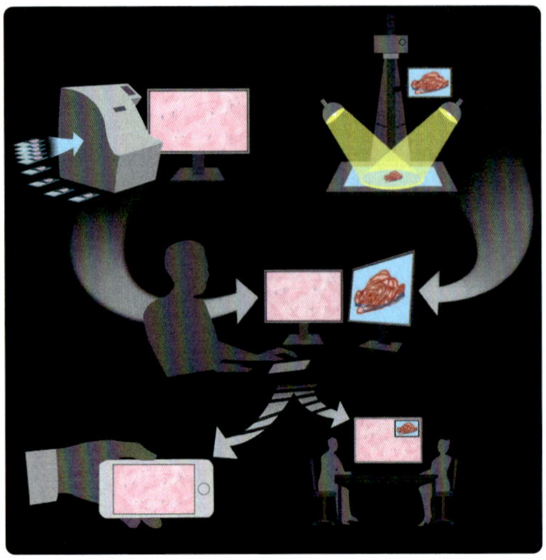

Telepathology: Wide Access

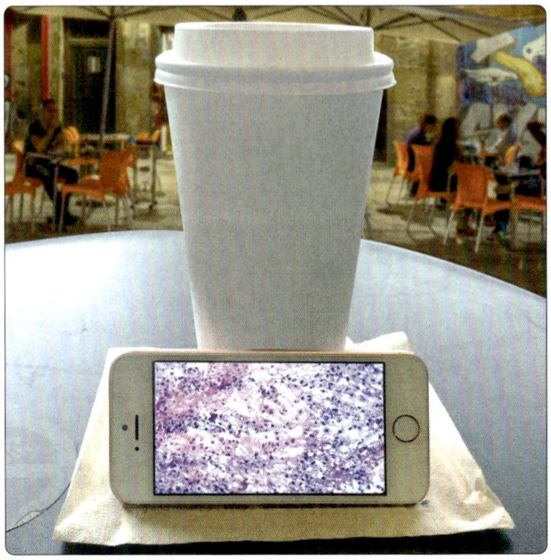

(Left) *A fully integrated telepathology system allows for capture and transmission of gross and microscopic images, as well as annotation and commentary by the interpreting pathologist. The images can then be sent to multiple types of screens for diverse uses.* **(Right)** *The ability to interpret microscopic images on screens frees pathologists from the need to be in a specific location with a microscope in order to render a diagnosis. In addition, multiple pathologists can view the same image from diverse sites.*

INTEGRATION OF TELEPATHOLOGY INTO INTRAOPERATIVE CONSULTATION

Gross Examination

- Qualified personnel on-site to are critical to successful and safe provision of services
  - Residents
    - Act as qualified prosectors
    - May be 1st responder on call, especially if attending pathologist lives in remote location
  - Pathology assistants or specialized technologists
    - May prosect specimen and prepare slides according to protocols (especially for small specimens) or under phone or video direction from pathologist
    - May be used in hospitals without regular on-site pathologist staffing
- In an ideal system, images of gross specimens are captured as digital photographs

Preparation of Slides

- Personnel on-site prepare cytologic or frozen section slides

Microscopic Examination

- Image capture remains "add-on" to workflow for on-site personnel
  - Robotic telepathology: Slide is placed on the microscope stage
  - Static image telepathology: Images are taken by camera
    - Usually requires at least pathology residency training to select diagnostic areas
  - Whole-slide imaging (WSI): Slides must be placed in scanner
- Attending pathologist
  - If pathologist is on-site, slides can be viewed directly via microscope or images can be viewed on screen
  - If pathologist is off-site, slides &/or images can be viewed according to system utilized
  - In either situation, pathologist can use telepathology for subspecialist or 2nd opinion on unusual or challenging cases

TYPES OF IMAGE-CAPTURE METHODS

Video Images

- Methods
  - Slide is viewed on microscope with digital or analog video camera
  - Video images are transferred to remote site by closed network or web-based sharing systems
  - Microscope stage movement and focus may be controlled by
    - On-site personnel under verbal direction of remote pathologist
    - Pathologist on-site, directing remote consultant's attention to selected areas
    - Off-site pathologist via robotic microscopy
  - Web-based sharing systems
    - Require computer at on-site video capture
    - Can use computer, phone, or handheld device (for commercially available systems with device applications)
- Advantages
  - All information available on slide is potentially available to off-site pathologist
  - If robotic microscope controlled by off-site pathologist is used, this method closely mimics pathologist being on-site
  - Viewing of images takes place in real time with communication between person on-site and pathologist
- Disadvantages
  - If on-site person controls microscope, it may be difficult to communicate best method of examining slide
  - Can be time consuming for off-site pathologist
  - Some robotic microscopes are "clunky" in practical operation
  - Images are not routinely saved

Static Digitized Images

- Methods
  - Static photographs are taken with digital camera, which may be
    - Fixed part of microscope
    - Camera attached to eyepiece
    - Phone or other camera-containing device attached to eyepiece
  - Photographs are transmitted to consultant, usually as JPEG attachments via
    - Email
    - Text message
    - Less commonly as image cache accessed from remote computer
- Advantages
  - Inexpensive
  - Fast
  - Recipient does not need special equipment or computer to review images
  - 1st-line pathologist can select and carefully capture areas of concern
    - Very focal findings
    - Cytology findings, particularly if focal or if smear is suboptimal
  - No requirement for real-time interaction with person in IOC room
    - Useful for cases in which rapid diagnosis is needed for expedited postoperative, but not necessarily intraoperative, management
  - Images can be kept as permanent file and attached to case in some laboratory information systems
- Disadvantages
  - Except for very small pieces of tissue, ability of consultant to evaluate entire specimen is limited
    - Absolutely dependent on prosector; subject to sampling error
  - Selection of images for review is influenced by expertise and bias of 1st-line pathologist
    - Subspecialty expertise may be needed for both selection and interpretation of key areas
  - Only portions of tissue are captured on slide and only at set magnifications

Whole-Slide Imaging

- Methods

- After preparation, entire slide is scanned, uploaded, and stored as digitized image on institution- or cloud-based server
- Digitized image can be viewed on computer by off-site pathologist

- Advantages
  - Does not require expertise to choose most diagnostic areas of slide
  - Provides closest experience to (and sometimes better than) on-site viewing
  - Specialized software allows viewing of slide at different magnifications
  - Real-time interaction with person on-site is not required
  - Image can be kept permanently, viewed at any time, and annotated for permanent section correlation
- Disadvantages
  - Scanners are expensive
  - Slide preparation extremely important
    - Clean, glue free
    - Placement of tissue centrally on glass
    - Minimal folds or other artifacts that vary thickness of tissue
    - Personnel must be well trained in using instrument
      - Not suitable for multiple users with minimal training &/or episodic experience
  - Cytology slides should be uniformly thin and may require 40x scanning
  - Time to scan slide dependent on size of tissue area and magnification
    - Scanning at 40x very slow (but usually not necessary)
  - Stored file sizes for WSI are extremely large
  - One image at a single focal depth does not capture information from entire thickness of tissue on slide
    - May be important when evaluating very small structures, such as mitotic figures
    - Advanced systems image slide at multiple focal depths (Z axis)
      - However, this greatly increases file size for each slide

REGULATORY ISSUES

CAP Accreditation Requirements for Telepathology

- CAP Laboratory Accreditation Checklist
  - As of 2016, there are sections on telepathology and remote data assessment, and WSI, both under "Laboratory General"
  - Telepathology modes defined
    - Static telepathology: Preselected still image(s)
    - Dynamic telepathology: Real-time viewing of images (includes robotic microscopy, video streaming, and desktop sharing)
    - Virtual slides/WSI: Digitization of entire slide
  - Checklist section applies to
    - Primary diagnoses made by telepathology
    - Frozen section diagnoses
    - Formal 2nd opinion consultations
    - Ancillary techniques in which pathologist participates in interpretation of images
    - Real-time evaluation of fine-needle aspiration specimens for triaging and preliminary diagnoses
  - Checklist items
    - GEN.50057: There is a method for the individual reviewing cases to ensure correct patient identification for slides/images and data files submitted for review
    - GEN.50614: The individual reviewing cases has access to pertinent clinical information at the time of slide/image(s) or remote data file review
    - GEN.50630: The laboratory validates telepathology systems used for clinical diagnostic purposes by performing its own validation studies, including approval for use by the laboratory director (or designee who meets CAP director qualifications) before the technology is used for the intended diagnostic purpose(s)
    - GEN.51728: The lab has a procedure addressing training requirements for all users of the telepathology system
    - GEN.52842: There are procedures in place to ensure that sites engaging in telepathology and remote data assessment provide reasonable confidentiality and security
    - GEN.52850: The telepathology records include diagnoses made and statements of adequacy assessment, preliminary diagnosis, or recommendations for additional studies provided at the time of evaluation
    - GEN.52860: The telepathology services are included in the laboratory's quality management program
    - GEN.52900: There are records showing that all users of the whole slide imaging system have been trained
    - GEN.52920: the laboratory validates whole slide imaging systems used for clinical diagnostic purposes by performing its own validation studies, including approval for use by the laboratory director (or designee who meets CAP director qualifications) before the technology is used for the intended diagnostic purpose(s)

United States Food and Drug Administration Regulations for Telepathology

- WSI has been approved as a class II diagnostic device in United States for primary pathology diagnosis
  - As of April 2017, this approval is limited to single vendor: Philips IntelliSite Pathology Solution (PIPS)
- WSI has been approved and is employed in Canada for primary pathology diagnosis
- IOC diagnosis in most cases can be reasonably regarded as preliminary in nature, subject to subsequent review in context of permanent and additional sections and, therefore, not a final primary diagnosis
  - Exceptions to this characterization would include specimens completely exhausted by protocol for intraoperative diagnosis &/or not retained for permanent section (e.g., Mohs surgery)
- Consensus guidelines for validation of WSI have been published and include
  - All laboratories using WSI clinically should implement their own validation studies
  - Validation should be appropriate to intended clinical use

Developments in Telepathology

Imaging System	Types	Year
Real-time imaging	Television microscopy	1952
	Dynamic-robotic telepathology	1986
Static image telepathology	Store and forward telepathology	1987
	Whole-slide imaging (automated)	1991
	Whole-slide imaging (operator directed)	1994
Multimodality telepathology	Hybrid dynamic robotic/static imaging	1989
	Whole-slide imaging dynamic robotic/static imaging	2011

Pantanowitz L et al: American Telemedicine Association clinical guidelines for telepathology. J Pathol Inform. 5(1):39, 2014.

Clinical Applications of Telepathology

Patient Care Application	Description
Frozen section interpretation	Remote interpretation of frozen section slides
Digital image analysis	Automated interpretation of assays (e.g., immunohistochemistry or in situ hybridization using algorithms); quantification (intensity or percent positivity); feature identification (e.g., mitotic figures, abnormal cells); computer-assisted diagnosis
Intrapractice	Consultation within practice (e.g., review by subspecialty experts)
Archiving	Fast and convenient slide image retrieval; backup documentation for medicolegal purposes; comparison with previous biopsies (also useful in intraoperative consultation); preservation of virtual slides for which tissue may be used for molecular testing
Diagnostic pathology report	Whole-slide image links (including frozen sections) in traditional and integrated pathology reports
Consultation/expert 2nd opinion	Expert 2nd opinion of challenging cases by national or international experts
Treatment protocols	Whole-slide images can be provided for central review for purpose of treatment protocols
Quality assurance	Conventional slide sharing and "re-reads"; can integrate with patient medical records for random case selection; easy access to archived frozen section slides for comparison with permanent sections &/or final diagnosis; tracking of slide review
Clinical conferences	Use of whole-slide images for case presentations of intraoperative and permanent section slides

Adapted from Hipp J et al: College of American Pathologists Digital Resource Guide. CAP Press, 2017.

    - Validation slides for IOC should employ intraoperatively prepared frozen sections or cytology preparations
  - Validation should emulate real-world environment
  - Validation can encompass entire WSI system (i.e., each component need not be separately validated)
  - 60 cases required for 1 application that reflect spectrum and complexity of case types
  - Qualified pathologist should be involved
  - Study should establish glass slide-digital image intraobserver variability
  - Wash-out periods between review of glass slide and digital image mandated
  - Validation should confirm that all material present on glass slide is included in digital image

Licensure

- Pathologists may make diagnoses on specimens from different institutions, different states, or different countries
- Licensure requirements vary by jurisdiction
- Requirements in both receiving and sending jurisdictions must be followed
- It is typical for pathologists performing telepathology consultations to be licensed in multiple states

Reimbursement

- At this time, diagnoses by telepathology are billable in same manner as direct on-site evaluation

SELECTED REFERENCES

1. Evans AJ et al: Implementation of whole slide imaging for clinical purposes: issues to consider from the perspective of early adopters. Arch Pathol Lab Med. 141(7):944-959, 2017
2. Farris AB et al: Whole slide imaging for analytical anatomic pathology and telepathology: practical applications today, promises, and perils. Arch Pathol Lab Med. 141(4):542-550, 2017
3. Hipp J (ed) et al: College of American Pathologists Digital Pathology Resource Guide. CAP Press, 2017
4. Pantanowitz L et al: American Telemedicine Association clinical guidelines for telepathology. J Pathol Inform. 5(1):39, 2014
5. Food and Drug Administration: Code of federal regulations title 21. http://www.accessdata.fda.gov/scripts/cdrh/cfdocs/cfcfr/CFRSearch.cfm?fr=860.3&SearchTerm=classification%20definitions. Updated June 1, 2013. Accessed December 5, 2013
6. Park S et al: The history of pathology informatics: A global perspective. J Pathol Inform. 4:7, 2013
7. CAP Inspection Update: Telepathology and Remote Data Assessment
8. FDA Approval Letter

(Left) *The live analog video-based telepathology system connecting Boston Logan Airport and the Massachusetts General Hospital in 1968 is widely considered to be the 1st working telepathology system in history. (Courtesy Massachusetts General Hospital, Archives and Special Collections.)* **(Right)** *The simplest and most readily available method of capturing a microscopic image is to use a camera, either attached to a microscope or as a mobile phone, to take a static photograph of a glass slide. (Courtesy R. Owings, MD.)*

1st Use of Live Telepathology

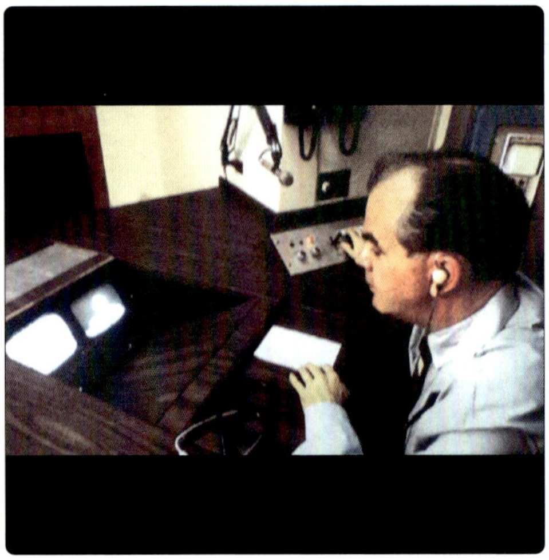

Static Image Capture Using Camera

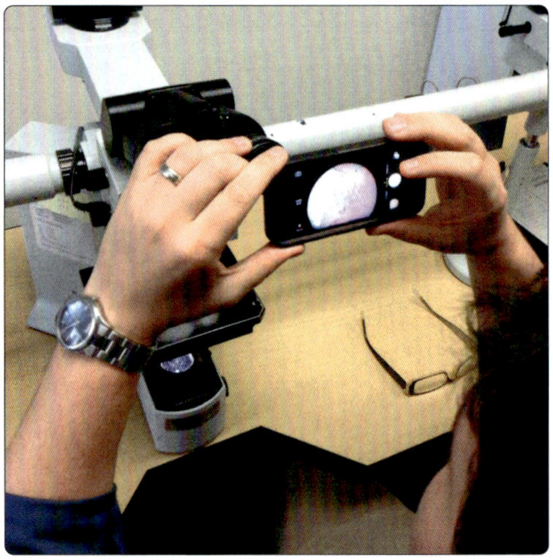

(Left) *Static photographs of slides are relatively small files that can easily be transferred via text or email messages. The images can be viewed on multiple devices, such as computer screens or handheld devices without the need for special programs.* **(Right)** *A static image is easily captured and viewed. However, only a small amount of information on a slide is conveyed, as only a portion of the tissue at 1 magnification is included. A skilled pathologist is often necessary to choose the diagnostic areas for photography.*

Viewing Images via Computer Screen

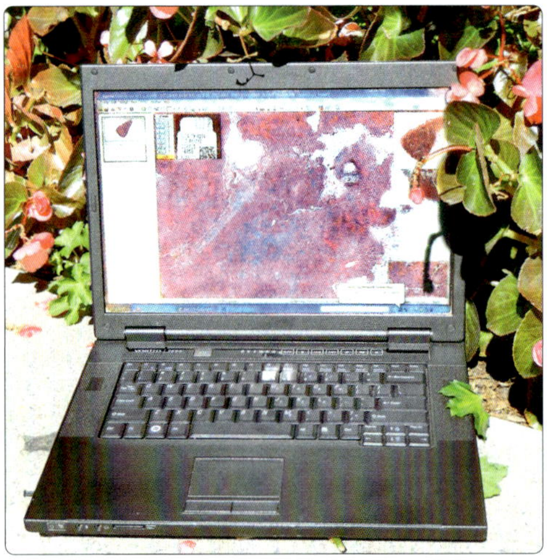

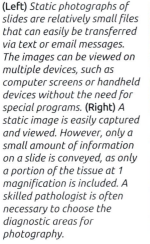

Static Image on Phone: Frozen Section

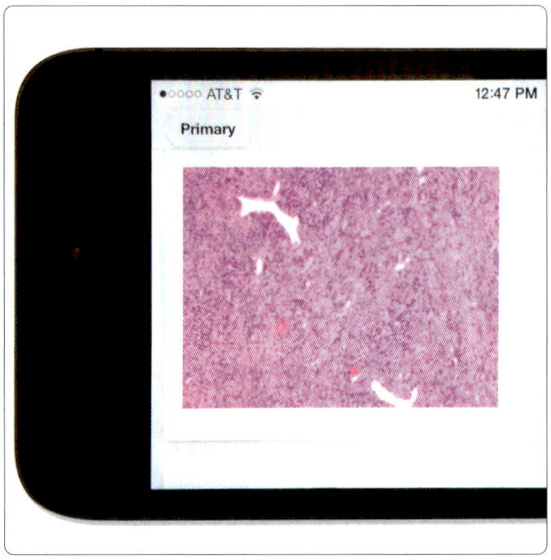

(Left) *This static photograph shows a readily identifiable adenocarcinoma of enteric origin that could be easily diagnosed by an experienced pathologist viewing the image. No special viewing software is required.* **(Right)** *Key features of cytologic preparations may be easier to capture with static images than with whole-slide imaging (WSI), as an experienced pathologist can work around air-dried, thick, or obscured areas to select optimal fields. However, this method is limited when the person taking the photographs lacks experience.*

Static Image: Frozen Section of Metastatic Colonic Adenocarcinoma

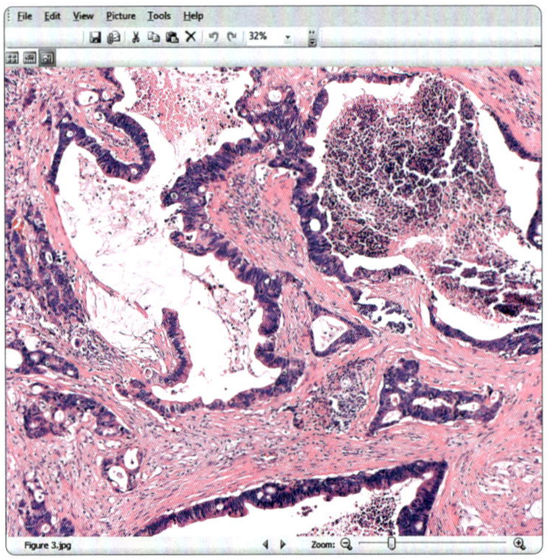

Static Image: Cytologic Preparation of Sarcoma

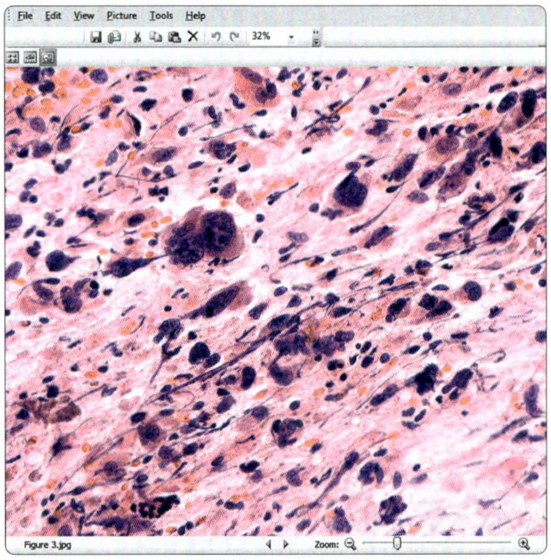

Robotic Telepathology

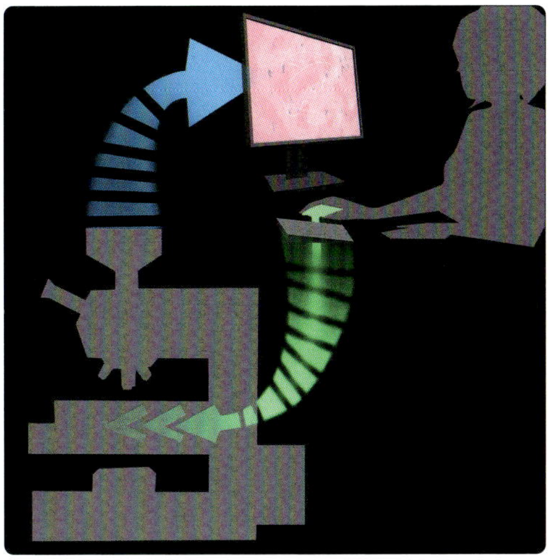

Web Meeting/Screen Sharing: Frozen Section of Metastatic Adenocarcinoma

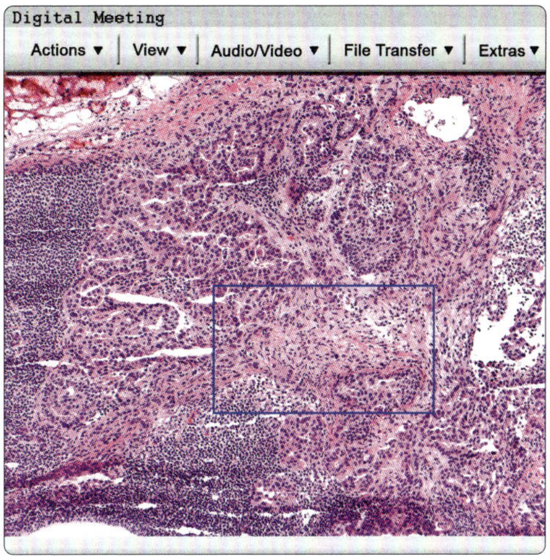

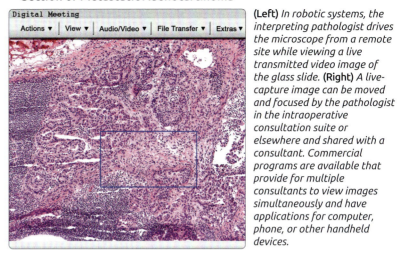

(Left) *In robotic systems, the interpreting pathologist drives the microscope from a remote site while viewing a live transmitted video image of the glass slide.* **(Right)** *A live-capture image can be moved and focused by the pathologist in the intraoperative consultation suite or elsewhere and shared with a consultant. Commercial programs are available that provide for multiple consultants to view images simultaneously and have applications for computer, phone, or other handheld devices.*

Whole-Slide Imaging

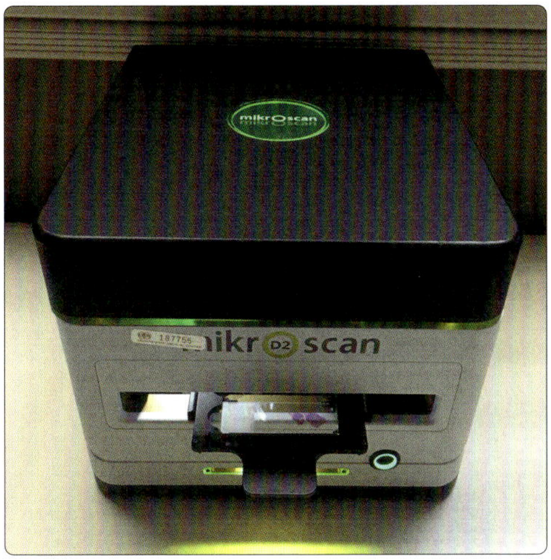

Whole-Slide Imaging: Frozen Section of Atypical Carcinoid Tumor

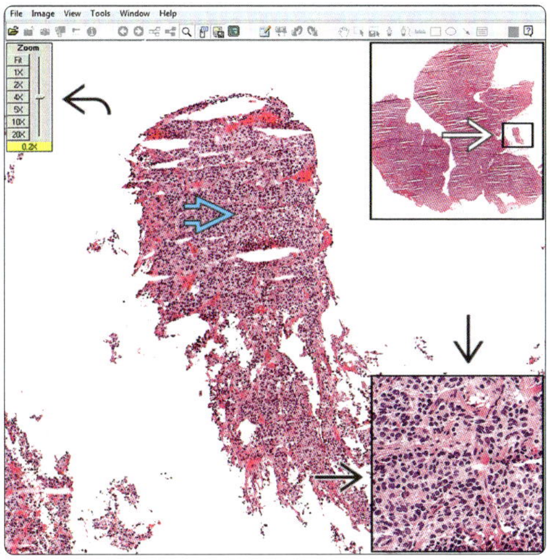

(Left) *WSI has the advantage of capturing almost all of the visual information in a glass slide. Special computer programs are required for viewing. The large files can be challenging to store and transfer.* **(Right)** *This WSI-viewing program provides different virtual magnifications. The upper inset shows the entire slide with the current area on the screen shown in a box. The site of the cursor is shown at higher magnification in the lower inset. This is a useful feature when quickly scanning at low magnification.*

Whole-Slide Imaging: Touch Prep of Malignant Melanoma

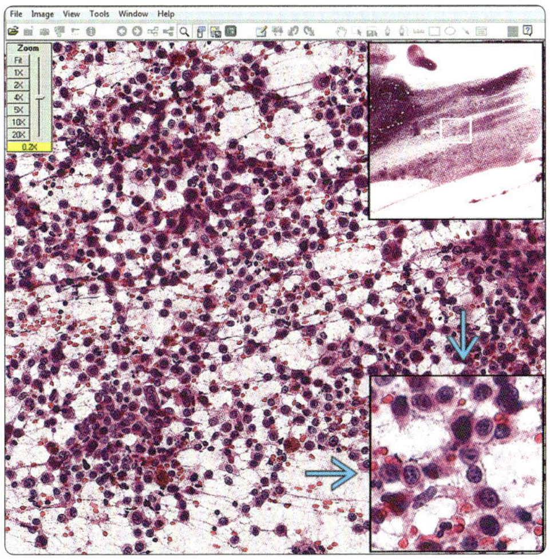

Whole-Slide Imaging: Future Uses

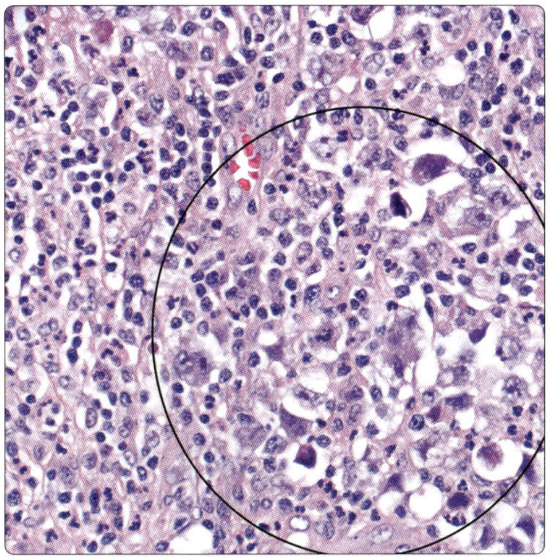

(Left) *WSI can be used effectively with cytology preparations if thinly smeared areas of uniform thickness are selected. Note pigmented malignant melanoma cells in a magnified area. Because each slide of a cytologic preparation is unique, WSI is particularly useful for documentation.* **(Right)** *As technology develops, image analysis can assist pathologists for diagnosis and reporting. In this example, a small cluster of Hodgkin cells in an extensive background of lymphocytes has been identified using an algorithm.*

SECTION 2

Methods

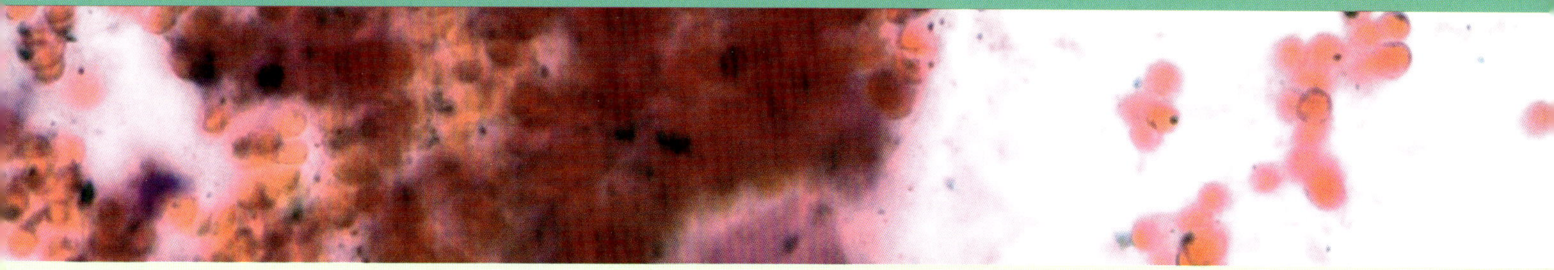

INTRODUCTION

Importance of Gross Examination

- Good gross evaluation often provides more information and can be more accurate than microscopic evaluation
  - **Large specimens**
    - Critical for optimal evaluation
      - Tissue most likely to yield critical important findings for intraoperative management must be identified
    - In some cases, gross examination is adequate for intraoperative consultation
      - Margins for colon carcinomas in absence of prior treatment
      - Margins for sarcomas in absence of prior treatment
      - Circumscribed thyroid nodules: Microscopic evaluation for focal capsular or vascular invasion best performed on permanent sections
      - Grossly determined bone resection margins for bone tumors more accurate than frozen sections
  - **Small specimens**
    - Often entirely frozen
    - Gross examination primarily for documentation

Objectives

- Document specimens received
  - Number of specimens
  - Identification of each specimen
- Determine important gross pathologic features
  - Appearance of tumors
    - Gross appearance often highly correlated with histologic type
  - Number of tumors
    - Distance of tumors from each other
  - Tumor size
    - Often best determined when tissue is fresh
  - Location of tumors
  - Gross distance from oriented margins prior to contraction (colon and skin)
- Select best areas for frozen section evaluation
  - Margins should be serially sectioned to identify closest approach to margin
  - Cystic ovarian tumors should be examined to identify most likely areas of invasive carcinoma
  - Uteri examined to identify deepest area of invasion
  - Best section for tumor identification is usually the interface with normal tissue
    - Central necrotic &/or fibrotic areas should be avoided
- Select best tissue for special studies
  - Central areas of tumor often fibrotic or necrotic
  - Most viable areas of tumor often at peripheral interface with normal tissue
  - Adjacent normal tissue should not be included for most assays

DOCUMENTATION

Small Specimens

- Gross description includes
  - Size of specimens
  - Number of fragments
  - Color of tissue
    - Red friable fragments may be fibrin and not tissue
  - Consistency (e.g., hard, firm, rubbery, soft)
  - Recognizable features (e.g., polyp, squamous mucosa, epithelium)

Large Specimens

- Gross description includes
  - Type of organs/tissue present
  - Size of each component
  - Location of any lesions (tumors, ulcers)
  - Distance of lesions from margins

ORIENTATION

Importance

- Correct orientation necessary to determine distance of malignancies from margins
  - Close or positive margins may be indication for additional removal of tissue in designated areas

Colon Carcinoma: Margins

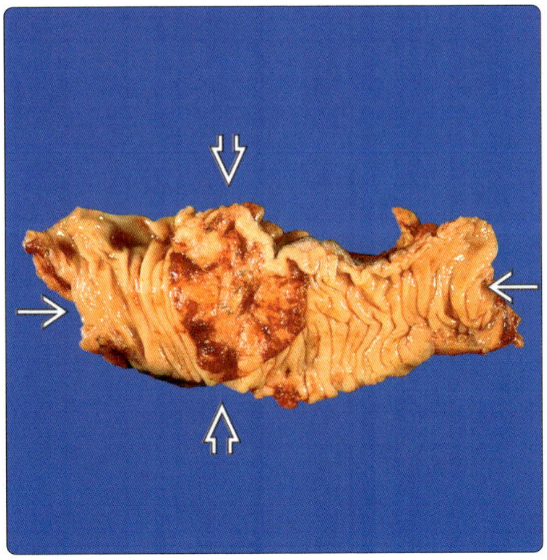

Rectal Carcinoma: Margins

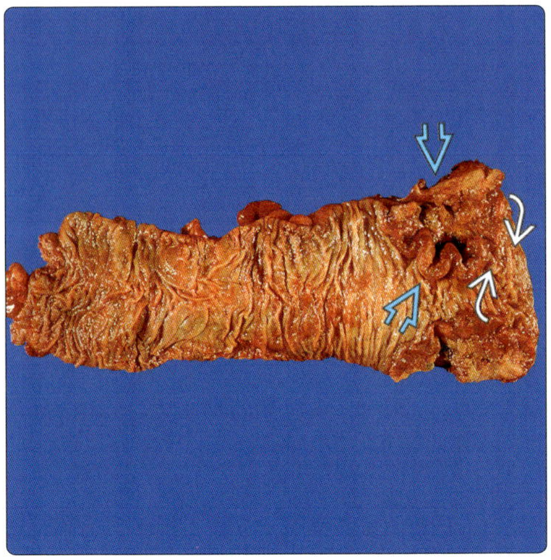

(Left) *This colon carcinoma ➡ is located far from the proximal and distal margins ➡. Gross examination is a reliable method to ensure colon margins are free of carcinoma. There is no need to examine normal margins with frozen sections.* **(Right)** *The proximity of a rectal cancer ⇨ from the distal margin ➡ may be used to assess the need for radiation therapy and is best determined grossly before muscle contraction. If there has been preoperative therapy, in some cases frozen sections are useful to evaluate the margin for carcinoma.*

- Surgeon should indicate if margin evaluation needed for intraoperative management
- Pathologist should always verify orientation provided by surgeon
  - Any questions about orientation should be addressed prior to further specimen processing

Techniques

- Sutures
  - Surgeons may place multiple sutures to indicate specific margins
  - Several methods are used to indicate margins identified by sutures
    - Different materials of different colors
    - Different lengths (e.g., short = superior margin; long = lateral margin; often used for breast specimens)
    - Tied suture vs. blanket stitch
    - Different numbers of surgical clips or commercial markers attached to sutures
  - Sutures of different colors should be documented before inking
    - Light-colored sutures may be difficult to distinguish after being inked
- Diagram
  - May be best method to indicate orientation for complex specimens
- Separate specimens
  - Each margin may be sent as separate excision

INKING MARGINS

Methods

- In general, ink should be applied to specimens prior to sectioning
- Specimen surface should be dry and clean (i.e., without gross blood)
- Gauze pads or cotton swabs used to apply ink
  - Avoid introducing ink into crevices or other areas of specimen that are not true margins
- For large complex specimens, it may be preferable to ink selective areas
  - Inking entire specimen may make later orientation and identification of structures difficult
  - Artifactual smearing of ink onto nonmargins can occur
  - Often possible to identify most important margins to examine by frozen section with consultation with surgeon
    - Only those margins need be inked for intraoperative consultation
    - Orientation of uninked specimen will be easier to determine by prosector
- Helpful for institutions to develop routine policies for correlation of colors with specific margins
  - Same color should always be used for same margin

PROCESSING

Imaging

- Information from preoperative imaging often helpful to guide gross examination
- Size, location, and number of lesions often known preoperatively
- If specimen (e.g., breast biopsy) undergoes imaging after excision, specimen radiograph should be available to pathologist
  - Radiograph helpful to identify lesion type (mass, calcifications, clip, radioactive seed), location, and radiologic distance to margins

Methods

- Standard methods for processing specimens should be used
- Surgeon should provide information about structures present and mark any that are not grossly evident
  - All anatomic structures must be identified prior to inking specimen
    - Ink can make it more difficult to identify structures and marking devices (i.e., clips or sutures)
- Minimal examination (e.g., not completely sectioning specimen) may lead to suboptimal evaluation
  - Additional lesions smaller than primary lesion may be missed
  - Closest approach of malignancy to margin may not be identified
- If purpose of examination is to take tissue for ancillary studies requiring nonfixed tissue, bisecting large complex specimen provides complete cross section of tumor and maintains ability to orient specimen
  - Thin, complete cross sections more likely to yield useful tumor tissue
    - Adjacent normal tissue should not be taken for nonhistologic types of studies
    - Important for assessing lymph-vascular invasion for many tumors
  - Center of tumor may fibrotic or necrotic
- Specimens must be examined on clean surface away from other specimens
  - Contamination from other specimens can create diagnostic errors
  - Scalpels, other blades, forceps, and probes must be new or meticulously cleaned if previously used
  - Gloves and other protective clothing must be clean
- Large, potentially cystic masses must be opened with care
  - Fluid under pressure can create deceptively firm to hard mass
  - Puncture can result in forceful expulsion of cyst contents with contamination of environment and prosector
  - Possible cysts should be opened carefully, preferably near sink or with abundant pads capable of absorbing any contents
    - Small nick should be made on surface away from prosector
- Specimens can change shape and size after excision
  - Colon
    - Colon segments can contract 40% within 10-20 minutes
    - Distances of rectal carcinomas to distal margin should be measured as soon as possible
      - This distance may be used to determine need for radiation therapy
  - Skeletal muscle
    - Skeletal muscle in resections can contract when cut with a blade (e.g., resections for sarcomas of thigh)

- This phenomenon can be quite alarming when 1st encountered
  - Skin
    - Contraction occurs within 5 minutes of excision
  - Breast
    - Excisions flatten spontaneously or due to compression during specimen radiography
- Sectioning
  - Sharp blades must be used
    - Dull blades difficult to use and may result in injury to prosector
      - Tissue may be crushed rather than cut
      - Difficult to obtain sections of optimal thinness for frozen section and fixation
  - Parallel sections preferable to multiple cuts in different planes
    - Preserves ability to orient specimen
    - Ensures entire specimen examined
    - However, perpendicular sections in different planes may be necessary to evaluate multiple margins of some specimens
  - Single large cut to bisect specimen may be initially adequate to identify tumor mass in order to identify tissue for ancillary testing
    - Best area of tumor can be identified (central or periphery)
    - If multiple areas of different gross appearance present, it may be helpful to take paired samples for histology and ancillary testing
    - Specimen orientation maintained for further dissection and photography
  - Hollow organs should be opened such that tumor mass not transected, when possible
    - Information from imaging or endoscopy may be helpful to identify location
    - Outer surface can be palpated to identify location of mass
    - Finger can be introduced (e.g., into colon segment) to identify mass
    - Opening all hollow organs often helpful to orient specimen and identify structures

IMPORTANT GROSS FEATURES

Size of Tumors

- Size should be carefully determined and recorded in fresh state
  - Final size should be correlated with microscopic appearance on permanent sections
- Important for staging of some tumors
  - May diminish slightly after fixation
  - May be difficult to determine after sectioning
  - May be difficult to determine if tissue is taken for special studies
    - Size prior to removing tissue must be documented

Distance of Malignancies From Margins

- Often used to determine adequacy of surgical resection
  - Adequate margin varies for different types of tumors, sites, and clinical settings
- Distance of rectal carcinomas from distal margin may be used to determine need for radiation therapy
- Gross distance from margins should always be correlated with microscopic appearance
  - Margin grossly far from malignancy should not be interpreted as positive on microscopic examination unless clear reason for discrepancy
    - Tumor has diffusely infiltrative pattern not appreciated grossly
    - Tumor present in tissue plane not seen grossly (e.g., esophageal adenocarcinoma present in muscularis propria at margin beneath grossly negative squamous mucosa)
    - 2nd smaller focus of tumor present at margin
  - Other possibilities should be considered before interpreting such margin as positive
    - Ink leakage into specimen fissures or artifactually introduced onto nonmargin surfaces
    - Tumor present in lymphatics that would not be indication for additional surgery (e.g., at bronchial margin)
    - Nonmalignant cells that could be misinterpreted as malignancy (e.g., atypical ductal hyperplasia in breast excision)

Multiple Tumors

- Multiple tumor masses may be present due to numerous reasons
  - Area of carcinoma in situ giving rise to multiple invasive cancers
  - Intralymphatic tumor giving rise to multiple metastatic sites
  - Fragmentation of single tumor due to piecemeal removal by surgeon
  - Multiple biologically separate tumors
    - More common in patients with germline mutations (e.g., breast cancer) or environmental exposures (e.g., skin carcinoma in sun damaged skin)
- Identification of multiple tumors important to recognize when taking tissue for ancillary studies and for margin evaluation

ILLUSTRATION

Photography

- Photograph of intact specimen useful for later documentation
  - Can be helpful to identify location of sections for margin evaluation
- Photographs of typical and unusual lesions useful for teaching
- Pathologic findings best demonstrated when specimen fresh

Diagrams

- Simple diagrams can be used to document important features
  - Location and relationship of structures and lesions present
  - Location and colors of inks
  - Sites where tissue has been sampled

TISSUE ALLOCATION

Documentation

- Distribution of all tissue from surgical specimen documented
- Size and types of tissue sent to other laboratories recorded
  - Laboratory, investigator, or other identifying information should be included
  - In rare cases, tissue may need to be retrieved if inappropriate tissue allocated or there is an unexpected diagnosis on permanent sections
- Tissue saved by means other than standard formalin fixation documented

Formalin Fixation

- In general, at least some tissue should be fixed in standard manner in formalin
  - Majority of studies of immunohistochemical markers have been performed on formalin-fixed tissue
- Formalin penetrates slowly and complete fixation may require many hours
  - Specimens should be serially sectioned to ensure all areas adequately exposed to fixative
  - If specimen large and complete fixation may be delayed, thin slices of tumor should be fixed quickly
  - It may be helpful to include normal tissue as control for immunohistochemical studies
    - For example, normal breast tissue can be combined with breast carcinoma as control for hormone receptors
- Ideally, fixation occurs within 1-2 hours after blood supply terminated
  - Biomolecules degrade at different rates
    - Phosphoproteins and mRNA can degrade within minutes
    - Other types of proteins and DNA may degrade after hours

Other Fixatives

- Tissue should be placed in other types of fixatives when appropriate
- Histologic features of lymphomas often best preserved in special fixatives

Electron Microscopy

- Tissue must be minced into small fragments (~ 1 mm x 1 mm x 1 mm) for rapid fixation
- Special fixation necessary to preserve ultrastructural detail

Flow Cytometry

- Tissue must be unfixed
- Tissue should be kept moist in saline or in culture medium

Cytogenetics

- Tissue must be unfixed and viable
- Tissue can be placed in sterile tissue culture medium for transfer to laboratory

Frozen Tissue

- Can be used for mRNA and DNA studies
- If diagnostic tissue is limited, tissue used for frozen section diagnosis can be kept frozen

Research

- Tissue can only be released for research if not required for care of patient
  - Only pathologist can make this determination
- Individuals requesting tissue must have approval from institutional human studies committee

INFECTION PRECAUTIONS

Gross Findings Suggestive of Infection

- If specimen has findings suspicious for infection on gross examination, special handling should be considered
  - Necrosis without discrete tumor mass
  - Lung consolidation
- Cytologic preparations should be used when possible
  - Minimizes risk of infection by tissue injury from blades
  - Avoids aerosolization during frozen section preparation
  - Minimizes contamination of equipment

Tissue From Patients With Known or Suspected Infectious Disease

- Surgeon should always provide information about patients with possible infections
- Tissue from patients with diseases that can be transferred percutaneously or by inhalation must be handled with caution
  - Hepatitis B and hepatitis C
  - HIV
  - Tuberculosis
- Diagnosis should be deferred to permanent sections on fixed tissue when possible
- Cytologic preparations should be used when possible
  - Unfixed slides should not be submitted to other laboratories for examination
- Tissue from patients known or suspected to have prion disease (e.g., Creutzfeldt-Jakob disease) should not be examined
  - Symptoms include rapidly progressive dementia
  - Tissue must undergo prolonged fixation in special fixatives to inactivate prions
  - Risk to personnel too high and potential benefit to patient with rapidly fatal disease too small to warrant examination

SELECTED REFERENCES

1. Blasco-Morente G et al: Study of shrinkage of cutaneous surgical specimens. J Cutan Pathol. 42(4):253-7, 2015
2. Anderson ME et al: Frozen section versus gross examination for bone marrow margin assessment during sarcoma resection. Clin Orthop Relat Res. 472(3):836-41, 2014
3. Mavromatis ID et al: Validity of intraoperative gross examination of myometrial invasion in patients with endometrial cancer: a meta-analysis. Acta Obstet Gynecol Scand. 91(7):779-93, 2012
4. Clingan R et al: Potential margin distortion in breast tissue by specimen mammography. Arch Surg. 138(12):1371-4, 2003
5. Graham RA et al: The pancake phenomenon contributes to the inaccuracy of margin assessment in patients with breast cancer. Am J Surg. 184(2):89-93, 2002
6. Goldstein NS et al: Disparate surgical margin lengths of colorectal resection specimens between in vivo and in vitro measurements. The effects of surgical resection and formalin fixation on organ shrinkage. Am J Clin Pathol. 111(3):349-51, 1999

(Left) *The rectosigmoid junction (located at the termination of complete serosa covering) is best determined by gross evaluation of the outer colonic surface. Carcinomas proximal to this point are in the sigmoid colon and in the rectum if distal.* **(Right)** *The ulceration marking the site of a polypectomy showing invasive carcinoma is difficult to see. Good communication with the surgeon is necessary to identify subtle lesions to ensure they have been removed. Two other polyps are present.*

Rectosigmoid Junction

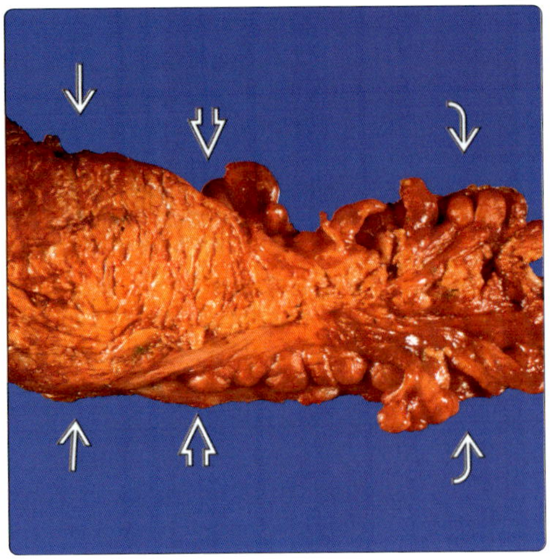

Difficult to Find Lesions

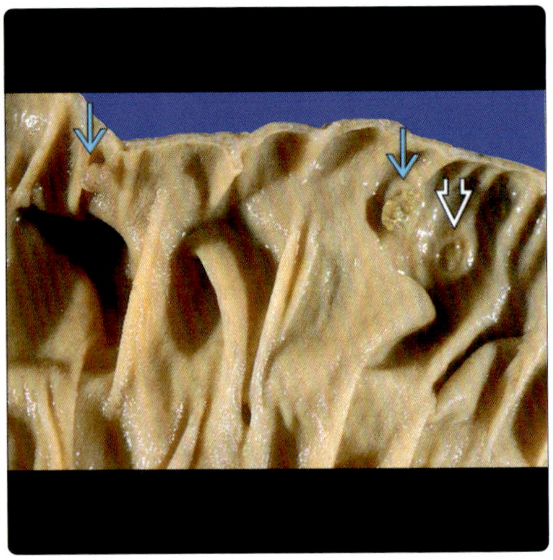

(Left) *Invasion of this colon carcinoma through the muscularis propria and into pericolonic fat is grossly evident. Involvement of the serosal surface by carcinoma is an important prognostic factor that should be evaluated grossly and documented microscopically.* **(Right)** *This carcinoid tumor of the small intestine has a distinct white homogeneous appearance and a rounded pushing border. The tumor has invaded into the lamina propria causing puckering of the overlying mucosa.*

Colon Carcinoma

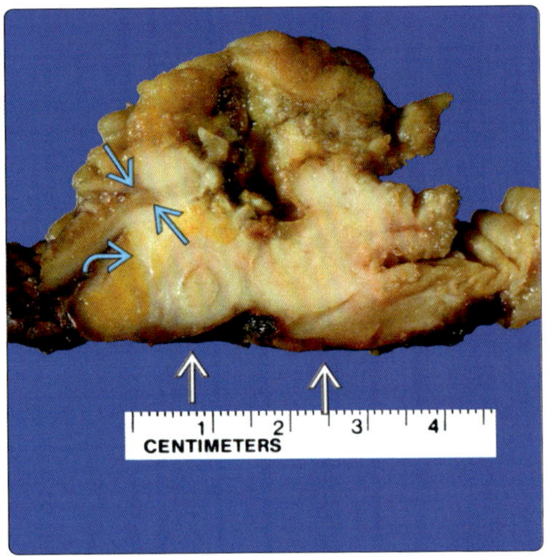

Carcinoid Tumor of Small Intestine

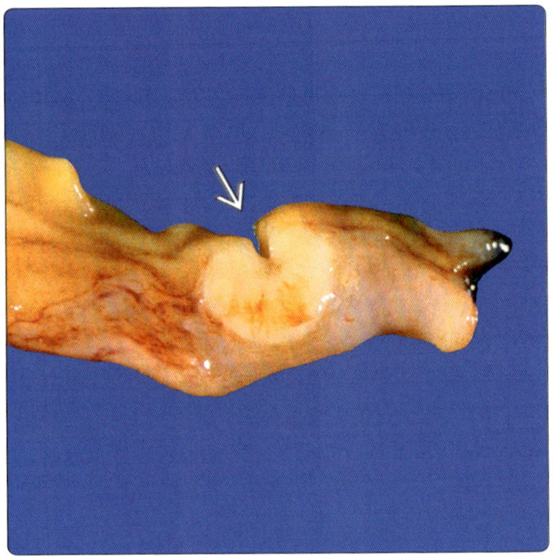

(Left) *Invasive carcinomas arising within Barrett mucosa can grow underneath an overlying normal-appearing squamous mucosa. It is important to evaluate a full-thickness margin specimen (both mucosa and muscularis) by frozen section.* **(Right)** *Signet ring cell carcinomas infiltrate the gastric wall, causing it to be thickened (linitis plastica). Mucosal lesions may not be present. Tumor involvement of margins is difficult to evaluate grossly. It is important that the frozen section includes full-thickness gastric wall.*

Esophageal Adenocarcinoma

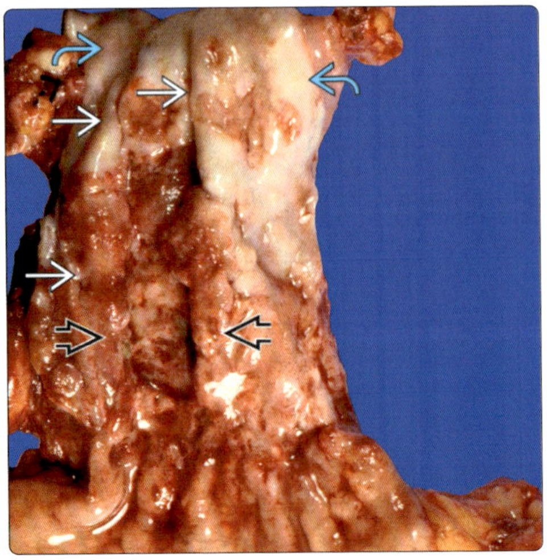

Gastric Signet Ring Cell Carcinoma

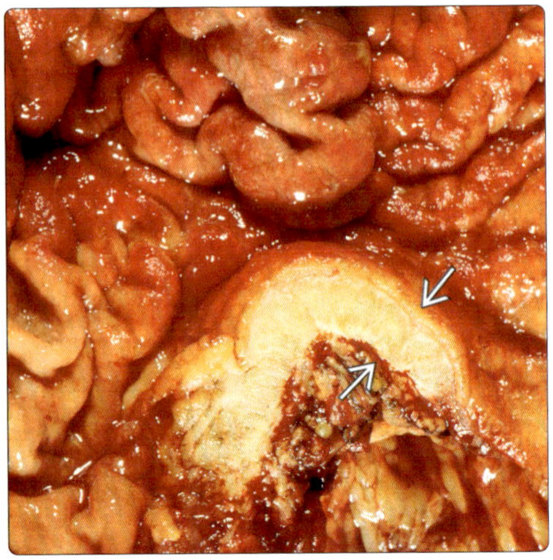

Metastatic Carcinoma to Lymph Node

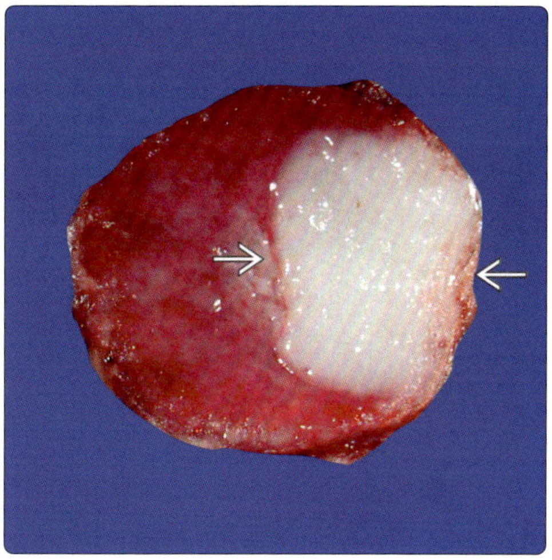

Lymphoma Involving Lymph Node

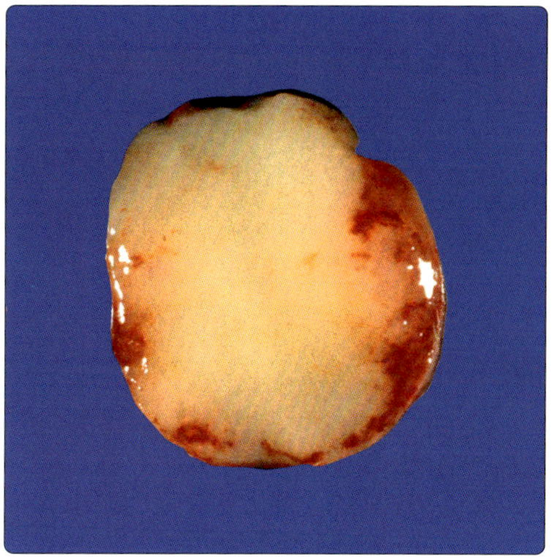

(Left) *Metastatic carcinoma ➡ usually forms a focal, firm, white mass in a lymph node. Larger metastases are easily detected grossly, but small macrometastases (2-3 mm) may only be evident on frozen section examination.* **(Right)** *Lymphomas typically diffusely involve nodes and have a fleshy homogeneous appearance. Cytologic preparations are preferred for the evaluation of histologic features and preserve tissue that can be used for ancillary studies.*

Radiation-Associated Angiosarcoma of Skin

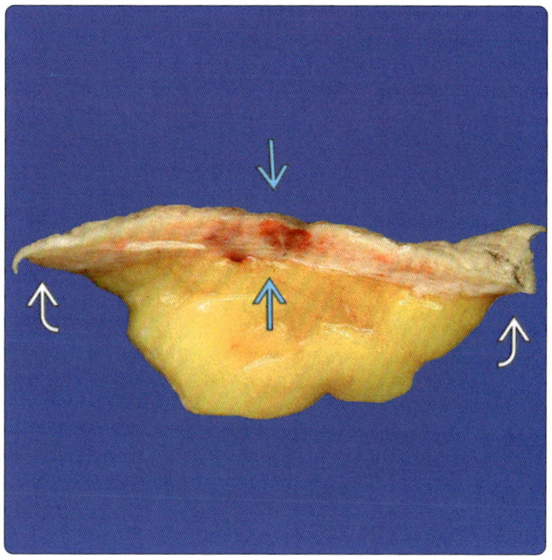

Endometrial Carcinoma

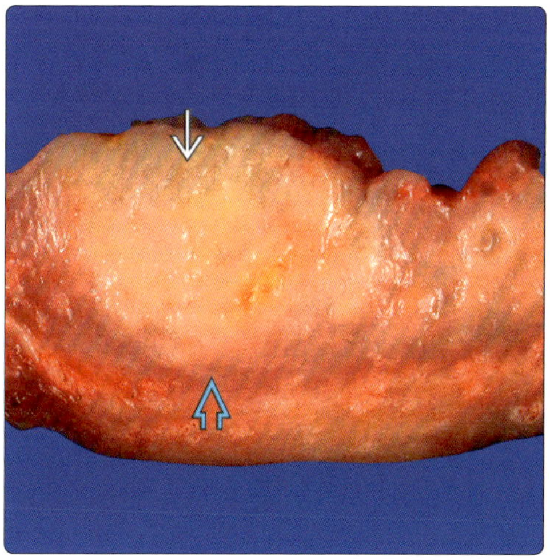

(Left) *This angiosarcoma ⇨ arose in breast skin after radiation treatment for breast carcinoma. It is important to be aware of the histologic type of tumor when evaluating margins by ➡ frozen section. (Courtesy I. Schaefer, MD.)* **(Right)** *Endometrial carcinomas ➡ are evaluated intraoperatively for depth of invasion. If the carcinoma invades to > 50% of the myometrium ⇨, a pelvic lymph node dissection may be performed. The deepest extent of invasion is determined grossly and confirmed by frozen section.*

Mucinous Cystic Ovarian Neoplasm

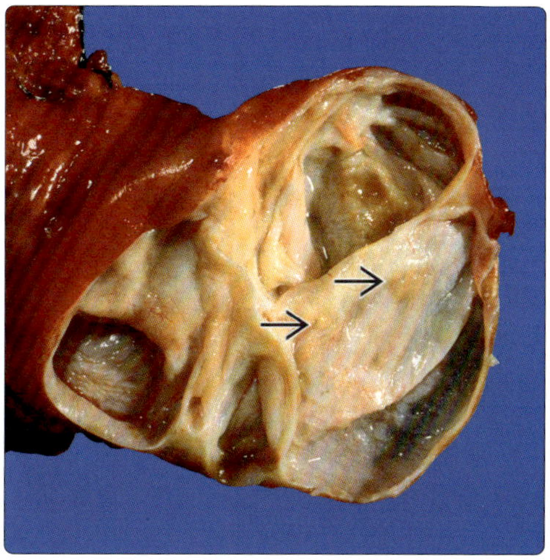

Ovarian Teratoma

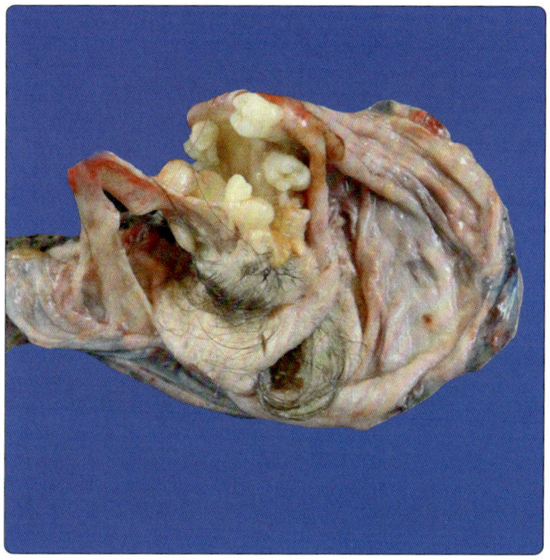

(Left) *It can be difficult to classify mucinous neoplasms on frozen section due to heterogeneity. All cystic spaces are opened and the inner surface examined for papillary excrescences ➡ or solid nodules that may be areas of carcinoma.* **(Right)** *Teratomas are common benign neoplasms of the ovary. The presence of teeth and hair clearly identify this cystic tumor as a teratoma. (Courtesy A. Sedlak, PA.)*

(Left) *This adenocarcinoma can be identified as a malignant lesion due to the invasion into adjacent lung parenchyma → and into a bronchus →. The absence of pleural involvement ➡ is an important prognostic factor and can be determined grossly.* **(Right)** *Carcinomas invading the pleura are fixed to it and typically cause puckering and retraction ➡. This area should be avoided for frozen section as this feature should be documented on permanent sections and considered for tumor classification and staging.*

Adenocarcinoma of Lung

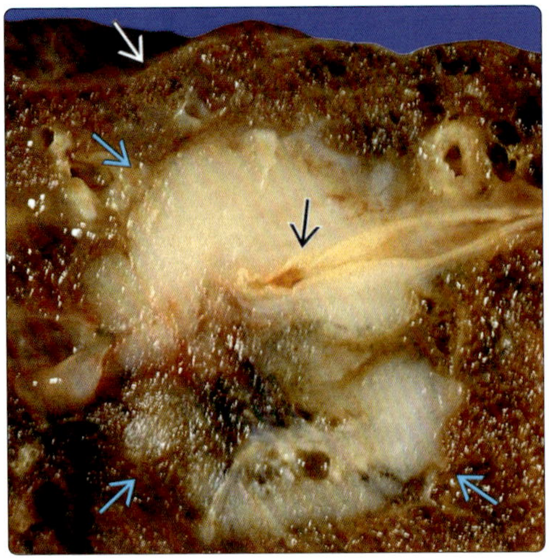

Pleural Invasion by Lung Carcinoma

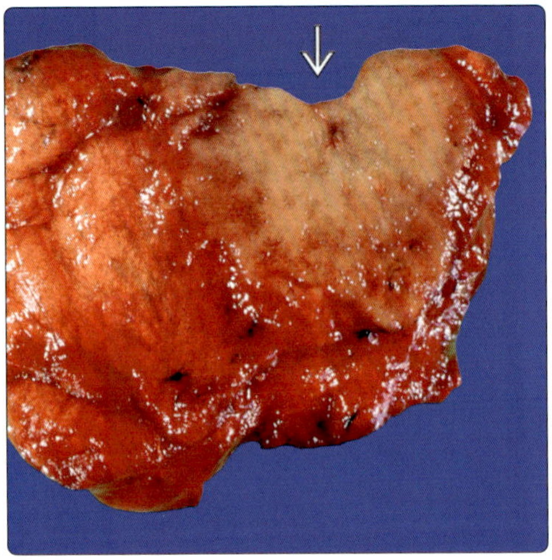

(Left) *Pulmonary squamous cell carcinomas are usually centrally located and often have central cavitation.* **(Right)** *Carcinoid tumors are generally well-circumscribed neoplasms and often have a yellow or white-yellow glistening cut surface. They can be located centrally or peripherally. (Courtesy G. Gray, MD.)*

Squamous Cell Carcinoma of Lung

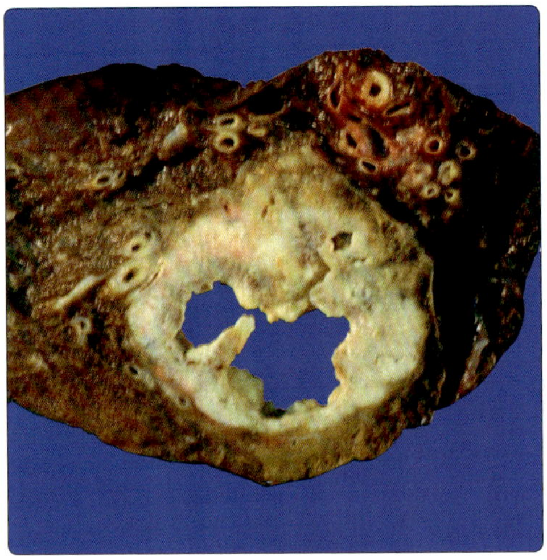

Carcinoid Tumor: Gross Appearance

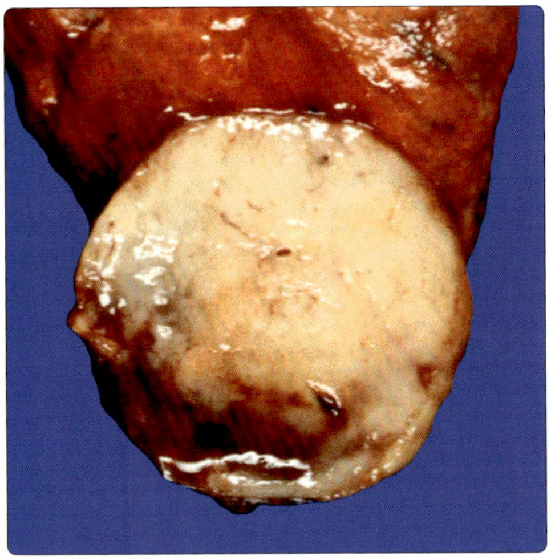

(Left) *Pulmonary hamartomas of the lung have a bulging, lobulated appearance due to the abundant cartilage. These tumors are easily recognized on gross examination.* **(Right)** *Squamous cell carcinomas are often located proximally in the lung and may involve the bronchial margin either as invasive carcinoma or carcinoma in situ. This invasive carcinoma → is present at the margin in the bronchial wall ➡. (Courtesy C. Gruessner, MD.)*

Pulmonary Hamartoma

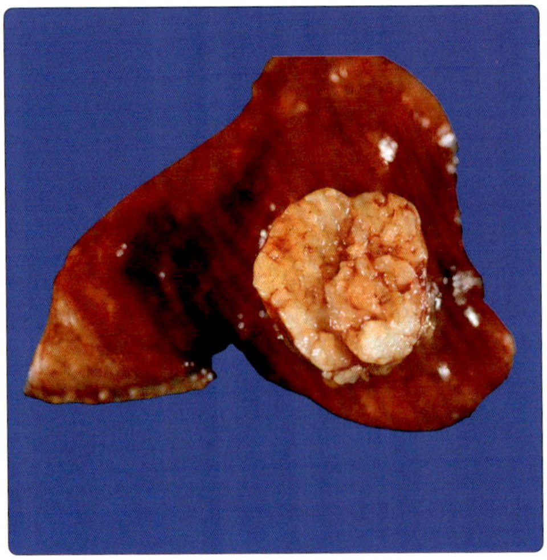

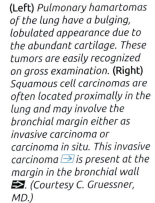

Squamous Cell Carcinoma at Bronchial Margin

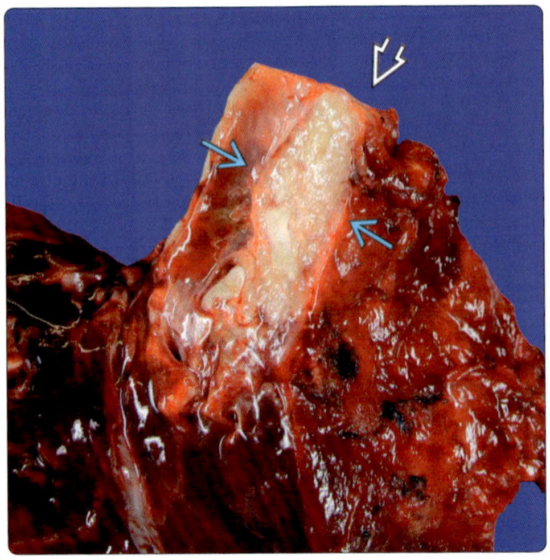

Renal Cell Carcinoma Involving Renal Vein

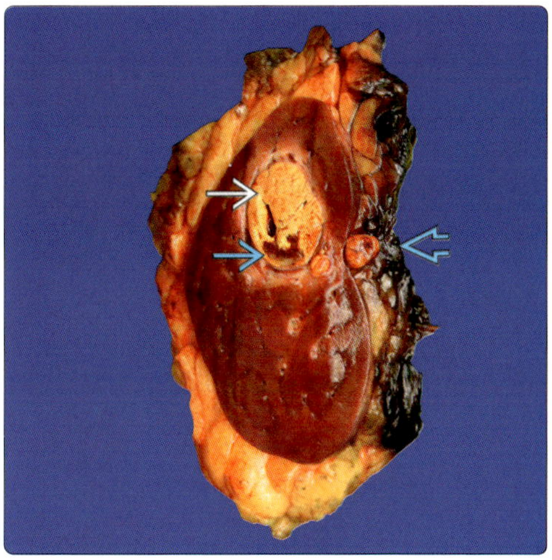

Ganglioneuroma of Adrenal Gland

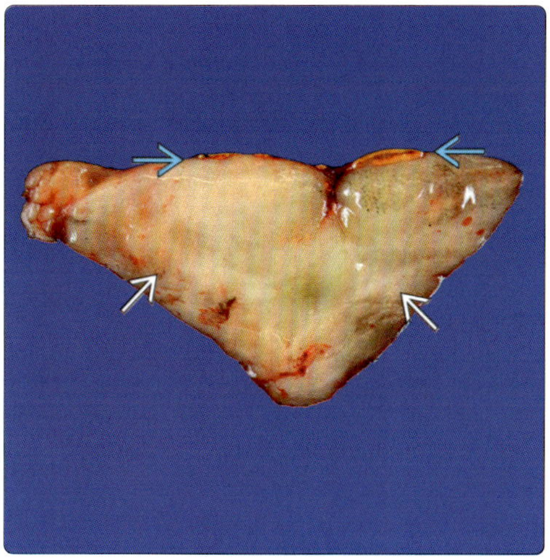

(Left) *The type of renal cell carcinoma can usually be determined grossly. This clear cell carcinoma has the characteristic golden yellow/orange color* ➡ *and blood lakes* ⇨. *The carcinoma has invaded into the renal vein* ⇨. *(Courtesy A. Christakis, MD.)* **(Right)** *This ganglioneuroma* ➡ *arose from the medulla of the adrenal gland* ⇨. *The fleshy gross appearance is distinct from the more common pheochromocytomas and cortical lesions of the adrenal gland. (Courtesy D. Poliferno, PA.)*

Thyroid Adenoma

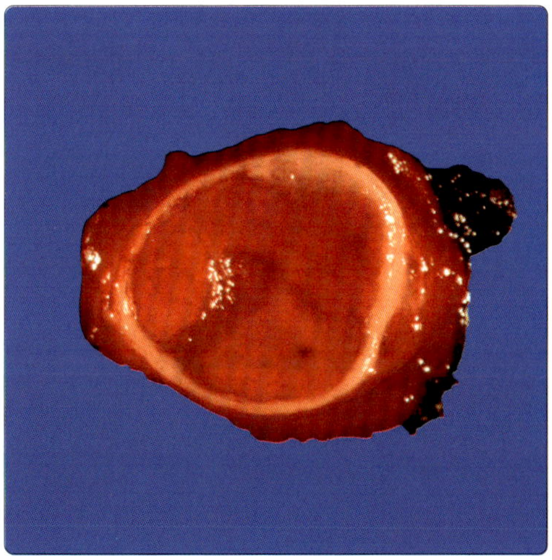

Papillary Thyroid Carcinoma

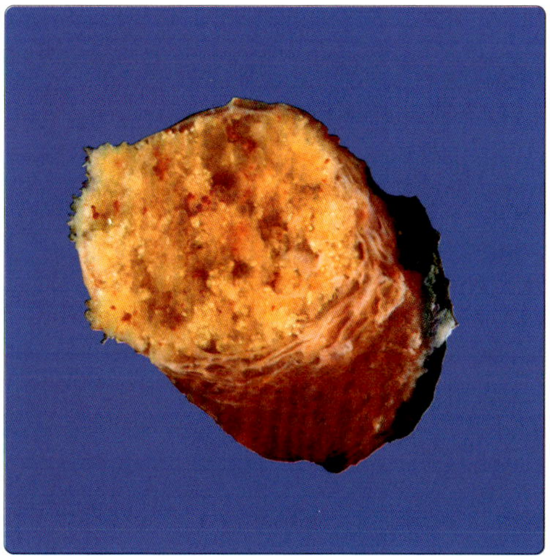

(Left) *This thyroid lesion has a thick capsule that must be completely examined microscopically for possible areas of invasion. This is generally not practical to attempt during an intraoperative consultation. It is preferable to diagnose this type of lesion on permanent sections.* **(Right)** *Papillary thyroid carcinoma has a distinct gross appearance. Most cancers will have been diagnosed by FNA prior to surgery. In this case, an intraoperative touch preparation could also confirm the diagnosis.*

Breast Specimen Inking

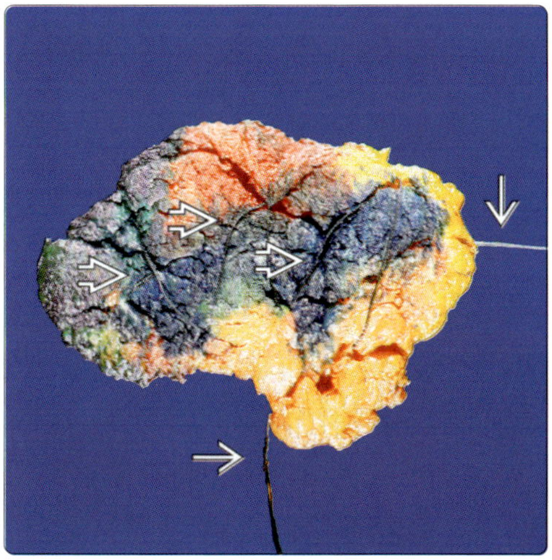

Breast Invasive Carcinoma

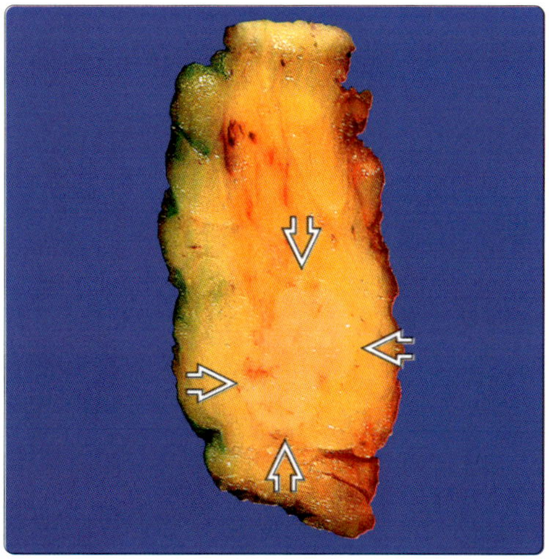

(Left) *This breast specimen has been oriented with 2 sutures of different lengths* ➡ *and a mattress stitch* ➡ *to identify an additional margin. The ink has smeared, which will make microscopic identification of margins difficult. Each margin section should be identified according to the gross orientation.* **(Right)** *The gross size* ➡ *of a carcinoma is an important prognostic factor for breast cancer, as well as others, and is best determined by palpation when the specimen is unfixed and before tumor tissue has been taken for special studies.*

INTRODUCTION AND GENERAL ISSUES

Applications

- Primary diagnosis
- Diagnosis in conjunction with conventional frozen section
- Confirmation of nodal metastasis or metastasis to other sites
- Confirmation of lesional tissue when there is limited material for diagnosis
- Confirmation of lesional tissue for triage for special studies &/or tissue banking

Advantages

- Contributes additional information over that provided by frozen section
  - Optimal preservation of nuclear and cellular detail
    - No ice crystal artifact
    - Complete nuclei are present
  - Evaluates cellular cohesion or lack thereof
  - Better demonstration of long cytoplasmic processes
  - 3-dimensional structure can be seen in some cases
- Easy sampling of multiple areas of specimen
- Speed of preparation
- Maximal preservation of tissue for permanent section diagnosis, ancillary studies, and investigational studies
- Minimizes exposure of personnel to potentially infectious agents (e.g., cases of granulomatous disease)
  - Avoids cryostat contamination
- Does not require special equipment (i.e., cryostat)
- Creates cytologic case record in files for comparison with future cytologic samples (e.g., fine-needle aspiration [FNA], effusions) from same patient

Disadvantages

- Requires specialized knowledge of cytopathology
- Lacks architectural information
  - In situ carcinoma is not clearly distinguishable from invasive carcinoma
- Some lesions are not amenable to cytologic examination
  - Paucicellular lesions
  - Lesions with dense stroma
- Some intraoperative questions are not amenable to cytologic examination
  - Margin evaluation when distance to margin is of importance
  - Margin evaluation if location of tumor is significant (e.g., bronchial resection margin)
  - Depth of invasion (e.g., endometrial carcinoma)

TECHNIQUE

Tissue Preparation

- Thinly slice through specimen to reveal best lesional areas
- If excessively bloody, blood should be blotted or gently scraped away

Touch Imprints

- **Most appropriate lesions**
  - Useful for highly cellular specimens that exfoliate easily
    - Lymph nodes
    - Lymphomas
    - Tumors not associated with desmoplastic stroma (especially small round blue cell tumors)
  - Can be used for specimens too small or too fragmented to be scraped to create smear preparations
- **Technique**
  - Touch clean and dry glass slide to freshly cut tissue surface for fraction of second
  - Avoid pressure or lateral movement
  - Immediately immerse in fixative for H&E or Papanicolaou staining
  - If air-dried slides are desired, slides must be thoroughly dried before staining
    - Drying requires several minutes
      - Heat source can be used to shorten drying time
    - Best technique for air-dried preparations
- **Advantages**
  - Cytoplasm tends to be better preserved than in scrape/smear technique
  - May show correlative architectural features (e.g., lymphoid follicles)

Pancreatic Adenocarcinoma Metastatic to Lymph Node

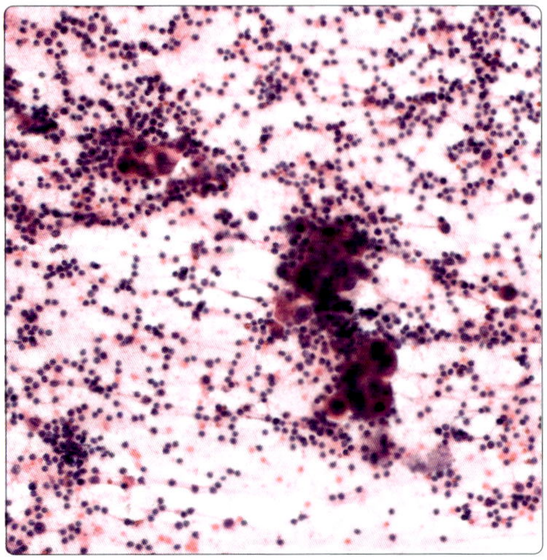

Pancreatic Adenocarcinoma Metastatic to Lymph Node

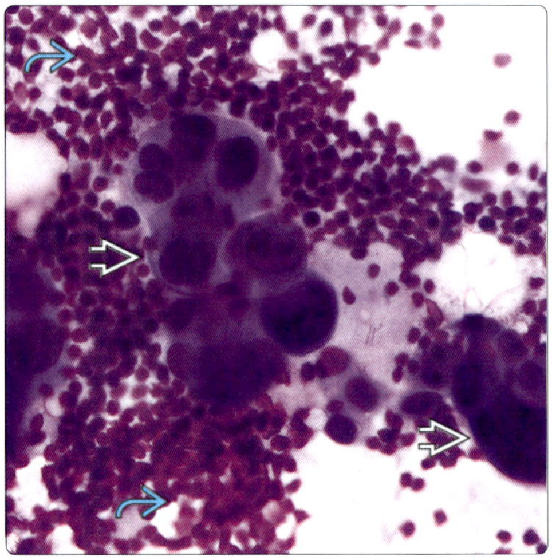

(Left) *This rapid-fixed H&E-stained preparation of pancreatic adenocarcinoma metastatic to a lymph node shows cohesive clusters of malignant cells. The tumor cells are large and have well-preserved nuclei with sharp chromatin detail and abundant cytoplasm.* **(Right)** *An air-dried smear stained with Wright-Giemsa accentuates the dual cell population of large cells of metastatic pancreatic adenocarcinoma* ➔ *in a background of small mature nodal lymphocytes* ➔.

- More likely to produce monolayers than cytologic smears
- **Caveats**
  - Multiple imprints on same slide should be avoided if slide is to be rapidly fixed
    - Only last imprint will be fixed optimally
    - Earlier imprints will show drying artifact
  - Multiple imprints work well for air-dried preparations

Smears

- **Most appropriate lesions**
  - Useful for less cellular or sclerotic lesions
    - Carcinomas in desmoplastic stroma
    - Bony specimens or heavily calcified specimens; may be only technique that will yield individual cells
- **Technique**
  - Scrape lesional cut surface 3-4x in same direction with clean, dry scalpel blade, accumulating semiliquid cell suspension on advancing edge of blade
    - Glass slide may be used instead of blade
    - Very gentle scraping should be used for soft cellular lesions
    - Additional or more forceful scraping may be required for fibrous paucicellular tumors
  - Cells can be directly smeared on 2nd slide
    - Angled blade or slide with cell suspension is drawn directly across length of 2nd slide, depositing streak of suspended cells
  - Alternatively, cell suspension can be smeared between 2 slides
    - Drop of semiliquid cell suspension is placed at center of slide
    - 2nd slide is opposed to 1st, compressing cell suspension between 2 slides
    - The 2 slides are separated in sliding motion, smearing suspension across both slides
  - Regardless of chosen technique, slides should be immediately immersed in fixative if H&E or Papanicolaou staining is planned
- **Advantages**
  - More effective at producing cellular smears from some specimens
  - More easily samples entire surface
    - Important if cytology is being used to evaluate metastasis to lymph node or margin status
- **Caveats**
  - Avoid excess scraping: Blade edge holds limited amount of suspension
  - Avoid excess manipulation: Smearing back and forth tends to damage cells (more cell damage is seen in "2-slide" method of smearing)
  - Some areas of slide may be too thick for interpretation

Squash

- **Most appropriate lesions**
  - Generally only applicable for soft tissue
  - Preferred technique of many neuropathologists, particularly for stereotactic biopsies
    - There is often too little tissue for smear preparations and tissue may not be sufficiently cellular for touch imprints
- **Technique**
  - Small (1 x 1 mm maximum) piece of abnormal tissue is separated from core or biopsy specimen
    - Larger fragment may smear off end of slide and not be able to be examined
    - If lesion is heterogeneous, multiple small fragments can be placed side-by-side
  - Using forceps, gently place tissue near labeled end of slide
    - Do not pinch or crush tissue
  - If there is significant liquid or blood, carefully dab corner of square of lens paper near tissue to absorb excess
  - Using another slide, firmly squash tissue and spread it along slide longitudinally
    - For very soft tissues, only gentle pressure is necessary
    - Too much pressure will rupture cells with little cytoplasm (e.g., lymphomas or medulloblastomas)
  - Separate 2 slides and immediately place in fixative
  - Both slides are stained and coverslipped
- **Advantages**
  - Best technique to demonstrate cells with long cytoplasmic processes
  - Shows 3-dimensional structure as well as single cell morphology
- **Caveats**
  - May help to perform squash over fixative jar to facilitate rapid fixation
  - If tissue is insufficiently soft, it may not be possible to use this technique

SLIDE STAINING TECHNIQUES

Rapid-Fixed: H&E or Rapid Pap

- Both techniques yield high quality nuclear detail and optimal cell preservation
- H&E preferred by most pathologists in intraoperative setting
  - More familiar to noncytopathologists
  - Facilitates correlation with tissue sections, especially concurrent frozen sections

Air-Dried: Romanowsky (Diff-Quik/Wright-Giemsa)

- Good for preservation of cytoplasmic detail and extracellular matrix (e.g., chondroid, osteoid, or colloid)
- Accentuates differences in cell populations (e.g., metastases to lymph nodes, or biphasic tumors)
- Familiar to hematopathologists for lymphoid lesions

DIAGNOSTIC FEATURES OF COMMONLY ENCOUNTERED TUMORS

Adenocarcinoma

- Cytology preparations usually of high cellularity
- Combination of clustered and dispersed epithelioid cells with anisonucleosis, vesicular chromatin, and variably prominent nucleoli
  - Abortive glandular structures, signet ring forms, or mucinous background may be apparent
- In organs where reactive changes that may simulate malignancy are common (lung, pancreaticobiliary), demonstration of dual cell population useful
  - Both tumor cells and reactive cells should be present as separate populations

- Appearance may vary greatly depending on degree of differentiation
- Well-differentiated carcinomas may closely simulate normal or reactive ductal or glandular epithelium
  - Form disordered sheets of cells (so-called drunken honeycomb appearance)
- Poorly differentiated carcinomas may simply be identifiable as carcinoma or "not otherwise specified" malignancy

Squamous Cell Carcinoma

- Clustered smear pattern
- "Generic" malignant nuclear features: Anisonucleosis, coarse chromatin
- Background of necrotic or keratinaceous debris may be present
  - Keratinization often not well manifested on smears
- Often dense, acidophilic cytoplasm
- Pitfall: May elicit foreign body giant cell reaction, creating confusion with granulomatous process

Well-Differentiated Neuroendocrine Tumor

- Shows similar features regardless of site of origin
- Dispersed smear pattern
- Round to ovoid, often plasmacytoid cells with scant to moderate cytoplasm
- Generally uniform nuclei with salt and pepper chromatin; nuclear size tends to be uniform within case (though may vary from case to case)

Small Cell Carcinoma

- Shows similar features regardless of site of origin
- Typically highly cellular with clustered pattern; crush artifact may be present in background
- When single cell pattern prominent, lymphoma often in differential diagnosis
- Dark basophilic cells, nuclei 2-3x size of lymphocyte
- Chromatin relatively fine; if present, nucleoli are small &/or indistinct
- Reciprocal molding characteristic and useful feature

Melanoma

- Dispersed smear pattern; typically dyscohesive
- Cells may be polygonal or (often) plasmacytoid with anisocytosis and prominent red nucleoli
- Multinucleation may be present
- Pigmentation and intranuclear cytoplasmic inclusions helpful for confirmation

Mesenchymal Tumors, Including Sarcoma

- Greatly variable appearance, depending on type, grade, cellularity, and matrix
- Patterns encountered
  - Pleomorphic
  - Epithelioid/round cell
  - Spindle cell
  - Giant cell rich
- Vigorous tissue scraping may be valuable to yield matrix or small tissue fragments

Lymphoproliferative Lesions

- **General considerations**
  - Most common use of intraoperative cytology is for detection and characterization of metastatic disease, most commonly to lymph node
    - Normal &/or reactive cellular components of lymph nodes must be distinguished from malignancies
  - When lymphoproliferative disease is suspected, intraoperative cytology is very useful for triage of limited tissue
  - Whenever possible, retention of lesional tissue in cell culture medium is desirable to preserve cells and for possible culture &/or flow cytometry
    - Especially important when differential diagnosis includes low- or intermediate-grade lymphoma and reactive conditions
- **Diagnostic features: Reactive patterns**
  - Polymorphous: Small mature lymphocytes with other elements (transformed lymphocytes, neutrophils, eosinophils, plasma cells, tingible body macrophages)
  - Monomorphous: Predominantly small mature lymphocytes; flow cytometry of potential high value
  - Granulomatous: Epithelioid histiocytes, multinucleated giant cells, lymphocytes, plasma cells
  - Suppurative: Intact and degenerated neutrophils
- **Diagnostic features of "small cell" lymphoma patterns**
  - Includes small lymphocytic lymphoma/chronic lymphocytic lymphoma, marginal cell lymphoma, mantle cell lymphoma, follicular lymphoma
  - Monotonous population of small mature lymphocytes; flow cytometry of potential high value
  - Coarse chromatin and nucleoli may be evident
  - Tingible body macrophages rare
- **Diagnostic features of "large cell" lymphoma patterns**
  - Includes follicular mixed lymphoma, diffuse large B-cell lymphoma, others
  - Mixed or monotonous population of large atypical cells, often with more open chromatin; immunoblastic cells
  - Tingible body macrophages may be frequent in high-grade lesions
  - When material is limited and cytology overtly malignant, tissue preservation for permanent section may be of higher value than flow cytometry
- **Diagnostic features of Hodgkin lymphoma**
  - Mixed cell population
  - Reed-Sternberg cell variants: Large, atypical cells; may be bi- or polylobated
    - Chromatin may be dark and coarse or more vesicular with large nucleoli
  - Background: Predominantly small mature lymphocytes but may have significant admixture of lymphocytes and neutrophils
  - Flow cytometry of limited value

SITE-SPECIFIC CONSIDERATIONS

Breast Carcinoma, Primary Tumor

- **General considerations**
  - Intraoperative evaluation of primary breast carcinoma now exceedingly rare; primary use is in sentinel lymph node evaluation
  - In unusual cases where clinically justified, primary value of intraoperative cytology is to preserve tissue in grossly suspicious but small lesion

- **Diagnostic features**
  - Clustered and dispersed cells
  - Often plasmacytoid in appearance with eccentric nuclei and moderate cytoplasm
  - Nuclei are typically large with dark/coarse chromatin; nucleoli variable
  - Cytoplasm usually eosinophilic; intracytoplasmic vacuoles may be evident, particularly lobular carcinoma
  - Histiocytoid features may be seen, especially in moderately or poorly differentiated lobular carcinoma

Breast Carcinoma, Sentinel Node

- **Gross examination of critical importance**
  - Intraoperative surgical management may rely not just on presence but also on extent of tumor
  - Node should be serially sectioned at < 0.2-cm intervals and all surfaces carefully examined
- **Technique for nodes with no macroscopic lesion identified**
  - Scrape all cut surfaces to make cell-rich semiliquid pooled smear(s)
  - If multiple nodes are sampled, use separate blades and make separate smear(s) for each node
- **Technique for nodes with gross lesion present**
  - Focus scrape preparation on gross target lesion to obtain higher concentration of lesional cells
  - If size of lesion is borderline (± 2 mm), prepare concurrent frozen section to better determine size
  - If lesion is cytologically indeterminate, prepare frozen section to assess
  - If multiple nodes are sampled, use separate blades and make separate smear(s) for each node
- **Diagnostic features**
  - Biphasic population of tumor cells and lymphocytes
  - Tumor cells show similar features to those listed for primary breast carcinoma

Thyroid

- **General considerations**
  - Intraoperative consultation most effective when used in conjunction with preoperative FNA results
    - Follicular lesions: Limited value due to need to assess tissue for capsular or vascular invasion
    - "Suspicious" or "atypical" lesions: Cytologic preparations are of high value for identifying papillary thyroid carcinoma
- **Diagnostic features of goiter/hyperplasia**
  - Variable cellularity and background colloid
  - Cells grouped in clusters or sheets
  - Small dark, round nuclei with coarse chromatin
  - Hürthle cells may be present
  - Cyst macrophages
- **Diagnostic features of follicular neoplasms**
  - Cellular aspirate with possible microfollicular pattern and scant colloid
  - Small dark, round nuclei with coarse chromatin
  - Hürthle cell population may predominate with single Hürtheloid cells prominent
  - Adenoma and carcinoma will show similar cytologic features
- **Diagnostic features of papillary carcinoma**
  - Cellularity may vary greatly depending on architectural pattern and degree of fibrosis
  - Large, often overlapping nuclei with irregular nuclear contours, nuclear grooves, open chromatin with small peripheral nucleoli, and (sometimes) intranuclear inclusions
    - Intranuclear inclusions are cytoplasmic invaginations that should be same color as cytoplasm
      - Can be mimicked by ice crystal artifact
  - Cytoplasm can vary greatly and be squamoid or Hürtheloid
  - Pitfalls
    - Intranuclear inclusions may be frequent in smears of hyalinizing trabecular tumor (hyalinizing trabecular adenoma)
    - Columnar cell variant of papillary carcinoma may show minimal nuclear features
    - Diffuse sclerosing variant of papillary carcinoma may show oncocytic (Hürtheloid) cytology and abundant lymphocytes, mimicking lymphocytic thyroiditis

Pancreaticobiliary

- **General considerations**
  - Primary intraprocedural role is confirming target tissue obtained by endoscopic ultrasound-guided biopsy
  - Cytology slides may be imprint preparations of core biopsies or FNA
  - Absence of malignancy does not mean target has been missed; communication with endoscopist is essential
- **Diagnostic considerations for primary site**
  - Adenocarcinoma variants
  - Chronic pancreatitis
  - Retention cysts, pseudocysts, and cystic neoplasms
  - Neuroendocrine neoplasms
- **Diagnostic considerations for lymph node**
  - Reactive/negative
  - Metastatic carcinoma or neuroendocrine tumor
  - Lymphoproliferative disorder

Liver

- **Uses**
  - Rapid confirmatory evaluation and preservation of tissue for metastatic lesions
  - Adjunct to histology for evaluation of primary lesions (hepatocellular carcinoma, cholangiocarcinoma)
- **Limitations**
  - Most intraoperative consultations for primary liver tumors involve margin assessment

Bone and Soft Tissue

- **Uses**
  - Adjunct to frozen section for confirmation of malignancy
  - Primary diagnosis, particularly for bone metastasis when material limited or too calcified to section in cryostat
- **Limitations**
  - Use for sarcoma margins limited (though employed in some centers)
  - May be used for bone marrow margins of bone lesions
    - Gross examination of specimen to determine distance from margin may be more accurate

Lung

- **Uses**
  - Rapid confirmation of gross metastatic disease or granulomas in lung or mediastinal lymph nodes
- **Limitations**
  - Appearance of reactive pneumocytes and bronchial cells may overlap with that of well-differentiated carcinomas
    - Any indeterminate case should undergo frozen section confirmation
  - Some carcinomas (particularly squamous) may elicit granulomatous reactions

Gynecologic

- **Uses**
  - Adjunct to frozen section for most ovarian tumors
    - Some tumors have very characteristic cytologic features
  - Adult granulosa cell tumor
    - Monotonous population of cells that may seem minimally atypical relative to frozen section, with very uniform nuclei
    - Scant cytoplasm, fine chromatin, and prominent nuclear grooves
  - Dysgerminoma
    - Large, polyhedral cells with clear or granular cytoplasm
    - Background of small mature lymphocytes
    - Granulomas may be present
- **Limitations**
  - Many aspects of intraoperative gynecologic consultation rely heavily on tumor architecture
  - Overlap of low-grade benign or borderline lesions with malignancy
  - Overlap of metastatic and primary tumors
  - Evaluating extent of invasion (e.g., of myometrium by endometrial adenocarcinoma) requires frozen section

Peritoneal Nodules

- **Uses**
  - Rapid assessment of metastatic carcinoma, sarcoma, or neuroendocrine tumor
- **Limitations**
  - Small nodules of adenocarcinoma from gastrointestinal tract, pancreaticobiliary origin, or gynecologic origin may be sclerotic
    - Frozen section may be preferred technique

Central Nervous System

- **Uses**
  - Rapid, tissue-sparing diagnosis of metastatic disease (carcinoma, melanoma), pituitary adenoma, craniopharyngioma
  - Aid adequacy assessment in stereotactic core needle biopsies
  - Adjunct to frozen section in diagnosis of primary central nervous system lesions
    - Normal vs. abnormal
    - Neoplastic vs. nonneoplastic
    - Type of neoplasm (glial vs. nonglial)
    - Grade of neoplasm
- Touch preparations
  - Best for lymphomas or pituitary adenomas
- Smear preparations
  - Best for metastatic carcinoma or meningioma
- Squash preparations
  - Glial tumors
    - Neural cells have long, intertangling processes that may not be well represented in touch preps or smears
  - Meningiomas and schwannomas
    - May be too fibrous to squash well
- **Limitations**
  - Architectural patterns important for some diagnoses (e.g., primary central nervous system lymphoma)
  - Some smear patterns may be nonspecific or subtle (e.g., inconspicuous macrophages in demyelinating disease)

HELPFUL DIAGNOSTIC CLUES BY PATTERN OR FEATURE

Tumors With Dispersed Pattern, Plasmacytoid Cells

- Plasma cell dyscrasia or plasmacytoid lymphoma
- Neuroendocrine tumors
- Breast carcinoma
- Melanoma
- Medullary thyroid carcinoma
- Pituitary adenoma

Tumors With Intranuclear Inclusions

- Papillary thyroid carcinoma
- Meningioma
- Melanoma
- Low-grade adenocarcinoma of lung (lepidic pattern carcinoma, previously bronchioloalveolar carcinoma)
- Hepatocellular carcinoma
- Renal cell carcinoma
- Glioblastoma

Lymphocyte-Rich Lesions That may Mimic Nodal Metastases

- Seminoma/dysgerminoma
- Medullary pattern carcinoma of breast or colon
- Lymphocytic thyroiditis
- Lymphoepithelial pattern of nonkeratinizing squamous cell carcinoma
- Thymic tissue and neoplasms
- Warthin tumor of salivary gland

SELECTED REFERENCES

1. Ye Q et al: Fine-needle aspiration versus frozen section in the evaluation of malignant thyroid nodules in patients with the diagnosis of suspicious for malignancy or malignancy by fine-needle aspiration. Arch Pathol Lab Med. 141(5):684-689, 2017
2. Jakubiak M et al: Fast cytological evaluation of lymphatic nodes obtained during transcervical extended mediastinal lymphadenectomy. Eur J Cardiothorac Surg. 43(2):297-301, 2013
3. Krishnani N et al: Intraoperative squash cytology: accuracy and impact on immediate surgical management of central nervous system tumours. Cytopathology. 23(5):308-14, 2012

Cytologic Preparation: Smear With Scalpel

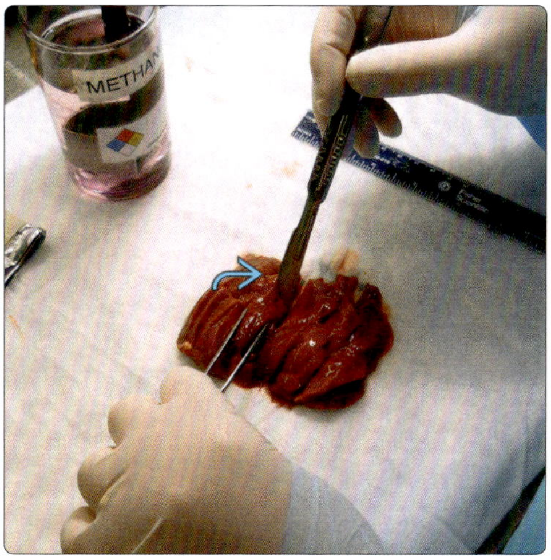

Cytologic Preparation: Smear With Scalpel

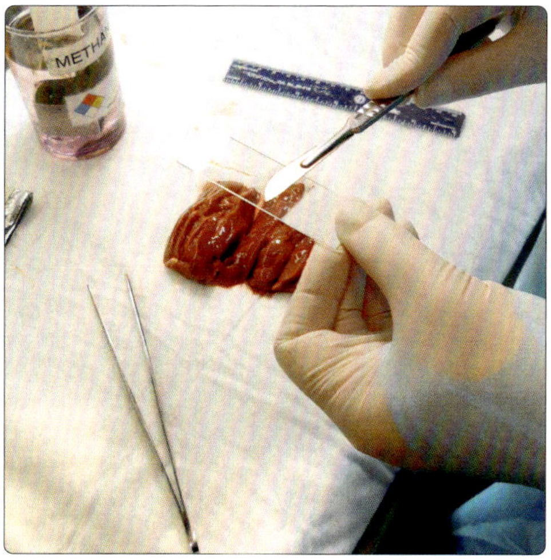

(Left) *The specimen is thinly sectioned to identify the area most representative of the lesion. A smear is made by scraping the surface of the lesion with a scalpel. This technique is appropriate for tissue that appears firm &/or calcified. An entire surface or multiple areas can be scraped.* **(Right)** *After scraping the tissue with the scalpel blade, the material is thinly smeared along the length of a glass slide. The slide should then be fixed immediately, unless an air-dried preparation is planned.*

Cytologic Preparation: Smear With Glass Slide

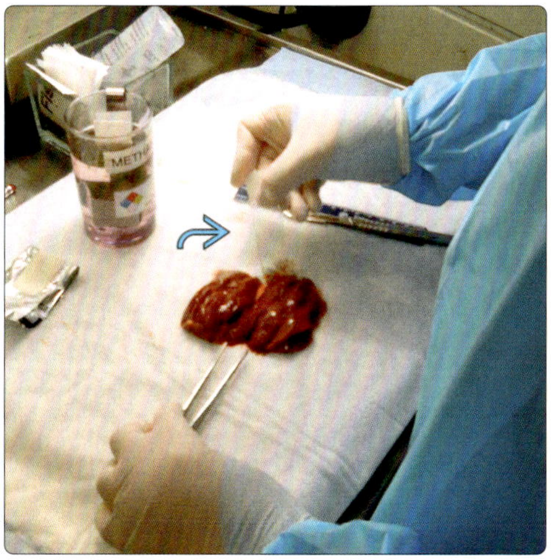

Cytologic Preparation: Touch Preparation

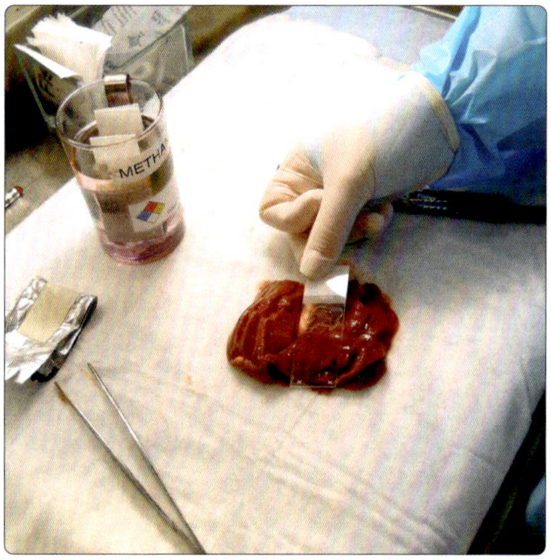

(Left) *Cytologic smears can be made by scraping the surface of the tissue with the edge of a glass slide. This technique is suitable for tumors with a fleshy appearance that likely will yield dyscohesive cells. It is also appropriate for necrotic tissue suspicious for an infectious process. The material is then smeared across another slide. Both slides can be stained.* **(Right)** *Touch preparations are made by gently touching a glass slide to the tissue. The slide is immediately fixed and then stained.*

Cytologic Preparation: Squash Preparation

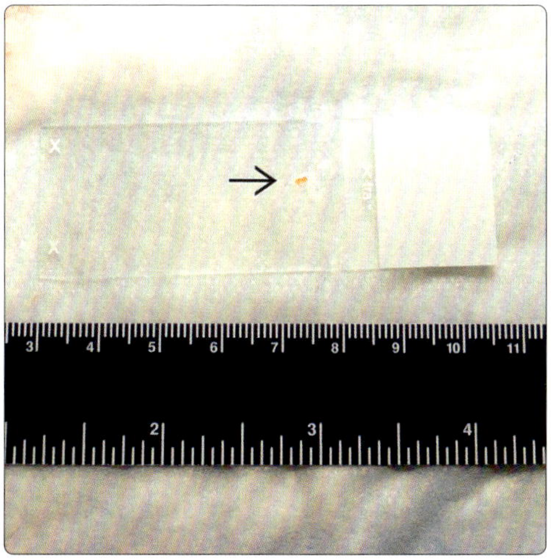

Cytologic Preparation: Squash Preparation

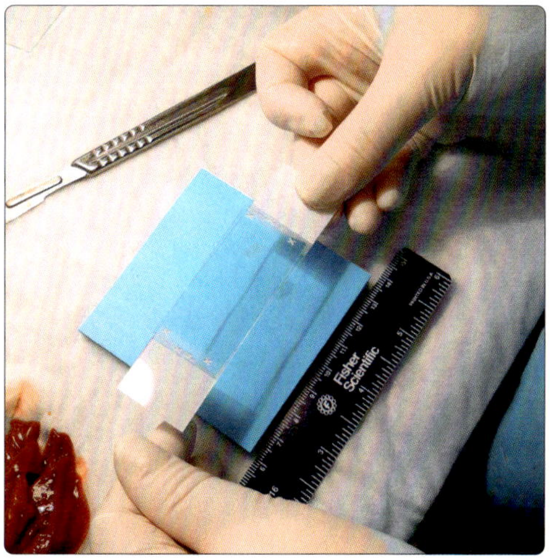

(Left) *Squash preparations can be used to examine tissue that is soft in consistency. This technique is generally only used for brain biopsies. A small (2-3 mm) fragment is gently placed near the frosted end of a slide. A drop of methanol can be placed next to the tissue to facilitate making the smear.* **(Right)** *To make a squash preparation, a 2nd slide (with the side to be labeled downward) is placed over the slide with the tissue and pressed firmly. The 2 slides are drawn apart in order to smear the tissue. The tissue is present on both slides.*

(Left) *When 2 slides ⇨ are used to smear or squash a specimen, tumor cells are present on each of the slides. Both slides should be stained for diagnostic use.* (Right) *Unless air-dried preparations are desired, slides should be immediately placed in a fixative. A delay of even a few seconds can result in significant artifact. It is helpful to have the fixative very close at hand. Air-dried slides may require several minutes for complete drying. Heat sources can be used to hasten complete drying.*

Cytologic Preparation: 2 Slides

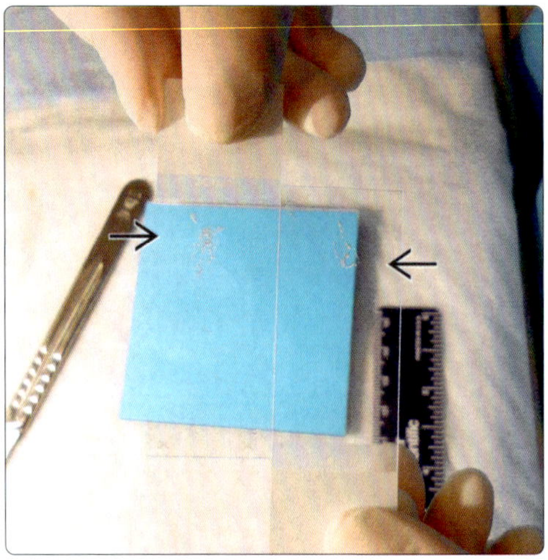

Cytologic Preparation: Immediate Fixation

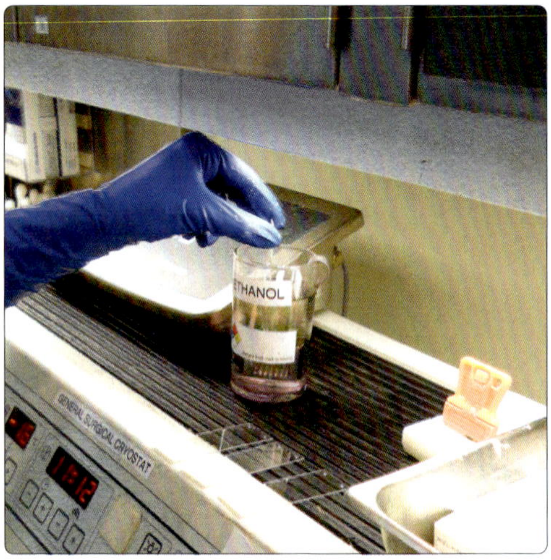

(Left) *Squash ⇨, smear ➡, and touch ➡ preparations each have advantages and disadvantages depending on the type of lesion. In many cases, multiple techniques can be used on the same specimen.* (Right) *Squash preparations reveal some types of underlying tissue structure ➡ as well as the morphology of single cells ⇨. This technique is particularly suitable for revealing elongated neural cell processes, which are more difficult to evaluate when tissue is examined in cross section on frozen section.*

Cytologic Preparations: Types

Squash Preparation

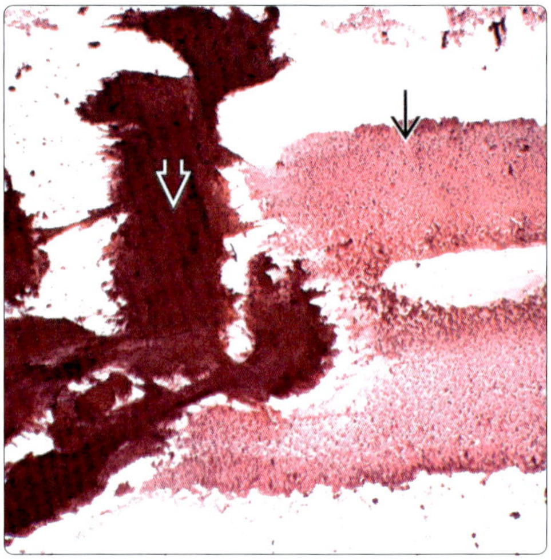

(Left) *Touch preparations are particularly suited to highly cellular tumors with little or no desmoplastic response, such as lymphomas or small blue cell tumors. The cells are easily dispersed from the tissue onto the slide, and the gentle handling results in minimal distortion of the cells.* (Right) *The process of smearing is a test of the cohesiveness of cells. For example, lymphomas and melanomas are seen as single cells and carcinomas as clumps of cells. Single cells are usually seen well.*

Touch Preparation

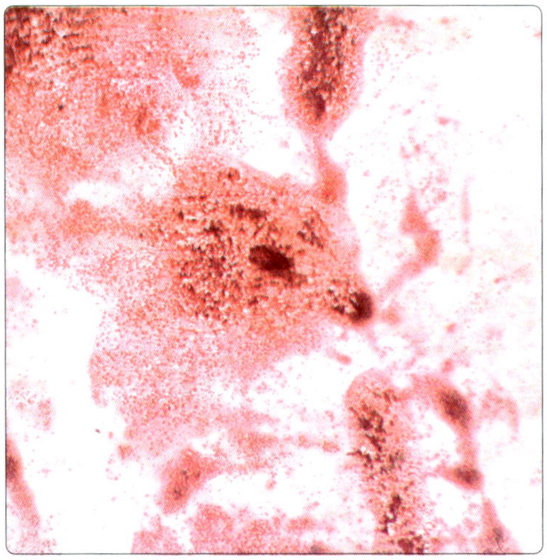

Cytologic Smear

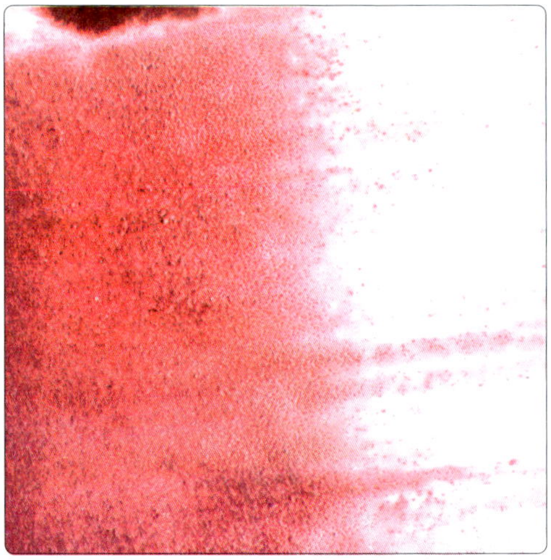

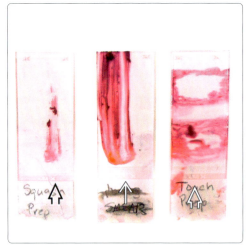

Adenocarcinoma: General Features

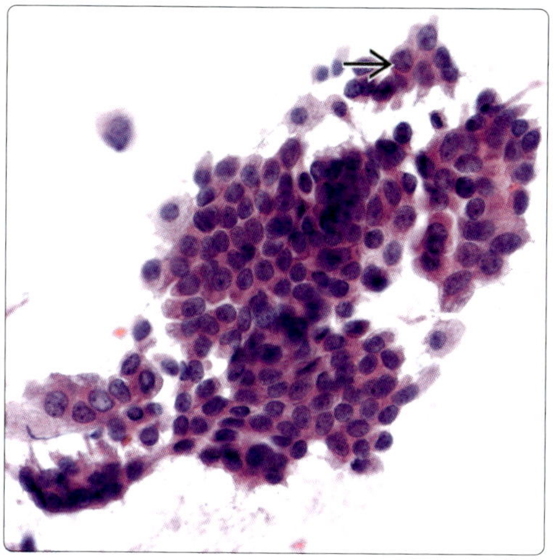

Adenocarcinoma: General Features

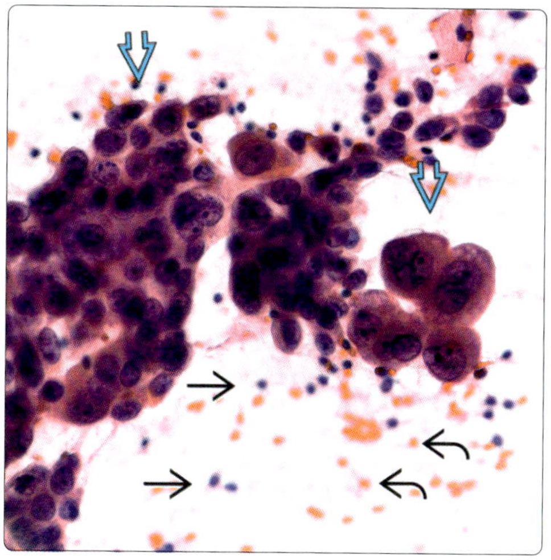

(Left) *This scrape prep of well-differentiated adenocarcinoma of the lung shows sheets of cohesive cells with large nuclei, moderate cytoplasm, mild anisonucleosis, and nuclear overlap. There is abortive gland formation →.* **(Right)** *This moderately differentiated adenocarcinoma → of the lung shows clusters of atypical epithelioid cells. The greater cell size is striking relative to background lymphocytes → and erythrocytes →. Anisonucleosis as well as nuclear crowding and overlap are prominent.*

Colonic Adenocarcinoma: General Features

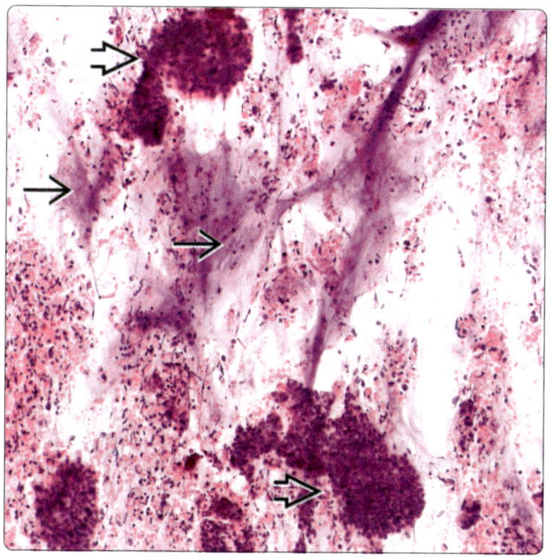

Colonic Adenocarcinoma

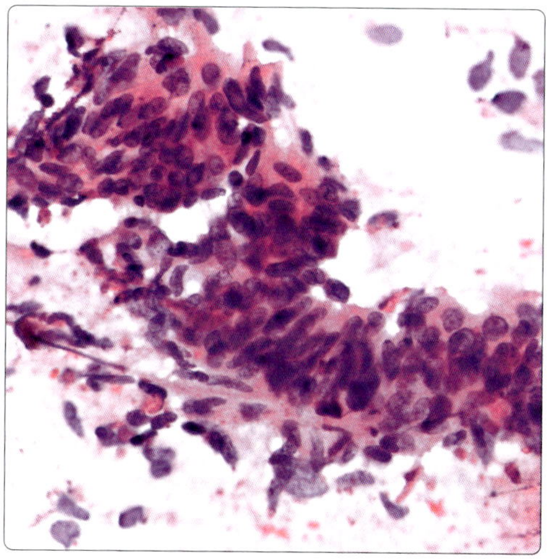

(Left) *Colonic adenocarcinoma often shows, in addition to clusters →, sheets of atypical epithelial cells and abundant background mucin →. A background of necrosis and inflammatory cells may also be seen.* **(Right)** *Colonic adenocarcinoma can have a "picket fence" arrangement of large, hyperchromatic nuclei with crowding and overlap. This pattern correlates with the tall columnar cells, forming gland-like structures seen in tissue sections.*

Mucinous Adenocarcinoma

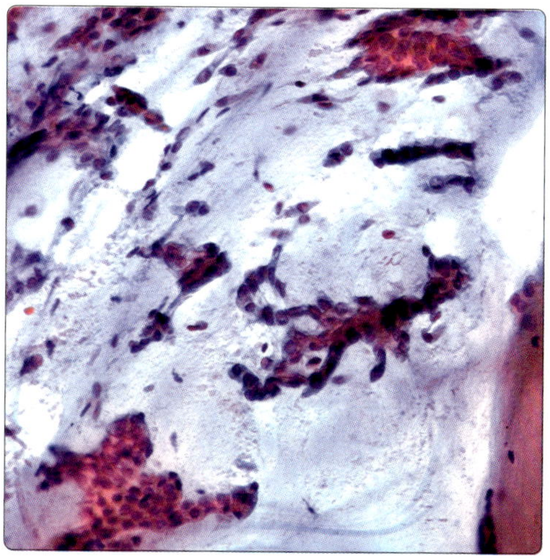

Pancreatic Signet Ring Cell Adenocarcinoma

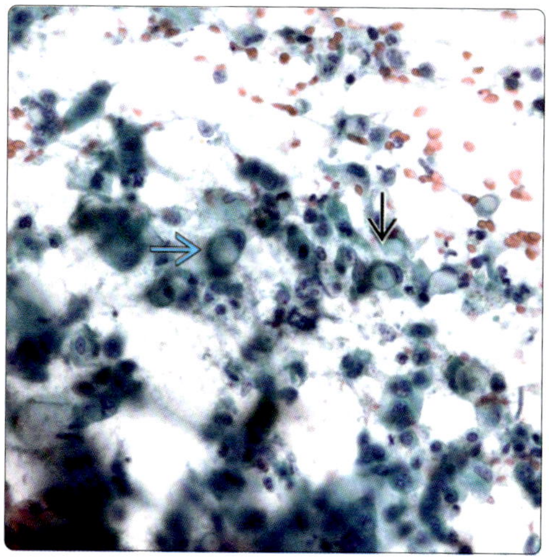

(Left) *Mucinous adenocarcinoma, regardless of origin, is typified by clusters of neoplastic epithelial cells floating in a background of blue-gray mucin. This example is from an endoscopic ultrasound-guided biopsy of the pancreas.* **(Right)** *This pancreatic adenocarcinoma shows clustered as well as solitary malignant epithelial cells with prominent intracytoplasmic vacuoles →, some with a target sign (central mucin droplet) →.*

(Left) *Squamous cell carcinoma usually shows a clustered growth pattern. Dense eosinophilic cytoplasm is typical, as are dark nuclei with coarse chromatin. Nucleoli may be variably prominent, usually less so than in adenocarcinoma. Keratin pearls are unusual in smears, but keratinous debris and cellular necrosis are common.* **(Right)** *This example of pulmonary squamous cell carcinoma shows clusters of cells with prominent intracytoplasmic keratinization and marked nuclear atypia.*

Squamous Cell Carcinoma

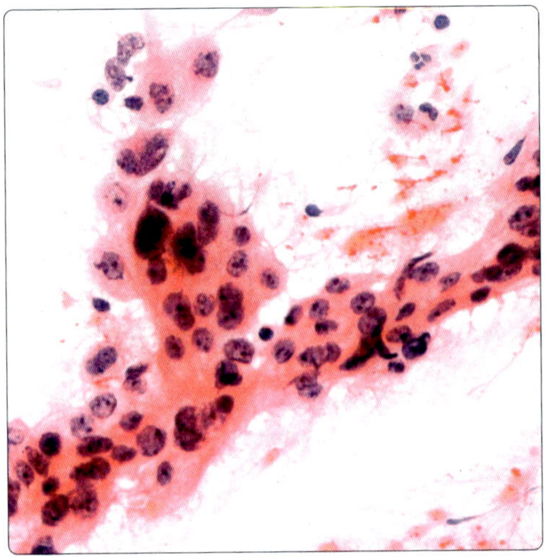

Squamous Cell Carcinoma

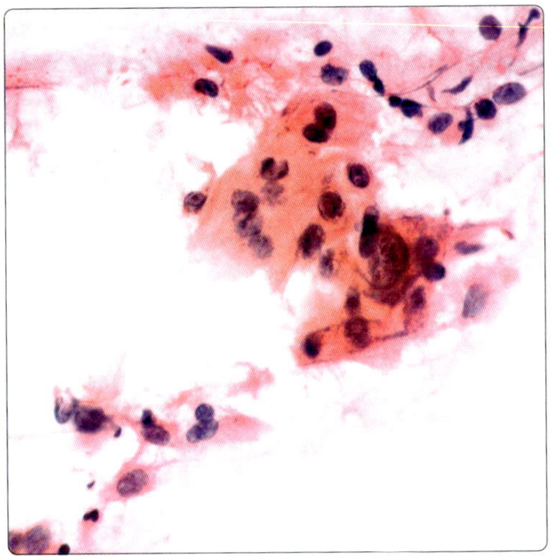

(Left) *This scrape preparation of metastatic well-differentiated neuroendocrine tumor of the small bowel shows dyscohesive, uniform plasmacytoid cells with large nuclei and endocrine (salt and pepper) chromatin.* **(Right)** *The nuclei in this lung carcinoid tumor are stripped of cytoplasm but maintain a dispersed pattern, nuclear uniformity, and endocrine pattern chromatin. The final diagnosis was atypical carcinoid. Distinguishing atypical vs. typical carcinoid is usually not possible on cytology preparations.*

Well-Differentiated Neuroendocrine Tumor

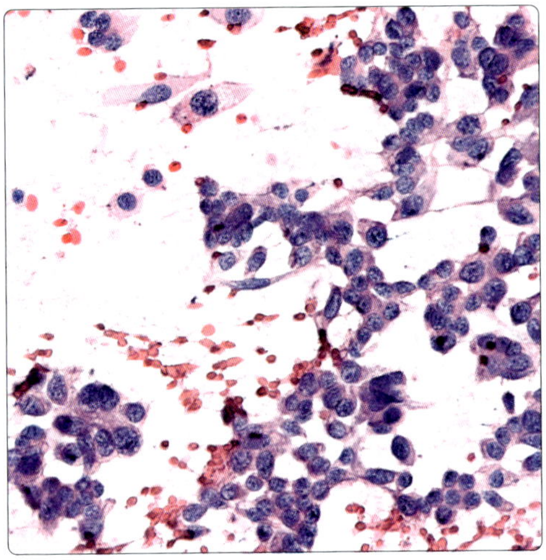

Atypical Carcinoid Tumor of Lung

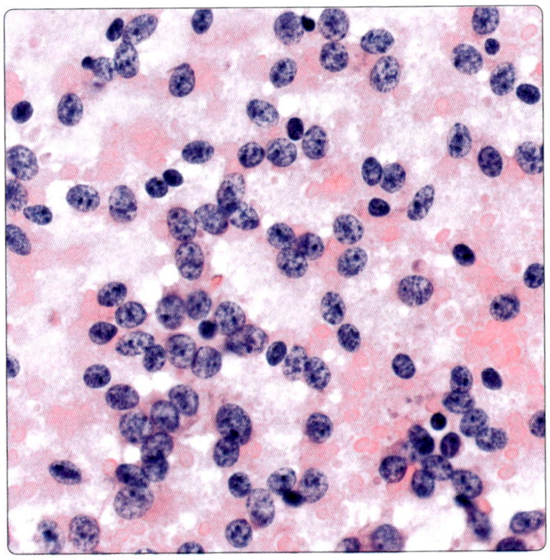

(Left) *Small cell carcinoma shows similar features regardless of site of origin. Dark cells with scant cytoplasm and nuclear molding are characteristic. Apoptosis and mitoses may be evident in larger clusters.* **(Right)** *This highly cellular scrape preparation shows small blue cells with extremely scant cytoplasm, malignant appearing nuclei, and apoptotic debris. The differential diagnosis includes carcinoma, melanoma, lymphoma, and sarcoma. The final diagnosis was sinonasal carcinoma.*

Small Cell Carcinoma

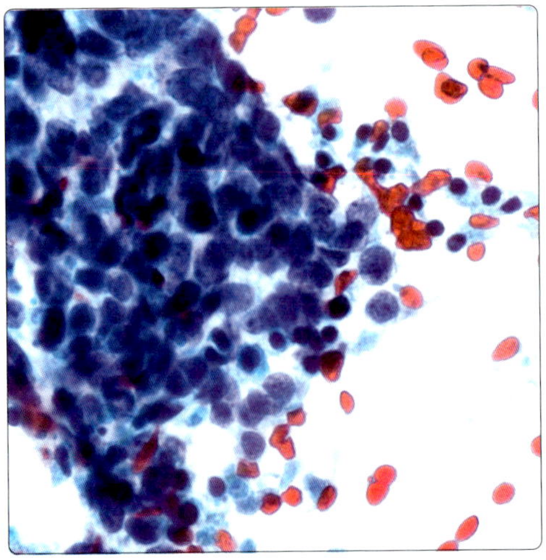

Sinonasal Undifferentiated Carcinoma

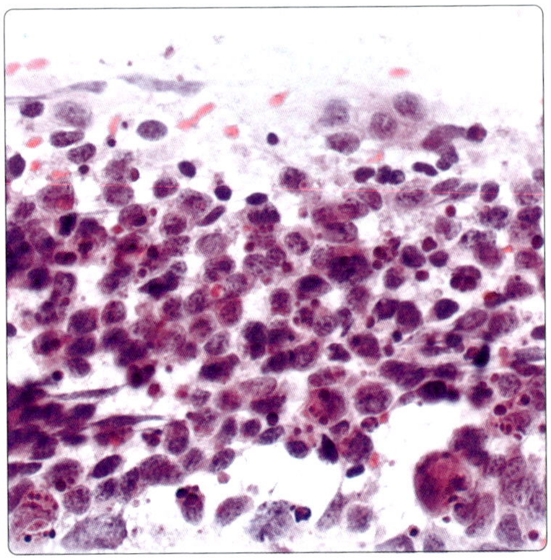

Ductal Carcinoma of Breast

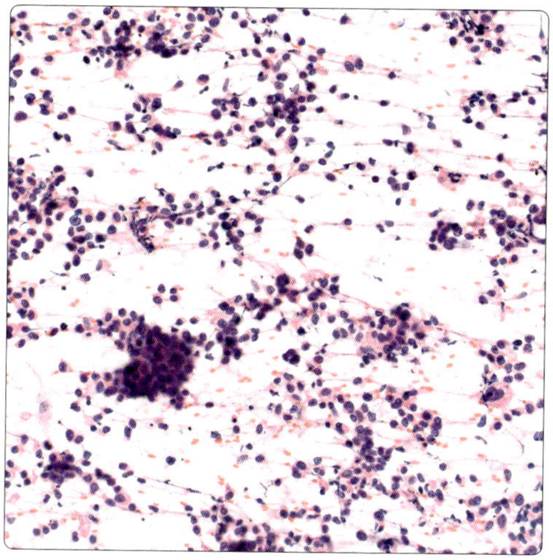

Ductal Carcinoma of Breast

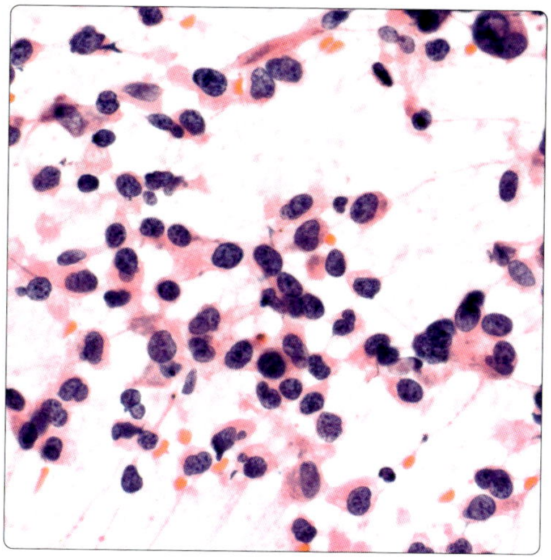

(Left) *Cytologic features of primary breast carcinoma include a high cellularity smear, uniform population of epithelial cells with nuclear atypia, and dyscohesion with single cells (which should be interpreted with caution in a vigorously scraped specimen). Requests for intraoperative primary diagnosis of breast carcinoma are, fortunately, rare.* **(Right)** *Scrape preparations from a breast mass show single atypical cells, some with eccentric nuclei, giving a plasmacytoid appearance, dark nuclei, and dense cytoplasm.*

Metastatic Ductal Carcinoma of Breast

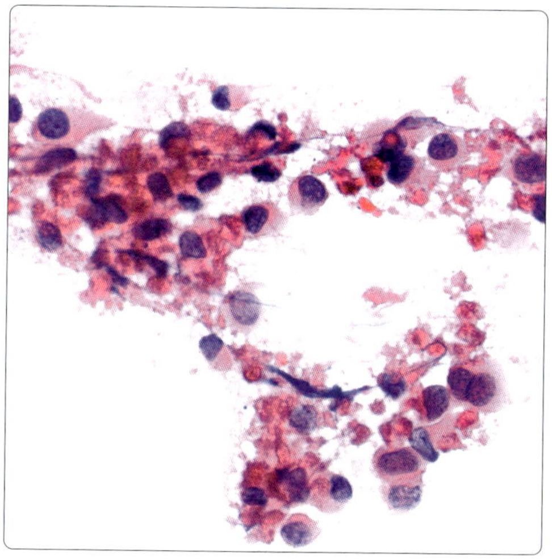

Thyroid: Nodular Hyperplasia (Goiter)

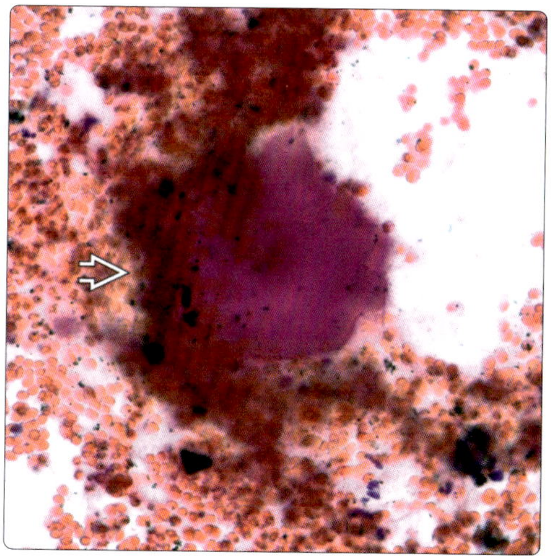

(Left) *Breast carcinoma usually retains its primary character in metastatic lesions. This is a case of metastatic breast carcinoma to the brain. The cells show large, eccentrically placed, dark nuclei and dense eosinophilic cytoplasm.* **(Right)** *Cytologic preparations are particularly helpful for thyroid lesions due to the excellent demonstration of colloid as well as nuclear features. Dense colloid appears as purple or pink amorphous material* ➲ *on H&E-stained scrape preparations.*

Thyroid: Nodular Hyperplasia (Goiter)

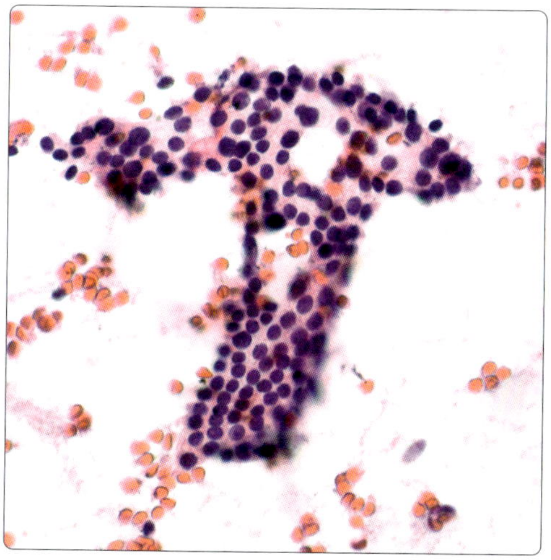

Thyroid: Follicular Lesion

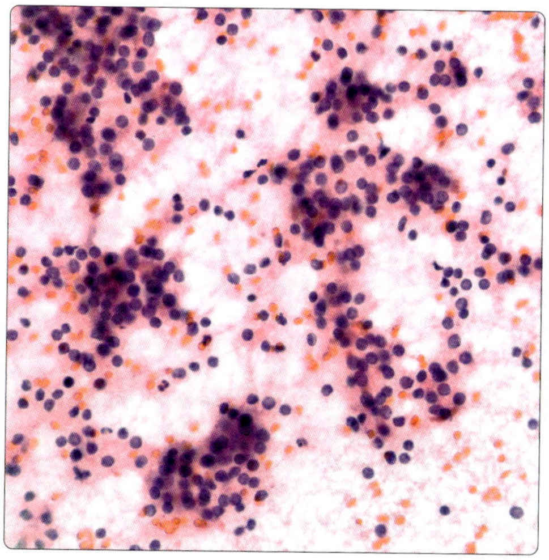

(Left) *In smears prepared from benign hyperplastic thyroid nodules, 2-dimensional sheets of follicular epithelial cells with uniform, small, round, dark nuclei are typical.* **(Right)** *Thyroid follicular lesions are characterized by high cellularity, a small/microfollicular pattern, and scant colloid. The cytologic differential diagnosis includes cellular hyperplastic nodule and follicular adenoma/carcinoma. The final diagnosis for this lesion was minimally invasive follicular carcinoma.*

(Left) *Hürthle cell neoplasms of the thyroid will show smear patterns similar to other follicular lesions and may also show prominent single cells. Hürthle cell features include a polygonal shape, central to slightly eccentric uniform large round nuclei, and often prominent nucleoli. Cytoplasm is dense and eosinophilic.* **(Right)** *Papillary thyroid carcinoma is characterized by sheets of epithelial cells with ovoid nuclei, grooves, and fine chromatin. Intranuclear inclusions are further confirmation.*

Thyroid: Hürthle Cell Neoplasm

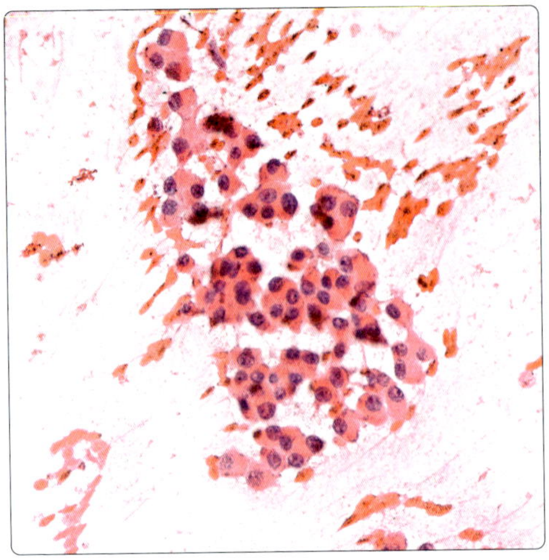

Papillary Thyroid Carcinoma

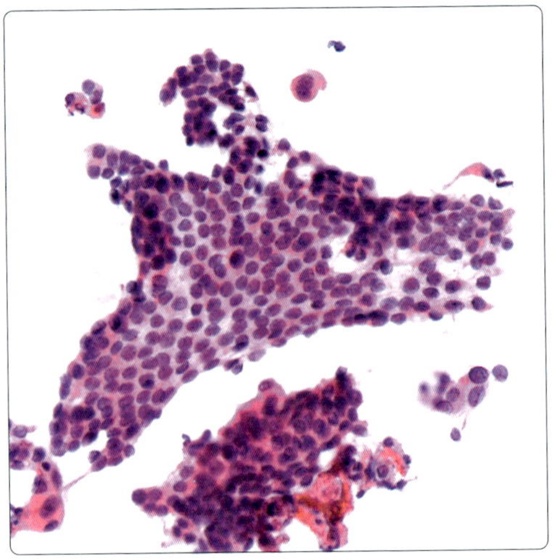

(Left) *Papillary thyroid carcinoma has characteristic nuclear features, including large ovoid nuclei with powdery fine chromatin, small distinct peripheral nucleoli, and intranuclear inclusions ⇨. Grooves are present but are often better demonstrated by focusing up and down.* **(Right)** *Metastases to the thyroid are rare. This is a case of lobular breast carcinoma metastasizing to a Hürthle cell adenoma as a "collision" tumor. Note the eccentric, hyperchromatic nuclei and cytoplasmic mucin vacuoles ➡.*

Papillary Thyroid Carcinoma

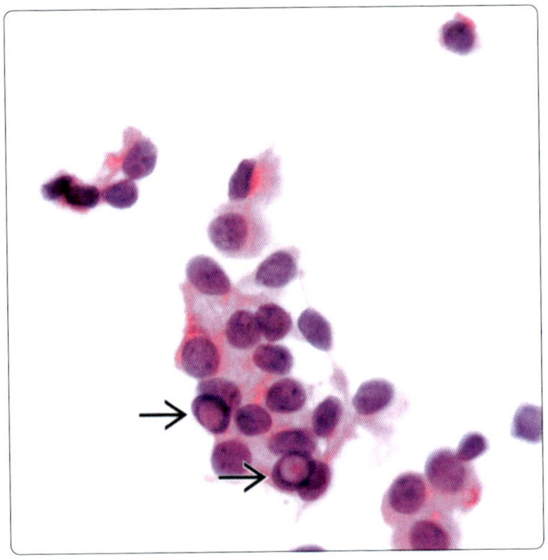

Thyroid: Metastatic Lobular Carcinoma of Breast

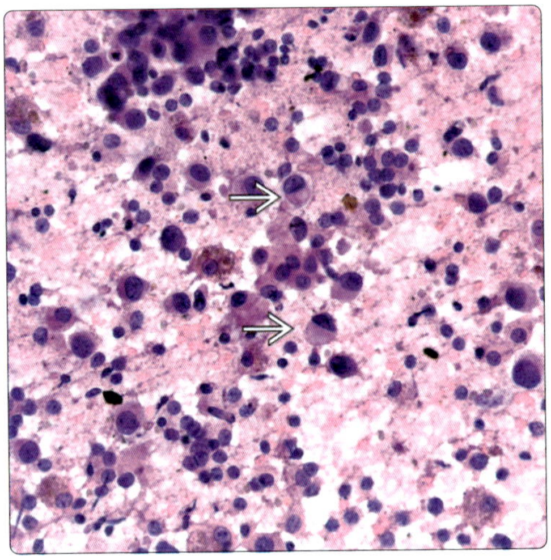

(Left) *These clustered epithelioid cells in thymoma demonstrate open chromatin, distinct nucleoli, and moderate anisonucleosis in a background of small mature lymphocytes.* **(Right)** *Epithelioid cells in thymoma may show growth as cohesive sheets with large nuclei, open chromatin, and prominent nucleoli. Nuclei are typically more uniform than in carcinomas, but in epithelioid-predominant lesions, the distinction may be difficult.*

Thymoma

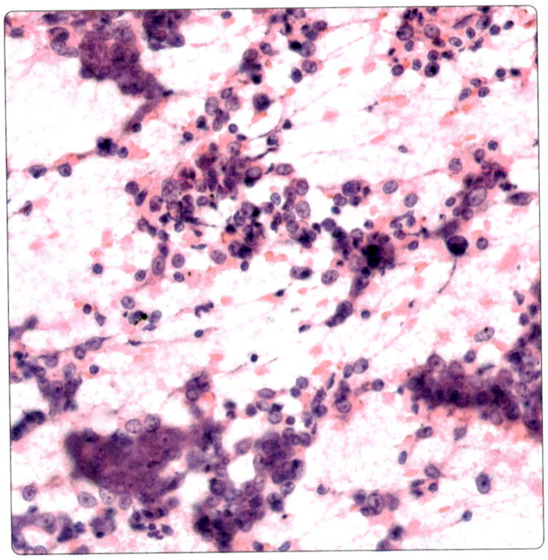

Thymoma

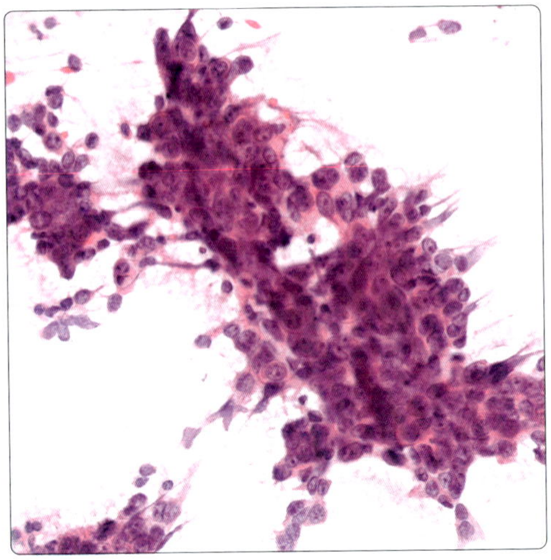

Malignant Melanoma

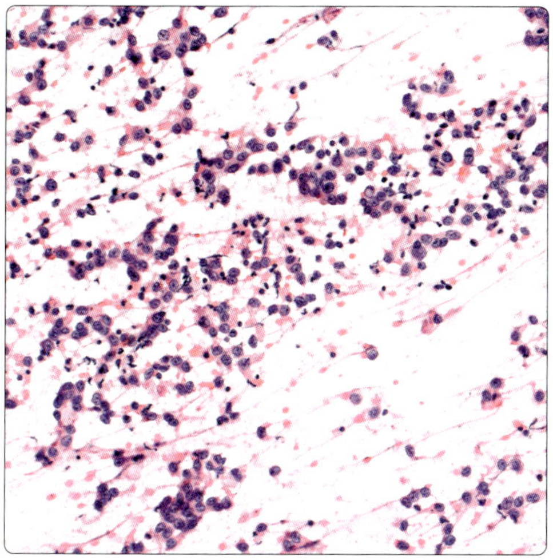

Malignant Melanoma

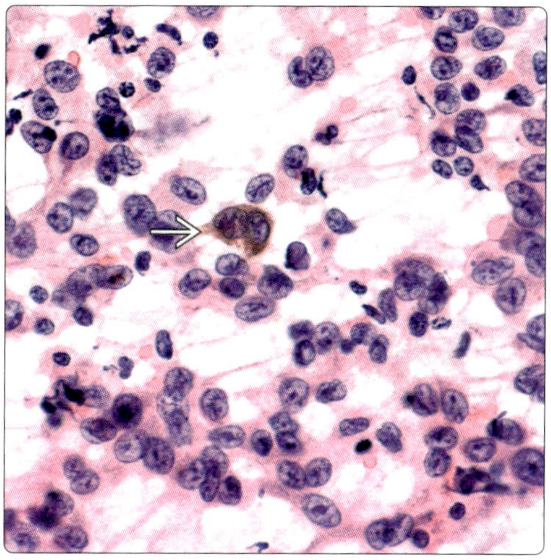

(Left) *Melanoma usually shows a dispersed cell pattern and plasmacytoid cells. A similar appearance can also be seen in breast carcinomas and neuroendocrine tumors. Features that would favor melanoma are melanin pigment, intranuclear cytoplasmic inclusions, multinucleated cells, and prominent red nucleoli.* **(Right)** *When present, pigmented cells with melanin granules ➡ help to establish a diagnosis of malignant melanoma. However, this feature is not always present, especially in metastatic melanoma.*

Malignant Melanoma

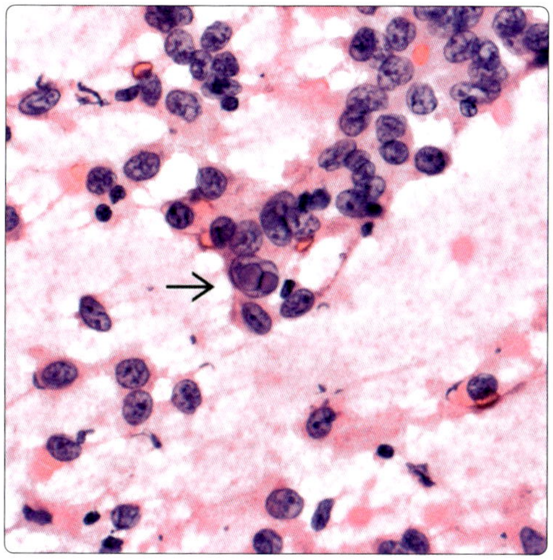

Undifferentiated Pleomorphic Sarcoma

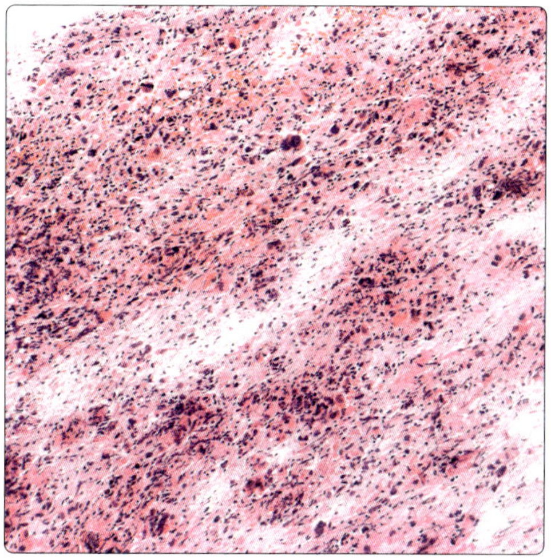

(Left) *Intranuclear cytoplasmic inclusions ➡ are a useful diagnostic feature of malignant melanoma. Although marked pleomorphism is often present, there is usually not a great degree of variation from cell to cell within a single tumor.* **(Right)** *This scrape preparation from a distal foot mass shows a cellular smear with clustered and individual cells, marked anisonucleosis, nuclear hyperchromasia, and variable cytoplasm. The dispersed nature of the cells favors sarcoma over carcinoma.*

Undifferentiated Pleomorphic Sarcoma

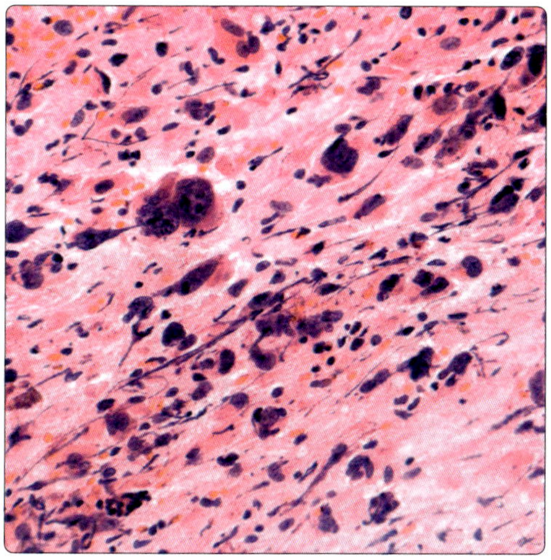

Osteosarcoma

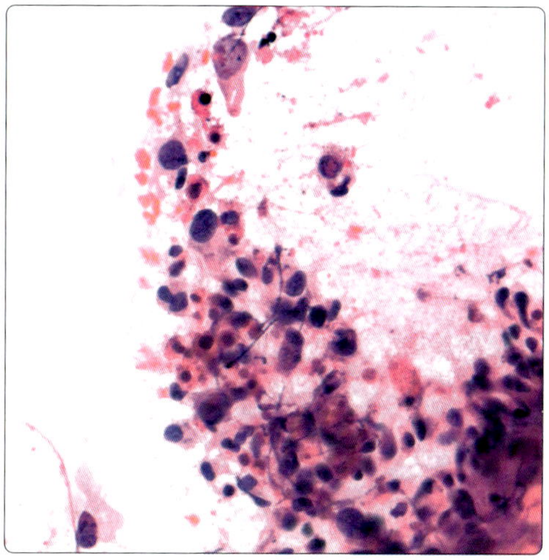

(Left) *Cytology preparations of high-grade sarcomas often show nonspecific but highly malignant features. Cells are often distributed both singly and in small clusters, and may show striking anaplasia. In this case, there is also a necrotic background.* **(Right)** *Intraoperative cytology may be particularly useful to document malignancy in cases of osteosarcoma when specimens are heavily calcified and frozen sections are not possible. This example shows single and clustered malignant cells, some apoptotic.*

Osteosarcoma

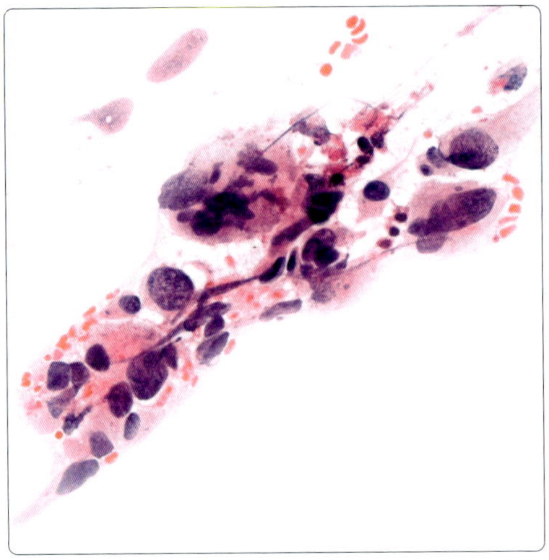

Osteosarcoma

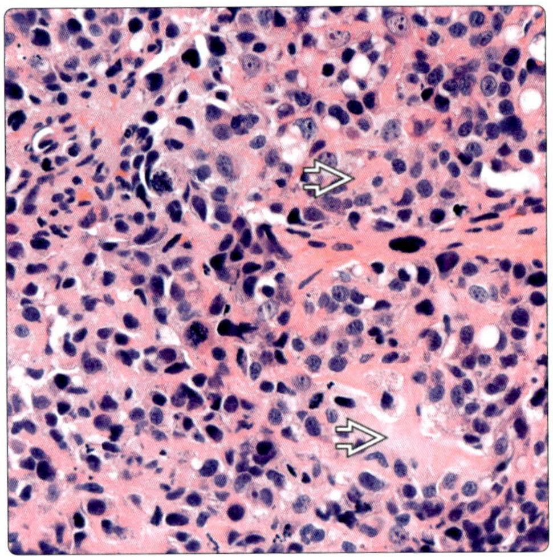

(Left) *Epithelioid cell morphology may be seen in osteosarcoma, which otherwise shows high-grade malignant cells with marked anisonucleosis and coarse chromatin. Osteoid may not be evident in touch preparations.* **(Right)** *Frozen section from an osteosarcoma shows epithelioid cells with anisonucleosis and coarse chromatin, the same cells that can be seen in a cytologic preparation. A frozen section has the advantage of also showing tissue architecture and intercellular osteoid deposition ➡.*

Solitary Fibrous Tumor/Hemangiopericytoma

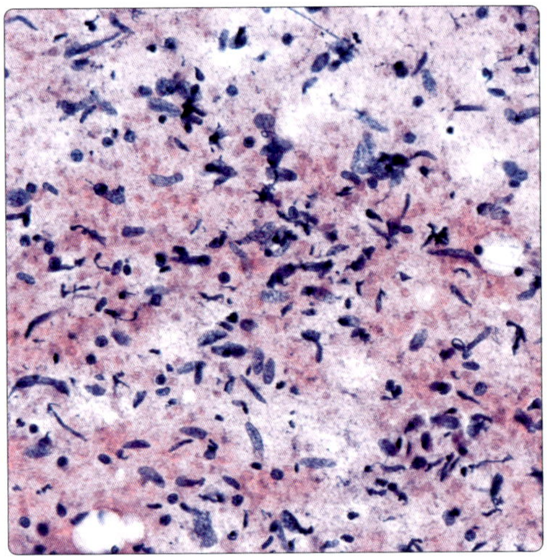

Solitary Fibrous Tumor/Hemangiopericytoma

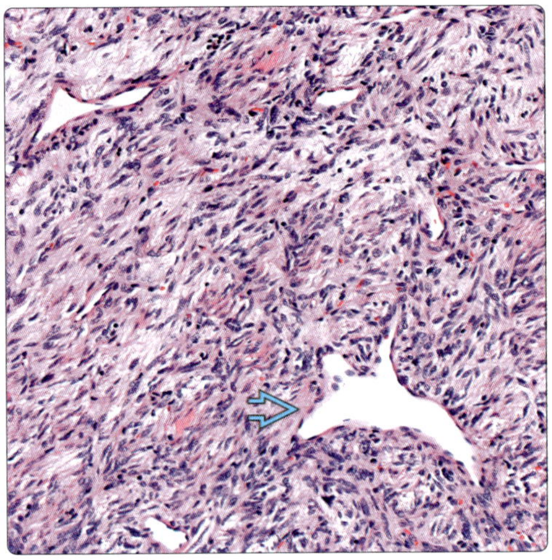

(Left) *Solitary fibrous tumor/hemangiopericytoma may yield preparations of low cellularity. A good scrape preparation shows large spindled nuclei in a hemorrhagic background.* **(Right)** *This permanent section of a solitary fibrous tumor/hemangiopericytoma shows spindle-shaped neoplastic cells that are also seen on cytologic scrape preparations. However, an advantage of a tissue section is that it also shows the staghorn vessels ➡ that are characteristic of this tumor.*

Solitary Fibrous Tumor/Hemangiopericytoma of Brain

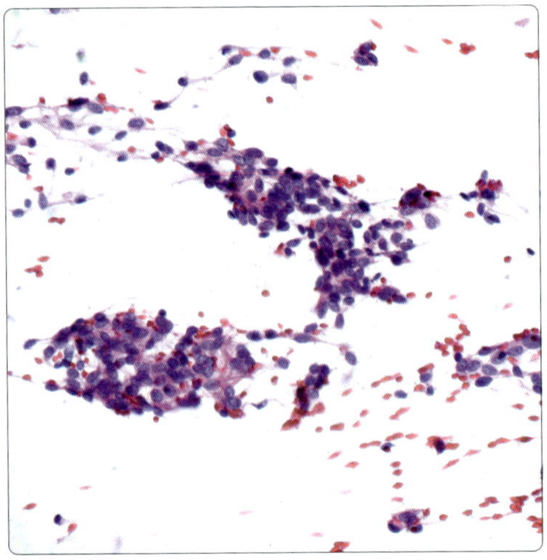

Gastrointestinal Stromal Tumor

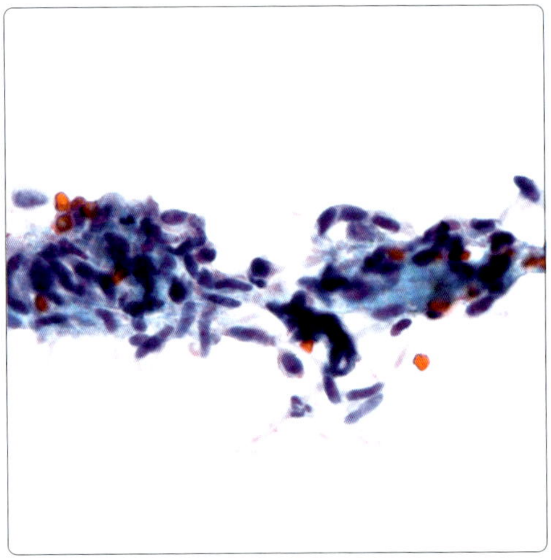

(Left) *This touch imprint shows groups of fusiform cells with relatively bland nuclei in a hemorrhagic background from a solitary fibrous tumor/hemangiopericytoma* **(Right)** *This gastrointestinal stromal tumor (GIST) shows a well-visualized cluster of uniform spindled cells. Cytologic preparations and fine-needle aspirations from spindle cell GISTs are often frustratingly paucicellular. Epithelioid GISTs may resemble carcinomas or lymphomas on cytologic preparations or frozen section.*

Schwannoma

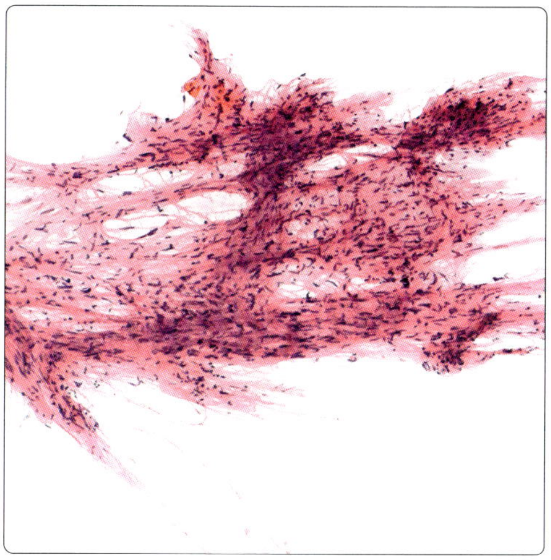

Schwannoma

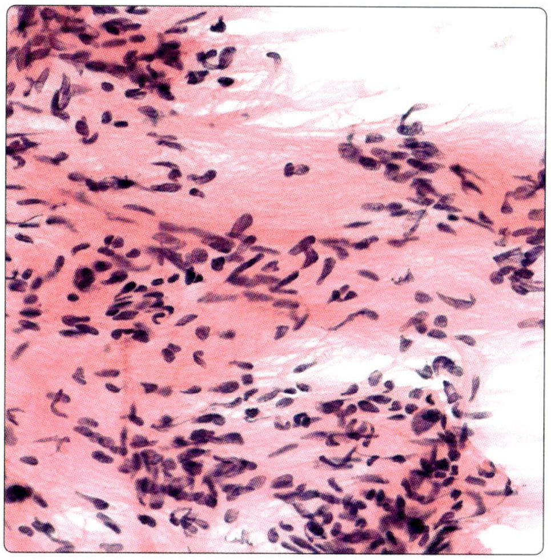

(Left) *Cytologic preparations from a schwannoma may require vigorous scraping. This example shows a large cluster of spindled cells in fibrillary stroma. There is only mild variability in nuclear size and chromatin pattern.* **(Right)** *Some schwannomas have a nondescript benign spindle cell appearance. This case shows more specific palisading of bland nuclei, some wavy, in a fibrillary background.*

Desmoplastic Small Round Cell Tumor

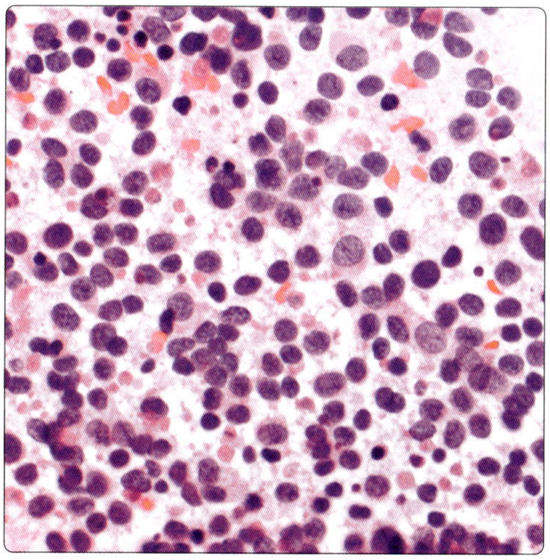

Desmoplastic Small Round Cell Tumor

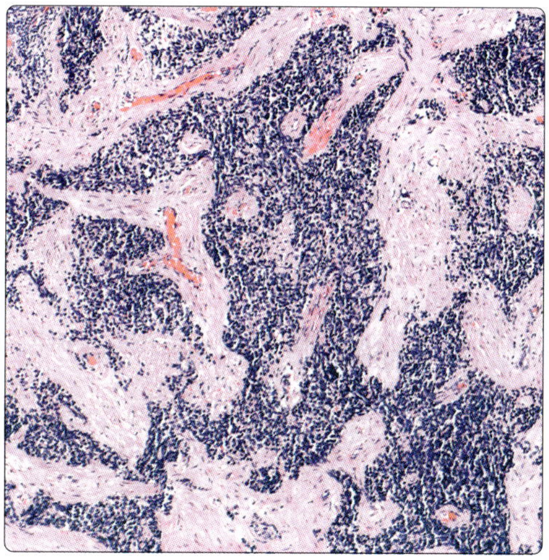

(Left) *Cytology preparations of desmoplastic small round cell tumors will show a dispersed pattern of malignant cells with dark nuclei and scant cytoplasm. The differential diagnosis includes Wilms tumor, Ewing family tumors, rhabdomyosarcoma, high-grade neuroendocrine carcinoma, and lymphoma. The clinical scenario may determine tissue triage based on cytologic findings.* **(Right)** *A frozen section shows small blue cells in desmoplastic stroma characteristic of desmoplastic small round cell tumor.*

Angiomatoid Malignant Fibrous Histiocytoma

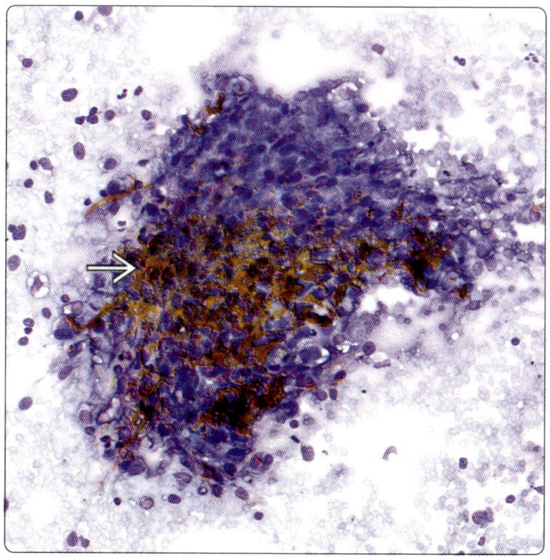

Angiomatoid Malignant Fibrous Histiocytoma

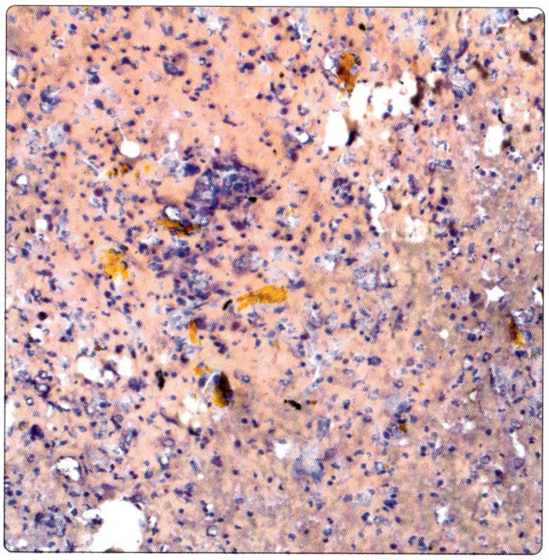

(Left) *This touch preparation of an axillary mass with a hemorrhagic center shows clusters of lesional cells with hematin pigment ➔. A diagnosis of angiomatoid fibrous histiocytoma was rendered on the basis of intraoperative gross and cytologic evaluation and confirmed on permanent sections.* **(Right)** *This angiomatoid malignant fibrous histiocytoma shows cell clusters comprised of spindled and epithelioid cells with moderate pleomorphism in a background of blood and hematoidin pigment.*

(Left) *This chordoma shows nested and solitary epithelioid cells with pale pink cytoplasm and low nuclear:cytoplasmic ratios in a myxoid background.* **(Right)** *A characteristic feature of chordoma are frequent cells with abundant bubbly cytoplasm ("physaliferous" cells).*

Chordoma

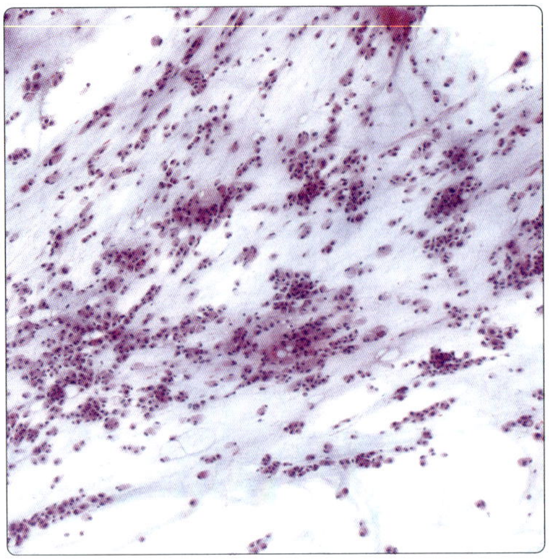

Chordoma

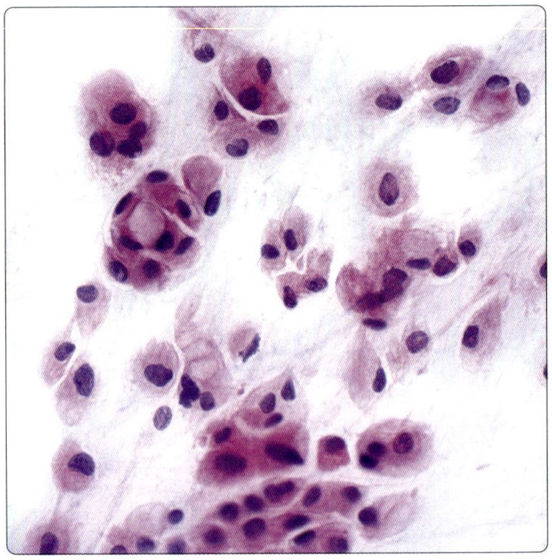

(Left) *Characteristic features of Langerhans cell histiocytosis are epithelioid/histiocytoid cells with "coffee bean" nuclei that have bland chromatin and prominent grooves. There are admixed inflammatory cells, including some eosinophils.* **(Right)** *This frozen section of Langerhans cell histiocytosis shows a predominant population of lesional cells with abundant cytoplasm and bland nuclei intermingled with smaller inflammatory cells.*

Langerhans Cell Histiocytosis

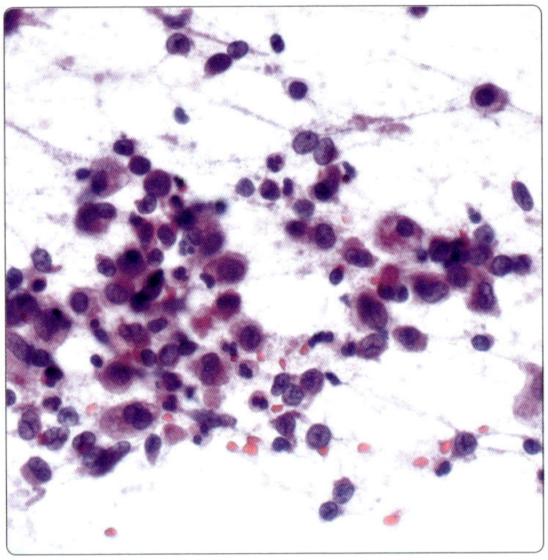

Langerhans Cell Histiocytosis

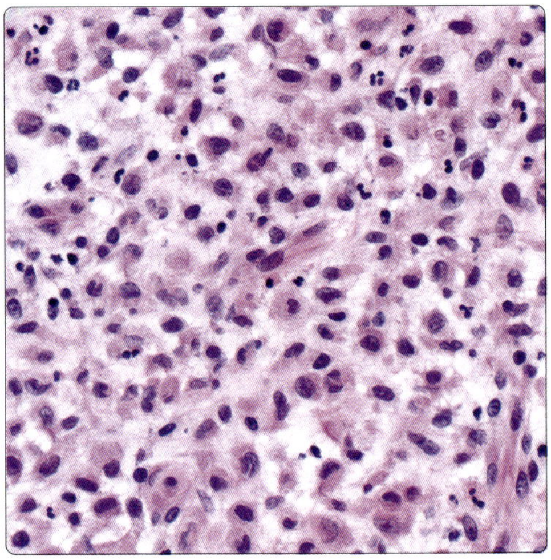

(Left) *Adult granulosa cell tumor cytologic preparations are characterized by highly uniform cells with round to ovoid nuclei, open chromatin, and prominent nuclear grooves. Often, the nuclei look more bland on cytologic preparations than on frozen section, which is a clue to the diagnosis.* **(Right)** *Renal cell carcinoma may show deceptively bland features. This touch prep of a bone metastasis shows a low nuclear:cytoplasmic ratio, pale cytoplasm, prominent nucleoli, and a bloody background (common).*

Adult Granulosa Cell Tumor of Ovary

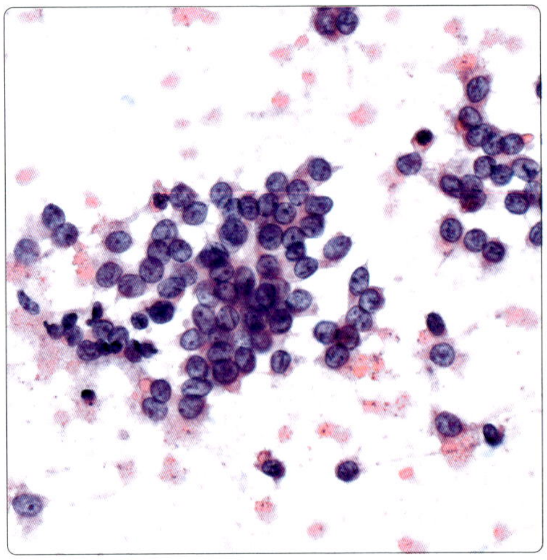

Renal Cell Carcinoma

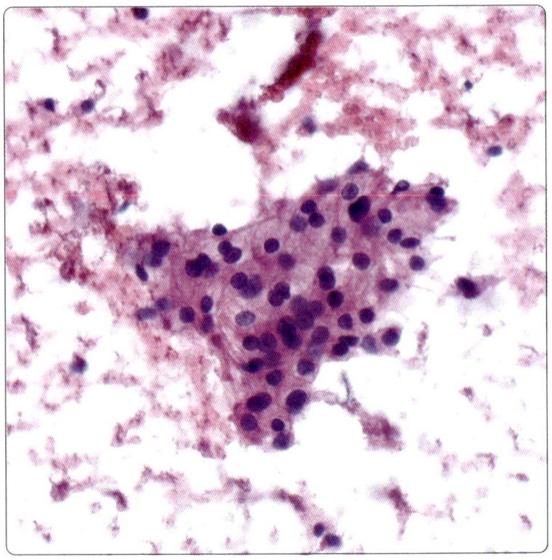

Lymph Node: Benign Reactive Changes

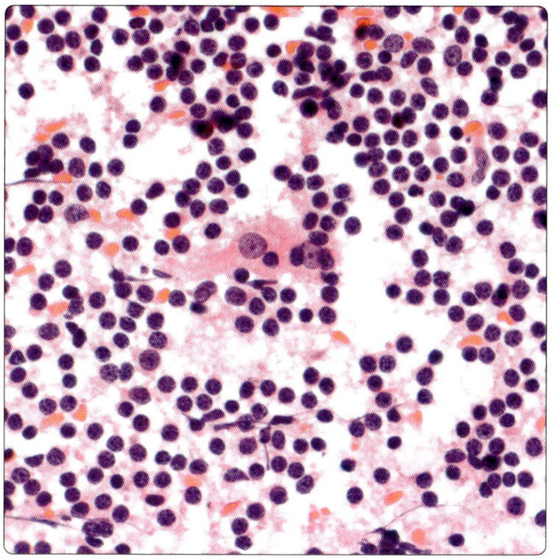

Lymph Node: Granuloma

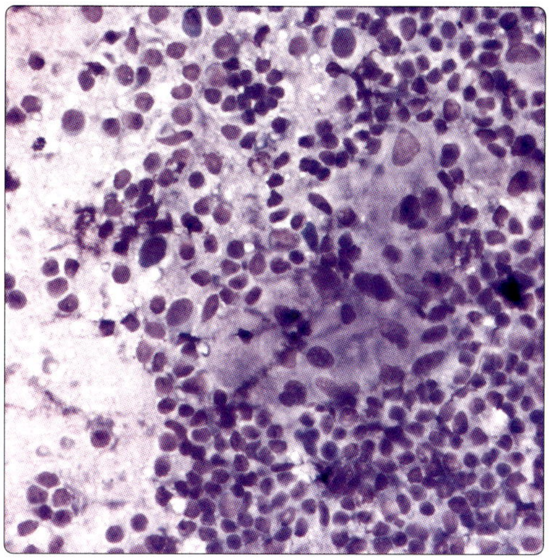

(Left) *This touch prep shows a population of small mature lymphocytes with admixed histiocytes in a reactive lymph node. Occasionally, the histiocytes may have ingested debris (tingible body macrophages). Plasma cells and neutrophils may be in evidence in some cases. A polymorphous background favors benignity but may be seen in some neoplasms.* **(Right)** *This air-dried, Romanowsky-stained slide from a lymph node shows nonnecrotic epithelioid granulomata in a background of small mature lymphocytes.*

Hodgkin Lymphoma

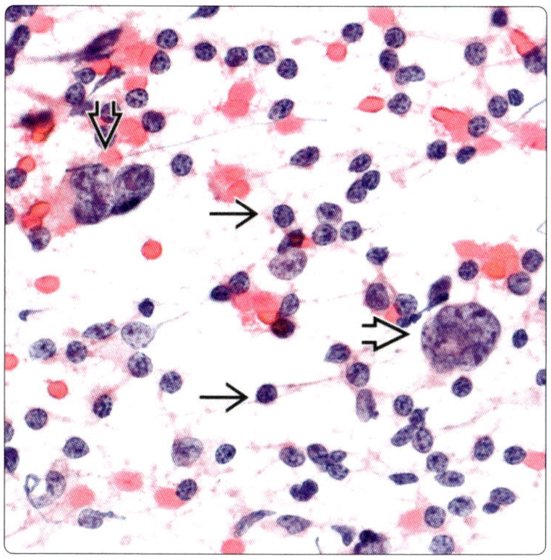

Hodgkin Lymphoma

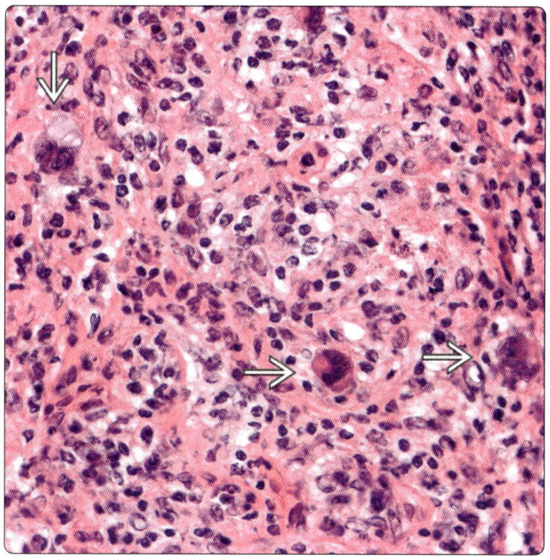

(Left) *Hodgkin lymphoma characteristically demonstrates a biphasic population of large, multinucleate/polylobate cells ⇨ in a background of small mature lymphocytes →. The background may be polymorphous (eosinophils, neutrophils, plasma cells), resembling a reactive process. In addition, neoplastic cells may be sparse, making diagnosis difficult in some cases.* **(Right)** *Hodgkin cells ➡ in a background of fibrosis and nonneoplastic lymphocytes are seen in this frozen section slide.*

Burkitt Lymphoma

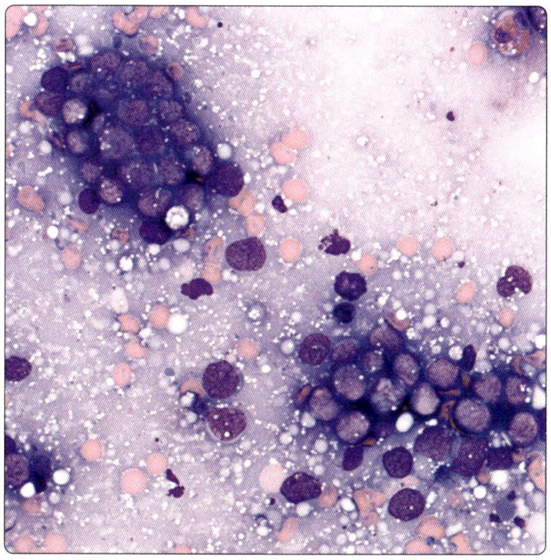

Diffuse Large B-Cell Lymphoma

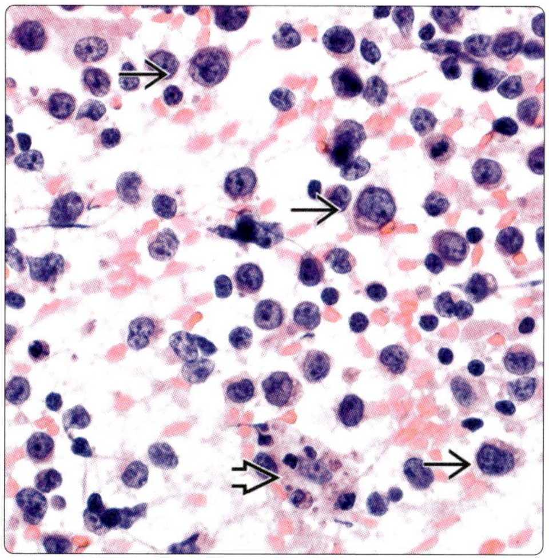

(Left) *On air-dried smears, Burkitt lymphomas show a monomorphic population of large, immature lymphoid cells, some with cytoplasmic vacuoles. Tingible body macrophages may be evident in the background.* **(Right)** *Touch imprints of large cell lymphomas will usually show a population of large atypical lymphoid cells →, some with clumped chromatin, in a background of small mature lymphocytes and tingible body macrophages ⇨. The latter may be seen both in reactive and high-grade neoplastic processes.*

(**Left**) *Lymphomas may be primarily sited in the brain. This lesion shows a dispersed smear pattern with atypical lymphoid cells, some having plasmacytoid features.* (**Right**) *Cytology preparations are highly useful and accurate for quick evaluation of pituitary adenoma. The specimens are often small and fragmented, making frozen section difficult. Plasmacytoid cells with round, enlarged nuclei, salt and pepper chromatin, and monomorphic cytoplasm are characteristic.*

Plasmablastic Lymphoma

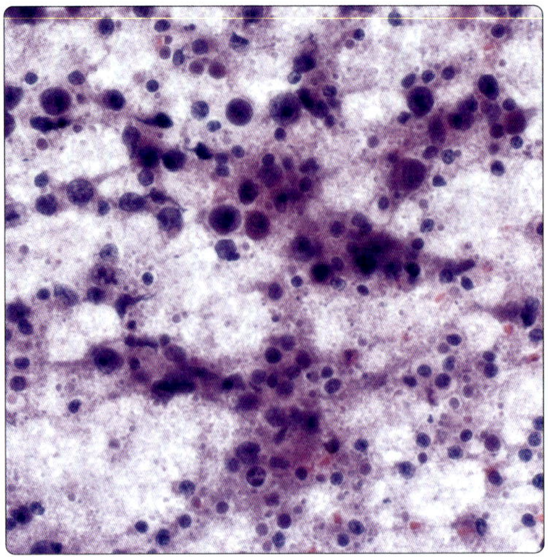

Pituitary Adenoma

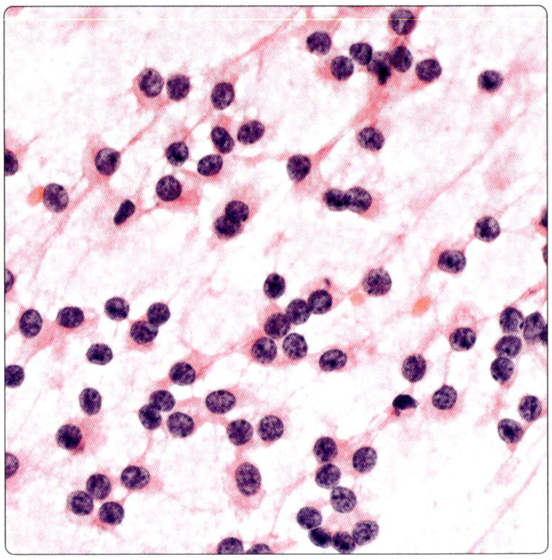

(**Left**) *This cellular specimen from a meningioma shows a monotonous population of epithelioid cells with bland nuclei, moderate nuclear:cytoplasmic ratios, and fibrillar processes that should not be mistaken as evidence of glial differentiation.* (**Right**) *Both the cellularity and cytologic appearance of meningioma will vary with the histologic type. The whorled appearance of cells in this meningothelial pattern is typical* ➪ *and intranuclear inclusions may be present.*

Meningioma

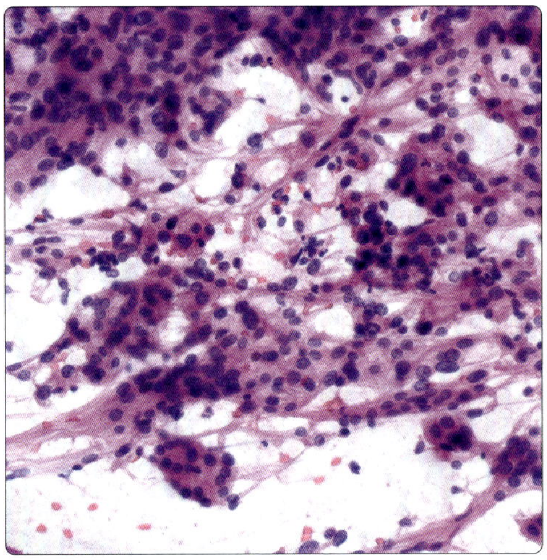

Meningioma

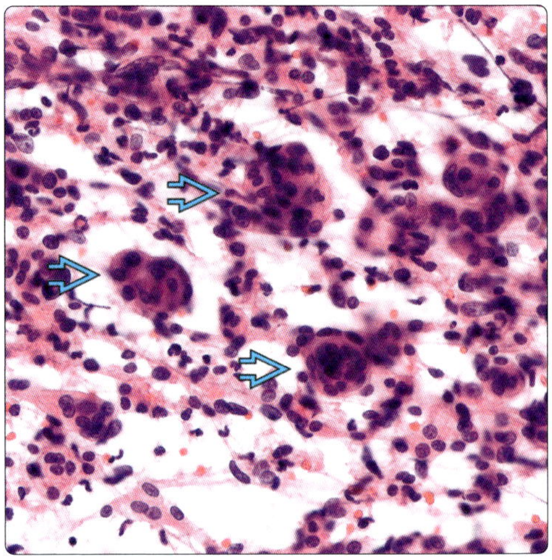

(**Left**) *Low-grade gliomas will present as hypercellular lesions with large, dark, but still somewhat uniform nuclei in a fibrillary background.* (**Right**) *Pilocytic astrocytoma shows mildly pleomorphic cells in a gliofibrillary background with prominent Rosenthal fibers.*

Oligodendroglioma

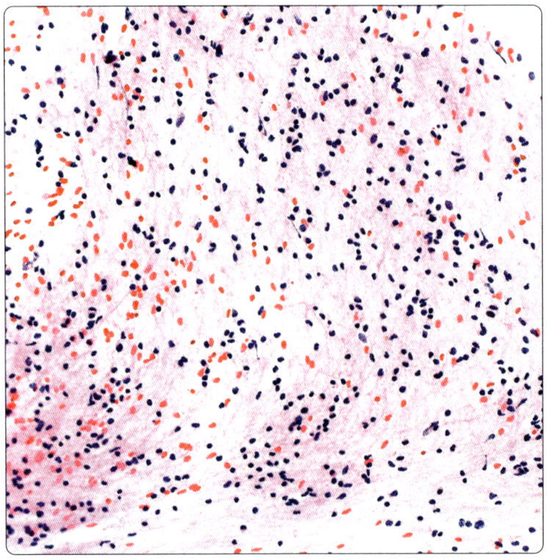

Pilocytic Astrocytoma

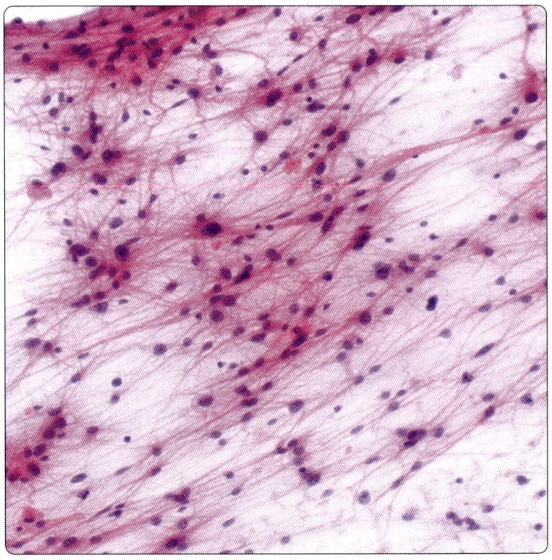

Glioblastoma Multiforme

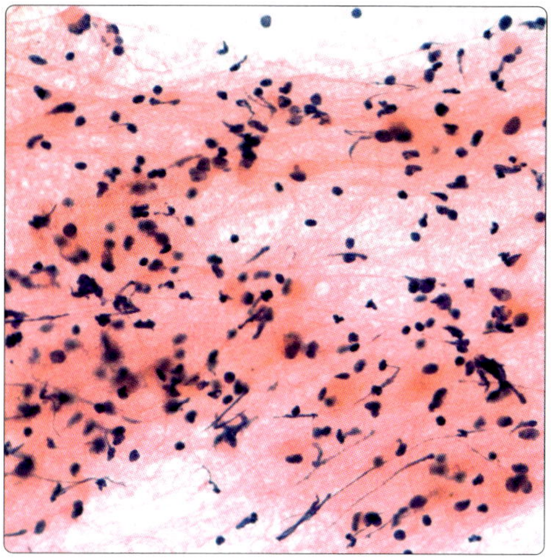

Glioblastoma Multiforme

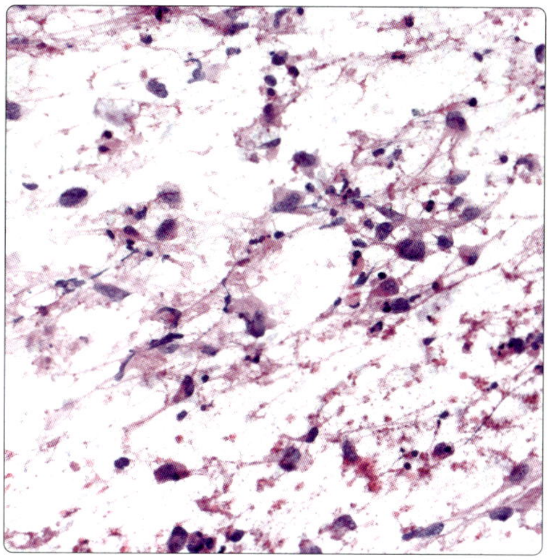

(Left) *High-grade gliomas are typically cellular with more atypical cells in a fibrillary background, often with some perivascular clustering. In glioblastoma, necrosis can be seen in some cytologic preparations.* **(Right)** *Central nervous system masses are often examined by squash preparations, as in this case. This glioblastoma multiforme shows marked nuclear pleomorphism and a necrotic background.*

Ependymoma

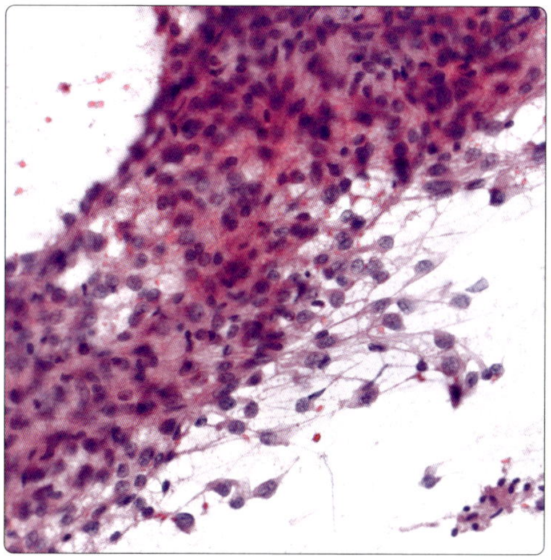

Craniopharyngioma

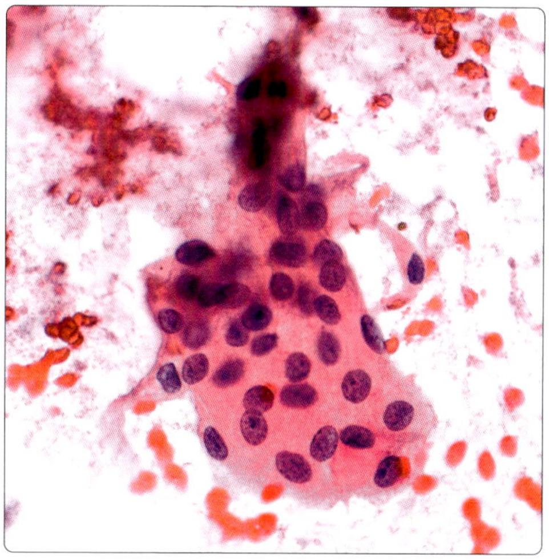

(Left) *This rather thick preparation from an ependymoma shows round to ovoid tumor cells with fibrillar processes. Rosettes may sometimes be observed, but were not seen in this case.* **(Right)** *Cells from craniopharyngioma usually have a squamoid appearance and can be keratinized. Necrotic debris may be seen in the background.*

Medulloblastoma

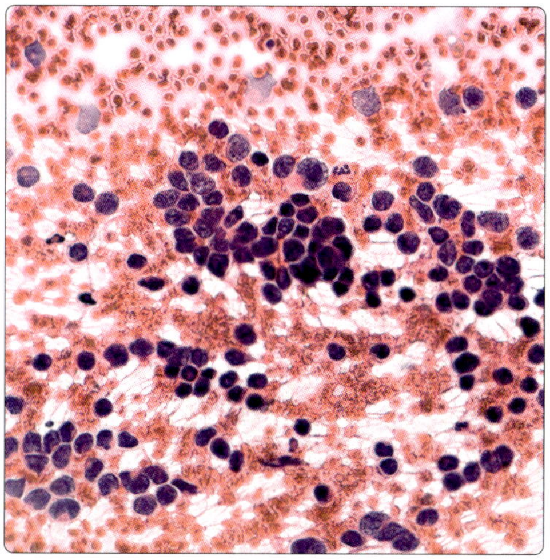

Brain Infarction

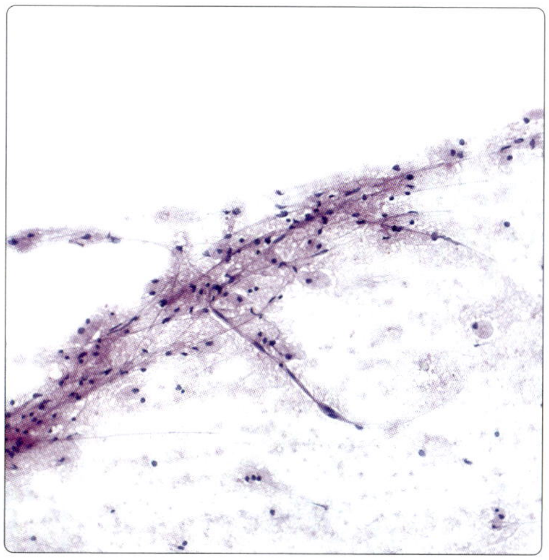

(Left) *Medulloblastoma will often be suspected preoperatively based on age and location. Cytologically, these tumors are similar to other small round blue cell tumors with dispersed growth pattern, scant cytoplasm, and dark nuclei.* **(Right)** *Not all intraoperative consultations are for neoplasms. Foam cells in a brain touch preparation should prompt consideration of nonneoplastic disease, such as in this case of infarction.*

INTRODUCTION

Purpose

- In order to cut thin sections < thickness of 1 cell for microscopic evaluation, tissues must be hardened
- Freezing tissue is rapid method that can be used to harden tissue sufficiently to allow thin sectioning
- A physical limitation to performing intraoperative consultations quickly is time required for tissue to freeze
  - Priority should be given to gross evaluation of specimen and selection of tissue for freezing
  - The sooner tissue starts freezing, the more quickly slides can be available for diagnosis
  - Less urgent tasks can be performed while tissue is freezing (e.g., writing detailed gross description or labeling slides)

METHOD

Selection of Tissue

- Good gross examination is required in order to select tissue most likely to yield most helpful diagnosis
- Orientation should be maintained when important
  - Skin sections should be perpendicular to epidermal surface
  - Colon sections should be perpendicular to mucosal surface
- Section should be ≤ 8 mm x 8 mm x 1-2 mm (thick) in size to freeze well
  - If more tissue needs to be frozen, section should be divided into multiple blocks
- If moist, tissue should be gently blotted dry
  - Minimizes freezing artifact
  - Do not use gauze or place tissue on gauze as this can introduce artifactual holes in tissue
- **Freezing permanently changes tissue**
  - Morphologic appearance of tissue is not same as tissue that has never been frozen
    - As water freezes, ice crystals form in tissue
    - Larger crystals form with time; tissue should be frozen as quickly as possible to minimize crystal size
    - Ice crystals disrupt cellular structures and these changes are not completely reversed with thawing
    - Chromatin pattern of nuclei often is indistinct
    - Nuclei can appear hyperchromatic compared to tissue that has not been frozen
  - Antigens can be altered by freezing, and this can change immunoreactivity patterns
    - Previously frozen tissue should be avoided for additional studies
    - If used, results should be interpreted with caution
  - Histochemical stains can be altered on previously frozen tissue
  - Small primary tumors should never be completely frozen for these reasons

Type of Tissue

- Any tissue that can be cut with scalpel can be cut by microtome for frozen section
- Bone and other calcified lesions cannot be cut
  - Scrape preparations from bone may be used to evaluate marrow margins on bones
  - Heavily calcified lesions are generally benign and need not be evaluated by frozen section intraoperatively
- Adipose tissue requires colder temperatures and is difficult to cut
  - If not important for diagnosis, fatty tissue should be dissected away from important areas of specimen
    - For example, lymph nodes should be dissected away from surrounding adipose tissue
- Tissue fixed in formalin does not adhere well to slides
  - If only immersed in formalin for short time and of sufficient size, it may be possible to cut a central section that has not yet been exposed to formalin
  - If it is necessary to examine fixed tissue, special coated slides must be used
- Tissue with suspected or known infectious disease should not be frozen unless absolutely necessary for patient management
  - High-risk infectious diseases for pathology personnel are HIV, hepatitis B, hepatitis C, and tuberculosis
  - Cytologic preparations should be used when possible

Cryostat

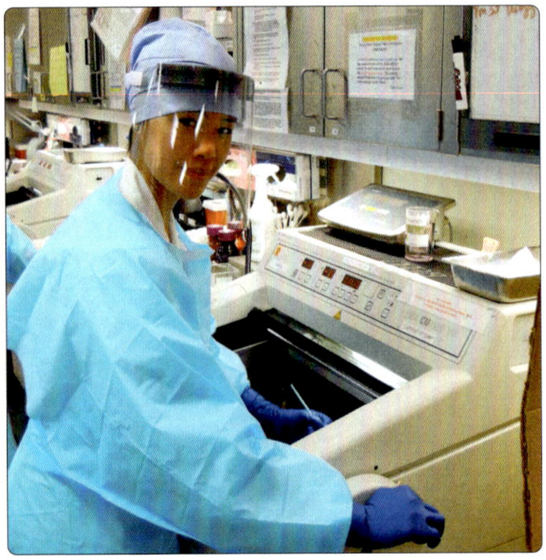

Frozen Section

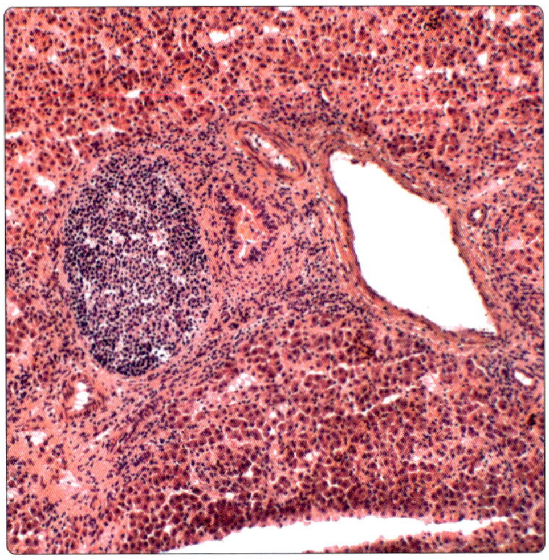

(Left) *Freezing is a rapid method to harden tissue in order to cut sections only a few microns thick that can be used for intraoperative pathologic diagnosis. (Courtesy V. Chan, BS.)* **(Right)** *Well selected, prepared, sectioned, and stained frozen sections can closely approximate the quality of a permanent section. However, a major limitation is that only a small amount of tissue can be frozen.*

- If frozen section is prepared, cryostat should be marked as contaminated and decontaminated after use

Terminology

- Chuck: Metal platform used for holding embedding medium and tissue for sectioning
- Base: Embedding medium placed and frozen on chuck to cushion and protect tissue
- Block: Tissue frozen on base and covered by additional embedding medium

Preparation of Block

- There are multiple methods of preparing a base of embedding medium according to particular cryostat and equipment used
  - Embedding medium is a liquid mixture that solidifies when frozen at appropriate temperature for cutting sections
    - Density is similar to tissue when frozen
    - Container must be kept capped when not in use
      - Alcohol can evaporate and adversely alter quality of compound
  - If specimen is very small, base can be precut and faced on cryostat to minimize amount of tissue lost to level block
- Tissue can be transferred to frozen base by touching base to tissue
- Orientation can be important for margin sections
  - Perpendicular margin sections should be placed such that inked margin is clearly visible at 1 edge
  - Orientation of en face margins should be recorded
    - If true margin is superficial aspect of tissue, 1st frozen section slide is true margin
    - Slides are labeled to indicate 1st and subsequent deeper levels
    - If true margin is embedded face down, 1st frozen section is not true margin
    - If positive, deeper levels can be obtained that are closer to true margin
- Multiple fragments should be grouped closely but not overlap
- Tissue should not extend beyond edge of chuck
- Thin sections can be rolled and embedded in cross section

Freezing Tissue

- Embedding medium is applied to completely cover tissue
  - Should not extend beyond chuck
    - If medium extends to back or stem of chuck, it must be removed or it will interfere in attaching chuck to cryostat
  - Can be kept cool in refrigerator to speed freezing process
  - Should form rim around tissue to aid in holding tissue and tethering section to chuck when cutting
- Chuck with covered tissue block is placed in cryostat to freeze
  - Some cryostats have rapid freezing cycles
  - Alternative methods use bath of isopentane
- Different types of tissues cut optimally at different temperatures
  - Majority of tissue: -10°C to -20°C
  - Very soft tissue (brain, spleen, adrenal gland, lymph node): -7°C to -10°C
  - Adipose tissue: -20°C to -40°C

Methods to Accelerate Freezing

- Heat extractor
  - Metal block that may be attached to handle that is kept cold in cryostat
  - After embedding medium is slightly cooled (and appears opaque), extractor can be placed on top of block
    - Do not use immediately as it will compress and distort tissue
    - Use of heat extractor creates flat surface
  - If extractor sticks to block, stem of chuck can be gently knocked against freezing plate
    - If block detaches from chuck, it can be reattached to new chuck with embedding medium
    - Small amount of oil on extractor can prevent sticking
- Cooling plate
  - Some cryostats have quick freeze option that cools plate
  - After embedding medium is opaque, block is placed face down on plate
- Rapid freezing aerosol spray
  - Sprays are available to cool face of block quickly
  - Not recommended due to increased risk of inhalation of infectious disease organisms or toxic fumes
    - Exposure to *Mycobacterium tuberculosis* is reported after use of this type of spray
  - If used, spray should be within cryostat with lid closed as much as possible to contain spray
    - Cryostat should be free of shavings that will contribute to contamination
  - Face masks should be worn

Sectioning on Cryostat

- Chuck is positioned in microtome such that blade 1st cuts most solid area of tissue
  - Solid areas of tissue should be positioned closest to blade
    - Adipose tissue should not be 1st portion of tissue cut
  - Epidermal or mucosal surfaces should be perpendicular to blade
  - Most important part of tissue should not be 1st area cut
    - Leading edge of section is area of tissue most likely to show artifacts of compression or folding
- Blade must be sharp and without nicks in order to create complete thin sections
  - Dull or nicked blades result in sections with chatter artifact &/or holes
- Block is trimmed or faced until complete section is obtained
  - Bases can be pre-faced prior to adding specimen to minimize tissue loss when facing block
  - Rough cut sections can be removed from blade with large brush or swab
    - Brush should always go in same direction as blade
    - If blade is brushed across or against cutting surface, this can cause blade to be nicked or dulled
  - Never remove by hand due to risk of severe laceration from blade
- Some cryostats use antiroll plate to hold cut tissue section flat against plate

- Tissue section is left slightly attached to block to prevent curling
- As alternative to antiroll plate, brush can be used
  - Tissue section is guided onto plate with brush at leading edge of tissue section
  - Section is left slightly attached to block to prevent curling
  - Brushes are kept cold within cryostat
- Glass slide is gently applied to surface of tissue section
  - Slides should be labeled with case number and a designation for frozen section
  - Label must be able to withstand solutions used for staining
- Frozen tissue rapidly melts onto room temperature slide

Fixation

- As soon as slides are prepared, they must be immediately placed in methanol
  - Methanol with slide holder should be within easy reach of cryostat
- Any delay results in significant air-drying artifact, which impedes interpretation

Disposition of Frozen Tissue

- Remaining tissue should be fixed in formalin and submitted for permanent section
  - If multiple chucks are present in cryostat, each one can be identified by labeling surface with a felt tip marker
- Frozen tissue block can be briefly immersed in formalin to cause slight melting and then removed with hand or ruler
  - Frozen tissue should not be removed using blade
  - Chuck is small, and tissue block is hard; force required to sever block can result in loss of control of blade and injury to nondominant hand
- Small frozen section remnants are wrapped in lens paper before being placed in labeled cassette
  - Excess embedding medium should be trimmed away
- Comparison of frozen section to permanent section is important quality assurance parameter
  - If there is difference in interpretation, surgeon must be notified and reason for discrepancy explained in pathology report
- If frozen tissue is required for ancillary studies, and additional tissue is not available for freezing, frozen section remnant can be retained for this purpose

Levels

- If very little tissue is present, initial levels should be shallow to ensure some tissue is captured before all tissue is sectioned
  - Sequential levels can be taken for staining rather than going deep into section
- If large section is present, or if multiple fragments are present, frozen section should be representative cross section of all tissue
  - After cutting and fixing, check to see that all tissue is represented on slide
    - If not, deeper levels should be taken
  - Important diagnostic information can be lost if some tissue is not present
- Deep levels can be helpful when examining margins to look for small areas of tumor near margin
  - Requires cutting deep into section and discarding some of intervening tissue
  - Deep levels should not be used for small biopsies of diagnostic tissue if tissue is limited
- At least 2 levels should be obtained for each frozen section

TROUBLESHOOTING

Section Shows Shatter (or Chatter) Artifact

- Appearance similar to venetian blind
- Block too cold
  - Block can be slightly warmed with thumb or palm
  - Section must be cut immediately because block will rapidly cool
    - A few sections may need to be discarded to get to level with optimum temperature for sectioning
  - Care must be taken to prevent cutting hand on blade
    - Move block as far from blade as possible
    - Lock handwheel to prevent block from moving
- Cryostat blade dull, nicked, or missing
  - Replace with new blade
- Tissue too hard
  - Fragments of bone or other calcified tissue may be too hard to section
  - Tissue that cannot be cut easily with scalpel should not be selected for frozen section
    - If possible, soft tissue should be separated away from hard tissue
- Section is not cut in continuous motion
  - Handwheel should be turned with smooth motion
  - Hesitation or stopping before completing section can result in tears

Sections Crumple Into Mass on Blade

- Block too warm
  - Leave block in cryostat longer
    - After initial sections, center of block may not be sufficiently cold
  - Use heat extractor or other mechanism to cool block rapidly
- Blade is at wrong angle
  - Angle should be adjusted to 30°
- Edge of section may not be transferring well to plate
  - Use brush to catch leading edge of section and guide onto plate
  - If there is excessive embedding medium, cut down to V shape around tissue
    - Tip of V is easier to catch with brush
  - If using plate to hold sections, check adjustment

Frozen Block Falls Off Chuck

- Block may be knocked off chuck by blade
  - Chuck may be loose, blade may be at wrong angle, or section width may be too thick
- Block may stick to heat extractor and detach from chuck
  - Drop of oil on surface of heat extractor will keep it from sticking to block
- Block can be reattached to new chuck using embedding medium
  - Allow to cool before trying to cut again

Comparison of Frozen Section and Cytologic Techniques

Feature	Frozen Section	Cytologic Preparation
Histologic advantages	Tissue structure seen, distance to margins can be evaluated	Excellent nuclear detail, cellular cohesion evident, extracellular material well seen (e.g., thyroid colloid)
Required equipment and maintenance	Substantial (cryostat)	Minimal (glass slides)
Time for preparation	> 5 minutes	< 1 minute
Sampling	Small portion of tissue optimal for evaluation; artifacts in tissue used are permanent	Wide surface of tissue can be sampled; all tissue saved for optimal fixation; some densely fibrotic or low-cellularity lesions may not be evaluable
Potential artifacts	Freezing (ice crystal), drying	Drying
Required expertise	Appearance is similar to permanent sections	Requires special expertise in cytopathology
Safety	Exposure to cryostat blade, possible exposure to infectious agents	Minimal risk for harm or contamination of equipment

Blade Does Not Cut Block

- Base is soft
- Bases prepared day before and left to go through freeze and thaw cycles overnight will be soft and crumbly
  - Blade may push embedding down rather than cutting through it
  - All bases should be newly prepared same day

Very Small Specimens

- It can be challenging to capture enough of small specimen for diagnosis
- Base can be pre-faced in cryostat to avoid loss of any tissue when facing tissue for frozen sections
- Tissue can be dipped in eosin to aid in identifying it when covered with embedding medium
  - Eosin does not interfere with normal staining
- Tissue can be placed in drop of embedding medium placed on top of cooled chuck ("wet embedding")
  - Heat extractor is held gently on top of embedding medium in order to not crush tissue before it is adequately frozen

Adipose Tissue

- Fatty tissue is very difficult to cut well
- If fatty tissue is not important for diagnosis, as much as possible should be trimmed away
- Block may cut better when colder than normal for frozen sections (< -20°C down to -50°C)
- If other methods do not work, thicker sections can be cut

Thick and Thin Sections

- Chuck or blade are loose
  - Stem of chuck must be firmly attached to cryostat
  - Blade must be firmly attached

Air-Drying Artifact

- After staining, cells look splayed out with smudgy chromatin and indistinct cell borders
  - Slides must be fixed immediately after sectioning

Ice Crystal Artifact

- Tissue is riddled with holes or looks compressed due to formation of large ice crystals
  - Tissue needs to be blotted dry before freezing
  - Specimen may be too large and therefore freezes slowly, allowing large crystals to form

Portion of Block Knocked Out by Blade

- May be due to loose chuck or blade
  - Make sure all attachments are secure
- May be due to large piece of tissue and uneven freezing
  - Tissue must be allowed to freeze completely before cutting
- Detached portion of tissue can be reattached to new base with embedding medium if tissue is important

Tears in Section

- May be due to staples, sutures, or bone in tissue
  - Remove hard objects from tissue
- Blade is nicked
  - Replace blade or move blade to undamaged portion

Tissue Does Not Adhere to Slide

- Tissue is very dense fibrous tissue or cartilage
  - Use charged slides
  - Be very gentle when staining slides and use minimal agitation

SELECTED REFERENCES

1. Nigam J et al: Comparative study of intra-operative cytology, frozen sections, and histology of tumor and tumor-like lesions of nose and paranasal sinuses. J Cytol. 30(1):13-7, 2013
2. Taxy JB: Frozen section and the surgical pathologist: a point of view. Arch Pathol Lab Med. 133(7):1135-8, 2009
3. Edgerton ME et al: Immunohistochemical performance of antibodies on previously frozen tissue. Appl Immunohistochem Mol Morphol. 8(3):244-8, 2000
4. Shidham V et al: Intraoperative scrape cytology: comparison with frozen sections, using receiver operating characteristic (ROC) curve. Diagn Cytopathol. 23(2):134-9, 2000

Preparing Base

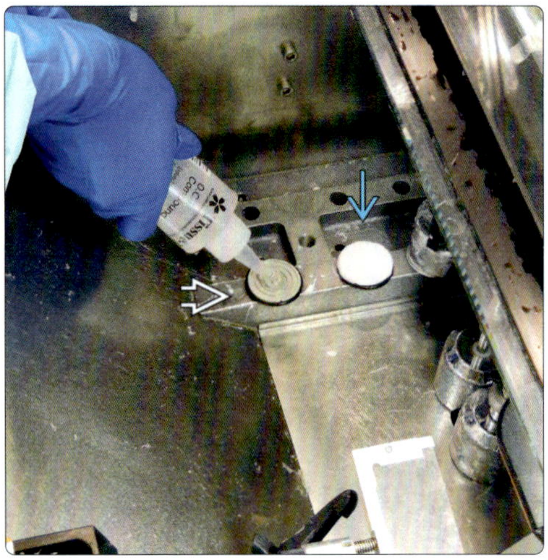

Chuck and Frozen Base

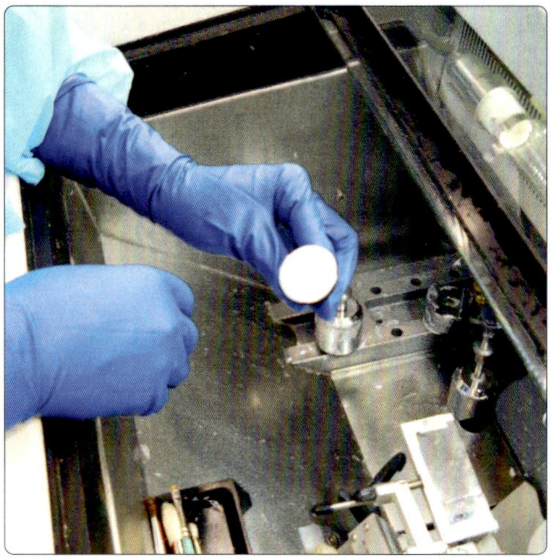

(Left) *The base is prepared by applying embedding medium to a precooled metal chuck* ➡ *in the cryostat. The embedding medium should completely cover the surface of the chuck but not drip over the sides. The medium forms a white opaque surface when frozen* ⇨. **(Right)** *The chuck and base are ready for use when the embedding medium is frozen. If the tissue is very small, the base can be pre-faced on the cryostat to create the correct angle to ensure no tissue is lost when frozen sections are cut.*

Size of Tissue

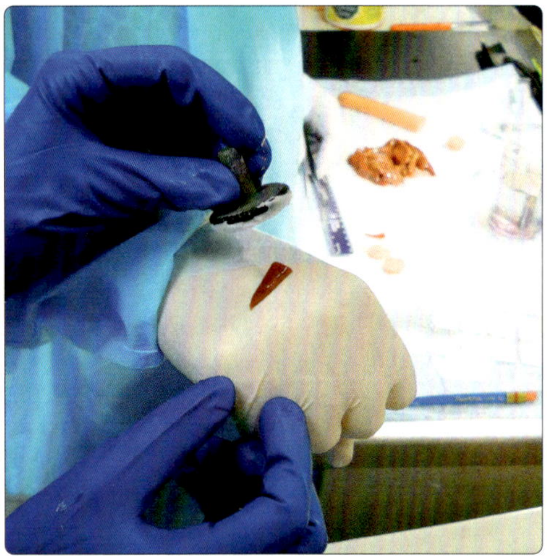

Embedding Medium

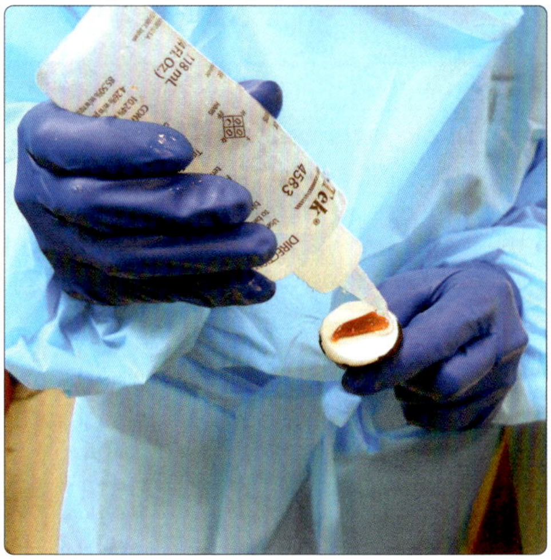

(Left) *The optimum size of tissue for freezing is ~ 8 mm x 8 mm and ≤ 2 mm in thickness. If moist, the tissue should be gently blotted dry. The specimen adheres readily to a chuck covered with frozen embedding medium to form a block.* **(Right)** *The tissue is completely covered by additional embedding medium. Only enough should be used to cover the tissue; it should not extend beyond the edges or onto the stem or back of the chuck. If necessary, excess medium should be removed after freezing.*

Heat Extractor

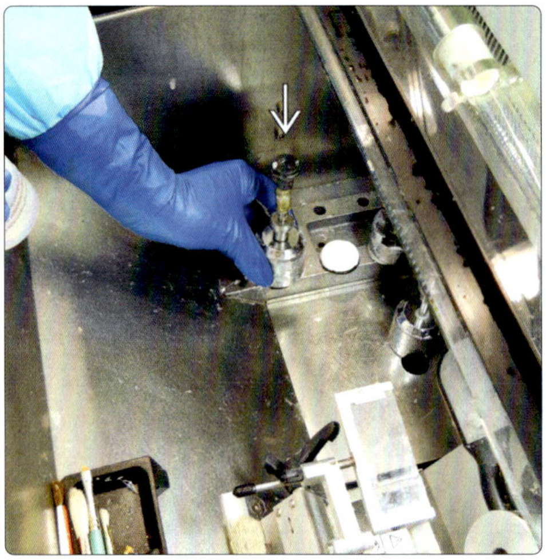

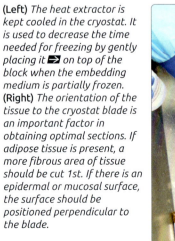

Orientation of Tissue and Blade

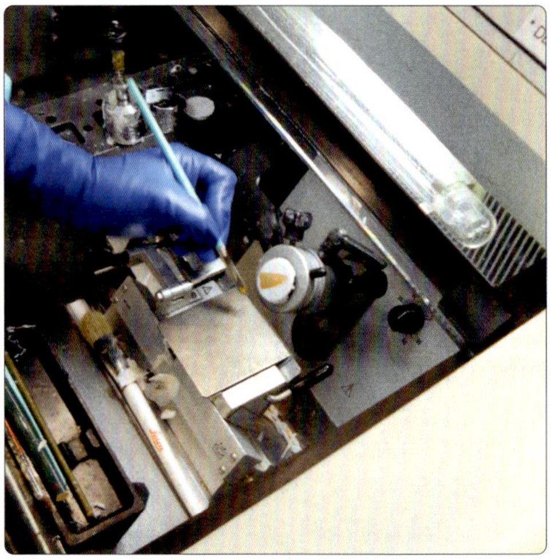

(Left) *The heat extractor is kept cooled in the cryostat. It is used to decrease the time needed for freezing by gently placing it* ➡ *on top of the block when the embedding medium is partially frozen.* **(Right)** *The orientation of the tissue to the cryostat blade is an important factor in obtaining optimal sections. If adipose tissue is present, a more fibrous area of tissue should be cut 1st. If there is an epidermal or mucosal surface, the surface should be positioned perpendicular to the blade.*

Cutting Sections

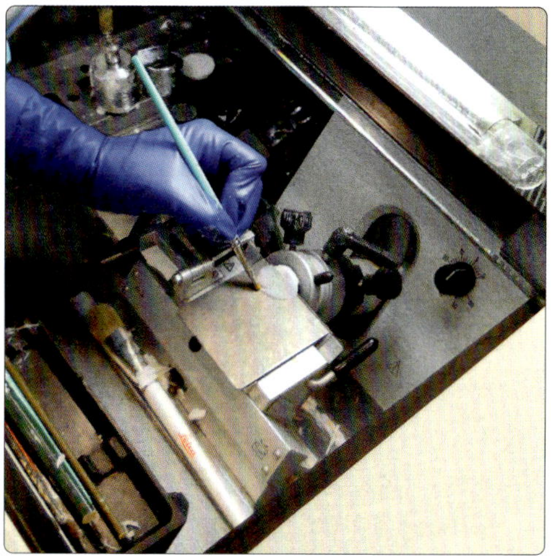

Picking Up Section

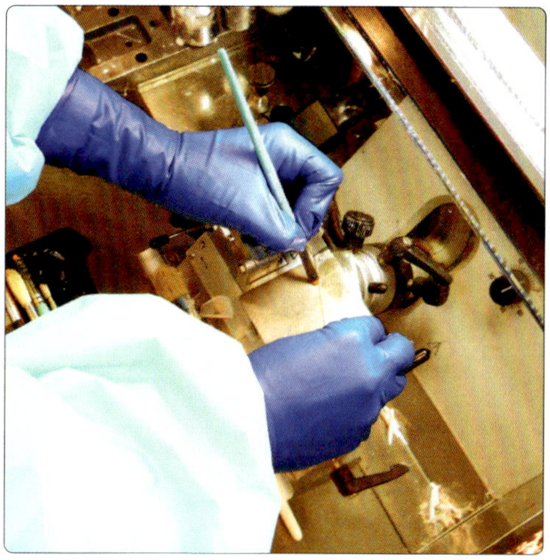

(Left) *As a section is cut, a fine brush is used to prevent the tissue from curling. If the specimen is brittle, causing shattering, a finger applied briefly to the block will warm it slightly. In some cryostats, a plate across the blade provides the same function as the brush.* **(Right)** *The section of tissue should be left slightly attached to the block to prevent the section from curling. A labeled room temperature slide is then applied gently to the tissue. The tissue rapidly melts onto the slide.*

Size of Tissue: Too Large

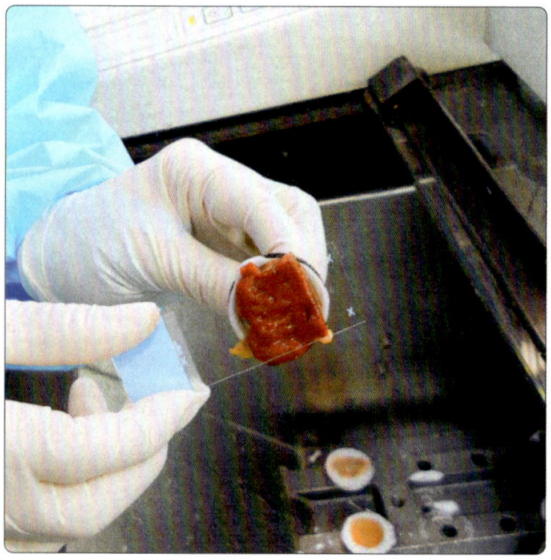

Poor Block Preparation

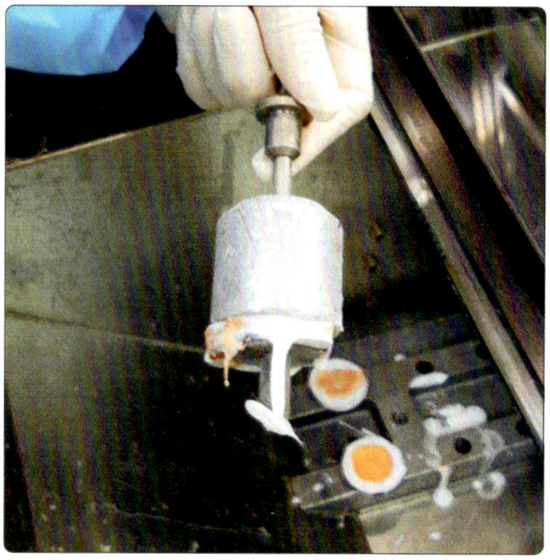

(Left) *This specimen is too large. It does not fit on the chuck and a cut section would not fit on a slide. The tissue would freeze slowly, which increases the likelihood of ice crystal artifact. The specimen should be cut into 2 pieces if it is necessary to examine all of the tissue.* **(Right)** *Too much embedding medium was applied onto the block and it has run off the edges and onto the back of the chuck. The excess medium must be removed with care in order for the chuck to fit securely onto the cryostat.*

Methanol Fixation

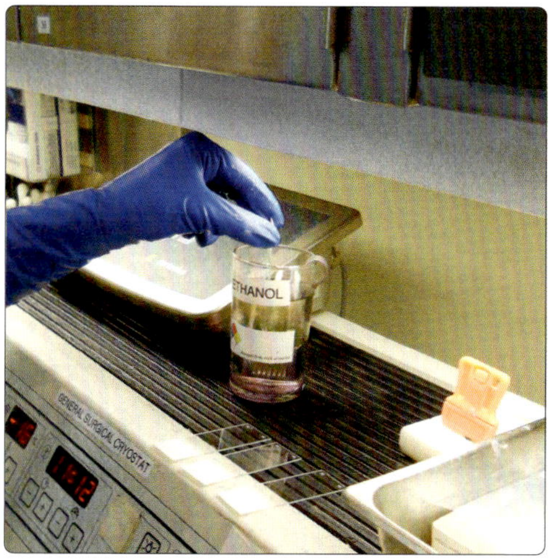

Identifying Tissue Blocks

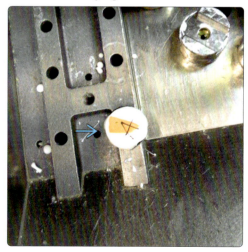

(Left) *It is very important to fix tissue sections as soon as possible. Any delay results in significant artifacts. A methanol container with a slide rack should be within easy reach of the cryostat.* **(Right)** *A single cryostat is often used for multiple frozen sections. Although each specimen should be returned to a labeled container as soon as possible after the slides are prepared, at times, this is not possible. Blocks are easily identified by marking the surface with a felt tip pen* ⇒.

Adipose Tissue

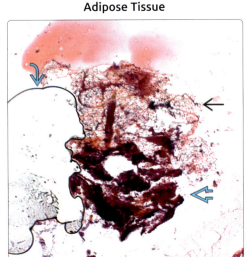

Chatter Artifact

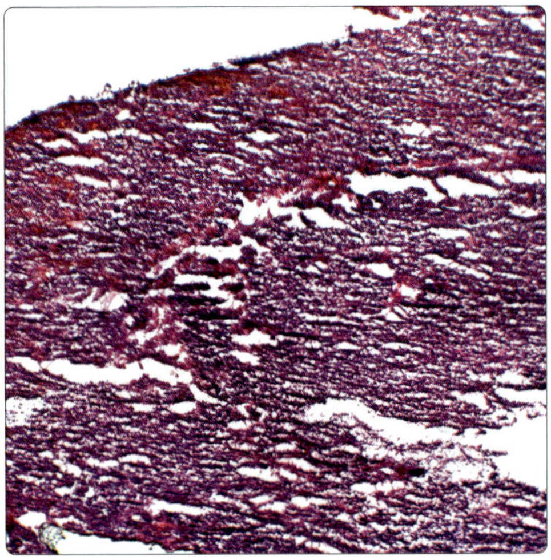

(Left) *Adipose tissue ➔ typically does not cut well. The tissue has crumpled ➔, causing thick areas, and air bubbles ➔ are under the coverslip. Adipose tissue requires colder temperatures. Setting the cryostat to evenly cut thicker sections may result in slides that can be interpreted.* **(Right)** *Dull blades &/or brittle tissue create a ripple effect. The normal architecture is disrupted and the cells distorted, precluding optimal interpretation. A similar appearance is created with ice crystal artifact.*

Freezing Artifact: Compression

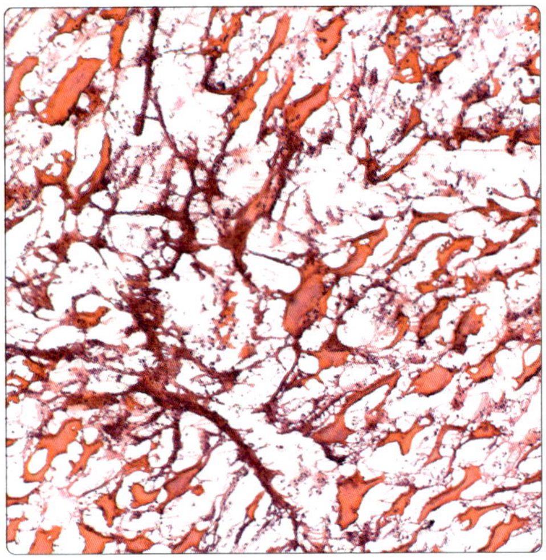

Metastatic Paraganglioma

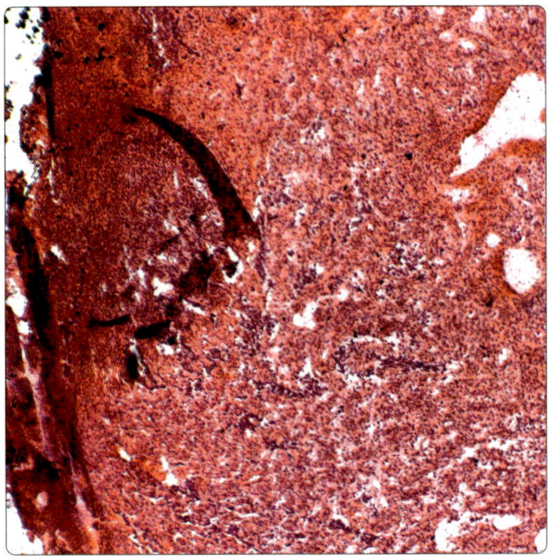

(Left) *This tissue is barely recognizable as skeletal muscle due to marked compression by ice crystals in the stroma. The specimen was likely too large and moist.* **(Right)** *This metastatic paraganglioma to a lymph node was misinterpreted as normal pancreatic tissue, as the section was cut too thickly, and the cellular detail was difficult to discern. Often, if additional slides are requested, the block has had time to freeze more completely, and the additional sections are of better quality.*

Shatter Artifact

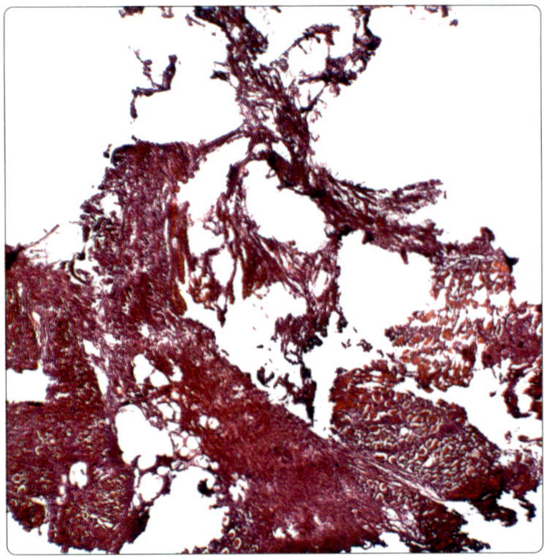

Air-Drying Artifact

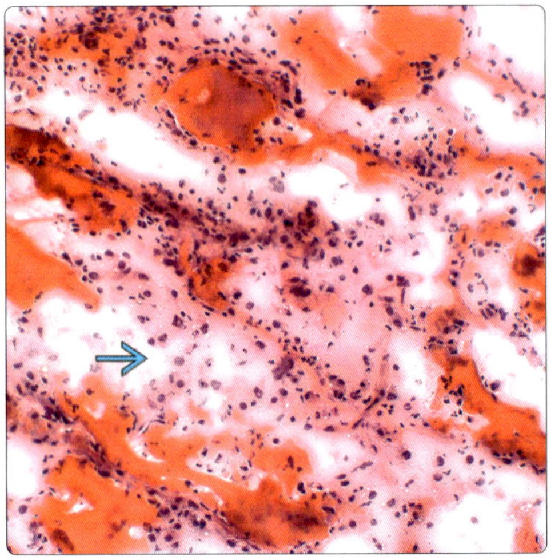

(Left) *Shattered or incomplete sections can occur for a variety of reasons. If the tissue contains calcified fragments, these should be separated out before freezing. Adipose tissue does not freeze well and should be dissected away when possible. Nicks in the blade can tear tissue.* **(Right)** *If the slides are not immediately immersed in methanol, the tissue dries, creating significant artifact. The nuclei appear enlarged and pale ➔. Additional slides should be cut and fixed appropriately.*

Nuclear Ice Crystal Artifact

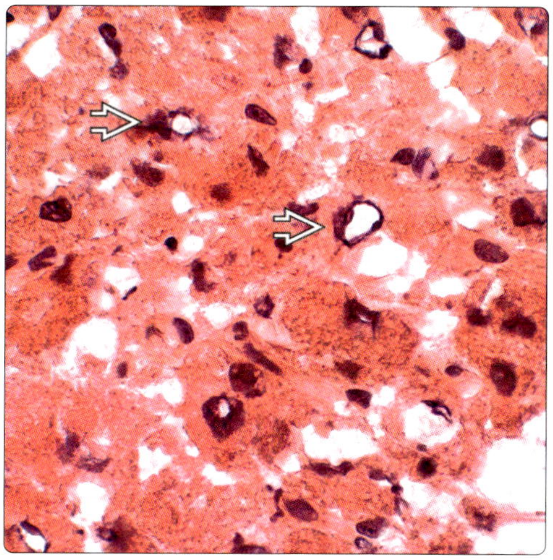

Permanent Section of Frozen Section Remnant

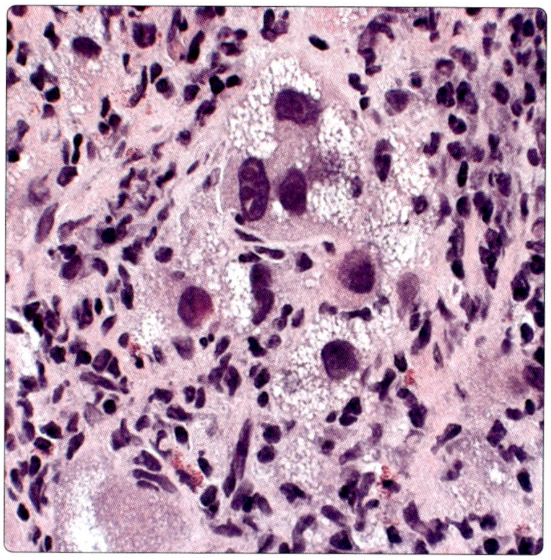

(Left) *Ice crystal artifact caused holes to form within nuclei ➔ in this hepatocellular carcinoma. Very thin sections can also accentuate the appearance of holes. This effect should not be confused with the nuclear clearing seen in papillary thyroid carcinomas and other tumors.* **(Right)** *Freezing creates changes in tissue that remain after formalin fixation and paraffin embedding. The nuclear features of this hepatocellular carcinoma are only somewhat better seen in this permanent section of the frozen section remnant.*

Organizing Pneumonia on Frozen Section

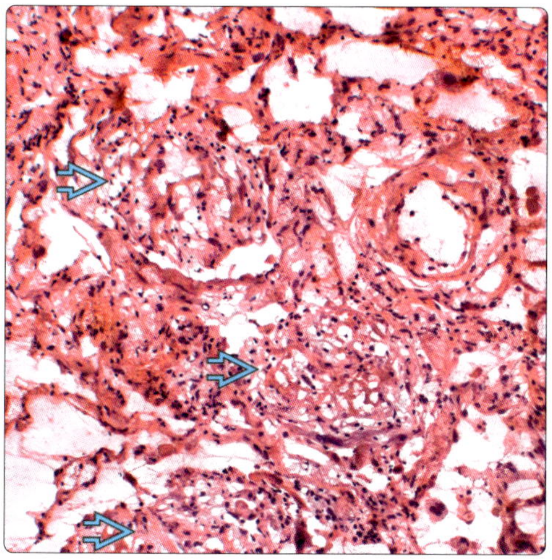

Organizing Pneumonia on Permanent Section of Frozen Section

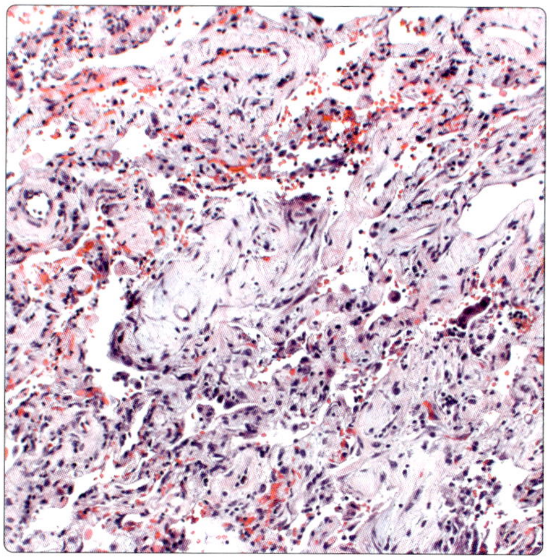

(Left) *Areas of loose fibrosis ➔ are present in alveolar spaces of this frozen section of a focal area of pneumonia. If the patient was immunocompromised and infection is a concern, unstained and fixed slides could be used for special stains for microorganisms.* **(Right)** *The frozen section remnant should be fixed and examined on permanent sections for quality control. The tissue is permanently altered. The nuclear detail is usually smudged. This is why an entire primary lesion should never be frozen.*

Adenomatoid Tumor on Frozen Section

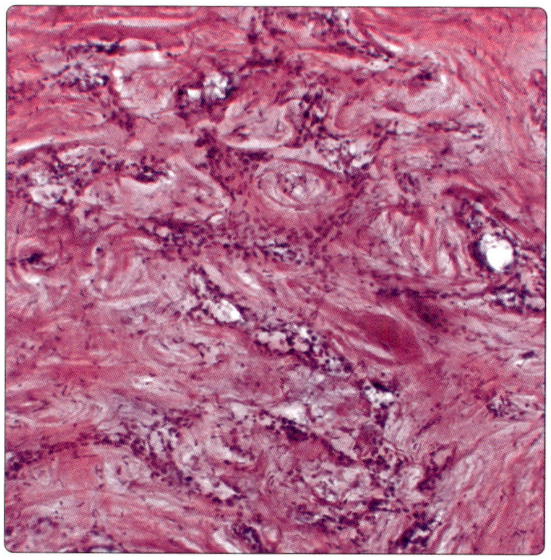

Adenomatoid Tumor on Permanent Section

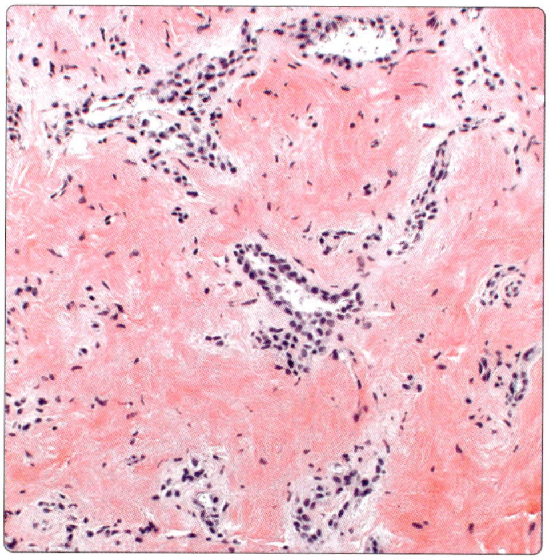

(Left) *This adenomatoid tumor of the peritoneum is hard to discern in this frozen section that is thickly cut and overstained. It could be easily mistaken for a metastatic carcinoma.* **(Right)** *The benign features of this adenomatoid tumor are more easily seen on this thinly sectioned and well-stained permanent section than on a prior frozen section. The nuclei are small, uniform, and bland. The surrounding tissue is paucicellular and dense rather then the cellular desmoplasia seen associated with invasive carcinomas.*

FIXATION AND STAINING OF SLIDES

Introduction

- Preparation of high-quality tissue sections is essential for accurate frozen section diagnosis
- Close attention to rapid and appropriate fixation, staining, and coverslipping can result in slides comparable to those obtained on formalin-fixed, paraffin-embedded permanent sections

SLIDES

Labeling

- Slides are labeled with surgical pathology number and subdesignation for specific frozen section
- Label slides before use to prevent specimen mix-ups
  - Unused labeled slides should be discarded
- Use pencil or other marker that will not be dissolved during staining process
- Label identifies side of slide onto which tissue will be placed

Plain Glass Slides

- Appropriate for majority of frozen sections and cytologic preparations
- Frozen section melts onto slide at room temperature

Coated or Charged Slides

- Used to help keep tissue on slide during staining
- Some tissue does not stick well to slides
  - Tissue exposed to formalin, however briefly
    - Tissue will have larger ice crystals due to lower freezing temperature
    - If piece of tissue is large enough, cut central section with minimal exposure to formalin
  - Cartilage
  - Cauterized tissue
- Unstained coated slides in fixative may be submitted to histology laboratory for special stains in some situations
  - If infectious disease is suspected, slides can be submitted for special stains that will be available in a few hours or early the following day

FIXATION

Types of Fixatives

- 95% ethanol, methanol, acetone, and combinations of fixatives can be used
- Very important to fix slide as soon as section is cut
  - Container of fixative should be kept at hand to allow immediate immersion
  - Prolonged time to fixation results in air drying and alters histologic appearance
    - Loss of nuclear detail with smudging of chromatin
    - Artifactual enlargement of cells and nuclei
    - Architecture not well preserved (cell borders obscured)
- Slides should be in fixative for at least 30-50 seconds
  - Longer fixation is not harmful
  - Fixative should be at room temperature for optimal effect

Air-Dried Slides

- Usually used for cytologic preparations
- Slides must be completely dry, which may take several minutes
  - Methods to heat slides can speed process
- Diff-Quik, rapid Papanicolaou, and other stains are used
- Brings out certain cytologic features
  - Cells appear larger, and this may aid in evaluation
  - Cytoplasmic features easier to visualize
  - Mucosubstances stained
  - Thyroid colloid preserved
- Could be potential infectious hazard if not stained and coverslipped
  - In general, such slides should be discarded when no longer needed for diagnosis

STAINS

Hematoxylin and Eosin

- Standard stain for frozen sections

Staining Slides

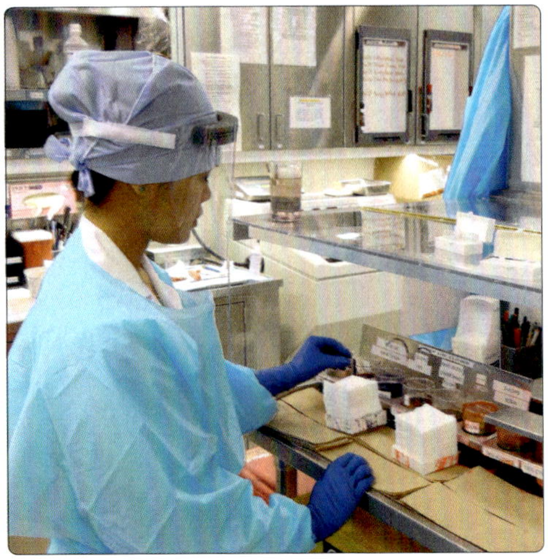

Staining Slides

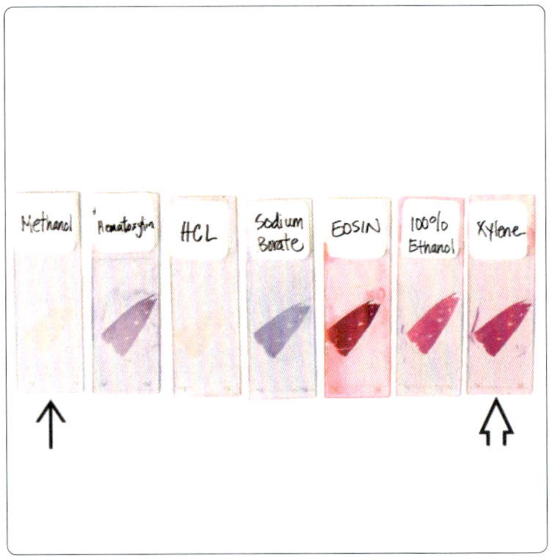

(Left) *Optimal staining is critical for diagnostic interpretation. Understanding the process is important in order to be able to troubleshoot and solve problems when they arise. (Courtesy V. Chan, BS.)* **(Right)** *H&E is the most common stain used for frozen sections. Multiple steps from the unstained tissue ⇒ to the final stained slide ⇒ are required to differentially stain the cellular components.*

- Often preferred because staining pattern is same as for permanent sections
- Hematoxylin for 60-90 seconds (cytologic preparations can be stained for 30 seconds)
  - Blot excess dye on absorbent material
  - Stains nuclei blue
    - Shade of blue should be appropriate to tissue (e.g., lymph nodes dark, adipose tissue light)
    - If inappropriate, stain longer or shorter time as appropriate
- Rinse in water until visible dye is removed
  - Blot excess water on absorbent material
  - Change water frequently between cases
- Acid alcohol (1% HCl in water) for ~ 1 second
  - "Differentiation" removes hematoxylin from nonnuclear components
  - Changes color from blue to purple
- Ammonia water (2% sodium borate) for ~ 2 seconds
  - "Bluing" restores pH to dye to enhance staining and restores color back to blue from purple
- Eosin for 2-4 seconds
  - Blot excess dye on absorbent material
  - Stains cytoplasm and other constituents pink to red
- Increasing concentrations of alcohol (95-100%): Dip for ~ 10 seconds in each concentration
  - Removes excess eosin and water from tissue
- Xylene: Dip until fluid runs clear
  - Leave slides in xylene until ready to coverslip to avoid drying artifact
  - Xylene has high index of refraction and renders tissues transparent

Toluidine Blue

- Used as alternative to hematoxylin and eosin (H&E)
  - May fade over time
  - Staining patterns are different than those seen with routine permanent sections
    - Less familiar to many pathologists
  - Less differential staining of cellular components compared to H&E
    - Nuclei: Deep purple to black
    - Cytoplasm of epithelial cells: Pale blue to purple
    - Elastic tissue: Green to blue
    - Mucosubstances: Faint purple
    - Mast cells: Granules are purple/red
    - Cartilage and collagen: May not be stained
- Rapid staining: Requires fewer steps and can be finished in ~ 1 minute
  - Toluidine blue for 6-10 seconds
  - Rinse in water
  - Dehydrate in acetone
  - Clear in xylene
  - Add coverslip

Diff-Quik

- Modified Wright-Giemsa/Romanowsky stain used primarily for air-dried cytologic preparations
  - These stains are proprietary combinations of methylene blue, eosin, and azure A
- Especially helpful in evaluation of cytologic detail
- Requires monolayers of cells as stain does not penetrate well
  - Touch preps may be more appropriate than smears
- Requires only 15-30 seconds depending on thickness of preparation
  - Manufacturer's instructions should be followed for staining

Rapid Papanicolaou Stain

- Used for cytologic preparations
  - Suitable for fixed or air-dried slides
- 2- to 3-minute staining time
- Multiple variants of this procedure are used

Oil Red O

- Stain to detect lipids
  - Lipids are extracted from tissue during normal processing for permanent sections
  - Lipids can only be detected in frozen tissue
- Uses
  - Normal parathyroid tissue vs. parathyroid adenoma
  - Renal tumors with cytoplasmic lipid vs. other tumors
- Currently, rarely used

Acetylcholinesterase

- Histochemical stain used to identify abnormal nerve fibers in lamina propria for evaluation of Hirschsprung disease

Other Histochemical Stains

- Rapid PAS-diastase, mucicarmine, and Alcian blue stains have been developed
- Not generally used

Immunohistochemical Stains

- Rapid (~ 20 minutes) procedures have been developed
- Need for such studies is too infrequent to make them useful for most laboratories

COVERSLIP

Size

- Usually supplied in small (square) and large (rectangular) sizes
- Choose coverslip that will cover tissue on slide

Placement of Coverslip

- Small drop of mounting medium is placed on edge of slide next to tissue
  - Too much mounting medium may smear onto coverslip and obscure tissue
  - Mounting medium on back of slide will cause slide to stick to microscope stage
    - If this happens, gauze dipped in xylene can be used to clean stage
- Coverslip is angled at edge of slide next to mounting medium
  - Edge of coverslip should touch both slide and mounting medium
  - Mounting medium should spread between slide and coverslip by capillary action
- Coverslip is eased onto slide as mounting medium spreads, being careful to not introduce bubbles

- Back and edges of slides are wiped &/or blotted to remove excess xylene and mounting medium

DISPOSITION

Storage

- Original frozen section slides should be preserved
- Good practice to store original frozen section slide with permanent slides for review at sign-out of case
- Comparison of frozen section slide and permanent section made from tissue remnant is useful
  - In some cases, finding is only present on frozen section and not on deeper levels on permanent section
    - If important finding is not present on all frozen section slides, best slide should be marked for use in later correlation
  - Quality assurance measure: Reevaluate frozen section diagnosis after review of entire case
    - If error found, should be documented in report and immediately communicated to surgeon and other treating physicians
    - Analysis of cause of errors is very useful teaching tool

TROUBLESHOOTING

Stain Too Pale

- Old stains
  - Replace stains periodically
- Too little time in hematoxylin or eosin
- Prolonged time in acid alcohol
  - Can cause pale nuclear staining
  - Reduce time in this solution
- Failure to dip in ammonia water
  - Necessary to restore pH and intensify staining
- Prolonged time in alcohol
  - Can result in poor staining
    - If coverslipping will be delayed, slides can be left in xylene without altering staining quality

Stain Too Dark

- Prolonged time in hematoxylin
  - Stain for shorter period of time
  - Increase time in acid alcohol
- Prolonged time in eosin
  - Decrease time in eosin
  - Increase time in each alcohol concentration

Precipitate is Present

- Dyes can precipitate over time
  - Hematoxylin may oxidize (sheen on surface)
- Can cause lack of sharpness of nuclear staining
  - Hematoxylin should be filtered or changed every day
  - If change is not practical, oxidized layer can be removed with paper towel

Slide Cloudy

- Xylene carryover into initial fixative
  - Xylene in hematoxylin looks like oil on surface of water
  - Change solutions frequently
  - Rinse slide holders in alcohol after use
- Water in xylene
  - Blot slides well after rinsing in water
  - Dehydrate well in alcohol, letting all fluid drain from slides after each concentration

Uneven Staining

- Insufficient dehydration leaving water in tissue
  - Increase time in alcohol concentrations to improve dehydration

Poor Nuclear Detail

- Slides may have not been fixed in methanol quickly enough
  - Air-drying artifact can occur with a delay of only 15 seconds
  - Results in smudgy chromatin and indistinct cell borders
  - Cut additional sections and fix quickly

Tissue Falls Off Slide

- Tissue may have been fixed in formalin
  - Use another specimen or deeper section that may not have touched formalin, if possible
  - Use coated slides
- Sclerotic tissue, bone or cartilage, or necrosis
  - Try coated slides &/or cytologic preparations
  - Tissue can be air dried briefly to improve cohesion
    - Artifacts will also be introduced
- Be very gentle when agitating slides during staining to avoid dislodging tissue
  - If tissue falls off during staining, it may not be possible to stain slide using normal procedure
    - Acid alcohol and ammonia water steps can be omitted
    - Tissue can be stained directly with toluidine blue or hematoxylin and coverslipped
    - Quality is suboptimal, but tissue may be identifiable
- In some cases, diagnosis may need to be deferred to permanent sections

Bubbles Under Coverslip

- Air may be allowed to enter during placement of coverslip
  - Thin mounting medium with 1-2 drops of xylene to facilitate spreading on slide
  - Additional xylene can be added at edges of coverslip to replace air
- Thick tissue sections can result in poor seal between slide and coverslip
  - Avoid cutting thick sections
  - Introduce additional xylene at edge of coverslip

Slide Sticky or Obscured by Mounting Medium

- Too much mounting medium used can result in smearing on slide
  - Use appropriate amount
  - Wipe away excess with xylene

SELECTED REFERENCES

1. Ammanagi AS et al: On-site toluidine blue staining and screening improves efficiency of fine-needle aspiration cytology reporting. Acta Cytol. 56(4):347-51, 2012
2. Martucciello G et al: A new rapid acetylcholinesterase histochemical method for the intraoperative diagnosis of Hirschsprung's disease and intestinal neuronal dysplasia. Eur J Pediatr Surg. 11(5):300-4, 2001
3. Humphreys TR et al: A pilot study comparing toluidine blue and hematoxylin and eosin staining of basal cell and squamous cell carcinoma during Mohs surgery. Dermatol Surg. 22(8):693-7, 1996

Unstained Tissue Section

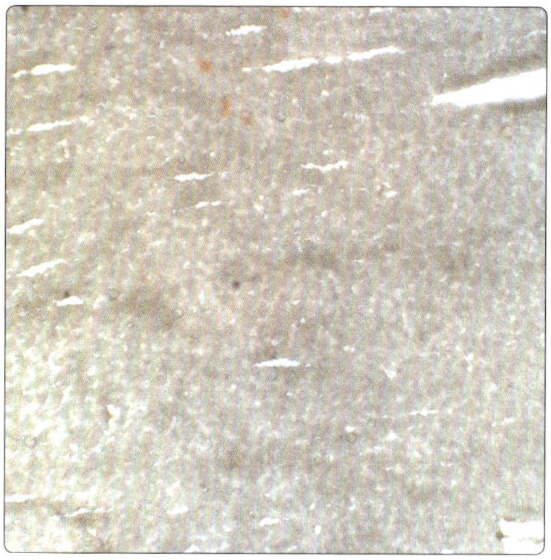

Hematoxylin Staining

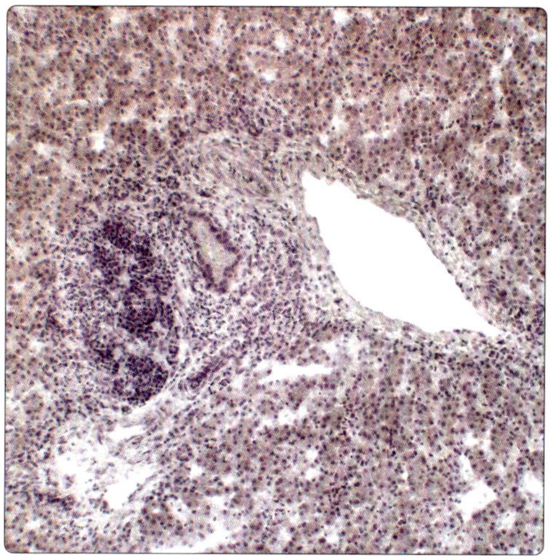

(Left) *Without differential staining of the various cellular components, tissues are colorless. Only the most obvious features of tissue structure can be discerned.* **(Right)** *Slides are 1st stained in hematoxylin for 60-90 seconds. Cytology specimens can be stained for a shorter period of time (30 seconds). This dye stains nuclei blue. After staining, the slides are rinsed in water to remove excess dye. If the final slides are too dark, they may have been left in this dye for too long a time.*

Acid Alcohol

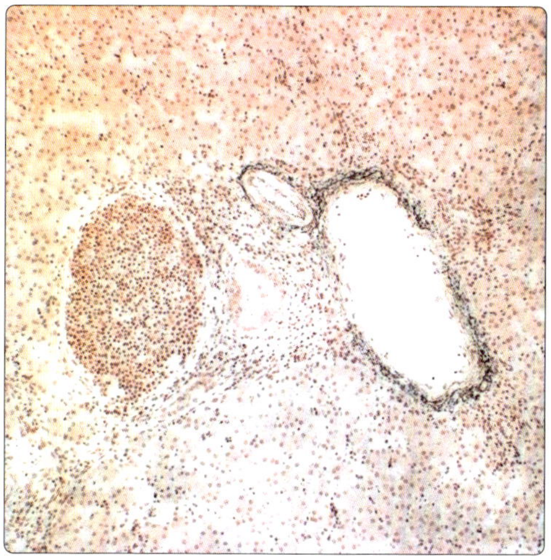

Ammonia Water

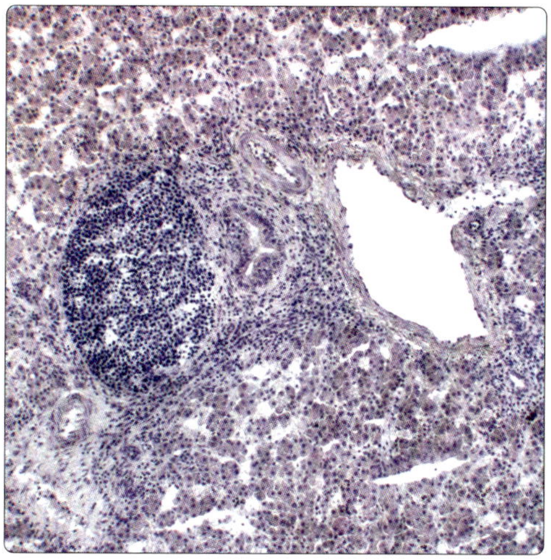

(Left) *Acid alcohol preferentially removes hematoxylin from nonnuclear components. This is termed "differentiation." Poorly stained nuclei can result from too long a period in acid alcohol or too little time in hematoxylin. The acidity changes the blue color to purple.* **(Right)** *Ammonia water (2% sodium borate) restores the basic pH after the treatment in acid alcohol. The color is changed from purple to blue and the staining intensity is enhanced (termed "bluing").*

Eosin

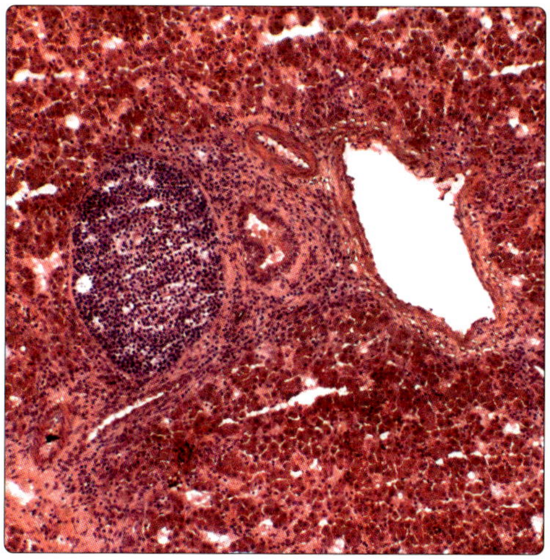

Hematoxylin and Eosin

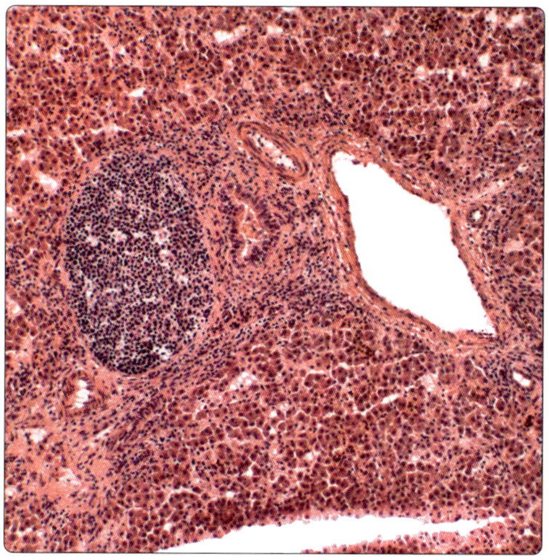

(Left) *Eosin stains cytoplasm and other cellular components from pink to red. The slides are then dehydrated in increasing concentrations of alcohol to remove the excess eosin and to remove water from the tissue.* **(Right)** *In the final step, slides are dipped in xylene. Xylene has a high index of refraction and renders tissues transparent. The cellular components can now be discerned clearly. Mounting media is now placed on the slide and a coverslip added. The slide can now be used for diagnosis.*

Oil Red O

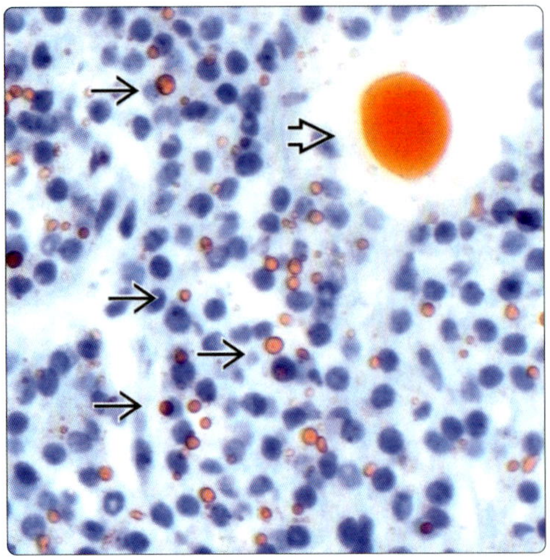

Oil Red O

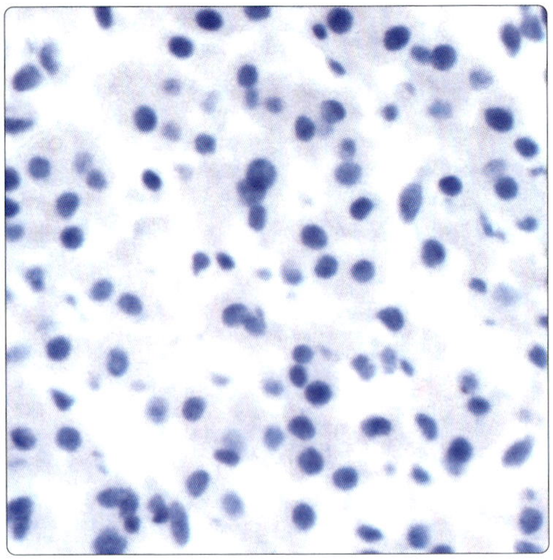

(Left) *Oil red O stain shows eosinophilic droplets of intracellular fat* ⇨ *and a large deposit of extracellular fat* ⇨ *in this parathyroid tissue. The presence of fat is typically more common in normal parathyroid glands and diminished or absent in hyperplasia and adenomas.* **(Right)** *This parathyroid lesion shows no intracellular fat on this oil red O stain. This is supporting evidence that this is hyperplasia or an adenoma. This stain can also be used to demonstrate lipid in renal tumors.*

Diff-Quik

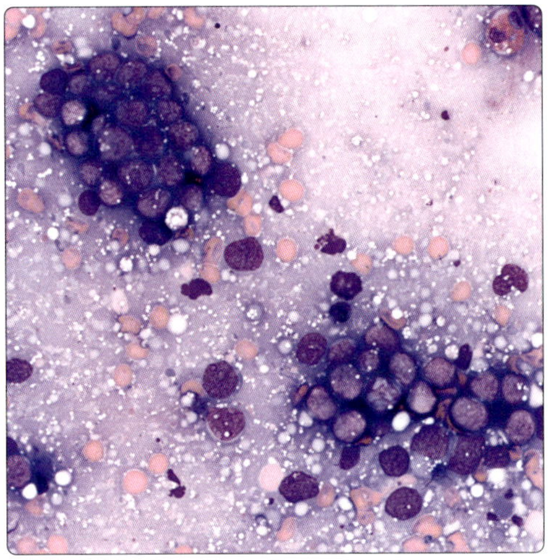

Diff-Quik

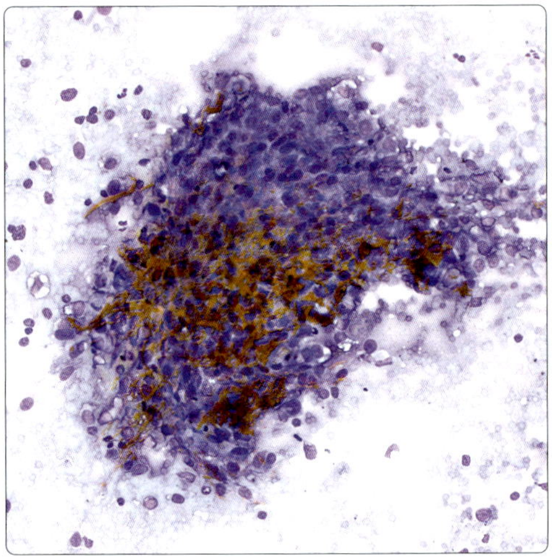

(Left) *Diff-Quik is a modification of the Wright-Giemsa stain that allows rapid staining of air-dried slides in seconds. Air drying causes the cells to spread out and appear larger than in preparations in which the tissue is fixed. The nuclear detail of this Burkitt lymphoma is well seen.* **(Right)** *In Diff-Quik stains, the nuclei are dark blue to purple. The cytoplasm is varying shades of blue, depending on the type of cell. The staining pattern is different than that seen in H&E on permanent sections.*

Diff-Quik

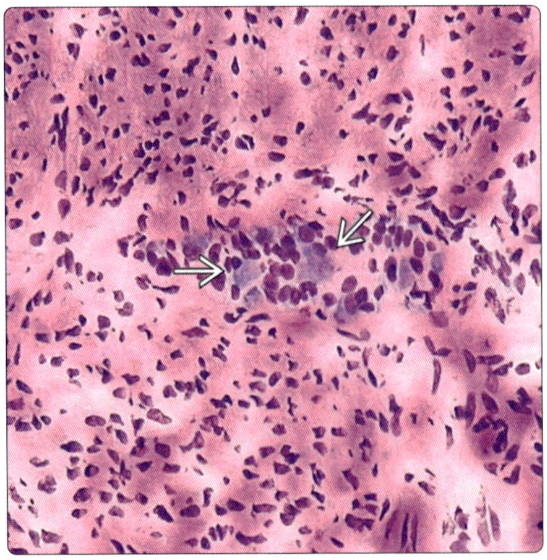

Acetylcholinesterase Stain

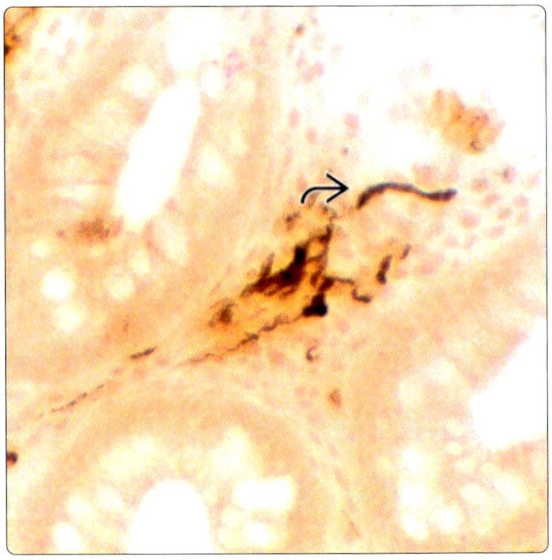

(Left) *Diff-Quik stain highlights ganglion cells* ➔ *by staining the cytoplasm a contrasting blue color on frozen section. This stain, as well as Giemsa stain, can be helpful in the evaluation of Hirschsprung disease. (Courtesy C. Mafnas, MD.)* **(Right)** *Acetylcholinesterase stain on frozen section accentuates prominent abnormal nerve fibers within the lamina propria* ↪ *and muscularis mucosa in cases of Hirschsprung disease. Such fibers are not present in these locations in the normal colon.*

Pale Staining

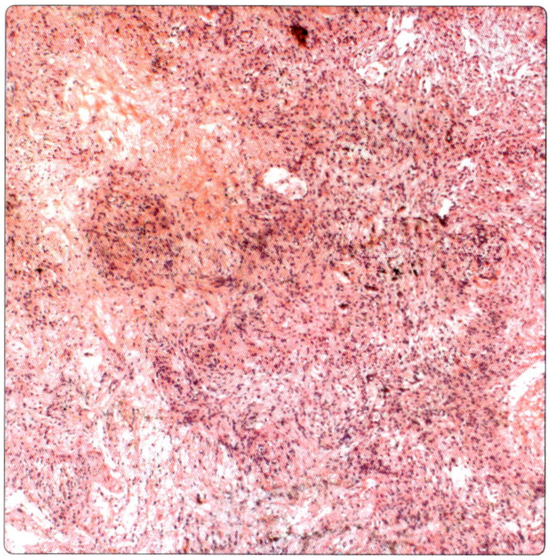

Hematoxylin Crystallization

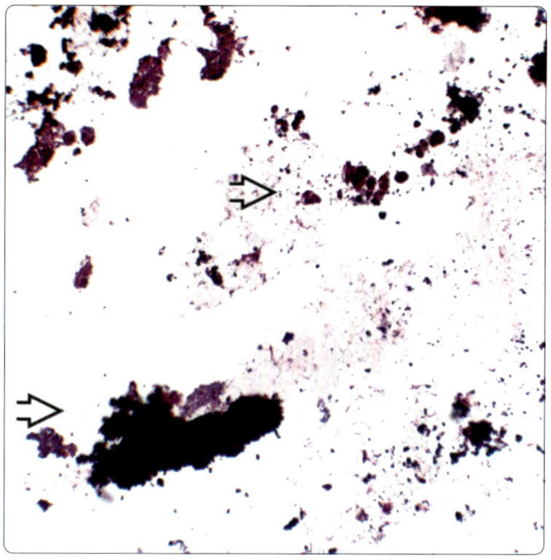

(Left) *Pale staining can be the result of old stains. Stains should be replaced periodically. If the stains are fresh, the tissue may require more time in hematoxylin or less time in acid alcohol to obtain a darker color.* **(Right)** *Hematoxylin can form crystals ⇨ that can obscure the features of the tissue being examined or may mimic microorganisms or calcifications. Stains should be changed and filtered frequently.*

Xylene Artifact

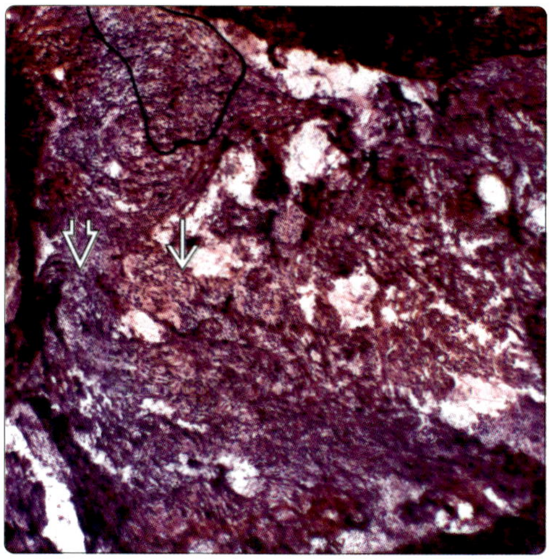

Bubbles

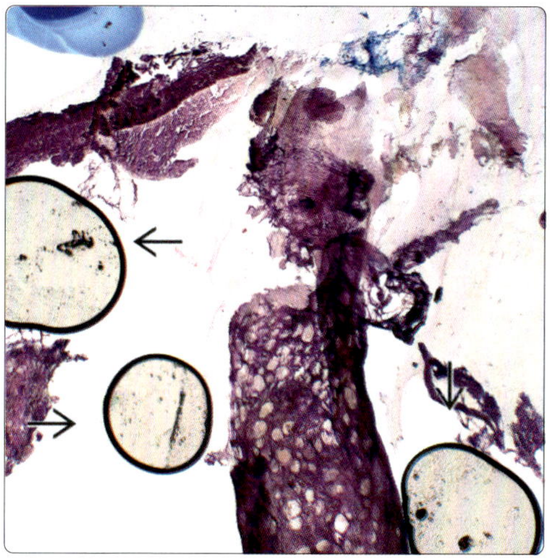

(Left) *Carry over of xylene into the fixative can create significant artifacts. Staining can be spotty, varying from dark ➡ to light ➡. The overall appearance of the tissue may be blurred. Slide holders should be rinsed in a large container of methanol before being reused to prevent carry over.* **(Right)** *It takes a bit of dexterity to prevent bubbles ⇨ from being trapped under the coverslip. Sufficient mounting medium (with an added drop of xylene) and holding the coverslip at 45° usually suffices.*

Uneven Staining

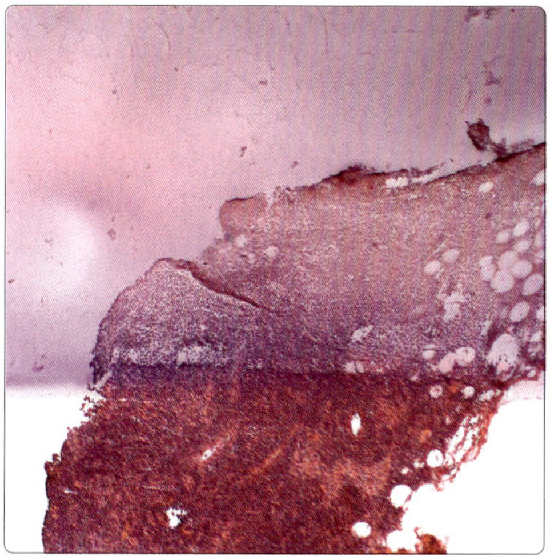

Multiple Artifacts

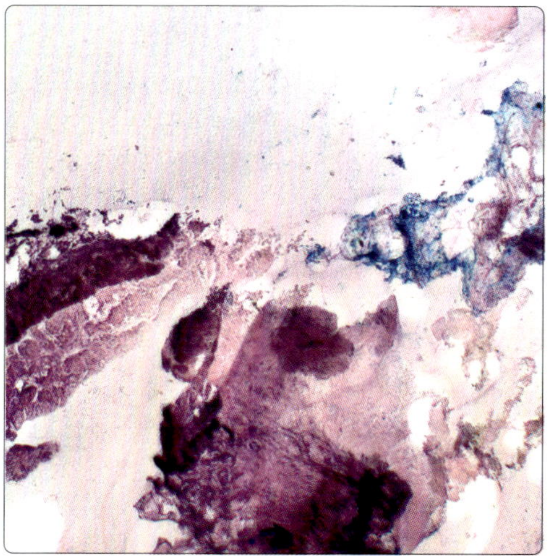

(Left) *The poor staining of this tissue section demonstrates how interpretation can be problematic when suboptimal. The top portion shows marked fading, possibly due to failure to submerge the slide in all of the staining reagents and failure to rinse away excess dye.* **(Right)** *This slide is essentially uninterpretable due to fragmentation, folding, and poor, irregular staining. It is preferable to prepare completely new slides rather than to potentially make an error trying to interpret a poor slide.*

BIOSPECIMEN COLLECTION

Reasons for Biospecimen Collection

- There are 3 main circumstances in which tissue is saved for purposes other than pathologic evaluation by routine formalin fixation and paraffin embedding
  - Diagnostic work-up performed for pathologic diagnosis requires special studies
    - Does not require additional patient permission
    - Tissue is linked to patient
    - Results of studies are included in patient's pathology report and are part of medical record
    - Studies are billed as part of diagnostic evaluation
  - Clinical protocol on which patient is enrolled requires tissue allocation
    - Patient provides permission as part of protocol
    - Tissue is linked to patient
    - Studies are performed on tissue as part of clinical protocol
    - Studies are supported by funding from protocol
    - Results of study are generally not included in patient's pathology report
      - Patient may or may not have access to results
  - Research protocols/tissue banking
    - If tissue would otherwise be discarded, general institutional permissions as part of surgical permission may be sufficient
      - Patients must give specific permission if tissue is linked to patient identifiers
    - Patients almost never have access to results
    - Support is provided by research protocols or by institution

Guidelines for Biospecimen Collection

- Multiple institutions provide information about biospecimen collection
  - International Society of Biologic and Environmental Repositories has issued recommended standard operating procedures (SOPs) for biospecimen collection
  - College of American Pathologists offers biorepository accreditation

Tissue Sampling

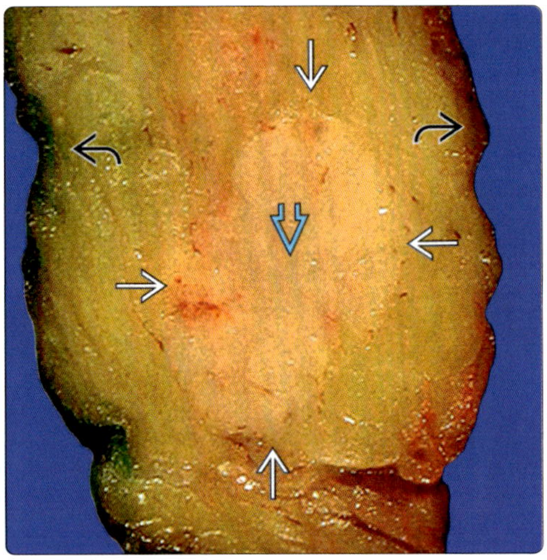

Freezing Tissue: Dry Ice

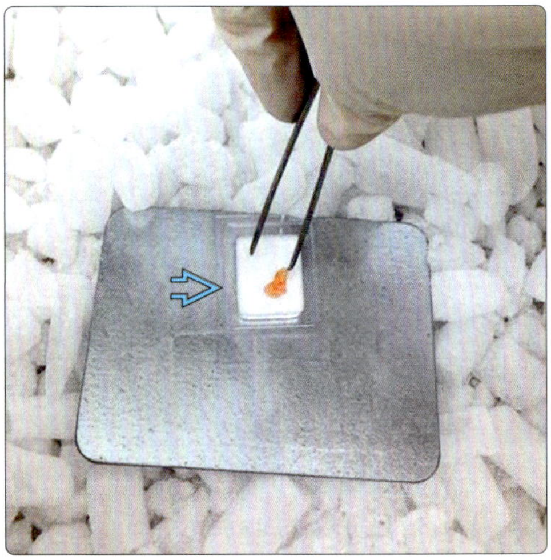

(Left) *The best location to take viable tumor is near the border of a carcinoma but not including normal tissue. The central portion of tumors is often necrotic or fibrotic. Other areas of the specimen of clinical importance, such as margins, must be preserved for patient care.* **(Right)** *Tissue frozen in cryoprotective embedding medium on a bed of dry ice can be sectioned on a cryostat to evaluate histologic features and to macrodissect the tissue if needed for molecular evaluation. (Courtesy L. Chichester, BS.)*

Freezing Tissue: Bath

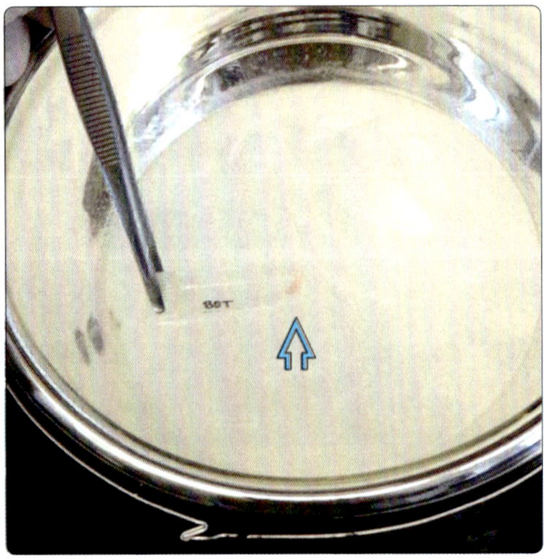

Frozen Tissue: Storage

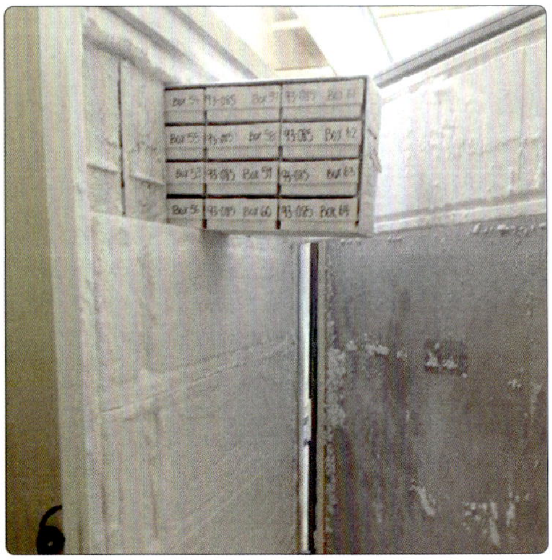

(Left) *Tissue that will be used primarily for assays without histologic evaluation can be frozen in a small tube in a liquid nitrogen or isopentane bath. (Courtesy L. Chichester, BS.)* **(Right)** *It is very important to have adequate storage for frozen tissue as well as robust mechanisms for documenting and retrieving specimens. (Courtesy L. Chichester, BS.)*

    - https://biospecimens.cancer.gov/bestpractices/Appendix6.pdf
  - National Cancer Institute (NCI) Biorepositories and Research Branch provides best practice documents, including NCI Best Practices Resources
    - https://biospecimens.cancer.gov/bestpractices
  - Biospecimen Reporting for Improved Study Quality guidelines provide list of information relevant to document biospecimens
- Important variables include following
  - **Preanalytical variables**
    - Related to sample procurement, processing, transportation, or storage
    - Preanalytic pathology information is acquired at time of specimen collection
  - **Analytical variables**
    - Related to performance of tests on biospecimen
    - It is responsibility of person or group conducting assays to collect this information
  - It is recommended that this information be available when studies using biospecimen are published

Role of Pathologist

- Pathologist should be notified prior to surgery that tissue is required for clinical protocol or research
  - Appropriate permission and Institutional Review Board (IRB) approval should be provided
  - For ongoing collection protocols, protocol for SOP should be developed and be available in intraoperative consultation room
    - SOP should be developed in conjunction with study team and pathology department to ensure that collection of tissue does not compromise patient care
  - Intraoperative consultation room is best location for identifying appropriate samples
    - Time for transfer of specimen after removal from patient can be minimized
      - System for transfer is available
    - Required equipment for specimen processing and documentation are available
    - Tissue can simultaneously be taken for patient care purposes and studies related to diagnosis
- Pathologist must ensure that patient is not harmed by taking of tissue
  - Pathologist is only person who can make informed decision about what tissue is necessary to examine for patient care
    - Pathologist can be important advocate for patient's best interests
  - Pathologist must be aware of any previous diagnosis, prior treatment, and purpose of current procedure in order to determine what tissue is required for optimal patient care
    - Minimal tissue to confirm diagnosis may be needed if there has been prior definitive diagnosis made
    - Patients with suspected malignancy, but without prior diagnosis, are at greatest risk for harm if tissue is taken that will not be available for microscopic evaluation
  - If there is any possibility of patient harm (e.g., by failure to make diagnosis on tissue given away for research studies), competing priorities for use of tissue should be discussed with patient's physician
- Pathologist should ensure that tissue taken is suitable for proposed studies
  - In some cases, frozen sections or cytologic preparations may be used to identify lesional tissue
    - If this is done solely for purpose of research study, study should provide financial support
  - Center portions of tumors are often ischemic resulting in fibrosis &/or necrosis
    - Most viable tumor tissue is at interface with normal tissue
  - Unless specifically requested, tumor/normal interface should not be taken for research
    - Intermingled tumor and normal tissue will confound results of nonmorphology-based assays
    - Adjacent normal tissue may contain prognostically important features (e.g., lymph-vascular invasion) and should be, in general, reserved for patient care
    - If tumor/normal interface is required for study, samples can be taken as long as they are very small relative to larger area of interface tissue
  - Tissue should not be taken that is needed to evaluate important prognostic factors
    - Margins
    - Lymph nodes
  - If normal tissue is requested, it should not include grossly evident tumor tissue
    - Normal tissue may be requested as control tissue (e.g., to evaluate for possible germline vs. somatic mutations)
    - If study only requires normal tissue, it is best to use specimens from patients without tumors (e.g., cosmetic procedures)
    - Some studies will want to have normal tissue adjacent to tumor and samples distant from tumor
- Pathologist must determine that tissue is only taken with appropriate permission and IRB approval
  - This information should be provided at time of request for tissue
- Pathologist must document type and amount of tissue taken for studies and destination of tissues
  - Tissue taken should be documented in gross description in pathology report
  - In some cases, it may be prudent to have recipient hold tissue until it is determined whether or not tissue is needed for diagnostic studies

Definitions

- Warm ischemic time
  - Time from cessation of blood flow to tissue until tissue drops below 37°C (body temperature)
  - When important, surgeon would need to document start of this time
- Cold ischemic time
  - Time after tissue drops below 37°C until tissue is fixed or frozen
    - Temperature should be lowered to 4°C by refrigerating or placing specimen on ice

  - Tissue is not considered fixed until fixative is in contact with lesion
    - Placement of intact specimens in fixative may not result in fixation of lesional tissue for many hours
- Ideally, ischemic times are as short as possible
  - When feasible, it is helpful to record these times for individual specimens to help determine quality of specimen
    - Ischemia can alter gene expression (mRNA levels) and cause protein degradation
    - DNA is more resistant to ischemia, but degradation can occur if prolonged

BIOMOLECULES

Protein

- Majority of proteins are stable for hours
  - Changes in protein expression can occur due to stresses during surgery, response to drugs, and hypoxia
- Many proteins can be identified in routine formalin-fixed tissue using immunohistochemistry
  - Formalin creates cross-links, which change conformation of protein and which may alter epitopes
  - Antibodies may or may not be adaptable for formalin-fixed tissue, depending on changes in epitope detected
- Frozen tissue may be preferred for some studies of proteins in their natural configuration
- Phosphorylated proteins are typically unstable
  - Phosphorylation and dephosphorylation can occur in response to ischemia
  - Rapid collection within 5 minutes and rapid freezing is important
  - Solutions containing phosphorylase and kinase inhibitors may be used

Other Cellular and Tissue Constituents

- Lipids, carbohydrates, minerals, and other biosubstances may be subject of study
  - Lipids generally do not persist after standard tissue processing
    - Fresh or frozen tissue may be required
  - Calcium deposits (e.g., in bone) may need to be removed in order to section tissue
    - Decalcifying agents can alter antigenicity of proteins and can degrade DNA
    - Fresh or frozen tissue may be required
    - Special microtomes that can section calcified tissues can be used

RNA

- Very unstable biomolecule
  - Levels of RNA can be increased or decreased during ischemia and temperature changes
  - Degradation can occur within minutes of ischemic time
- Special fixatives are available that can stabilize RNA
- Some analytic techniques have been optimized to detect smaller RNA fragments present in formalin-fixed tissue

DNA

- Most stable biomolecule
- Majority of studies can be performed on fresh, frozen, or formalin-fixed tissue
  - Main source of damage is from certain types of fixatives that cause DNA damage (e.g., Bouins fixative)
  - Similar results are obtained from formalin-fixed, paraffin-embedded tissue and frozen or fresh tissue
    - Amplicon length is shorter when formalin-fixed tissue is used
- Formalin fixation and storage have been associated with low-frequency transitions (C > T/G > A) that may complicate interpretation of sequencing results, especially at low levels of input template

Viable Cells

- Viable cells may be needed for treatment protocols to establish long-term cell lines, patient-derived xenograft models, or for short-term culture and karyotyping
- Cells that will be used to treat patient, or other patients, must be collected under very strict sterile conditions
  - In general, protocols should provide for cells or tissues to be removed in operating room
- Cells that will be used for long- or short-term culture can be allocated by pathologist using sterile conditions
- Cells can remain viable for up to 48 hours at room temperature
  - Cells should either be placed into culture or frozen in liquid nitrogen within this time period

METHODS

Freezing

- Tissue frozen for diagnosis in cryoprotective gel (embedding medium) can be saved frozen
  - Cryostats typically undergo freeze/thaw cycles to prevent frost build-up
    - Therefore, tissues cannot be stored in cryostat overnight
    - Tissue should be removed to another storage facility without thawing
  - Tissue can be removed from embedding medium by rinsing with buffer
- Snap freezing
  - Tissue in vial is placed in liquid nitrogen or in isopentane maintained at -20°C
  - Isopentane cooled on dry ice can be used when liquid nitrogen is not available
  - Only small (< 1 cm in at least 1 dimension) fragments of tissue should be frozen
    - Center portion of large fragments may freeze at slower rate
  - Tissue should be frozen for at least 2 or 3 minutes
    - Tissue can remain in isopentane for long periods of time
  - Tissue may be snap frozen and retained in aluminum foil to reduce drying

Viable Cells

- Depending on downstream protocol, tissue may be placed in culture medium or sterile saline
  - Dimethyl sulfoxide or glycerol may be added as cryoprotectant if samples will be retained in liquid nitrogen

Tissue Allocation for Studies Not for Diagnosis

Critical Steps
(1) Determine if Institutional Review Board Approval has been obtained
(2) Determine if there is approval for patient identifiers to accompany specimen
(3) Determine type and amount of tissue requested
(4) Determine if this tissue can be taken without compromising care of patient
(5) Obtain tissue and place in appropriate fixative or freeze
(6) Document type of tissue, amount of tissue, and where tissue will be located
(7) In some cases, it may be appropriate to request that tissue not be processed until final diagnosis is rendered

Recommended Preanalytical Pathologic Data Elements for Biospecimens

Element	Examples
Anatomical site	Organ or type of tissue
Sample type	Fine-needle biopsy, core-needle biopsy, incisional biopsy, excision
Pathology diagnosis	Tumor type or normal tissue
Date and time biospecimen is removed from patient	This is information that would need to be provided by surgeon/clinician
Date and time biospecimen is placed into initial stabilization	If stabilization is performed by pathologist, this information can be provided
Collection mechanism	Tissue section, needle biopsy, or cytologic preparation
Type of initial stabilization	Frozen (include temperature) or fixation (include type)

These elements are included in the Biospecimen Reporting for Improved Study Quality guidelines.

Special Fixatives

- QIAGEN Allprotect Tissue Reagent (QIAGEN, Valencia, CA, USA)
  - Preserves DNA, RNA, and protein in fresh tissue for up to 1 week at room temperature and 1 year in refrigerator
- Invitrogen RNAlater can be used to stabilize mRNA
  - Rapidly penetrates tissue and inactivates RNase to stabilize RNA
  - Tissue section should be < 0.5 cm in at least 1 dimension
  - Tissue is submerged in 5 volumes of Invitrogen RNAlater solution in cryogenic vial
  - Vial should be transferred as soon as possible (ideally within 1 hour) to 4°C refrigerator
    - Specimen should be kept at 4°C from 4 hours to overnight to allow fixative to penetrate tissue
    - Tissue can be stored at 4°C for 1 month, at 25°C for 1 week, or at -20°C indefinitely
  - Morphologic features of tissues are maintained and are similar to traditional formalin-fixed tissues

Imprint on Nitrocellulose Paper

- Cross section of fresh tissue is imprinted onto nitrocellulose paper
- Cells are dried and do not require fixation or refrigeration
- DNA and RNA can be recovered from cells

SELECTED REFERENCES

1. Caixeiro NJ et al: Quality assessment and preservation of RNA from biobank tissue specimens: a systematic review. J Clin Pathol. 69(3):260-5, 2016
2. Chalfin HJ et al: Role of biobanking in urology: a review. BJU Int. 118(6):864-868, 2016
3. Gaignaux A et al: A biospecimen proficiency testing program for biobank accreditation: four years of experience. Biopreserv Biobank. 14(5):429-439, 2016
4. Han HS et al: Molecular testing and the pathologist's role in clinical trials of breast cancer. Clin Breast Cancer. 16(3):166-79, 2016
5. Lewis C et al: Building a 'repository of science': the importance of integrating biobanks within molecular pathology programmes. Eur J Cancer. 67:191-199, 2016
6. Lee SM et al: Pre-analytical determination of the effect of extended warm or cold ischaemia on RNA stability in the human ileum mucosa. PLoS One. 10(9):e0138214, 2015
7. Miles G et al: Genetic testing and tissue banking for personalized oncology: analytical and institutional factors. Semin Oncol. 42(5):713-23, 2015
8. Poste G et al: The national biomarker development alliance: confronting the poor productivity of biomarker research and development. Expert Rev Mol Diagn. 15(2):211-8, 2015
9. Riondino S et al: Ensuring sample quality for biomarker discovery studies - use of ICT tools to trace biosample life-cycle. Cancer Genomics Proteomics. 12(6):291-9, 2015
10. Zhou JH et al: Biobanking in genomic medicine. Arch Pathol Lab Med. 139(6):812-8, 2015
11. Chen G et al: Cytosine deamination is a major cause of baseline noise in next-generation sequencing. Mol Diagn Ther. 18(5):587-93, 2014
12. Robb JA et al: A call to standardize preanalytic data elements for biospecimens. Arch Pathol Lab Med. 138(4):526-37, 2014
13. True LD: Methodological requirements for valid tissue-based biomarker studies that can be used in clinical practice. Virchows Arch. 464(3):257-63, 2014
14. Yong WH et al: A practical approach to clinical and research biobanking. Methods Mol Biol. 1180:137-62, 2014
15. College of American Pathologists biorepository accreditation. https://biospecimens.cancer.gov/bestpractices/Appendix6.pdf
16. National Cancer Institute Biorepositories and Research Branch Best Practice Resources. https://biospecimens.cancer.gov/bestpractices

SURGICAL/CLINICAL CONSIDERATIONS

Goal of Consultation

- To identify radioactive seed placed to mark breast lesion or abnormal lymph node
  - Radioactive seed must be stored in safe, secure place until eventual disposal

Effect on Institutional Practices

- United States Nuclear Regulatory Commission and its Agreement States authorize institutions to perform this procedure
- Institution must document that all radioactive seeds are placed and recovered according to best practices
- If seeds cannot be located, are not properly documented, or are inappropriately discarded, institutional permission to use radioactive seeds may be withdrawn

Clinical Setting

- Nonpalpable breast lesions detected by imaging must be identified in order for surgeon to locate and excise them
- Most common procedure has been for radiologist to place wire at site of lesion
  - Major disadvantage to this technique is that wire must be placed prior to surgery on same day
    - It can be difficult to coordinate radiology and surgical schedules
  - Many patients find placement of wire and waiting with wire protruding from their breast until surgery uncomfortable
- Alternative technique is for radiologist to place radioactive seed at site of lesion
  - Seeds can be placed days to weeks prior to removal
    - State law may determine length of time seed can remain prior to removal
  - Patients generally find this technique less painful and more convenient
  - Surgery can take place when convenient for patient and surgeon

Emerging Alternative Nonradioactive Localizing Procedures

- There are several disadvantages of radioactive seeds
  - Safety concerns about radioactivity require special handling and disposal of seeds
  - Regulations may limit time seed can remain within patient
  - Nonradioactive alternative would be desirable
- SAVI SCOUT radar localization system (Cianna Medical, Aliso Viejo, CA) is nonradioactive infrared (IR)-activated electromagnetic wave reflector
- Magseed (Endomagnetics, Inc., Austin, TX) is device for magnetic seed localization
- LOCalizer (Health Beacons, Concord, MA) is radiofrequency identification tag that uses radiowaves to transfer information ranging from 1 serial number to several pages of data

SPECIMEN EVALUATION

Probes

- Pathology department should be equipped with same type of gamma probe used by surgeon to localize seed
  - These probes have narrow tips (10-15 mm), allowing exact location of seed to be identified
  - They are designed to detect type of radioactivity emitted by seed
- Typical laboratory radiation detectors can detect presence of radioactivity but have wide tips and cannot determine location specifically enough within specimen
  - Geiger counter: Detects alpha particles, beta particles, and gamma rays
  - Sodium iodide survey meter: Detects gamma rays

Radioactive Seed

- Cylindrical seed measures 4.5 x 0.8 mm and consists of titanium capsule surrounding internal core filament containing iodine-125
  - Seeds are longer than clips placed by radiologists to mark core needle biopsy sites but shorter than surgical clips

Equipment in OR Consultation Suite

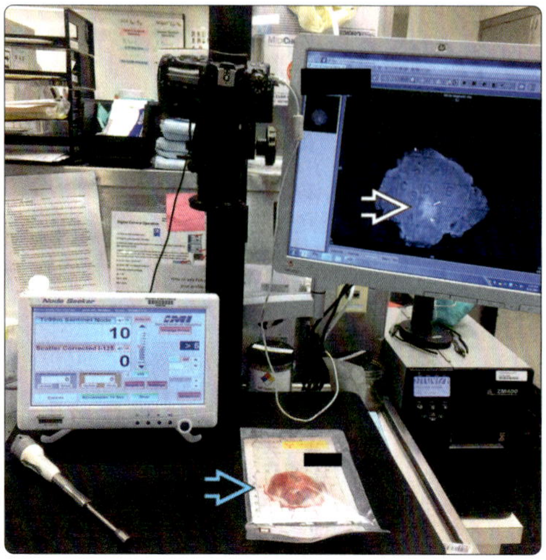

Specimen Sealed to Radiolucent Grid

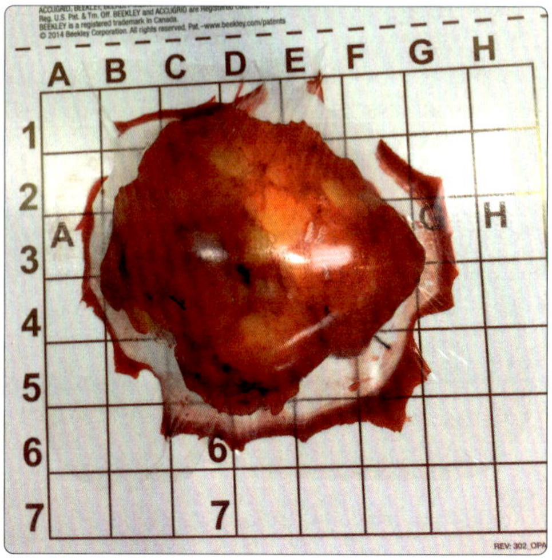

(Left) *The radioactive seed localized specimen is placed on a grid, radiographed, and sent to pathology in a sealed bag* ➔. *The digital image is reviewed in order to confirm that the seed and the biopsy clip* ➔ *are contained within the specimen and to identify their exact coordinates.* **(Right)** *The specimen is sealed to a radiolucent grid, which prevents loss of the seed and biopsy clip and facilitates their localization. The specimen radiograph will show the seed and clip within the specimen and the location according to the grid coordinates.*

Gross

- Surgeon must document that seed has been removed from patient using probe
  - Seed must be documented to be within specimen
- Specimen radiograph is taken to document location of seed, any clips present, and any findings by imaging
- Specimen radiograph must be provided to pathologist along with information that seed is present in specimen
- Occasionally, seed is displaced from specimen during surgery
  - Surgeon should retrieve seed and send it to pathology
  - Seed should not be replaced in specimen or radiographed on top of specimen
    - These practices can lead to confusion about original location of seed and can make localization of seed more difficult for pathologist
    - It is preferable for surgeon to place seed in separate specimen container and send seed in container to pathology
  - Pathologist must be aware that seed is not within specimen, as this increases possibility of seed being lost

Safety Procedures

- No special gloves, aprons, or face shields are necessary for handling seeds
  - Radiation level is very low

REPORTING

Specimen Radiograph

- Seed must be identified in specimen

Disposition of Radioactive Seed

- Retrieved seed is immediately placed in specimen container with patient identifier and caution labels
  - Seed can then be placed in shielded container for temporary storage
  - Seed must eventually be returned to nuclear medicine or radiation safety department for appropriate disposal
- Radioactive material tracking form provides documentation of seed transport from pathology laboratory to the recovering department
  - Identification, retrieval, and disposition of seed is documented in final pathology report

PITFALLS

Displacement of Radioactive Seed During Surgery or Specimen Processing

- Surgeon may transect core site resulting in extrusion of seed from specimen
- Sodium iodide survey meter or Geiger counter can be used for surveying large area in order to find displaced seed

Loss of Radioactive Seed

- All seeds placed in patients at institution must eventually be recovered and documented
- Loss of seed in operating room or during specimen processing can result in loss of institutional license to use seeds
- Procedures to prevent loss of seed should be implemented
  - Surgeon must document seed in specimen using gamma probe and by specimen radiography
  - Specimen is transported to pathology department in secure specimen container
  - Pathologist documents presence of seed in specimen container before opening container using probe
    - Specimen is carefully sectioned using probe to identify seed
  - Limiting range of where seed travels between patient and where seed will be removed from specimen is of value
    - If laboratory workflow allows, it is best to identify and remove seed in operating room consultation room next to operating room and to designate specific grossing bench for these specimens
    - All items that come in contact with specimen should be retained at grossing bench until seed is successfully obtained to avoid inadvertently discarding it into sharps container or medical waste container

Transection of Radioactive Seed

- Likelihood of transection is considered to be very low due to titanium encapsulation
  - It is possible to sever outer coating with scalpel if seed is immobilized with forceps
  - Forceps should be used carefully and scissors avoided when processing specimen
- Institutional office responsible for radiation safety should be contacted in event that seed is damaged
- Alternative specimen processing may be necessary in order to allow radioactivity within tissue to safely decay and to avoid contamination of equipment, especially if internal core filament is transected

Mistaking Core Needle Biopsy Clip for Radioactive Seed

- Some clips have cylindrical shape but are shorter than seeds
- Once removed, gamma probe must always be used to document cylindrical object is radioactive seed

SELECTED REFERENCES

1. Hayes MK: Update on preoperative breast localization. Radiol Clin North Am. 55(3):591-603, 2017
2. Gilcrease MZ et al: Transection of radioactive seeds in breast specimens. Am J Surg Pathol. 40(10):1375-1379, 2016
3. Goudreau SH et al: Preoperative radioactive seed localization for nonpalpable breast lesions: technique, pitfalls, and solutions. Radiographics. 35(5):1319-34, 2015

(**Left**) *The gamma probe is applied to the specimen at the grid coordinates suggested by the specimen radiograph. The presence of the seed is confirmed by the readings on a monitor* → *. Standard personal protective garb (gloves and apron) are sufficient for protection as the radiation level is very low.* (**Right**) *The immobilized specimen is carefully sliced with a knife* → *at the expected location of the seed. Ideally, the seed* → *is identified with a single slice into the specimen. The seed is marking a hemorrhagic core needle biopsy site.*

Gamma Probe Identification of Radioactive Seed

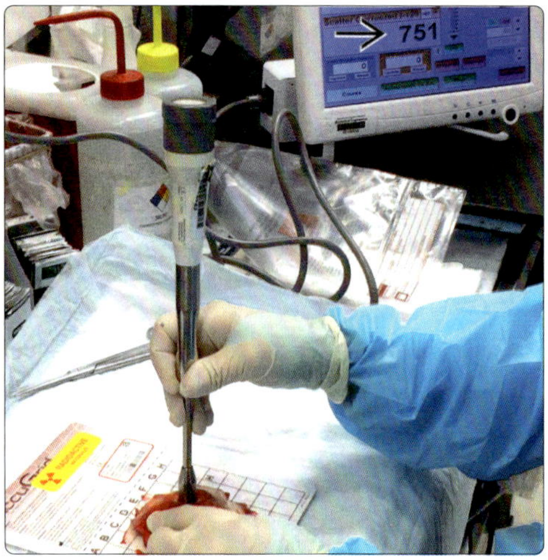

Radioactive Seed Retrieval From Specimen

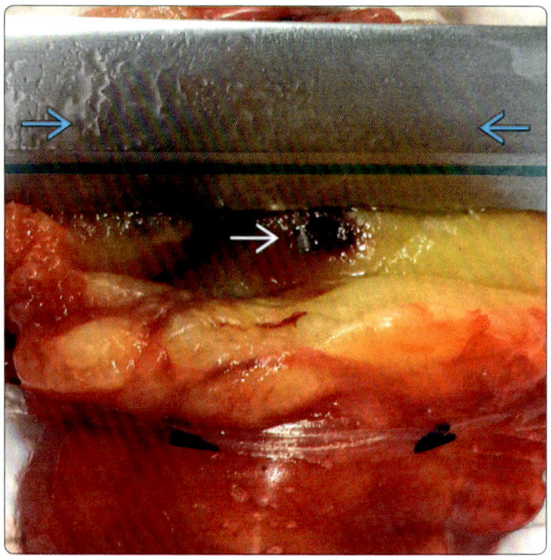

(**Left**) *The seed* → *is usually found in association with the lesion or biopsy site and the biopsy clip. It can be removed with the gentle use of forceps.* (**Right**) *The seed measures 4.5 x 0.8 mm. It is larger than biopsy clips and smaller than surgical clips. In this case, there is a portion of the gel from the biopsy site attached to the seed.*

Radioactive Seed Retrieval

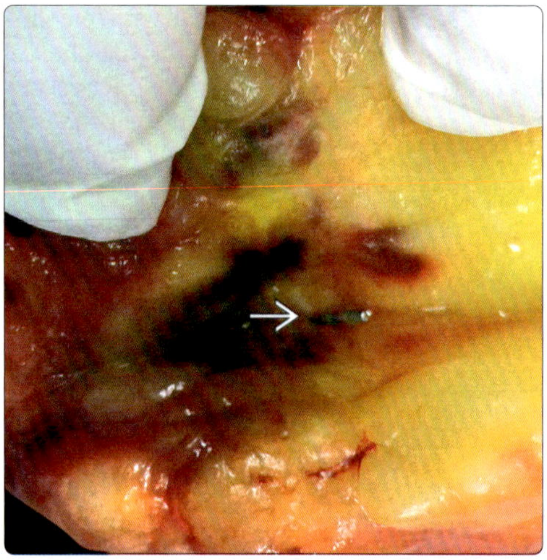

Radioactive Seed

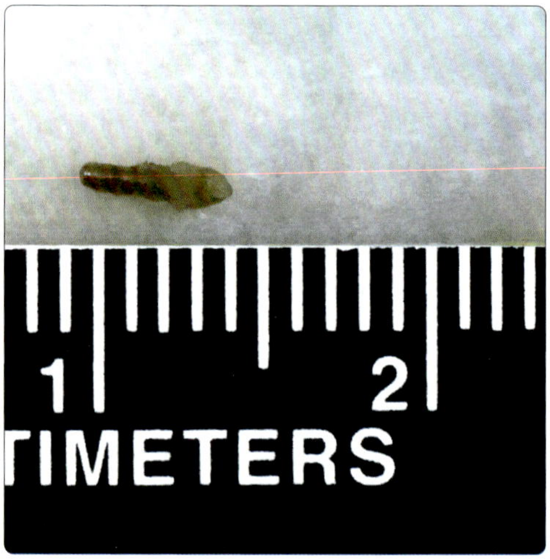

(**Left**) *The seed is collected in a glass vial or other container that can be labeled with the patient's name, the surgical pathology number, and a radiation safety caution sticker.* (**Right**) *The location of the seed in the specimen should be marked for the prosector who will process the specimen. In this case, the site has been marked by hooking a paperclip through the tissue.*

Radioactive Seed Collection

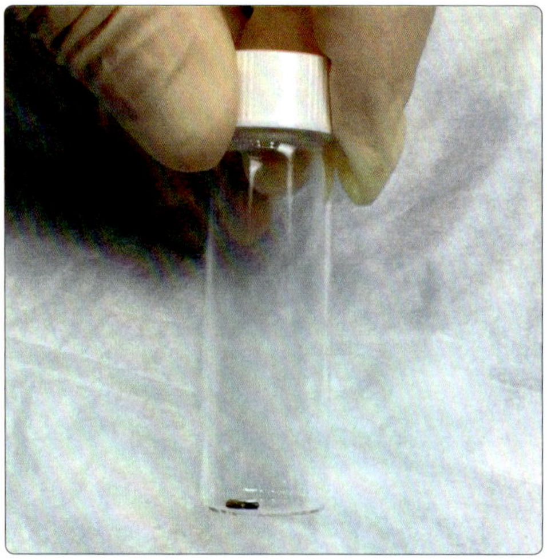

Marking Site of Radioactive Seed Removal

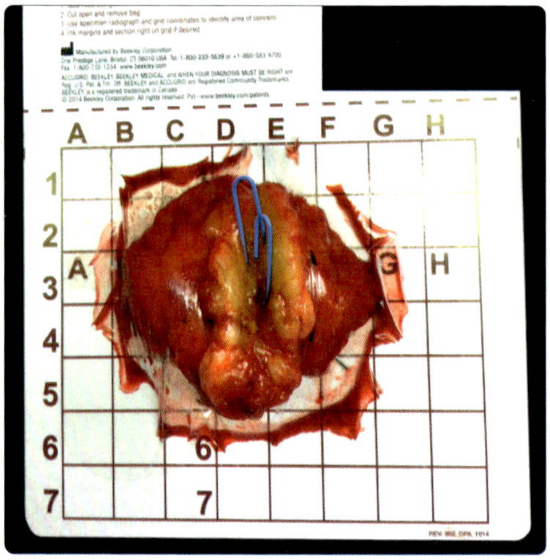

Radioactive Seed: Radiologic Appearance

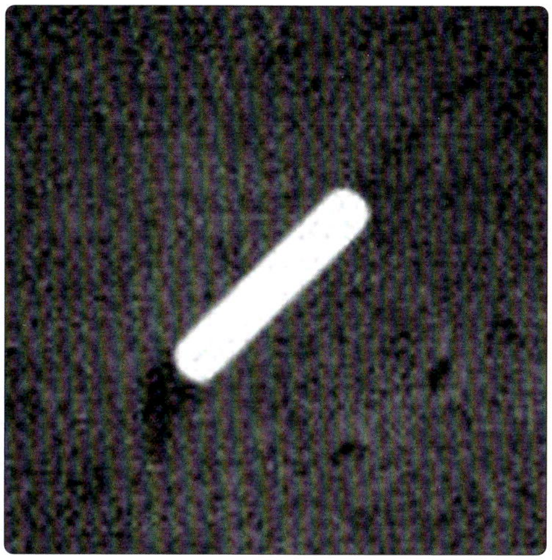

Specimen Radiograph: 2 Seeds Bracketing Calcifications

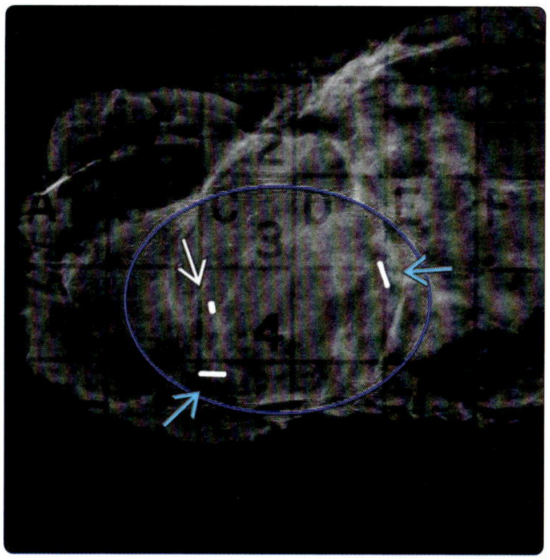

(Left) *A radioactive seed is a long cylinder. Clips placed by radiologists to mark core needle biopsy sites can also be cylindrical but are smaller in size. A seed is generally smaller than surgical clips.* **(Right)** *In this specimen radiograph, 2 seeds* ➙ *have been placed to bracket a larger area of dispersed calcifications. A clip* ➙ *is present and marks the site of a prior core needle biopsy. Note that the clip is also cylindrical but is smaller than the seeds.*

Specimen Radiograph: Clip Marking Calcifications and Seed

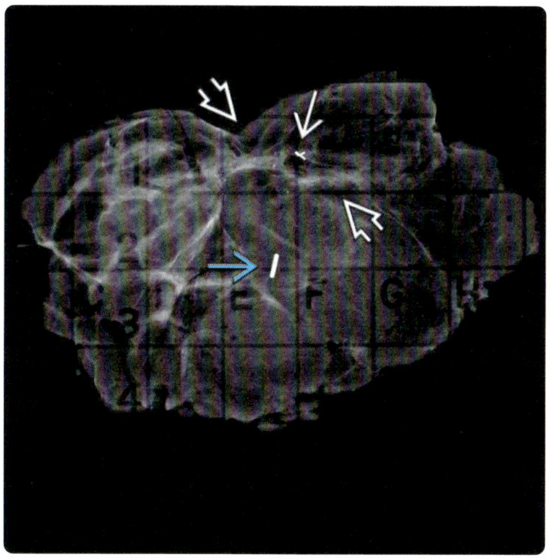

Specimen Radiograph Showing 2 Clips and 2 Seeds

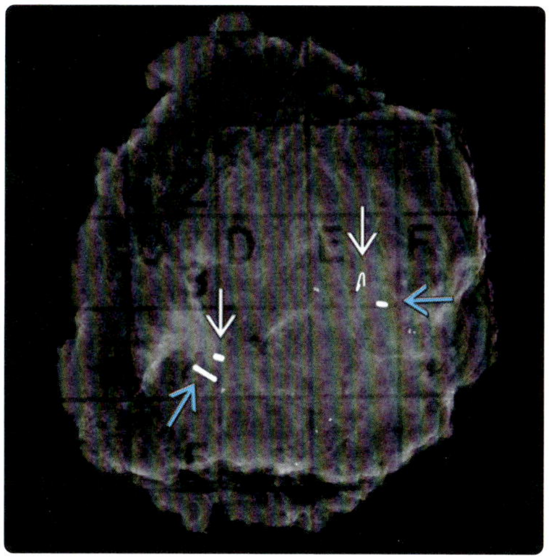

(Left) *The clip* ➙ *marking the site of a prior core needle biopsy is adjacent to the targeted cluster of calcifications* ➙*. The seed* ➙ *is slightly displaced from this area.* **(Right)** *In this specimen, 2 seeds* ➙ *have been used to mark the sites of 2 masses marked by clips* ➙ *from prior core needle biopsies. Note that one of the seeds appears smaller due to the angle of the seed in the specimen.*

Savi Scout and Clip

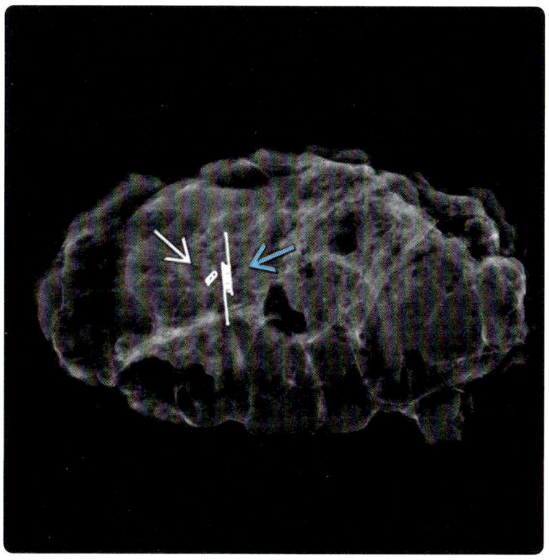

Savi Scout and Clip

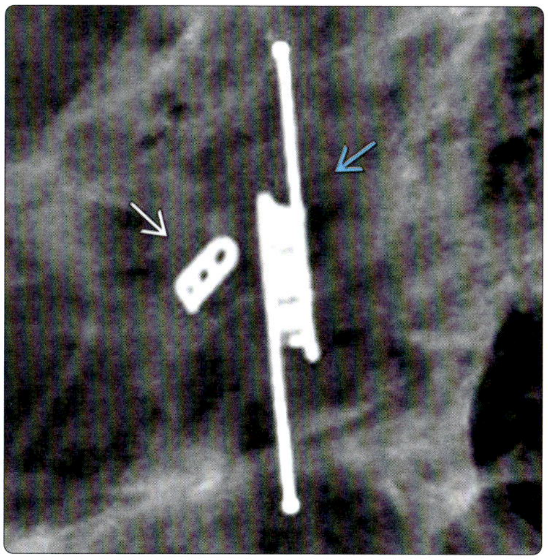

(Left) *The Savi Scout* ➙ *is a nonradioactive marker that can be used to identify the location of a clip* ➙*. The device can be disposed with other medical waste.* **(Right)** *The Savi Scout* ➙ *can be placed in the breast to allow the surgeon to identify the location of a clip* ➙*.*

MOLECULAR METHODS TO DETECT LYMPH NODE METASTASES

Purpose

- Intraoperative detection of lymph node metastases can be important for management of patients with cancer
  - Resection for possible cure may not be attempted for sites such as pancreas or lung
  - Complete axillary dissection may be performed for metastatic breast cancer
  - Removal of additional nodes after positive node is identified may not be required for staging (e.g., lung) and often increases morbidity
- Molecular methods have been proposed as alternative to frozen section for intraoperative diagnosis of metastases

Potential Advantages Compared to Histopathology

- Can detect very minimal tumor involvement in lymph nodes
- Does not require pathologist to interpret findings

Potential Disadvantages Compared to Histopathology

- Detection of very rare tumor cells in lymph nodes may not have clinical significance
- Difficult to determine size of metastasis
  - Number of mRNA copies detected correlates to some extent with size of metastasis but may not be as accurate as histology
  - May not be able to accurately discriminate between macrometastases, micrometastases, and isolated tumor cells
- Requires purchase and maintenance of specific equipment in intraoperative consultation room
- Requires training of personnel to perform and interpret assay
- Does not detect diseases other than carcinoma expressing selected marker(s)
  - Infections
  - Carcinomas not expressing selected marker(s)
  - Other types of malignancies (e.g., lymphoma, melanoma)
- Does not detect extranodal extension of carcinomas
- Results on whole nodes (i.e., without histologic confirmation) will need to be adopted for current staging systems
  - Reported as (-), (+), and (++)

TYPE OF MOLECULAR TECHNIQUES

RT-PCR

- Probes for mRNA transcripts are used to amplify corresponding sequences from RNA prepared from lymph nodes
- Method using cytokeratin 19 and mammaglobin was commercially available
  - Marketed by Veridex, LLC (GeneSearch Breast Lymph Node Test Kit) from 2007-2010
  - Withdrawn in American and European markets due to limited sales

One-Step Nucleic Acid Amplification (OSNA)

- Lysate is made from lymph node tissue and inserted into proprietary device
- RT loop-mediated isothermic amplification is used to detect targeted sequence
- Assay is completely automated
- Commercial system uses 6 primers to amplify mRNA for cytokeratin 19
  - Marketed by Sysmex Corporation in Hyogo, Japan (LYNOAMP)
  - Adopted in ~ 290 hospitals worldwide, including over 10% of hospitals in United Kingdom
  - Not used widely in United States

ACCURACY

Tissue Allocation

- If both molecular technique and histopathology are used, nodal tissue must be divided
- Small metastases typically enter through afferent lymphatic and are localized to 1 portion of node
- Bisection of node with small metastasis can result in tumor cells being present in only 1/2 of node in up to 50% of cases

Lymph Node: Histopathology

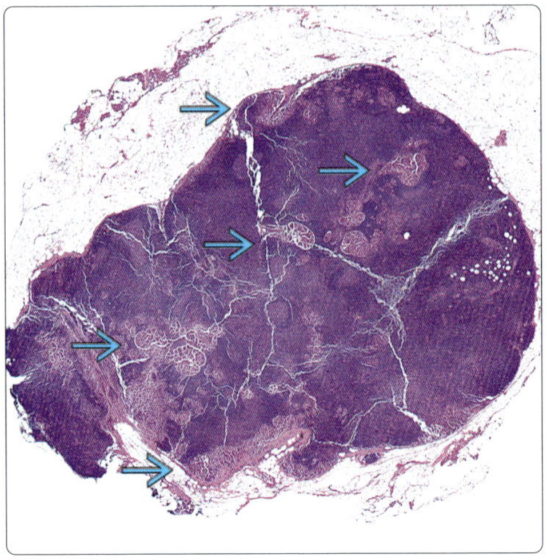

Lymph Node: Molecular Assay

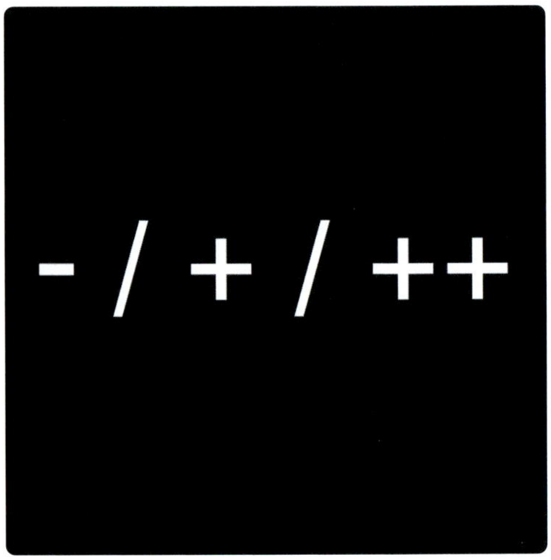

(Left) *Histopathologic evaluation of lymph nodes can determine the presence and size of metastasis* ➔ *and if there is extranodal invasion. This information can alter the subsequent intraoperative management of the patient. In addition, other disease processes can be detected (e.g., infection, sarcoidosis).* **(Right)** *Molecular assays detect the presence of mRNA transcripts in nodal tissue. The results are reported as thresholds for the amount of mRNA corresponding to a specific gene or genes expressed by epithelial cells.*

- This unequal distribution of tumor makes comparison of 2 techniques for detection of small metastases difficult
- Best allocation procedure for comparisons is to alternate thin slices to each technique
  - Highly dependent on skill of prosector
- If both histopathology and molecular methods are used, discrepancies may be difficult to resolve
  - For example, there are multiple possibilities for negative result on histopathology and positive molecular test
    - Molecular result may be false-positive result
    - Molecular method may detect minimal tumor involvement not detected by histopathology
    - Molecular method may detect macrometastasis that was missed by histopathology due to tissue allocation
    - Therefore, appropriate node classification could be N0, N0 (i+), N1mi, or N1

False-Positive Results for Molecular Assays

- Estimated to be ~ 2.5% of cases if tissue allocation is excluded as cause
- Potential reasons
  - Contamination of specimen with epithelial cells
  - Leaky transcription of epithelial genes from nonepithelial cells
  - Benign epithelial inclusions
- Clinical significance
  - Would result in patient being inappropriately identified as having metastatic disease
  - Could result in inappropriate surgery, staging, and treatment

False-Negative Results for Molecular Assays

- Estimated to be ~ 8% if tissue allocation is excluded as cause
- Potential reasons
  - Some carcinomas do not express transcript detected by assay
    - ~ 2% of carcinomas do not express CK19
  - Necrotic tumor
  - Cautery artifact
- Clinical significance
  - Would result in patient being inappropriately identified as not having metastatic disease
  - Could result in inappropriate surgery, staging, and treatment

TURNAROUND TIME

Histologic Examination

- Typically reported within ~ 20 minutes of specimen delivery
- Examination of additional nodes could take more time

Molecular Methods

- Average total time for transport, sample preparation, and amplification is 40 minutes
- Depends on number and size of nodes

COST

Histopathology

- No additional costs if intraoperative consultation is offered by facility

Molecular Techniques

- Initial cost for equipment
- Ongoing cost of reagents
- Training of personnel to perform assay and interpret results

CLINICAL IMPLICATIONS

Sentinel Lymph Nodes in Breast Cancer

- Numerous studies have compared one-step nucleic acid amplification (OSNA) to pathologic assessment of sentinel nodes in breast cancer
  - Pooled analysis shows OSNA has high specificity (94.8%), concordance rate (93.8%), and negative predictive value (97.6%)
- However, clinical utility of OSNA in this setting is questionable
- Recent clinical trials have shown that carefully selected women with positive sentinel nodes do not benefit from completion axillary dissection
- Utilization of intraoperative assessment of sentinel nodes has declined
- Detection of very small metastases (< 0.2 cm) has little prognostic significance
- Most important goal of sentinel lymph node assessment is to accurately identify macrometastases (> 0.2 cm)
  - Criticism of OSNA is that original cut-off for macrometastases (> 5,000 cytokeratin 19 mRNA copies) was set too low
  - Up to 20% of patients would be incorrectly classified as having macrometastatic disease and possibly overtreated
  - This threshold has been employed in most studies

Lung Cancer

- Surgery for cure may not be performed or delayed if metastatic disease is discovered in contralateral lymph node
- Prognostic significance of metastatic disease only detected by molecular methods needs to be investigated
- If keratin expression is used, contamination of sample by pleural mesothelial cells (due to pleural adhesions) should be considered

Other Malignant Tumors

- Studies have investigated the application of OSNA to a variety of other cancers, including gastric, colorectal, thyroid, uterine, and head and neck cancers
- Test performance (sensitivity, specificity, concordance, positive predictive value, and negative predictive value) is generally similar to that of breast cancer
- Caution is advised in application of OSNA to gynecologic cancer given possibility of benign inclusions in pelvic nodes

SELECTED REFERENCES

1. Tamaki Y: One-step nucleic acid amplification (OSNA): where do we go with it? Int J Clin Oncol. 22(1):3-10, 2017
2. Nakagawa K et al: The novel one-step nucleic acid amplification (OSNA) assay for the diagnosis of lymph node metastasis in patients with non-small cell lung cancer (NSCLC): results of a multicenter prospective study. Lung Cancer. 97:1-7, 2016
3. Yamamoto H et al: OSNA-assisted molecular staging in colorectal cancer: a prospective multicenter trial in Japan. Ann Surg Oncol. 23(2):391-6, 2016

SECTION 3

Contents

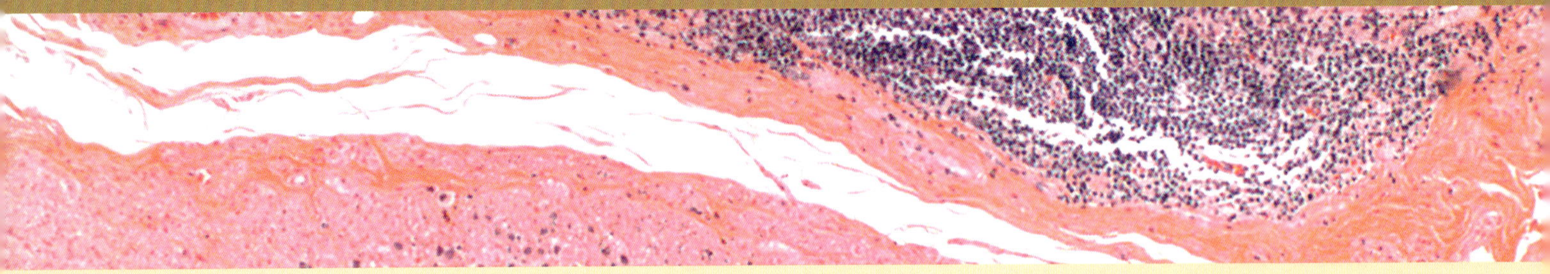

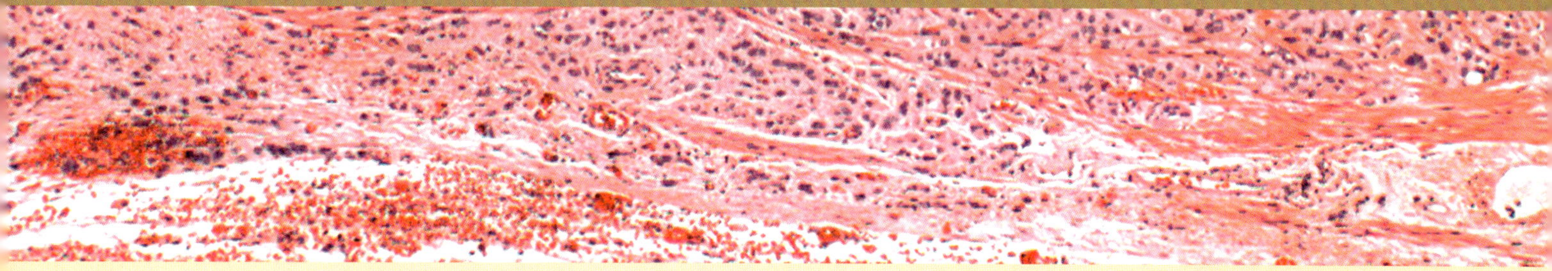

Contents

SURGICAL/CLINICAL CONSIDERATIONS

Goal of Consultation

- Diagnose mass in adrenal or at another site of paraganglia
  - Evaluate mass for malignancy
- Intraoperative diagnosis may not be needed to guide surgical management in many cases
  - Tissue may be taken for ancillary studies for some tumors

Change in Patient Management

- Additional surgery may be performed if malignancy is diagnosed

Clinical Setting

- Adrenal lesions may be detected due to functional tumors causing clinical syndromes or as image-detected masses
- Majority of tumors are cortical adenomas
  - ~ 15% are detected due to clinical syndromes
    - Cushing syndrome: Excess cortisol
    - Conn syndrome: Excess aldosterone
    - Virilization or feminization: Excess sex steroids
  - Many nonfunctional tumors are found as "incidentalomas" on imaging performed for unrelated symptoms
- Pheochromocytomas are usually detected by clinical symptoms
  - Paroxysmal hypertension, tachycardia, diaphoresis, and headache
  - Diagnosis confirmed by plasma or urine tests for catecholamines and metanephrines
- Adrenal gland may be removed as part of radical nephrectomy for renal cell carcinoma
  - Incidental adrenal lesions are usually small adenomas
  - Metastatic renal cell carcinoma to adrenal is less common
- Bilateral gland involvement can be due to adrenal cortical hyperplasia, hereditary pheochromocytoma, or metastases
- Tumors arise less commonly from other paraganglia
  - Most common are carotid body (at bifurcation of carotid artery) and organ of Zuckerkandl (at bifurcation of aorta or origin of inferior mesenteric artery)
  - May be detected due to clinical symptoms or by presence of mass by palpation or imaging

SPECIMEN EVALUATION

Gross

- **Complete excision**
  - Ink outer surface
  - Serially section through gland at 3-mm intervals
  - Identify all masses present
    - Cortical and medullary tumors can generally be identified based on gross appearance
    - Number
    - Size
    - Location: Arising in cortex or medulla or extraadrenal with secondary adrenal involvement
    - Border: Circumscribed or infiltrative
    - Color
    - Necrosis
  - Evaluate adjacent adrenal tissue
    - Normal: Golden yellow cortex ~ 3 mm, central pearly gray medulla
    - Cortical hyperplasia: Diffuse or nodular enlargement of cortex
    - Cortical atrophy: Cortex < 2 mm in thickness, fibrous thickening of capsule
    - Medullary hyperplasia: Diffuse or nodular enlargement of medulla
  - Assess involvement of adjacent tissues or organs if present
- **Needle biopsy**
  - Biopsies may be submitted to determine if adequate tissue for diagnosis is present
  - Document number and size

Frozen Section

- Small representative section of lesion may be frozen

Cortical Adenoma: Gross Appearance

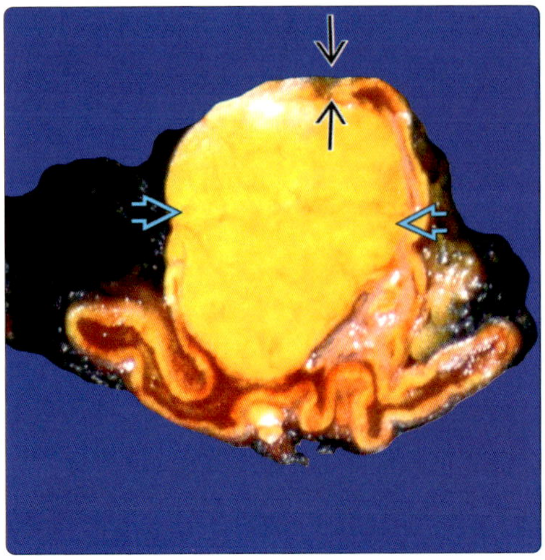

Pheochromocytoma: Gross Appearance

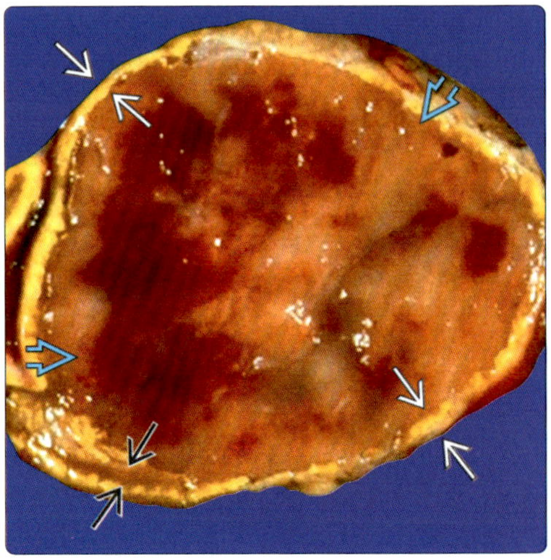

(Left) *The most common tumor of the adrenal is a benign adenoma ⇨ arising from the cortex ⇨. Many are yellow-orange in color, as is the cortex, due to the high steroid content. Cortical carcinomas are very rare.* **(Right)** *The adrenal medulla is the largest organ of the paraganglionic system. The most common tumor of this system, pheochromocytoma ⇨, arises in the medulla ⇨ and is surrounded by normal adrenal cortex ➡.*

- Only lesions > 1 cm in size should be examined by frozen section
- Entire lesion should never be frozen

Cytology

- Cytological examination may be very helpful for diagnosis
  - Origin of adrenal tumors (cortical or medullary)
  - Diagnosis of metastatic tumors

MOST COMMON DIAGNOSES

Adrenal Cortical Adenoma

- Well-circumscribed mass arising from cortex
  - Usually unilateral and solitary
- Majority < 5 cm
  - Carcinomas are usually larger
- Tumor cells arranged in nesting/alveolar pattern, short cords, anastomosing trabeculae, or mixture of patterns
  - Mitotic figures absent or rare
  - Necrosis uncommon
- Cushing syndrome
  - Moderately sized adenomas with bright yellow color
  - Cause suppression of ACTH by producing cortisol
    - Results in atrophy of normal gland
- Conn syndrome
  - Often small (< 2 cm) and pale in color
  - Overproduce aldosterone
    - Normal gland is not affected
- Adenomas associated with virilization or feminization
  - Typically large (> 10 cm) and tan-white to brown
- Nonfunctioning adenomas
  - May be small or large
  - Geographic or mottled zones of dark pigmentation may be present

Adrenal Cortical Carcinoma

- Bulky tumors with red-brown fleshy, firm appearance
  - Typically unilateral and large
    - If bilateral, consider contralateral metastasis
- Histologically diverse
  - May resemble normal adrenal
  - Patternless sheets or nests of cells
  - Broad trabeculae and fine sinusoids
  - Clear to eosinophilic cytoplasm
  - Nuclei range from bland to highly atypical
  - Variable mitotic rate
- It is not possible to predict malignant behavior with certainty
- High nuclear pleomorphism, chromatin irregularities, and prominent nucleoli favor carcinoma

Pheochromocytoma and Paraganglioma

- Paraganglia are distributed symmetrically from base of skull to pelvis
  - Most common site for neoplasm is adrenal medulla
  - Other sites include
    - Carotid body (at bifurcation of carotid artery)
    - Organ of Zuckerkandl (at bifurcation of aorta or origin of inferior mesenteric artery)
    - Glomus tympanicum (middle ear)
    - Glomus jugulare (jugular foramen)
  - Increased malignant potential is observed for head and neck sites
- Typically yellow-white to red-brown circumscribed tumors 5-8 cm in size
  - May have necrosis, hemorrhage, or cystic degeneration
- ~ 10% are bilateral
- In adrenal, these tumors arise from medulla
  - ~ 30% are associated with hereditary syndromes
    - At least 10 susceptibility genes have been identified
    - Medullary hyperplasia may be present (increased thickness &/or multiple nodules)
- Cells have nested zellballen pattern
  - Basophilic cytoplasm; bizarre, isolated, atypical nuclei
  - Zellballen are surrounded by inconspicuous glial-type sustentacular cells
- ~ 10% will have malignant behavior (locally invasive with metastases)
  - Difficult to predict this group based on histologic features
  - Features associated with, but not diagnostic of, malignant behavior include
    - Large nests or diffuse growth
    - Central or confluent tumor necrosis
    - High cellularity
    - Spindle cell pattern
    - High mitotic rate (> 3 mitoses/10 HPF)
    - Vascular or capsular invasion

Metastasis

- Majority of metastatic carcinomas are from lung or kidney
  - More likely to be bilateral
- May be difficult to determine origin of primary tumor

Myelolipoma

- Well-circumscribed, soft, tan-yellow to focally red-brown mass
  - Resembles adipose tissue with focal fibrous areas
- Lesion is within adrenal gland and may compress it
- Tumor consists of adipose tissue and bone marrow elements
- 20% associated with tuberous sclerosis

Adrenal Cortical Hyperplasia

- Diffuse: Uniform increase in thickness of cortex
  - Most commonly due to pituitary Cushing disease (pituitary adenoma producing ACTH)
- Nodular: Multiple nodules in both glands
  - Most commonly primary hyperplasia (etiology unknown)

Primary Pigmented Adrenal Cortical Disease

- Bilateral adrenal involvement with multiple pigmented (black, brown, or red) nodules of cortical hyperplasia
  - Clinical history of Cushing syndrome
  - 90% of cases associated with Carney complex

Adrenal Cyst

- Usually small and unilocular and filled with serous or serosanguineous fluid
  - May arise from blood vessels or lymphatics
- Some are pseudocysts without identifiable lining

Distinguishing Between Adrenal Cortical Adenoma and Adrenal Cortical Carcinoma

Criteria	Adenoma	Carcinoma
Mitoses	Rare to absent	> 5/50 HPF, may be atypical
Venous invasion	Absent	Present
Weight	< 50 g	> 100 g
Necrosis	Absent	Present with confluent necrosis
Hormone production	Often functional	Usually nonfunctional
Color	Variable	Variable; does not differentiate from adenoma
Borders	Well circumscribed	Invasive
Hemorrhage	Absent	Frequent
Necrosis	Absent	Frequent
Capsular invasion	Absent	Usually present
Invasion into adjacent tissues	Absent	Usually present
Intratumoral fibrosis	May be present	Usually present
Myxomatous degeneration	May be present	Usually present
Nuclear atypia	May have nuclear atypia	Nuclear atypia usually present
Diffuse architecture (patternless sheets of cells)	Usually absent	May be present

Adjacent Neoplasm Compressing Adrenal

- Identification of normal adrenal is crucial to confirm lesion did not arise from adrenal
- Lymphomas can arise from adjacent nodes and surround adrenal
- Tissue for ancillary studies to identify tumor may be helpful

Pediatric Tumors

- All very rare
- More likely to be neuroblastoma, ganglioneuroblastoma, or ganglioneuroma than cortical tumors or pheochromocytoma
- **Neuroblastoma**
  - Soft and hemorrhagic with frequent areas of necrosis
  - Cysts may be present
  - May invade into surrounding tissue
- **Ganglioneuroma and ganglioneuroblastoma**
  - Firmer, white to tan, and may have areas of calcification
  - If there are gross areas resembling neuroblastoma, these should be sampled for ancillary testing
- Eligibility for treatment protocols is often based on results of ancillary testing
  - Nonfixed tissue may be required for cytogenetic studies, molecular studies (frozen), and electron microscopy

REPORTING

Frozen Section

- Presence or absence of neoplasm
- Specific diagnosis when possible
  - If definitive diagnosis of adenoma or carcinoma or pheochromocytoma can be made, this should be reported
- Report if invasion into large vessels or adjacent structures is identified
- There is no need to report margins

Cytology

- Report diagnosis when possible

PITFALLS

Benign vs. Malignant Cortical Neoplasms

- No single feature is diagnostic of carcinoma
- Usually not distinction that needs to be made intraoperatively

Adenoma vs. Metastatic Renal Cell Carcinoma

- Cytoplasm of adrenal adenoma cells is vacuolated, whereas cytoplasm of renal cell carcinoma should be clear
  - May be more evident on cytologic preparations
- **Caution**: It may be very difficult to differentiate these neoplasms, specially on frozen section

Cortical Neoplasm vs. Pheochromocytoma

- Pheochromocytoma has nested and zellballen pattern with basophilic cytoplasm and bizarre, isolated, atypical nuclei
  - Pheochromocytoma has usually been diagnosed preoperatively
- **Caution**
  - Occasionally, these tumors have similar histopathological appearance
  - Adrenal cortical neoplasms may also have intranuclear inclusions

SELECTED REFERENCES

1. Lam A: Lipomatous tumours in adrenal gland: WHO updates and clinical implications. Endocr Relat Cancer. 24(3):R65-R79, 2017
2. Martínez Manzano Á et al: Calcified adrenal pseudocyst: a rare pathology. Cir Esp. ePub, 2017
3. Yamazaki Y et al: Histopathological classification of cross-sectional image negative hyperaldosteronism. J Clin Endocrinol Metab. jc20162986, 2016
4. Phitayakorn R et al: Perioperative considerations in patients with adrenal tumors. J Surg Oncol. 106(5):604-10, 2012

Cortical Adenoma: Gross Appearance Associated With Cushing Syndrome

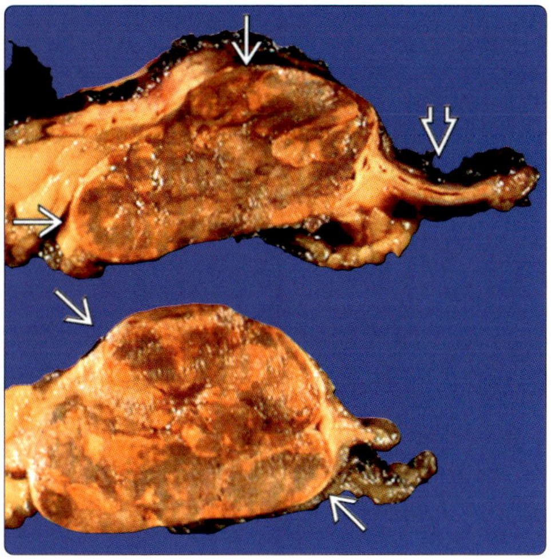

Cortical Adenoma: Gross Appearance Associated With Cushing Syndrome

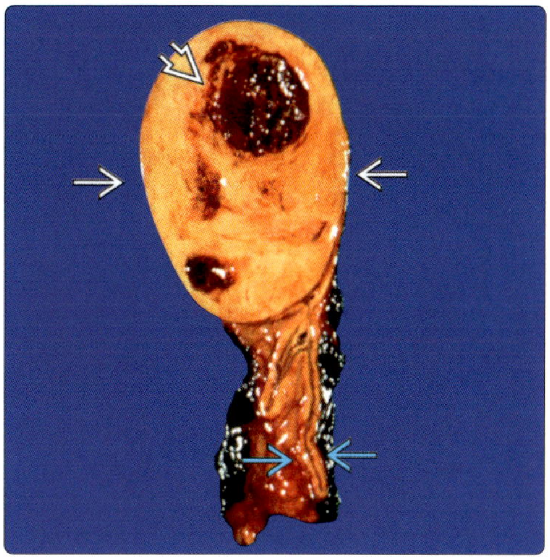

(Left) *Cortisol-producing adenomas ➡ cause downregulation of ACTH, which, in turn, causes atrophy of the normal adrenal cortex ➡. The mottled appearance with areas of dark discoloration is due to the compact eosinophilic cytoplasm of the tumor cells, lipid depletion, and increased lipofuscin pigment.* **(Right)** *This cortisol-secreting adenoma ➡ shows the typical well-circumscribed, golden-yellow appearance with an old hemorrhage ➡. The cortex of the normal adrenal gland is atrophied ➡.*

Cortical Adenoma: Pigment

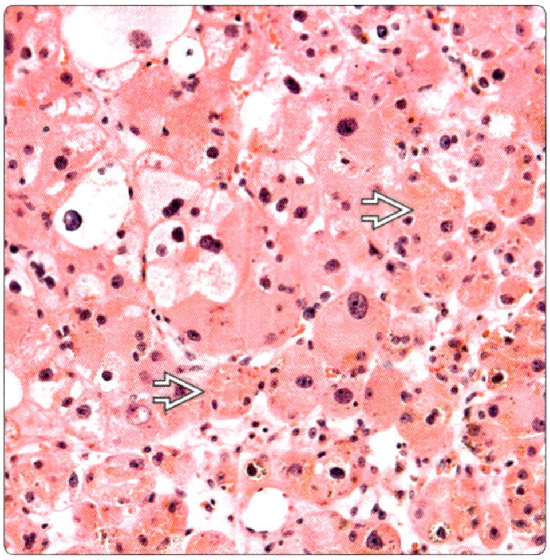

Cortical Adenoma: Cytoplasmic Clearing

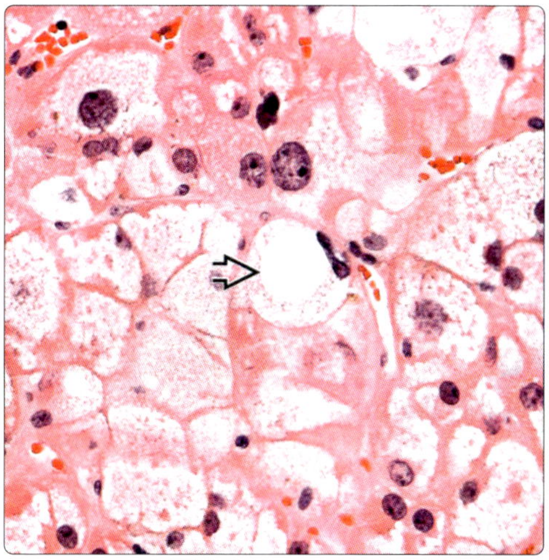

(Left) *The tumor cells in cortisol-producing adrenal adenomas are arranged in a solid pattern with cytoplasmic lipofuscin pigment ➡, gradation in cell size, and a varying amount of lipid. Nuclear pleomorphism can be present but is not an indication of malignancy.* **(Right)** *In this cortisol-producing adenoma, the tumor cells are arranged in short cords or clusters. Individual tumor cells contain abundant lipid, which appears as numerous clear vacuoles ➡. There is variation in nuclear size.*

Cortical Adenoma: Gross Appearance Associated With Virilization

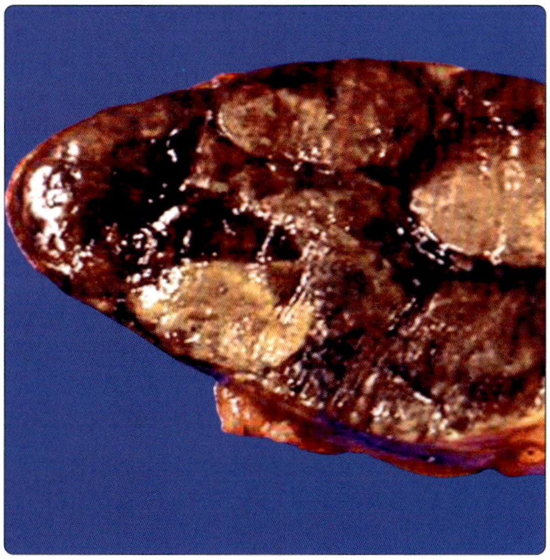

Cortical Adenoma: Oncocytic Cells

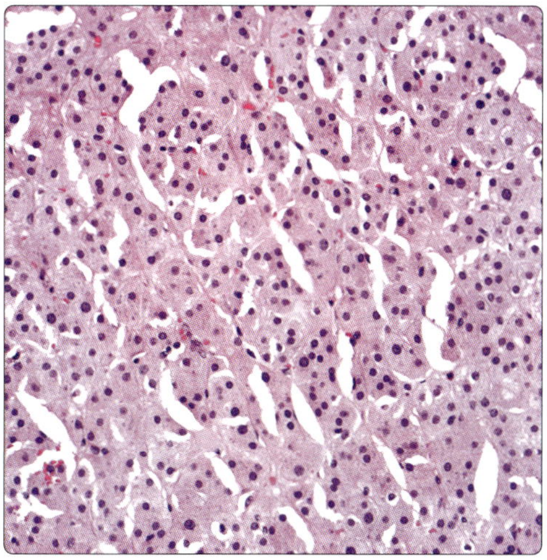

(Left) *Cortical adenomas associated with virilization or feminization are generally large (> 1,000 g). This cortical adenoma has a mottled appearance with areas of dark discoloration due to lipid depletion, hemorrhage, and increased lipofuscin pigment.* **(Right)** *This adrenal cortical adenoma was detected due to secretion of sex steroids and consists of eosinophilic cells with abundant cytoplasm. This pattern resemble the cells in the zona reticularis, the cells that normally produce sex steroids.*

(Left) *Adrenal cortical adenomas are well circumscribed and generally limited to the adrenal gland. Areas of hemorrhage may be present ➡. In contrast, adrenal cortical carcinomas are generally much larger (> 6 cm), and the normal gland may be difficult to identify.* **(Right)** *This adrenal cortical adenoma has a well-circumscribed border with a thick fibrous capsule ⇨. Capsular invasion can be seen in some benign tumors and is not a definitive predictor of malignant behavior.*

Cortical Adenoma: Gross Appearance, Hemorrhage

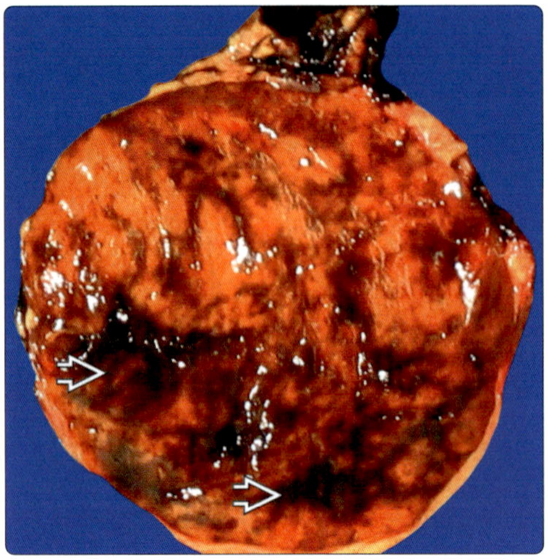

Cortical Adenoma: Capsule

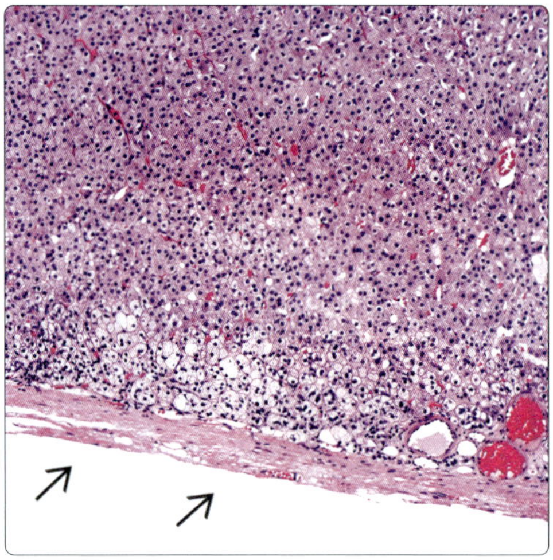

(Left) *Aldosterone-producing tumors ➡ are generally smaller and paler in color compared to adenomas that produce cortisol. The zona glomerulosa (the zone of aldosterone-producing cells) ⇨ in the adjacent adrenal gland is also often increased in thickness.* **(Right)** *This aldosterone-secreting adenoma shows a typical nesting pattern as well as large lipid-rich cells with finely vacuolated cytoplasm, which are usually the predominant cell type.*

Cortical Adenoma: Gross Appearance Associated With Conn Syndrome

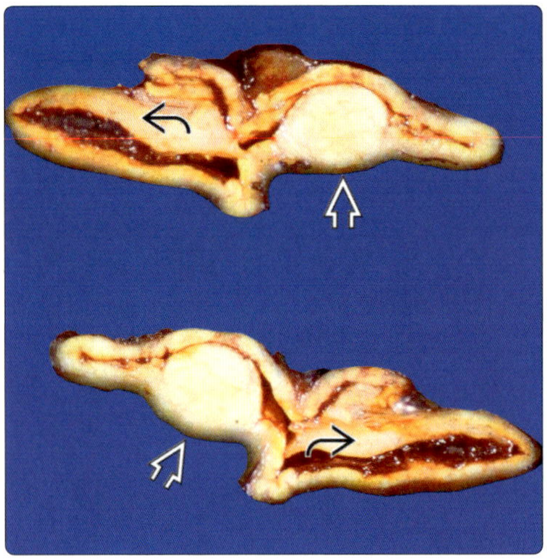

Cortical Adenoma: Lipid-Rich Cells

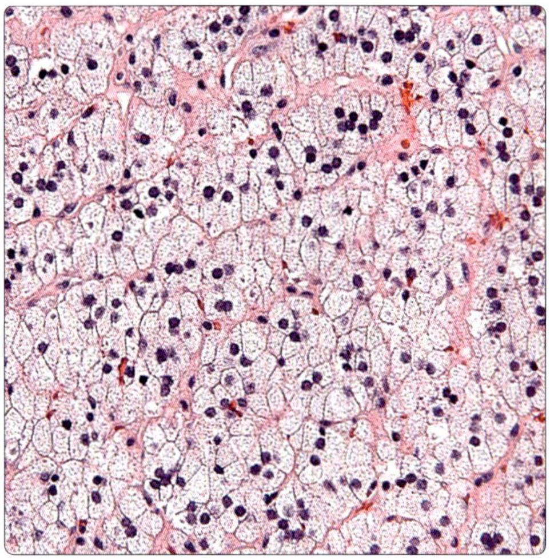

(Left) *This cortisol-producing adrenal cortical adenoma is composed of large cells with eosinophilic cytoplasm and enlarged hyperchromatic nuclei. Prominent intranuclear inclusions ⇨ can be present.* **(Right)** *More than 90% of adrenal masses in patients with renal cell carcinoma are benign adenomas or hyperplasia. A metastasis grossly can closely resemble a cortical adenoma. However, the cells of renal cell carcinoma have clear cytoplasm ⇨ rather than the finely reticulated cytoplasm seen in adenomas.*

Cortical Adenoma: Oncocytic Cells With Nuclear Pseudoinclusions

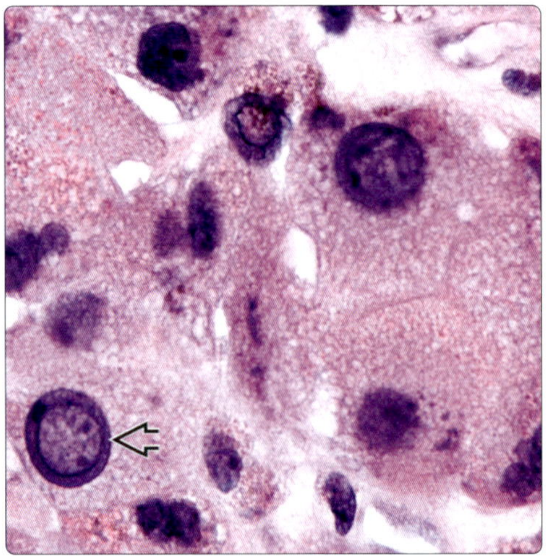

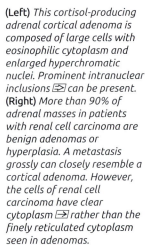

Metastatic Renal Cell Carcinoma: Clear Cytoplasm

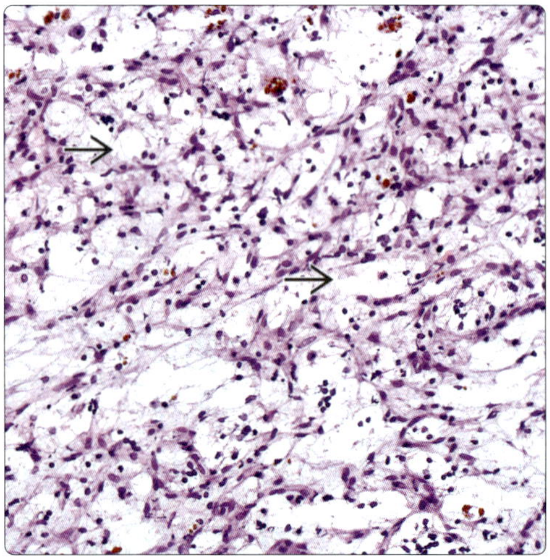

Cortical Carcinoma: Gross Appearance

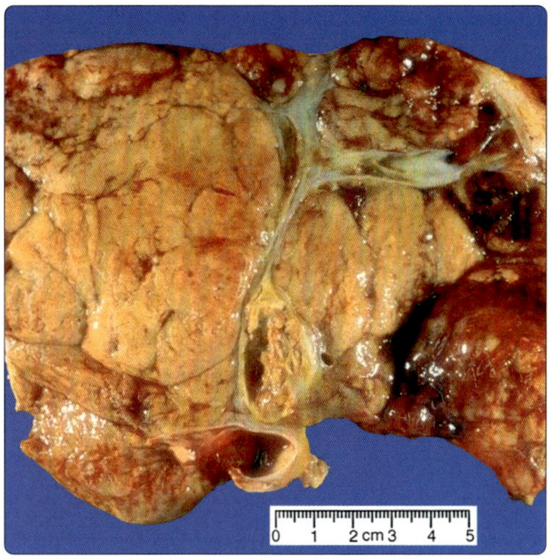

Cortical Carcinoma: Gross Appearance

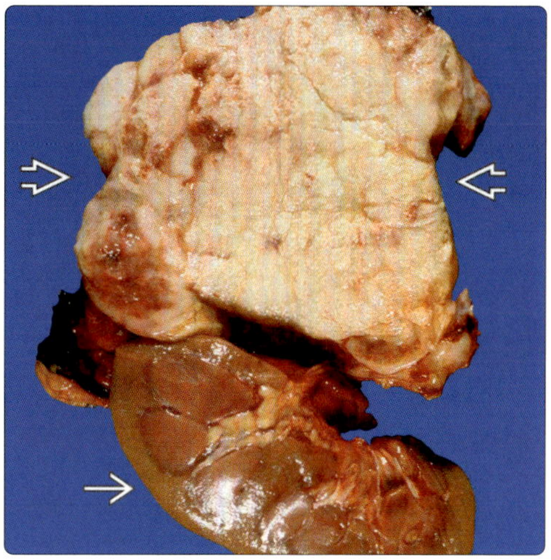

(Left) *This adrenal cortical carcinoma forms an irregularly shaped, bulky, unilateral mass and has a light brown, variegated, cut surface. There is also extensive necrosis, degenerative changes, hemorrhage, and calcification. More than 90% of tumors weighing > 50 g behave in a malignant fashion.* **(Right)** *This adrenal cortical carcinoma ➡ has been excised with a radical nephrectomy ➡. The tumor forms a large fleshy mass with areas of necrosis. The residual adrenal gland cannot be seen.*

Cortical Carcinoma: Gross Appearance

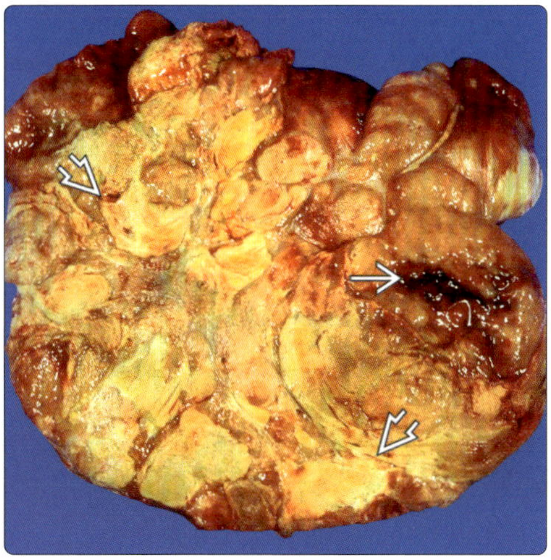

Cortical Carcinoma: Cytologic Preparation

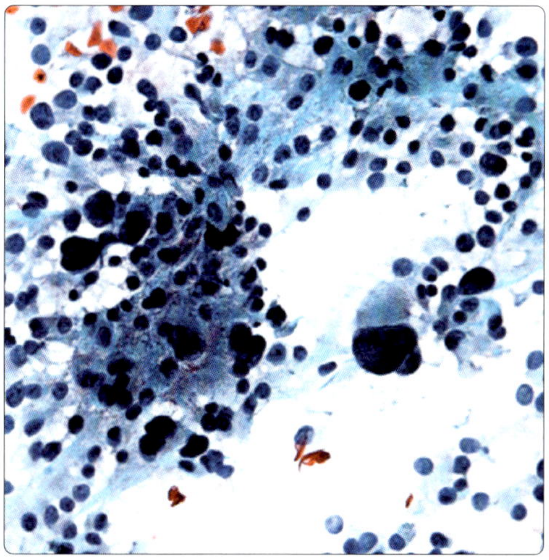

(Left) *This rare pediatric adrenal cortical carcinoma has a yellow, pink, to light brown variegated cut surface with extensive areas of necrosis ➡, degenerative changes, and hemorrhagic areas ➡. Neuroblastoma and ganglioneuroma are more common tumors in this age group.* **(Right)** *Cytologic diagnosis of adrenal cortical carcinoma can be challenging. The degree of nuclear pleomorphism and nuclear irregularity shown in this cytologic preparation favors carcinoma, confirmed on permanent sections.*

Cortical Neoplasm

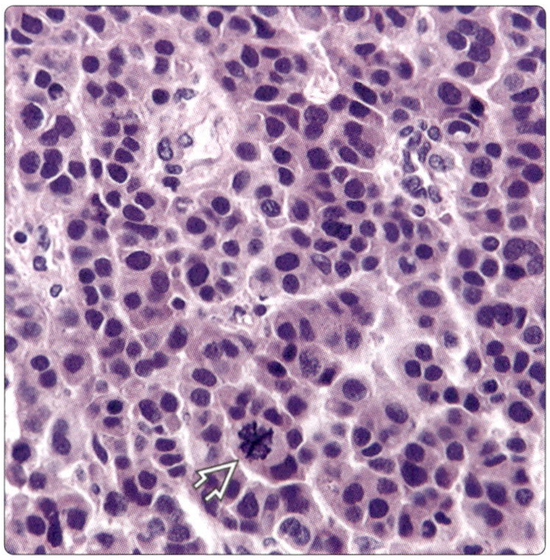

Cortical Carcinoma: Vascular Invasion

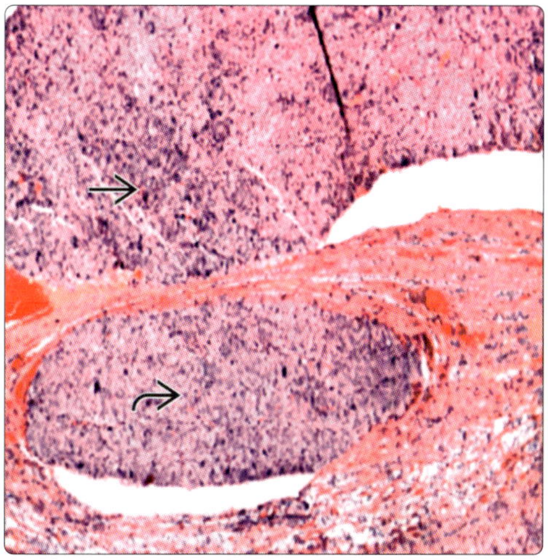

(Left) *It is difficult to predict the clinical behavior of cortical tumors, although high-risk lesions can be identified. A high mitotic rate, especially when combined with the presence of atypical mitoses ➡, is generally seen only in malignant tumors.* **(Right)** *A tumor embolus ➡ attached to the wall of a large vein with a muscular coat is seen adjacent to adrenal cortical carcinoma ➡. This finding is generally seen only in adrenal cortical tumors behaving in a malignant fashion.*

Pheochromocytoma: Anatomic Location

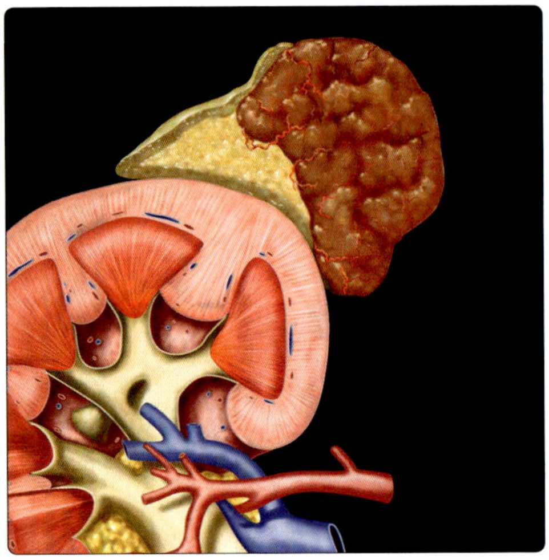

Pheochromocytoma and Medullary Hyperplasia: Gross Appearance

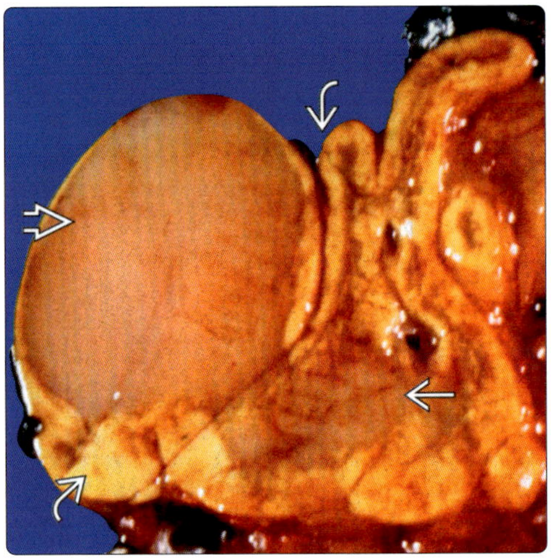

(Left) *Over 1/3 of pheochromocytomas are associated with germline mutations, including MEN2, von Hippel Lindau, and familial pheochromocytoma. The association is stronger if the patient is < 18 years of age (~ 60%) and if involvement is bilateral (~ 85%).* **(Right)** *This small pheochromocytoma is gray-pink and homogeneous, which distinguishes it from the bright yellow cortex. The presence of medullary hyperplasia in the adjacent gland suggests that the patient may have a germline mutation.*

Pheochromocytoma: Gross Appearance With Central Necrosis

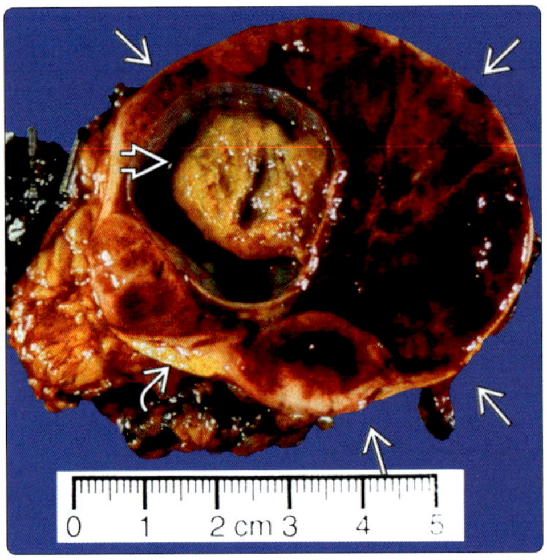

Pheochromocytoma: Gross Appearance With Hemorrhage

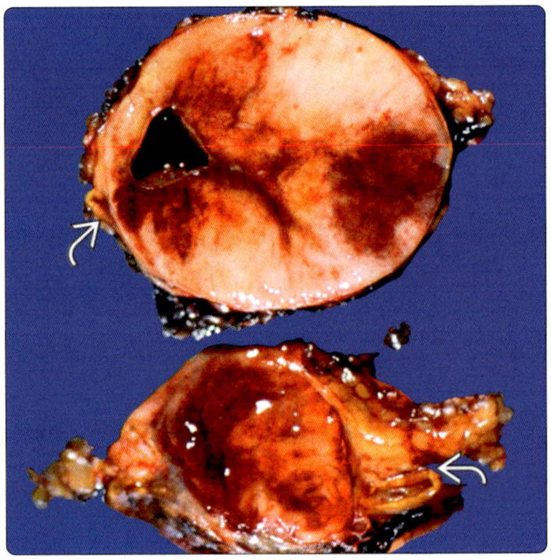

(Left) *This well-circumscribed adrenal pheochromocytoma has a central area of necrosis and hemorrhage. A small area of residual cortex is present. Central necrosis is more common in tumors that metastasize but is not a definitive criterion for malignancy.* **(Right)** *This well-circumscribed adrenal pheochromocytoma has areas of hemorrhage. The gross appearance of pheochromocytomas is variable and may mimic other tumors. A small area of residual adrenal cortex is present.*

Pheochromocytoma: Cytologic Appearance

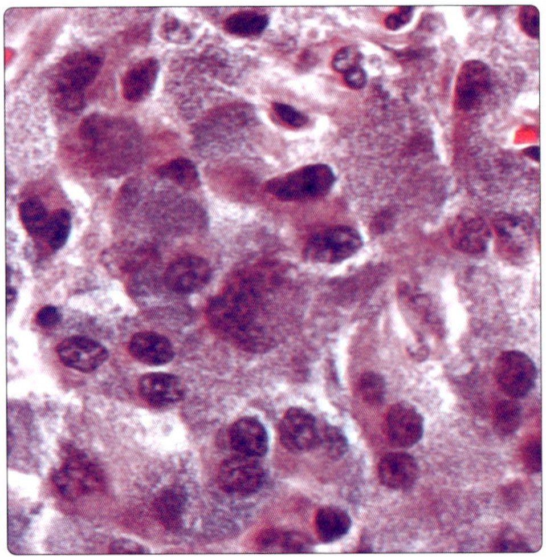

Pheochromocytoma: Hyaline Globules

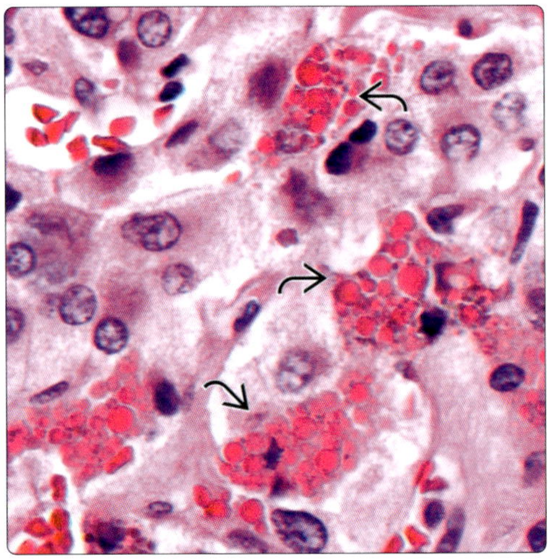

(Left) *Pheochromocytoma may contain cells with ample basophilic, amphophilic, or clear cytoplasm. This tumor shows the characteristic basophilic granular cytoplasm of some of these tumors. Nuclear pleomorphism is not a strong predictor of malignant behavior.* **(Right)** *An individual pheochromocytoma can contain a mixed population of small cells and large cells with prominent nucleoli. Hyaline globules are present in some pheochromocytomas but may also be present in some adrenal cortical tumors.*

Pheochromocytoma With Medullary Hyperplasia: Gross Appearance

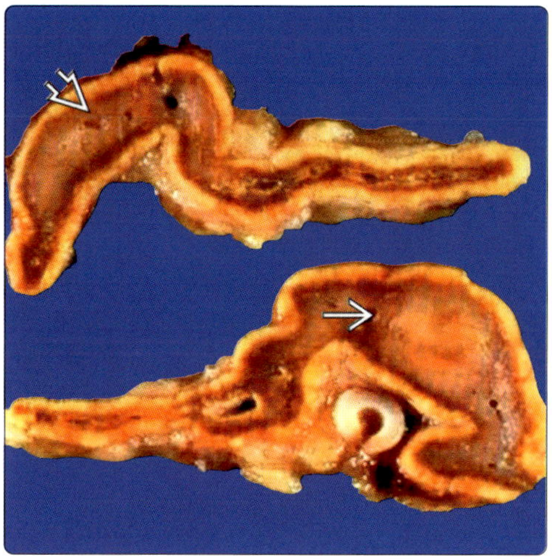

Pheochromocytoma: Cellular Pleomorphism

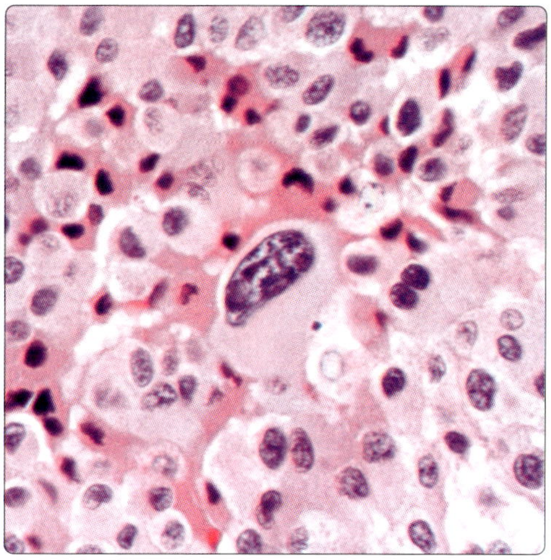

(Left) *This adrenal gland shows both MEN2-associated adrenal medullary hyperplasia ⇨ and a small pheochromocytoma ➡. Adrenal medullary hyperplasia is a characteristic finding in patients with MEN2. Tumors may be bilateral.* **(Right)** *The growth of this pheochromocytoma is patternless with thin fibrous septa and lacks the more usual zellballen cellular arrangement. There is marked variability in cell size with scattered pleomorphic cells surrounded by smaller tumor cells.*

Pheochromocytoma: Mitoses

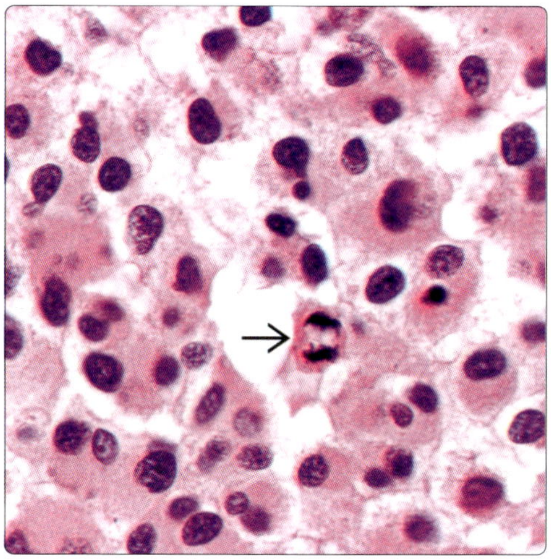

Pheochromocytoma: Atypical Mitosis

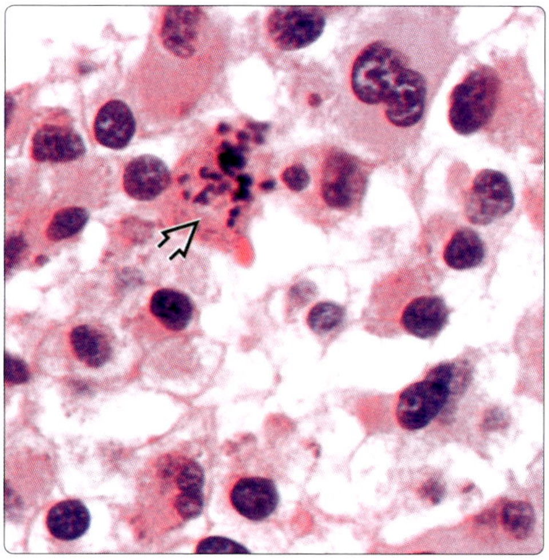

(Left) *Although the classic pattern of pheochromocytoma is a zellballen pattern, numerous variants and combined patterns exist, including diffuse growth, large zellballen, spindle cells, and cell cords. Mitotic figures → may be present.* **(Right)** *Malignant behavior is difficult to predict for pheochromocytomas. This malignant tumor showed an increased mitotic rate, atypical mitotic figures ⇨, and a diffuse growth pattern composed of compact eosinophilic cells.*

Pheochromocytoma: Proliferation

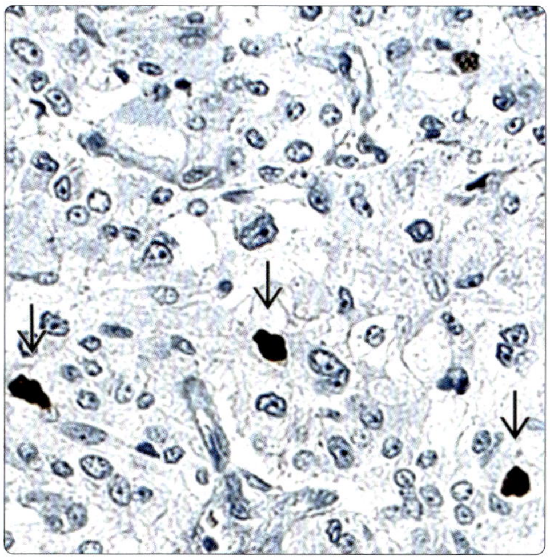

Paraganglioma Metastatic to Liver: Gross Appearance

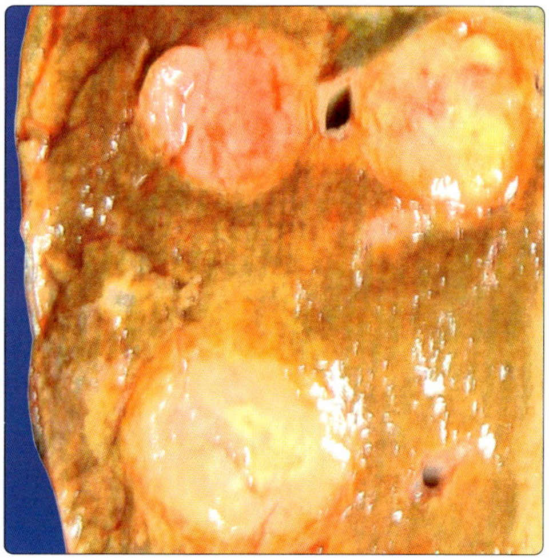

(Left) *Primary and metastatic pheochromocytomas usually have low proliferation. Increased proliferation detected by mitotic count or Ki-67(+) cells → is rare and, when present, may be associated with aggressive behavior.* **(Right)** *It is difficult to predict malignant behavior in paragangliomas. Ultimately, the only definite criterion for malignancy is the finding of metastases. These liver metastases occurred in a patient with a hereditary SDHB-associated malignant middle ear paraganglioma.*

Contents

(**Left**) *This paraganglioma was the cause of paroxysmal hypertension in a young patient. The tumor is fairly well circumscribed and tan with a thin fibrous pseudocapsule and areas of degenerative changes.* (**Right**) *The typical tumor cells of a paraganglioma have round to oval nuclei and eosinophilic, finely granular cytoplasm. The cells are organized into nests of cells (zellballen) that are surrounded by sustentacular cells. Nuclear atypia may be present but is not an indication of malignancy.*

Paraganglioma: Gross Appearance

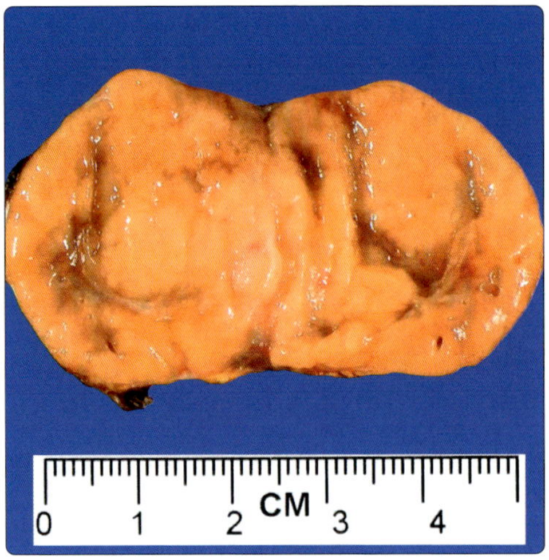

Middle Ear Paraganglioma

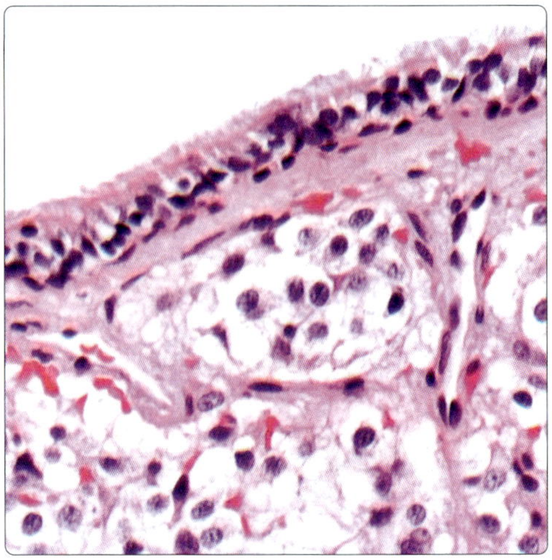

(**Left**) *Sustentacular cells* ➔ *are glial-type cells that have features of nonmyelin-forming Schwann cells. They are found in paragangliomas and some types of carcinoid tumors. They are less frequent in paragangliomas that exhibit malignant behavior. They are occasionally present in metastatic tumors.* (**Right**) *The spindle-shaped sustentacular cells* ➔ *surrounding the zellballen of a paraganglioma are more easily seen using an immunohistochemical study for S100.*

Paraganglioma

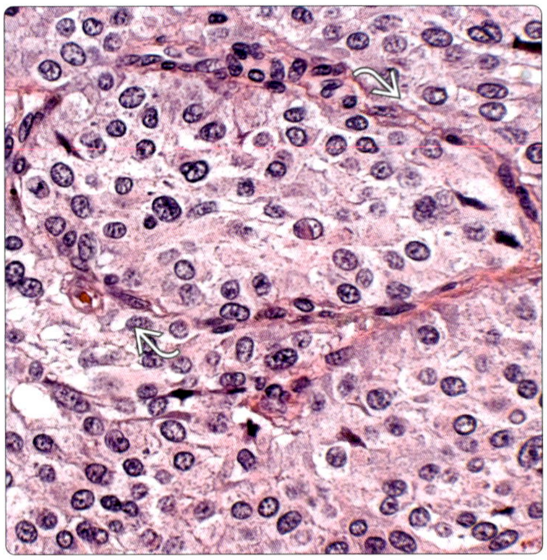

Paraganglioma: Sustentacular Cells

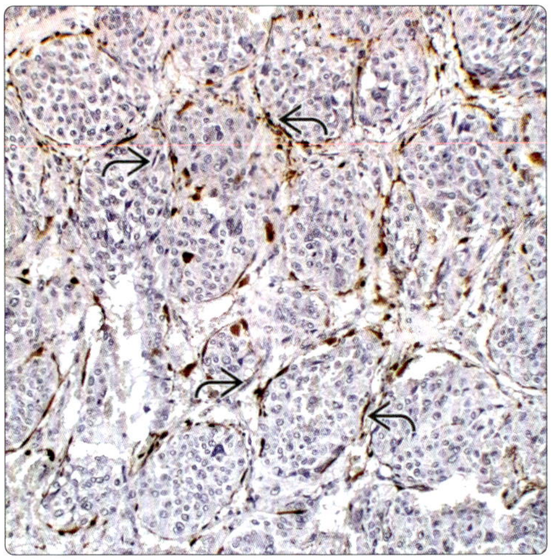

(**Left**) *Scattered cells with marked increase in nuclear size* ➔*, bizarre forms, and irregular nuclear membranes can be seen in paragangliomas but are not indicative of malignant behavior.* (**Right**) *Only a small subset of paragangliomas behave in a malignant fashion. It is very difficult to predict this group based on the histologic appearance. Although this paraganglioma invades into adjacent adipose tissue, this is not an indication of definitive malignant behavior and metastasis.*

Paraganglioma: Pleomorphic Cells

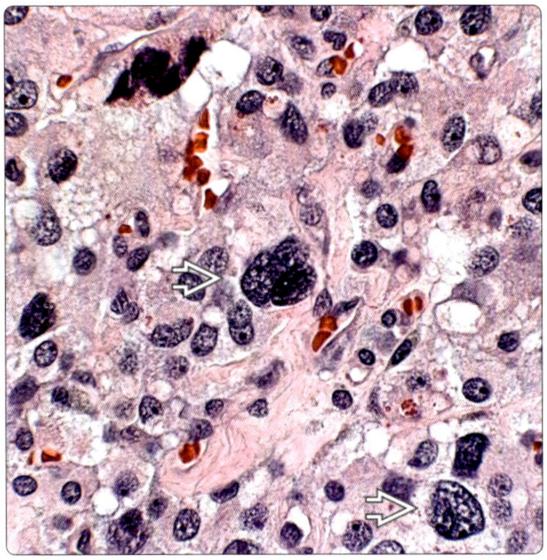

Paraganglioma: Invasion

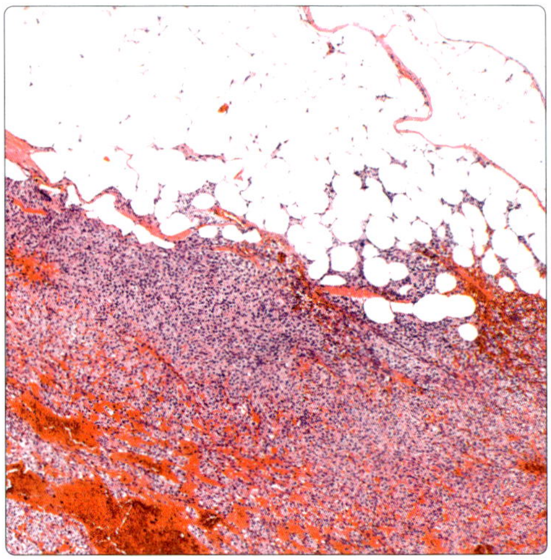

Primary Pigmented Nodular Adrenal Disease: Gross Appearance

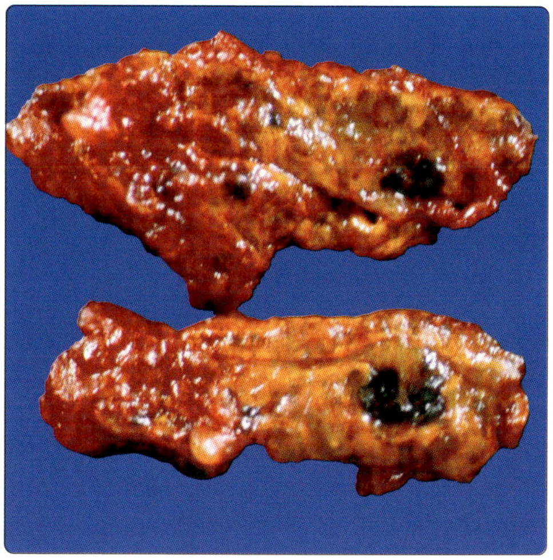

Adrenal Myelolipoma: Gross Appearance

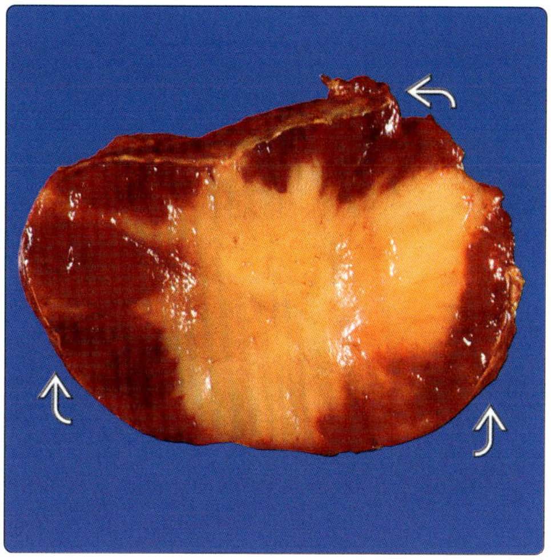

(Left) *The adrenal gland in primary pigmented nodular adrenal disease is studded with pigmented micronodules and occasional macronodules due to the confluence of smaller nodules. The outer surface has an irregular contour. Almost all cases are associated with Carney complex.* **(Right)** *Myelolipomas form well-circumscribed masses within the adrenal gland. A thin rim of normal adrenal ➔ can be seen around the edge. The yellow areas correspond to adipose tissue and the red areas to bone marrow elements.*

Adrenal Pseudocyst: Gross Appearance

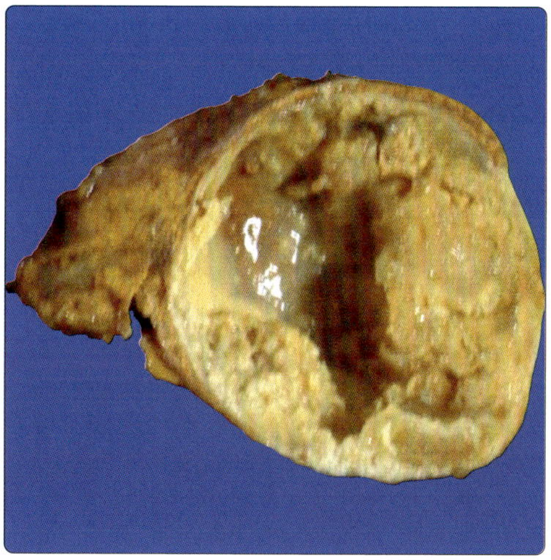

Adrenal Pseudocyst: Gross Appearance

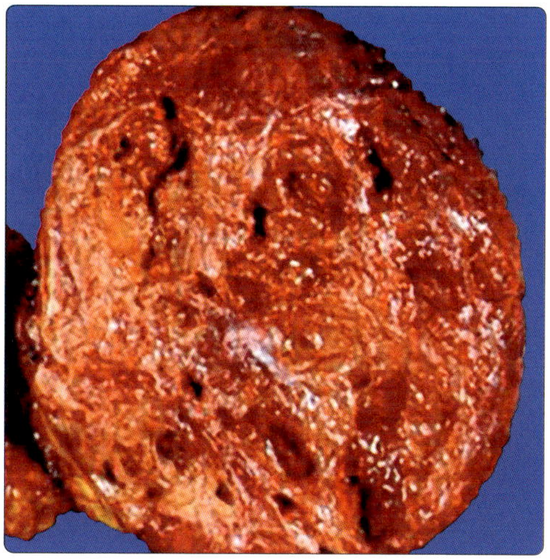

(Left) *Adrenal pseudocysts are usually unilocular, lack epithelial or endothelial lining cells, and have a thick fibrous wall. Calcification, chronic inflammation, and hemosiderin-laden macrophages are often present in the cyst wall. True adrenal cysts can arise from blood vessels or lymphatics.* **(Right)** *This pseudocyst of the adrenal developed in an adrenal cortical adenoma. The cyst is completely filled by red-tan fibrin due to extensive hemorrhage into the cyst.*

Extraadrenal Liposarcoma: Gross Appearance

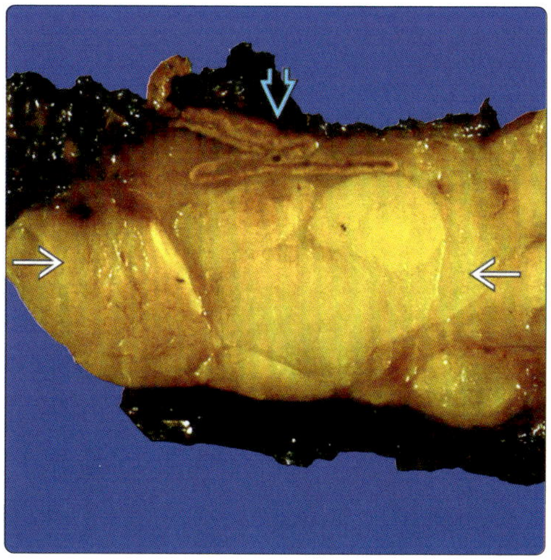

Metastatic Carcinoma to Adrenal Gland: Gross Appearance

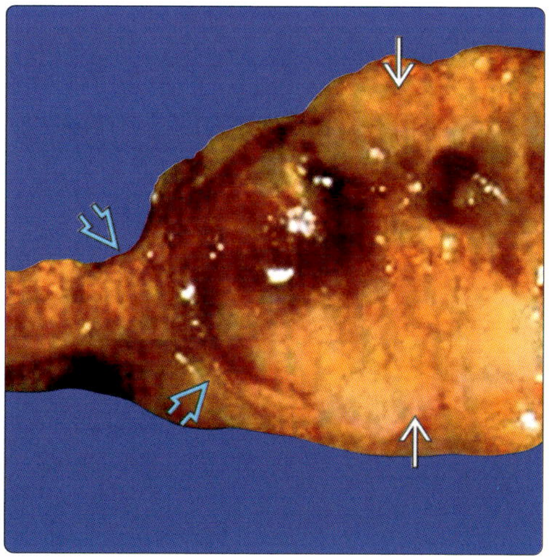

(Left) *This retroperitoneal liposarcoma ➔ was originally thought to be an adrenal tumor, as it partially encases the gland ⇨. Tumors adjacent to the adrenal may be sarcomas or lymphomas or other unusual tumors.* **(Right)** *Carcinoma usually metastasizes to both adrenal glands. The gross appearance depends on the primary site. A metastasis ➔ lacks the specific gross features of adrenal tumors and is often necrotic. In this case, a small remnant of adrenal cortex is present ⇨.*

SURGICAL/CLINICAL CONSIDERATIONS

Goal of Consultation

- Provide diagnosis for mediastinal mass

Change in Patient Management

- If thymoma, teratoma, or seminoma is confirmed, mass will be resected
- If lymphoma is confirmed or suspected, complete resection is not necessary
  - Role of intraoperative consultation: Confirm sufficient tissue is obtained for diagnosis and ancillary studies
- If carcinoma confirmed, surgeon may debulk tumor, but complete resection is usually not possible
  - Role of intraoperative consultation: Ensure diagnostic tissue has been obtained

Clinical Setting

- Age, gender, symptoms, and imaging findings usually suggest most likely diagnosis
- Surgical intent is to resect likely thymomas, germ cell tumors, and benign lesions
- In other settings, surgical intent is to obtain sufficient tissue for diagnosis
  - Locally invasive tumors that do not appear to be resectable
  - Suspected lymphoma or metastatic carcinoma
- Posterior mediastinal masses are less common
  - Majority are neurogenic tumors (e.g., schwannoma) or enteric cysts

SPECIMEN EVALUATION

Gross

- Biopsies
  - Describe size, color, consistency (soft, firm)
- Resections
  - Describe outer appearance (circumscribed, irregular, ragged), encapsulation, and color
    - Note any adherent structures, such as pleura or pericardium
  - Maintain orientation if provided
  - Ink outer surface according to orientation and serially section
  - Note lesions, including size, color, shape (circumscribed or infiltrating), fibrous bands, calcification, necrosis, and cysts

Frozen Section

- Biopsies
  - If small, entire specimen can be frozen
  - If lymphoma suspected and specimen large enough, consider saving nonfrozen tissue
    - Cytologic examination should be considered
    - Alternatively, request additional fresh tissue
- Resections
  - Representative section frozen for diagnosis
- Margins on resections
  - Often difficult to evaluate in thymic lesions
    - High false-negative and false-positive rates

Cytology

- Can be helpful if lymphoma suspected
  - May be difficult to distinguish low-grade lymphoma from thymoma or lymphocyte-rich carcinoma

MOST COMMON DIAGNOSES

Thymoma

- Most common anterior mediastinal tumor
- Usually occur in adults (age: 30-50); very rare in children
- 1/3 to 1/2 are asymptomatic, and mass is found incidentally by imaging
- 1/3 of patients have autoimmune disorder
  - Myasthenia gravis: 30-40%
    - Conversely, ~ 10% of patients with this condition have thymoma
  - Cushing syndrome
- Well-circumscribed, solid, yellow/gray mass
  - Majority have thick capsule
  - Lobules are separated by fibrous septa
  - Cystic degeneration is common

(Left) *Thymoma is the most common neoplasm of the anterior mediastinum. The tumor grows as an encapsulated, circumscribed, tan, fleshy mass. The fine, white septa ⇒ separating the lobules are characteristic.* **(Right)** *Some thymomas contain such prominent intervening fibrous septa ⇒ that the characteristic microscopic lobularity of these tumors is readily apparent grossly.*

Thymoma

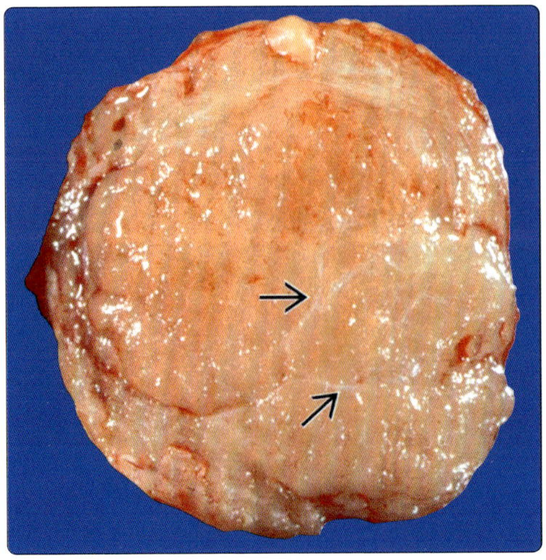

Fibrous Septa in Thymoma

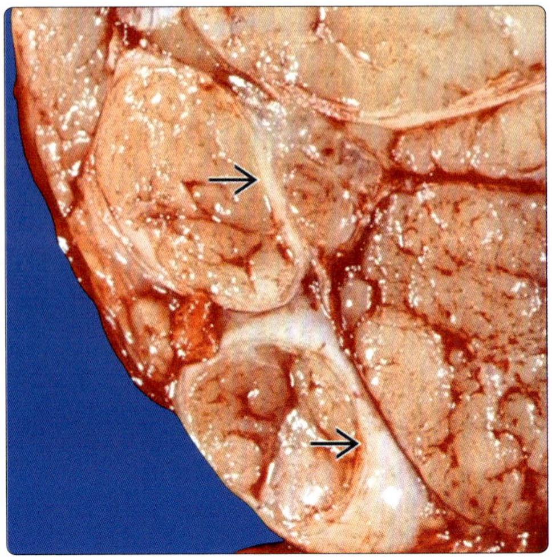

- Invasion into adjacent soft tissue is important prognostic factor
  - Any histologic type can be locally invasive
- Hassall corpuscles may be absent or rare
- Variety of morphologic types
  - Spindle cell
    - Must be distinguished from sarcomas
    - Generally lack nuclear pleomorphism, mitoses, and necrosis
    - Often associated with cystic change
  - Lymphocyte rich
    - May be difficult to distinguish from lymphoma
    - Mitoses and necrosis are usually absent
    - Medullary zones consist of circumscribed areas of dispersed lymphocytes resulting in area that appears paler than surrounding tumor
  - Mixed lymphoepithelial
  - Rich in epithelial cells (atypical thymoma)
    - Should be distinguished from metastatic carcinoma
    - Epithelioid cells can have abundant cytoplasm and large nuclei with prominent nucleoli
    - Mitoses may be present
    - Squamous foci can be present
    - Cells usually grow in sheets with background of small lymphocytes
    - Retraction away from blood vessels is characteristic

Thymic Carcinoma

- Preoperative evaluation typically demonstrates large, aggressive, and infiltrative mass
  - Alternatively, preexisting stable mass (thymoma) may show sudden rapid growth
- Most common histologic type is poorly differentiated, nonkeratinizing squamous cell carcinoma (lymphoepithelial-like carcinoma)
  - Numerous other histologic types occur, including basaloid, clear cell, spindle cell, mucinous, mucoepidermoid, neuroendocrine, and papillary
  - Overtly malignant cytology
  - Necrosis is common

Lymphoma

- Most cases represent mediastinal involvement by systemic lymphoma, but primary mediastinal lymphomas occur
  - Involvement of multiple nodal sites favors systemic lymphoma
- May be difficult to distinguish from lymphocyte-rich thymoma in some cases
- Features favoring lymphoma
  - Atypical lymphocytes
  - Mitoses
  - Necrosis
  - Infiltration into adipose tissue
  - Lack of fibrous bands
    - Exception: Hodgkin lymphoma, nodular sclerosis type
  - Lack of circumscription
- **Hodgkin lymphoma, nodular sclerosis type**
  - Most common form of Hodgkin lymphoma
  - Generally occur in young adults
  - Characteristic Reed-Sternberg cells and increased eosinophils may be identified
  - Associated changes can make diagnosis difficult
    - Sclerosis, granulomas, and thymic cysts can obscure tumor cells
- **Diffuse large B-cell lymphoma**
  - Most common in adult women
    - Associated with superior vena cava syndrome
  - Large, necrotic mediastinal mass
  - Can be associated with extensive sclerosis obscuring tumor cells
    - Can mimic carcinoma with desmoplasia
  - Arises in thymus
    - Entrapped thymic tissue may be present
- **Lymphoblastic lymphoma**
  - Most common in children and adolescents
    - Rapidly enlarging anterior mediastinal mass that may cause pleural effusion, airway obstruction, &/or superior vena cava syndrome
  - Intraoperative diagnosis may be needed to initiate immediate treatment
  - Small to medium-sized cells
    - Convoluted or regular nuclear membranes
    - Inconspicuous nucleoli
    - Frequent mitotic figures
    - Interspersed tingible body macrophages can confer starry-sky appearance
  - Crush artifact may make diagnosis difficult

Germ Cell Tumors

- 10-20% of mediastinal masses
- Usually occur in young adult men or children
  - Elevated serum markers may be present (AFP, PLAP, hCG), depending on type of tumor
- **Primary mediastinal teratoma**
  - Most common germ cell tumor in mediastinum
  - Composed of varying amounts of tissue from at least 2 of 3 embryonic germ cell layers: Ectoderm, mesoderm, endoderm
  - Mature teratoma
    - No immature elements; vast majority are benign
  - Immature teratoma
    - Contains immature elements and has malignant potential
  - Usually cystic; rupture of cysts can result in florid granulomatous inflammatory reaction
- **Primary mediastinal seminoma**
  - 2nd most common germ cell tumor in mediastinum
  - Histologically very similar to testicular seminoma or ovarian dysgerminoma
    - Metastatic testicular seminoma to mediastinum is very unlikely in absence of retroperitoneal lymph node metastases
  - Associated changes can make diagnosis difficult
    - Extensive stromal sclerosis can result in crush artifact and may obscure tumor cells
    - Granulomas can obscure tumor cells
    - Often associated with cystic change in thymus
- **Primary nonseminomatous mediastinal germ cell tumors**
  - May be composed of pure or mixed elements of embryonal carcinoma, yolk sac carcinoma, choriocarcinoma, and others
  - Usually locally advanced and not resected

- Intent of surgery is to obtain sufficient tissue for diagnosis

Neuroendocrine Carcinoma

- Most examples represent local extension or metastatic disease from another primary
- Less common is neuroendocrine carcinoma of thymus
- Histologic findings are similar to other neuroendocrine tumors
  - May be well, moderately, or poorly differentiated

Mesenchymal (Soft Tissue) Tumors

- **Solitary fibrous tumor**
  - Most common mesenchymal tumor of mediastinum
  - Monomorphic spindle cell neoplasm with abundant collagen and often prominent staghorn vasculature
  - Can be difficult to distinguish from spindle cell thymoma
    - Both treated with complete excision, if possible
- **Synovial sarcoma**
  - Cellular monomorphic spindle cell neoplasm with mitotic activity
  - Biphasic variants contain well-formed to poorly formed glandular elements
  - May be impossible to distinguish from spindle cell thymoma on frozen section

Benign Lesions

- **Idiopathic sclerosing mediastinitis**
  - Most common in adults 30-45 years of age; men more common than women
    - May be associated with histoplasmosis or tuberculosis
    - Other cases associated with autoimmune disease, sarcoidosis, radiation, or drug use
    - However, many cases do not have identifiable cause
  - Sclerosis that may envelop nerves and blood vessels and inflammatory cells
  - Overtly malignant cells or atypical nests/sheets are not seen
- **Castleman disease**
  - Longitudinal section of small vessel traversing lymphoid follicle (lollipop sign) is helpful if present
  - May not be possible to distinguish from lymphoma on frozen section
- **Thymic cysts**
  - Multiple cysts are often associated with chronic inflammation, fibrosis, and hemorrhage
  - Cysts are lined by low cuboidal, squamous, or columnar epithelium
  - Fibrosis, chronic inflammation, and granulomas may be present
  - Cysts are also seen in association with Hodgkin lymphoma, seminoma, thymic carcinoma, thymoma, seminoma, and yolk sac tumor
- **Thyroid or parathyroid**
  - Normal glandular tissue can be found in mediastinum
- **Thymic hyperplasia**
  - Increase in size beyond that typical for patient age
  - Germinal centers may be present (lymphoid hyperplasia)
  - Can be associated with myasthenia gravis or other autoimmune disorders

Metastatic Carcinoma

- Previous history of carcinoma of lung, breast, or other sites is important

REPORTING

Frozen Section

- Diagnosis should be rendered if possible because immediate treatment options may be affected
- Histologically malignant lesions may need to be deferred for ancillary testing
- If lymphoma suspected, request additional fresh tissue for ancillary studies, if needed

PITFALLS

Small Blue Cells With Crush Artifact

- Normal lymphocytes and tumors without desmoplastic stroma are easily crushed during biopsy
  - May be difficult to distinguish lymphoma, small cell carcinoma, and carcinoid tumor from lymphocytes
    - Diagnosis of small cell carcinoma should only be made if mitoses &/or necrosis are present
- If cellular morphology cannot be discerned, additional tissue should be requested

Sclerosing Lesions

- Multiple benign and malignant lesions of mediastinum are associated with dense collagenous stroma
- Stroma can obscure diagnostic cells &/or result in crush artifact, making interpretation difficult or impossible on frozen section

Granulomatous Inflammation

- Tumors and infections can result in formation of granulomas
  - Typical lesions are Hodgkin lymphoma, seminoma, or mycobacterial or fungal infections
- Granulomatous inflammation alone usually does not form large masses
- Multiple frozen sections may be necessary to find diagnostic areas

Thymic Cysts

- Neoplasms can be associated with cystic change in thymus
- Cysts may need to be sampled extensively to rule out tumor

Hassall Corpuscles vs. Metastatic Carcinoma

- Normal Hassall corpuscles consist of nests of squamous cells in thymus
- Cells with keratohyaline granules are often present

SELECTED REFERENCES

1. Detterbeck FC et al: Which way is up? Policies and procedures for surgeons and pathologists regarding resection specimens of thymic malignancy. J Thorac Oncol. 6(7 Suppl 3):S1730-8, 2011
2. Marchevsky A et al: Policies and reporting guidelines for small biopsy specimens of mediastinal masses. J Thorac Oncol. 6(7 Suppl 3):S1724-9, 2011
3. de Montpréville VT et al: Frozen section diagnosis and surgical biopsy of lymph nodes, tumors and pseudotumors of the mediastinum. Eur J Cardiothorac Surg. 13(2):190-5, 1998
4. Jüttner FM et al: Pitfalls in intraoperative frozen section histology of mediastinal neoplasms. Eur J Cardiothorac Surg. 4(11):584-6, 1990

Thymoma

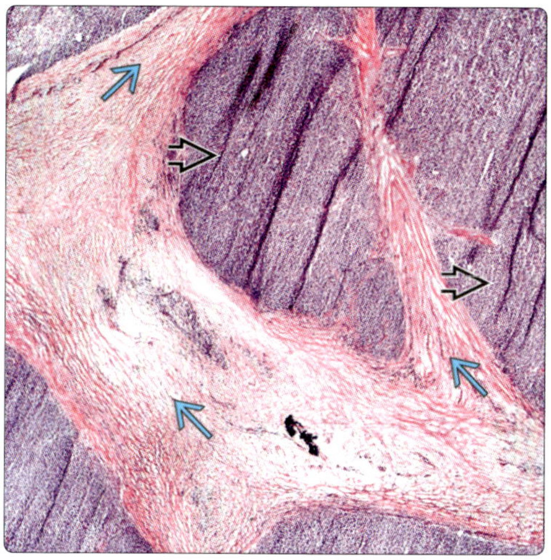

Lymphocyte-Predominant Thymoma

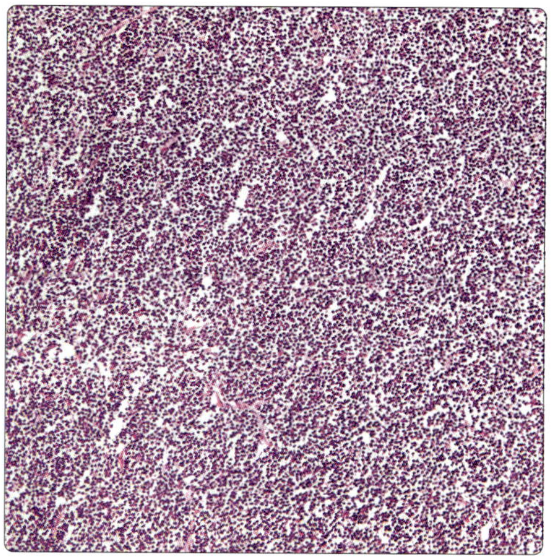

(Left) *Thymomas typically have a marked nodular architecture with large lobules of neoplastic cells separated by variably thickened fibrous septa. The septa would not be typical of lymphomas.* **(Right)** *In many thymomas, the lymphocytic component is so prominent and diffuse that it may be impossible to distinguish these tumors from a lymphoma, particularly on a small intraoperative biopsy. Other typical features of thymoma must be sought out to assist in making the diagnosis.*

Lymphocyte-Predominant Thymoma

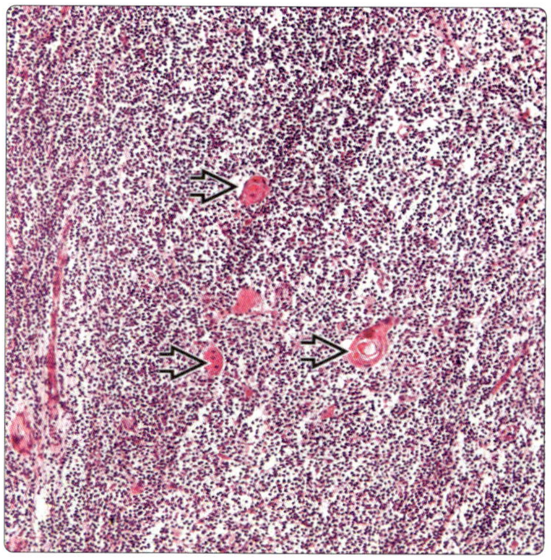

Epithelial-Predominant Thymoma

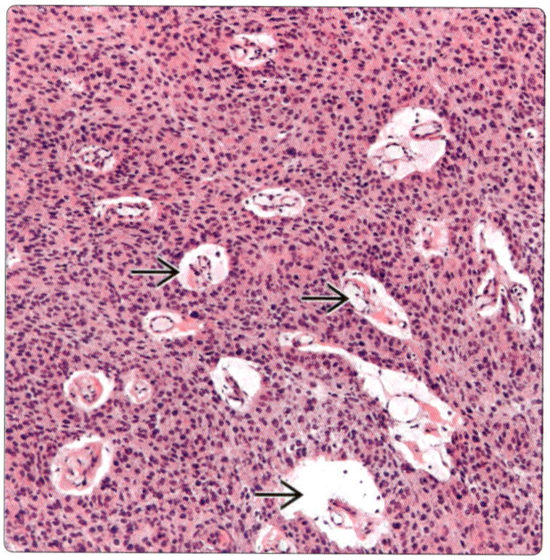

(Left) *Although they are much more commonly seen in normal nonneoplastic or hyperplastic thymus, the focal presence of Hassall corpuscles in an expansile lymphoid neoplasm supports the diagnosis of thymoma. These structures are identified by their pink, squamoid morphology.* **(Right)** *Some thymomas consist of pink epithelioid cells, spindle cells, or a mixture of both. Marked cytologic atypia is not seen. Perivascular retraction space artifact is a useful finding that suggests thymoma.*

Thymic Neuroendocrine Carcinoma

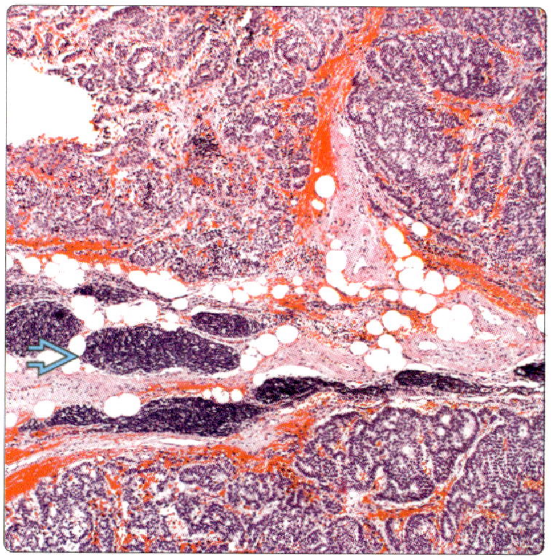

Thymic Hyperplasia

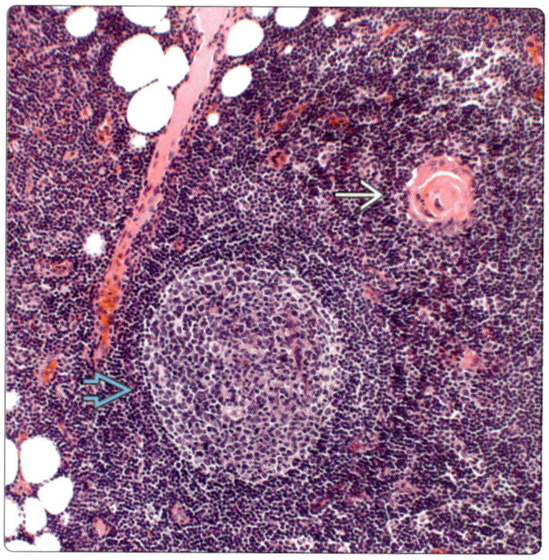

(Left) *The most common thymic carcinoma is poorly differentiated lymphoepithelioma-like squamous cell carcinoma, but a variety of other types occur as well. It may be difficult to distinguish them from metastatic carcinoma. This case of neuroendocrine thymic carcinoma surrounds an area of residual normal thymus.* **(Right)** *Germinal centers are generally not seen in the thymus. This case of lymphocytic thymic hyperplasia can be recognized due to the presence of Hassall corpuscles.*

(Left) *The architecture of nodular sclerosis Hodgkin lymphoma (NSHL) somewhat resembles a thymoma, except that the lobularity is often more vaguely defined and irregular. The sclerotic collagen is also more patchy or zonal rather than in well-formed septa and can be so prominent as to obscure tumor cells.* (Right) *Clues to an NSHL diagnosis in cases with extensive sclerosis, multiple granulomas, or cystic change include increased eosinophils* ⇨ *and the presence of Reed-Sternberg cells* ⇨*, which may vary from focal to numerous.*

Nodular Sclerosis Hodgkin Lymphoma

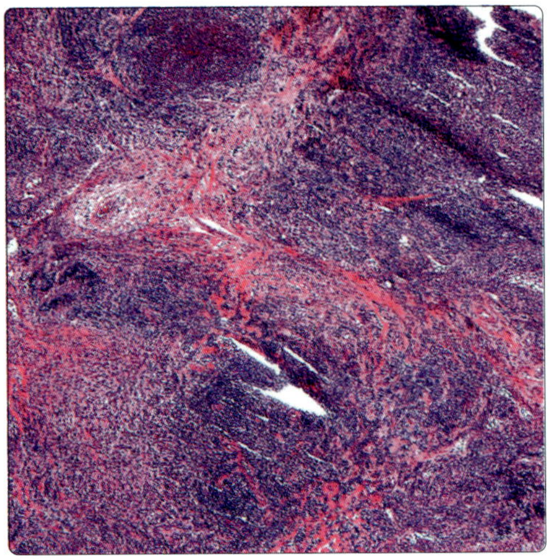

Nodular Sclerosis Hodgkin Lymphoma

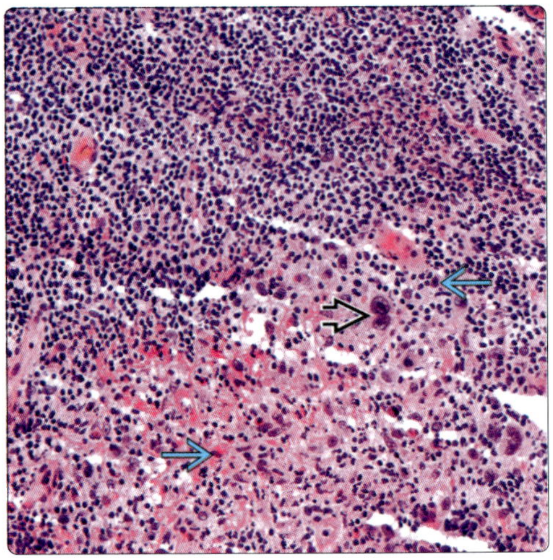

(Left) *Hodgkin lymphoma and germ cell tumors can be associated with thymic cysts. When cysts* ➡ *rupture, the inflammatory reaction to spilled cyst contents* ⇨ *can obscure the diagnostic cells. In this case, scattered Reed-Sternberg cells are present* ⇨*.* (Right) *Children and young adults with mediastinal lymphoblastic lymphoma can present with a medical emergency due to obstructive symptoms. Sheets of small cells with hyperchromatic nuclei, a high mitotic rate, and necrosis are usually seen.*

Hodgkin Lymphoma

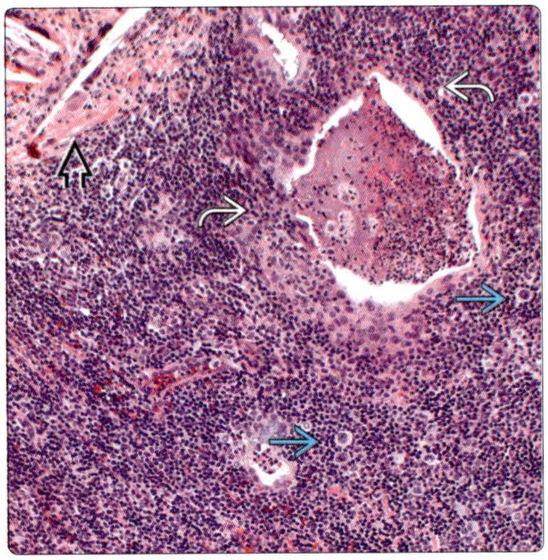

Lymphoblastic Lymphoma

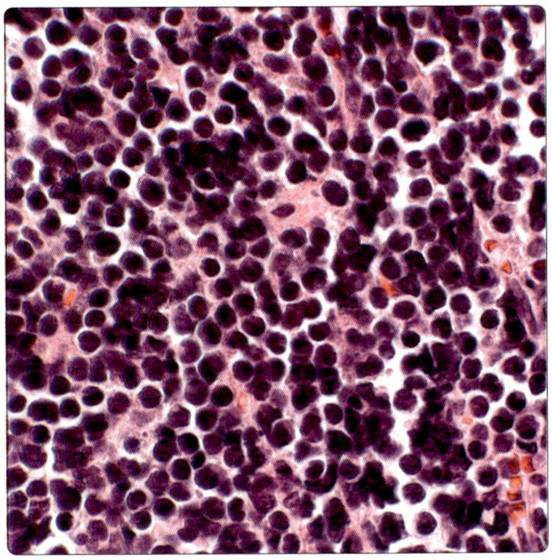

(Left) *Large B-cell lymphomas of the mediastinum are frequently associated with marked sclerosis. Crushing of the tumor cells can make diagnosis very difficult on frozen section. Areas of intact tumor cells* ⇨ *may be difficult to find.* (Right) *Sclerosing mediastinitis cannot be diagnosed with certainty on frozen section. Hodgkin lymphoma and B-cell lymphoma can also have a similar appearance. It may be prudent to take tissue for ancillary studies in all cases. In this case, no tumor was identified.*

Mediastinal Large B-Cell Lymphoma

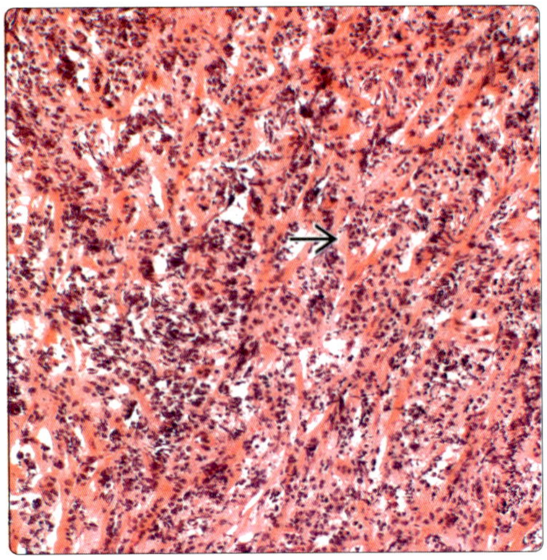

Sclerosing Mediastinitis

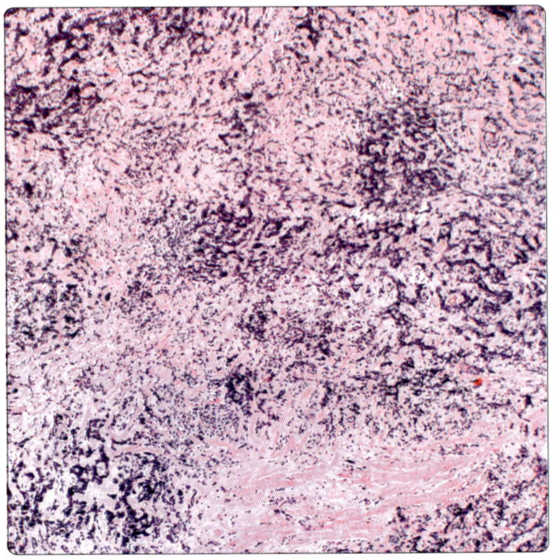

Thymic Cyst

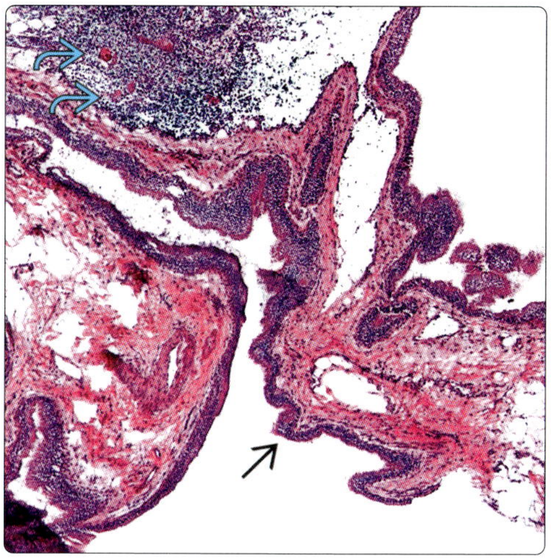

Mediastinal Teratoma

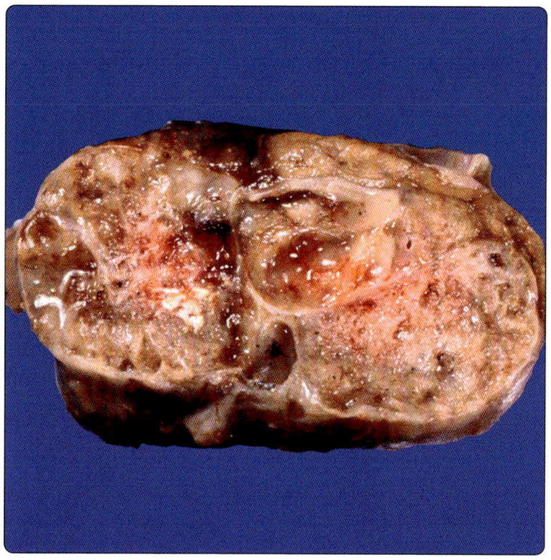

(Left) Thymic cysts are lined by ciliated, respiratory-type epithelium →. Thymic tissue may be present in the wall with Hassall corpuscles ↷. Hodgkin lymphoma and seminoma are associated with cysts. The tissue within the walls should be examined for diagnostic cells. (Right) As in other body sites, teratomas in the mediastinum often form multiple cysts that are evident on gross examination. Unusual intracystic findings include hair and even teeth. These tumors are most common in young males.

Teratoma

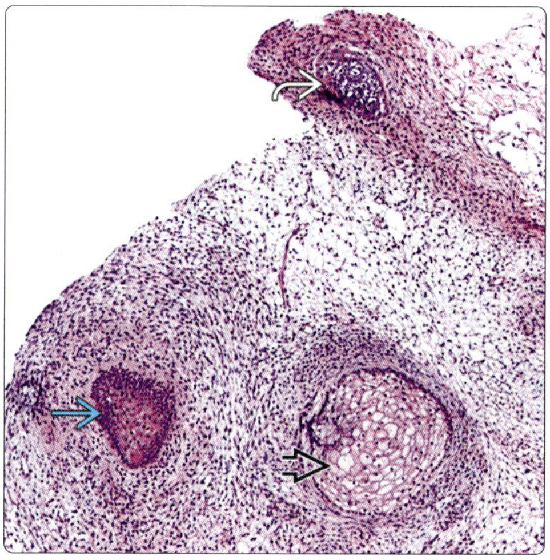

Teratoma

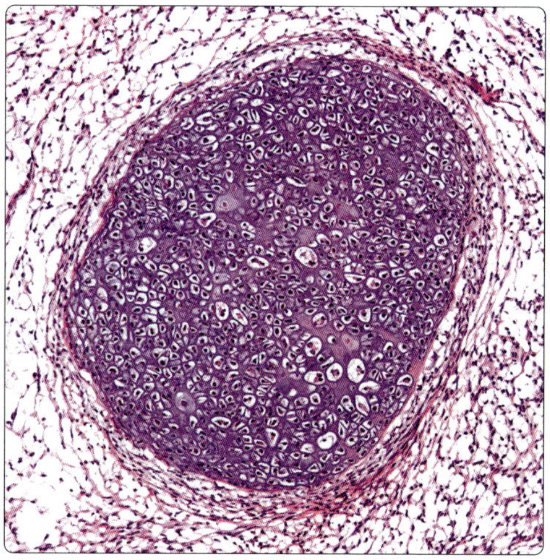

(Left) The key to identifying a teratoma is recognition of a mixture of tissues from at least 2 of the 3 embryonic germ cell layers. Some of the more common findings include squamous →, sebaceous ↷, and cartilaginous ⇨ tissues. Notably, pancreatic tissue is also disproportionately more common in mediastinal teratomas. (Right) The cartilage seen in teratomas is immature and often highly cellular. This appearance is common and should not be misinterpreted as chondrosarcoma.

Mediastinal Seminoma

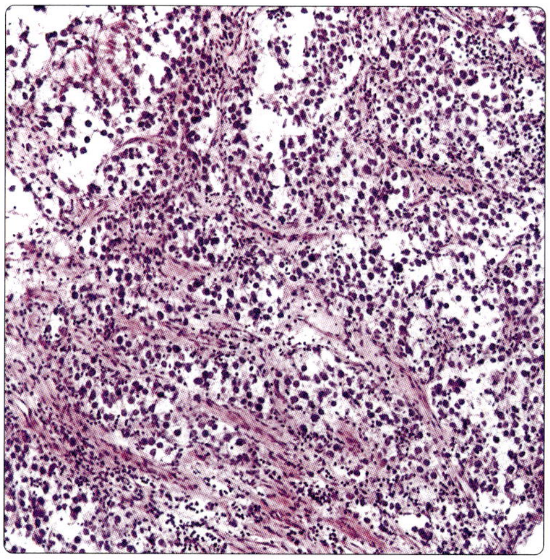

Mediastinal Seminoma

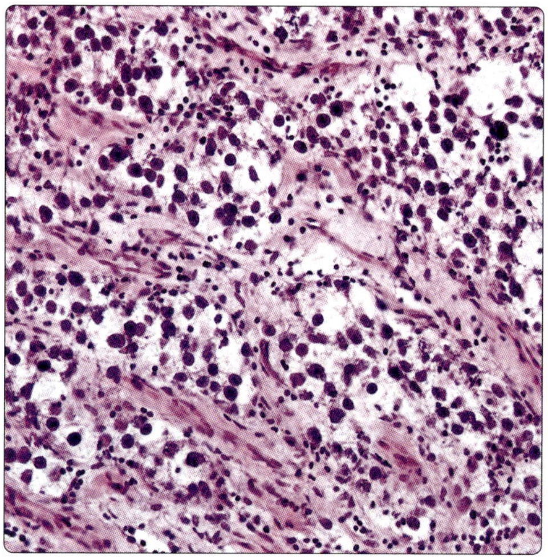

(Left) Mediastinal seminoma is essentially identical histologically to its testicular and ovarian counterparts (dysgerminoma). The tumor cells are often quite nested but may form sheets, and the thin septa contain a variable number of lymphocytes. (Right) The tumor cells of seminoma are monomorphic and demonstrate prominent clear cytoplasm. Characteristically, large central nucleoli are present. Multinucleated giant cells or frank granuloma formation may also be seen.

SURGICAL/CLINICAL CONSIDERATIONS

Goal of Consultation

- Determine if appendiceal carcinoma or carcinoid is present
- Determine if proximal margin is free of carcinoid or if low-grade appendiceal mucinous neoplasm (LAMN) is present

Change in Patient Management

- Right hemicolectomy may be performed
  - Invasive carcinoma requires additional surgery for nodal staging
  - Proximal margin positive for LAMN or carcinoid requires additional surgery for tumor free margins

Clinical Setting

- Appendix may be sent for intraoperative consultation in following settings
  - Dilated appendix suspicious for LAMN
  - Serosal nodularity in resections being performed for acute appendicitis
- If right colectomy is planned based on clinical and imaging findings, examination of appendix will not change clinical management

SPECIMEN EVALUATION

Gross

- Outer surface is examined for exudates, mucin pools, and nodularity suspicious for tumor
- Proximal margin is identified and removed as en face margin
- Tip of appendix is transected longitudinally
  - Tip is examined for masses, abnormalities in wall thickness, and luminal contents
  - Mesoappendix examined for masses &/or mucin
- Remainder of appendix is serially sectioned

Frozen Section

- If gross lesion is suspicious for malignancy, representative section is frozen for diagnosis

Low-Grade Appendiceal Mucinous Neoplasm: Gross Appearance

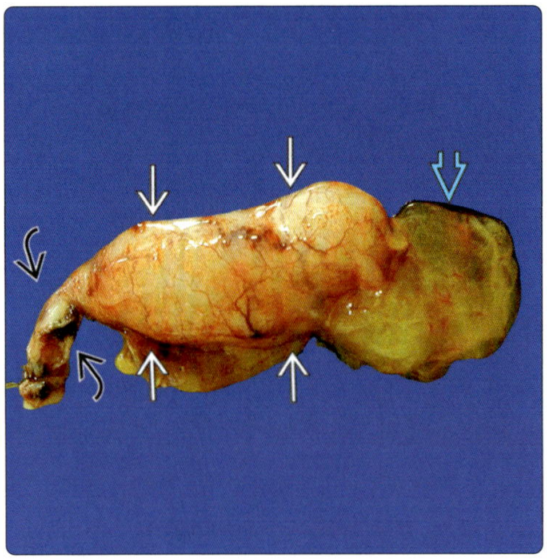

Low-Grade Appendiceal Mucinous Neoplasm: Mucin

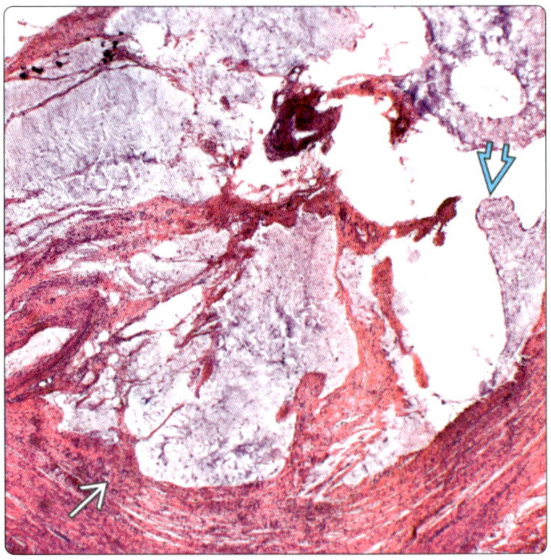

(Left) *Low-grade appendiceal mucinous neoplasms (LAMNs) cause marked luminal distension ➔ compared to the normal appendix ➚. Rupture can lead to extravasation of mucin ⇨ into the peritoneal cavity and possible pseudomyxoma peritonei.* **(Right)** *Dissecting pools of acellular mucin ➔ are present in LAMN. Epithelial cells ⇨ may be scant and cytologically low grade. Clusters of high-grade malignant cells floating in mucin pools are diagnostic of mucinous adenocarcinoma.*

Low-Grade Appendiceal Mucinous Neoplasm: Mucin

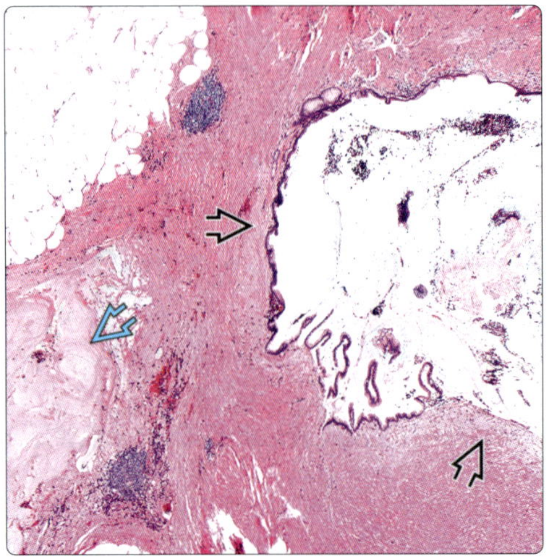

Low-Grade Appendiceal Mucinous Neoplasm: Muscularis Mucosa

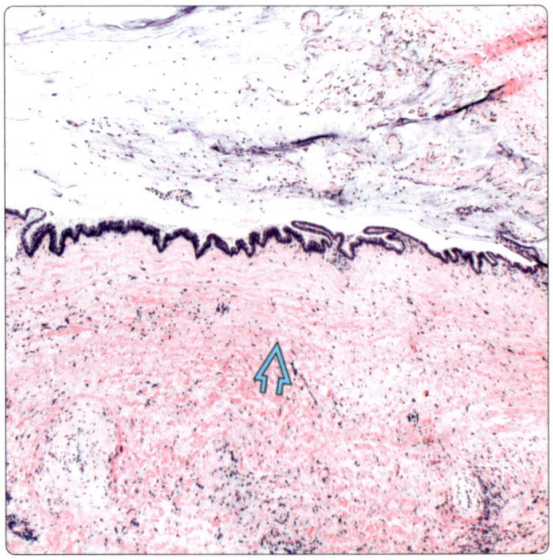

(Left) *LAMNs show cystic dilation and an expansile, pushing border ⇨ that often extends deep into the muscularis propria. Acellular mucin pools ⇨ are characteristic of LAMN.* **(Right)** *LAMNs are composed of hypermucinous dysplastic epithelium. Unlike mucinous cystadenoma, the muscularis mucosa ⇨ in LAMN is disrupted and mucin pools may be present in the appendiceal wall and/or serosa.*

MOST COMMON DIAGNOSES

Conventional Adenocarcinoma

- Similar to colonic counterpart
- Typically arises in association with tubular or villous adenomas of appendix
- Minority arise in association with serrated polyps

Mucinous Neoplasms

- **Mucinous cystadenoma**
  - May cause dilation of appendix
    - Lumen lined by dysplastic epithelium
    - Intact muscularis mucosae with no mucin extravasation
- **Low-grade appendiceal mucinous neoplasm (LAMN)**
  - Markedly dilated lumen
  - Tall columnar mucinous epithelium with (usually low grade) dysplastic nuclei
  - Epithelium often surrounded by thick collagenous, hyalinized stroma, ± calcifications
  - Mucin extravasation into muscularis propria &/or serosa
  - May be associated with extraappendiceal mucin
- **Mucinous adenocarcinoma**
  - Rare
  - Infiltrative lesion with tumor cells floating in pools of extracellular mucin
  - May be associated with synchronous peritoneal disease
  - Resembles mucinous adenocarcinomas seen at extraappendiceal sites in GI tract

Neuroendocrine Tumors

- Most common appendiceal tumor
  - Incidental findings in ~ 0.5-1.0% of appendectomies performed for appendicitis
  - Well-differentiated neuroendocrine tumors may have insular, trabecular, or tubular patterns
  - Tubular carcinoids can be mistaken for adenocarcinoma
- Usually arise at tip and form bulbous swelling
  - Firm, yellow to white, and circumscribed

Goblet Cell Carcinoid

- Distinctive neoplasm of appendix
  - Staged and treated as adenocarcinoma
    - Subset transforms to higher grade lesion [adenocarcinoma ex goblet cell carcinoid (GCC)]
- Causes diffuse thickening of wall
  - Rarely diagnosed intraoperatively
- Well-differentiated, crypt-like glandular structures invade appendiceal wall
  - Mitoses are rare
- No precursor lesion present in mucosa

Acute Appendicitis

- Seldom sent for intraoperative consultation
- Entire appendix may be enlarged, congested, and edematous
- Purulent exudate may be present on serosa
- Lumen may be obstructed
  - Fecalith, foreign body, parasite

Endometriosis

- Wall of appendix may be thickened and hemorrhagic
- Endometrial glands are associated with endometrial stroma and hemosiderin deposits

Fibrous Obliteration of Lumen

- Tip of appendix can be fibrotic and lumen obliterated
- Appearance can grossly mimic tumor involvement

REPORTING

Frozen Section

- Report definite invasive adenocarcinoma when present
  - Report GCC, if possible
- When LAMN is present, report "favor LAMN" with caveat that final diagnosis requires evaluation of entire appendix
- Report "well-differentiated neuroendocrine tumor" when present
  - Important not to mistake tubular carcinoids for invasive adenocarcinoma
  - Comment on mesoappendix invasion if present

PITFALLS

Tumor Obscured by Inflammation

- GCCs often present as acute appendicitis
- Tumor cells may be obscured by inflammation

Endometriosis Mistaken for Adenocarcinoma

- Characteristic endometrial stroma should be present
- Adenocarcinomas have greater nuclear atypia

Tubular Carcinoid Mistaken for Adenocarcinoma

- Tubular carcinoids are not associated with mucosal precursor lesion
  - Adenocarcinomas are often associated with polyps
- Well-differentiated conventional adenocarcinomas have greater nuclear atypia than carcinoids

Lymphoid Cells Within Lymphatics Mistaken for Neuroendocrine Tumors

- Lymphatics distended by lymphocytes is common finding in appendix
- Filled lymphatics can mimic trabecular pattern reminiscent of neuroendocrine tumors

Mucin Extravasation in Inflammatory Disorders Mistaken for LAMN

- Acute appendicitis or diverticulitis with tissue destruction may lead to mucin extravasation
- Dysplastic mucinous lining epithelium must be present for diagnosis of LAMN

SELECTED REFERENCES

1. Rouzbahman M et al: Mucinous tumours of appendix and ovary: an overview and evaluation of current practice. J Clin Pathol. 67(3):193-7, 2013
2. Tirumani SH et al: Mucinous neoplasms of the appendix: a current comprehensive clinicopathologic and imaging review. Cancer Imaging. 13:14-25, 2013
3. Carr NJ et al: Pathology and prognosis in pseudomyxoma peritonei: a review of 274 cases. J Clin Pathol. 65(10):919-23, 2012
4. Timofeev J et al: Appendiceal pathology at the time of oophorectomy for ovarian neoplasms. Obstet Gynecol. 116(6):1348-53, 2010

(Left) *The majority of cases of pseudomyxoma peritonei originate from primary appendiceal mucinous neoplasms. This appendix is obscured by a gelatinous mass of mucin.* **(Right)** *An infiltrative tumor pattern is needed for a definitive diagnosis of mucinous adenocarcinoma. This specimen shows a mucinous adenocarcinoma with cystic dilation ⇨ of the lumen. An area of carcinoma has invaded beyond the thick fibrous rim ↷ into periappendiceal adipose tissue ⇨.*

Pseudomyxoma Peritonei: Gross Appearance

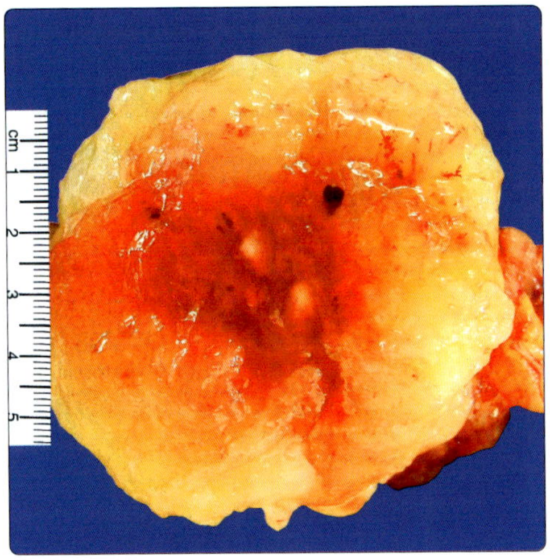

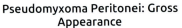

Mucinous Adenocarcinoma: Gross Appearance

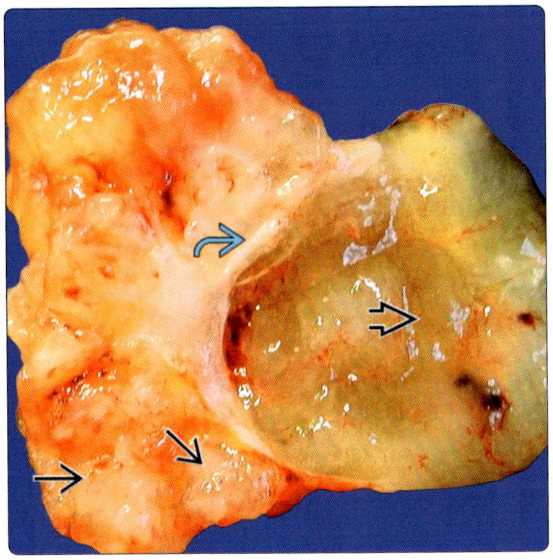

(Left) *Mucinous cystadenomas are lined by tall columnar mucinous epithelium with nuclear hyperchromasia and stratification. The muscularis mucosa ⇨ is intact and there is no mucin extravasation into the appendiceal wall.* **(Right)** *Acellular mucin extravasation into mesoappendix and serosa is associated with a low risk of recurrence and pseudomyxoma peritonei. The risk is higher in cases in which tumor cells are present in association with extravasated mucin.*

Mucinous Cystadenoma of Appendix

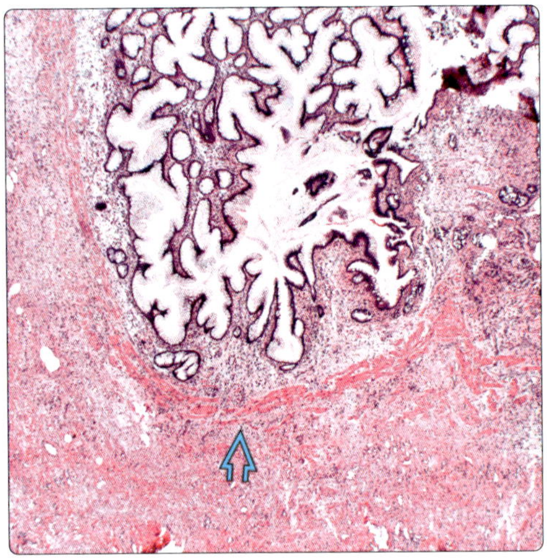

Acellular Mucin in Mesoappendix

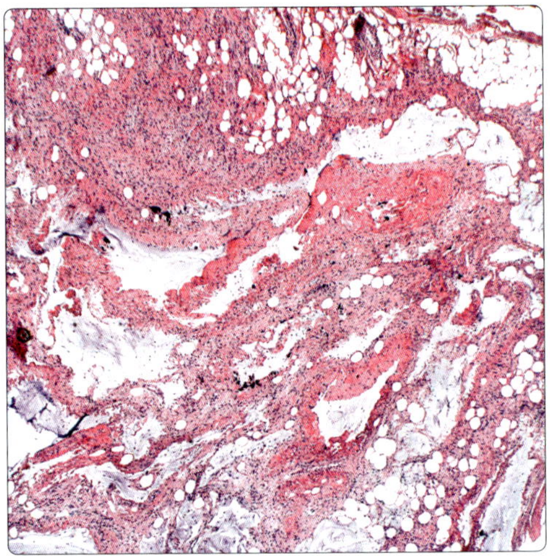

(Left) *Carcinoid tumors ⇨ are common incidental findings in the appendix. In this case, the clinical lesion was a ruptured appendiceal diverticulum ↷.* **(Right)** *Goblet cell carcinoids are unique tumors that occur almost exclusively in the appendix and are characterized by tumor nests that mimic normal crypts ⇨. They are composed of both mucinous and endocrine cells. No mucosal precursor lesion is present in these tumors. These tumors may give rise to signet ring cell and poorly differentiated adenocarcinomas.*

Carcinoid Tumor of Appendix

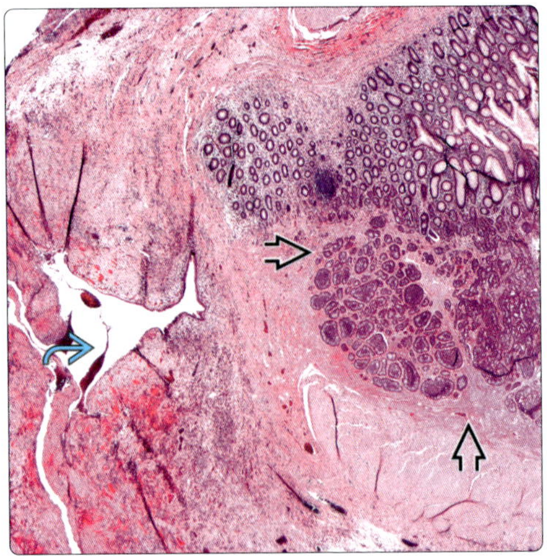

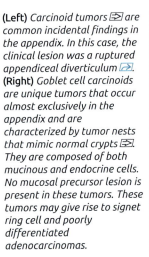

Goblet Cell Carcinoid of Appendix

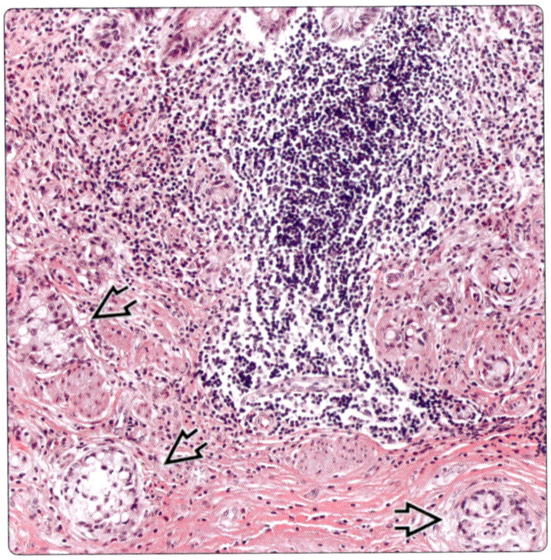

Contents

Serrated Polyp of Appendix

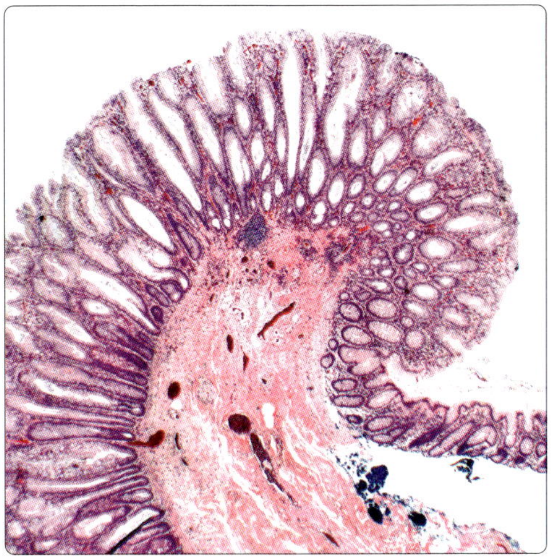

Metastatic Lobular Carcinoma of Breast to Appendix

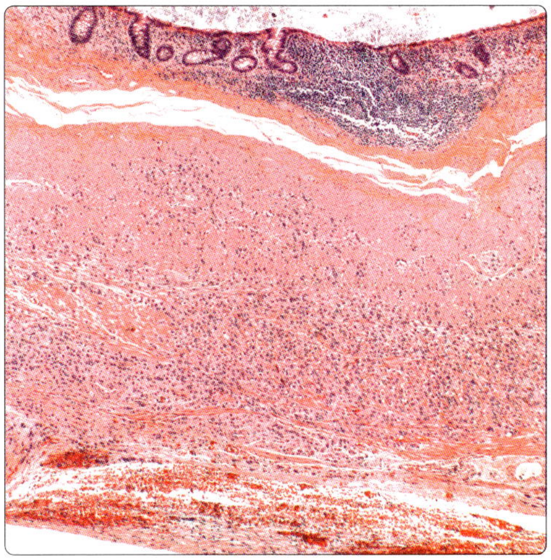

(Left) *This serrated polyp was present at the orifice of the appendix. Frozen section was requested to ensure the entire polyp had been removed. Adenocarcinomas of the appendix are typically associated with polyps.* **(Right)** *Metastases to the appendix are rare. This lobular breast cancer in the muscularis would need to be distinguished from a primary signet ring cell carcinoma or a signet ring cell metastatic from another site.*

Appendix: Distended Lymphatics

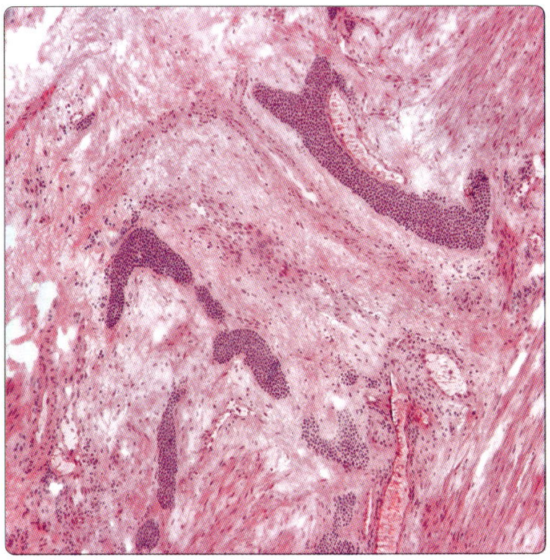

Endometriosis

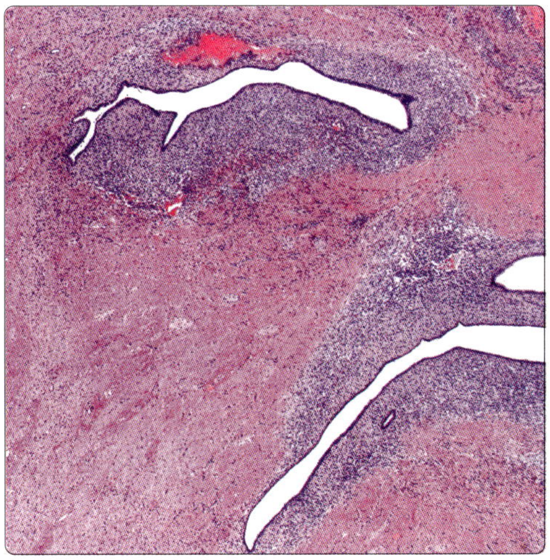

(Left) *Lymphatics plugged with lymphoid cells can mimic the nested and trabecular architecture of neuroendocrine tumors. However, this is a common normal finding in the appendix.* **(Right)** *Endometriosis can involve the body or tip of the appendix. Although the muscularis and mesoappendix are typically involved, the mucosa is not. The glands are lined by tall columnar cells surrounded by endometrial stroma and hemosiderin-laden macrophages.*

Appendix: Fibrous Obliteration

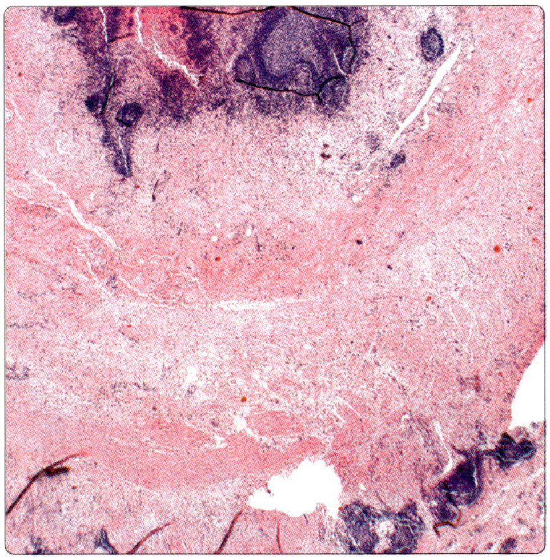

Acute Appendicitis

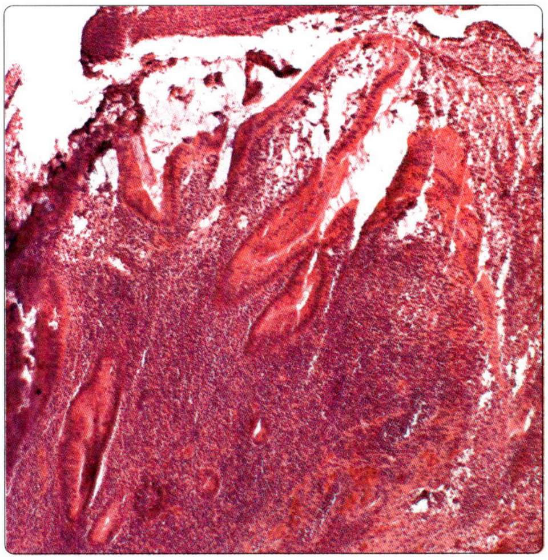

(Left) *The tip of the appendix often undergoes fibrous obliteration. If prominent, the fibrosis can grossly mimic a carcinoid tumor. The wall is markedly thickened and the lumen may be absent.* **(Right)** *The appendix is most commonly removed due to appendicitis and intraoperative consultation is rarely necessary. In this case, the appendix was markedly enlarged due to the inflammation and edema, raising concern about a possible neoplasm.*

SURGICAL/CLINICAL CONSIDERATIONS

Goal of Consultation

- Determine if bone lesion is benign/reactive or malignant
- Evaluate margins after definitive resection of malignant bone tumor

Change in Patient Management

- Reactive lesions may be followed clinically or excised
- Benign neoplasms are often excised or curetted without need to document negative margins
- Low-grade malignancies are resected, often widely (if possible) and with margin assessment
  - Complete curettage may also be attempted in some well-localized tumors
- High-grade malignancies may be treated with radiation/chemotherapy prior to resection or resected before treatment
- Positive bony &/or marrow margins may generate additional resection or possibly closure and subsequent adjuvant therapy

Clinical Setting

- Patient age ranges from pediatric to adult
- Lytic &/or blastic lesions identified on radiograph
  - May be incidentally discovered on plain film during evaluation for other conditions
- Bone destruction &/or soft tissue invasion often apparent in locally aggressive &/or malignant tumors
- Malignancies are more likely than benign lesions to cause pain

SPECIMEN EVALUATION

Radiograph

- Review of appropriate patient radiographs or radiologic reports prior to receipt of specimen is highly recommended
  - Radiologist's differential diagnosis is essential for correlation with pathologic findings
  - Can often identify whether or not lesion is growing aggressively
- Knowing specific bone as well as anatomic region of bone involved is diagnostically useful information
- Identification of aggressive growth pattern radiographically can be essential in helping classify low-grade bone malignancy intraoperatively

Gross

- Bone specimens sent for intraoperative consultation and diagnosis are almost invariably composed of small fragments of soft tissue and bone
- Intraoperative margins sent for bone tumors are either peripheral soft tissue margins or intramedullary marrow margins

Frozen Section

- Separate hard bony fragments from soft tissue fragments
- Softer bony fragments can be frozen, but harder bone may damage cryostat blade &/or distort frozen section
  - Tissue that can be cut easily with scalpel blade can generally be sectioned on cryostat
- All tissue should be frozen unless entire lesion has been curetted and sent to pathology
  - If completely curetted, representative tissue from specimen usually suffices
    - These specimens are usually from presumptively benign lesions

Cytology

- Touch prep slides of lesional tissue may be helpful if metastatic carcinoma is suspected

MOST COMMON DIAGNOSES

Metastasis

- Far more common than primary bone tumors
- Carcinoma is most common, but melanoma, sarcoma, or lymphoma may also spread to bone
- Must always be considered in patients > 45 years of age
  - Patients often have history of cancer elsewhere as well as prior metastatic disease (e.g., to lymph nodes, lung)
- Any bone may be involved
  - Most often proximal humerus, proximal femur, or spine

Metastatic Carcinoma

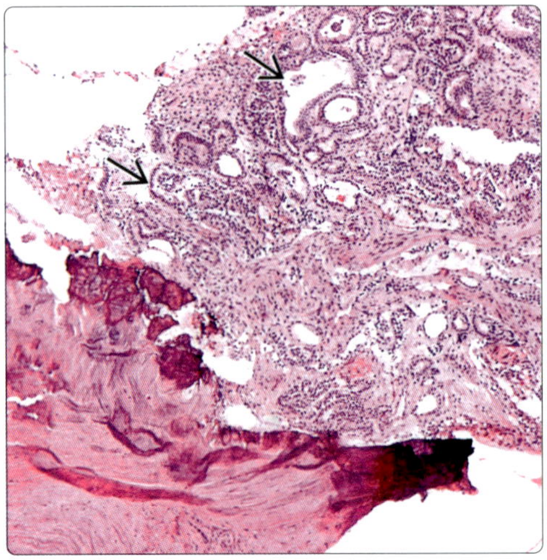

Metastatic Carcinoma

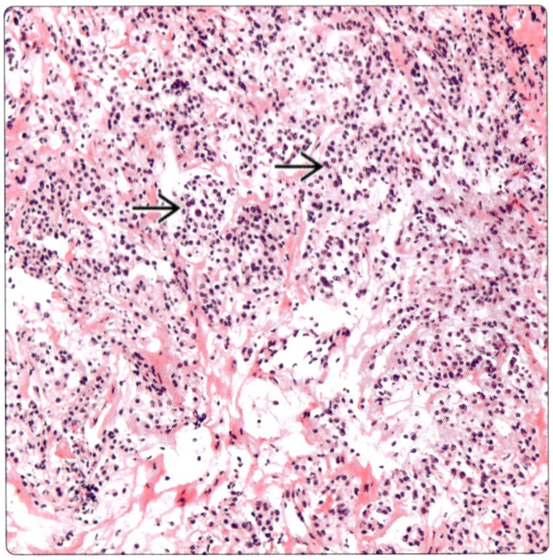

(Left) *The morphology of metastatic carcinoma varies widely depending on the type of primary tumor and degree of differentiation. This metastatic adenocarcinoma displays well-formed glandular elements ⇒.* **(Right)** *Some metastatic carcinomas can be subtle and easily missed. Identification of an abnormal architectural pattern that is not seen in normal bone (e.g., vague tumor cell nesting ⇒ or epithelioid cells in cohesive sheets) is critical.*

- Histologic appearance depends on primary tumor
  - Usually adenocarcinoma (most common primary sites include breast, lung, kidney, prostate, liver, and thyroid)
    - Some metastatic carcinomas (particularly from prostate) are osteoblastic and produce focal to abundant woven bone
  - Amount of tumor present may be relatively limited compared to size of lytic lesion
    - Metastases can stimulate osteoclasts to resorb bone
    - Multiple sections may need to be examined to identify metastatic cells
- Immunohistochemical studies performed on permanent sections may be necessary for classification if no primary site is known
  - Decalcification can diminish immunoreactivity for some antigens
  - If possible, softer areas of tumor should be separated and not decalcified

Osteosarcoma

- Most commonly seen in young patients 10-20 years of age
  - 2nd peak occurs in patients > 50 years of age who have predisposing condition (e.g., radiation, Paget disease)
- Imaging often shows large permeative and destructive lesion in metaphysis/diaphysis of long bone, most commonly around region of knee (~ 50% of cases)
- Most cases show sheets of frankly malignant cells with high level of mitotic activity
- Diagnosis depends upon identification of pink seams of osteoid or immature bone directly produced by malignant cells
- Some tumors may show focal or prominent cartilaginous differentiation, leading to possible confusion with chondrosarcoma
  - Younger age and presence of cellular sheets of malignant cells (± osteoid) favor osteosarcoma
- Other variant morphologies include fibroblastic (spindled), small cell, clear cell, telangiectatic, and giant cell rich

Enchondroma

- Often painless unless associated with fracture
- Imaging often shows small, well-circumscribed lesion without locally aggressive features in diaphysis/metaphysis of long bones
- In long bones: Generally composed of fragments and nodules of bland hyaline cartilage, often with thin, pink seam of peripheral bone
  - Chondrocyte cellularity is often low and with minimal or no nuclear atypia
- In small bones of hands and feet: Often much more cellular and may demonstrate mild nuclear atypia and myxoid matrix degeneration
  - Clinical and radiologic correlation to evaluate for pathologic cortical bone disruption and soft tissue extension is most helpful in excluding chondrosarcoma
- In some cases, it can be extremely difficult, if not impossible, to histologically distinguish enchondroma from low-grade chondrosarcoma
  - Correlation with imaging is often critical in making this distinction
  - In ambiguous cases, a diagnosis of "low-grade cartilaginous lesion, final diagnosis deferred to permanent sections" is appropriate
  - Any subsequent curetted tissue should be submitted for permanent histologic evaluation

Chondrosarcoma

- Often painful
- Imaging generally shows irregular, large, and destructive tumor, often with cortical disruption and soft tissue extension, involving metaphysis/diaphysis of long bones
  - Clear cell chondrosarcoma (variant) characteristically arises in epiphysis of long bones
- Cellularity and chondrocyte nuclear atypia vary widely depending on grade, but most cases show higher degree of both than seen in benign cartilage or enchondroma
  - Chondrocyte necrosis and prominent matrix degeneration are also more common in chondrosarcoma
- Chondrosarcoma of small bones of hands and feet is very rare and requires evidence of true bony or soft tissue invasion for diagnosis
- Dedifferentiated chondrosarcoma may show cellular, noncartilaginous high-grade sarcoma or neoplastic cartilage or both, depending on what portion of tumor is sampled at time of frozen section

Ewing Sarcoma

- Most common in patients < 20 years of age
- Painful, enlarging mass, often with soft tissue swelling
- Imaging shows large, poorly defined destructive tumor most often centered in metaphysis or diaphysis of long bones or flat bones of pelvis
- This is a type of small round blue cell tumor consisting of sheets of monomorphic small round cells with scanty cytoplasm within variably fibrous background
  - Most cells have finely distributed chromatin and inconspicuous nucleoli
- Necrosis is often abundant
- Diagnosis of "malignant small round blue cell tumor, final diagnosis deferred to permanent sections" is often appropriate
  - Must exclude other morphologically similar neoplasms, such as small cell osteosarcoma, mesenchymal chondrosarcoma, or lymphoma
  - Confirmatory ancillary testing (IHC, FISH, etc.) is required on permanent sections

Giant Cell Tumor

- Typically occur in adults (age range: 25-45 years)
- Localization to epiphysis of long bone is characteristic, similar to chondroblastoma and clear cell chondrosarcoma
  - Also shows metaphyseal extension in many cases
- Tumor is often locally aggressive and may show limited soft tissue extension
- Composed of sheets of multinucleated osteoclast-like giant cells in background of bland, monomorphic ovoid, or spindled stromal cells
  - Giant cells may be very large (> 50 nuclei)
  - Stromal cells should **not** show malignant cytologic features or atypical mitoses

- Evidence of frank malignancy should raise possibility of other tumors, such as metastatic carcinoma, osteosarcoma, dedifferentiated chondrosarcoma, etc.
- May contain areas of aneurysmal bone cyst (ABC)
  - Epiphyseal location suggests secondary ABC over primary ABC

Chondroblastoma

- Typically occurs in skeletally immature patients with open growth plates (age range: 10-25 years)
- Localization to epiphysis or apophysis of long bone is characteristic
- Imaging shows well-defined tumor of variable size, often with sclerotic margins
- Contains large number of osteoclast-like giant cells, similar to giant cell tumor
- Predominant cell type (chondroblast) is generally pink, epithelioid, and contains nucleus that is sometimes grooved
- Identification of stromal chicken-wire calcification and fragments of cartilage is common
- Chondroblastoma can be distinguished from giant cell tumor
  - Young age, epithelioid "fried egg" cells with grooved nuclei, chicken-wire calcification, and presence of cartilage all favor chondroblastoma
- May contain areas of ABC

Fibrous Dysplasia

- Most common in young to middle-aged patients; often asymptomatic
- May present as solitary or multiple lesions (either within same or different bones)
  - Most common in long bones
  - Other sites (e.g., ribs and craniofacial bones) may be involved
- Imaging shows well-circumscribed intramedullary tumor, most commonly in diaphysis and metadiaphysis
- Composed of mixture of fibroblasts and immature (woven) bone trabeculae
  - Spindled fibroblasts are bland and may demonstrate storiform growth pattern
    - Stroma is often collagenous but may be myxoid
  - Woven bone trabeculae are characteristically irregularly shaped, discontinuous, and often lack osteoblastic rimming
  - Woven bone production can be focal in some tumors and may not be sampled, potentially leading to diagnostic difficulty
- Does not demonstrate infiltrative or permeative growth pattern through preexisting lamellar bone (this finding suggests low-grade osteosarcoma)

Aneurysmal Bone Cyst (ABC)

- Most commonly arise in young patients (< 20 years) in metaphyseal region of long bones
- Imaging generally shows expansile, lytic, and cystic lesion, often with fluid levels due to blood
- Composed of variably thick cyst walls containing bland, spindled to ovoid cells; scattered giant cells; and focal seams of osteoid
  - Frankly malignant cells are inconsistent with diagnosis and may suggest telangiectatic osteosarcoma
- Epiphyseal lesions with appearance of ABC are usually different tumors (giant cell tumor, chondroblastoma, etc.) with secondary ABC

Osteomyelitis

- Patients often complain of pain and systemic symptoms
- Can easily mimic neoplasm on imaging
- Early osteomyelitis shows fragments of mature lamellar bone associated with granulation tissue, necrotic bone, and collections of acute inflammatory cells
- Chronic osteomyelitis often shows intertrabecular loose fibrosis and more prominent plasma cell infiltrate
  - Fibrous dysplasia and low-grade osteosarcoma show cellular spindle cell proliferation rather than loose fibrosis
  - Plasma cell neoplasms contain sheets of plasma cells and lack granulation tissue

Langerhans Cell Histiocytosis (Eosinophilic Granuloma)

- Usually presents in first 3 decades of life
  - May be solitary (eosinophilic granuloma) or multifocal
    - Systemic disease involves multiple organ systems and frequently occurs in first 2 years of life
- Most common in craniofacial bones but can involve any bone
- Imaging usually shows small, well-defined lesion (may have punched-out appearance)
- Composed of irregular sheets and nests of pink histiocytic cells (Langerhans cells) within typically prominent mixed chronic inflammatory infiltrate
  - Langerhans cell nuclei are generally ovoid with nuclear grooves (coffee bean-shaped) or notched
  - Eosinophils are variably prominent and may show eosinophilic abscess formation
    - Reactive germinal centers may be present
  - Inflammation may be prominent and obscure diagnostic Langerhans cells

Metaphyseal Fibrous Defect (Nonossifying Fibroma/Fibrous Cortical Defect)

- Most common in 2nd decade of life
- Imaging shows small, well-demarcated, cortical-based lesion in metaphysis of long bone
- Painless and asymptomatic, unless large or associated with fracture
- Composed of bland, spindled fibroblasts in storiform growth pattern associated with scattered multinucleated osteoclast-like giant cells
  - Number of giant cells may be striking, but sheets of giant cells are not seen (as in giant cell tumor)
- Xanthomatous change and chronic inflammation are commonly identified

Plasma Cell Neoplasm

- Includes solitary plasmacytoma, multiple myeloma, and lymphomas with plasmacytic/plasmablastic differentiation
- Very common primary malignant bone tumors
- Most patients are middle aged or older

- May present as localized lesion (plasmacytoma) or as component of widespread disease (plasma cell myeloma)
- Composed of sheets of plasma cells demonstrating varying degrees of nuclear atypia
  - Poorly differentiated plasma cells may be difficult to distinguish from carcinoma, and clinical/radiographic correlation or even deferral may be required
    - Touch preps may be helpful in evaluation of cells

Lymphoma

- Most commonly represents involvement of bone by systemic disease, although primary lymphomas of bone occur rarely
- Usually occurs in adults, but age range is wide
- Imaging shows large, destructive mass often centered in metadiaphysis of long bone
  - May extend to form soft tissue mass
- Histologic appearance depends upon type of lymphoma, but most form dyscohesive sheets of variably monomorphic round cells and would be classified as small round blue cell tumors
  - Well-formed cohesive nests and aggregates are not generally seen as in carcinoma
- Evaluation may be hindered by extensive crush artifact or necrosis, and more tissue should be requested for evaluation in this situation
- Diagnosis of "atypical lymphoid infiltrate" or "malignant neoplasm, suggestive of lymphoma, final diagnosis deferred to permanent sections" is usually satisfactory
  - Further ancillary testing and morphologic evaluation is often necessary
  - Ancillary studies should be sent when possible [flow cytometric analysis, frozen tissue (molecular studies), special fixatives]

REPORTING

Frozen Section

- Specific diagnosis is always preferred but is not always possible
  - Additional sampling and ancillary studies may be required
- Most critical distinction is between benign and malignant
  - If malignant, distinguishing between low-grade and high-grade process is also important
  - Diagnosis of "low-grade neoplasm, final diagnosis deferred to permanent sections" may be necessary if distinction between benign and low-grade malignant lesion is not possible
- Ensure that sample received is adequate for subsequent evaluation on permanent sections
  - If not, request more tissue be sent
- Diagnosis of small round blue cell tumor implies malignancy (likely high grade) and almost always requires deferral of final diagnosis to permanent sections
  - Final classification usually requires ancillary studies

PITFALLS

Overdiagnosing Giant Cell Tumor

- Most bone tumors contain multinucleated osteoclast-like giant cells
- Location, age, and radiographic appearance are paramount for making diagnosis
- Giant cell tumor is reasonably considered in setting of epiphyseal bone lesion demonstrating sheets of multinucleated giant cells with no malignant stromal cell atypia

Low-Grade Chondrosarcoma vs. Enchondroma

- Can be extremely difficult if not impossible to distinguish histologically
- Clinical behavior and radiographs are critical in helping make distinction
  - Cortical erosion/destruction &/or soft tissue extension support chondrosarcoma
  - Enchondroma is typically small, well localized, and more likely to be found incidentally
- Diagnosis of "low-grade cartilaginous neoplasm, final diagnosis deferred to permanent sections" is acceptable in cases with little to no supportive clinicoradiologic information

Misinterpreting Fracture Callus as Malignancy

- Pathologic fracture can coexist in benign or malignant lesions
- Fracture is often known or suspected clinically
  - Preexisting history of trauma to area is often available
- Fracture callus is composed of hypercellular cartilage admixed with woven bone formation and fibroconnective tissue, often in relatively linear array (along original fracture line)
  - Hypercellular cartilage may raise possibility of chondrosarcoma, but overall context essentially precludes that diagnosis
- Identification of fracture in patients > 45 years of age should prompt careful search for metastatic carcinoma
- Exuberant fracture callus may clinically simulate (rare) true bone neoplasm due to apparent bony expansion

Small Focus of Metastatic Carcinoma Not Seen

- High level of suspicion for metastatic carcinoma must be maintained in any patient > 45 years of age, particularly if history of carcinoma exists
- Often component of reactive stromal myofibroblastic proliferation is associated with metastatic carcinoma
  - Its sole presence may indicate that additional sections should be cut in case diagnostic tissue is focal
- All remaining tissue should be submitted for frozen section evaluation if there is clinical suspicion for metastatic disease and no diagnostic findings are found on initial evaluation

Biopsy Not Representative of Lesion

- Reactive soft tissue overlying bone may be unintentionally sampled instead of true lesion
  - What appears to be chronic osteomyelitis may actually be adjacent reactive and inflamed fibroblastic tissue overlying true neoplasm
- Clinical and imaging findings help guide interpretation

SELECTED REFERENCES

1. Bhaker P et al: Role of intraoperative pathology consultation in skeletal tumors and tumor-like lesions. Sarcoma. 2014:902104, 2014
2. Sezak M et al: Feasibility and clinical utility of intraoperative consultation with frozen section in osseous lesions. Virchows Arch. 461(2):195-204, 2012

(Left) *The identification of cellular sheets of malignant cells directly associated with osteoid* ⇨ *or immature (woven) bone formation is characteristic of osteosarcoma. The majority of these tumors are large, destructive lesions and occur predominantly in teenagers around the region of the knee.* **(Right)** *Most osteosarcomas are high-grade malignancies with obvious nuclear pleomorphism and numerous mitoses* ⇨*. However, some tumors may show less pleomorphism. Note the pink osteoid deposition* ⇨*.*

Osteosarcoma: Bone Formation

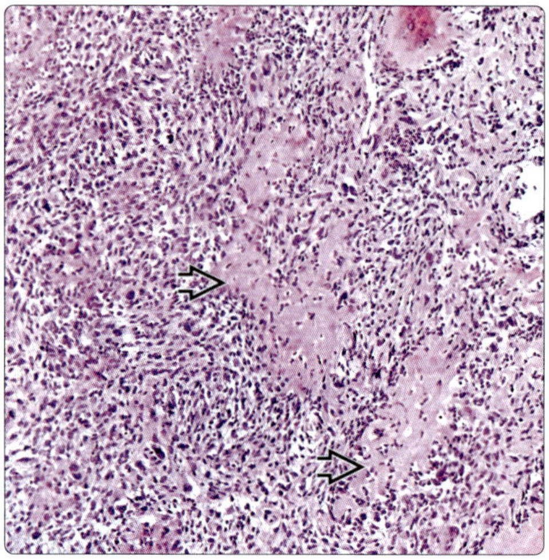

Osteosarcoma: Cytologic Features

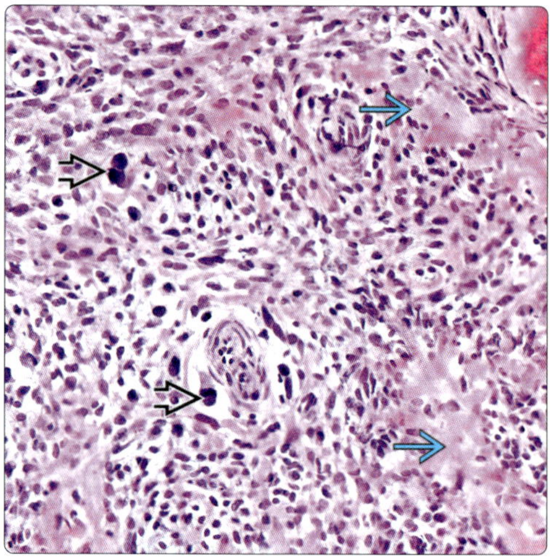

(Left) *In some osteosarcomas, osteoid and immature (woven) bone production are not present or not seen on the frozen section. Clinical and radiographic information often aid in diagnosis in these cases, and additional tissue may need to be procured by surgeon. In older patients, an undifferentiated pleomorphic sarcoma of bone must also be considered.* **(Right)** *Low-grade cartilaginous neoplasms (e.g., enchondroma) can be difficult to distinguish on frozen section and often require radiographic correlation.*

Osteosarcoma: Lack of Bone Formation

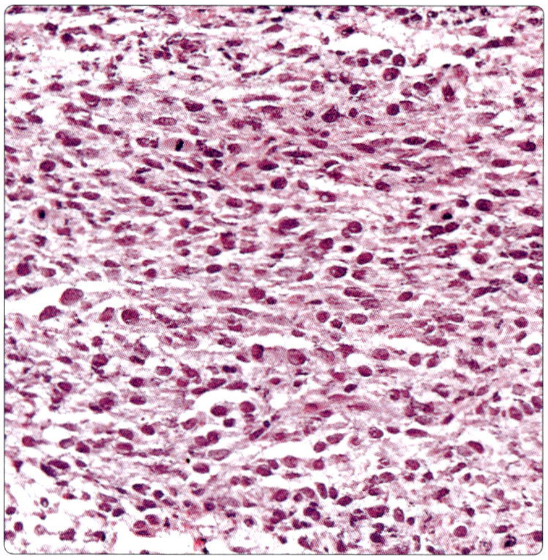

Low-Grade Cartilaginous Neoplasms

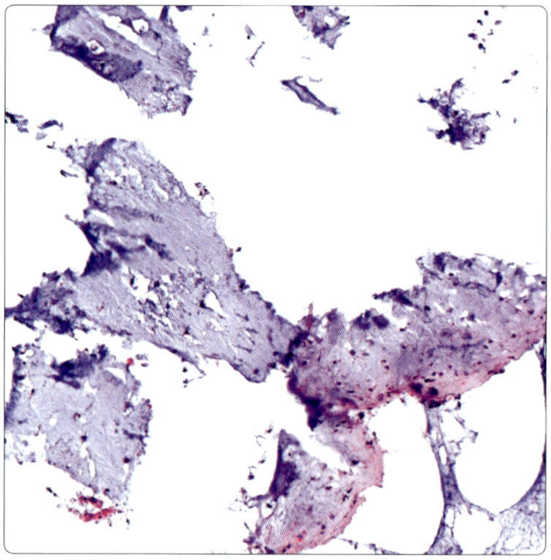

(Left) *Enchondromas often show a thin rim of pink bone* → *around the cartilaginous lobules. Cellularity is usually lower than is seen in low-grade chondrosarcomas. However, enchondromas of the small bones often show a higher degree of cellularity* ⇨ *and may be overdiagnosed as malignant.* **(Right)** *Ewing sarcoma is a type of small round blue cell tumor and is generally characterized by sheets of small cells with scant, pink to clear cytoplasm. This tumor occurs in pediatric patients, and necrosis is common.*

Enchondroma

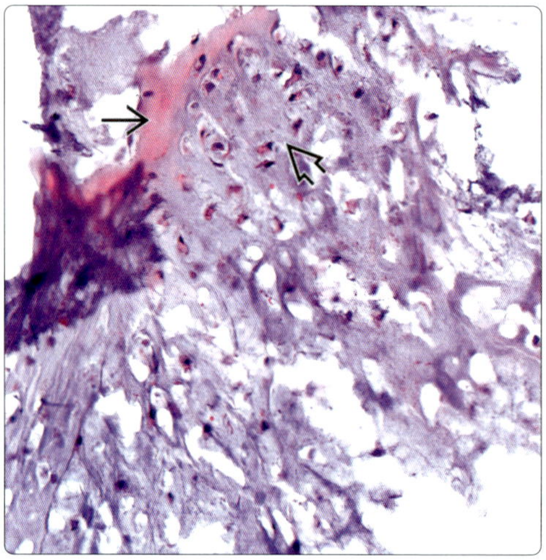

Ewing Sarcoma

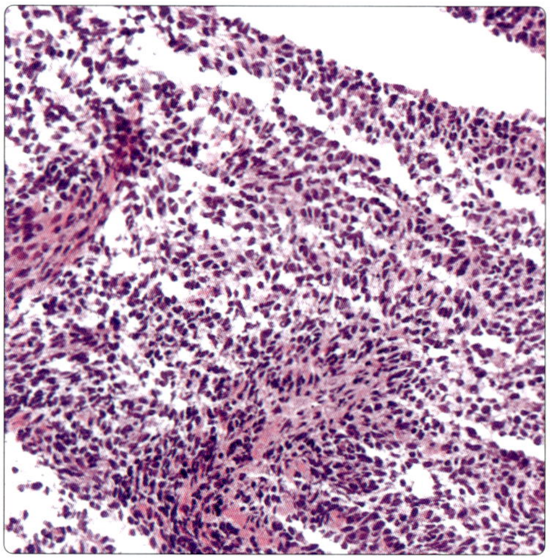

Ewing Sarcoma: Crush Artifact

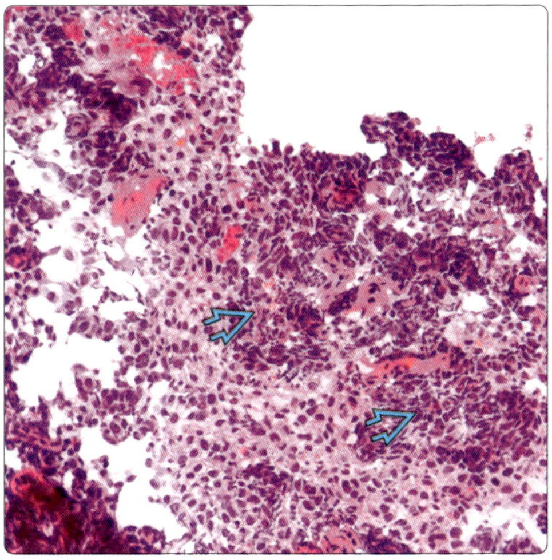

Giant Cell Tumor of Bone

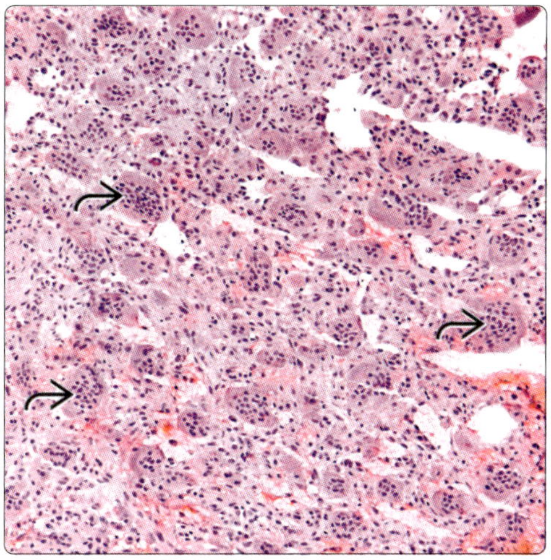

(Left) *As with most small round blue cell tumors, the cells of Ewing sarcoma may be easily disrupted during the biopsy. This image shows areas of crush artifact, which resemble aggregates of small lymphocytes.* **(Right)** *Although most bone lesions contain scattered osteoclast-like giant cells, a true giant cell tumor of bone often shows diffuse sheets of these cells. Correlation with age (typically 25-45 years) and epiphyseal location is also very useful in establishing the diagnosis.*

Giant Cell Tumor of Bone

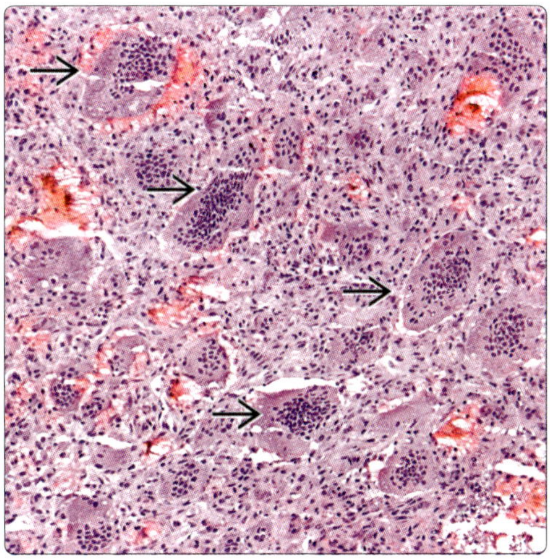

Chondroblastoma

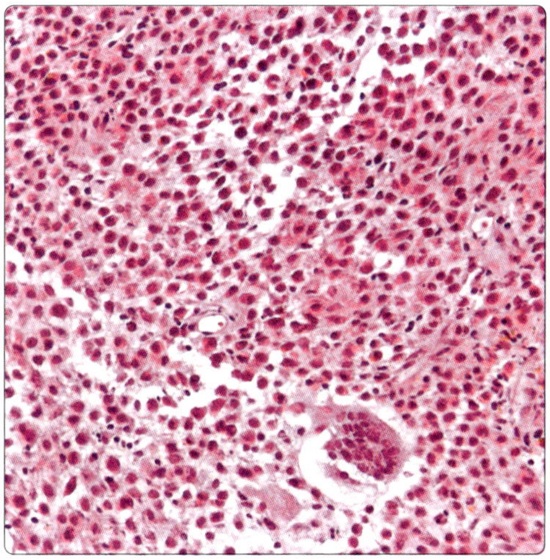

(Left) *The osteoclast-like giant cells in a giant cell tumor of bone also have the tendency to grow quite large and may demonstrate 50-100 nuclei. Also note that the admixed stromal cells are not malignant. If malignant, this finding would suggest other diagnoses.* **(Right)** *Although chondroblastoma shares some histologic similarities with giant cell tumor, the constituent cells of the former are more round, plump, and eosinophilic. They may even show cytoplasmic clearing (fried egg morphology).*

Chondroblastoma: Calcification

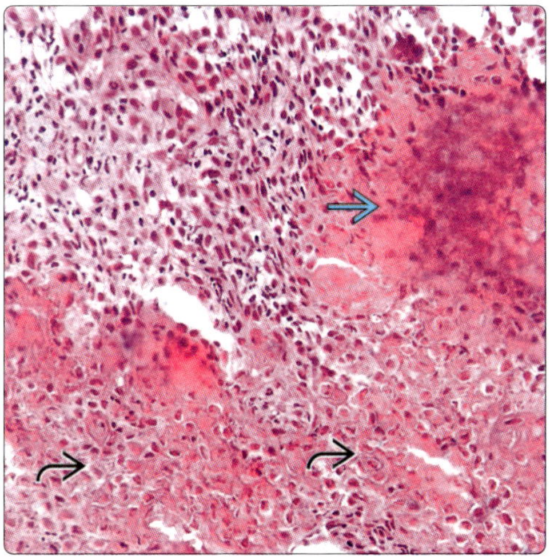

Chondroblastoma: Cartilage

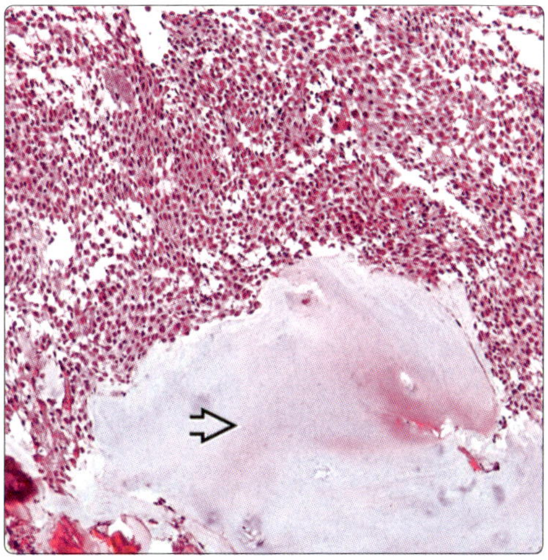

(Left) *Foci of calcification are common in chondroblastoma, particularly when the calcification is deposited both between and around the cells (chicken-wire pattern). This pattern, however, is usually better appreciated on permanent sections.* **(Right)** *Fragments of cartilage are also found in many cases of chondroblastoma. This finding is not typical of giant cell tumor of bone. Also note the sheet of round, plump, and pink cells that characterizes this tumor.*

(Left) *Classic fibrous dysplasia is composed of bland stromal spindle cells within a fibromyxoid stroma admixed with irregular fragments of immature (woven) bone. It is important to be aware that some areas within fibrous dysplasia may show absolutely no bone formation.* **(Right)** *The irregular bone fragments in fibrous dysplasia are characteristically immature (cellular with no lamellae) and usually do not show osteoblastic rimming; however, some cases show focal rimming. Note the bland stromal cells.*

Fibrous Dysplasia

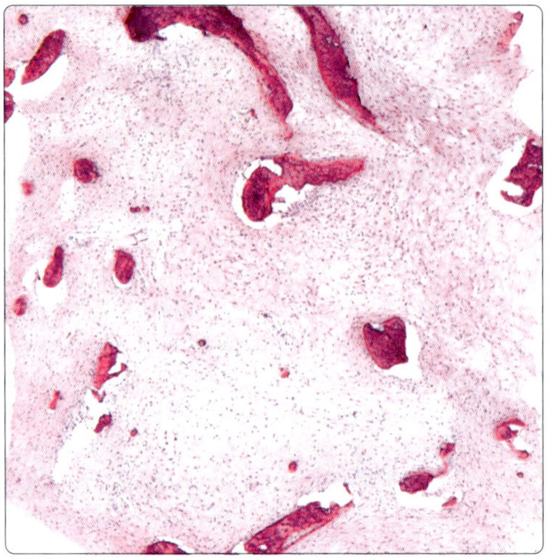

Fibrous Dysplasia: Immature Bone

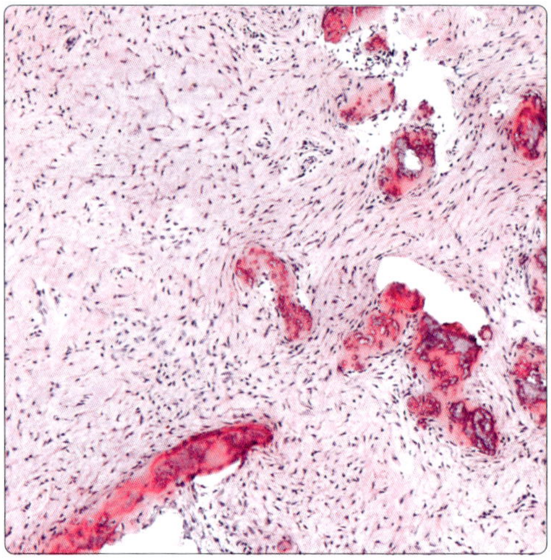

(Left) *Classic aneurysmal bone cyst shows thin ribbons ⇨ of cyst lining composed of loosely cellular bland spindled cells and scattered osteoclast giant cells →. Importantly, there is no malignant nuclear atypia.* **(Right)** *Some cases of osteomyelitis will show a variably prominent neutrophilic infiltrate → in addition to chronic inflammation. Granulation tissue with reactive stromal capillaries ⇨ is also often present. No cytologic or cellular patterns typical of malignancy are seen.*

Aneurysmal Bone Cyst

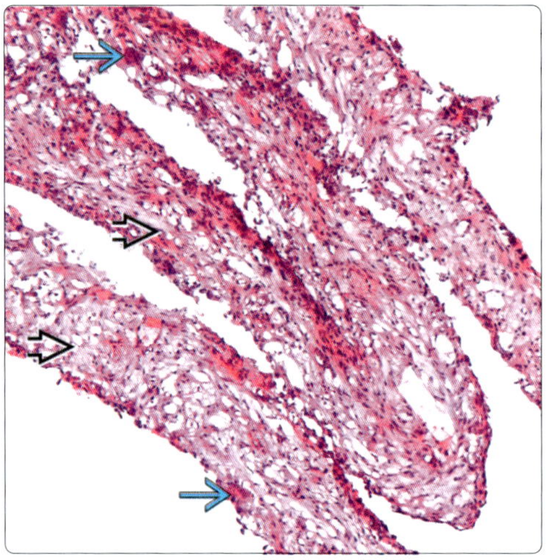

Osteomyelitis

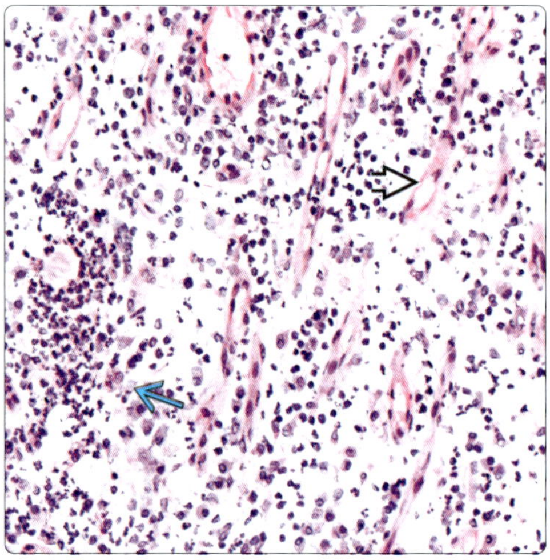

(Left) *In some cases of chronic osteomyelitis, the plasma cell infiltrate may be striking and mimic a plasma cell neoplasm. However, in osteomyelitis, the plasma cells are intermingled with other inflammatory cells, and they are generally not cytologically atypical.* **(Right)** *Evidence of fracture may be seen in the setting of a benign or malignant lesion. It is often characterized histologically by a relatively linear arrangement of hypercellular cartilage, immature bone formation →, and bland fibroconnective tissue ⇨.*

Chronic Osteomyelitis

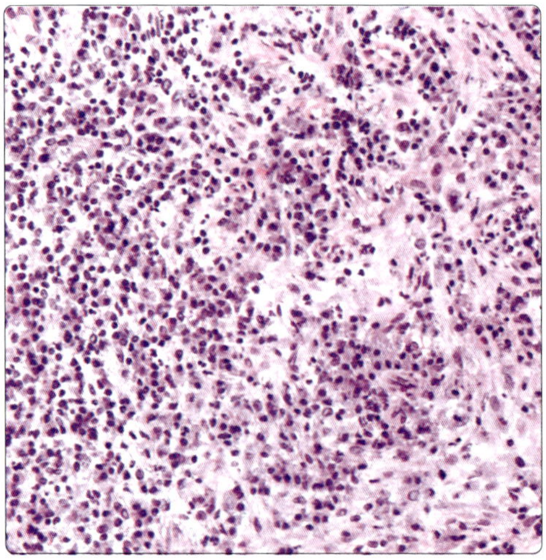

Fracture Callus

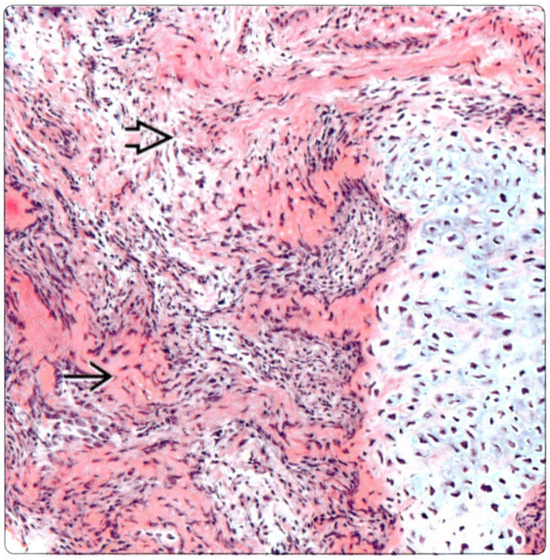

Langerhans Cell Histiocytosis

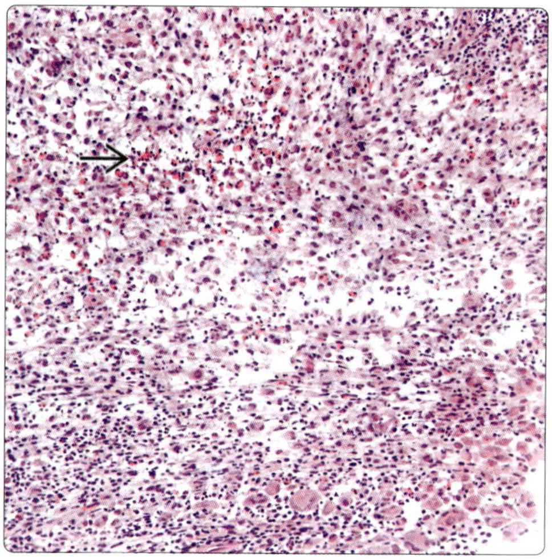

Langerhans Cell Histiocytosis: Cytology

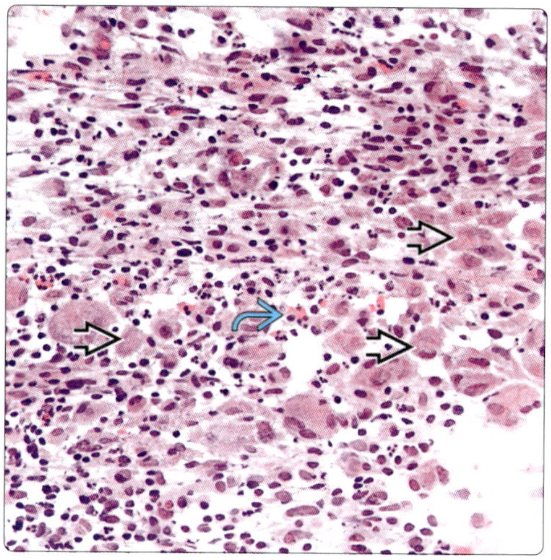

(Left) *Langerhans cell histiocytosis (eosinophilic granuloma of bone) may be easily confused with a florid inflammatory process, such as osteomyelitis. It is composed of aggregates and small sheets of pink histiocytoid cells in a background of chronic inflammatory cells, particularly eosinophils → (often abundant).* **(Right)** *The diagnostic Langerhans cells ⇨ are round, pink, and contain an indented (coffee bean-shaped) or grooved nucleus. Inflammatory cells, including eosinophils ↪, are present.*

Metaphyseal Fibrous Defect

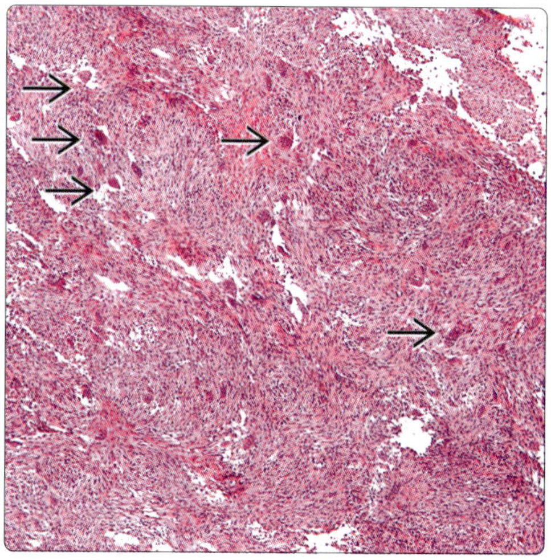

Metaphyseal Fibrous Defect: Inflammatory Cells

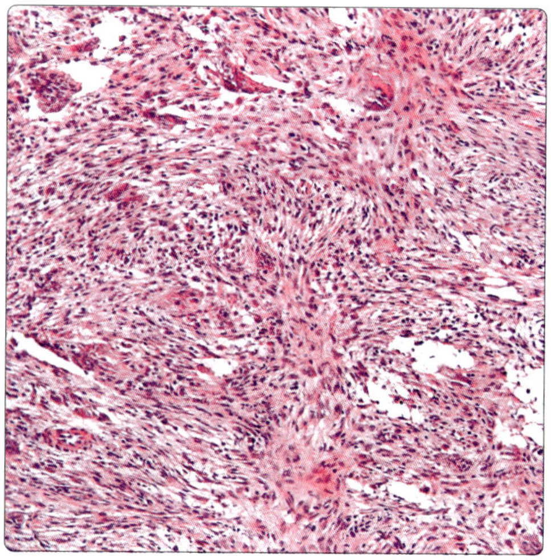

(Left) *Metaphyseal fibrous defect (also referred to as nonossifying fibroma or fibrous cortical defect) is characterized by a cellular proliferation of bland spindle cells forming broad whorls (storiform growth pattern) with admixed osteoclast-like giant cells. Note that the giant cells → may be prominent in number, but they do not form sheets as seen in giant cell tumor.* **(Right)** *An admixed chronic inflammatory component (lymphocytes, histiocytes) is common in metaphyseal fibrous defect.*

Plasma Cell Neoplasm

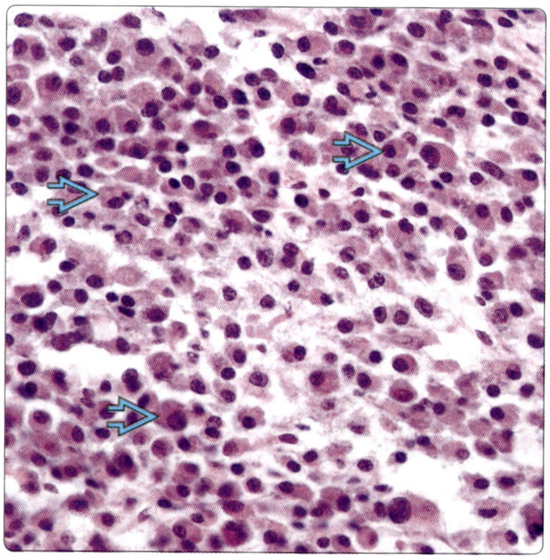

Lymphoma

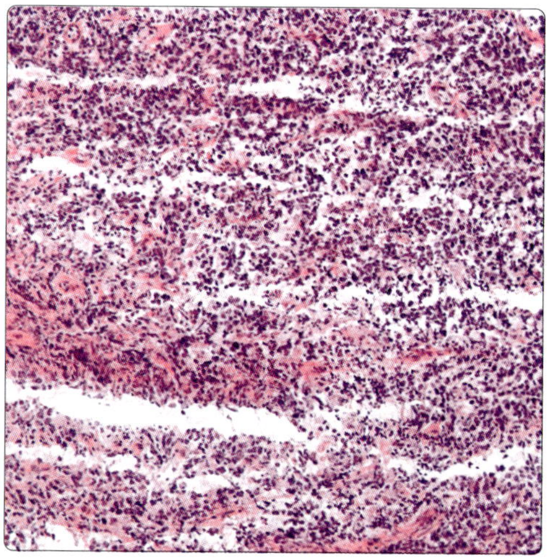

(Left) *Plasma cell neoplasms (including solitary plasmacytoma of bone and plasma cell myeloma) are all composed of sheets of neoplastic plasma cells (identified by their eccentric nuclei ⇨ and perinuclear hof). The plasma cells of myeloma may show more profound cytologic atypia and can mimic carcinoma.* **(Right)** *Diffuse sheets of dyscohesive cells are typical of most lymphomas, but subtyping often requires ancillary testing. Necrosis is often prominent in high-grade lymphomas.*

(Left) *Axial CT of the spine in a patient with prostate carcinoma shows a metastasis that is both lytic and densely blastic. Lytic lesions predominate in most cases of metastatic carcinoma and are usually multiple.* (Right) *Lateral radiograph shows a typical case of an osteosarcoma in the proximal fibula near the knee in a young person. The mass contains osteoid matrix and has a prominent "sunburst" periosteal reaction as well as matrix formation in the soft tissue mass.*

Blastic/Lytic Metastasis

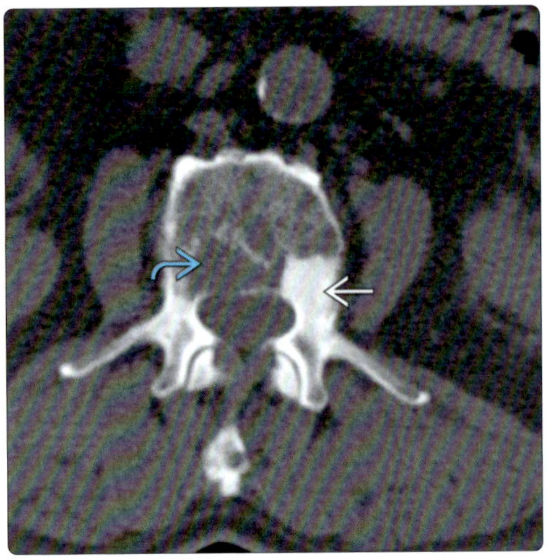

Osteosarcoma

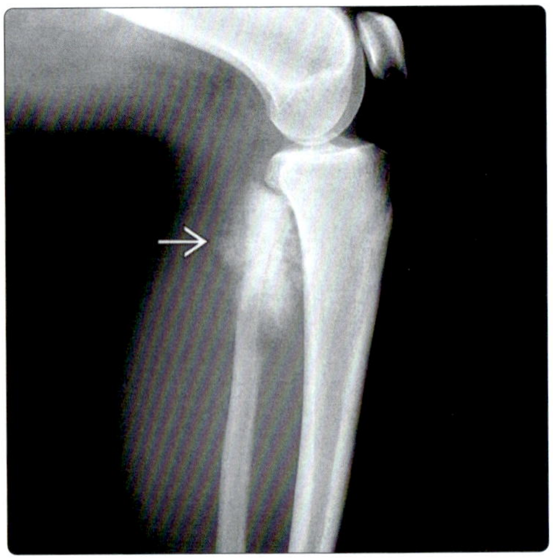

(Left) *AP radiograph demonstrates the typical well-localized "stippled" chondroid matrix of an enchondroma with rings and arcs. The metaphyseal location is typical for this diagnosis, and there is no cortical erosion/destruction or soft tissue extension.* (Right) *Axial CT shows a mass arising from the neural arch containing ringed and stippled calcifications, a typical appearance for chondroid tumor matrix. Given the large size, this tumor is most consistent with a chondrosarcoma.*

Enchondroma

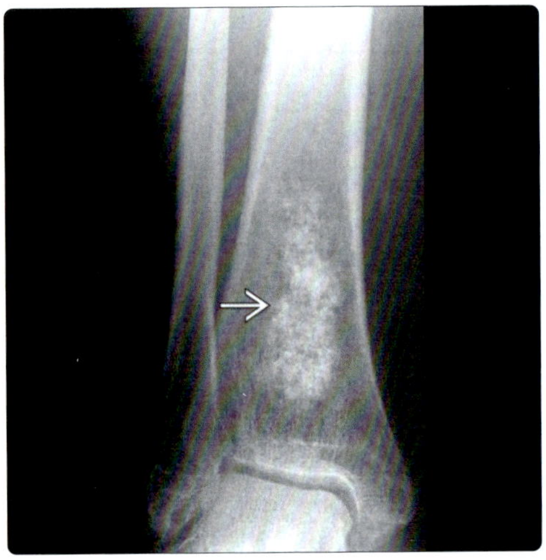

Chondrosarcoma

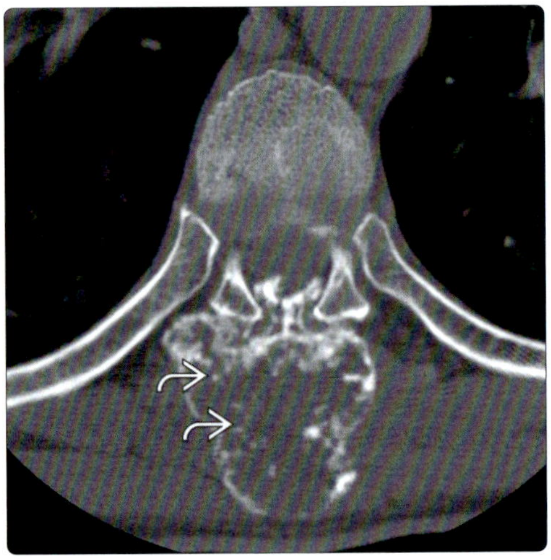

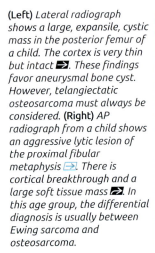

(Left) *Lateral radiograph shows a large, expansile, cystic mass in the posterior femur of a child. The cortex is very thin but intact. These findings favor aneurysmal bone cyst. However, telangiectatic osteosarcoma must always be considered.* (Right) *AP radiograph from a child shows an aggressive lytic lesion of the proximal fibular metaphysis. There is cortical breakthrough and a large soft tissue mass. In this age group, the differential diagnosis is usually between Ewing sarcoma and osteosarcoma.*

Aneurysmal Bone Cyst

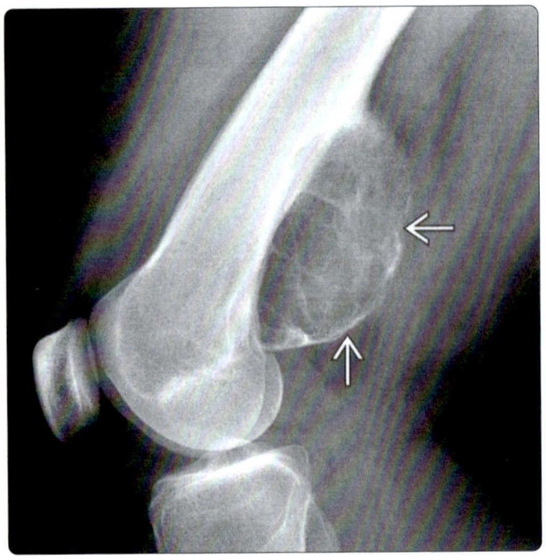

Ewing Sarcoma

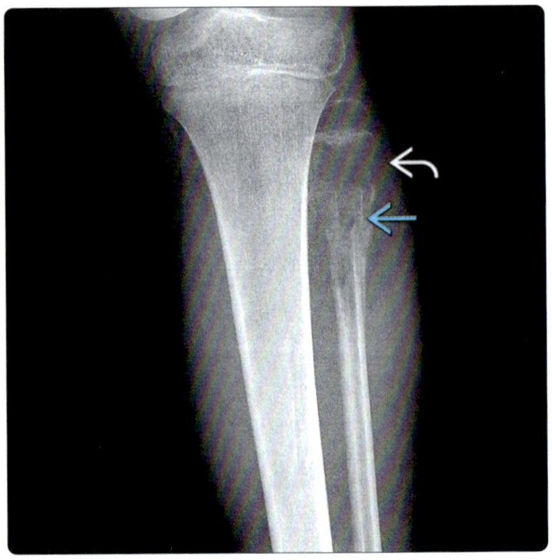

Giant Cell Tumor of Bone

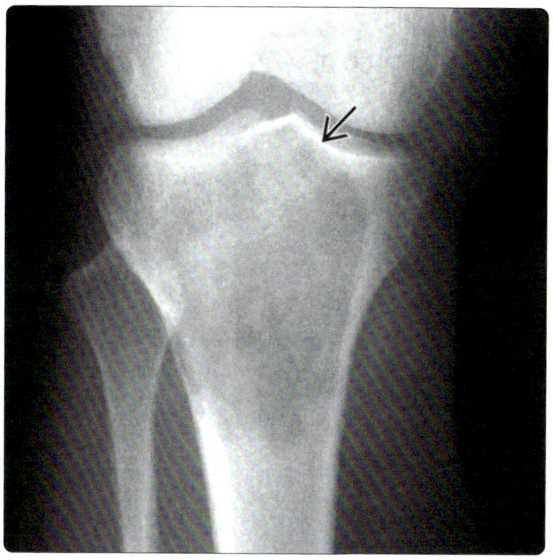

Chondroblastoma

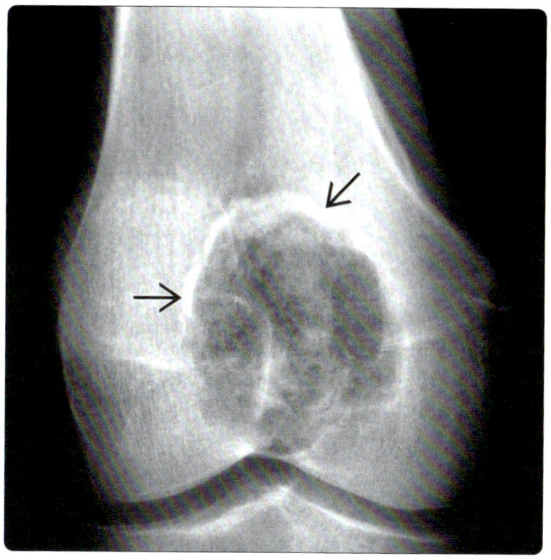

(Left) *AP radiograph shows a classic giant cell tumor of the proximal tibia. Here, the lesion is completely lytic and somewhat eccentrically placed, centered in the metaphysis and extending into the epiphysis and subarticular surface. Note the lack of a sclerotic margin.* **(Right)** *AP radiograph shows a very well-circumscribed lytic lesion with a sclerotic border involving the epiphysis and metaphysis. These findings are typical of chondroblastoma.*

Fibrous Dysplasia

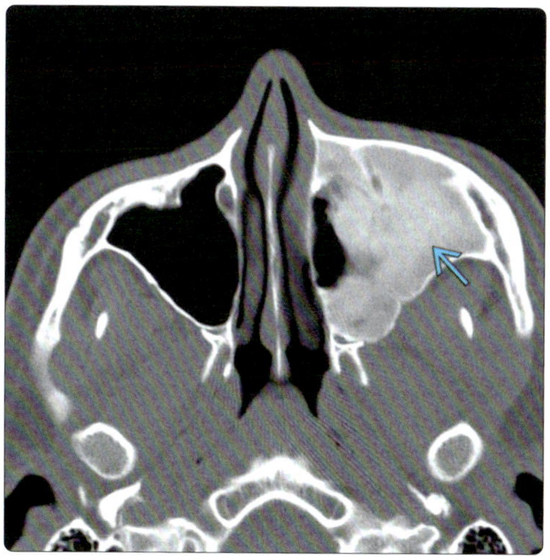

Langerhans Cell Histiocytosis (Eosinophilic Granuloma)

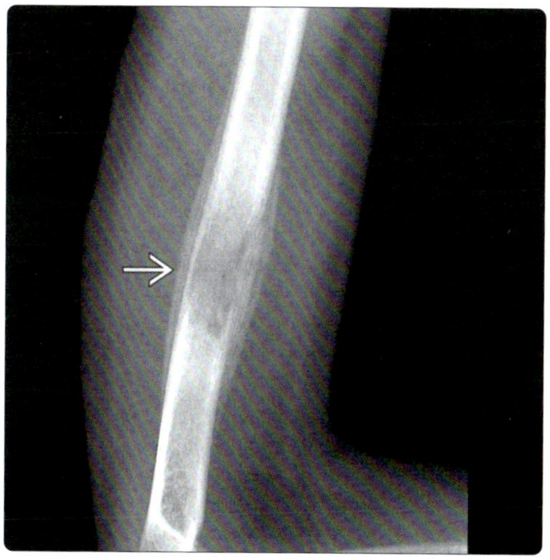

(Left) *Axial CT of the sinus demonstrates the characteristic ground-glass appearance of fibrous dysplasia. This finding can also be appreciated on MR. In long bones, fibrous dysplasia generally lacks aggressive features.* **(Right)** *Lateral radiograph in a child shows a highly permeative diaphyseal lesion with a prominent periosteal reaction. Given these findings, the differential diagnosis is often between Ewing sarcoma and Langerhans cell histiocytosis.*

Metaphyseal Fibrous Defect (Nonossifying Fibroma)

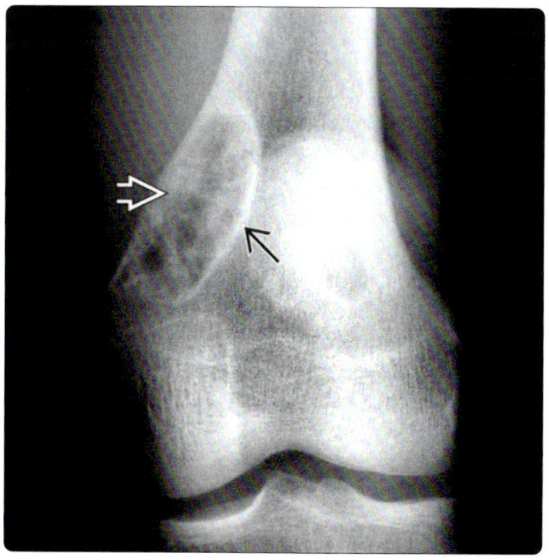

Plasma Cell Myeloma

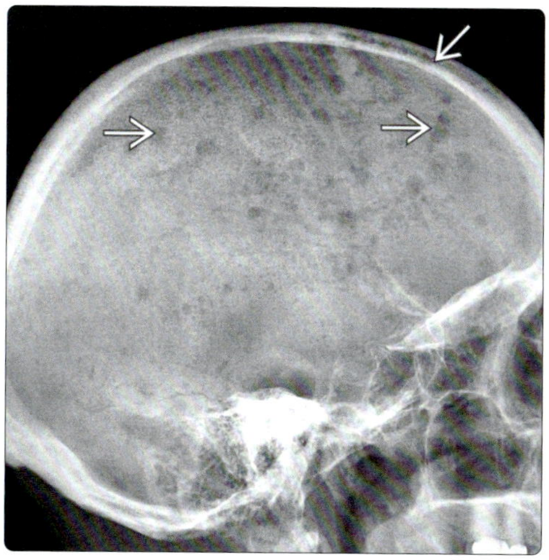

(Left) *AP radiograph shows a typical metaphyseal fibrous defect in a young adult. Note that the lesion is well circumscribed, metaphyseal, and cortically based. It demonstrates a densely sclerotic margin, supporting a benign nature.* **(Right)** *Lateral radiograph from a skeletal survey demonstrates numerous punched-out lytic bone lesions in the skull. This is commonly seen in advanced cases of plasma cell myeloma, but metastatic carcinoma can also have this appearance.*

SURGICAL/CLINICAL CONSIDERATIONS

Goal of Consultation

- Determine if carcinoma is present
  - Tissue may be taken for ancillary studies that require unfixed tissue in some cases, but only if invasive carcinoma is identified
  - Margin evaluation may be requested by surgeon

Change in Patient Management

- Additional tissue may be taken to achieve negative margins &/or lymph nodes may be sampled
- **Caution**
  - Primary diagnosis by frozen section is not recommended
    - False-positive and false-negative results are rare but do occur
  - Preferable to make diagnosis by core needle biopsy or small excisional biopsy on permanent sections
    - There are many options that should be discussed with patient before definitive surgery
      - Type of surgery (breast conservation or mastectomy)
      - Nodal sampling (sentinel node biopsy or axillary dissection)
      - Neoadjuvant therapy (chemotherapy or hormonal therapy)
- There are only rare situations in which patients benefit from primary intraoperative diagnosis of breast lesion

SPECIMEN EVALUATION

Specimen Radiograph

- If performed, specimen radiograph should be provided to pathologist
- Radiograph is reviewed to determine type of lesion, presence of clips, and presence of wire or radioactive seed
- Distance to 4 of the 6 margins can be evaluated
- If obvious mass forming lesion (> 1 cm) is not present, evaluation should be deferred to permanent sections

Gross

- Specimen orientation provided by surgeon is identified (e.g., by sutures or ink color)
- If not previously inked, specimen is inked according to orientation
  - If inked by surgeon, correct orientation according to color is verified
- Specimen is serially sectioned
  - Majority of carcinomas have typical gritty texture (like cutting a water chestnut)
  - Other types of carcinoma can be firm (not hard) or mucinous
- Gross lesions are identified by palpation of a discrete firm to hard mass
  - If > 1 cm, frozen section may be considered if result will change intraoperative decisions
    - However, sufficient tumor must be available for permanent section evaluation and ancillary studies
  - Gross lesions < 1 cm should not be frozen
    - Sufficient nonfrozen tissue may not be available for diagnosis and ancillary studies
    - Diagnostic errors are most likely for small lesions
- Tissue without a gross lesion should not be frozen
  - Frozen section artifact &/or loss of tissue during slide preparation may preclude definitive diagnosis even on permanent sections
- Tissue from diagnostic specimen should never be taken for ancillary studies or research unless there is a definitive diagnosis of invasive carcinoma

Frozen Section

- Should be a small representative section of lesion > 1 cm in size (not including adjacent breast tissue)
  - Entire lesion should never be frozen

Cytology

- Touch preparations or scrape cytology may be performed on lesions > 1 cm that are suspicious for invasive carcinoma

Invasive Carcinoma: Irregular Mass on Mammography

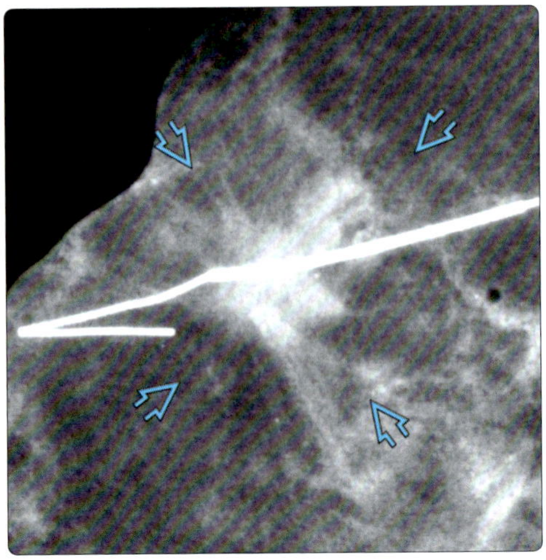

Invasive Carcinoma: Gross Appearance of Irregular Mass

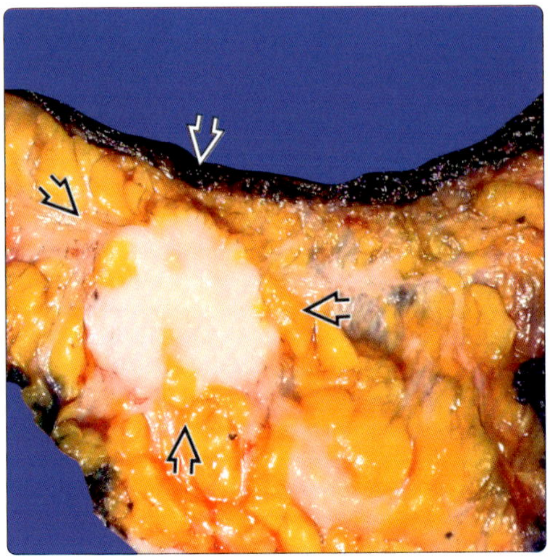

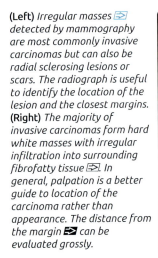

(Left) *Irregular masses ⇨ detected by mammography are most commonly invasive carcinomas but can also be radial sclerosing lesions or scars. The radiograph is useful to identify the location of the lesion and the closest margins.* **(Right)** *The majority of invasive carcinomas form hard white masses with irregular infiltration into surrounding fibrofatty tissue ⇨. In general, palpation is a better guide to location of the carcinoma rather than appearance. The distance from the margin ➡ can be evaluated grossly.*

MOST COMMON DIAGNOSES

Invasive Carcinoma With Irregular Borders

- Majority of breast cancers grow as masses that irregularly invade adjacent tissue
  - Hard consistency
  - Borders palpated as a distinct edge or shelf delineating cancer from normal tissue
- Size is carefully recorded to nearest mm
  - Size by palpation is more accurate than size by visual inspection

Invasive Carcinoma With Circumscribed Borders

- Most common are mucinous and "triple negative" (negative for hormone receptors and HER2) carcinomas
- Flat or concave surface rather than bulging like fibroadenoma
  - White and firm rather than hard
- Size is carefully recorded to nearest mm

Invasive Lobular Carcinoma

- Majority form hard, irregular mass similar to carcinomas of no special type ("ductal" carcinomas)
- Minority form subtle diffuse tissue thickening
  - Involved adipose tissue may have pale white color compared to normal yellow fat
- Size is carefully recorded to nearest mm when possible

Ductal Carcinoma In Situ

- Majority of cases are not grossly visible
- A few cases of high-grade ductal carcinoma in situ (DCIS) form ill-defined firm masses
  - Punctate (comedo-like) necrosis may be extruded if tissue is gently compressed
- Breast tissue without clearly defined mass should not be frozen
  - It can be difficult to distinguish high-grade DCIS from invasive carcinoma on frozen section
    - DCIS, lobular carcinoma in situ, and apocrine metaplasia in sclerosing adenosis can closely mimic invasive carcinoma
  - Freezing artifact &/or tissue loss can complicate diagnosis on permanent sections

Fibroadenoma

- White, circumscribed mass with bulging surface with clefts
- Infarction with necrosis can occur during pregnancy

Phyllodes Tumor

- Usually circumscribed: High-grade lesions may have infiltrative borders
- Size is usually larger and clefts more prominent than fibroadenomas

Sarcoma

- Very rare primary lesion in breast
- Angiosarcoma is most common type
- Form poorly defined, hemorrhagic firm, but usually not hard, large gross lesions

Radial Sclerosing Lesion

- Irregular white mass by imaging and visual examination
  - Radiating arms are long relative to central nidus

Core Needle Biopsy Site

- Most typically an area of hemorrhage with adjacent fat necrosis
- Gel pledgets placed at time of biopsy may resemble rice, gray gelatin, or have other appearances
- Metallic clips are very small and can be difficult to identify
  - Location should be evident in specimen radiograph

Silicone Granuloma

- Silicone bleeds through implants, even in absence of rupture
- Silicone granuloma can form very hard lobulated mass, closely resembling carcinoma grossly
- Lesion consists of histiocytes filled with silicone
  - Silicone is often refractile but does not polarize

REPORTING

Frozen Section

- If definitive diagnosis of invasive carcinoma can be made, this should be reported
  - No need to report histologic type or grade

Cytology

- Reported as positive or negative
- In some cases, definitive diagnosis of invasion may be required to determine if nodes should be sampled

PITFALLS

False-Negative Diagnoses

- Rare (< 10%) if only lesions suspicious for invasive carcinoma undergo examination
- Mammographically detected carcinomas are typically small
- Invasive lobular carcinomas can be difficult to identify

False-Positive Diagnoses

- Rare (< 1%) if only lesions highly suspicious for invasive carcinoma undergo examination
- **Sclerosing adenosis**
  - Most common lesion mistaken for invasive carcinoma
  - Closely mimics invasive carcinoma when involved by carcinoma in situ or apocrine metaplasia
  - Tubules are generally closely packed and back to back
  - Borders are generally circumscribed or lobulated
- **Granular cell tumor**
  - Gross appearance can be very similar to invasive carcinoma
  - Cells have abundant granular cytoplasm and regular round nuclei
- **Nonbreast malignancies**
  - Lymphoma, melanoma, and metastatic carcinoma can mimic primary breast carcinoma
  - Important to recognize, as treatment is generally not surgical
  - Clinical history of prior tumor is very helpful

SELECTED REFERENCES

1. Manfrin E et al: Intra-operative frozen section technique for breast cancer: end of an era. Pathologica. 103(6):325-30, 2011

Contents

(Left) *Grade I carcinomas consist of well-formed tubules in a reactive desmoplastic stroma and can be difficult to distinguish from adenosis on frozen sections. Invasion around normal epithelium is an important clue.* (Right) *Grade III carcinomas typically consist of sheets of cells with pleomorphic nuclei that are clearly malignant. There is often a lymphocytic infiltrate and necrosis. In the absence of ductal carcinoma in situ (DCIS), the possibility of lymphoma, melanoma, or metastatic carcinoma should be considered.*

Grade I Invasive Carcinoma

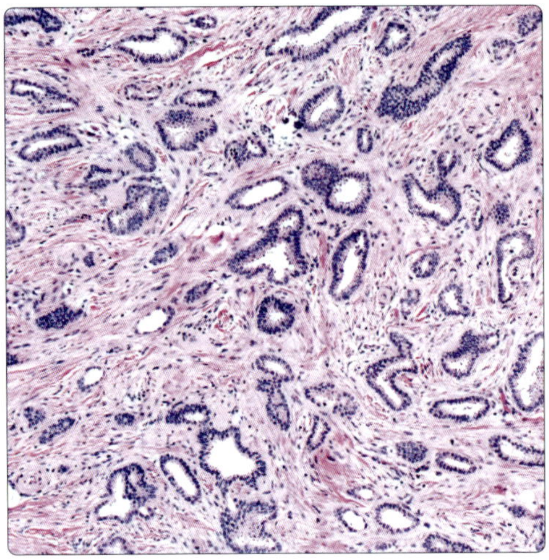

Grade III Invasive Carcinoma

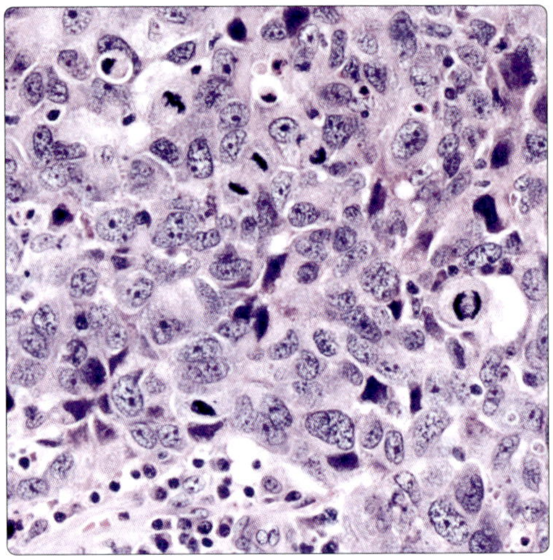

(Left) *Circumscribed masses ➙ are usually benign lesions such as fibroadenomas or nodular adenosis. Some invasive carcinomas also form rounded masses. In this case, the carcinoma is clearly at the margin as shown by the specimen radiograph.* (Right) *A minority of invasive carcinomas have pushing circumscribed margins ➙ and grossly resemble benign lesions such as fibroadenomas. Mucinous carcinomas and carcinomas negative for hormone receptors and HER2 often have this appearance.*

Invasive Carcinoma: Circumscribed Mass on Mammography

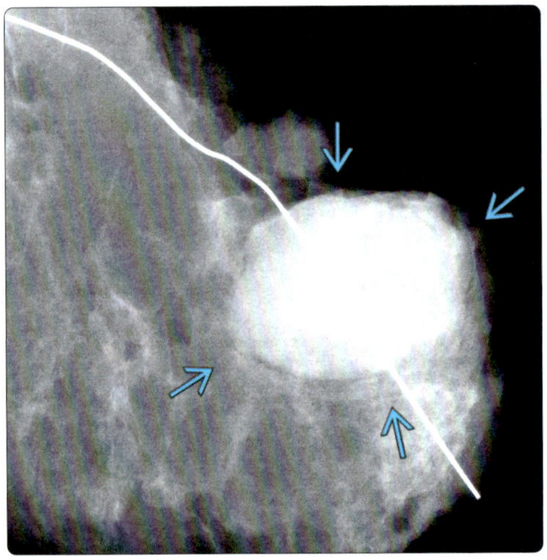

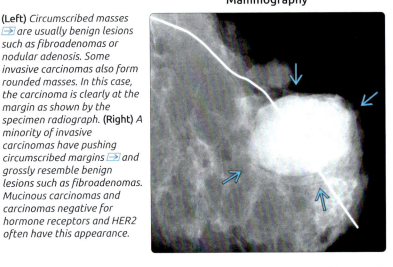

Invasive Carcinoma: Gross Appearance of Circumscribed Mass

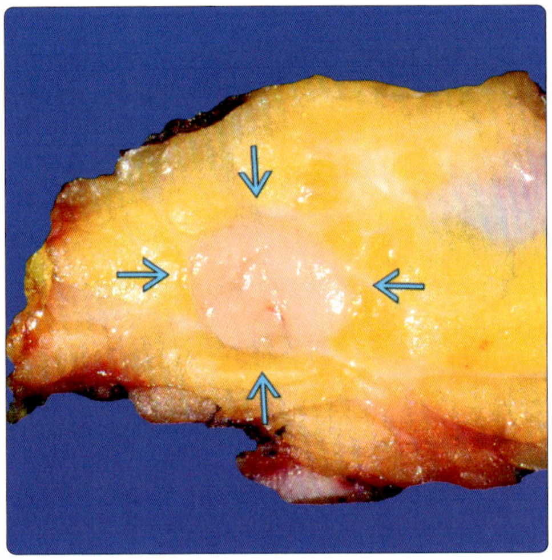

(Left) *Although many invasive lobular carcinomas form irregular masses on mammography, some have a very subtle appearance as architectural distortion without formation of a discrete mass ➙.* (Right) *This invasive lobular carcinoma infiltrates in adipose tissue with little to no desmoplastic response. These carcinomas can be difficult to detect on mammography and by gross examination. Identification on frozen section can be particularly difficult.*

Invasive Lobular Carcinoma: Architectural Distortion on Mammography

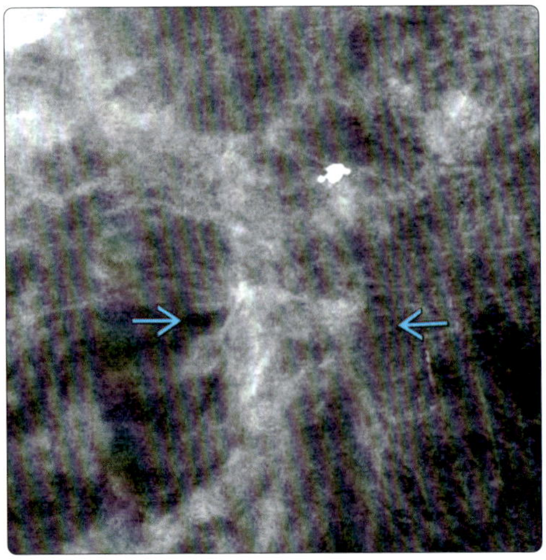

Invasive Lobular Carcinoma

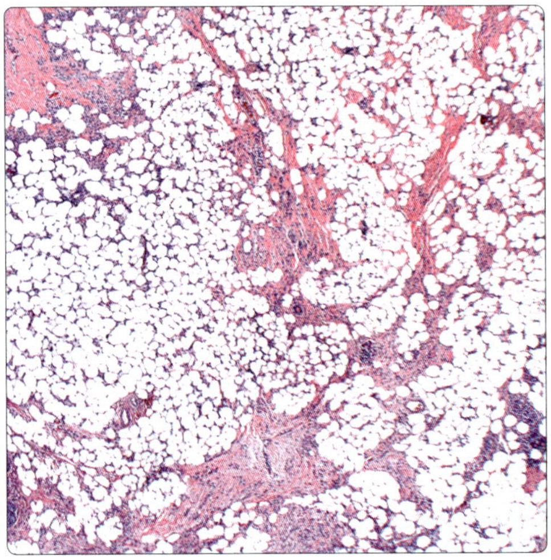

Invasive Carcinoma: Freezing Artifact

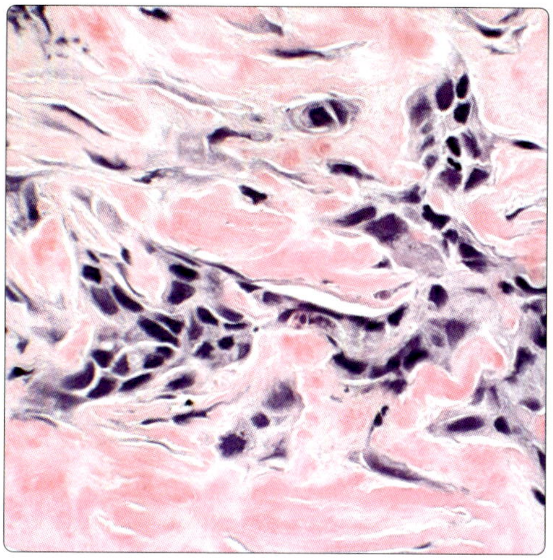

Invasive Carcinoma: Permanent Section

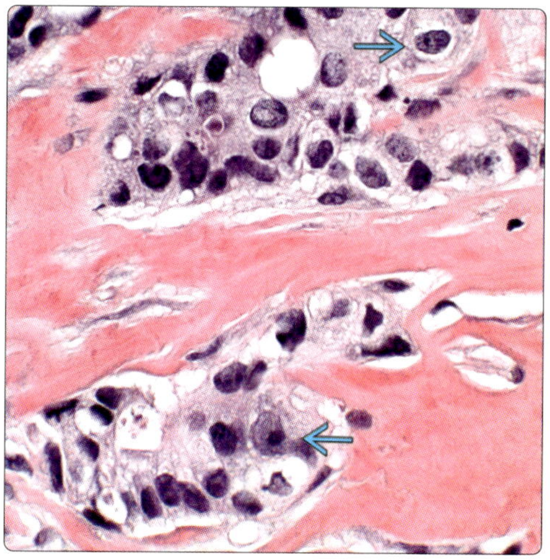

(Left) *This invasive carcinoma can be recognized due to the irregular infiltrative pattern in stroma and the nuclear pleomorphism. However, the nuclear detail is smudged and nucleoli cannot be seen.* **(Right)** *Grading is an important prognostic factor for breast carcinoma and is also used for determining stage. It is critical to see nuclear detail including nucleoli →. Freezing artifact can obscure nuclear detail and should be avoided whenever possible.*

Invasive Carcinoma: Freezing Artifact

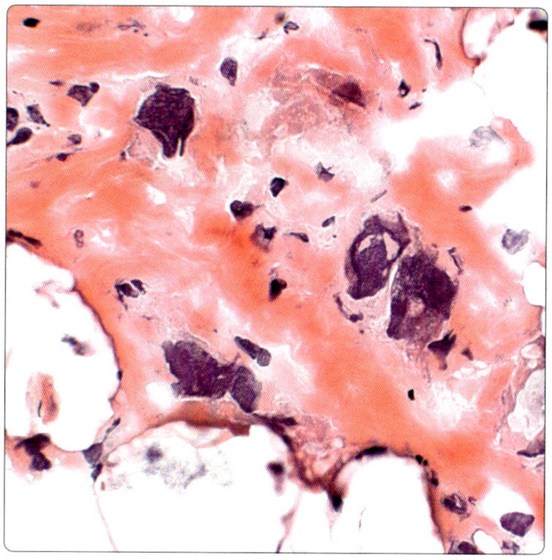

Normal Breast Tissue: Freezing Artifact

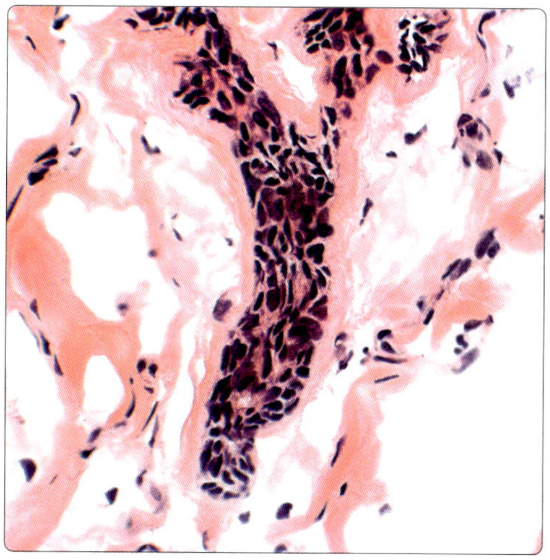

(Left) *Frozen section artifact in this invasive carcinoma has resulted in the nuclei appearing enlarged and irregular with a smudged chromatin pattern. Marked artifact such as this precludes accurate nuclear classification for grading.* **(Right)** *This is a normal duct on frozen section. The nuclei are hyperchromatic, and the chromatin pattern is homogeneous and dense.*

Invasive Carcinoma: Frozen Section and Cautery Artifact

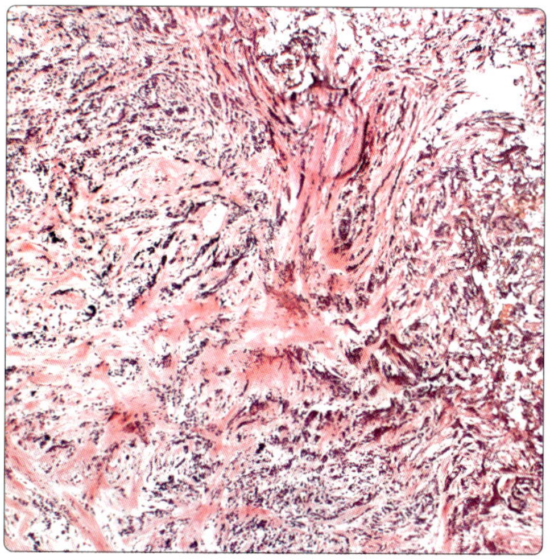

Invasive Carcinoma: Frozen Section

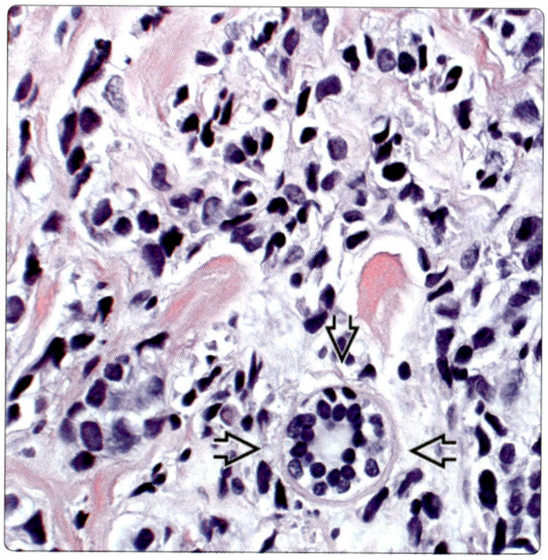

(Left) *This frozen section shows marked frozen section and cautery artifact. Although the overall pattern appears infiltrative, it would be difficult to know with certainty if the numerous epithelial elements are invasive carcinoma or extensive sclerosing adenosis.* **(Right)** *This invasive carcinoma is more easily diagnosed by recognizing that the tumor infiltrates around a normal tubule ⇨. Compared to the normal cells, the nuclei of the carcinoma cells are larger and irregular in shape and lack myoepithelial cells.*

(Left) *Radial sclerosing lesions can form irregular masses on mammography. In general, the length of the spiculations are longer in comparison to the central nidus as compared to irregular invasive carcinomas. These lesions should be evaluated on permanent sections and not by frozen section.* **(Right)** *Radial sclerosing lesions form irregular masses* → *and can closely mimic invasive carcinomas radiographically, grossly, and microscopically. Unlike a carcinoma, only the central nidus of the lesion is firm to hard.*

Radial Sclerosing Lesion: Mammographic Appearance

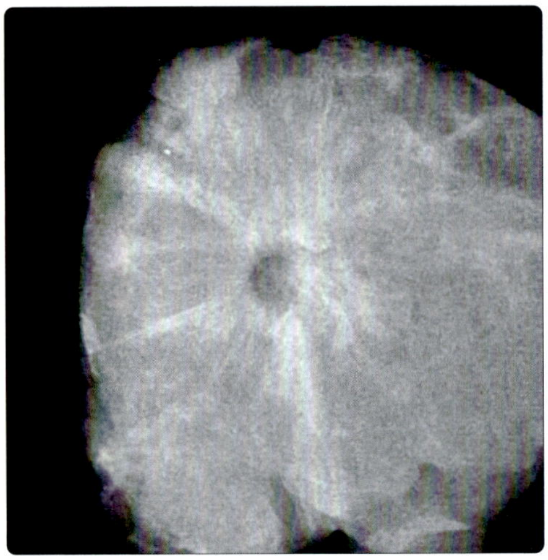

Radial Sclerosing Lesion: Gross Appearance

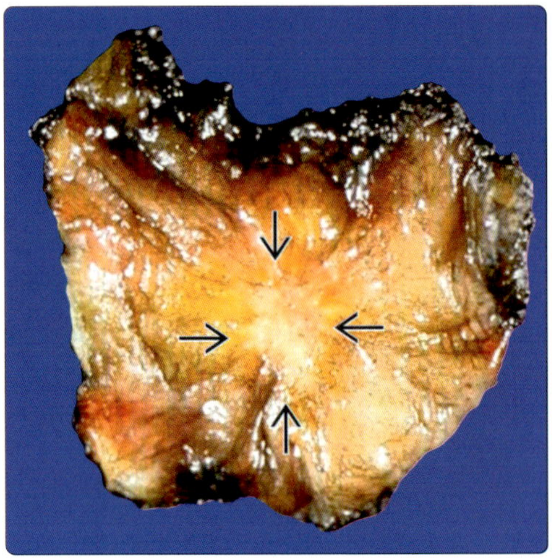

(Left) *A radial sclerosing lesion has a central area of compressed glands in dense stroma that closely resembles invasive carcinoma. The stroma is typically denser and less cellular than that seen in desmoplasia associated with carcinomas. A myoepithelial cell layer is present.* **(Right)** *Metallic clips are placed to mark the site of image-guided core needle biopsies. The presence of the clip must be documented by specimen radiography. Clips are small* ⇨ *and easily dislodged and lost during sectioning of the specimen.*

Radial Sclerosing Lesion

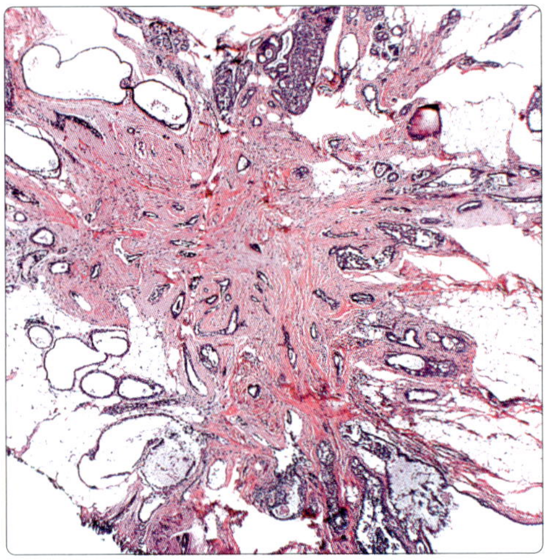

Clip at Core Needle Biopsy Site

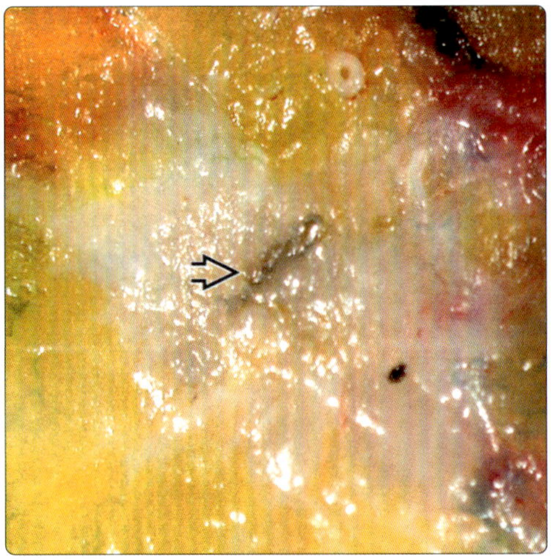

(Left) *A biopsy cavity* → *may be present if a carcinoma has been excised. The surrounding fibrosis and fat necrosis* ⇨ *may be difficult to distinguish from residual carcinoma. The closest margin suspicious for residual invasive carcinoma may be frozen in selected cases.* **(Right)** *Biodegradable material may be placed in the cavity created by a core needle biopsy to help mark the site and allow detection by ultrasonography. The gel pledgets* ⇨ *have a variety of appearances, including white rice-sized pellets, gray gelatin, or pink collagen.*

Excisional Site

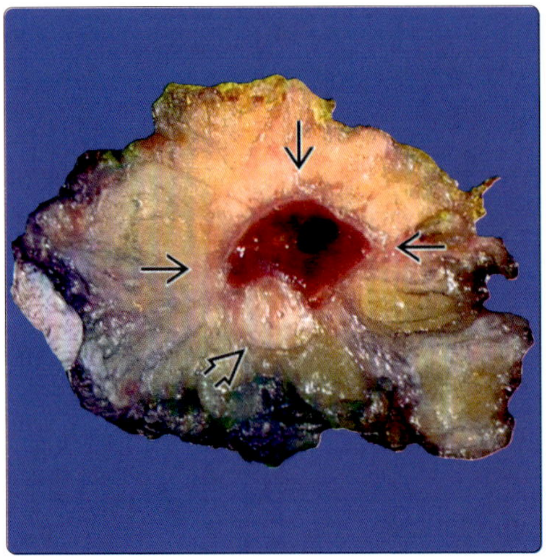

Gel Pledgets at Core Needle Biopsy Site

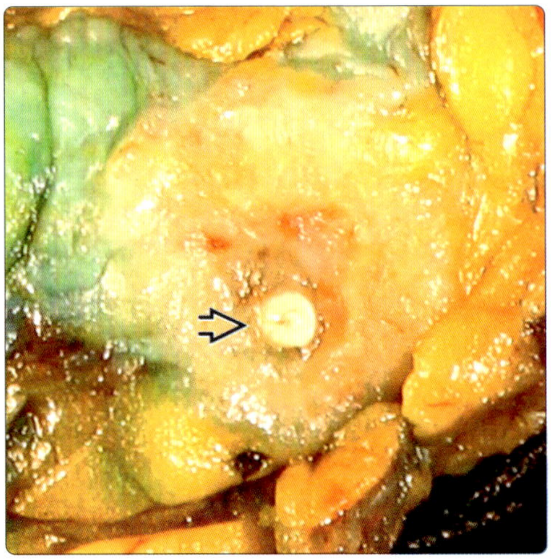

Nodular Sclerosing Adenosis

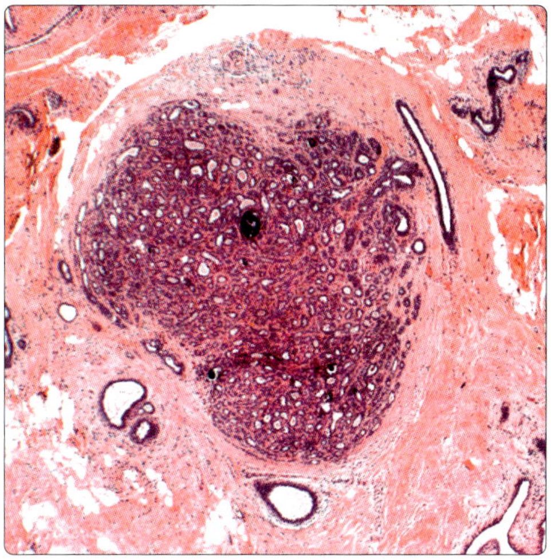

Sclerosing Adenosis Involved by Carcinoma In Situ

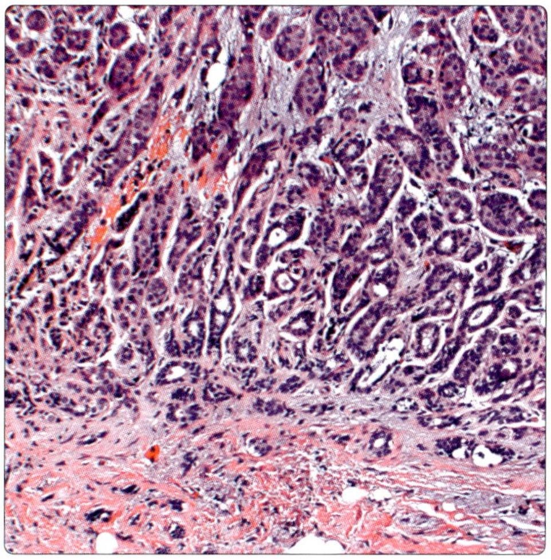

(Left) *Sclerosing adenosis is the lesion most commonly mistaken for invasive carcinoma. Unlike carcinoma, the tubules are in an organized back-to-back pattern, the stroma is sparse &/or very dense, and the borders are typically circumscribed.* **(Right)** *Sclerosing adenosis closely mimics invasive carcinoma when involved by DCIS (as in this case), lobular carcinoma in situ, or apocrine metaplasia. In general, these lesions should not be evaluated by frozen section.*

Fibroadenoma: Gross Appearance

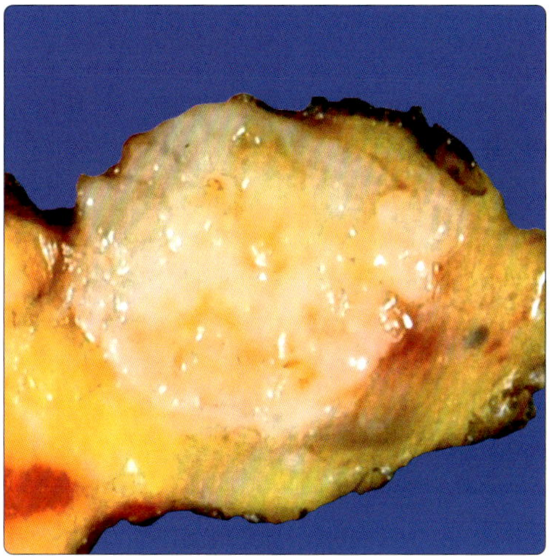

Fibroadenoma

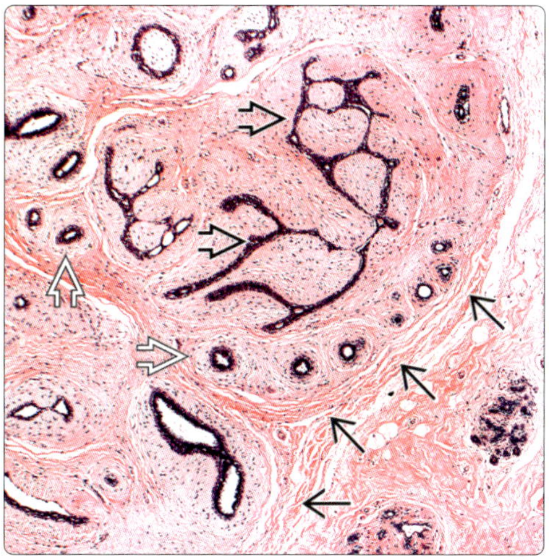

(Left) *Fibroadenomas form well-circumscribed rubbery white masses and typically bulge from the cut surface. Slit-like spaces correspond to areas of stromal growth pushing against and distorting ducts.* **(Right)** *Fibroadenomas are proliferations of intralobular stroma. The borders are well circumscribed and pushing* ➔*. The associated epithelium is typically pushed and distorted by the stroma (intracanalicular pattern* ➔*) but can also be surrounded by stroma (pericanalicular pattern* ➔*).*

Phyllodes Tumor: Gross Appearance

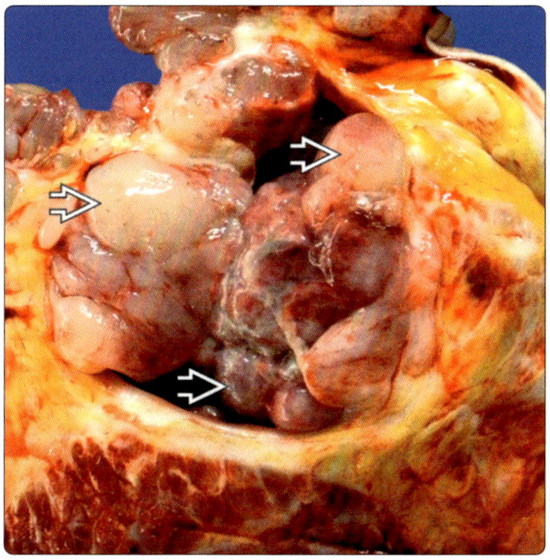

Phyllodes Tumor

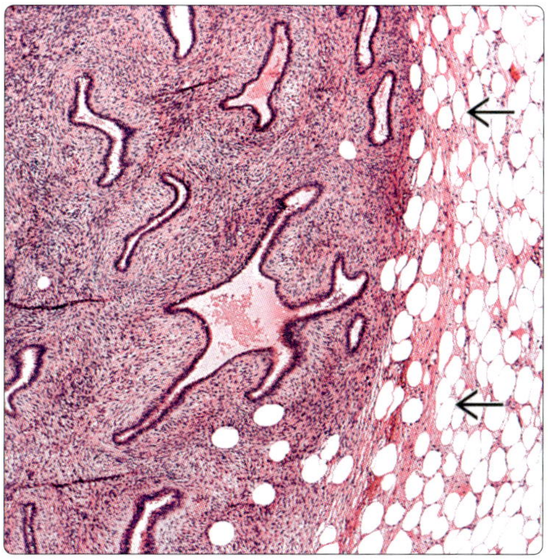

(Left) *Phyllodes tumors are usually larger than fibroadenomas. Stromal overgrowth results in the leaf-like (phyllodes) pattern of balls of tumor covered by epithelium* ➔ *within a cystic space.* **(Right)** *The stroma of phyllodes tumors is highly cellular, and mitoses are typically present. In higher-grade tumors, the associated benign epithelium may be scant or absent, and infiltration into surrounding breast tissue* ➔ *is present. Wide margins are preferable to completely resect high-grade tumors.*

SURGICAL/CLINICAL CONSIDERATIONS

Goal of Consultation

- Identify positive or close margins for carcinoma

Change in Patient Management

- Utility of intraoperative evaluation of margins depends on practice parameters at different institutions
- **Breast-conserving surgery**
  - Specimen may consist of single oriented excision or excision with separate cavity shave margins
  - If intraoperative assessment suggests close or positive margins, additional tissue may be removed to obtain clear margins
- **Mastectomy**
  - Deep margin is muscle fascia
    - Surgeon removes muscle only when carcinoma invades into it
    - Generally evident by imaging, clinical examination, or during operation
    - Radiation rather than additional surgery is treatment for positive deep margin
  - Superficial margin is contiguous with skin flaps
    - In majority of patients, breast ducts and lobules do not extend into subcutaneous tissue
    - In minority of patients, normal breast tissue &/or carcinoma may be present in flaps
    - Benefit of additional surgery or radiation therapy for close margin unclear
  - Nipple margin of nipple-sparing mastectomy
    - Submitted separately by surgeon or taken as section of nipple base by pathologist
    - If ductal carcinoma in situ (DCIS) or invasive carcinoma present, nipple may be excised
  - Intraoperative assessment of deep and superficial margins rarely performed

Clinical Setting

- For breast-conserving surgery, the contemporary 10-year local recurrence rate ranges from 5-10%
- A positive margin is associated with 2x increase in risk of local recurrence
- Until recently, there was no universal agreement as to what constitutes an adequate negative margin
  - Recent consensus guidelines define negative margins as no ink on invasive cancer or DCIS in setting of breast-conserving surgery for early-stage breast cancer
  - For cases of DCIS only, adequate margin defined as > 2 mm
- Routine practice of obtaining wider negative margins widths does not appear to further reduce local recurrence rates
- Surgical removal of all subclinical disease may not be required to achieve local control
  - Radiation therapy and systemic therapy play important roles in reducing local recurrence
- Biologic subtype of carcinoma influences local recurrence
- Majority of invasive carcinomas can be palpated by surgeon and easily completely resected
  - Evaluation of margins for invasive carcinoma can generally be performed by gross examination
  - Gross margins cannot be reliably assessed for diffusely infiltrative carcinomas (e.g., lobular carcinoma) and carcinomas treated with neoadjuvant therapy
- DCIS frequent cause of close or positive margins
  - Usually not grossly evident
  - Margin involvement can be very focal
  - Diagnosis by frozen section can be very difficult
    - May be in fatty tissue that does not freeze well, and technically adequate sections may be difficult to produce
    - Can be difficult to distinguish from usual hyperplasia, atypical ductal hyperplasia, and lobular carcinoma in situ on frozen section
    - Evaluating entire surface of excisional specimen by frozen section generally not practical in time allotted for breast surgery
- Surgeon should understand that negative margins by intraoperative evaluation may be close or positive in final evaluation

Specimen Radiograph: Mass With Clip and Wire

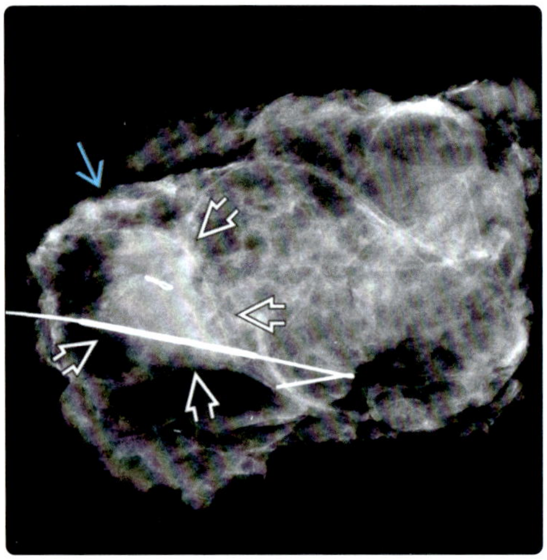

Margin Inks: Gross Appearance

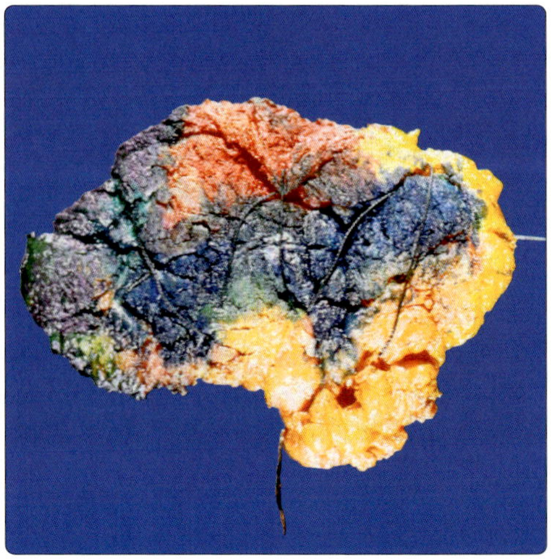

(Left) *Specimen radiograph is essential in order to identify the types of lesions present (masses, calcifications, clips, or radioactive seeds) and their relationship to margins. In this case, the closest approach of an invasive carcinoma ➔ (with a clip) to a margin ➔ can be correlated with gross findings.* **(Right)** *The specimen should be oriented such that 6 margins can be identified and inked with separate colors or otherwise identified. The surgeon has also identified a margin that cannot be further excised with a whip stitch (e.g., skin or muscle fascia).*

SPECIMEN EVALUATION

Gross

- Excisions
  - For wire or seed localized excisions, specimen radiograph should be provided
    - Identify lesions present: Masses, calcifications, clips, radioactive seeds
    - Identify relationship of lesions to 4 margins present on radiograph
      - 2nd radiograph may be taken to identify remaining 2 margins
  - Specimen should be oriented to identify 6 margins
    - Inks can be used to identify margins if frozen section is to be performed
    - If cytology preparations planned, specimen is not inked
  - Surgeon should identify any margins that cannot undergo reexcision (e.g., skin or muscle fascia)
  - Specimen serially sectioned (2-3 mm)
    - Gross lesions correlated with radiologic findings
    - Distance of invasive carcinomas to margins recorded
    - Areas suspicious for margin involvement identified

Frozen Section

- Excisions
  - Most suspicious area(s) for involvement by carcinoma may be taken as small perpendicular section
    - Areas of adipose tissue should be avoided as tissue will not freeze well
  - En face sections not recommended as distance of carcinoma to margin cannot be assessed

Cytology

- Scrape preparations can be taken from the 6 margins
- If surface cauterized, may be difficult to obtain cells that can be interpreted

Possible Emerging Technologies

- MarginProbe System (Dune Medical Devices, Paoli, PA, USA)
  - FDA-approved for clinical use for margin analysis in breast-conserving surgery
  - Hand-held probe measures electrical properties of breast tissue using radiofrequency spectroscopy
  - Either specimen or biopsy cavity can be evaluated
    - Involved margins can be excised and new margin tested
  - Reported high false-positive and false-negative rates may limit usefulness
- Near-infrared optical imaging
  - Optical imaging systems are paired with fluorescent contrast agents to assess optical properties of tissue
  - Can detect cancer cells at surgical margins with relatively good sensitivity and specificity
  - Images would likely be interpreted by pathologists

REPORTING

Gross Examination

- Distance of grossly evident invasive carcinomas can be reported to each margin

Frozen Section

- Information about histologic type of prior carcinoma is essential for optimal evaluation
  - Invasive lobular carcinoma can be very difficult to detect by frozen section
- Excisions
  - Positive margins reported when ink on carcinoma
    - Invasive carcinoma or DCIS at margin should be specified
  - Close margins are reported as distance of invasive carcinoma or DCIS from margin

Cytology

- Margins reported as positive or negative

PITFALLS

False-Negative Diagnoses

- **Tissue with involved margins not examined**
  - Generally not possible to examine all margin tissue by frozen section
  - Surgeons should understand that status of margins can change after examination of additional tissue on permanent sections
- **DCIS misinterpreted as hyperplasia**
  - DCIS can be difficult to diagnose in frozen sections containing artifact or thickly cut due to adipose tissue
  - High-grade DCIS easier to recognize when high-grade nuclei ± necrosis present
  - Low-grade DCIS may not be recognizable if there is significant artifact
- **Cautery artifact**
  - Cautery can preclude ability to diagnose breast lesions
- **Invasive lobular carcinoma mistaken for inflammatory cells**
  - Grade I and II lobular carcinomas can closely resemble lymphocytes or histiocytes
  - Lobular carcinoma within biopsy site changes can be difficult to identify

False-Positive Diagnoses

- **Atypical ductal hyperplasia mistaken for DCIS**
  - Lesions can be difficult to distinguish even on permanent sections
- **Ink leakage into tissue cracks**
  - Care must be taken to prevent smearing of ink in areas not identified as margin
- **Inflammatory cells mistaken for invasive lobular carcinoma**
  - Lymphocytes and small histiocytes can infiltrate tissue in linear arrays

SELECTED REFERENCES

1. Gray RJ et al: Intraoperative margin management in breast-conserving surgery: a systematic review of the literature. Ann Surg Oncol. ePub, 2017
2. Schnitt SJ: Evaluation of margins in invasive carcinoma and ductal carcinoma in situ: the pathologist's perspective. Breast. ePub, 2017
3. Keating J et al: Identification of breast cancer margins using intraoperative near-infrared imaging. J Surg Oncol. 113(5):508-14, 2016
4. Butler-Henderson K et al: Intraoperative assessment of margins in breast conserving therapy: a systematic review. Breast. 23(2):112-9, 2014
5. Esbona K et al: Intraoperative imprint cytology and frozen section pathology for margin assessment in breast conservation surgery: a systematic review. Ann Surg Oncol. 19(10):3236-45, 2012

(Left) *This invasive carcinoma* ⇨ *is close to, but not present at, the yellow inked margin* ➡ *and far from the remaining margins. However, DCIS could be present at the margin and is not usually visible by gross examination or by imaging.* **(Right)** *A perpendicular margin* ➡ *has been selected for frozen section in order to show the closest approach of this invasive carcinoma* ⇨ *to the margin. The tissue selected for frozen section should be small and consist of fibrous tissue in order to freeze well and avoid freezing artifacts.*

Evaluation of Margins: Gross Appearance

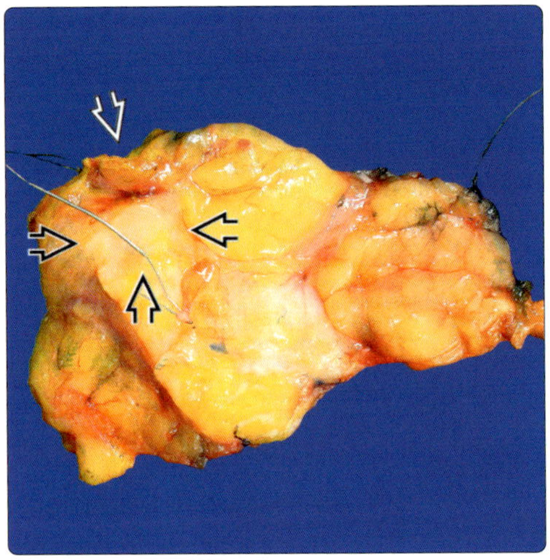

Perpendicular Margin: Gross Appearance

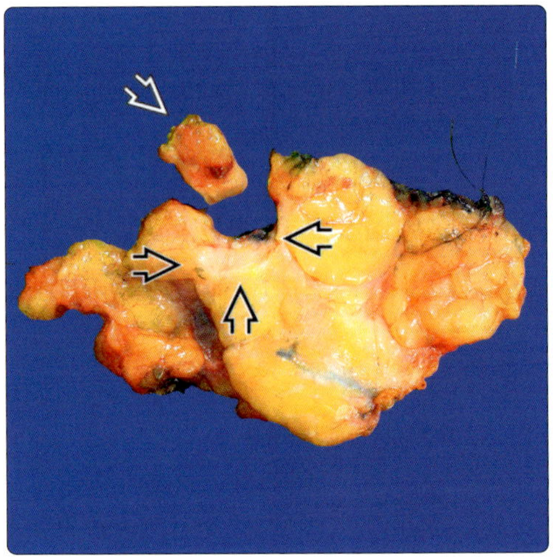

(Left) *Breast tissue often consists predominantly of adipose tissue, which does not freeze well. Fragmentation and folding of the tissue may result in poor staining and bubbles under the coverslip. Although invasive carcinoma is at the margin* ⇨*, this would be very difficult to diagnose in this section.* **(Right)** *This ductal carcinoma in situ (DCIS)* ⇨ *appears to be close to a black inked margin* →*. However, this appears to be ink leakage into a tissue crevice. The DCIS is farther away from the outer edge of the tissue, which may be the true margin* ⇨*.*

Breast Margin: Freezing Artifact

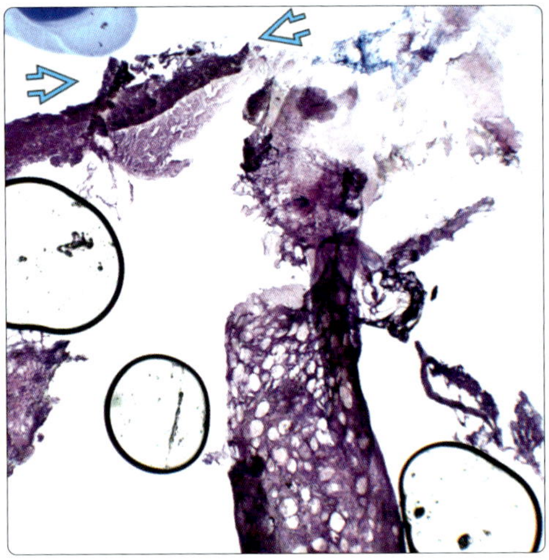

Breast Margin: Ink Leakage

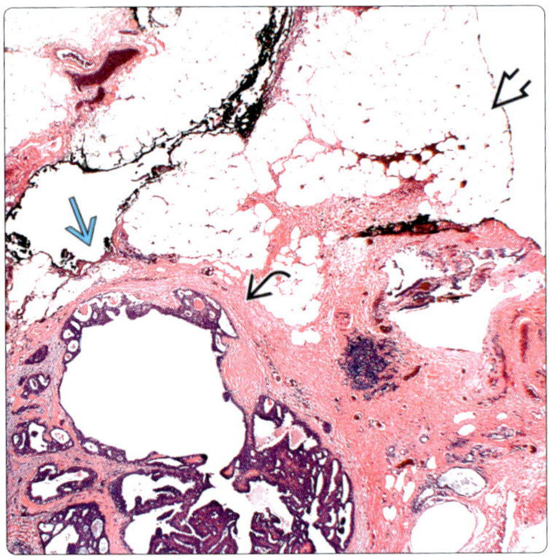

(Left) *Due to tissue disruption, it is difficult to determine if this is invasive or in situ carcinoma* ⇨ *at the margin, and if this is true margin involvement or artifact. Correlation with gross and imaging findings is important.* **(Right)** *Invasive low-grade lobular carcinoma has been transected at the margin* →*. This can occur because these carcinomas frequently do not form an obvious mass that can be palpated by the surgeon. The small cells with scant cytoplasm are difficult to identify as tumor cells on frozen section.*

Breast Margin: Positive for Carcinoma

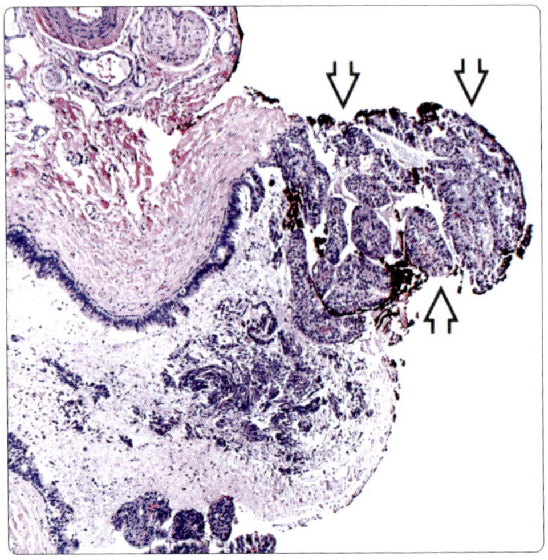

Breast Margin: Invasive Lobular Carcinoma

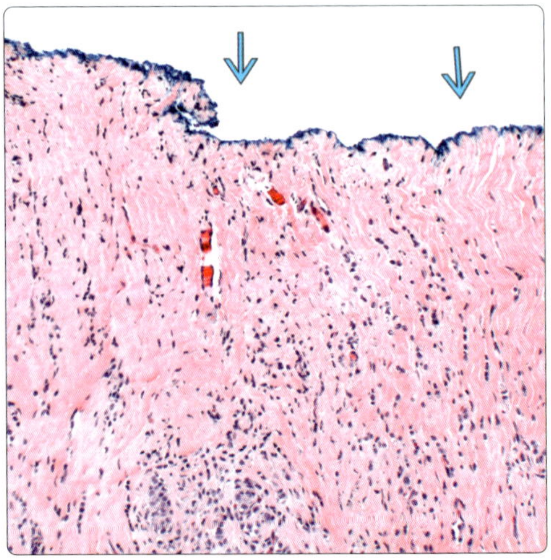

Breast Margin: Cautery Artifact

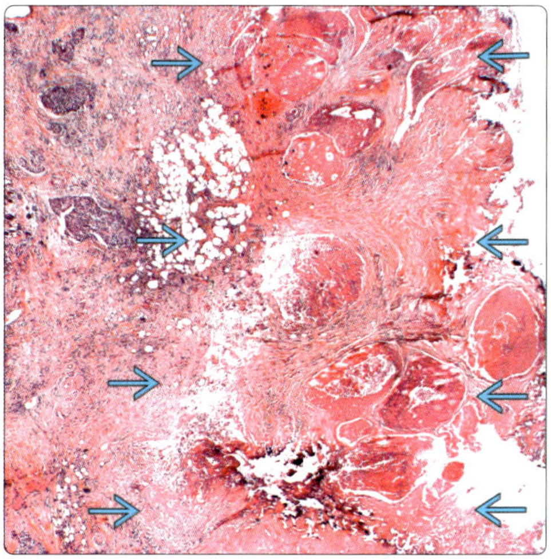

Breast Margin: Cautery Artifact

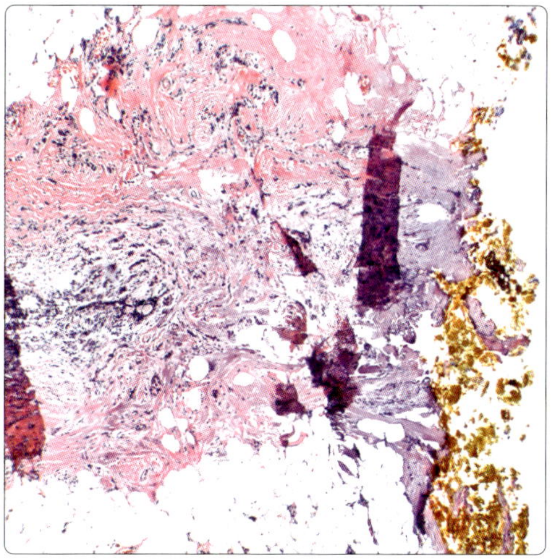

(Left) *The edge of a breast specimen is often heavily cauterized for 1-3 mm* → *. This can make evaluation of the tissue at the margin very difficult, if not impossible.* **(Right)** *This invasive carcinoma is present at the yellow inked margin. It is difficult to recognize the carcinoma due to crush and cautery artifact.*

Breast Margin: Cautery Artifact

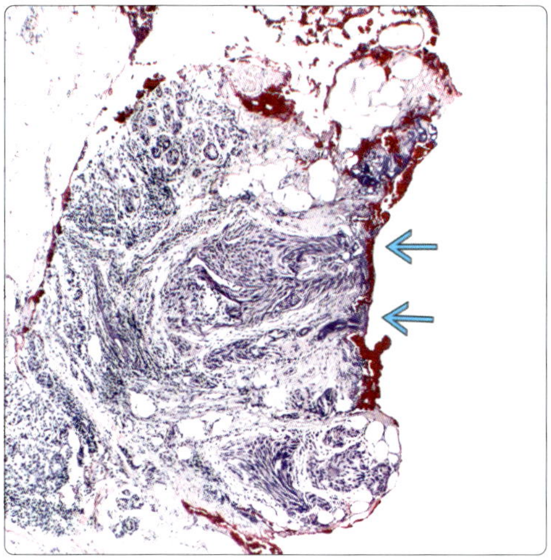

Breast Margin: DCIS

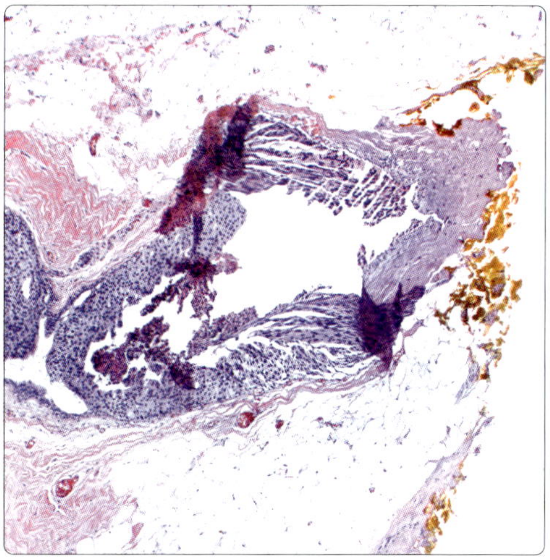

(Left) *DCIS is present at the red inked margin* → *. Although the cautery artifact demonstrates that this is a true surgical margin and not ink leakage, it also makes interpretation more difficult.* **(Right)** *This area of DCIS is very close, but not quite at the yellow inked margin. However, this finding does not exclude DCIS in the remaining tissue as the involved duct may have crossed the margin outside of this plane of section.*

Breast Margin: Cautery Artifact

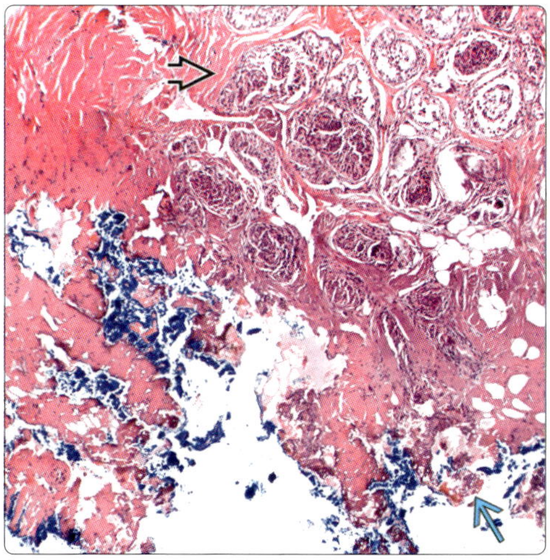

Breast Margin: DCIS

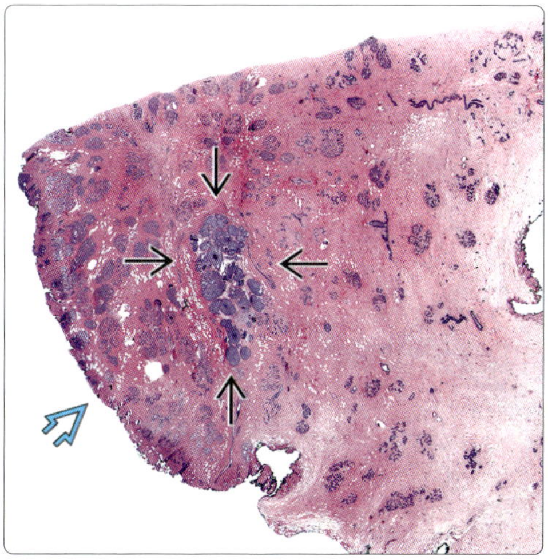

(Left) *The area of DCIS at the margin* → *is heavily cauterized and difficult to identify. DCIS in the same area but farther away from the margin can be recognized* ⇨ *. This margin would be difficult to evaluate on frozen section, which must be performed on small tissue specimens in order to freeze well.* **(Right)** *This focus of DCIS* → *is 3 mm from the closest margin* ⇨ *. This is an adequate negative margin according to recent guidelines (> 2 mm).*

SURGICAL/CLINICAL CONSIDERATIONS

Goal of Consultation

- To identify invasive carcinoma or ductal carcinoma in situ (DCIS) in nipple margin of skin- and nipple-sparing mastectomy

Change in Patient Management

- If nipple margin is reported as positive, surgeon will likely remove nipple papilla or entire nipple areola complex during procedure
- **Caution**
  - It is important to report whether cancer is located in lactiferous sinuses, nipple dermis, or in breast tissue away from nipple

Clinical Setting

- Nipple-sparing mastectomy is defined as resection of breast tissue with preservation of entire skin envelop, including nipple areola complex
  - Introduced as alternative to standard mastectomy in early 2000s
  - Used for both prophylactic and therapeutic mastectomies
  - Facilitates single-stage breast reconstruction in selected patients
- Preservation of skin and nipple is associated with improved cosmetic outcomes and psychosexual benefits
  - Patients avoid additional surgical procedures required for nipple reconstruction
- Plane of resection is generally through or just below smooth muscle of areola
  - In some techniques, core of nipple tissue above smooth muscle layer is also removed
- Nipple-sparing mastectomy is oncologically safe option for carefully selected patients
  - Suggested patient selection criteria
    - No clinical or imaging evidence of nipple involvement
    - Tumor is < 5 cm in size
    - Tumor is located > 2 cm from nipple
    - Tumor is ER positive and HER2 negative
    - DCIS is not extensive
    - Clinically negative axilla
  - Number of eligible women has expanded with increasing experience with this surgical technique
  - Nipple margin involvement in therapeutic mastectomies is reported to be 0-14% in studies with strict patient selection criteria
  - Majority of nipples excised for positive margin contain no residual malignancy
    - In some institutions, radiation to nipple is used as alternative to additional surgery
  - Locoregional recurrence rate is low (< 5%), and majority occur in chest wall away from nipple
    - Rate of recurrence in preserved nipple areola complex is < 1%
    - Recurrence as DCIS involving nipple skin (Paget disease) has been reported
    - Current follow-up is relatively short as this is new technique
- Intraoperative frozen section analysis of nipple base margin may or may not be performed depending on institutional preferences
  - Intraoperative diagnosis facilitates reconstructive planning and prevents additional surgery
  - High specificity and moderate sensitivity
  - May not be indicated for prophylactic mastectomy given rarity of positive nipple margins
- Finding of invasive carcinoma or DCIS in nipple margin specimen is indication for removal of nipple
  - Finding of lobular carcinoma in situ (LCIS) may or may not result in removal of nipple

SPECIMEN EVALUATION

Gross

- **Nipple margin submitted as separate specimen by surgeon**
  - Generally consists of 1 or multiple small fragments of tissue
  - Typically not full en face section of nipple base
  - Specimen is usually too small to be oriented

Types of Mastectomies

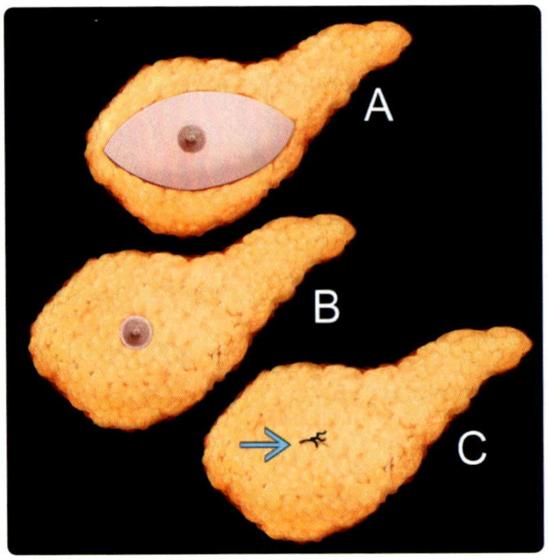

Nipple-Sparing Mastectomy

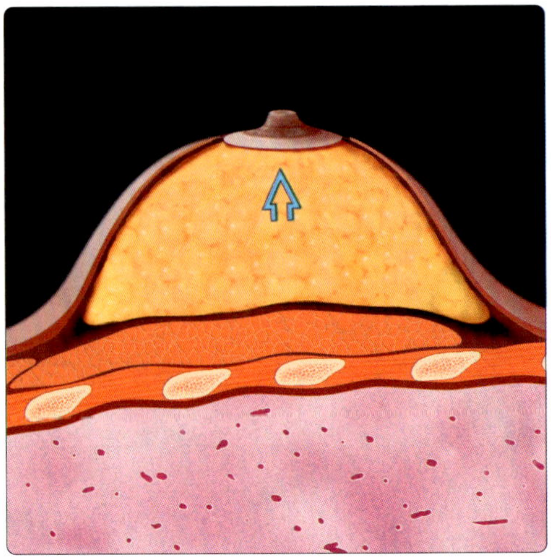

(Left) *(A) A traditional mastectomy removes the nipple and a surrounding ellipse of skin. (B) A skin-sparing mastectomy removes the nipple and only a small portion of surrounding skin. (C) A nipple- and skin-sparing mastectomy removes only breast tissue. The location of the nipple is typically marked with a suture ➡.* **(Right)** *The base of the nipple ➡ is an important margin of a nipple-sparing mastectomy. The margin may be involved by either invasive carcinoma or carcinoma in situ.*

- May contain tissue from within nipple ("nipple core biopsy"), superficial retroareolar tissue, or deeper breast tissue
- **Nipple margin taken by pathologist from mastectomy specimen**
  - Nipple site is often marked by suture and can be designated with ink
  - Nipple margin can be evaluated by en face or perpendicular sections
    - En face sections are better able to sample all of lactiferous sinuses
      - It may be difficult to obtain full en face section due to retraction of major ducts at this site
    - Perpendicular sections can evaluate distance of carcinoma from nipple margin
      - Generally requires at least 2-3 blocks of tissue
  - Distance of carcinoma from designated nipple margin is documented on subsequent processing of mastectomy specimen

Frozen Section

- All tissue considered to be nipple margin should be frozen for evaluation
- Any tumor in unoriented specimen is considered positive margin

REPORTING

Gross Examination

- Gross identification of tumor at margin of mastectomy should be reported
  - This would be highly unusual finding

Frozen Section

- Type of carcinoma: Invasive carcinoma, DCIS, or LCIS
  - Nipple adenomas, large duct papillomas, and syringomatous adenomas are other lesions that occur at nipple
    - These lesions are highly unlikely to be present in nipple margin specimen due to careful clinical and radiologic selection of women with normal nipples for this procedure
- Location of carcinoma: Involving lactiferous sinuses, areolar tissue, or breast tissue
- Relationship to inked margin, if applicable

PITFALLS

False-Negative Diagnoses

- **Sampling error: Tissue with involved margins not examined**
  - Tissue submitted by surgeon typically does not include entire nipple base
  - Additional tissue sampled from designated nipple margin of mastectomy may reveal carcinoma
- **Interpretation error: DCIS or LCIS misinterpreted as hyperplasia**
  - Intraductal proliferations can be difficult lesions to interpret on frozen sections
- **Freezing and crush artifact**
  - Can make diagnosis of cancer challenging

False-Positive Diagnoses

- **Hyperplasia or atypical hyperplasia mistaken for carcinoma in situ**
  - Caution is advised in reporting positive findings for equivocal frozen sections in order to avoid morbidity of unnecessary nipple areola complex excision

SELECTED REFERENCES

1. Alperovich M et al: Nipple-sparing mastectomy and sub-areolar biopsy: to freeze or not to freeze? evaluating the role of sub-areolar intraoperative frozen section. Breast J. 22(1):18-23, 2016
2. Headon HL et al: The oncological safety of nipple-sparing mastectomy: a systematic review of the literature with a pooled analysis of 12,358 procedures. Arch Plast Surg. 43(4):328-38, 2016
3. Tang R et al: Positive nipple nargins in nipple-sparing mastectomies: rates, management, and oncologic safety. J Am Coll Surg. 222(6):1149-55, 2016
4. Duarte GM et al: Accuracy of frozen section, imprint cytology, and permanent histology of sub-nipple tissue for predicting occult nipple involvement in patients with breast carcinoma. Breast Cancer Res Treat. 153(3):557-63, 2015
5. Morales Piato JR et al: Improved frozen section examination of the retroareolar margin for prediction of nipple involvement in breast cancer. Eur J Surg Oncol. 41(8):986-90, 2015

Nipple-Sparing Mastectomy

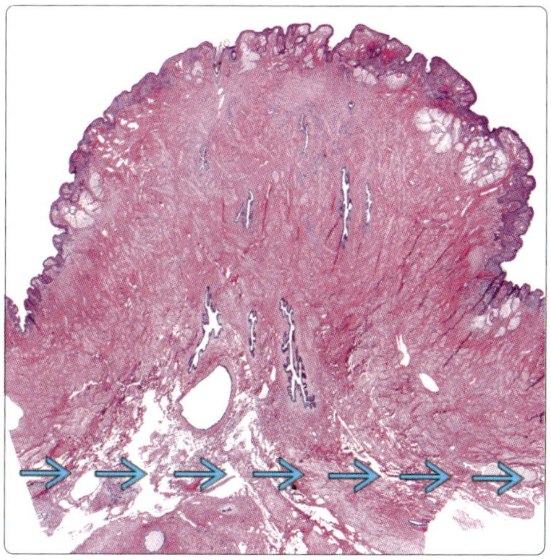

Nipple Base: Lactiferous Sinuses

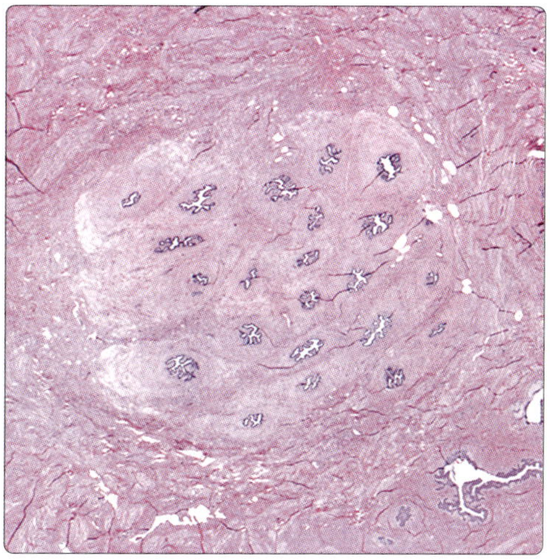

(Left) *The line of resection for a nipple-sparing mastectomy is along the base of the nipple* ➡*. Although some surgeons attempt to remove a "core" of nipple tissue above this line, in general, lactiferous sinuses and adjacent lobules (in some women) above the smooth muscle are not removed.* **(Right)** *An ideal nipple margin would include a cross section of all ~ 15-20 lactiferous sinuses. In practice, the margin submitted for evaluation typically includes < 5 of the major sinuses.*

Contents

(Left) DCIS is present involving a lactiferous sinus at the base of the nipple. If a nipple-sparing mastectomy was performed, the DCIS in the nipple would not be removed. Recurrence as Paget disease has been reported after nipple-sparing mastectomy. (Right) The location of the nipple base on the mastectomy is usually indicated by a suture. An en face margin can be taken. Alternatively, the area of the base can be inked and perpendicular sections taken. In this case, DCIS is close to a green inked margin.

DCIS Involving Lactiferous Sinus

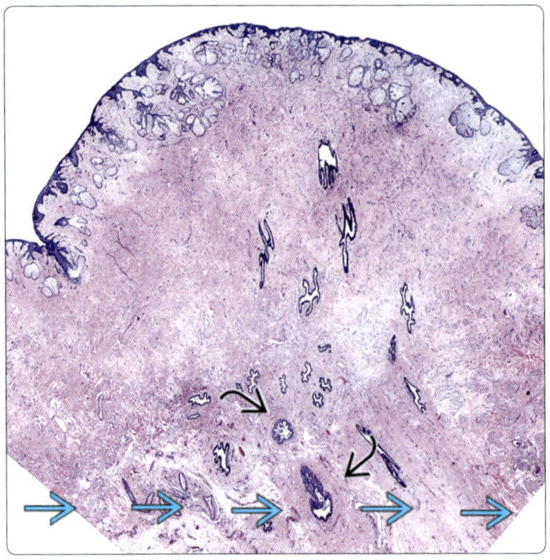

Nipple Margin: Perpendicular From Mastectomy

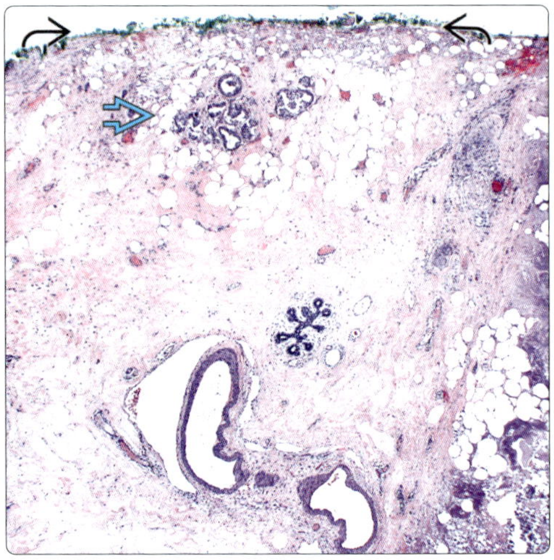

(Left) A nipple margin provided by the surgeon typically consists of 1 or multiple small fragments of tissue. It is often not possible to orient the specimen. The tissue should contain lactiferous sinuses. Cautery and crush artifact often make interpretation difficult. (Right) Lactiferous sinuses can be difficult to evaluate for in situ carcinoma due to the convoluted shape being conducive to tangential sectioning. In this case, there is also crush artifact leading to cellular dyscohesion.

Nipple Margin: Submitted as Separate Specimen by Surgeon

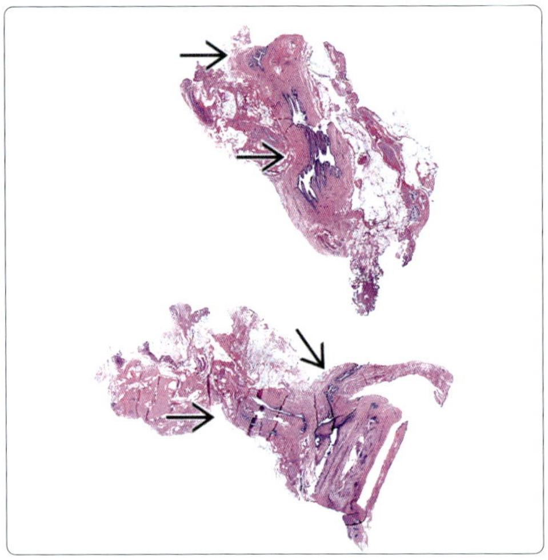

Lactiferous Sinus With Crush Artifact

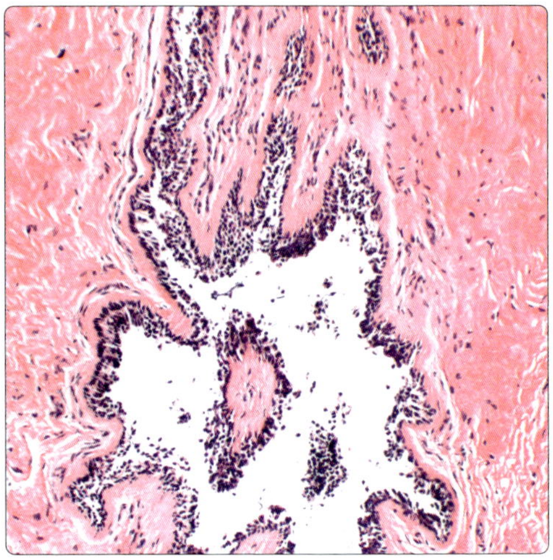

(Left) A small focus of invasive carcinoma is present in a fragmented nipple base margin specimen. Lactiferous sinuses are present and document that the carcinoma is present within nipple tissue. (Right) This invasive lobular carcinoma is present in the nipple adjacent to lactiferous sinuses. It would be very difficult to diagnose this type of nipple involvement on frozen section.

Nipple Margin: Invasive Carcinoma

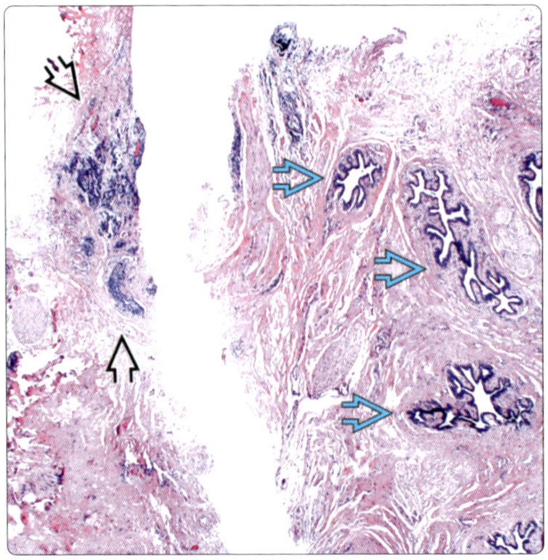

Nipple Margin: Invasive Lobular Carcinoma

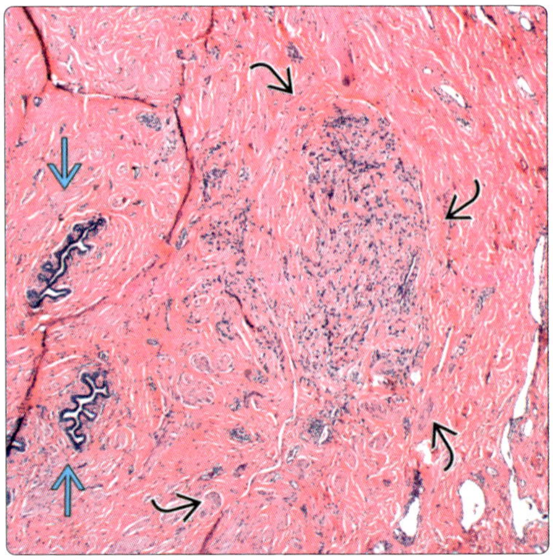

DCIS Involving Lactiferous Sinus

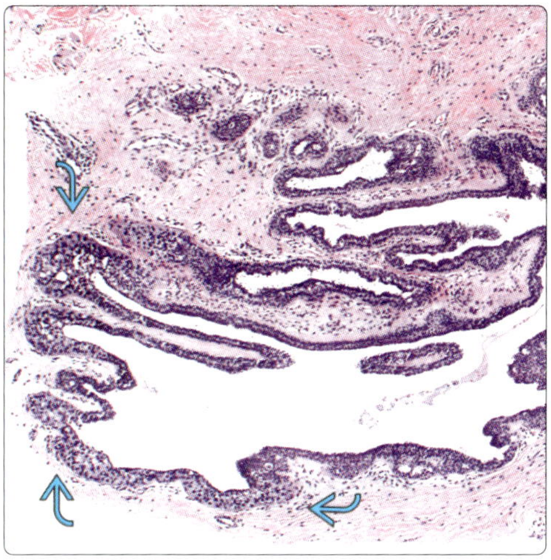

Nipple Margin

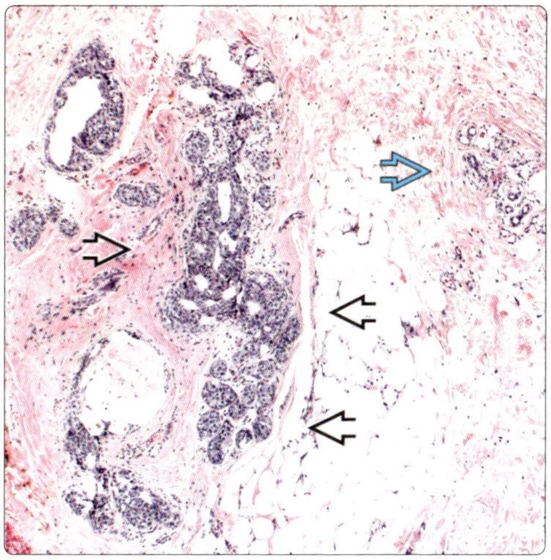

(Left) *DCIS is present in a clinging pattern along a portion of a lactiferous sinus. It may not be possible to distinguish DCIS from ADH in a margin specimen alone without reference to the type and location of DCIS elsewhere in the breast.* **(Right)** *DCIS is present in tissue submitted by the surgeon as the nipple margin. However, the presence of a lobule and adipose tissue show that the tissue is deep to the nipple. This finding may not be as predictive of nipple involvement as compared to a true sample of nipple tissue.*

Flat Epithelial Atypia Involving Lactiferous Sinus

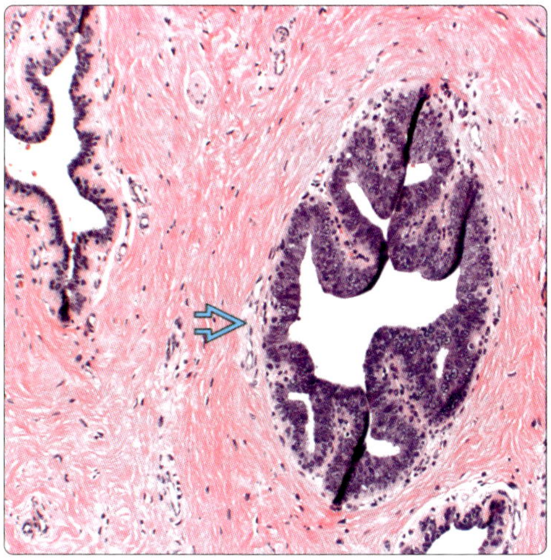

Nipple Margin: Atypical Lobular Hyperplasia

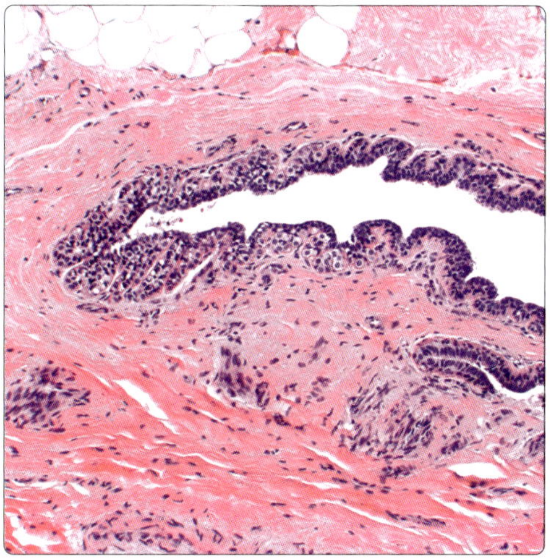

(Left) *This lactiferous sinus is involved by flat epithelial atypia. It would be important to compare this area to areas of DCIS to determine if this is likely to be an extension of DCIS or a separate lesion.* **(Right)** *Atypical lobular hyperplasia may be difficult to detect in a lactiferous sinus on a frozen section. This finding may be an indication for removal of the nipple for a prophylactic mastectomy but possibly not for a woman with cancer.*

Lymph-Vascular Invasion in Nipple

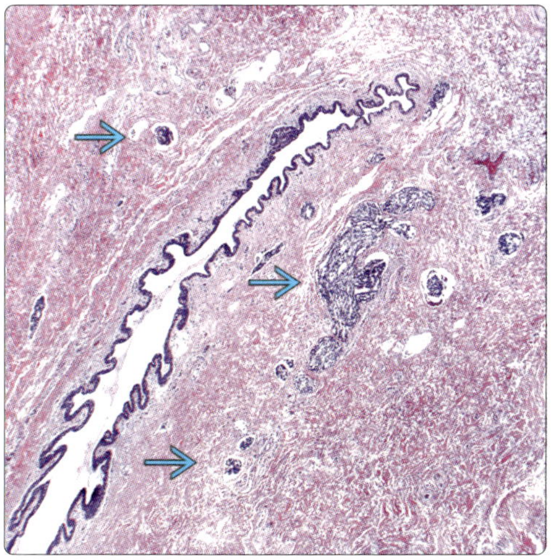

Nipple Margin With Epithelial Displacement

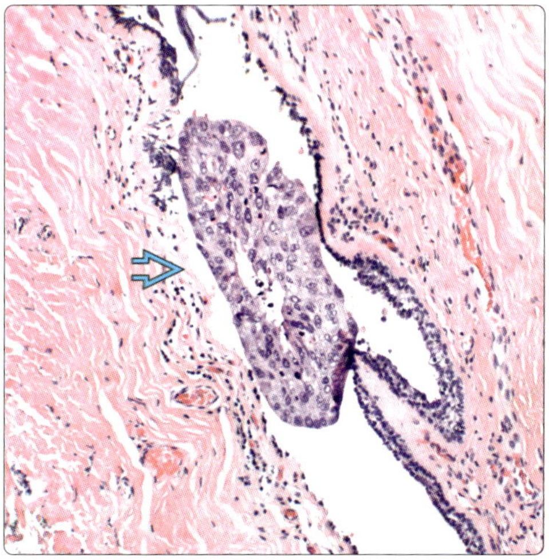

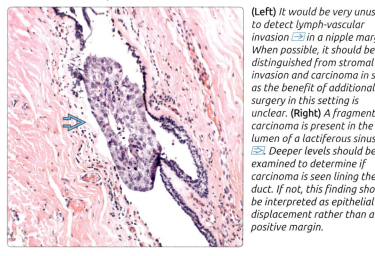

(Left) *It would be very unusual to detect lymph-vascular invasion in a nipple margin. When possible, it should be distinguished from stromal invasion and carcinoma in situ, as the benefit of additional surgery in this setting is unclear.* **(Right)** *A fragment of carcinoma is present in the lumen of a lactiferous sinus. Deeper levels should be examined to determine if carcinoma is seen lining the duct. If not, this finding should be interpreted as epithelial displacement rather than a positive margin.*

SURGICAL/CLINICAL CONSIDERATIONS

Goal of Consultation

- Confirm diagnosis for treatment planning

Change in Patient Management

- Specific diagnosis can guide further treatment
  - If procedure is primarily to establish diagnosis, no additional sampling is necessary
  - If carcinoid, limited (sleeve) resection may be performed
  - If small cell carcinoma, patient will likely receive chemotherapy without surgery
  - Other types of carcinoma may be considered for presurgical chemotherapy &/or radiation therapy

SPECIMEN EVALUATION

Gross

- Typically small fragments of unoriented tissue

Frozen Section

- Entire specimen is usually frozen

MOST COMMON DIAGNOSES

Squamous Cell Carcinoma

- Evidence of keratinization is helpful

Carcinoid Tumor

- Endobronchial location is classic
- Monomorphic nuclear cytology and nested/acinar/trabecular growth patterns should be seen

Salivary Gland-Like Neoplasm

- Includes pleomorphic adenoma, adenoid cystic carcinoma, mucoepidermoid carcinoma, and others

Small Cell Carcinoma

- Small cells with scant cytoplasm (lymphocyte-like); crush artifact common
- Mitoses, apoptotic cells, and necrosis should be seen

REPORTING

Frozen Section

- If specific diagnosis cannot be rendered at time of frozen section, descriptive diagnosis (e.g., positive for carcinoma/malignancy) is indicated
  - Diagnosis of small cell carcinoma should be rendered, if possible
- Deferring diagnosis to permanent sections may be necessary in difficult cases

PITFALLS

Small Blue Cells With Crush Artifact

- Differential diagnosis includes
  - Small cell carcinoma: Do not diagnose unless mitoses &/or necrosis is present
  - Carcinoid tumor: Characteristic growth patterns support diagnosis
  - Lymphoma: Sheets of atypical lymphocytes ± necrosis
  - Reactive lymphocytes: Germinal center formation is reassuring
- Additional biopsies should be requested if interpretation is not possible

Overdiagnosing Carcinoma

- Reactive mucosal endothelial cells or lymphocytes can mimic invasive carcinoma
  - Overlying epithelium is usually not dysplastic
- Squamous cell carcinoma in situ may be difficult to distinguish from invasive carcinoma in small unoriented biopsies
  - In situ carcinomas generally not treated by surgery
- Be wary of biopsies that are too superficial; request more tissue to get adequate sample of lesion

SELECTED REFERENCES

1. Gupta R et al: What can we learn from the errors in the frozen section diagnosis of pulmonary carcinoid tumors? an evidence-based approach. Hum Pathol. 40(1):1-9, 2009

Squamous Cell Carcinoma

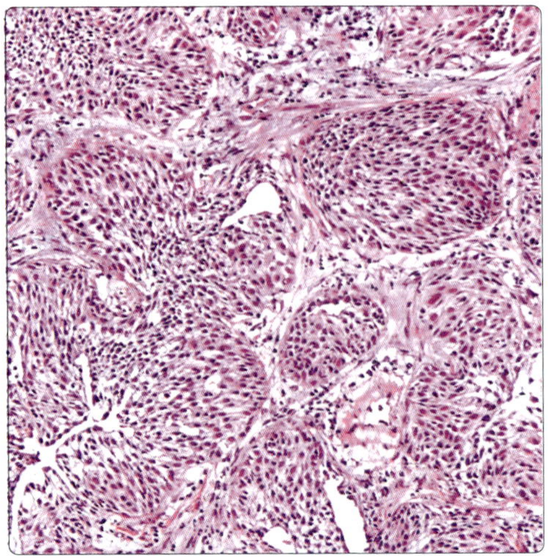

Squamous Cell Carcinoma: Keratin

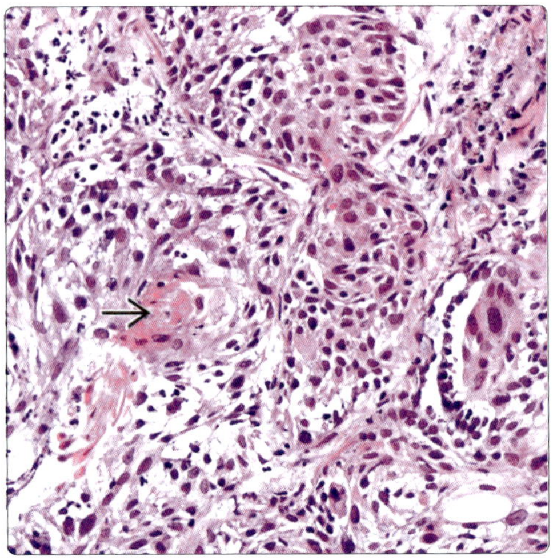

(Left) *Squamous cell carcinoma (SCC) may involve the bronchus or trachea. Almost all SCCs of the trachea are primary to that site, but most SCCs of the mainstem bronchus are extensions from the lung.* **(Right)** *SCC of the bronchus and trachea has the same histologic findings as SCC at other sites. Demonstration of keratin production ⇒ or origin from overlying squamous dysplasia can be very helpful to confirm the diagnosis.*

Adenocarcinoma

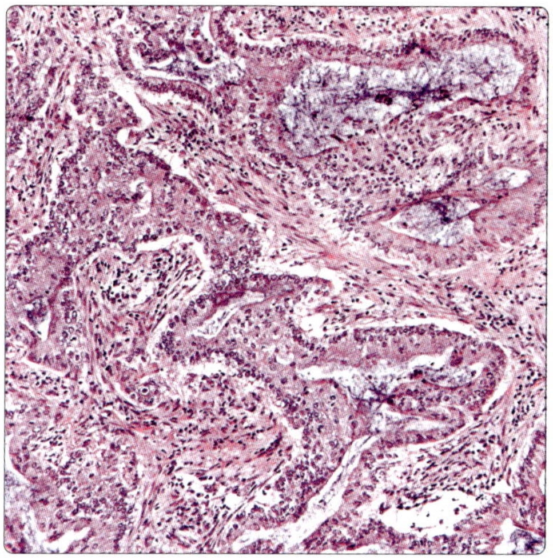

Adenoid Cystic Carcinoma

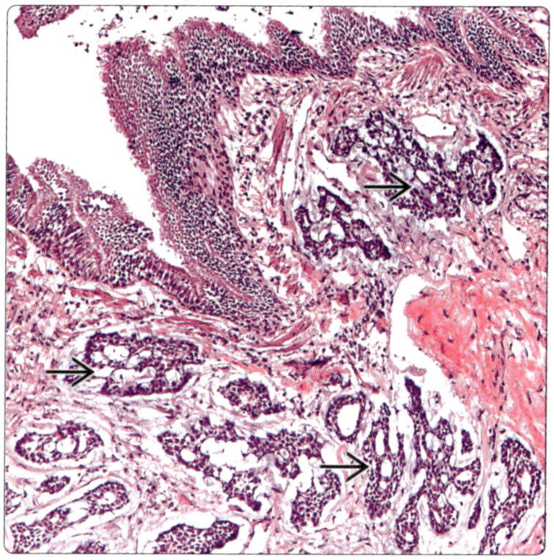

(Left) *Conventional adenocarcinoma, as seen in the lung, is very uncommon in the bronchus and trachea unless there is local extension. Most adenocarcinomas of the bronchus are of salivary-type origin or metastatic (e.g., from the colon).* **(Right)** *The bronchial submucosal glands can give rise to tumors that are identical to those seen in the salivary gland. Adenoid cystic carcinoma (shown here, with Swiss cheese pattern →), pleomorphic adenoma, and mucoepidermoid carcinoma are the more common types.*

Carcinoid Tumor

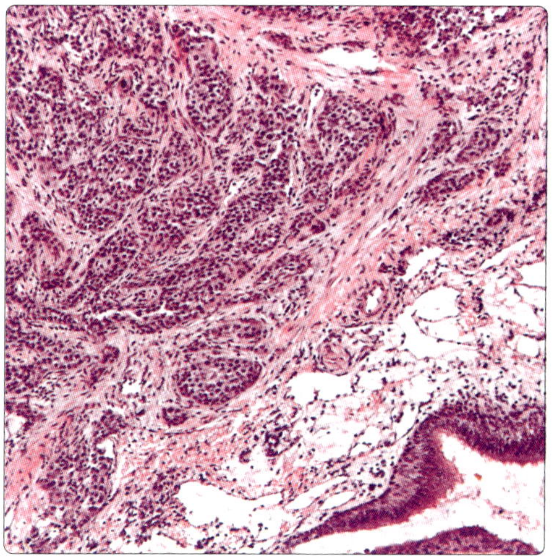

Carcinoid Tumor

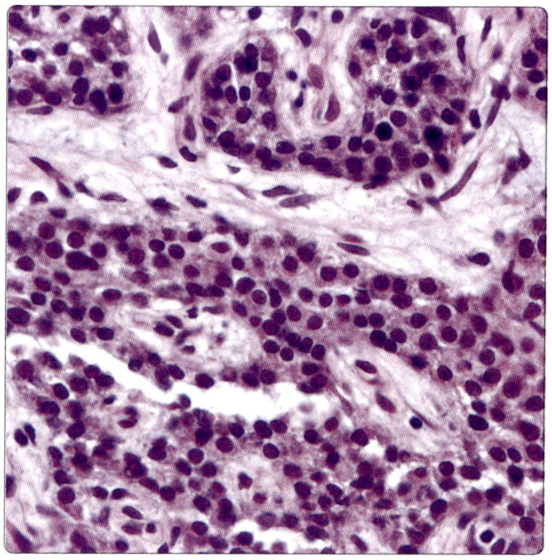

(Left) *Endobronchial origin with an exophytic pushing growth pattern is a common presentation for pulmonary carcinoid tumors. These tumors are characterized by nests, trabeculae, sheets, and acini of monomorphic epithelioid cells.* **(Right)** *Small, monomorphic cells and nuclei within the context of a classic architectural growth pattern are helpful in diagnosing a carcinoid tumor. Note how the characteristic salt and pepper nuclear chromatin pattern may not be present on frozen section preparations.*

Small Cell Carcinoma

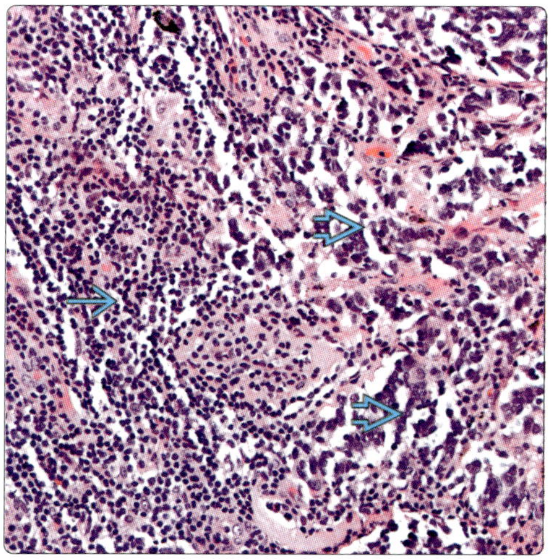

Reactive Endothelial Cells

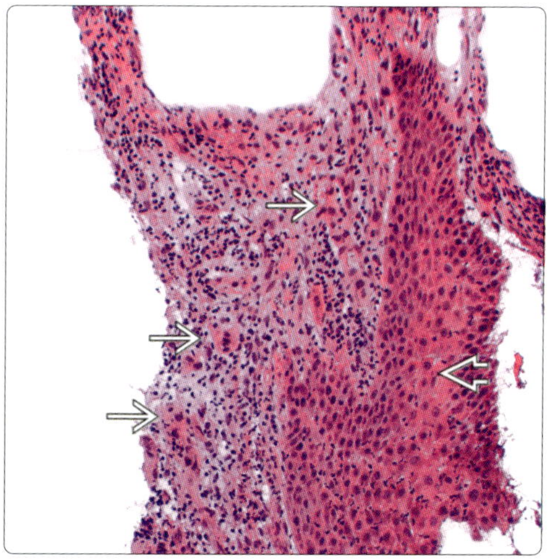

(Left) *Small cell carcinoma ⇒ can be difficult to distinguish from lymphocytes →. Tumor cells should show numerous mitoses and necrosis. If there is extensive crush artifact, a definite diagnosis may not be possible.* **(Right)** *In cases of infection or inflammation, submucosal capillaries may show prominent reactive endothelial cells → that mimic small nests of invasive carcinoma. Note that the overlying epithelium ⇒ is metaplastic, not dysplastic. Whether or not there is a mass at the site of the biopsy is also important.*

SURGICAL/CLINICAL CONSIDERATIONS

Goal of Consultation

- Diagnosis to determine appropriate intraoperative and postoperative treatment
  - Resection (e.g., pilocytic astrocytoma, ependymoma, metastasis, medulloblastoma)
  - Biopsy for diagnosis followed by treatment with radiotherapy or chemotherapy (e.g., diffuse infiltrating pontine glioma) or steroids (demyelinating disorder)
- Proper handling of tissue for ancillary studies (i.e., molecular studies, electron microscopy, microbiologic culture)

Change in Patient Management

- Immediate intraoperative planning
- Diagnostic tissue allocation for additional studies

Clinical Setting

- 3 main clinical scenarios require tissue sampling
  - Patients with symptoms and signs of increased intracranial pressure, such as nausea and vomiting
    - Urgent surgery to prevent impending herniation
  - Patients with chronic or subacute symptoms, such as ataxia and seizures
    - Biopsy to diagnose slow-growing or insidious process
  - Patients with specific cranial nerve palsies or hearing loss indicative of
    - Subarachnoid involvement by inflammatory or metastatic infiltrates
    - Local pressure by mass lesions, such as vestibular schwannomas
    - Biopsy to diagnose disease process
- Previous history is paramount
  - Adults: History of systemic malignancy, such as carcinoma, lymphoma, or demyelinating disease
  - Pediatric: History of leukemia or extracranial solid neoplasm
    - History of posterior fossa radiation
      - A medulloblastoma survivor is at risk for secondary glioblastoma multiforme (GBM)

Neuroimaging

- Review of imaging studies is important to determine most likely differential diagnosis for lesion
- **Neuroanatomic localization**
  - Cerebellar hemisphere
    - Metastases and hemangioblastomas in adults
    - Pilocytic astrocytomas and some subtypes of medulloblastoma in children
  - Cerebellar midline: Medulloblastomas in children
  - 4th ventricle: Ependymomas in children, subependymomas in adults
  - Cerebellopontine angle: Choroid plexus tumors and ependymomas in children
    - Vestibular schwannomas and meningiomas in adults
    - Dermoid cyst in adults or children
- **Signal characteristics**
  - Cysts with mural nodules in pilocytic astrocytomas, hemangioblastomas
  - Contrast enhancement in pilocytic astrocytomas and medulloblastomas (heterogeneous), metastases, and abscesses (rim pattern)
  - Decreased diffusion in infarcts, hemorrhages
  - Ill-defined, nonenhancing hemispheric lesions in low-grade gliomas
  - Rim enhancing after contrast administration in glioblastomas, lymphomas, toxoplasmosis

SPECIMEN EVALUATION

Gross

- Usually very few distinctive macroscopic features
  - Gliomas: Soft, gray-translucent, gelatinous texture
  - Pilocytic astrocytomas: Firm, rubbery, white-tan
  - Choroid plexus tumors: Papillary fronds, prominent vasculature
  - Hemangioblastomas: Vascular, hemorrhagic
  - Vestibular schwannomas, meningiomas: Firm, fibrous, or rubbery, gray-tan; difficult to smear
  - Abscesses: Purulent, sometimes with fibrous wall
  - Many lesions are hemorrhagic (nonspecific)

Diffuse Intrinsic Pontine Glioma: MR Appearance

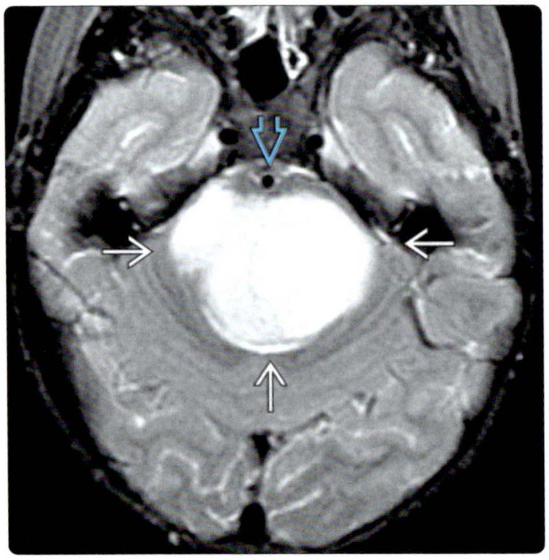

Cerebellum and Brainstem Gliomas

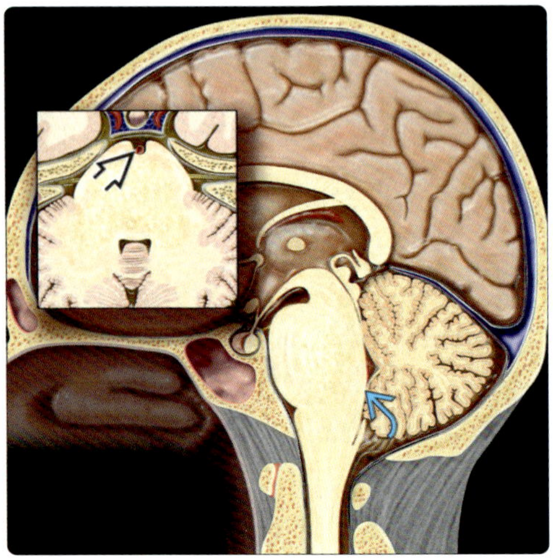

(Left) *Axial T2WI MR of the brainstem shows a diffuse intrinsic pontine glioma (DIPG) with marked expansion and hyperintensity of the pons ➡. Note the tumor wrapping around the basilar artery ⇨, a growth pattern typical of DIPGs. DIPGs are usually fibrillary and have a poor outcome despite therapy.* **(Right)** *Glial tumors are the most common primary tumor of the cerebellum and brainstem. This DIPG compresses the 4th ventricle ↗ and surrounds the basilar artery ⇨.*

- Distinguish lesional from normal for frozen section and smear preparation
  - Brainstem, cerebellar tissue: Soft pink-white, easily smeared as thin uniform film
  - Meningeal tissue: Membranous, vascular, does not smear well
  - White matter: Pearly white, sticky, but smears well
  - Metastases: Granular or mucoid, pink, gray, tan-yellow, or hemorrhagic, depending on type; smears in clumps
  - Gliomas: Usually more gray and mucoid, smears well or in strings
  - Reactive brain tissue: Smears well; however, reactive astrocytes often hold tissue together giving it clouds in sky pattern

Frozen Section

- Important not to use entire specimen (may be only specimen received)
  - Do smear cytologic prep first
  - Use ~ 1 mm of tissue from both ends of core biopsy to represent proximal and distal to lesion
- Frozen method
  - Perch tissue to be frozen on small bead of embedding medium; do not cover with medium
  - If core biopsy, bisect sample longitudinally, not perpendicularly, after ends were taken for smears, and freeze 1/2
  - Freeze quickly with light touch of metal heat extractor or cryospray to avoid ice crystals in tissue
  - Step section carefully into block when making slides
- In some cases, cytologic preparations only may be preferable
  - Small specimens, suspected infectious disease, or calcified lesions

Cytology

- Smear (squash) for soft specimens, works for most samples
- 2 or 3 < 1-mm pieces put next to each other may be used to represent different sites on same slide
- Touch preparation for firm/fibrous/calcified lesions
- Scan entire slide, as lesions may be heterogeneous

Allocation for Special Studies

- Glial tumors, some metastatic tumors (lung, colon)
  - Reserve frozen tissue for molecular studies
  - Required by some cancer centers for clinical trial eligibility
  - Flow cytometry for lymphoma
- Infectious specimens
  - Tissue should be sent for microbiologic cultures
  - Sterile tissue sent directly from operating room is preferable for this purpose

MOST COMMON DIAGNOSES

Diffuse Intrinsic Pontine (Brainstem) Glioma

- Frozen section
  - Yield varies on the target and navigation
    - Amount of tissue is usually small due to location
    - Nondiagnostic or inconclusive samples due to heterogeneity are common
  - Morphologic features can range from diffuse astrocytoma to frank GBM
    - Diffuse low-grade appearance does not exclude high-grade features elsewhere
    - Small amount of tissue often limits further molecular analysis
- Smear
  - Hyperchromatic, ovoid or fusiform nuclei
  - Various degrees of atypia and pleomorphism
  - Mitotic activity
  - Fibrillary background
  - No Rosenthal fibers or eosinophilic granular bodies
  - Microvascular proliferation
  - Necrosis
- Difficulties
  - Usually extremely small samples
    - Frozen should be performed only when necessary to confirm lesional tissue
    - Most of the tissue should be reserved for molecular analysis
    - Can be surrounded by reactive gliosis

Juvenile Pilocytic Astrocytoma

- Frozen section
  - Dense areas with fibrillary background containing Rosenthal fibers and eosinophilic granular bodies, alternating with loose, microcystic regions
    - Rosenthal fibers are thick, eosinophilic twisted fibers (made up of intermediate filaments)
  - Oval nuclei with occasional pleomorphism, rare or no mitoses
  - Frequent microvascular proliferation of no prognostic significance
  - Necrosis rare (suggests alternative diagnosis)
- Smear
  - Clear bipolar cytomorphology, multinucleated cells ("coins on the plate") can be present
  - Network of coarse Rosenthal fibers in background and eosinophilic granular bodies
  - Knots of microvascular proliferation should not be mistaken for microvascular proliferation in GBM
  - Mitotic figures can be present; however, abundant mitoses are unusual and warrant caution
- Difficulties
  - If sample very small, may not have all diagnostic features
  - If uncertain, can be reported as "astrocytoma with piloid features"

Medulloblastoma

- Frozen section
  - Small round blue cell tumor with broad sheets of solid tumor
  - Single cell apoptosis and geographic necrosis
  - High mitotic rate, though may depend on staining quality
  - Variable features
    - Homer Wright rosettes (classic medulloblastoma)
    - Connective tissue septa creating nodular pattern (desmoplastic medulloblastoma)
    - Large bizarre cells with prominent nucleoli (anaplastic/large cell medulloblastoma)

Contents

  - Nodular or desmoplastic architecture suggests sonic hedgehog subtype
  - Not necessary to distinguish variants intraoperatively
- Smear
  - Uniform, oval or carrot-shaped nuclei with little cytoplasm, usually conspicuous mitotic figures
  - Dirty necrotic background with nuclear fragments
- Difficulties
  - Indistinguishable from atypical teratoid/rhabdoid tumor (AT/RT) on intraoperative consultation
  - Report as "small blue cell tumor, diagnosis deferred to permanent sections"
  - If smear is too aggressive, nuclei may disrupt in chromatin clumps and streaks
  - Normal hypercellular granular cell layer of cerebellar cortex may cause problems
    - Cells are smaller and lack mitoses
    - Scattered Purkinje cells can be helpful
- Sufficient amount of tumor tissue should be reserved for molecular studies

Atypical Teratoid/Rhabdoid Tumor (AT/RT)

- Frozen section
  - "Small blue cell tumor" without rosettes or desmoplastic nodules
  - Variably conspicuous rhabdoid cells with abundant, dense, eosinophilic cytoplasm
    - May not always be present
  - Occasional clear cells and "cannibal" cells (one cell engulfing another)
- Smear
  - Predominantly uniform, oval or carrot-shaped nuclei with little cytoplasm
  - Rhabdoid cells better seen on smear than frozen section
  - Apoptotic cells and (usually) high mitotic rate
- Difficulties
  - Indistinguishable from other malignant small round blue cell tumors on intraoperative consultation
  - Report as "small blue cell tumor, diagnosis deferred to permanent sections"
  - Abundant rhabdoid cells can also be seen in metastatic rhabdomyosarcoma

Ependymoma

- Frozen section
  - Variably cellular with perivascular pseudorosettes, ependymal tubules or canals, and small intracytoplasmic vacuoles (lumina)
  - Microvascular proliferation of no prognostic significance (WHO grade II)
  - Marked cytologic atypia, mitoses, and necrosis indicate anaplastic ependymoma (WHO grade III)
- Smear
  - Glial tumor cells with uniform oval nuclei, often with small nucleoli and slightly granular chromatin
  - Cytoplasmic processes, radially arranged around blood vessels, ± vascular cell proliferation
- Difficulties
  - Must establish diagnosis with reasonable certainty, as resection is definitive therapy (unlike medulloblastoma or AT/RT)
  - Grading is not reliable due to tumor heterogeneity and is not predictive of outcome
  - Report as "ependymoma, grading deferred to permanent sections" (unless obviously anaplastic)
  - Molecular studies are superior to histologic grading

Schwannoma

- Frozen section
  - Spindle cell neoplasm with Antoni A and B areas
    - Antoni A areas consist of linear arrays of palisades of Schwann cell nuclei (Verocay bodies)
    - Antoni B areas have looser stroma and myxoid stroma
  - Variable nuclear size and shape but predominantly fusiform
  - Hyalinized vessels, macrophages, and other degenerative changes
- Smear
  - Often tough to smear, as tissue stays in clumps; little may come off on touch prep
  - Irregular, angulated groups of spindle cells
  - Thick hyalinized blood vessels
- Difficulties
  - May be indistinguishable from fibroblastic meningioma or solitary fibroblastic tumor

Hemangioblastoma

- Frozen section
  - Multivacuolated cells (oil red O positive) amid fine capillary stroma
  - Often striking nuclear atypia without mitoses
  - Microcystic changes
  - Numerous small blood vessels may be prominent feature
- Smear
  - Lipidized stromal tumor cells and fine capillaries
  - Nuclear atypia (high nuclear:cytoplasmic ratio, hyperchromasia, irregular nuclear outlines)
- Difficulties
  - Strong resemblance to metastatic renal clear cell carcinoma
  - In patients with von Hippel-Lindau disease, both lesions can occur in same patient

Choroid Plexus Tumors

- Frozen section and smear
  - Papilloma
    - Well-formed papillary structures with benign cuboidal or ciliated epithelium
    - Usually adults
  - Atypical papilloma
    - More complex configurations of epithelial structures with solid areas and nuclear atypia
  - Choroid plexus carcinoma
    - Very atypical, often solid, pleomorphic with necrosis
    - Often in small children, in which metastatic carcinoma would be unusual
    - Indistinguishable from metastatic adenocarcinoma

Other Neoplasms

- **Metastases**
  - Histology can vary highly based on primary site
    - Often dedifferentiated

  - Most commonly adenocarcinomas of lung, breast, and melanoma
  - May present as hemorrhage, particularly melanoma and renal cell carcinoma
- **Lymphoma**
  - Large lymphoid cells with prominent nucleoli
  - Karyorrhectic debris and mitoses
  - Usually in background of lymphoglandular bodies
    - Round, pale, basophilic cytoplasmic fragments of lymphocytes measuring 2-7 µm
  - Rarely occurs in isolation in posterior fossa
- **Desmoplastic infantile astrocytoma and ganglioglioma**
  - Marked collagenous/fibroblastic component with inconspicuous astrocytes &/or ganglion cells
  - Often growing on meningeal surface and attached to overlying dura
  - Usually, but not exclusively, low grade
- **Glioneuronal tumors**
  - Dysembryoplastic neuroepithelial tumor
    - Unusual in cerebellum, may have macrocystic component
    - Small round neurocytic or oligodendrocyte-like nuclei in single file or nodular growth pattern
    - Scattered ganglion cells "floating" in microcystic spaces
    - Low grade/hamartomatous
  - Rosetted glioneuronal tumor of 4th ventricle
    - Small neurocytic cells forming rosettes with islands of neuropil in center
    - No mitotic activity

Demyelinating Disease

- **Progressive multifocal leukoencephalopathy**
  - Occurs in immunosuppression (AIDS, transplant recipients, and, rarely, due to immunomodulating drugs), due to reactivation of John Cunningham (JC) virus infection
  - Frozen section and smear
    - Some large, smudgy, glial cell nuclei (viral cytopathic change) and numerous foamy macrophages
    - Variable perivascular lymphocytic infiltrates composed of small lymphocytes
- **Multiple sclerosis**
  - Only biopsied when rare acute tumefactive (tumor-like) single lesion is present
  - Frozen section and smear
    - Foamy macrophages and sometimes atypical, reactive astrocytes
    - May have large astrocytes with peculiar mitoses (Creutzfeldt cells)
    - Variable perivascular lymphocytic infiltrates
- Important to recognize so resection is not performed

Abscesses and Infections

- **Bacterial abscess**
  - Aerobic/anaerobic
    - Neutrophils, necrotic debris, fibrovascular wall
    - Organism not usually visible
    - Tissue for microbiologic culture should be sent (if not sent from operating room)
    - Report as "abscess contents, favor bacterial"
    - Recommendation to send sterile material for microbiology is warranted in report
  - Mycobacterial
    - Lymphocytes, epithelioid histiocytes, giant cells, necrotic debris
    - Tissue for acid-fast bacilli smear and culture should be sent (if not sent from operating room)
    - Report as "necrotizing granuloma, suggest sterile material be sent for microbiology"
- **Fungal infections**
  - Variable acute/chronic inflammatory infiltrates, depending on organism and host immune status
  - Hemorrhage accompanies angioinvasive fungi, such as *Aspergillus*
  - Organism often seen on frozen section or smear
  - Report as "fungal infection, suggest sterile material be sent for microbiology"
- **Toxoplasmosis**
  - Frequent in HIV and may mimic lymphoma or glioblastoma on imaging
  - Necrotic debris mixed with neutrophils and macrophages
  - Look for bradyzoite cysts given that tachyzoites are easily mistaken for karyorrhectic debris
    - Thin-walled cysts varying in size from 5-70 µm
    - Filled with crescent-shaped bradyzoites
  - Important to recognize to avoid further resection
- **Cerebellitis**
  - Tumor-like lesion may be present on imaging mimicking neoplasm
  - Occurs in children
  - Extensive lymphocytic inflammation and disruption of normal architecture
  - Presumed viral, though inclusions not seen

Hemorrhages

- Usually related to hypertension or amyloid angiopathy, especially in older patients
- May result from vascular malformations, such as cavernous angiomas or developmental venous anomalies
- Rarely biopsied unless imaging characteristics are atypical or expansion (growth) of lesion occurs
- Can be due to metastatic disease (adults) or acute leukemia (children)

Infarcts

- May be embolic or from localized atherosclerosis of posterior circulation
- Rarely biopsied, unless imaging characteristics are atypical

REPORTING

Frozen Section

- For core biopsies, adequacy for diagnosis is main question; definitive diagnosis may be deferred
- Open biopsy may alter management significantly if unexpected results (toxoplasmosis vs. lymphoma)
- Intraoperative planning depends on distinction between
  - Ependymoma, medulloblastoma, pilocytic astrocytoma where maximum safe resection is attempted
    - Ependymoma: Surgery is critical modality as tumor is resistant to radiation and therapy

    - Medulloblastoma and AT/RT can be treated with adjuvant therapy; therefore, surgery may not need to be as aggressive
  - Diffuse infiltrating pontine glioma, lymphoma
    - Biopsy followed by radiation and chemotherapy
  - Tumor (requiring allocation for molecular oncology) and infection (allocation for microbiology)

Cytology

- Important adjunct to diagnosis of
  - Pilocytic astrocytoma (bipolar cytomorphology, Rosenthal fibers) in astrocytic lesion with microvascular proliferation, so as not to overgrade
  - Small blue cell tumor with little cytoplasm (medulloblastoma, AT/RT) vs. ependymoma (cell processes around vessels)
  - Lymphoma

PITFALLS

Presence of Macrophages

- Strong indicator of nonneoplastic diagnosis (e.g., demyelination, infection)
  - May be seen, however, in treated high-grade tumors

Superficial Biopsy of Meninges

- If only superficial biopsy of meninges is mistakenly taken, arachnoid cell hyperplasia, which is a reactive process to underlying tumor, can mimic a meningioma

Presence of Rosenthal Fibers

- Seen in slow-growing or longstanding lesions, including nonneoplastic (e.g., close to craniopharyngioma or cysts)
- By itself, does not imply pilocytic astrocytoma; reactive brain surrounding a lesion can contain abundant Rosenthal fibers
- Conversely, when not seen in small biopsies, may make diagnosis of pilocytic astrocytoma difficult (report as "astrocytoma with piloid features")

Microvascular Proliferation

- Criterion for anaplasia (grade III or IV) in diffuse astrocytomas but **not** in pilocytic astrocytomas or ependymomas
- If tumor classification is equivocal at time of intraoperative consultation, best to defer grading unless mitoses &/or necrosis are seen in addition to microvascular proliferation

Necrosis Following Radiotherapy

- Grading of low-grade or anaplastic gliomas may be complicated by radiotherapy-induced necrosis, mimicking glioblastoma
- Clues are vessels with fibrinoid or hyaline wall changes
- Report as "glioma with effects of treatment, grading deferred to permanent sections"

Keratin Debris

- Epidermoid and dermoid cyst can be filled with amorphous keratin debris without obvious epithelial lining
- Should not be confused with necrosis in malignant glioma or abscess

SELECTED REFERENCES

1. Somerset HL et al: Approach to the intraoperative consultation for neurosurgical specimens. Adv Anat Pathol. 18(6):446-9, 2011
2. Takei H et al: Cytomorphologic characteristics, differential diagnosis and utility during intraoperative consultation for medulloblastoma. Acta Cytol. 51(2):183-92, 2007
3. Uematsu Y et al: The usefulness and problem of intraoperative rapid diagnosis in surgical neuropathology. Brain Tumor Pathol. 24(2):47-52, 2007
4. Parwani AV et al: Atypical teratoid/rhabdoid tumor of the brain: cytopathologic characteristics and differential diagnosis. Cancer. 105(2):65-70, 2005
5. Zagzag D et al: Demyelinating disease versus tumor in surgical neuropathology. Clues to a correct pathological diagnosis. Am J Surg Pathol. 17(6):537-45, 1993

Diffuse Intrinsic Pontine Glioma: Frozen Section Appearance

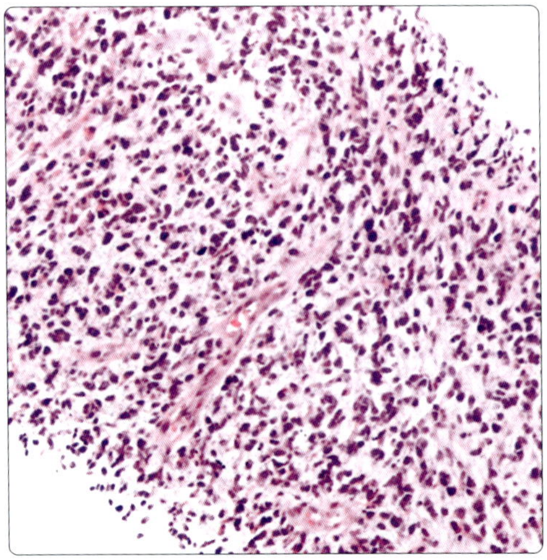

Diffuse Intrinsic Pontine Glioma: Cytologic Appearance

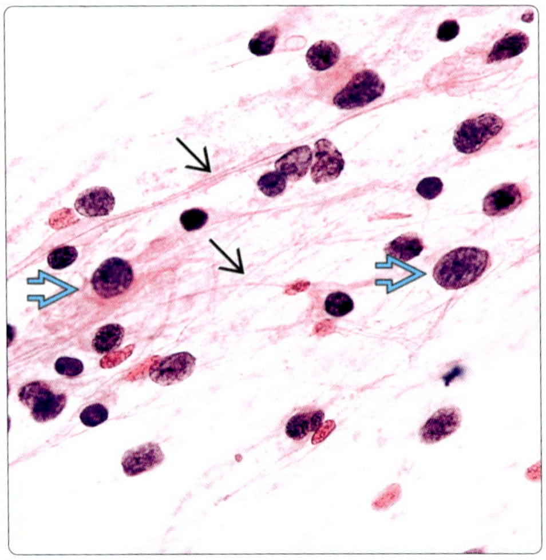

(Left) *Core needle biopsy of a diffuse intrinsic pontine glioma has anaplastic features, including high cellularity and mitotic activity on frozen section. Necrosis should not be present unless there has been prior radiotherapy.* **(Right)** *Infiltrating astrocytoma is characterized by irregular, dark, hyperchromatic, ovoid or fusiform nuclei with inconspicuous nucleoli* ⇨ *sitting in a fibrillar background* ➙.

Juvenile Pilocytic Astrocytoma: MR Appearance

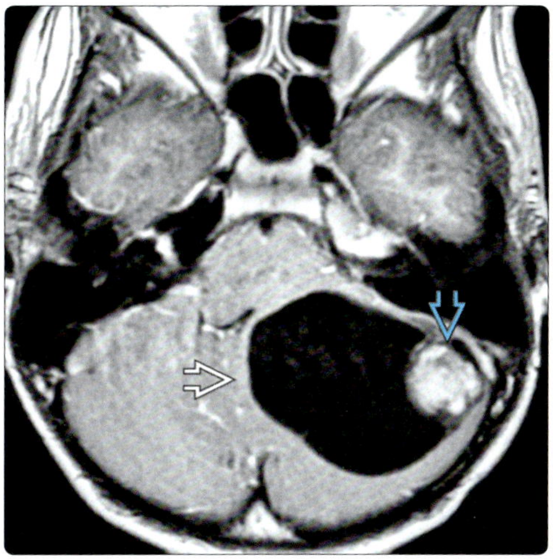

Juvenile Pilocytic Astrocytoma

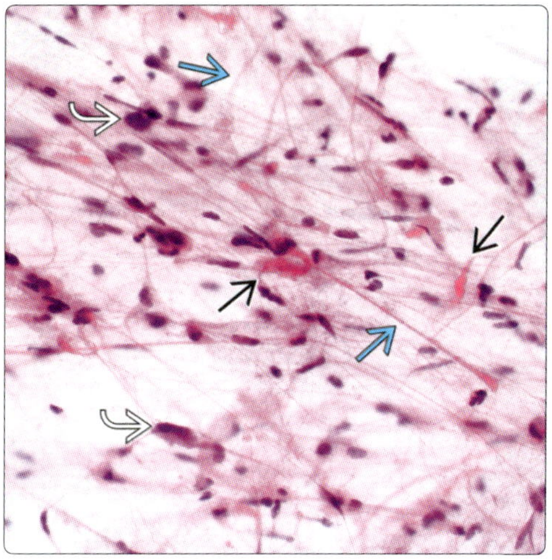

(Left) *Axial T1WI MR with contrast shows the classic cyst with mural nodule appearance of cerebellar juvenile pilocytic astrocytoma. Note the typical intense enhancement of the nodule ➾ with no enhancement of the cyst wall ➾. Mass effect on the 4th ventricle with associated hydrocephalus is common.* **(Right)** *Juvenile pilocytic astrocytoma shows elongated nuclei and numerous hair-like (piloid) processes ➙. Pleomorphic cells can be present ➦ but are not concerning. Rosenthal fibers ➙ confirm the diagnosis.*

Juvenile Pilocytic Astrocytoma

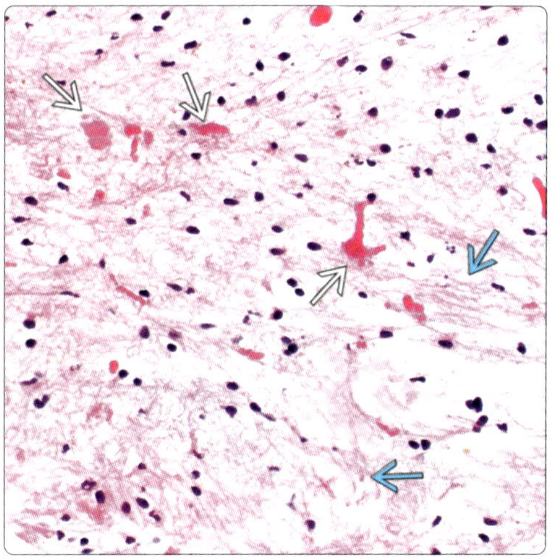

Juvenile Pilocytic Astrocytoma

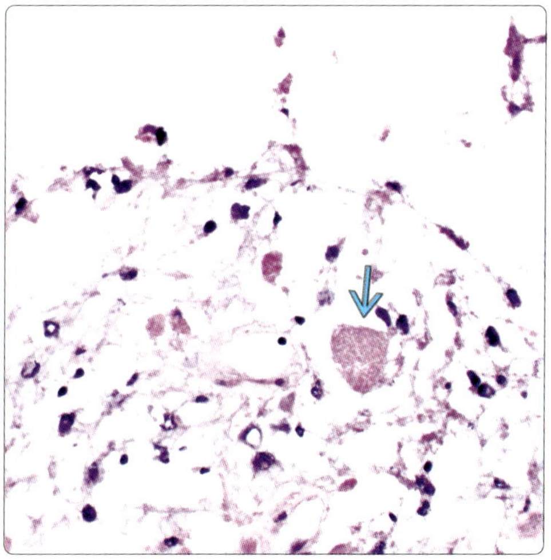

(Left) *A frozen section of a juvenile pilocytic astrocytoma often shows a moderately cellular neoplasm composed of small glial cells. The background can be quite fibrillary ➙, and Rosenthal material ➙ can vary in abundance.* **(Right)** *In some areas, juvenile pilocytic astrocytoma can be paucicellular and fibrillary, and eosinophilic granular bodies ➙, rather than Rosenthal fibers, can be observed.*

Capillary Hemangioma

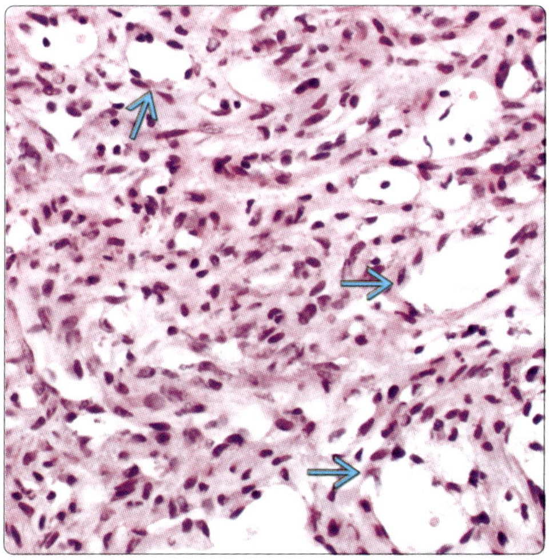

Metastatic Renal Cell Carcinoma

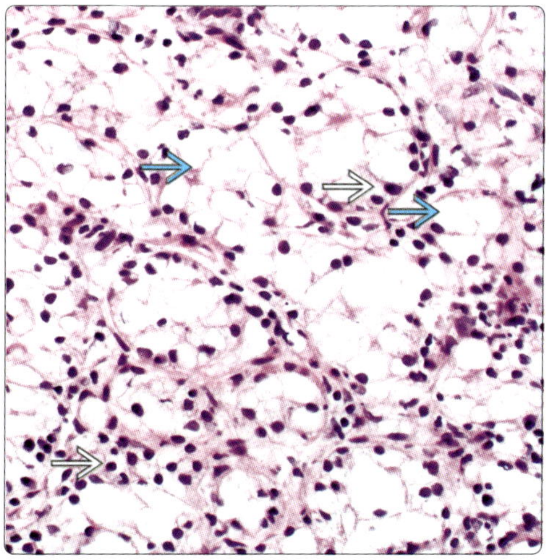

(Left) *Vascular lesions can be challenging to distinguish from gliomas or metastatic tumors in the brain. Capillary hemangioma is characterized by numerous small vascular channels ➙ that resemble a microvascular proliferation. However, a glial or epithelial neoplastic component is absent.* **(Right)** *Metastatic RCC is composed of bland cells with small nuclei ➙ and abundant clear cytoplasm ➙. The lesion can be markedly hypervascular or hemorrhagic, and the differential includes hemangioblastoma. Both can occur in von Hippel-Lindau.*

Medulloblastoma: Location

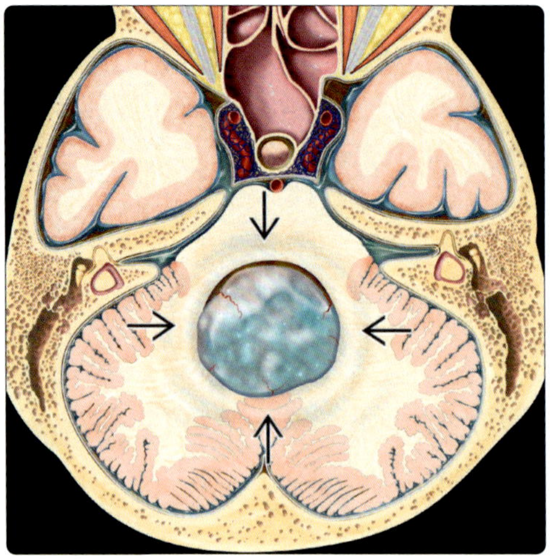

Medulloblastoma: MR Appearance

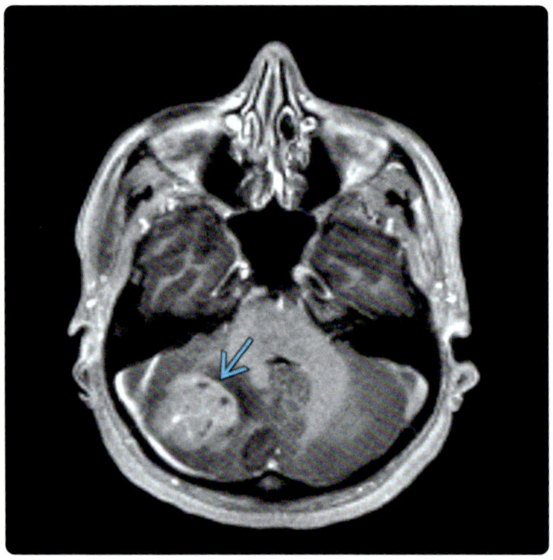

(Left) *Axial view of the cerebellum shows a spherical tumor centered in the 4th ventricle →, the typical location for medulloblastoma. This tumor occurs most frequently in children 5-10 years of age and in young adults. It is rarely seen in adults over the age of 35.* **(Right)** *The majority of medulloblastomas arise from the vermis (75%) and most are irregularly enhancing (90%). This image shows a cerebellar hemispheric lesion on axial T1 postcontrast MR without definite enhancement →, which was a medulloblastoma.*

Medulloblastoma: Cytologic Features

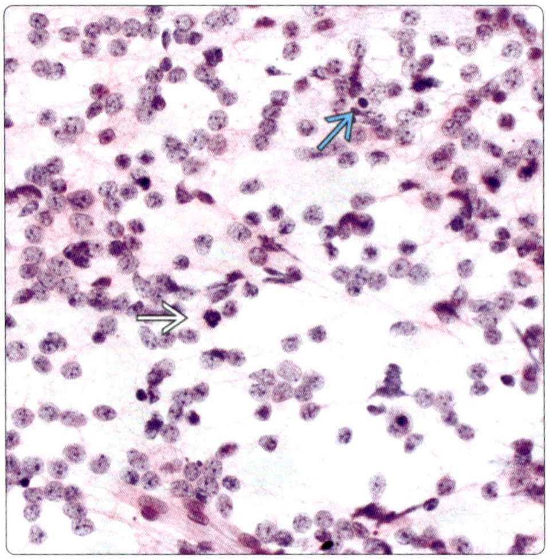

Medulloblastoma: Cytologic Features

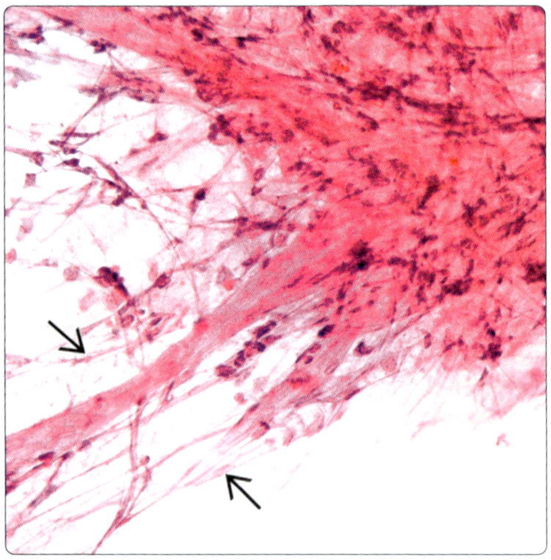

(Left) *Smear of a medulloblastoma shows a single layer of monomorphic small round blue cells. Mitosis → or apoptotic bodies → can easily be observed.* **(Right)** *Medulloblastomas are subject to possible smear artifact if the preparation is done aggressively. The nuclear chromatin can be smeared →, which may render the slide very difficult to interpret. Touch preparations may avoid this artifact.*

Medulloblastoma

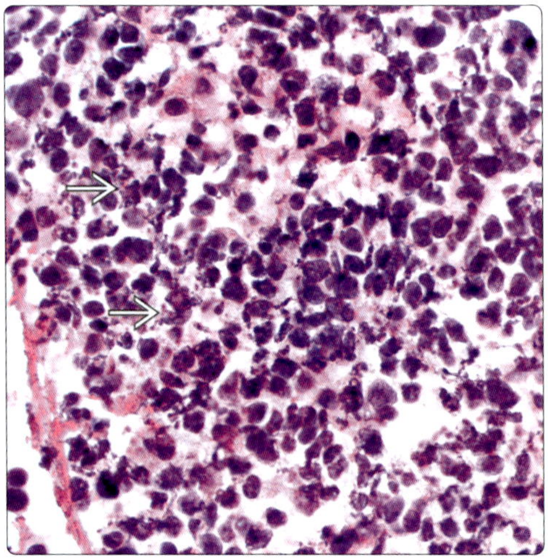

Medulloblastoma

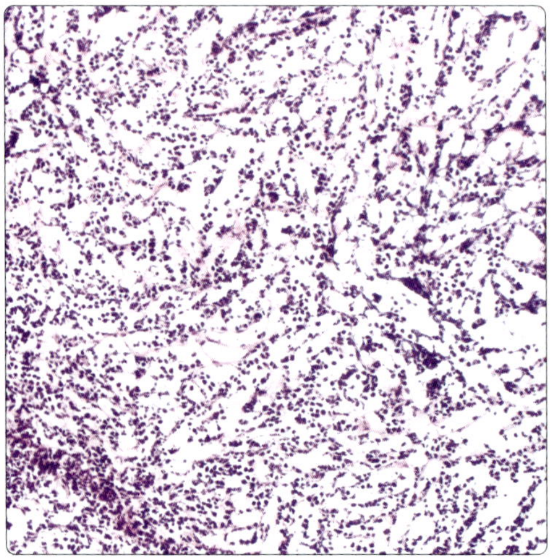

(Left) *Frozen section of a medulloblastoma shows freezing artifact causing cells to appear fragmented →. The nuclear detail is much less clear than in a cytologic preparation. Intraoperative distinction from atypical teratoid/rhabdoid tumor (AT/RT) is not possible, as this requires immunostaining for INI1/SNF5.* **(Right)** *On a frozen section of medulloblastoma, neuropil and architectural features, such as pale nodules, could be difficult to observe due to freezing artifacts. Only sheets of small round blue cells are noted.*

Ependymoma: MR Appearance

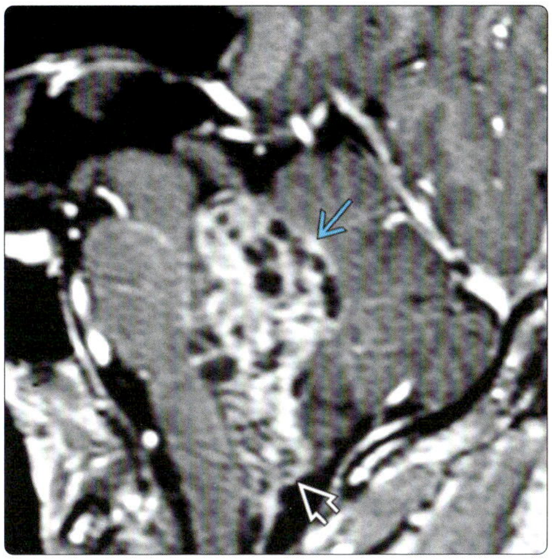

Ependymoma: Gross Appearance

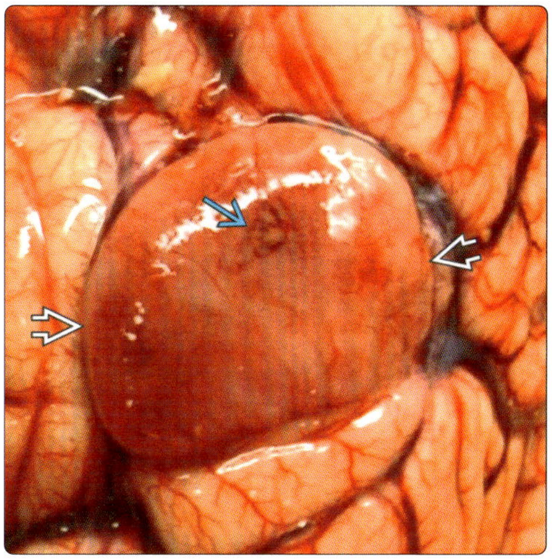

(Left) *Sagittal T1WI C+ FS MR shows a classic ependymoma extending from the 4th ventricle into the cisterna magna. The appearance of cystic areas intermixed with an enhancing solid tumor is typical.* **(Right)** *A gross specimen of an ependymoma metastasis to the surface of the brain shows a mushroom-like pink lesion with a smooth glistening surface and a focus of necrosis.*

Ependymoma: Cytologic Features

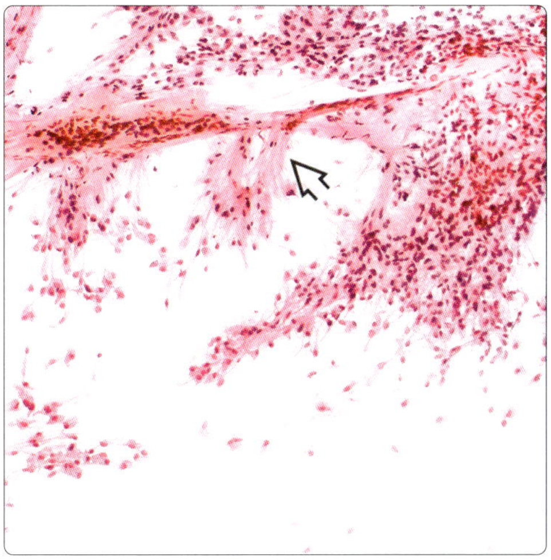

Ependymoma

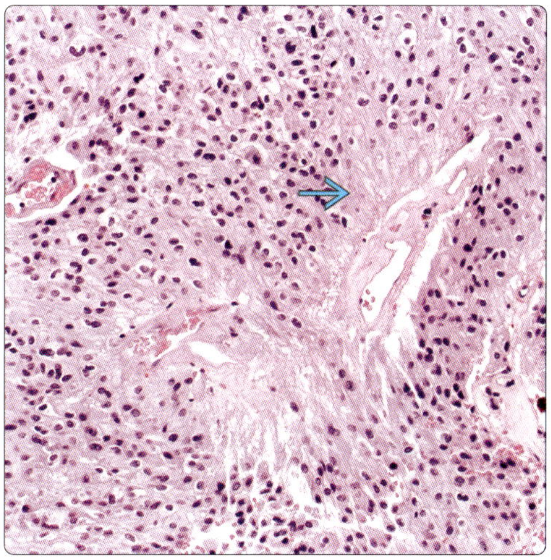

(Left) *Typical features of an ependymoma on a smear are uniform oval nuclei with fibrillary cytoplasm and cells extending to blood vessel basal lamina (perivascular pseudorosettes). Nuclear features are bland, and microvascular proliferation, mitoses, and necrosis are absent in this WHO grade II tumor.* **(Right)** *Ependymoma shows perivascular arrays of fibrillary cells, forming perivascular pseudorosettes around a blood vessel. The nuclei are uniform and bland.*

Atypical Teratoid/Rhabdoid Tumor

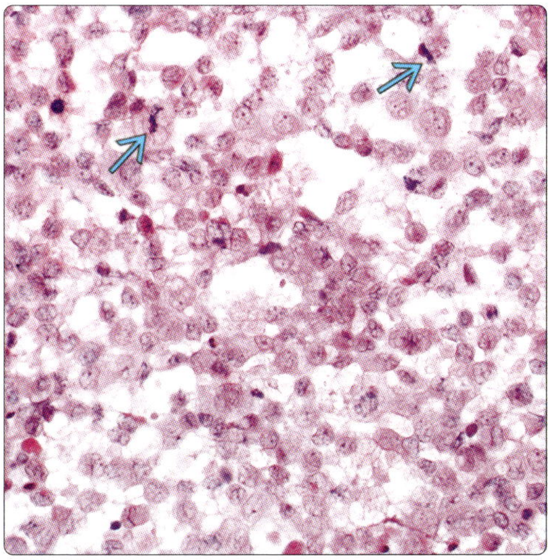

Atypical Teratoid/Rhabdoid Tumor

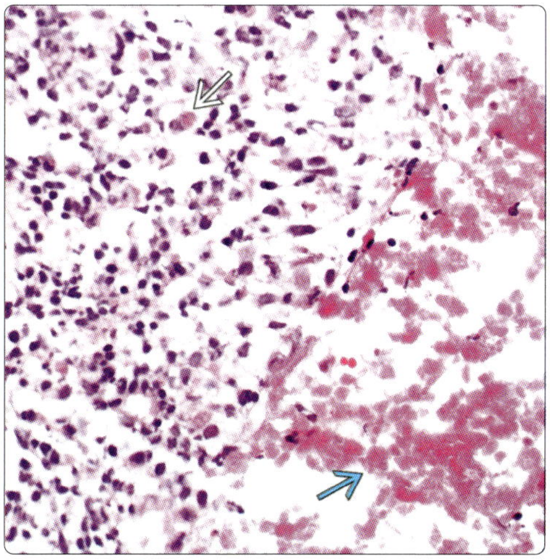

(Left) *Smear of an atypical teratoid/rhabdoid tumor (AT/RT) in a 7-week-old infant shows a hypercellular tumor composed of large pleomorphic cells with large nuclei, prominent nucleoli, and abundant pink cytoplasm. Mitotic figures are abundant.* **(Right)** *On frozen section, rhabdoid features of an AT/RT are less prominent, though cells with pink cytoplasm can be noted. Necrosis is also prominent.*

(Left) *Hemangioblastomas are characterized by multivacuolated stromal cells filled with lipid. These cells occasionally have pleomorphic hyperdense nuclei* → *of no prognostic significance. The vacuolated stromal cells lie alongside fine capillaries.* **(Right)** *The appearance of hemangioblastoma in tissue sections shows lobules of vacuolated stromal cells* →*, some with enlarged nuclei that are crisscrossed with fine capillaries* →*. The tumor closely resembles clear cell carcinoma of the kidney.*

Hemangioblastoma: Cytologic Features

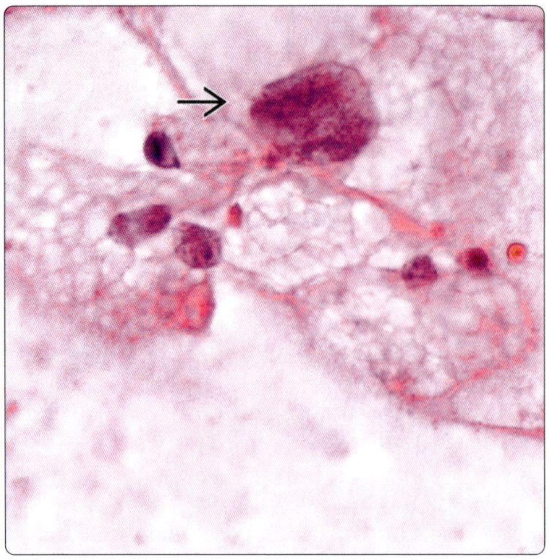

Hemangioblastoma

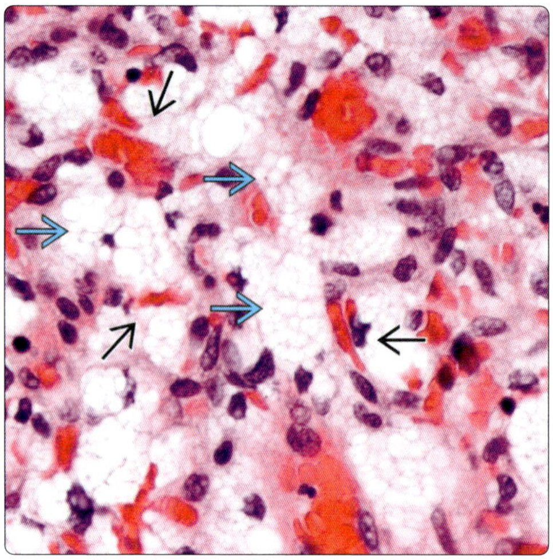

(Left) *The typical cytologic appearance of a schwannoma on a smear consists of dense syncytial groupings of spindled cells and thick hyalinized vessels. The dense stroma can make it difficult to prepare suitable cytologic preparations from these tumors.* **(Right)** *Schwannomas are composed of relatively monomorphic spindle cells with cigar-shaped nuclei, which are often arranged in palisading* → *groups flanking an anuclear zone composed of cellular processes* → *forming Verocay bodies.*

Schwannoma: Cytologic Features

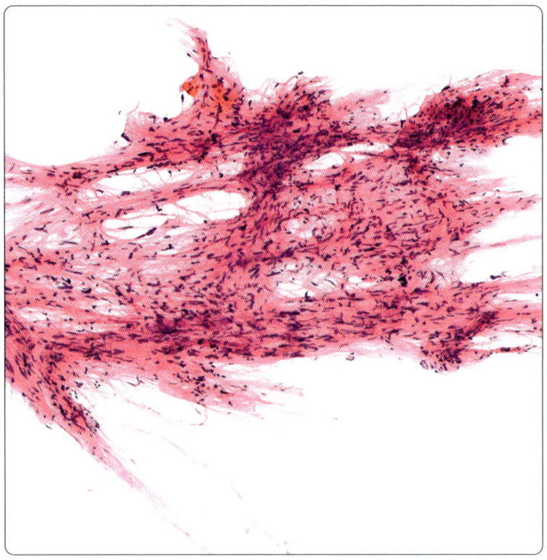

Schwannoma

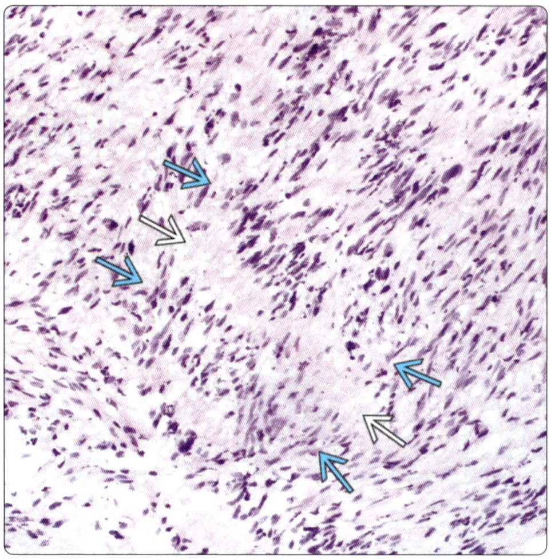

(Left) *Coronal T1WI MR with contrast shows 2 separate rim-enhancing masses* → *with intervening signal abnormality in the cerebellar hemisphere. The differential diagnosis includes metastatic tumor and high-grade glioma.* **(Right)** *A bacterial abscess shows normal cerebellar cortex (granule cells, Purkinje cells* →*, and molecular layer) intermingled with neutrophilic infiltrates amid cellular debris* →*. Material must be sent from the OR in sterile fashion for culture and sensitivity.*

Cerebellar Abscess: MR Appearance

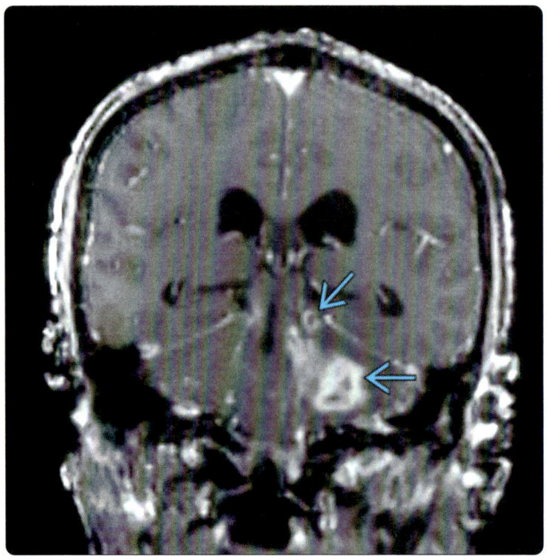

Cerebellar Abscess

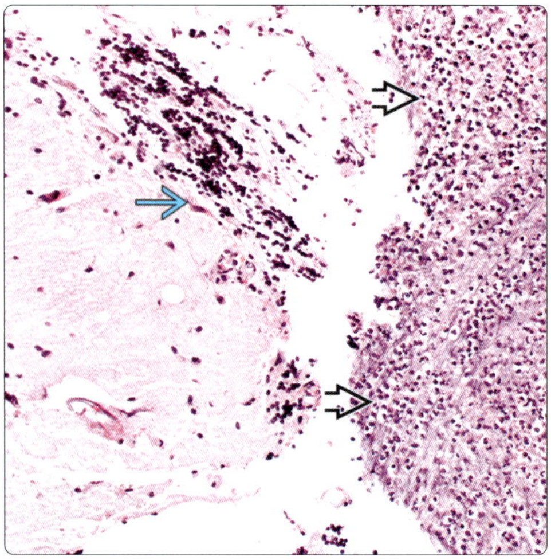

Medulloblastoma: MR Appearance

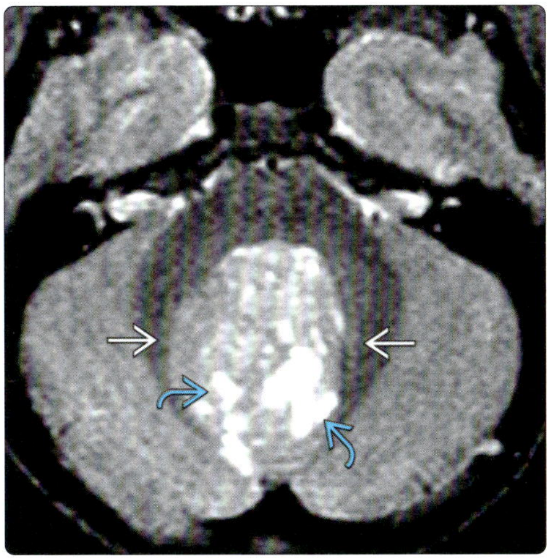

Medulloblastoma

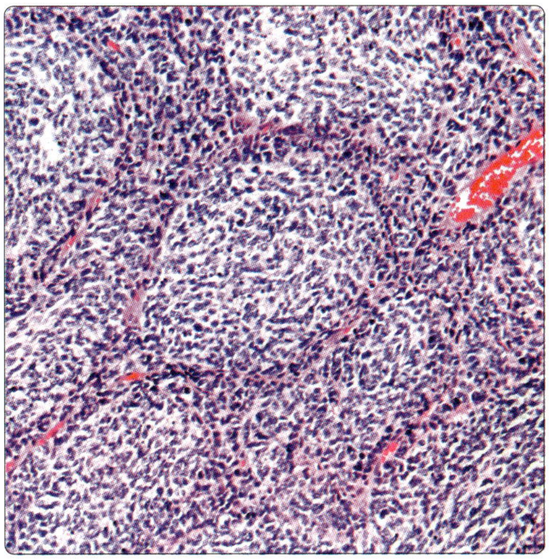

(Left) *Axial FLAIR MR of a medulloblastoma shows a heterogeneous, high signal intensity mass with well-defined borders in the region of the 4th ventricle . Note the multiple intratumoral cysts .* **(Right)** *The typical appearance of a desmoplastic medulloblastoma is round or oval clusters of cells with more cytoplasm (neuropil-like space between nuclei) surrounded by less differentiated cells. This is appearance is suggestive of the sonic hedgehog type of medulloblastoma.*

Ependymoma: Location

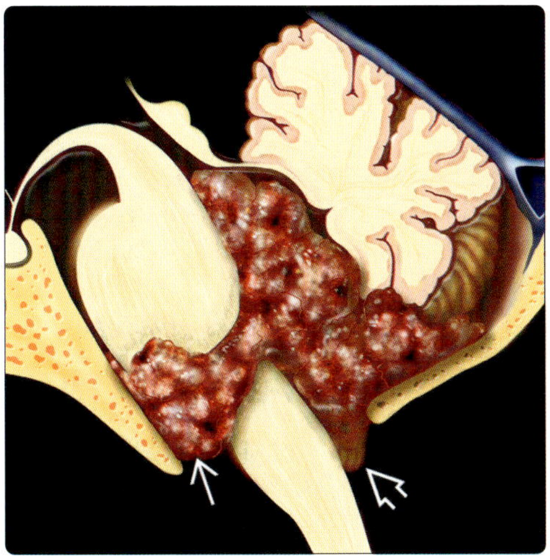

Hemangioblastoma: Gross Appearance

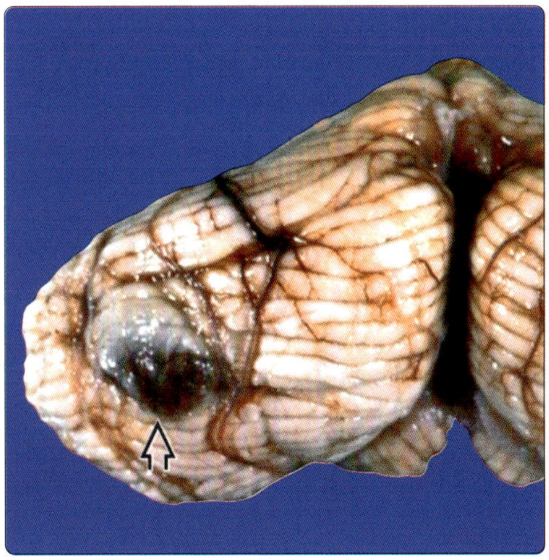

(Left) *Sagittal section shows an ependymoma extending through the 4th ventricle outlet foramina into the cisterna magna and cerebellopontine angle . This plastic pattern of growth is typical of ependymoma in this location and increases the difficulty of surgical resection.* **(Right)** *Gross pathology shows a solitary hemangioblastoma of the cerebellar hemisphere. The well-delineated, very vascular-appearing tumor nodule abuts the pia. (Courtesy E. Ross, MD.)*

Pilocytic Astrocytoma: Location

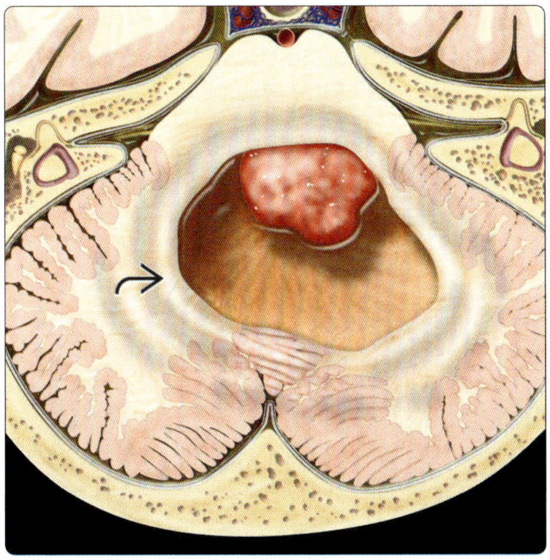

Multiple Hemangioblastomas: Location

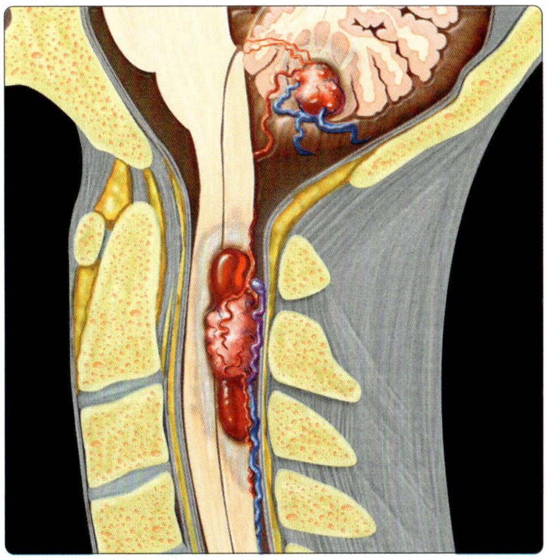

(Left) *Section of cerebellum and pons shows a large cystic lesion with a mural nodule, causing compression of adjacent parenchyma and obliteration of the 4th ventricle (not visible). This is the typical appearance of a pilocytic astrocytoma.* **(Right)** *Patients with von Hippel-Lindau disease may have multiple highly vascular hemangioblastomas in the cerebellum and spinal cord. These tumors abut the meninges and have significant intraparenchymal components.*

SURGICAL/CLINICAL CONSIDERATIONS

Goal of Consultation

- Determine if diagnostic tissue is present
- Assist neurosurgeon to decide whether gross total resection should be attempted (glioma, metastasis) or whether biopsy alone is sufficient to determine neoadjuvant therapy (lymphoma)
- Allow for proper handling of tissue for ancillary studies (i.e., molecular studies, electron microscopy, microbiologic culture)
  - Determine if sufficient tissue is available for research studies (e.g., tumor banking, primary cell lines, patient derived xenografts)

Change in Patient Management

- If specimen does not show diagnostic tissue, additional samples should be requested
- Margins are rarely assessed, neurosurgeon may submit sample to assess whether tissue is normal
- In nonneoplastic conditions, often specific diagnosis cannot be determined on frozen section
  - Sufficient tissue should be obtained for ancillary studies for eventual diagnosis on permanent sections

Clinical Setting

- Patients with new and sudden neurologic symptoms often require tissue sampling
  - Patients presenting with symptoms, nondiagnostic imaging studies, and focal lesion require diagnosis
    - New onset of seizures
    - Localizing signs (e.g., hemiparesis, language difficulty)
    - Signs and symptoms of increased intracranial pressure
  - Patients with known systemic illnesses and suspected brain involvement require diagnosis
    - Primary systemic malignancy with suspicion for metastatic carcinoma
    - Bone marrow transplant or other immunocompromised states at risk for infection
  - Patients with diseases that require tissue sampling for ancillary studies but do not require intraoperative diagnosis
    - Dementing illness, including Creutzfeldt-Jakob disease
      - Frozen tissue is saved for molecular analysis, remaining tissue is treated with formic acid
    - Vasculitis: Levels on paraffin block are more useful for diagnosis of focal lesions

SPECIMEN EVALUATION

Neuroimaging Findings

- Imaging findings are very helpful in suggesting most likely diagnosis and duration
  - Neuroanatomic localization and signal characteristics
  - Mass effect, cystic/solid nature, presence of hydrocephalus, thinning of overlying bone, loss of cerebral parenchymal volume

Clinical Presentation

- Combination of imaging features and clinical presentation can narrow differential diagnosis and help to determine whether sample is representative of disease or whether additional samples should be requested
- Pathologist uses this information to determine if specimen is sufficient for diagnosis
  - Diagnostic sample: Highly cellular neoplasm in patient who presents with centrally necrotic cerebral tumor
  - Nondiagnostic sample: Rare atypical cells in patient who presents with centrally necrotic cerebral tumor

Gross

- Usually very few distinctive macroscopic characteristics
  - Gliomas: Gray-translucent, soft, gelatinous texture
  - Metastatic carcinoma: Red or tan, gritty consistency
  - Abscesses: Purulent, sometimes with fibrous wall
- Distinguish lesional tissue from normal
  - Normal cortex: Gray, soft consistency
  - Normal white matter: Chalky white, homogeneous, soft consistency

Glioblastoma Multiforme: Gross Appearance

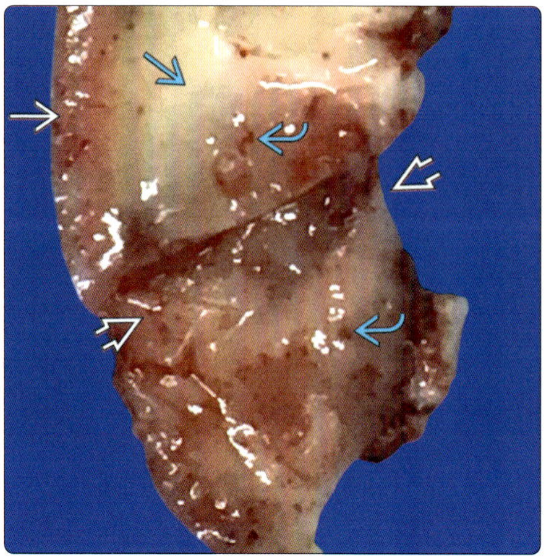

Glioblastoma Multiforme: Cytologic Appearance

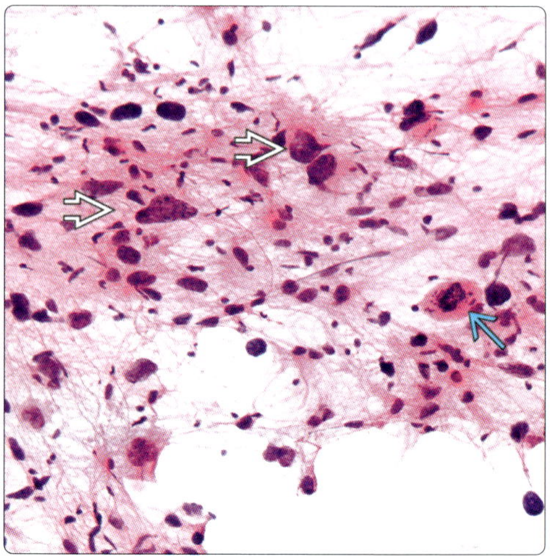

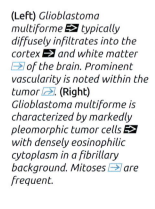

(Left) *Glioblastoma multiforme typically diffusely infiltrates into the cortex and white matter of the brain. Prominent vascularity is noted within the tumor.* **(Right)** *Glioblastoma multiforme is characterized by markedly pleomorphic tumor cells with densely eosinophilic cytoplasm in a fibrillary background. Mitoses are frequent.*

Frozen Section

- Important to not use entire specimen as additional tissue may not be available for other studies
- Minute portion of specimen is taken for cytologic preparation
  - If core biopsy is provided, small fragment from each end of core is used
  - If large specimen is provided, several small fragments should be reserved for smear preparation
- Frozen section method
  - Tissue to be frozen is perched on small bead of embedding medium but not covered with medium
  - Tissue is frozen quickly with light touch of metal heat extractor or cryospray to avoid ice crystals in tissue
  - Block is carefully step-sectioned to preserve tissue when making slides
- In some cases, cytologic preparations without frozen sections may be preferable
  - Very small specimens, suspected infection, or specimens with calcifications

Cytologic Preparations

- Smear method
  - 1-3 pinhead-sized fragments are placed 1/3 of way down on glass slide
    - In general, the smaller the fragment, the better the smear
  - 2nd slide is used to gently smear tissue on slide
    - Slides are held above fixative container to avoid any delay in fixation
  - Glass slides should not be pushed too hard together trying to smear tissue
  - Slides are placed immediately in fixative to avoid drying artifact
- Smear characteristics: Consistency of tissue between glass slides can be very informative as to nature of lesion
  - Schwannomas and fibroblastic meningiomas are firm and difficult to smear
  - Crunching "sand" between glass suggests calcifications
  - Soft, highly cellular tumors, such as pituitary adenomas, smear easily in single cell layer
- Touch preparation method
  - Use for firm/calcified/fibrous lesions
  - Tissue is gently and rapidly touched (held gently in forceps) once to slide surface
  - Slide is placed immediately in fixative to avoid drying artifact
- After staining, slide is inspected to identify how evenly tissue has been smeared
- Entire slide is carefully reviewed, as lesions may be heterogeneous
  - Diagnostic cells sometimes can be pulled out toward end of smear

MOST COMMON DIAGNOSES

Diffuse Astrocytoma (WHO Grade II)

- Frozen section
  - Cellularity slightly > normal brain with mild cytologic atypia
  - Elongated nuclei in infiltrating cells in white matter
  - Perineuronal satellitosis in cortex
  - Mitoses very rare and no necrosis or vascular proliferation
- Smear
  - Fibrillary background clearer than in frozen
  - Individual cytologically atypical nuclei (hyperchromatic, irregularly shaped, enlarged compared to normal glia)
- Difficulties
  - Findings must correlate with neuroimaging
    - Diffuse astrocytoma is noncontrast enhancing
    - Enhancement implies higher grade
    - Infiltrating edges of high-grade tumors are identical to low-grade tumors
  - Distinction from reactive processes, such as encephalitis, may require special studies

Oligodendroglioma (WHO Grade II)

- Frozen section
  - Uniform, round nuclei
  - Satellitosis around cortical neurons, subpial tumor cell accumulation
  - Branching capillary network (chicken-wire vasculature)
  - Often, microcalcifications, microcysts
  - May have microvascular proliferation and rare mitoses but no necrosis
- Smear
  - Fine fibrillary background
  - Uniform, round "naked" nuclei (no cytoplasmic processes, in contrast to astrocytomas)
- Difficulties
  - Typical perinuclear halos ("fried eggs") require formalin fixation, therefore not present on intraoperative preparations
    - Often not distinguishable from diffuse astrocytoma
    - Report as "glioma without anaplastic features"
  - As for diffuse astrocytomas, must correlate with imaging to make sure sample is not from infiltrating edge of higher grade tumor

Ependymoma (WHO Grades II and III)

- Frozen section
  - Variably cellular with perivascular pseudorosettes, ependymal tubules or canals, and small intracytoplasmic vacuoles (lumina)
    - Presence of ependymal differentiation is highly variable and often difficult to identify on frozen section
  - Foci of hypercellularity suggest anaplasia
  - Necrosis can be present in grade II and grade III tumors
  - Higher degree of pleomorphism and mitotic activity may indicate anaplasia
    - Grade does not have to be rendered on frozen section and has overall poor prognostic value
    - Sufficient tissue for molecular testing is important
  - Microvascular proliferation of no prognostic significance
  - Evidence of ependymal differentiation may be scarce in anaplastic tumors, making distinction from high-grade glioma or primitive neuroectodermal tumor (PNET) challenging on frozen section

- Some ependymomas may have areas of subependymoma (i.e., mixed ependymoma/subependymoma tumor)
- Smear
  - Glial tumor cells with uniform oval nuclei, often with small nucleoli
  - Cytoplasmic processes, radially arranged around blood vessels, ± vascular cell proliferation
  - Occasional intracytoplasmic lumina as well as cilia and terminal bars (blepharoplasts) in tubules
- Difficulties
  - Important to distinguish from astrocytoma, as gross total resection is preferred treatment for ependymoma

Anaplastic Astrocytoma (WHO Grade III)

- Frozen section and smear
  - More cellularity and nuclear pleomorphism than grade II astrocytoma
  - Mitotic activity
  - No necrosis or microvascular proliferation
- Difficulties
  - May be indistinguishable from anaplastic oligodendroglioma or glioblastoma
  - Report of "high-grade glioma" is sufficient

Anaplastic Oligodendroglioma (WHO Grade III)

- Frozen section and smear
  - More cellularity and nuclear pleomorphism than grade II oligodendroglioma
  - Brisk mitotic activity is common
  - May have necrosis, microvascular proliferation
- Difficulties
  - May be indistinguishable from anaplastic astrocytoma or glioblastoma
  - Report of "high-grade glioma" is sufficient

Glioblastoma Multiforme (WHO Grade IV)

- Frozen section
  - Dense cellularity, pleomorphism, mitotic activity in excess of lower grades
  - Tumor cells may have spindled, epithelioid, gemistocytic, small cell, &/or giant cells
    - Glioblastoma multiforme (GBM) variants: Gliosarcoma, small cell GBM, giant cell GBM, granular cell GBM
      - Unnecessary to distinguish variants on frozen section
  - Glomeruloid microvascular proliferation and endothelial hyperplasia
  - Necrosis with peripheral nuclear palisading
- Smear
  - Cytologically malignant cells (hyperchromasia, high nuclear:cytoplasmic ratio, irregular nuclear outline, mitoses)
  - Coarse fibrillary background
  - Knotted and blind-ending glomeruloid vessels and necrosis
- Difficulties
  - Occasionally, epithelioid features mimic carcinoma
  - If only necrotic tissue received, cannot distinguish from necrotic metastasis or lymphoma, infarct, or inflammatory process

Glioneuronal Tumors

- **Ganglioglioma**
  - Usually indolent tumor of childhood, arising in temporal lobe, can present with seizure and have cystic appearance
  - Smear and frozen
    - Atypical ganglion cells scattered among variably pleomorphic astrocytoma nuclei, fibrillary or myxoid background
    - Perivascular lymphocytic cuffs
    - Defer grade, unless obvious anaplasia (mitoses, microvascular proliferation, or necrosis)
- **Dysembryoplastic neuroepithelial tumor**
  - Low-grade, multinodular, cystic tumor of superficial cortex of young patients
    - Can present with seizures
  - Smear and frozen
    - Small round neurocytic or oligodendrocyte-like nuclei in single file or nodular growth pattern
    - Scattered ganglion cells "floating" in microcystic spaces or myxoid background
    - May have cortical disorganization and abnormal neuronal cytomorphology (cortical dysplasia) at interface with brain
- **Central neurocytoma**
  - Low grade, usually arising in ventricles but may be extraventricular
  - Strictly speaking, neurocytic tumor but with astrocytic features detectable in some cases
  - Smear and frozen
    - Small round neurocytic or oligodendrocyte-like cells
      - Often with perinuclear halos and fine capillary network
  - May be impossible to distinguish from oligodendroglioma on frozen

Supratentorial Primitive Neuroectodermal Tumor

- Smear and frozen section: Small blue cells with high apoptotic and mitotic indices
- Frozen section: Well or poorly formed tumor cell rosettes with fibrillary centers
- May be difficult to distinguish from small cell GBM, anaplastic oligodendroglioma, or lymphoma on limited biopsy

Other Primary Neuroepithelial Tumors

- **Pleomorphic xanthoastrocytoma**
  - Superficial cortical lesion, often with cyst, in young adults
  - Frozen section and smear
    - Bizarre ganglioid and astrocytic cells, some with foamy cytoplasm
    - Eosinophilic granular bodies in background
  - Definitive diagnosis may require ancillary studies (*BRAF* gene analysis, immunohistochemistry)
- **Subependymal giant cell tumor of tuberous sclerosis**
  - Bulky, nodular tumor in floor of lateral ventricle
  - Usually, patient has stigmata of tuberous sclerosis (cortical tubers, sebaceous hyperplasia, subungual nodules, Lisch nodules, "ash-leaf" spots)
  - Frozen section and smear: Bizarre cytomorphology with large cells having ganglioid and astrocytic features

- **Pilomyxoid astrocytoma**
  - Often large optic pathway tumors of childhood
  - Smear and frozen
    - Bipolar glial cells in myxoid background
    - No Rosenthal fibers or eosinophilic granular bodies
- **Chordoid glioma of 3rd ventricle**
  - Circumscribed enhancing mass in hypothalamus/anterior 3rd ventricle
  - Histologically bland but gross total resection rarely possible due to location
  - Smear and frozen section
    - Glial epithelioid cells in cords, myxoid background
    - Dense lymphoplasmacytic infiltrate
- **Choroid plexus tumors**
  - Papilloma
    - Frozen section: Well-formed papillary structures with benign cuboidal or ciliated epithelium
    - Smear: Papillary structures well seen
  - Choroid plexus carcinoma
    - Frozen and smear: Very atypical, indistinguishable from metastatic adenocarcinoma
- Pineal region tumors
  - Pineoblastoma: Virtually identical to PNET on smear and frozen section
  - Pineocytoma: Uniform round neurocytic cells, abundant neuropil, no mitoses
  - Pineal parenchymal tumor: Hypercellular, nodular architecture, composed of round neurocytic cells, often nodular, with some mitotic activity

Craniopharyngioma

- Suprasellar mass in children or young adults
- Heterogeneous and lobulated on imaging with calcification
- Smear: Squamoid or basaloid epithelium, "wet" keratin, calcium, foreign body giant cells
- Frozen section: Nests of basaloid epithelium and stellate reticulum amid keratin
- Difficulties
  - Adjacent brain may have gliosis and Rosenthal fibers, mimicking pilocytic astrocytoma
  - If only keratin contents received, may not be distinguishable from dermoid or epidermoid cysts

Germ Cell Tumors

- Usually midline (suprasellar, pineal region) in children and young adults
- Frozen section and smear: Pure germinoma, pure teratoma, or mixed with choriocarcinomatous and endodermal sinus elements (identical to gonadal or other extragonadal tumors)
- Important to recognize germinoma component intraoperatively
  - Nongerminomatous germ cell tumors respond less well to adjuvant therapy
    - More extensive resection would likely be attempted

Metastases

- Often multifocal, circumscribed, at gray-white junction or in meninges
- Common sites of origin
  - Lung, breast, kidney, skin (melanoma), gastrointestinal tract
  - Appearances similar to primaries
    - Glands or large epithelioid cells typical of breast, non-small cell lung, colon
    - Pigment in melanoma
      - Not always abundant
    - Clear cells characteristic of renal cell
  - Prostate, thyroid extremely rare
  - Tumor diathesis (nuclear and cytoplasmic debris) on smear
- Difficulties
  - Extensive hemorrhage, particularly in renal cell carcinoma, melanoma, choriocarcinoma
    - May obscure tumor cells
  - Extensive necrosis in colonic carcinoma
    - Can mimic glioblastoma
  - Glioblastomas with epithelioid or sarcomatous areas mimic carcinoma or sarcoma
  - Small cell carcinoma may mimic small cell glioblastoma or PNET

Primary Central Nervous System Lymphoma

- Periventricular, sometimes multifocal, in elderly or immunocompromised hosts
- Almost always diffuse large B-cell type
  - Usually does not infiltrate into brain parenchyma
  - Dyscohesive large nuclei with prominent nucleoli on smear and frozen section
  - Perivascular and patchy distribution with variable involvement of blood vessels
- Difficulties
  - If patient has received steroids, tumor may be almost completely necrotic
  - Important to recognize lymphoma
    - Resection not indicated and can actually be harmful
    - Allocate material for ancillary studies (flow cytometry, molecular studies)

Demyelinating Disease

- **Multiple sclerosis**
  - Rarely biopsied, only in setting of acute tumefactive demyelination
  - Frozen section and smear
    - Macrophages, atypical reactive astrocytes
    - Variable perivascular lymphocytic infiltrates
- **Progressive multifocal leukoencephalopathy**
  - Occurs in immunosuppression
  - Due to reactivation of JC virus infection
  - Frozen section and smear
    - Large smudgy glial cell nuclei (viral cytopathic change) and macrophages
    - Variable perivascular lymphocytic infiltrates

Abscesses and Infections

- **Bacterial infections**
  - **Aerobic/anaerobic**
    - Neutrophils, necrotic debris, fibrovascular wall, but organisms are usually not visible
    - Portion of specimen should be sent for microbiologic culture (if not sent from operating room)
    - Report as "abscess contents, favor bacterial, suggest sterile material be sent for microbiology"

- **Mycobacterial**
  - Lymphocytes, epithelioid histiocytes, giant cells, necrotic debris
  - Portion of specimen should be sent for acid-fast bacilli smear and culture (if not sent from operating room)
  - Report as "necrotizing granuloma, suggest sterile material be sent for microbiology"
- **Fungal infections**
  - Variable acute/chronic inflammatory infiltrates, depending on organism and host immune status
  - Hemorrhage accompanies angioinvasive fungi, such as *Aspergillus*
  - Organisms often seen on frozen section or smear
  - Report as "fungal infection, recommend sterile material be sent for microbiology"
- **Viral infections**
  - Herpes simplex (HSV) 1 and 2
    - Affects mesial temporal lobes, often asymmetrically
    - Only biopsied if poor response to antiviral therapy or if asymmetric with mass effect
    - Smear and frozen: Macrophages, lymphocytes, microglial nodules (microglia surrounding individually necrotic neurons), ± viral cytopathic effect (giant cells rarely seen, in contrast to cutaneous HSV)
    - Immunohistochemical studies on permanent sections and CSF titers are diagnostic
    - Saving frozen tissue for work-up of other infectious agent if HSV turns out to be negative may be helpful

Hemorrhage

- Usually related to hypertension or amyloid angiopathy, especially in older patients
- May result from vascular malformations, such as cavernous angiomas or developmental venous anomalies
- Rarely biopsied, unless imaging characteristics are atypical or expansion (growth) of lesion occurs
- Important to exclude hemorrhagic metastases by generous sampling of blood clot for paraffin sections

Infarct

- May be embolic or from localized atherosclerosis of posterior circulation
- Rarely biopsied, unless imaging characteristics are atypical

REPORTING

Frozen Section

- For core biopsies, adequacy for diagnosis is main question; definite diagnosis may be deferred
- Open biopsy may alter management significantly if unexpected results (e.g., toxoplasmosis vs. lymphoma)
- Intraoperative planning depends on distinction between
  - Ependymoma of any grade (requiring resection) from PNET (treated with radiation and chemotherapy)
  - Germ cell tumor (treated with radiation and chemotherapy) and nongerminomatous germ cell tumor (treated with more extensive resection in addition to radiation and chemotherapy)
  - Tumor (requiring allocation for molecular oncology) and infection (allocation for microbiology)

Cytology

- Important adjunct to diagnosis of
  - Small blue cell tumor with little cytoplasm (PNET, metastasis) vs. ependymoma (cell processes around vessels)
  - Pilocytic astrocytoma (bipolar cytomorphology, Rosenthal fibers) in astrocytic lesion with microvascular proliferation, so as not to overgrade
  - Lymphoma and germ cell tumor

PITFALLS

Presence of Macrophages

- Strong indicator of nonneoplastic diagnosis
  - Demyelination, infection, infarct
  - Reconsider diagnosis of tumor; however, they may be present in gliomas treated with radiation

Microvascular Proliferation

- Defined as multilayered vascular cell nuclei surrounded by basal lamina
- Difficult to identify in smear preparations where thickness is uncontrolled
- Of value in grading of astrocytomas but not in ependymomas and oligodendrogliomas
- Occasionally seen in metastatic neoplasms

Necrosis Following Radiotherapy

- Usually accompanied by other evidence, e.g., vascular wall fibrinoid change or hyalinization, endothelial atypia
- In treated low-grade gliomas, necrosis may not indicate anaplastic progression
- Report as "glioma with necrosis and radiation changes, grading deferred," unless obvious high-grade features (pleomorphism, vascular proliferation, mitotic activity) present
- If no cellular component is identified, report as inadequate

Presence of Rosenthal Fibers

- Seen in slow-growing or longstanding lesions, including nonneoplastic lesions
- By itself, does not imply pilocytic astrocytoma
  - Conversely, when not seen in small biopsies, may make diagnosis of pilocytic astrocytoma difficult

Small Round Blue Cell Tumor

- Differential includes lymphoma, small cell GBM, PNET/medulloblastoma, anaplastic oligodendroglioma, or metastatic neuroendocrine/small cell carcinoma
- Reasonable to defer to permanent sections
- Part of specimen should be sent for flow cytometry to exclude lymphoma

SELECTED REFERENCES

1. Somerset HL et al: Approach to the intraoperative consultation for neurosurgical specimens. Adv Anat Pathol. 18(6):446-9, 2011
2. Uematsu Y et al: The usefulness and problem of intraoperative rapid diagnosis in surgical neuropathology. Brain Tumor Pathol. 24(2):47-52, 2007

Glioblastoma Multiforme: Location

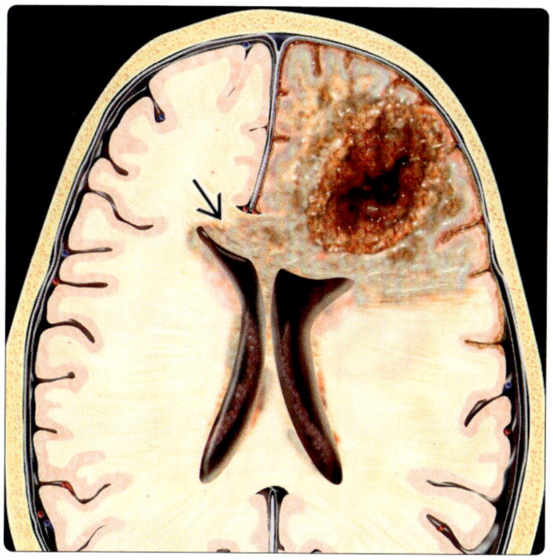

Glioblastoma Multiforme: Cytologic Features

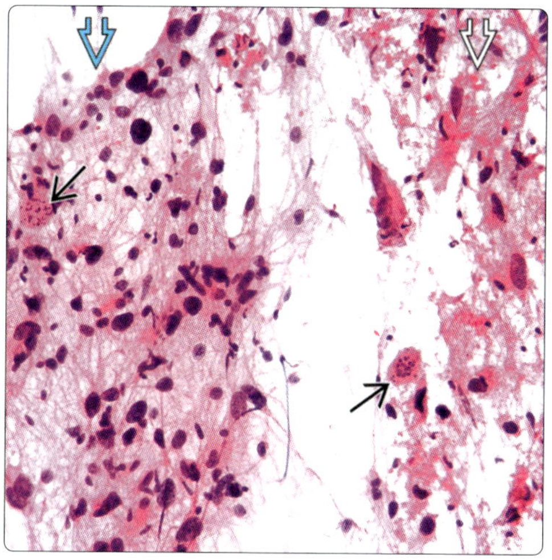

(Left) *Glioblastoma is the most common and most aggressive brain tumor, illustrated here as a large mass with a hemorrhagic and necrotic center and extending across the corpus callosum ⇒, causing midline shift.* **(Right)** *Viable tumor cells with an astrocytic phenotype ⇒ are present in contrast to necrotic cells and debris ⇒ frequently seen in glioblastomas. Note the fibrillary background and frequent mitoses ⇒.*

Glioblastoma Multiforme: Frozen Section

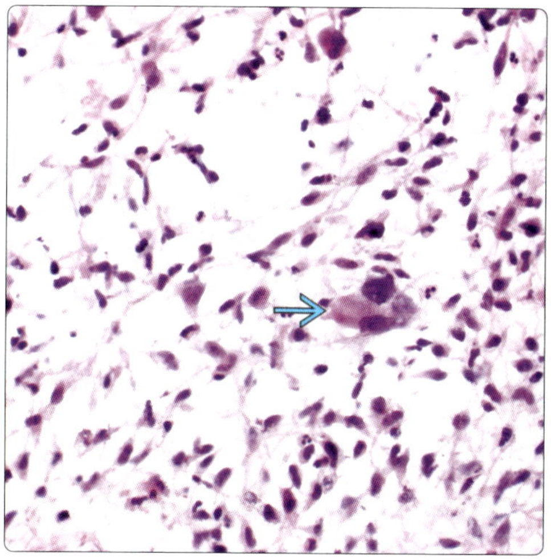

Glioblastoma Multiforme: Necrosis

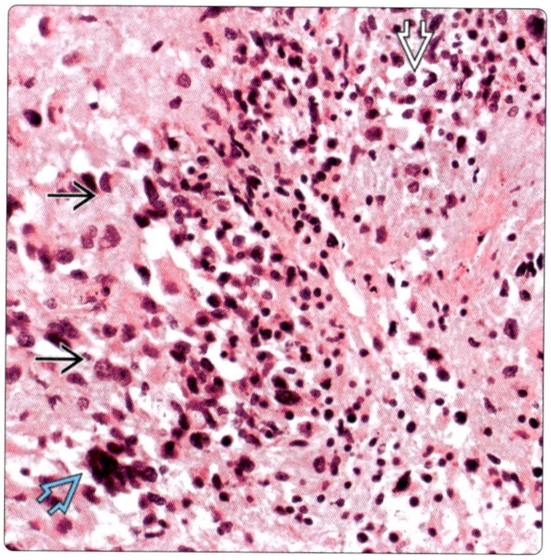

(Left) *Marked atypia and pleomorphism are typically observed in glioblastoma multiforme on frozen section. Pleomorphic multinucleated cells can be easily recognized ⇒ in the fibrillary astrocytic background.* **(Right)** *Tissue sections of glioblastoma show pleomorphic tumor cells ⇒, a row of loosely palisading tumor nuclei ⇒, and necrosis ⇒. There is a great variation in the degree of pleomorphism from tumor to tumor and in different areas within a given tumor.*

Glioblastoma Multiforme: Microvascular Proliferation

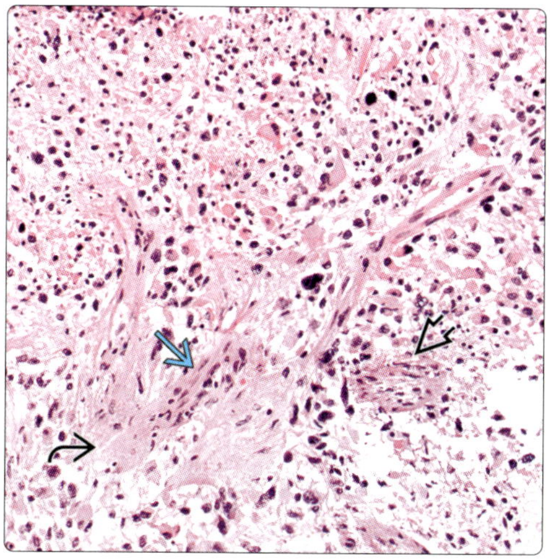

Glioblastoma Multiforme: Microvascular Proliferation

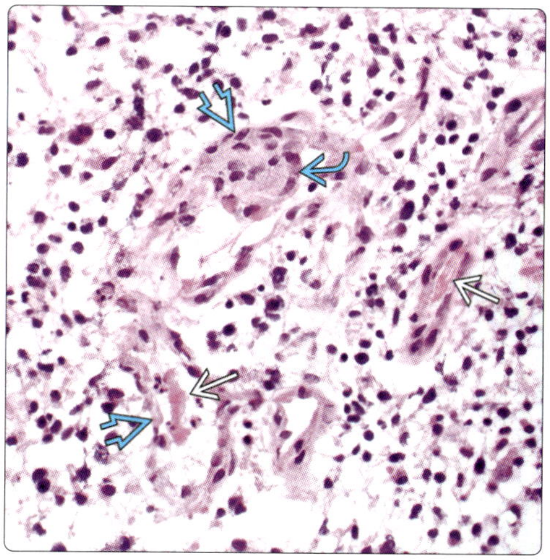

(Left) *Frozen tissue sections of glioblastoma may show microvascular proliferation ⇒ with thickened, hypercellular vessels, occasionally forming knots ⇒. Some vessels may have fibrinoid changes in their walls ⇒. Note the pleomorphism and necrosis in the tumor.* **(Right)** *Microvascular proliferation ⇒ with endothelial hyperplasia ⇒ is a hallmark of glioblastoma multiforme. Microvascular thrombi ⇒ are strongly associated with IDH1/2 wild-type tumors.*

(Left) *T2-weighted MR of a diffuse astrocytoma shows an ill-defined mass with signal abnormality in the right temporal lobe ⇨. The mass did not enhance with contrast.* **(Right)** *Diffuse astrocytoma is shown as an expansile tumor in the temporal lobe with extensive infiltration and effacement of normal architecture. The inset shows an axial section illustrating compression of midbrain structures by the tumor that obliterates basal cisterns →.*

Diffuse Astrocytoma: MR Appearance

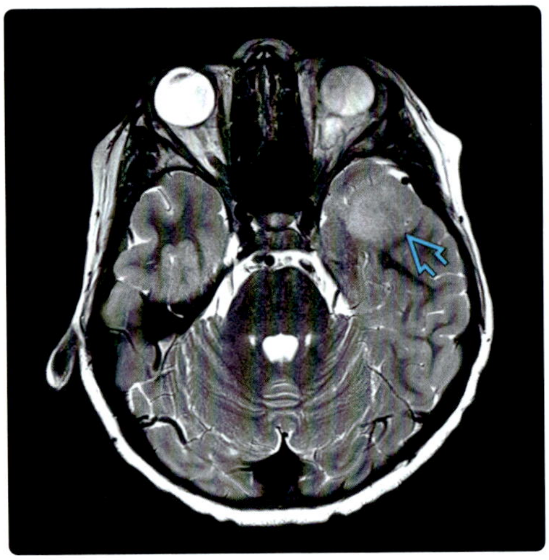

Diffuse Astrocytoma, WHO Grade II: Location

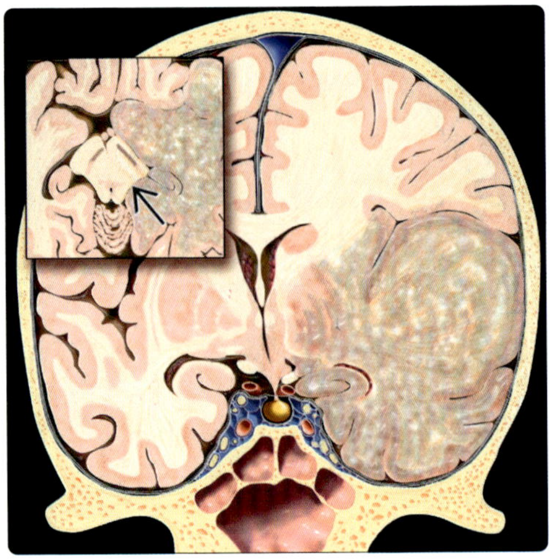

(Left) *A smear shows neoplastic astrocytes with moderate atypia in this diffuse astrocytoma. Features distinguishing tumor from reactive gliosis include fibrillary processes pointing in all directions and a high nuclear:cytoplasmic ratio.* **(Right)** *Smear of a diffuse astrocytoma shows slightly enlarged "naked" oval glial nuclei ⇨ surrounding a capillary →. (Courtesy R. Hewlett, PhD.)*

Diffuse Astrocytoma: Cytologic Features

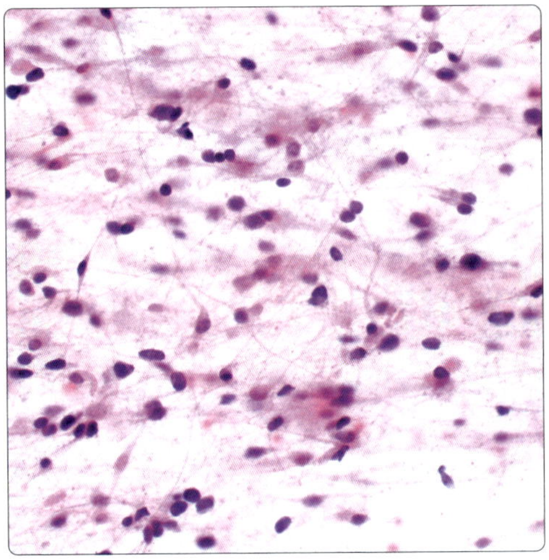

Astrocytoma, WHO Grade II: Cytologic Features

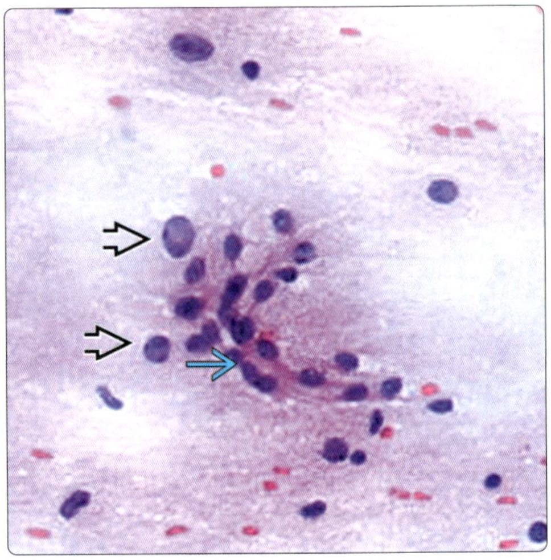

(Left) *Tissue section of a diffuse astrocytoma shows satellitosis of tumor nuclei around neurons ⇨ and capillaries →. (Courtesy R. Hewlett, PhD.)* **(Right)** *This diffuse astrocytoma is moderately hypercellular, and nuclear atypia is seen. Tumor cells infiltrate along a blood vessel →. However, microvascular proliferation or necrosis are not present.*

Astrocytoma, WHO Grade II

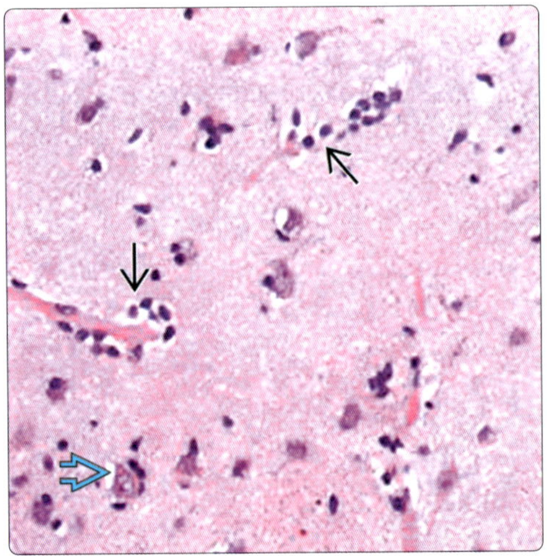

Diffuse Astrocytoma

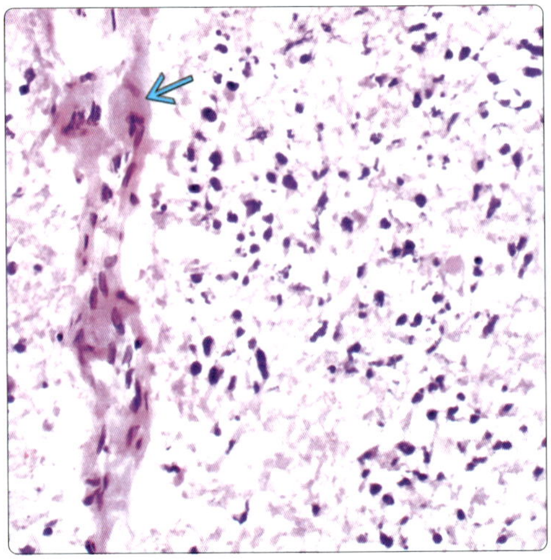

Gemistocytic Astrocytoma: Cytologic Features

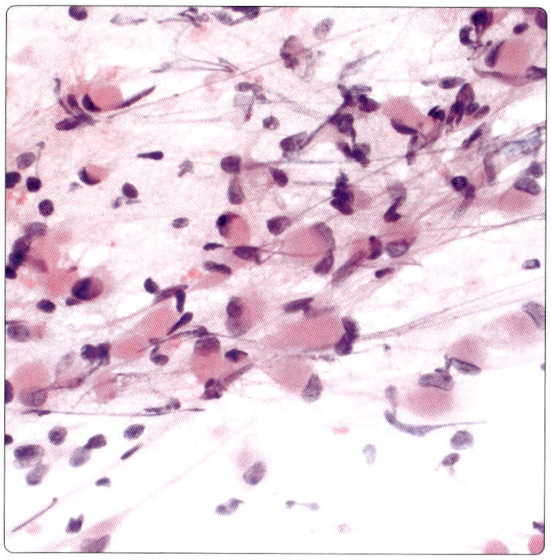

Gemistocytic Astrocytoma

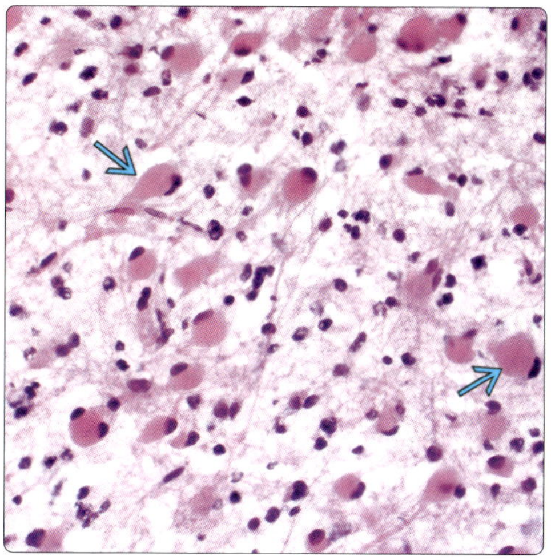

(Left) *Pleomorphic fibrillary cells with abundant densely pink cytoplasm are characteristic of gemistocytic astrocytoma. Compared to reactive gliosis, nuclei are larger and atypical, and cells have fewer processes.* **(Right)** *This gemistocytic astrocytoma is hypercellular and is composed of gemistocytic astrocytes ⇒ infiltrating though the brain.*

Oligodendroglioma: Gross Appearance

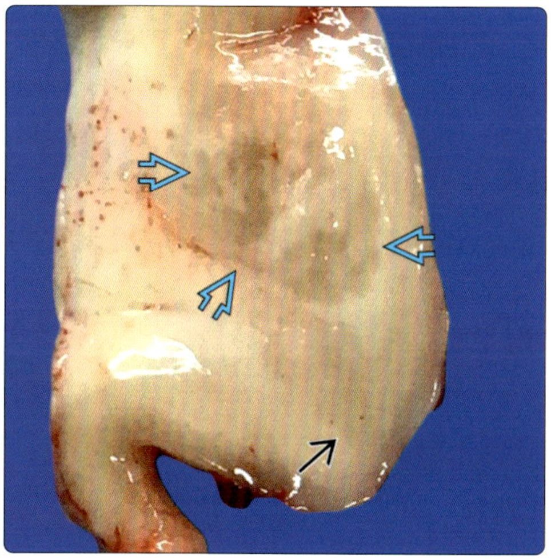

Oligodendroglioma: Cytologic Features

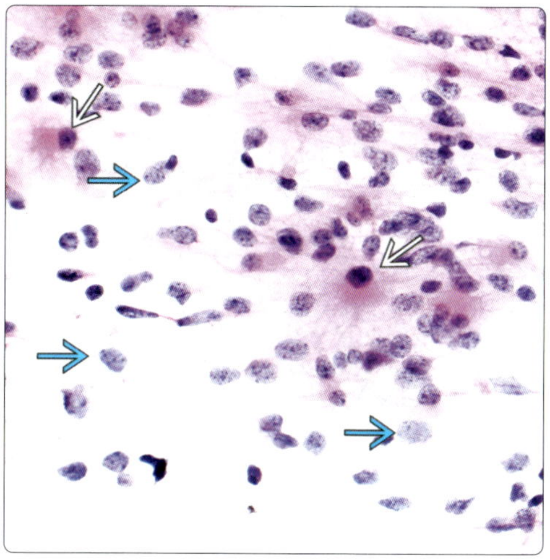

(Left) *Oligodendroglioma has an ill-defined gross appearance ⇒. However, attenuation of the normal white matter with slightly grayish irregular growth can be noted on the gross specimen. The cortex is also involved by tumor ⇒.* **(Right)** *Smear of an oligodendroglioma shows round monomorphic cells with fine chromatin and a minimal amount of cytoplasm ⇒. Reactive astrocytes are present ⇒. These cells should not be mistaken for an astrocytic component.*

Oligodendroglioma: Frozen Section

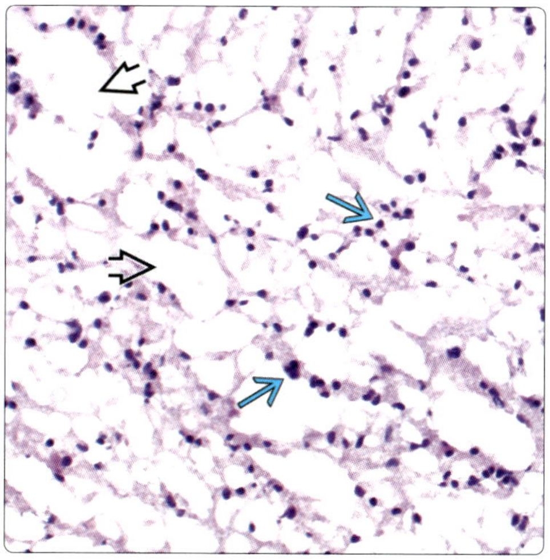

Oligodendroglioma, WHO Grade II

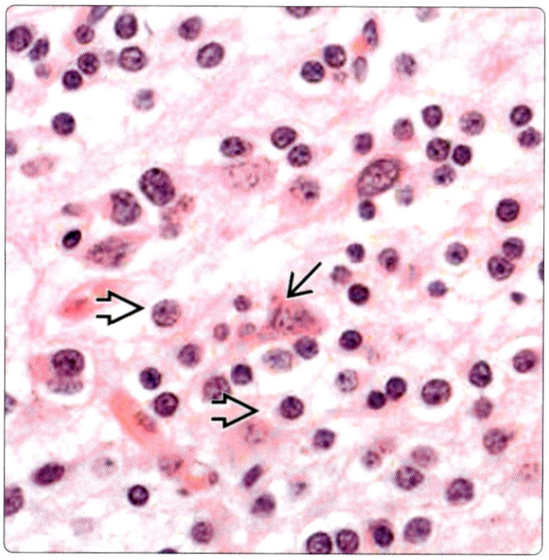

(Left) *Frozen sections of oligodendroglioma are often less informative than smears due to cerebral edema causing freezing artifacts ⇒. However, the tumor is clearly hypercellular, composed of small cells with uniform nuclei ⇒.* **(Right)** *Oligodendroglioma is characterized by uniform round nuclei ⇒ with dusty chromatin, perinuclear haloes, and no visible cytoplasm. Tumor cells surround cortical neurons ⇒. Halos are an artifact of formalin fixation and are not seen on smears or frozen sections. (Courtesy R. Hewlett, PhD.)*

Anaplastic Oligodendroglioma, WHO Grade III

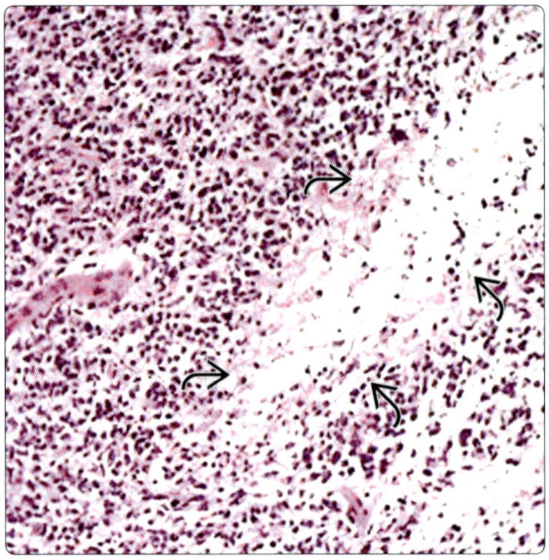

Anaplastic Oligodendroglioma, WHO Grade III

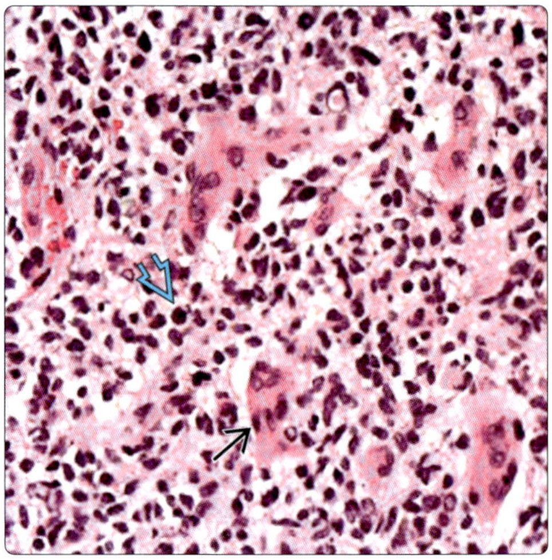

(Left) *Features of a grade III anaplastic oligodendroglioma are a high density of uniform, round oligodendroglial cells and geographic focus of necrosis* ↪. *(Courtesy R. Hewlett, PhD.)* **(Right)** *Brisk mitotic activity* ⇨ *and microvascular proliferation* →, *as well as mild to moderate pleomorphism, are features of a grade III oligodendroglioma. Perinuclear halos may be less conspicuous than in grade II tumors. (Courtesy R. Hewlett, PhD.)*

Primitive Neuroectodermal Tumor: Cytologic Features

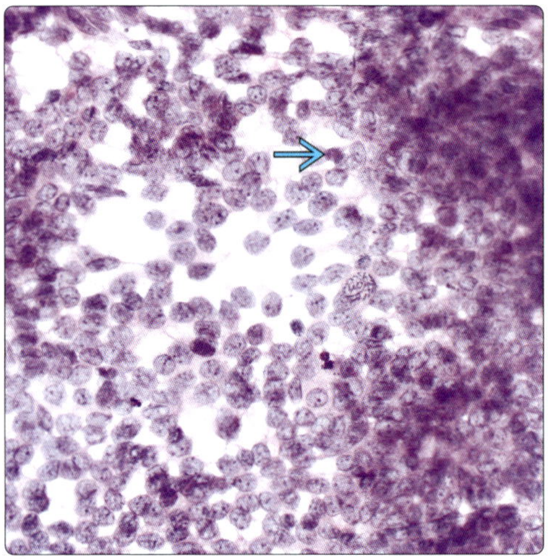

Primitive Neuroectodermal Tumor

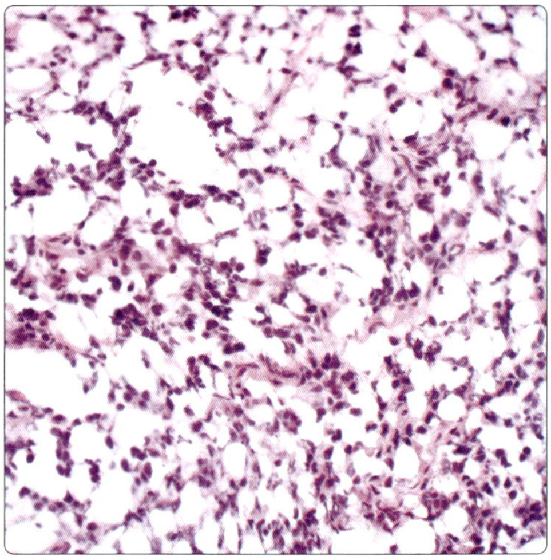

(Left) *PNETs are small round blue cell tumors with high cellularity, high nuclear:cytoplasmic ratio, mitotic activity, and lack of cellular processes* →. *It may be impossible to distinguish these tumors from lymphoma or metastatic neuroendocrine tumor.* **(Right)** *Frozen section of PNET shows sheets of small round blue cells with no recognizable architectural pattern. Diffuse sheets may distinguish PNET from lymphoma, which tends to be perivascular and shows patchy brain involvement.*

Pineal Parenchymal Tumor of Intermediate Differentiation

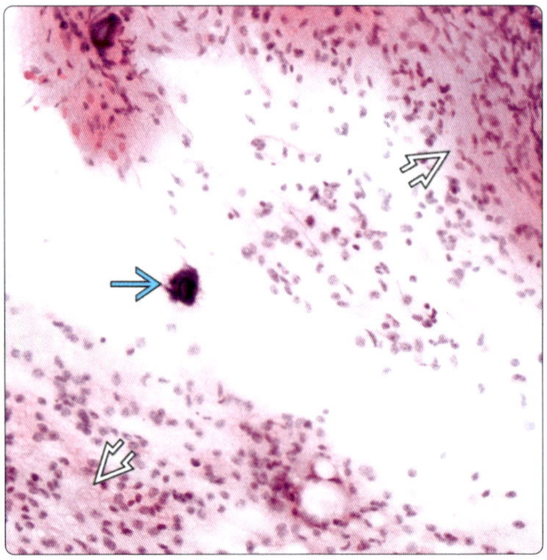

Pineal Parenchymal Tumor of Intermediate Differentiation

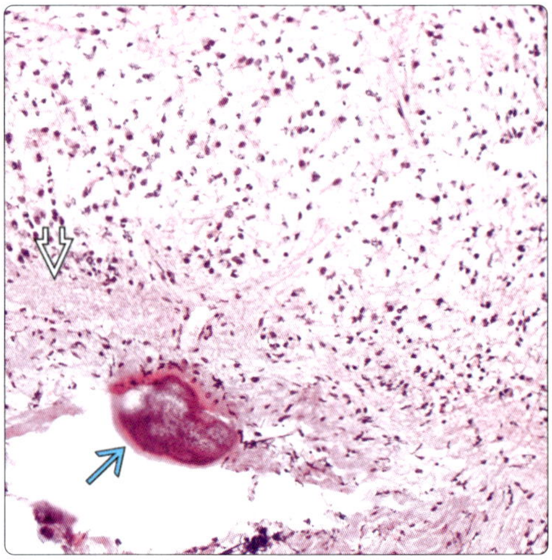

(Left) *Parenchymal tumors can range from pineoblastoma, which is a PNET, to pineocytoma. PPTIDs show higher cellularity than pineocytoma, but less cellularity than PNET. Calcifications* → *are often seen in pineal tumors, and cells are embedded in some neuropil* ⇨. **(Right)** *PPTID is a moderately hypercellular tumor composed of relatively small neurocytic cells in vague nodules with scant islands of neuropil* ⇨. *Calcification* → *is noted.*

Pleomorphic Xanthoastrocytoma: MR Appearance

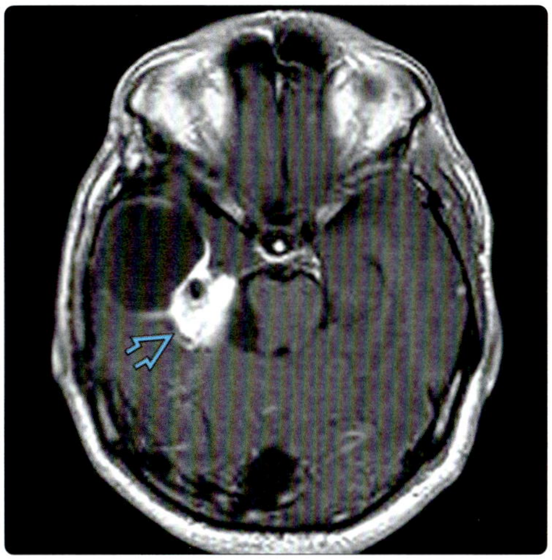

Pleomorphic Xanthoastrocytoma

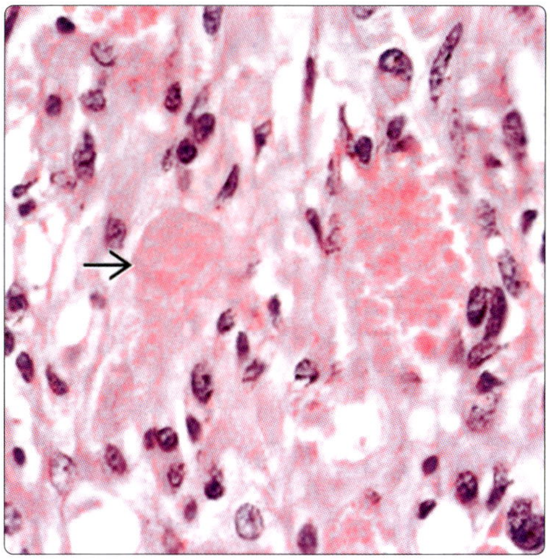

(Left) *This T1-weighted MR of a cystic temporal lobe lesion with an enhancing mural nodule* ➩ *is in a teenager with seizures. This site also harbors gangliogliomas and dysembryoplastic neuroepithelial tumors, which, along with PXA, may have a developmental (dysplastic) component. (Courtesy R. Hewlett, PhD.)* **(Right)** *Tumor cells are enlarged, bizarre, and have foamy cytoplasm in PXA. Eosinophilic granular bodies* ➩ *are common. Mitoses are rare. (Courtesy R. Hewlett, PhD.)*

Ganglioglioma: Cytologic Features

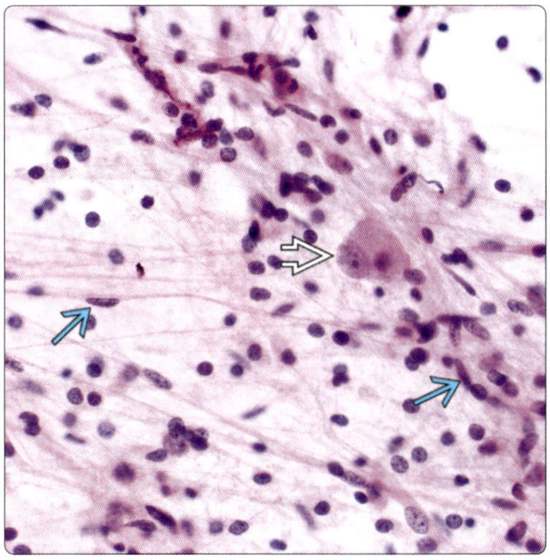

Ganglioglioma

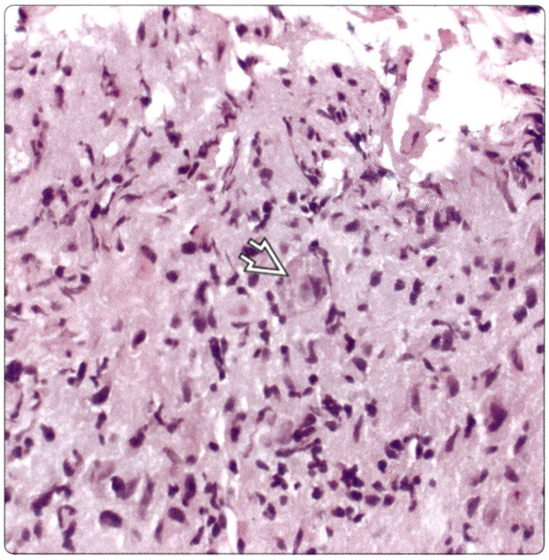

(Left) *Smear of a ganglioglioma shows a mixture of glial cells with long processes* ➩ *and a binucleated ganglionic cell* ➩*, characteristic of ganglioglioma.* **(Right)** *Ganglionic cells* ➩ *can be noted in the mixture of more elongated glial cells in a ganglioglioma. These tumors often harbor BRAF V600E mutations.*

Chordoid Glioma

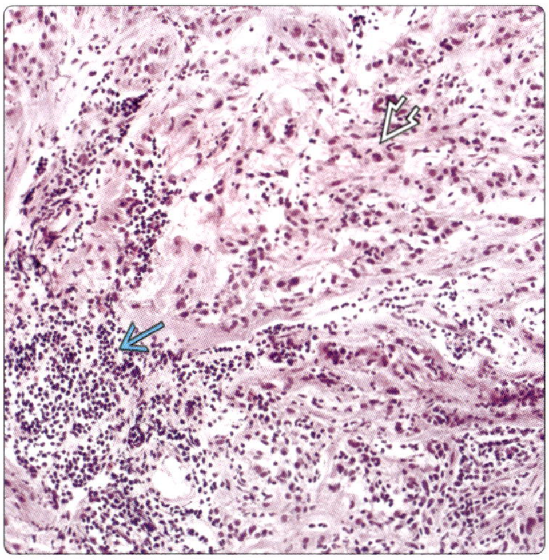

Metastatic Lung Carcinoma

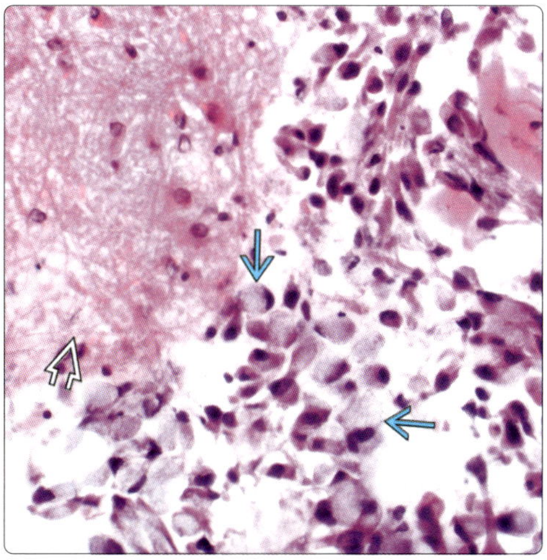

(Left) *Chordoid glioma can be difficult to diagnose due to the rich inflammatory infiltrate* ➩ *and the paucity of tumor cells in the frozen section material in some cases. Intermediate-size tumor cells with abundant pink cytoplasm are characteristic* ➩*.* **(Right)** *This metastatic mucinous lung adenocarcinoma to the brain is composed of pleomorphic signet ring cells* ➩*. Necrosis is often prominent in metastatic lesions* ➩*.*

(Left) *Normal pituitary gland is characterized by nests of small neuroendocrine cells ➡ separated by fibrous stroma ➡.* (Right) *Squamous epithelium lining cystic spaces or as part of solid nests is characteristic of a craniopharyngioma. Note the edematous appearance (stellate reticulum) ➡ as well as well-defined whorls of dense keratin ➡.*

Normal Pituitary Gland

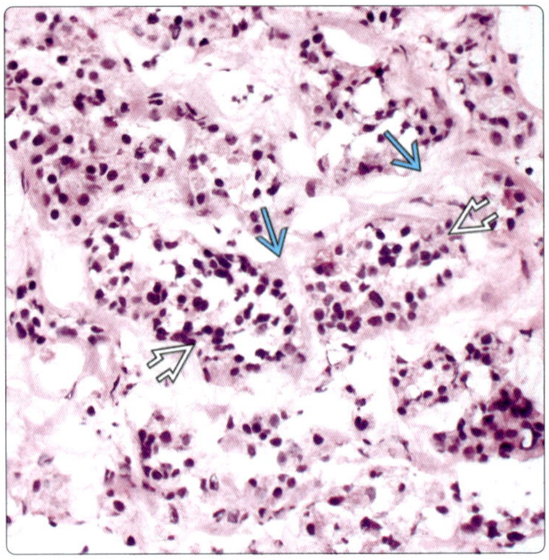

Craniopharyngioma

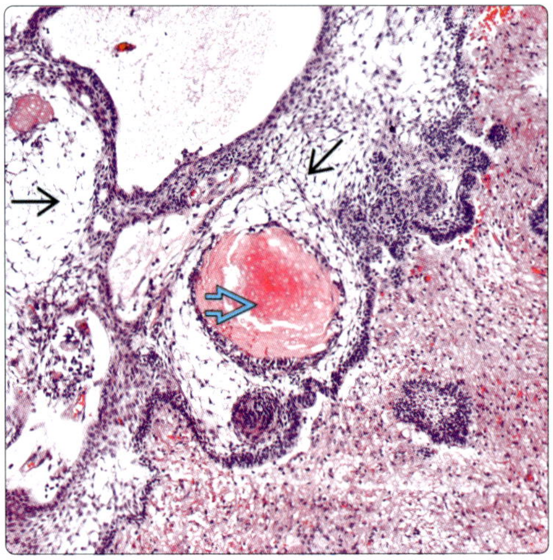

(Left) *Smear of a germ cell tumor shows a cluster of large cells with large nuclei and prominent nucleoli ➡ and distinct cell borders. Lymphocytes ➡ are inconspicuous in this case but are often abundant.* (Right) *A mixture of large tumor cells with prominent nucleoli ➡ is characteristic for a germ cell tumor. Tumor cells can be extremely scant in the background of heavy inflammation ➡, and diagnosis on frozen may not be possible.*

Germinoma: Cytologic Features

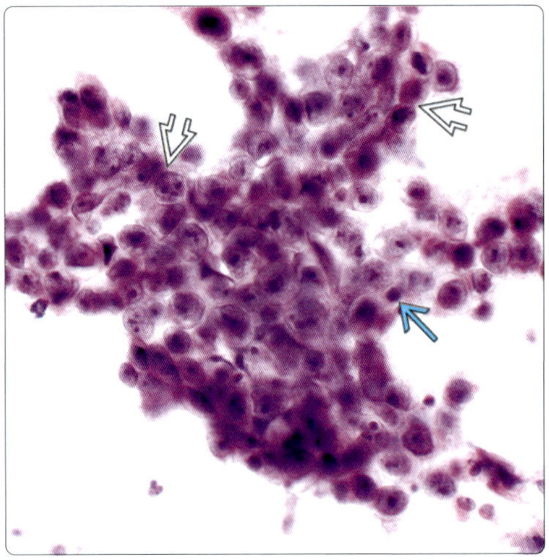

Germinoma: Frozen Section

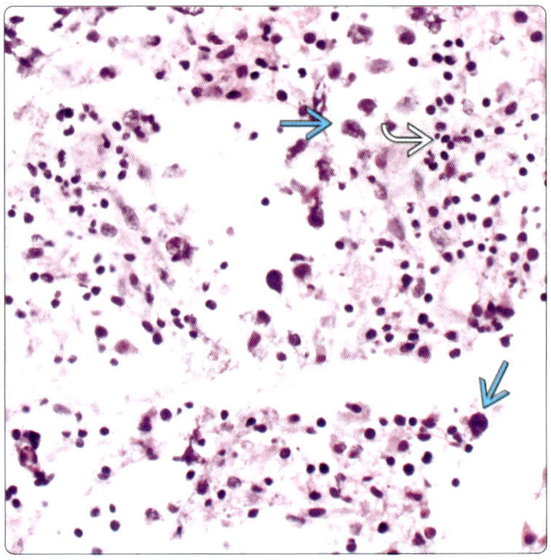

(Left) *Large, relatively uniform cells with high nuclear:cytoplasmic ratio and scant cytoplasm lacking cellular processes are typical for lymphoma, usually diffuse large B-cell type. Mitotic figures can be seen ➡.* (Right) *Patchy involvement of the brain is characteristic for central nervous system diffuse large B-cell lymphoma. A blood vessel is obscured by tumor cells in this section. However, a perivascular space is filled with lymphoma cells ➡.*

Central Nervous System Lymphoma: Cytologic Features

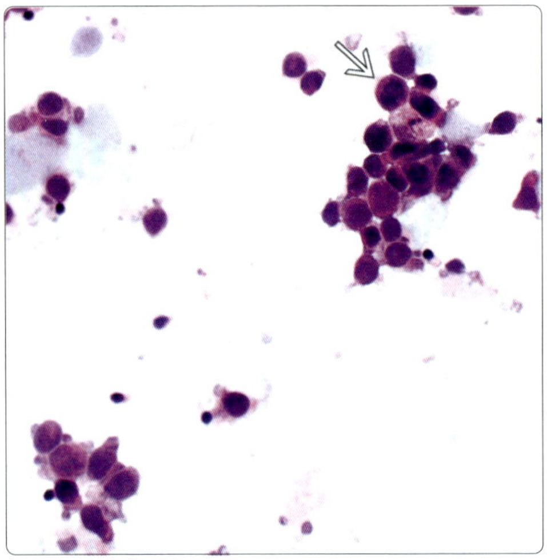

Central Nervous System Lymphoma: Frozen Section

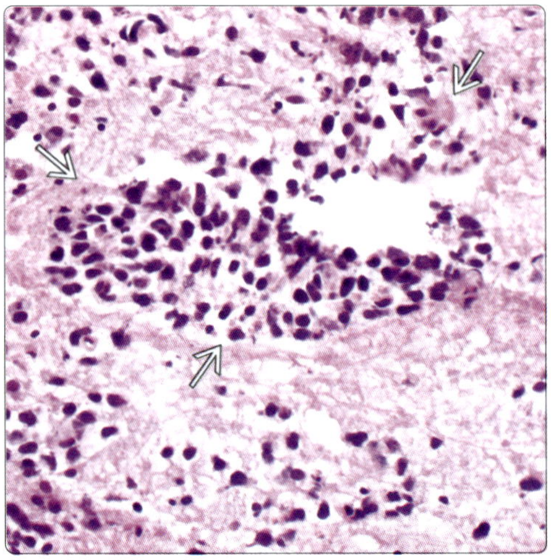

Multiple Sclerosis: Perivascular Lymphocytes

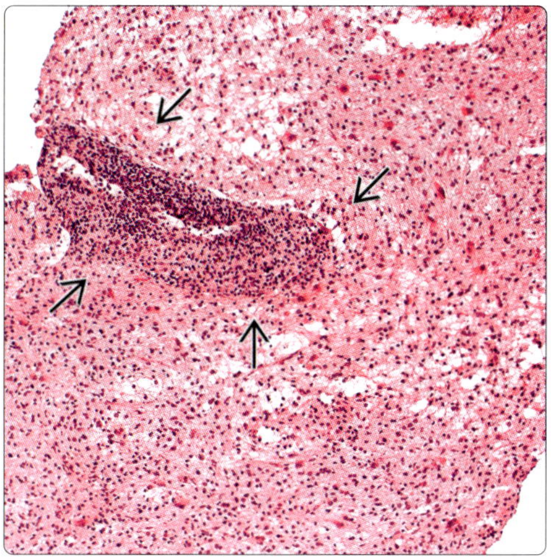

Multiple Sclerosis: Perivascular Lymphocytes

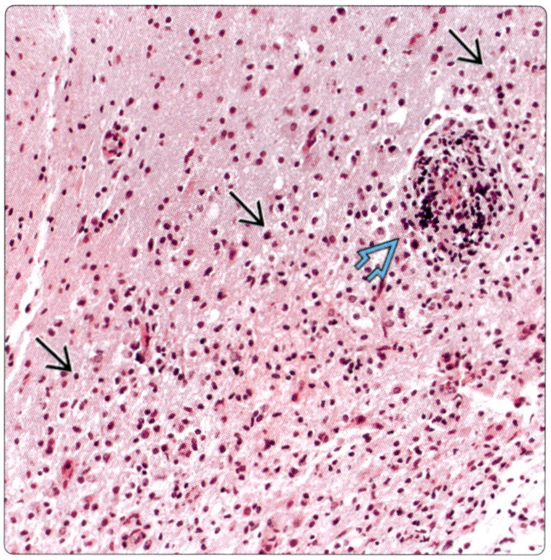

(Left) *A helpful feature in distinguishing an acute lesion of demyelination from glioma in a patient with multiple sclerosis is the presence of perivascular small lymphocytes* →*.* **(Right)** *Perivascular lymphocytic cuffs* ⇨ *are often at the margin of the demyelinative plaques* → *seen in multiple sclerosis. This interface is helpful in distinguishing this process from the infiltrative edge of a glioma.*

Acute Tumefactive Multiple Sclerosis

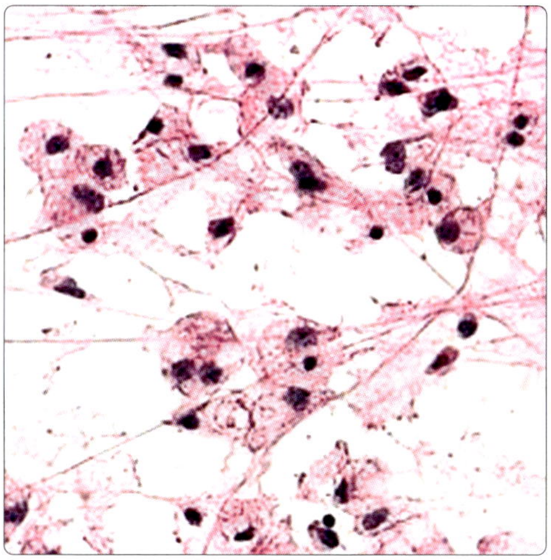

Reactive Gliosis

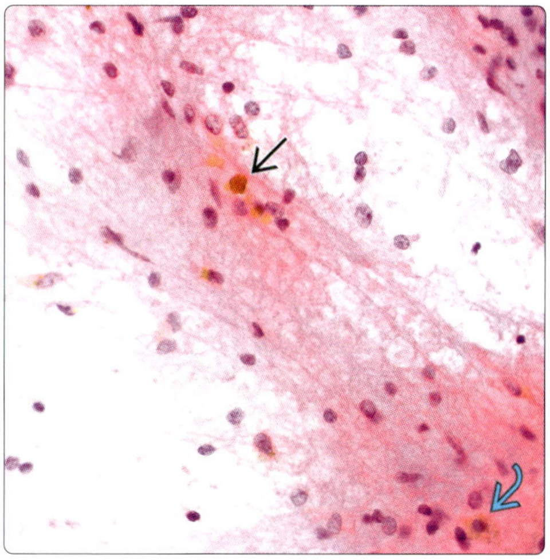

(Left) *Foamy macrophages are present amid preserved axons in a case of multiple sclerosis. Macrophages are rarely seen in untreated brain tumors & when present, suggest a reactive lesion. Axonal preservation is a hallmark of demyelination, & recognition of this process is crucial to avoid inappropriate resection. (Courtesy R. Hewlett, PhD.)* **(Right)** *Reactive astrocytes lack atypia, pleomorphism, & mitotic activity. Glial processes are not prominent. In this case, hemosiderin* → *& hemosiderin-laden macrophages* ↷ *are noted.*

Cerebral Abscess

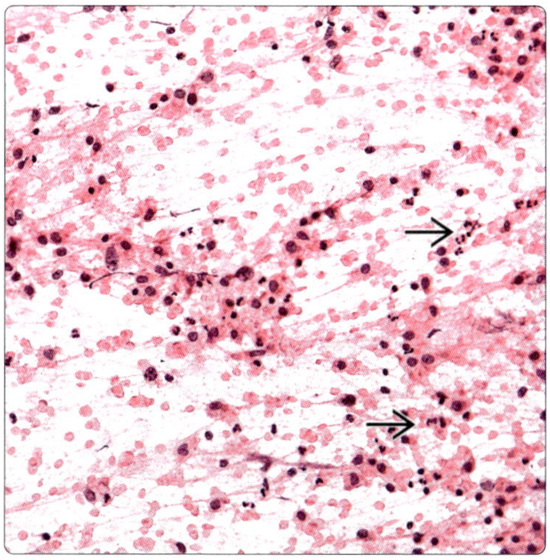

Cerebral Abscess: Gram Stain

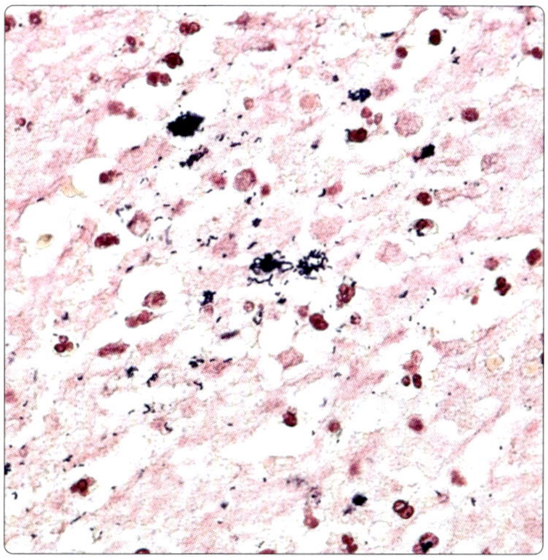

(Left) *Although abscesses are seldom biopsied, necrosis and numerous neutrophils* →*, particularly with hypersegmented nuclei, should raise that possibility when seen on a smear. Organisms are usually not seen on H&E.* **(Right)** *Special stains, such as Gram stain, are necessary to see bacteria in the necroinflammatory debris from the center of an abscess. Material should always be sent in sterile fashion for microbiologic culture, which allows proper identification of organisms and their sensitivity to antibiotics.*

SURGICAL/CLINICAL CONSIDERATIONS

Goal of Consultation

- To determine if biopsy is sufficient to establish or change diagnosis
- To identify malformation on gross examination
- To determine if tumor is present

Change in Patient Management

- If tumor is diagnosed, additional tissue may be removed as gross total resection can be curative for low-grade tumors

Clinical Setting

- Eligible patients
  - Patients with pharmacoresistant epilepsy, who have failed several drug regimens
    - Patients with uncontrolled or poorly controlled seizures have significant increased risk of sudden unexpected death in epilepsy (SUDEP)
  - Patients with mesial temporal sclerosis to remove sclerosed hippocampus
  - Patients with vascular malformations causing seizures
  - Specific conditions such as Rasmussen encephalitis or tuberous sclerosis complex
- Surgery is performed to remove lesion causing seizures
  - ~ 5-10% of patients with seizures undergo surgery
  - After surgery, ~ 60% of patients are seizure free, depending on etiology and extent of resection
  - Patients whose seizures persist after surgery have increased risk of SUDEP
- Majority of epileptogenic lesions are in temporal lobe (64%), followed by frontal lobe (16%), parietal lobe (9%), and occipital lobe (6%)
- It is important for pathologist to be aware of radiologic findings before intraoperative consultation
  - If radiologic correlate for seizure focus is seen
  - Differential diagnosis based on imaging appearance
- It is important for pathologist to be aware of clinical information before intraoperative consultation
  - Clinical diagnosis
  - Presence of electrodes inserted in cortex to identify seizure focus

Dysembryoplastic Neuroepithelial Tumor: MR Appearance

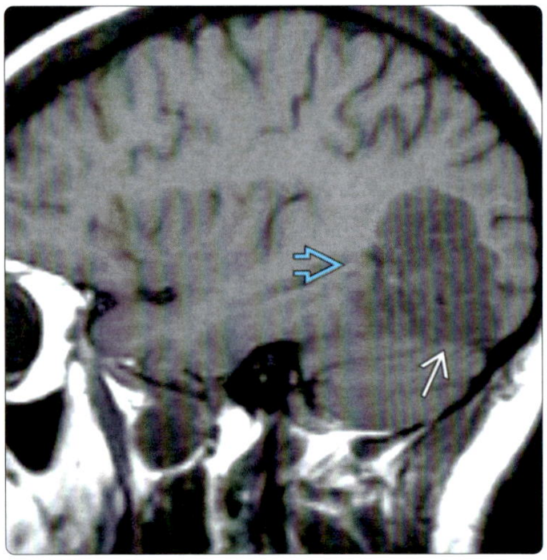

Dysembryoplastic Neuroepithelial Tumor: Gross Appearance

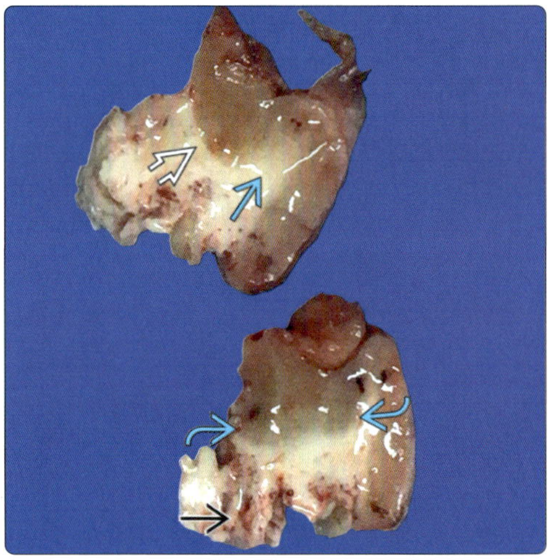

(Left) *Sagittal T1 MR in a young adult with seizures shows characteristic bubbly appearance of a dysembryoplastic neuroepithelial tumor (DNET). The tumor involves gray and white matter. These WHO grade I neoplasms have an excellent prognosis with surgical resection. (From DI: Brain, 3e.)* **(Right)** *This cortex removed for seizures shows that the normal gray-white border gradually becomes blurred due to grayish expansive DNET involving the white matter. Hemorrhage is perioperative.*

Hippocampal Sclerosis: MR Appearance

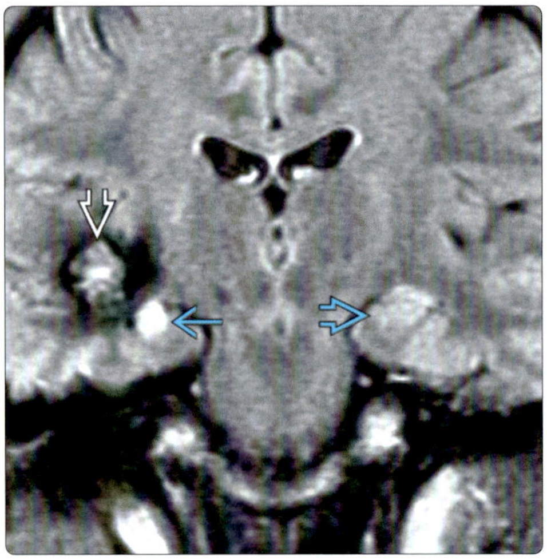

Hippocampal Sclerosis: Gliosis

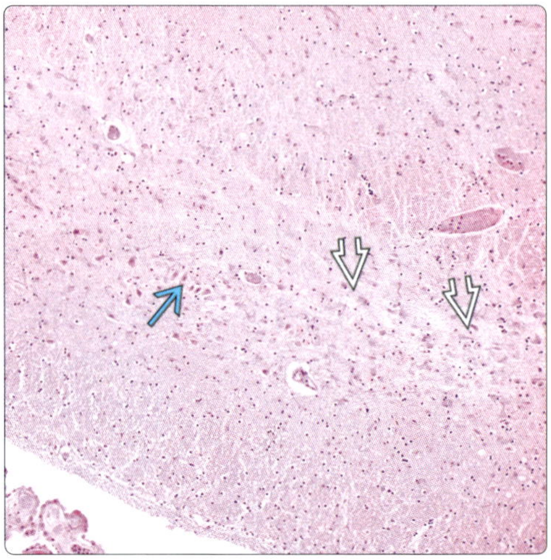

(Left) *Coronal FLAIR MR in a patient with chronic seizures and a large right temporal lobe cavernous malformation shows mesial sclerosis characterized by a gliotic shrunken hippocampus. The contralateral hippocampus has preserved volume and shape. (From DI: Brain, 3e.)* **(Right)** *Dense gliosis is a hallmark of specimens from patients with chronic seizures. Rare neurons of the hippocampus are preserved. In this area of the brain, the majority of the section is densely populated with reactive astrocytes.*

- Can produce reactive changes (small hemorrhages along needle tract, histiocytic reaction) and mild leptomeningeal inflammation
- Prior embolization of vascular lesions

Classification by Etiology

- Congenital
  - Alteration in brain structure from abnormal development
    - Hemimegalencephaly
    - Tuberous sclerosis complex
    - Focal cortical dysplasia
  - Intrauterine trauma (hypoxia, hemorrhage)
- Acquired postnatally
  - Trauma
  - Neoplasm
    - Low-grade glioneuronal tumors
    - Isocitrate dehydrogenase 1 and 2 mutated tumors
      - Associated with increased seizure activity
      - Majority of grade II and III oligodendrogliomas, astrocytomas, and secondary glioblastomas
    - Metastasis
  - Infection
  - Seizures from other causes

SPECIMEN EVALUATION

Gross

- Small biopsy of suspicious focus can be sent for frozen section evaluation.
- Some lesions have distinct gross features
  - Tuber: Firm, gliotic, and white on cut surface
  - Dysembryoplastic neuroepithelial tumor (DNET): Gelatinous with mucoid material
  - Low-grade glioma and ganglioglioma: Firm and chalky-white or tan, with loss of gray-white matter junction
  - Infiltrating glioma: Tan ill-defined mass with blurring of gray-white matter junction
  - Cortical lesions: Can show polymicrogyria or pachygyria
- Resections can be large, including entire temporal lobe and hippocampus
- Cortical specimens should be oriented, if possible, and cut thinly perpendicular to cortical surface to evaluate thickness of cortex, gray-white matter junction, and characteristics of white matter
- Hippocampus, if taken en bloc, can be oriented along long axis and cut perpendicular to long axis
- Amygdala is usually fragmented and cannot be properly oriented
- Many seizure-associated lesions can be calcified
  - Decalcification should be avoided as it has deleterious effects on quality of DNA

Frozen Section

- If small and abnormal in appearance, specimen is frozen similar to evaluation for tumor
  - Minute portion is taken for cytologic preparation
    - Small fragment from each end of core needle biopsy is removed for cytologic smears
  - Remaining tissue to be frozen is perched on small bead of embedding medium but not covered with medium
    - Tissue is frozen quickly with light touch of heat extractor or cryospray to avoid ice crystal artifact
    - Block is carefully step sectioned to preserve tissue
- If specimen is large or lobectomy, specimen is carefully sectioned, examined grossly, and areas of abnormal appearance frozen
- If no suspicious lesions are identified grossly, it is preferable to not freeze normal appearing tissue
  - For example, focal cortical dysplasia is best diagnosed on permanent sections

Cytology

- If suspicious for neoplasm, smear should be prepared as for other cerebral hemisphere tumors
- **Smear method**
  - 1-3 pinhead-sized fragments are placed 1/3 of way down on glass slide
  - 2nd slide is used to gently smear tissue on slide
    - Slides are held above fixative container to avoid any delay in fixation
    - Excessive force that would crush tissue should not be used when making smear
  - Slides are placed immediately in fixative to avoid drying artifact
- **Touch preparation method**
  - Use for firm, calcified, or fibrous lesions
  - Tissue is held gently in forceps and rapidly touched once to slide surface
  - Slide is placed immediately into formalin to avoid drying artifact

MOST COMMON DIAGNOSES

Tumors (~ 80% of Total)

- Most frequent cause of seizures is tumor
  - Most common types: Ganglioglioma, low-grade astrocytoma, low-grade glial/glioneuronal neoplasm, DNET, low-grade oligodendroglioma, low-grade mixed glioma
    - Infiltrating low-grade gliomas can be difficult to diagnose due to low cellularity
    - Gangliogliomas can be difficult to distinguish from cortical dysplasias with numerous dysplastic and balloon neurons
    - Myxoid matrix of DNET may not be well preserved on frozen section

Metastasis

- Acute seizures are presenting symptom in ~ 30% of patients with metastatic disease
- Usually located in gray-white junction

Malformation of Cortical Development/Focal Cortical Dysplasia (~ 20% of Total)

- Frozen section is not usually requested for diagnosis
- Proper orientation and sectioning is absolutely critical for final diagnosis
  - Sectioning must be performed perpendicular to cortical surface to enable proper evaluation of cortical layers
- Hamartia are small glioneuronal lesions
  - Should not be mistaken for infiltrating oligodendroglioma

Gliosis (~ 5% of Total)

- Majority of chronic epilepsy samples show diffuse reactive gliosis, which is often subpial
- Gliotic scar from old trauma can be seizure focus
- Presence of hemosiderin in superficial layers may suggest previous trauma

Vascular Malformations (~ 4% of Total)

- Arteriovenous malformation (AVM) is most common cause of seizure due to vascular abnormality
  - Usually supratentorial and follows middle cerebral artery territory
  - AVMs can be embolized before surgery
- Cavernous angiomas are most common vascular lesions causing intractable seizures
  - Honeycomb pattern on cut surface but often small
  - Hemorrhages and calcifications are common
  - 20-40% of patients have multiple lesions
- Malignant vascular tumors are exceedingly rare

Hippocampal Sclerosis (Mesial Temporal Sclerosis) (~ 1-2%)

- Usually readily identified by imaging
- Frozen section is generally not required for confirmation
  - However gross examination and proper orientation and sectioning is critical for final diagnosis
  - Identified grossly as small and firm hippocampus

Tuberous Sclerosis Complex

- Tuberous sclerosis complex (TSC) due to germline mutations in *TSC1* (codes for hamartin protein) and *TSC2* (codes for tuberin protein)
- 3 types of brain tumors
  - Cortical tubers
    - May cause seizures
    - Grossly form chalky-white, firm fibrous masses in white matter
      - Surface is smooth
    - Consist of abnormal neuronal forms including balloon cells and dysplastic neurons
  - Subependymal nodules
  - Giant cell astrocytoma

Rasmussen Encephalitis

- Also termed chronic focal encephalitis
  - Rare inflammatory neurological disease affecting 1 hemisphere
  - Results in frequent and severe seizures
- Cortical tissue is infiltrated by T cells
  - Perivascular inflammation without vascular destruction is typical
  - Reactive gliosis can be present
- Hemispherectomy for Rasmussen encephalitis is rarely evaluated on frozen section

Porencephaly

- Rare condition with cysts or cavities in cerebral hemispheres
- Can be caused by abnormal development, direct damage, inflammation, or hemorrhage
- Can be associated with seizures

Hemimegalencephaly

- Hamartomatous malformation resulting in increase in size of one hemisphere
- Hemispherectomy or functional hemispherectomy may be necessary to control seizures

REPORTING

Gross Examination

- Report size and orientation of specimen
- Thickness of cortex and gray-white matter border (sharp vs. blurred)
- Small and firm gliotic hippocampus confirms mesial temporal sclerosis (hippocampal sclerosis)
- Gyral abnormalities including poly/pachy micro-/macrogyria should be reported
- Tuber in TSC can be diagnosed grossly

Frozen section

- Tumors and other specific lesions reported when possible
  - Focal cortical dysplasia is usually not possible to accurately classify on frozen and diagnosis should be deferred to permanent sections

PITFALLS

Over and Underdiagnosis

- Long-standing seizures are associated with gliosis and reactive astrocytes
- Tumors can be overdiagnosed due to these chronic changes and dysplastic changes in malformations
  - Gliosis can resemble gemistocytic astrocytoma
  - Rosenthal fibers associated with reactive gliosis can resemble pilocytic astrocytoma
  - Hamartia can resemble infiltrating oligodendroglioma
- It can be difficult to identify tumors in presence of chronic changes
  - Low-grade glioneuronal tumors can be difficult to distinguish from dysplasia

Sampling Error

- Tissue next to tumor may be gliotic
- Resection sample can be large and may not be sufficiently sampled for frozen section

Multiple Lesions Present or Multifocal Disease

- ~ 14% of patients have multifocal lesions that could be cause of seizures
- Only 1 of 2 lesions may be identified by preoperative tests
- Some tumors can be multifocal (e.g., DNET)

SELECTED REFERENCES

1. Chen H et al: Mutant IDH1 and seizures in patients with glioma. Neurology. 88(19):1805-1813, 2017
2. Prayson RA: Utilization of frozen sections in the evaluation of chronic epilepsy-related cases. Ann Diagn Pathol. 17(1):145-9, 2013

Tuberous Sclerosis Complex: Brain Tumors

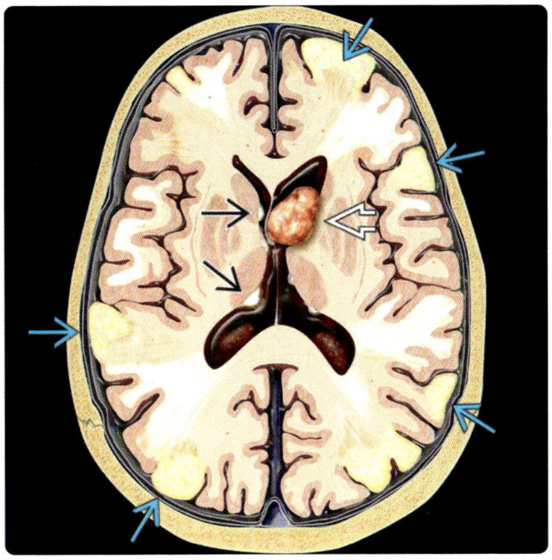

Tuberous Sclerosis Complex: MR Appearance

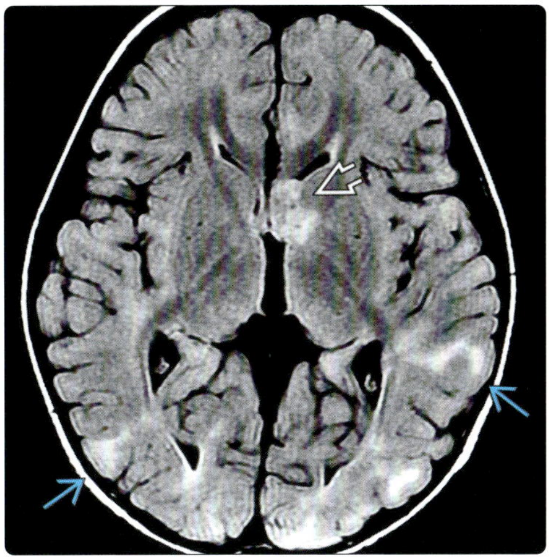

(Left) *The typical brain involvement in tuberous sclerosis includes subependymal giant cell astrocytoma* ➡ *in the foramen of Monro, subependymal nodules* → *, and cortical/subcortical tubers* ⇨ *. (From DI: Brain, 3e.)* **(Right)** *This MR study in a 14-year-old boy with tuberous sclerosis complex shows a well-demarcated subependymal giant cell astrocytoma* ➡ *and multiple hyperintense cortical tubers with expanded gyri and poor gray-white differentiation* ⇨ *. (From DI: Brain, 3e.)*

Cortical Tuber: Gross Appearance

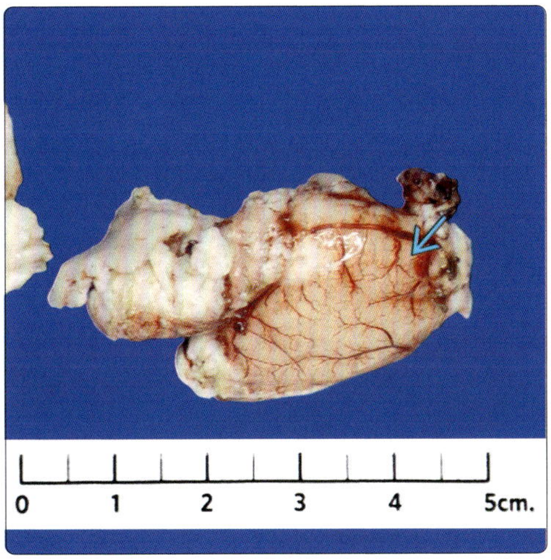

Cortical Tuber: Gross Appearance

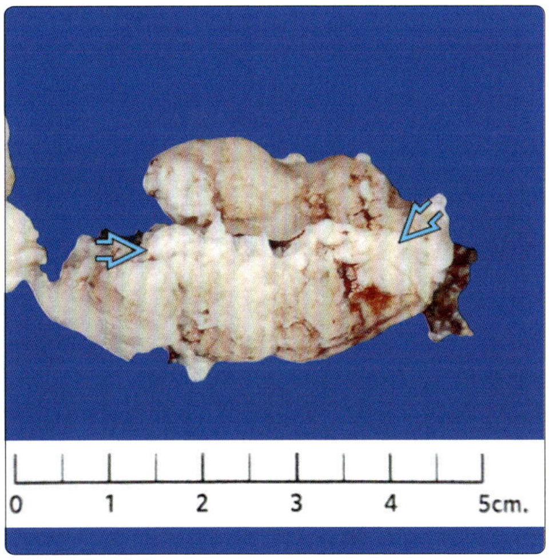

(Left) *This tuber associated with tuberous sclerosis complex forms a firm white mass and has an abnormal surface* ⇨ *including a cobblestone-like lesion, lack of a gyral pattern, and a smooth surface.* **(Right)** *This cortical tuber was removed en bloc. The base of the tuber shows chalky densely gliotic white matter* ⇨ *at the site of resection.*

Cortical Tuber: Balloon Cells

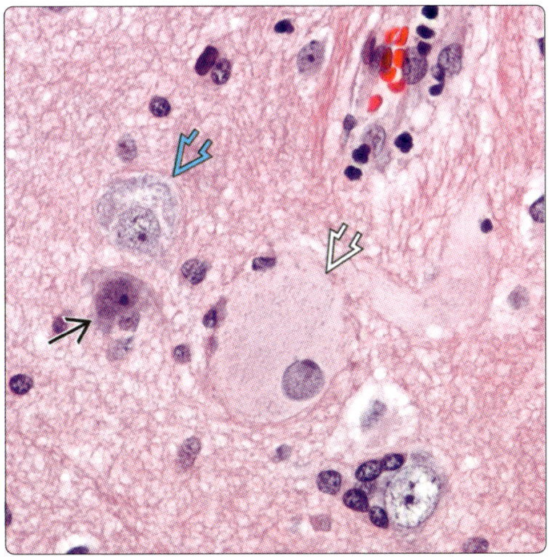

Long Standing Seizures: Microcalcifications

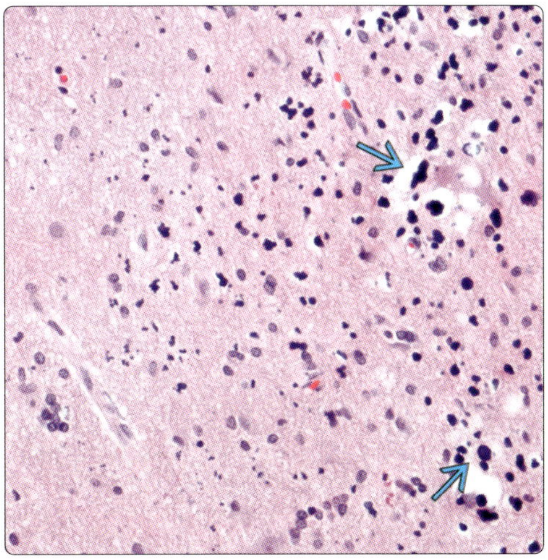

(Left) *Cortical tubers contain variety of abnormal neuronal forms, including balloon cells* ➡ *with abundant pink cytoplasm. In addition, dysplastic neurons* ⇨ *are present. A relatively normal neuron* → *is shown for comparison.* **(Right)** *Epileptogenic lesions, both neoplastic and nonneoplastic, are often accompanied by microcalcifications* ⇨ *.*

Rasmussen Encephalitis: MR Appearance

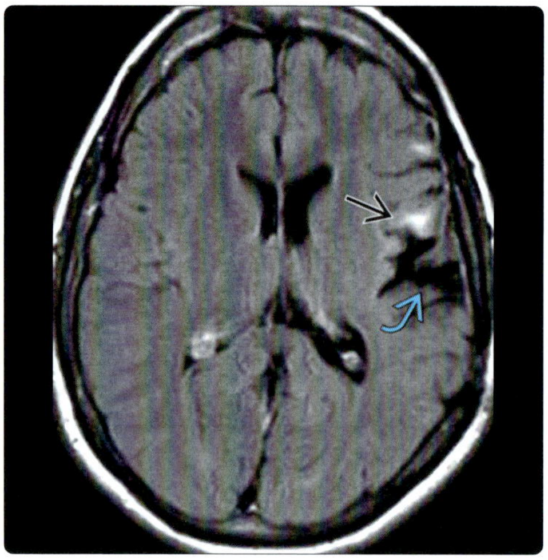

Rasmussen Encephalitis: Perivascular Inflammation

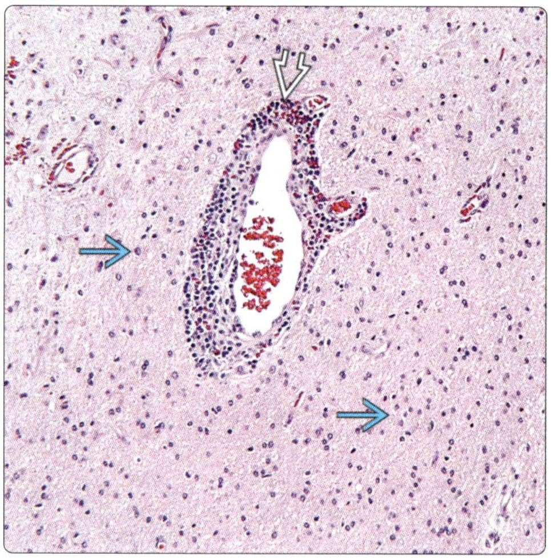

(Left) *Axial FLAIR MR in a patient with Rasmussen encephalitis shows prominence of left perisylvian fissure ➾ due to volume loss. There is associated subcortical gliosis ➔ in the frontal operculum. (From DI: Brain, 3e.)* **(Right)** *Hypercellular diffusely inflamed brain tissue is characteristic for Rasmussen encephalitis. One entire hemisphere is usually affected. Perivascular inflammation ➡ without vascular destruction is typically seen. Reactive gliosis ➔ can also be noted.*

Rasmussen Encephalitis: Cortical Gliosis

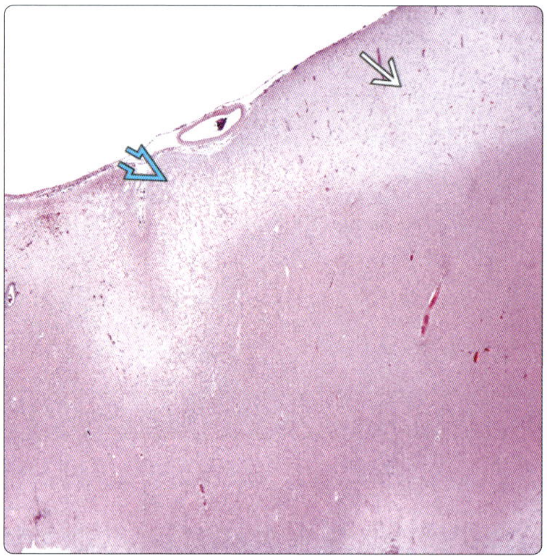

Microglial Nodule

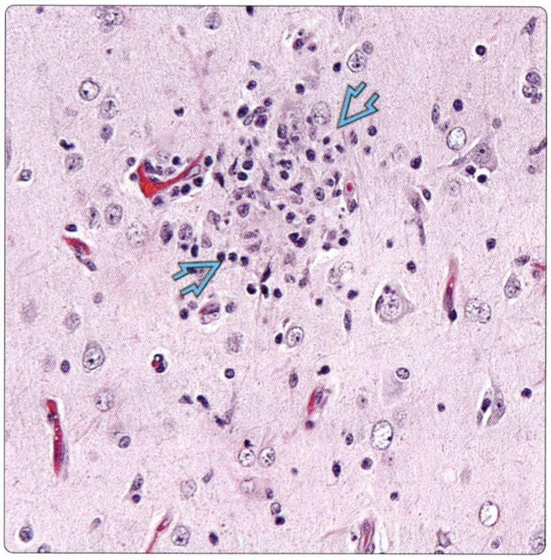

(Left) *Diffuse cortical gliosis ➡ with vacuolization ➔ in extreme cases, such as this case of Rasmussen encephalitis, is a result of long-standing seizure activity.* **(Right)** *Cortical microglial nodule ➔ has to be distinguished from hamartomas. Differential is broad and includes Rasmussen encephalitis and viral infection.*

Porencephalic Cyst: MR Appearance

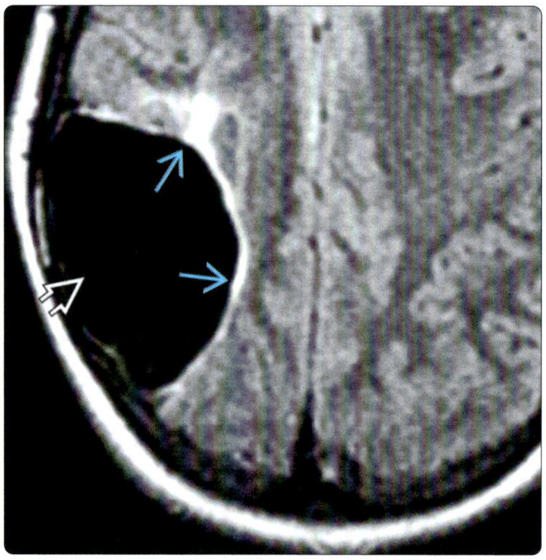

Porencephaly: Gross Appearance

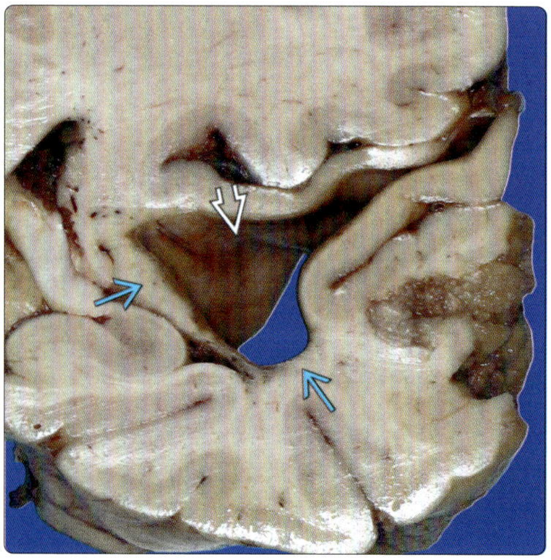

(Left) *Axial FLAIR MR shows fluid within a right parietal lesion ➡. This classic porencephalic cyst is lined by hyperintense gliotic white matter ➔. (From DI: Brain, 3e.)* **(Right)** *Seizures can be result of pre-, peri- or postnatal trauma that can result in scarring and loss of brain parenchyma. A large cavity ➡ is shown in the temporal lobe in this case of porencephaly. Surrounding tissue shows reactive gliosis ➔ and cortical neurons can be disorganized and appear dysplastic.*

Hemimegalencephaly: MR Appearance

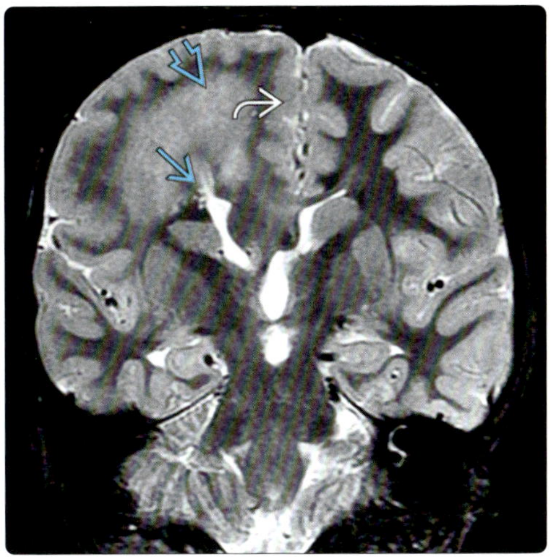

Neuronal Cytomegaly

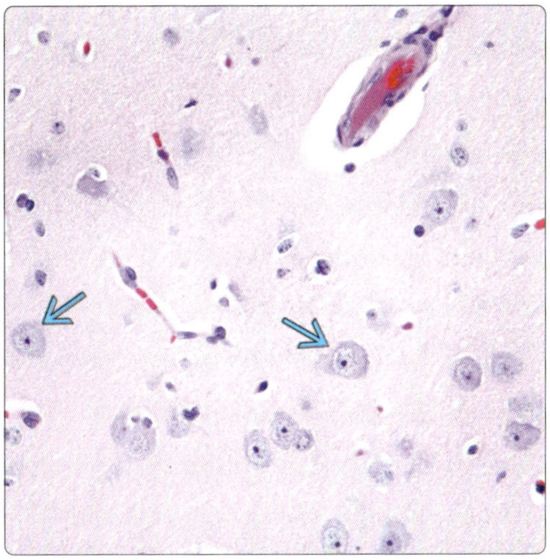

(Left) *Coronal T2WI of hemimegalencephaly shows the right hemisphere is enlarged, pushing across the midline. The ipsilateral frontal horn is deformed and pointed. Gliosis of the deep white matter is noted. (From DI: Brain, 3e.)* **(Right)** *Neuronal cytomegaly with large haphazardly arranged neurons is observed in variety of epileptogenic lesions, including focal cortical dysplasia and disorders of development, such as hemimegalencephaly.*

Focal Cortical Dysplasia: MR Appearance

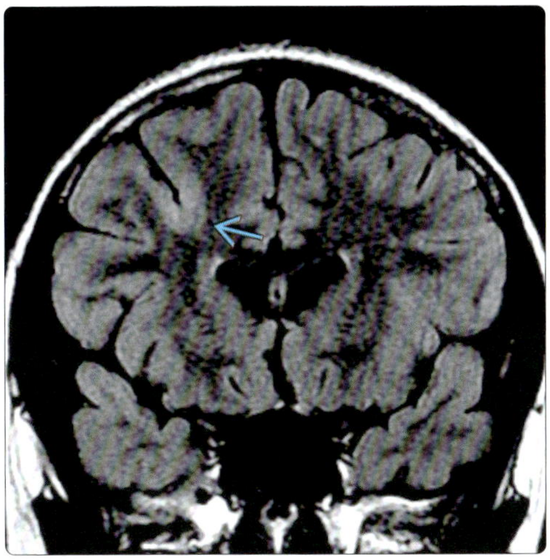

Focal Cortical Dysplasia: Gross Appearance

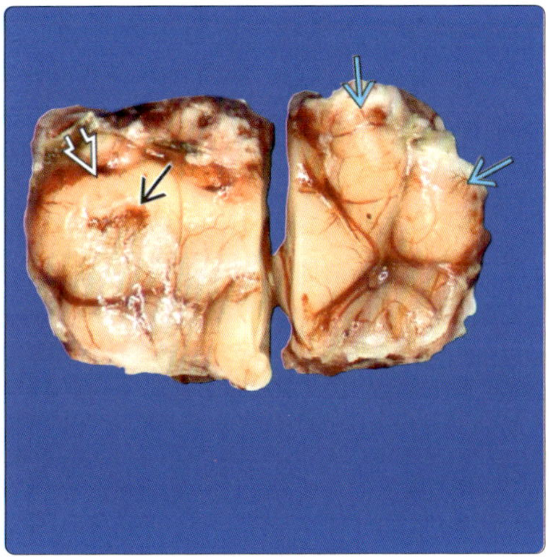

(Left) *An MR study in a 16-year-old girl with medically refractory epilepsy shows hyperintense, thickened cortex & gray-white matter blurring at the bottom of an abnormally deep sulcus. This is a typical display for "bottom-of-the-sulcus" morphology of focal cortical dysplasia. (From DI: Pediatrics, 3e.)* **(Right)** *The cortical surface shows a slightly enlarged gyrus in the site where a preoperative electrode was placed and detected a seizure focus associated with an underlying cortical dysplasia. Neighboring gyri are normal.*

Focal Cortical Dysplasia: Hamartia

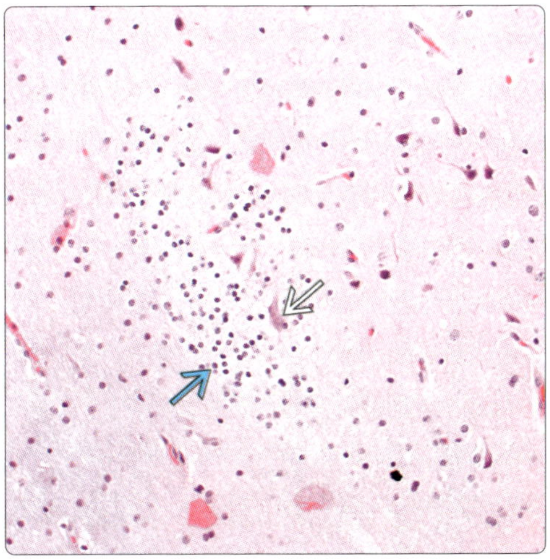

Long Standing Seizure Effect: Reactive Astrocytes

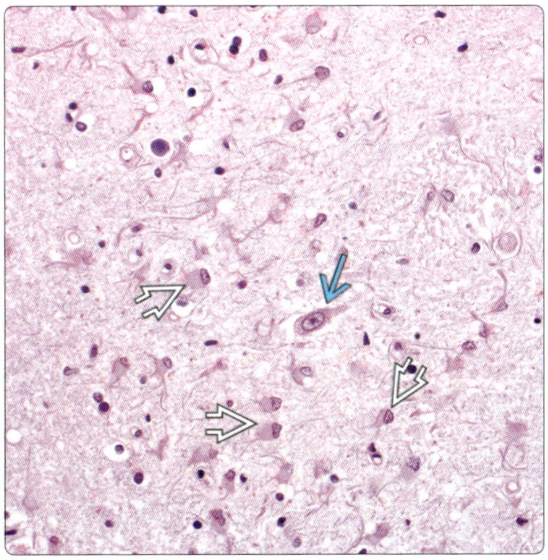

(Left) *Hamartia (a small glioneuronal lesion) can be identified in a dysplastic cortical specimen. Small neurocytic cells with perinuclear halo-surrounding neurons should not be mistaken for an infiltrating oligodendroglioma.* **(Right)** *Long-standing seizures invariably result in massive loss of neurons, which are replaced by reactive astrocytes. Abundant reactive astrocytes should not be mistaken for infiltrating gemistocytic astrocytoma on frozen section.*

SURGICAL/CLINICAL CONSIDERATIONS

Goals of Consultation

- Verify that lesion (identified by prior biopsy) is present in resected segment
- Evaluate proximal/distal margins
  - Measure distance to distal margin in low rectal resections
- Evaluate specimens resected for clinically benign disease if there are intraoperative findings suspicious for malignancy

Change in Patient Management

- If margin is positive or very close to tumor, additional colon may be resected
- If unexpected malignancy is detected, more extensive resection may be performed

Clinical Setting

- Carcinomas and large polyps are typically identified prior to surgical resection
- In majority of cases, margins can be adequately evaluated by gross examination
- If margin is close or difficult to evaluate due to prior treatment, intraoperative consultation may be requested
- Patients undergoing surgery for benign inflammatory bowel disease may have intraoperative findings of concern for malignancy
  - Abscesses, strictures, fistula tracts, &/or perforation can mimic malignancy

SPECIMEN EVALUATION

Gross

- Identify colon segment according to structures present
  - Right colectomy: Terminal ileum, cecum, appendix, ascending colon
  - Transverse colon: Colon with mesentery
  - Sigmoid colon: Colon with mesentery
  - Sigmoid/rectum: Mesentery on proximal sigmoid portion; distal portion lacks mesentery
    - Lesions are often close to distal margin due to proximity to sphincter muscles
      - Sparing anal sphincter, when possible, reduces morbidity to patients
    - Location of lesions as being in sigmoid, at sigmoid/rectal junction, or in rectum is determined
  - Abdominoperineal resection: Sigmoid, rectum, and anus
- Outer surface is examined for following features
  - Gross involvement by carcinoma
    - Perforation may be associated with hemorrhage or exudate
  - Puckering of serosa in area of colonic mass
    - Usually indicates carcinoma has invaded visceral peritoneum
  - Metastatic lesions to serosa
    - Often multiple; associated with serosal adhesions
  - Tattoo ink may be present, marking site of prior polypectomy
  - Completeness of mesorectal envelope for low anterior resections
    - Alterations introduced during processing should be distinguished from appearance of specimen when received
      - Any changes should be documented in gross description of specimen
    - Assessment of mesorectal envelope can be made in final report and should not be made intraoperatively
- Distal, proximal, mesenteric, and radial margins are inked as appropriate
- Specimen is palpated to identify site of lesion and any grossly involved lymph nodes
- Colon is opened with blunt-tipped scissors, avoiding transecting lesions
  - Stapled margins are completely opened by cutting as close to staple line as possible
- Mucosa can be gently rinsed with saline, if necessary
- All lesions and their relationship to margins are identified
  - Bowel segments can contract up to 40% within 10-20 minutes after excision

Colon Adenocarcinoma: Proximal and Distal Margins

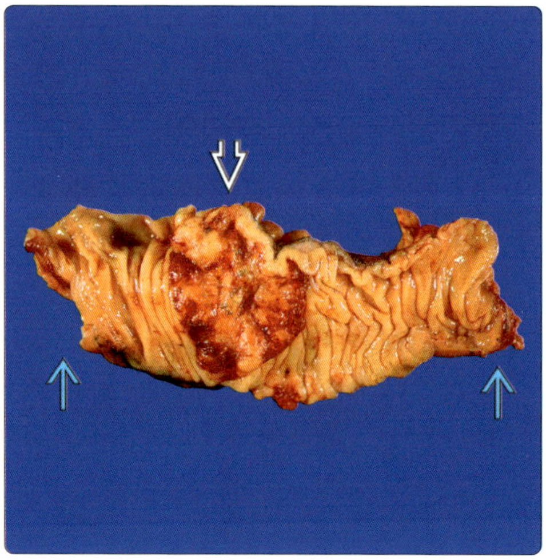

Rectal Adenoma: Distal Margin

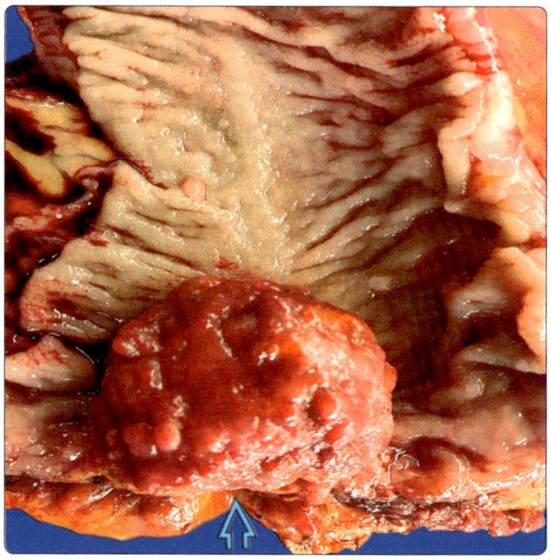

(Left) *In sites away from the rectum, carcinomas ➡ can be resected with widely free proximal and distal margins ➡. Frozen section is unnecessary if the mucosa at the resection margins appears normal on gross examination.* **(Right)** *The distal margin is often close for rectal tumors because the amount of colon that can be removed and spare the anal sphincter is limited. The muscularis propria retracts and the margin ➡ can appear erroneously close to the lesion. A perpendicular section is helpful to determine clearance from margin.*

Completeness of Mesorectal Envelope

Feature	Complete	Nearly Complete	Incomplete
Bulk	Substantial	Moderate	Little
Mesorectal Surface	Smooth	Irregular	Irregular
Defects	None > 5 mm	Present > 5 mm but not to muscularis propria	Present and extend to muscularis propria
Coning	None	May be present	Present

Bosch SL et al: The importance of the pathologist's role in assessment of the quality of the mesorectum. Curr Colorectal Cancer Rep. 8(2):90-98, 2012.

- Distances to margins are measured and recorded as soon as possible
- If no lesion is apparent, surgeon should be contacted
  - If lesion was polyp that was previously biopsied, site of polyp may be subtle area of mucosal ulceration or tattoo ink
- If surgeon wishes to view specimen in operating room, specimen should be transferred to clean surgical drape or pad
  - Specimen must be placed in appropriately labeled container for transfer

Frozen Section

- Perpendicular sections are taken if carcinoma or tumor bed is present near margin on gross examination
  - Very narrow negative margins may be adequate in some settings
- Ensure full-thickness sections for frozen section to avoid missing small foci of tumor deep in muscularis propria
- Frozen section may be taken in area most suspicious for malignancy in cases without prior diagnosis of malignancy

MOST COMMON DIAGNOSES

Adenocarcinoma

- Colon carcinomas are generally easily recognizable as elevated mass or ulceration with surrounding induration
- Typical carcinoma shows glands with tall columnar cells and extensive dirty necrosis
  - Less common histologic types are mucinous, medullary, and signet ring cell
- Margins can be evaluated and reported grossly if > 1.0 cm away from tumor
- Carcinomas that have responded well to treatment may show only subtle gross findings
  - Small ulcer, fibrosis/scarring, abnormal mucosal appearance, mucin, tattoo ink
  - Changes in benign cells can mimic malignancy
    - Regenerative changes in surface mucosa
    - Nuclear atypia in stromal cells
    - Ulceration, necrosis, or mucin in absence of residual viable tumor cells

Polyp

- May be pedunculated or sessile
- Large adenomas or serrated polyps may require surgical resection
  - Frozen sections of polyps are generally not necessary or recommended
- Distance to margin is only relevant information to be provided in these cases

Metastasis to Colon

- Metastases arise from intralymphatic growth in pericolonic adipose tissue or infiltration into colon from peritoneal deposits
- Can present as intraluminal mass mimicking colon primary

Endometriosis

- Clinically mimics cancer due to induration/stricture
- Endometrial glands deep in muscularis propria may be mistaken for cancer
- Presence of endometrial stroma around glandular epithelium is helpful in avoiding misdiagnosis

Diverticulitis

- Cancers can arise in colon involved with diverticular disease
- Inflammation and fibrosis related to diverticulitis may mimic cancer
- Frozen section diagnosis may be requested if "inflammatory mass" is close to resection margin

REPORTING

Gross

- Presence of lesion can be determined by gross examination
  - e.g., "2.4 cm ulcerated mass is present"
- Margins for colonic carcinomas can be reliably assessed by gross examination if there is no prior treatment
  - e.g., "Mass is 1 cm from closest distal margin"
- Distance of low sigmoid/rectal carcinomas from distal margin should be reported as accurately as possible

Frozen Section

- Margins
  - Positive or negative for tumor involvement
  - If tumor bed after treatment is present at margin, this can be reported
    - If acellular mucin is present in initial sections, deeper levels to detect possible tumor cells may be helpful

SELECTED REFERENCES

1. Mukkai Krishnamurty D et al: Importance of surgical margins in rectal cancer. J Surg Oncol. 113(3):323-32, 2016
2. Gomes RM et al: Role of intraoperative frozen section for assessing distal resection margin after anterior resection. Int J Colorectal Dis. 30(8):1081-9, 2015
3. Goldstein NS et al: Disparate surgical margin lengths of colorectal resection specimens between in vivo and in vitro measurements. The effects of surgical resection and formalin fixation on organ shrinkage. Am J Clin Pathol. 111(3):349-51, 1999

(**Left**) *The sigmoid colon is completely intraperitoneal and the root of the mesentery is a true radial margin of resection; however, this margin is rarely involved by carcinoma. The serosal surfaces are not surgical margins.* (**Right**) *The anterior surface of the upper rectum is covered with peritoneum . The posterior surface in the upper 1/2 and the entire circumference in the lower 1/2 of the rectum is a true soft tissue radial margin*

Sigmoid Colon: Mesenteric Margin

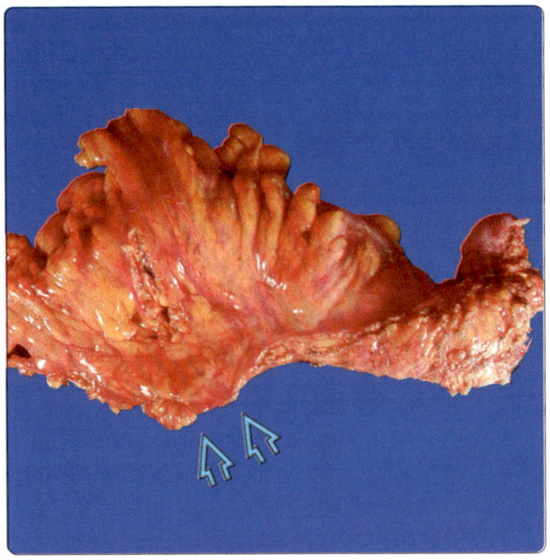

Rectum: Peritoneal Coverings

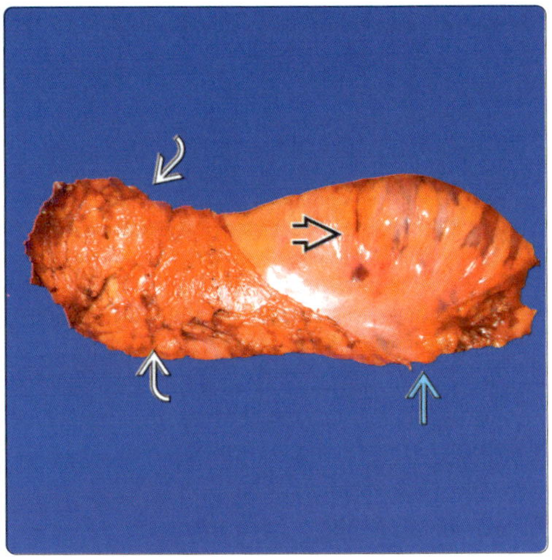

(**Left**) *This colon carcinoma has invaded through the muscularis propria , perforated the visceral peritoneum, and caused retraction of the serosa . This is an important prognostic factor but is not a surgical margin.* (**Right**) *It is not uncommon for patients to have > 1 colon carcinoma and for the carcinomas to be associated with polyps. It is important to completely open and carefully examine the margins for lesions in addition to the lesion for which the resection was intended.*

Colon Carcinoma: Serosal Surface

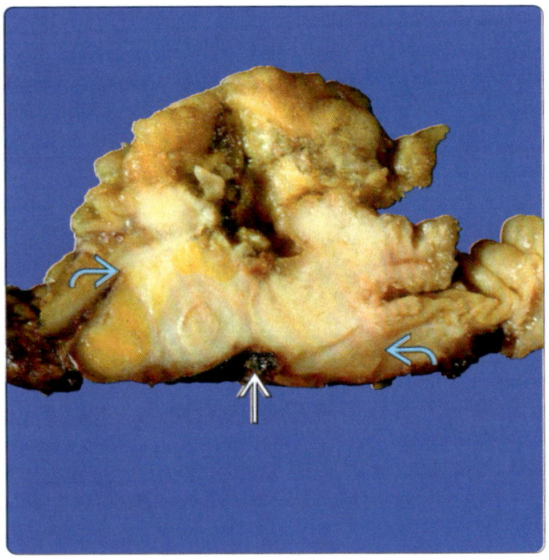

Multiple Colon Carcinomas: Gross Appearance

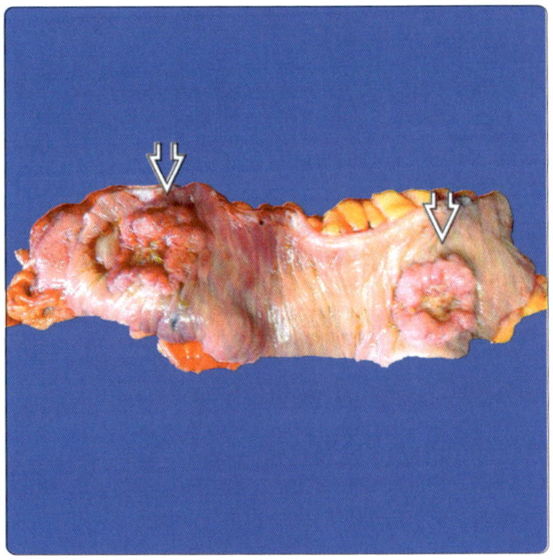

(**Left**) *Rectal cancers are treated with neoadjuvant chemoradiation, and treatment may lead to marked or complete regression . The distal margin is evaluated for subtle changes indicative of tumor bed or residual carcinoma and a frozen section performed if abnormal.* (**Right**) *The surface mucosa of the colon is ulcerated while the submucosa shows dense fibrosis consistent with tumor bed site without residual carcinoma. It can be difficult to evaluate margins in this setting.*

Postneoadjuvant Rectal Carcinoma: Gross Appearance

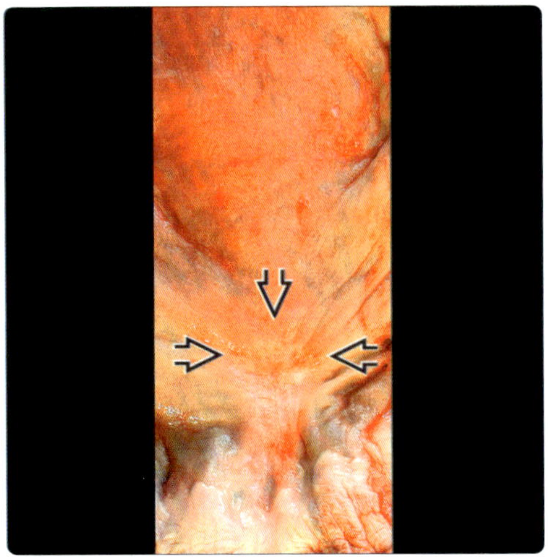

Tumor Bed in Colon After Neoadjuvant Therapy

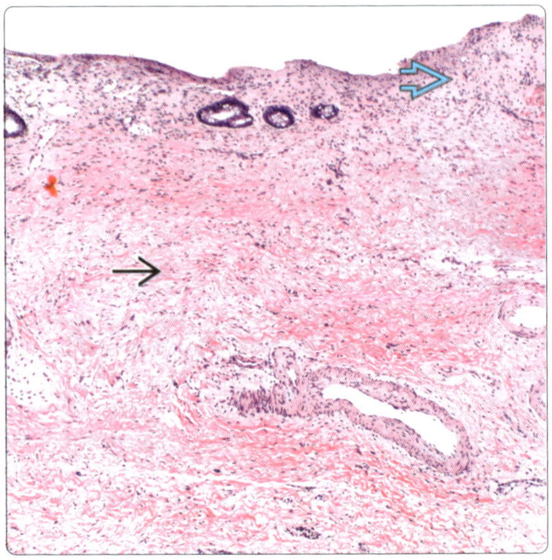

Polypectomy Site With Tattoo: Gross Appearance

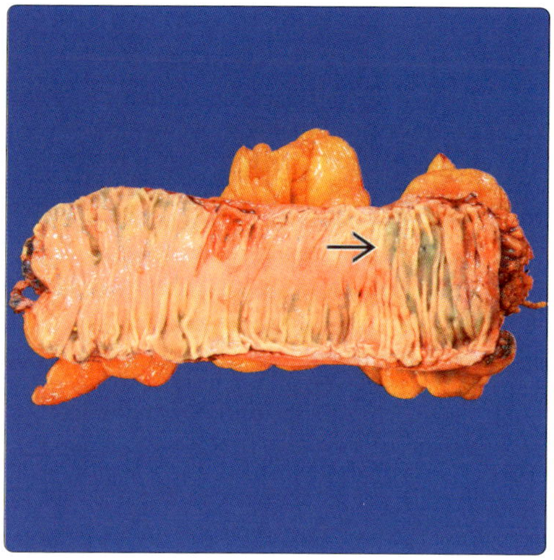

Tattoo Pigment

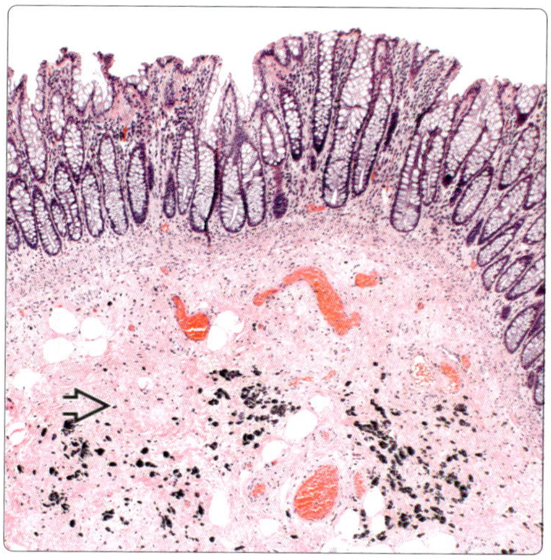

(Left) *At the time of polypectomy, tattoo pigment may be injected to mark the site. The gross examination should document any residual polyp or biopsy site in this area. Tattoo pigment can also sometimes be seen on the serosal surface.* **(Right)** *Tattoo pigment may be injected next to the site of a polyp biopsy. The pigment may be seen grossly as dark discoloration of the serosa and on microscopy as black pigment in the colonic wall.*

Resection After Prior Polypectomy: Gross Appearance

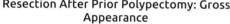

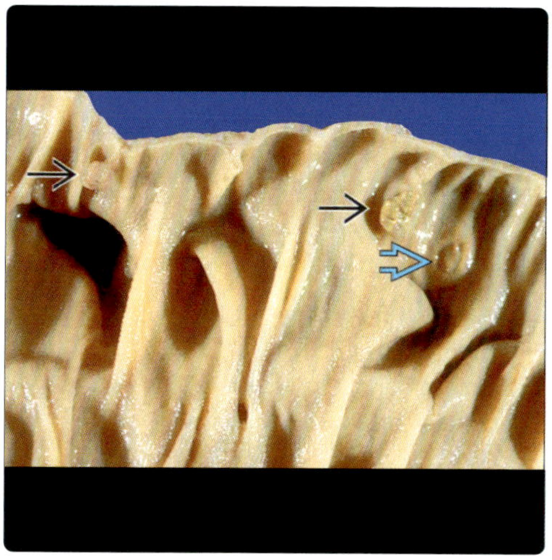

Endometriosis

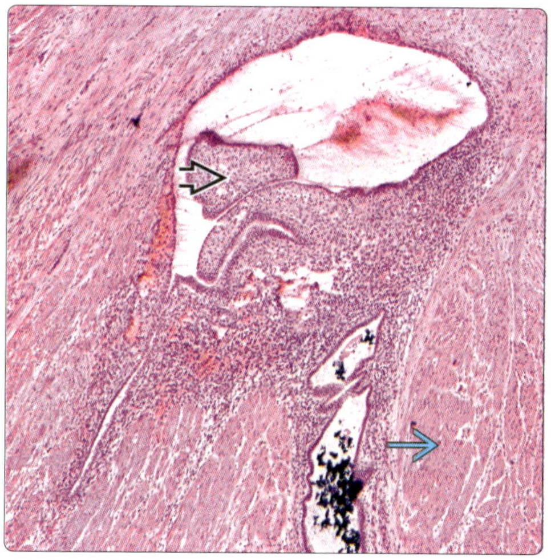

(Left) *This colonic resection was undertaken after a prior polypectomy revealed a small area of invasive carcinoma in a polyp. There is only a small ulceration present at the prior biopsy site, which could be very difficult to find on gross examination. Two other small polyps are also present.* **(Right)** *Endometriosis involving the colonic wall may cause stricture mimicking cancer. Benign endometrial glands and stroma are present deep in the muscularis propria in this example*

Cecal Carcinoma With Perforation: Gross Appearance

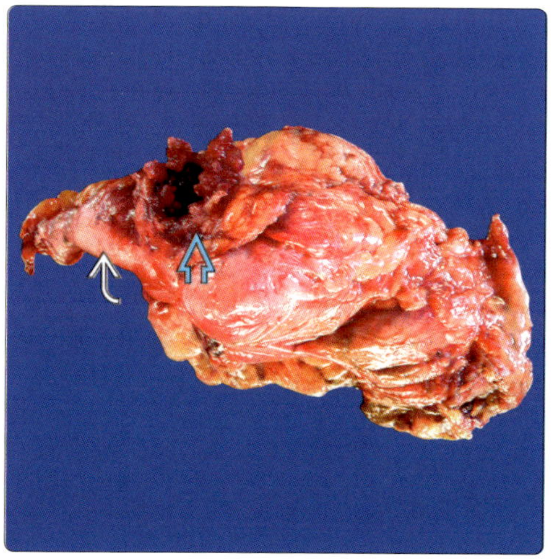

Bowel Perforation

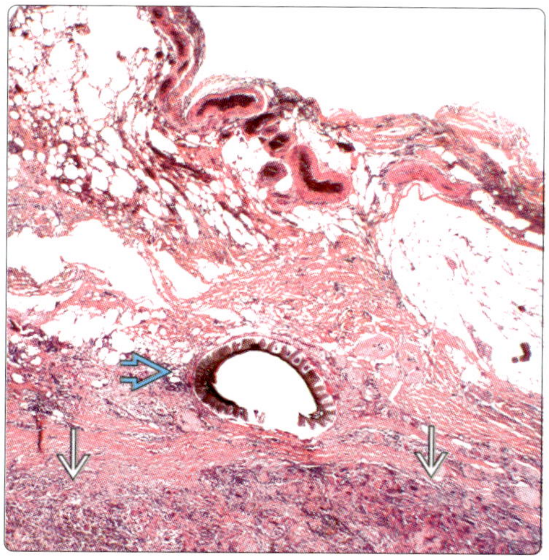

(Left) *This cecal carcinoma has perforated the wall. It is important to note whether the appendix is normal in tumors involving the cecum to rule out a primary appendiceal neoplasm with extension into the cecum* **(Right)** *After a bowel perforation, bowel contents can be found in the serosa and the accompanying inflammation can result in adhesions. In this case, there is both barium and plant material.*

SURGICAL/CLINICAL CONSIDERATIONS

Goal of Consultation

- Identify appropriate anastomotic site in Hirschsprung disease (HD) pull-through or ostomy takedown operation
  - Should be located within normally ganglionated bowel and proximal to transition zone (TZ)
- Establishing diagnosis of HD is best made on permanent suction rectal biopsies performed prior to pull-through surgery
  - Intraoperative consultation for this purpose should be strongly avoided

Change in Patient Management

- Surgeon submits biopsies for frozen section from distal-most portion of bowel thought to have normal innervation
  - If no ganglion cells are observed, additional (more proximal) biopsies sent until normal colon is identified
  - Additional biopsies are not necessary if tissue is diagnostic of normal bowel
- Although intraoperative error rate is low, consequences of erroneous diagnosis can have significant clinical impact on child

Clinical Setting

- HD (a.k.a. colonic aganglionosis) results from failure of neural crest cells to colonize entire length of colon
  - Ganglion cells are absent in distal intestine, resulting in inability of colon to contract and relax normally
- Often presents shortly after birth
  - Failure to pass meconium, abdominal distention, chronic constipation
  - Contrast enema reveals megacolon (proximally) with funnel-shaped TZ and thin distal aganglionic segment
- Colon can be involved to varying extents
  - Ultrashort-segment HD: Distal rectum (terminal 1-4 cm) in ~ 30% of cases
  - Short-segment HD: Rectosigmoid in ~ 45% of cases
  - Long-segment HD: Proximal colon to splenic flexure
  - Entire colon: < 10% of cases
  - Zonal colonic aganglionosis (skip-segment HD) is rare
  - Small bowel involvement is rare
- Aganglionic segment must be resected to restore normal colonic function

SPECIMEN EVALUATION

Gross: Intraoperative Biopsy for Frozen Section

- Full-thickness colonic biopsies or seromuscular biopsies preferred for intraoperative diagnosis
  - Recommended minimum dimensions
    - 1 cm in length
    - 3-5 mm in depth

Gross: Pull-Through Specimen

- May be submitted for frozen section evaluation of proximal margin
  - Entire proximal margin is submitted as en face section
- Several methods of sectioning may be utilized for processing remainder of specimen for permanent sections
  - Cut a full-length longitudinal strip, 3-4 mm in width
    - Cut strip into cassette-sized pieces with proximal ends inked, submit into multiple cassettes
    - Or ink proximal end, roll strip into coil, and place into single cassette
  - Take full-thickness circumferential sections rather than longitudinal sections along length of bowel segment
    - Roll strips into coils, submit into sequential cassettes
    - Include a strip from proximal resection margin
    - Easier to envision the often irregular interface between ganglionated and aganglionated regions

Gross: Diagnostic Suction Rectal Biopsies

- Performed prior to pull-through operation to establish diagnosis of HD on permanent sections
  - Attempting to make primary diagnosis of HD at intraoperative consultation should be discouraged
- Recommended that biopsies be taken at multiple levels (1 cm, 2 cm, and 3 cm) proximal to dentate line
- Skeletal muscle, transitional or squamous epithelium present indicates that biopsy is too distal for adequate evaluation

Normal Colon: Myenteric Plexus With Ganglion Cells

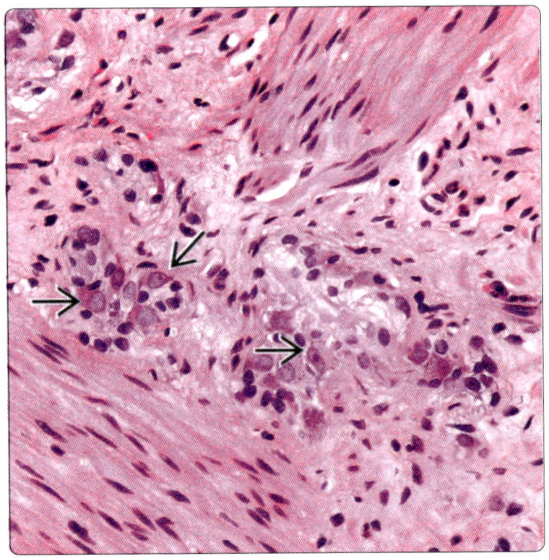

Hirschsprung Disease: Myenteric Plexus Without Ganglion Cells

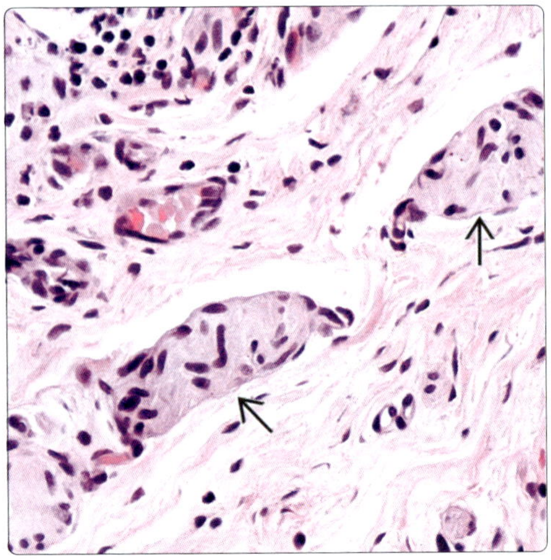

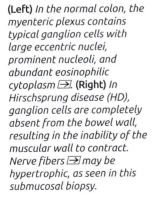

(Left) *In the normal colon, the myenteric plexus contains typical ganglion cells with large eccentric nuclei, prominent nucleoli, and abundant eosinophilic cytoplasm* ➡. **(Right)** *In Hirschsprung disease (HD), ganglion cells are completely absent from the bowel wall, resulting in the inability of the muscular wall to contract. Nerve fibers* ➡ *may be hypertrophic, as seen in this submucosal biopsy.*

- Distal-most rectum can be aganglionic normally
- Adequate biopsy specimens: Thickness of submucosa at least 1/3 total thickness
- Multiple deeper sections at each level must be evaluated to ensure aganglionosis
  - Prominent nerve fibers usually accompany HD
- Stains that may be used on permanent sections to evaluate for HD
  - Calretinin
    - Intrinsic nerve fibers and ganglion cells stain positively in lamina propria, muscularis mucosa, and submucosa of normal bowel
    - Negative in HD (large extrinsic nerve trunks may still stain positively)
    - Mast cells also stain positively with calretinin
  - High-affinity choline transporter
    - Like acetylcholinesterase (AChE) stain, shows increased density of nerves within muscularis mucosa and deep lamina propria
    - Can be performed on frozen or formalin-fixed paraffin-embedded tissue
  - Succinic dehydrogenase
    - Marker exclusively for ganglion cells

Frozen Section: Intraoperative Biopsies

- Orient sections perpendicular to serosal surface
  - Should include entire longitudinal muscular layer and most of circular layer
    - Including both layers is necessary to visualize myenteric plexus located between layers
    - Surgeon may provide suture or ink to aid in orientation
- Multiple levels of each block should be examined
  - At least 4 and up to 10 sections are usually sufficient for evaluation
- Thicker sections (6 μm) may be helpful
- Giemsa or Diff-Quik stains may be easier to interpret
  - Cytoplasm of ganglion cells is stained contrasting blue color
- Total colonic HD: Frozen sections of appendix not recommended
  - Possible skip lesions or hypoganglionosis
  - Smaller ganglion cells than rectum, may be distorted
  - Terminal ileal biopsies recommended instead
- **Reliability**
  - False-negative diagnosis: 3% (true ganglion cells not detected)
    - Surgeon will take additional biopsies that are more proximal
    - Harm to patient may be minimal, although more colon may be resected
  - False-positive diagnosis: 3% (nonganglion cells reported as ganglion cells)
    - Leaving aganglionic section of colon in patient may have significant clinical consequences

Frozen Section: Acetylcholinesterase Histochemistry

- Cholinergic nerve fibers of aganglionic colon are more prominent than in normal colon
  - Fibers contain increased amount of AChE
  - Diagnostic features can be seen in superficial layers of colon
- Rapid technique for AChE has been developed but is only used in some institutions
  - Requires frozen tissue
  - Stains prominent AChE-positive fibers within muscularis mucosa and often lamina propria
    - Normal pattern: Absence of fibers or minimal presence in muscularis mucosae or immediately subjacent submucosa
    - Abnormal pattern: Many nerve fibers in muscularis mucosae and extending into lamina propria
- **Reliability**
  - Has been reported to increase rate of definitive diagnosis from 83-95%
  - Sensitivity reported up to 100% with specificity ranging from 91-96%
    - False-negative diagnosis: Majority in neonatal period or in patients with total colonic aganglionosis
    - False-positive diagnosis: Can also occur

MOST COMMON DIAGNOSES

Normal Colon

- Meissner (submucosal) plexus is located deep to mucosa
  - Ganglion cells are fewer in number in this area
- Auerbach (myenteric) plexus is located in muscularis plexus
  - Located between longitudinal and circumferential muscularis propria layers
  - Ganglion cells are more abundant and larger
- Ganglion cells
  - Identified by large size, polygonal shape, abundant eosinophilic cytoplasm, round eccentric nuclei, large eosinophilic nucleoli
  - Organized in neural units
    - 2-10 ganglion cells are arrayed in semicircle around neural tissue
  - Should be present in normal numbers
- Normal nerve trunks range: 10-20 μm
  - Nerve fiber hypertrophy should not be seen

Hirschsprung Disease

- Absence of ganglion cells in both Meissner and Auerbach plexuses
  - Loss generally correlates between both plexuses
- Nerve fiber hypertrophy
  - ≥ 40-μm-submucosal nerve fiber diameter in majority of biopsies of infants
    - Older children and adults may normally have enteric nerve fibers of this thickness
  - May not be present in cases of total colonic aganglionosis
    - Nerves may be hypoplastic or absent in this case
- Abnormal cholinergic nerve fibers as detected by AChE histochemistry

Transition Zone

- Intervening funnel-shaped region located between dilated proximal colon (normally ganglionated) and nondilated distal segment (aganglionic)
  - ≤ 5 cm in length in shorter segment HD
  - May be > 5 cm in length in longer segment HD

- Difficult to detect by imaging in neonates early in disease process
- TZ needs to be removed surgically for successful treatment
  - Distal zone of normal innervation is not evenly circumferential
    - Partial circumferential aganglionosis
      - Ganglion cells may extend 2-3 cm farther on portion of bowel circumference, usually antimesenteric; therefore, anastomotic site should be ~ 3 cm proximal to most distal biopsy with ganglion cells
    - Multiple biopsies are preferred to ensure that anastomosis is within normal colon
- Ganglion cells can be sparse
  - Myenteric plexus may be hypoganglionated
    - Nerve fiber hypertrophy may be present
  - Submucosal plexus may be hyperganglionated
- Eosinophilic and mast cell infiltrates may be present and can be mistaken for ganglion cells

Intestinal Neuronal Dysplasia

- Submucosal hyperganglionosis (intestinal neuronal dysplasia type B) has been reported in proximal gut of 20-75% of HD colons

Pseudoobstruction

- Dysmotility disorder without mechanical obstruction
- Often due to myopathic process

REPORTING

Frozen Section

- Presence or absence of ganglion cells
  - If present, report normal or reduced numbers
- Status of nerve trunks: Presence or absence of nerve fiber hypertrophy
- Report if specimen is of inadequate size or thickness
- Circumferential frozen section of proximal margin recommended to help avoid TZ pull-through

PITFALLS

Failure to Recognize Immature Ganglion Cells

- Immature ganglion cells are present in premature neonates
  - Smaller than mature ganglion cells
  - Cytoplasm is scant, eccentric, and pear-shaped without stippled Nissl substance
  - Nucleoli less conspicuous
  - Can be mistaken for other cells such as lymphocytes or histiocytes
- Ganglion cells mature later in submucosal plexus
  - Myenteric plexus is preferred for evaluation
- Some mature ganglion cells should be present but may be sparse

Transition Zone Biopsies

- Presence of sparse ganglion cells &/or nerve fiber hypertrophy concerning for TZ should be reported

Misidentification of Cells as Ganglion Cells

- Mast cells, smooth muscle cells, or reactive stromal cells may be misinterpreted as ganglion cells
- Endothelial cells can appear enlarged and are often present near neural units
- Inflammation can cause reactive changes in stromal cells, endothelial cells, plasma cells, and lymphocytes
  - Cells can appear enlarged with large nucleoli and resemble ganglion cells
  - If histologic features are obscured by inflammation, interpretation on frozen section may be difficult
- Eccentric nuclei and neural units can help to distinguish ganglion cells from these other cell types

Long-Segment HD

- HD involving long segment of colon, entire colon, or total enteric HD can have different features compared to short-segment HD
- Biopsies often lack characteristic nerve fiber hypertrophy seen in short-segment HD

Superficial Biopsies

- Suction biopsy with only mucosa submucosa may not be sufficient for frozen section evaluation
  - Fewer ganglion cells are present in normal Meissner plexus and may be difficult to identify on frozen section
- Discordance rates compared to permanent sections are high (> 50%)

Inadequate Evaluation of Frozen Section Block

- Multiple sections (up to 10) may be required to detect ganglion cells
  - Each block should be sectioned deeply unless ganglion cells are clearly identified
- Sections that are too thick or thin can make identification of ganglion cells difficult

SELECTED REFERENCES

1. Kovach AE et al: Ganglion cells are frequently present in pediatric mucosal colorectal biopsies. Pediatr Dev Pathol. 1093526617704594, 2017
2. Mohanty S et al: Appendicular biopsy in total colonic aganglionosis: a histologically challenging and inadvisable practice. Pediatr Dev Pathol. 20(4):277-287, 2017
3. Moore SW: Advances in understanding functional variations in the Hirschsprung disease spectrum (variant Hirschsprung disease). Pediatr Surg Int. 33(3):285-298, 2017
4. Terra SA et al: A critical appraisal of the morphological criteria for diagnosing intestinal neuronal dysplasia type B. Mod Pathol. 30(7):978-985, 2017
5. Kapur RP: Histology of the transition zone in hirschsprung disease. Am J Surg Pathol. 40(12):1637-1646, 2016
6. Swaminathan M et al: Intestinal neuronal dysplasia-like submucosal ganglion cell hyperplasia at the proximal margins of hirschsprung disease resections. Pediatr Dev Pathol. 18(6):466-76, 2015
7. Rabah R: Total colonic aganglionosis: case report, practical diagnostic approach and pitfalls. Arch Pathol Lab Med. 134(10):1467-73, 2010
8. Kapur RP: Practical pathology and genetics of Hirschsprung's disease. Semin Pediatr Surg. 18(4):212-23, 2009
9. Staines WA et al: Fast evaluation of intraoperative biopsies for ganglia in Hirschsprung's disease. J Pediatr Surg. 42(12):2067-70, 2007
10. Shayan K et al: Reliability of intraoperative frozen sections in the management of Hirschsprung's disease. J Pediatr Surg. 39(9):1345-8, 2004

Normal Colon: Myenteric Plexus

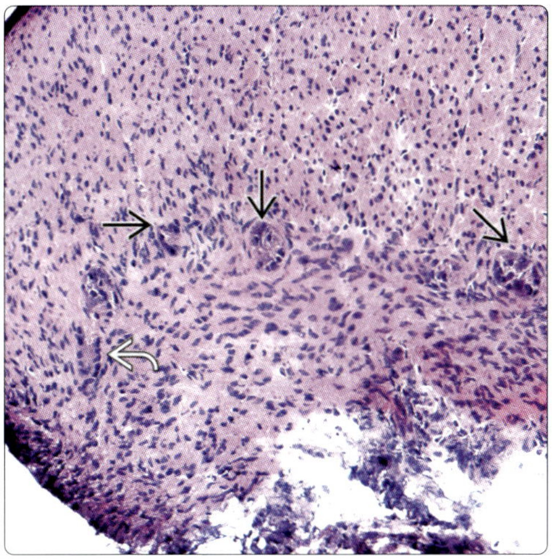

Normal Colon: Neural Unit

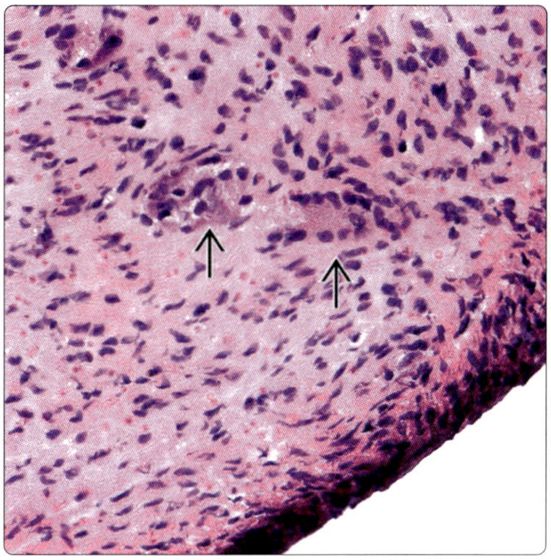

(Left) *Ganglion cells are most easily detected in the myenteric plexus on frozen section. These cells are recognized as large, plump cells arranged in clusters or aligned in semicircular patterns (neural units). If only sparse cells are seen, the biopsy may be from the transitional zone.* **(Right)** *Ganglion cells have dark, round, eccentric nuclei and abundant eosinophilic cytoplasm. They are often arranged in semicircular or horseshoe-shaped clusters. Nucleoli are not evident in this frozen section.*

Normal Colon: Ganglion Cells on Frozen Section

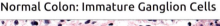

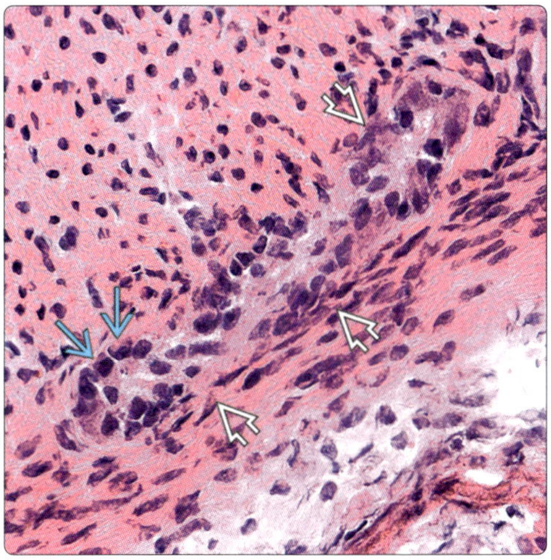

Normal Colon: Ganglion Cells on Permanent Section

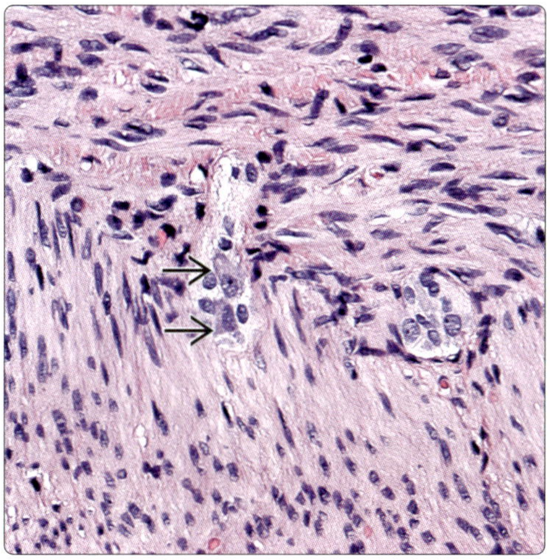

(Left) *This biopsy of a normal infant colon shows ganglion cells arranged in neural units with large, round, eccentric nuclei. Nucleoli are seen in some of the ganglion cells but tend to be less conspicuous on frozen sections of young children.* **(Right)** *Permanent sections of a normal colon demonstrate the classic features of ganglion cells, which include abundant eccentric cytoplasm with Nissl substance, large nuclei, and prominent nucleoli. These features may not be as crisp or distinct on frozen section.*

Normal Colon: Immature Ganglion Cells

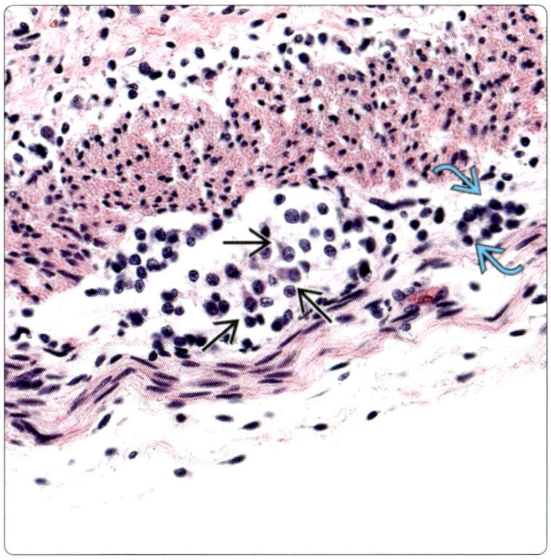

Hirschsprung Disease: Nerve Fiber Hypertrophy

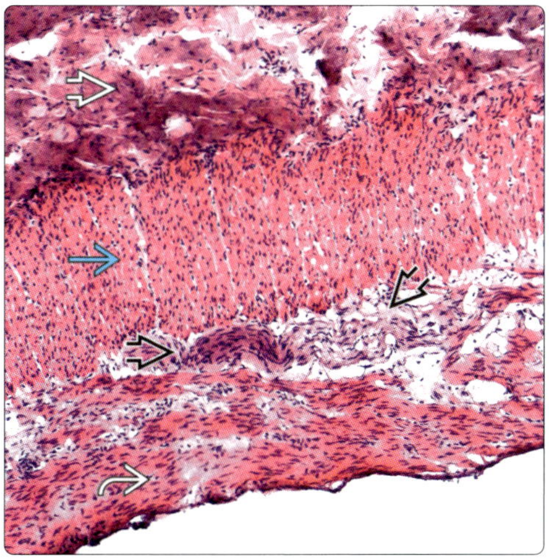

(Left) *Ganglion cells of premature infants can be challenging to identify, as they contain small nuclei, inconspicuous to absent nucleoli, and less abundant cytoplasm than mature cells. Clusters and circular arrangements can aid in their identification.* **(Right)** *This frozen section of an HD bowel shows submucosal, inner muscular, and outer muscular layers of the bowel wall. Significant nerve fiber hypertrophy is present in the myenteric plexus. No ganglion cells are seen.*

(Left) *In this frozen section of HD, ganglion cells are absent from the myenteric plexus. Although nerve fiber hypertrophy is often present, it is not seen in this case ⇨.* **(Right)** *Total colonic HD and, in this case, total enteric HD are rare. A pitfall to avoid is that long-segment HD may lack the characteristic nerve fiber hypertrophy in the myenteric plexus → usually seen in short-segment disease.*

Hirschsprung Disease: Myenteric Plexus

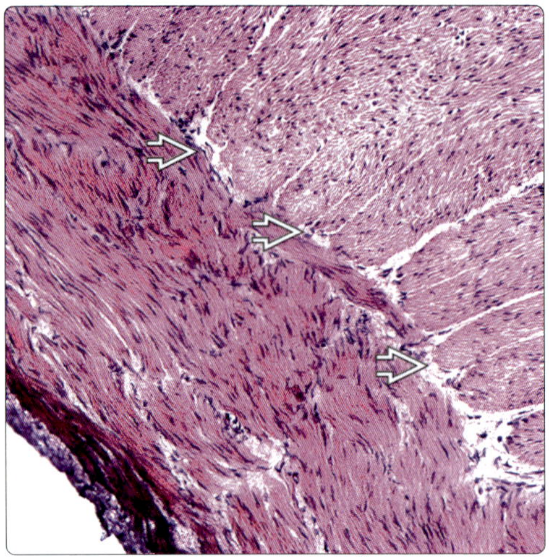

Hirschsprung Disease: Long Segment

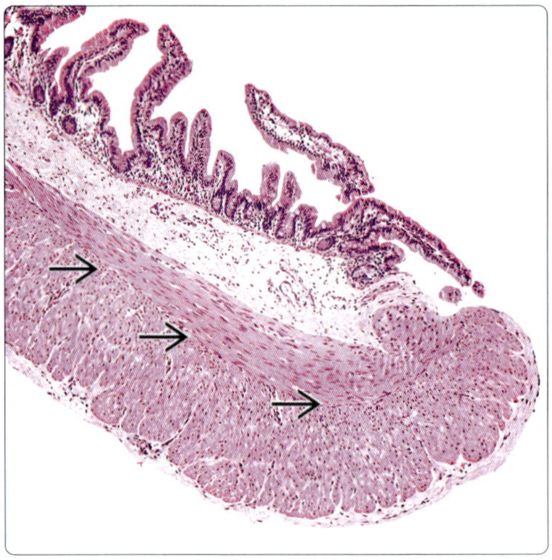

(Left) *Diff-Quik stain highlights ganglion cells ⇨ by staining the cytoplasm a contrasting blue color on frozen section. This stain can be helpful in the evaluation of HD. (Courtesy C. Mafnas, MD.)* **(Right)** *An acetylcholinesterase stain performed on frozen section tissue accentuates prominent abnormal nerve fibers within the lamina propria ↷ and muscularis mucosa in cases of HD. Such fibers are not present in these locations in the normally ganglionated colon.*

Normal Colon: Diff-Quik Stain

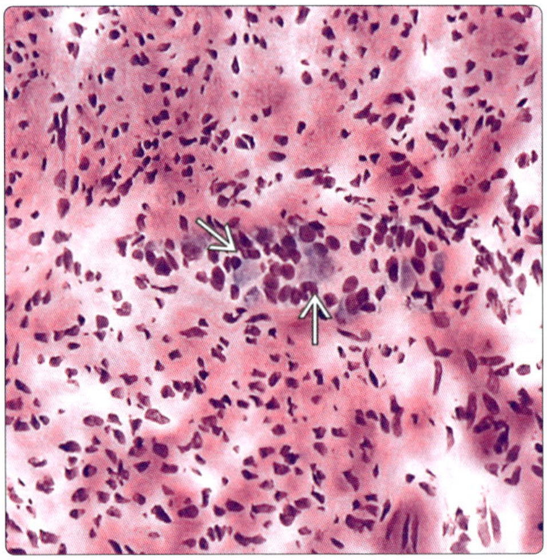

Hirschsprung Disease: Acetylcholinesterase Histochemical Stain

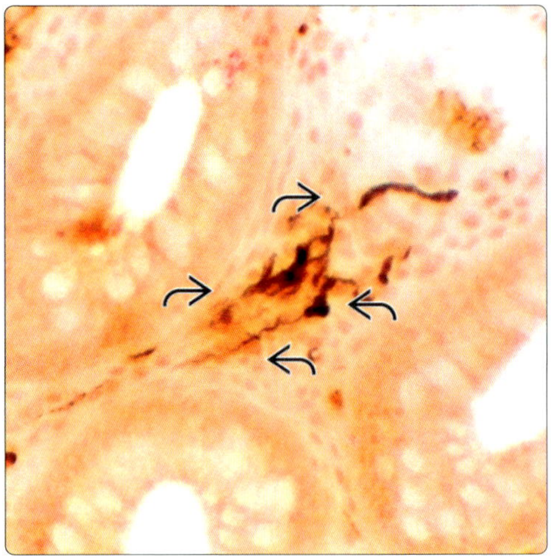

(Left) *Calretinin highlights intrinsic nerve fibers within the lamina propria, muscularis mucosa, and submucosa of a normal colon →. Ganglion cells and mast cells are also positive for calretinin.* **(Right)** *An immunohistochemical study for calretinin demonstrates the absence of intrinsic nerve fibers in the lamina propria and muscularis mucosa in this mucosal biopsy of HD. Occasional mast cells are positive, providing an internal control →. Larger extrinsic nerve fibers may be weakly positive ⇨.*

Normal Colon: Immunohistochemical Study for Calretinin

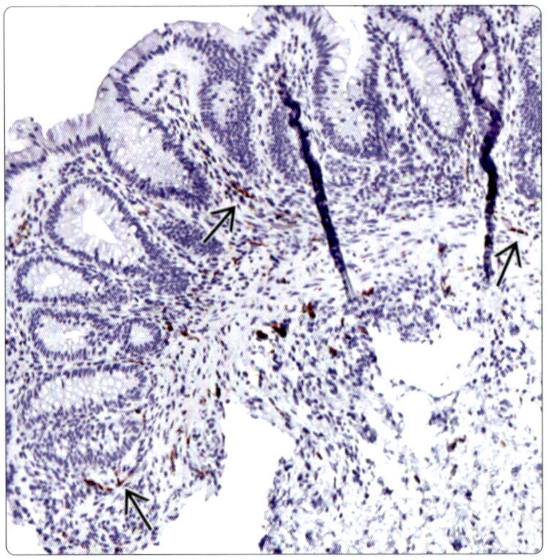

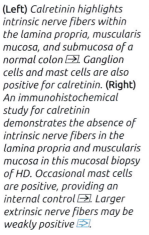

Hirschsprung Disease: Immunohistochemical Study for Calretinin

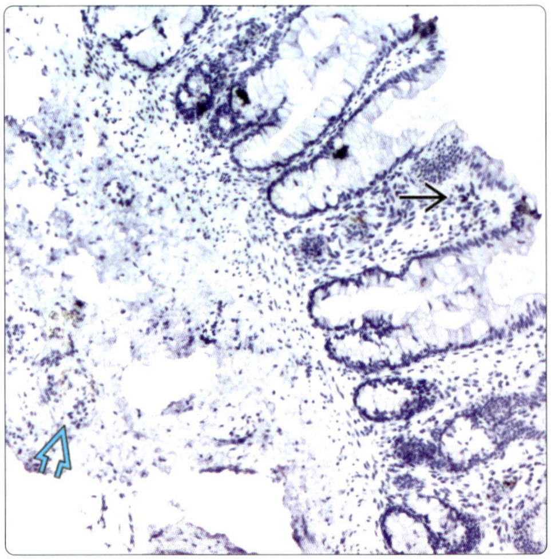

Seromuscular Colonic Biopsy for Frozen Section

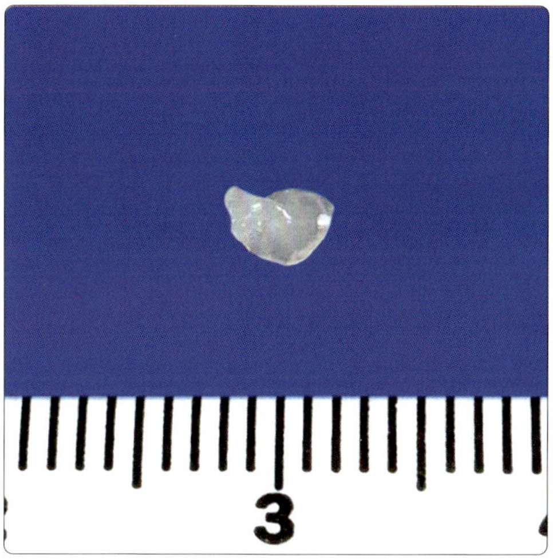

Seromuscular Colonic Biopsy for Frozen Section

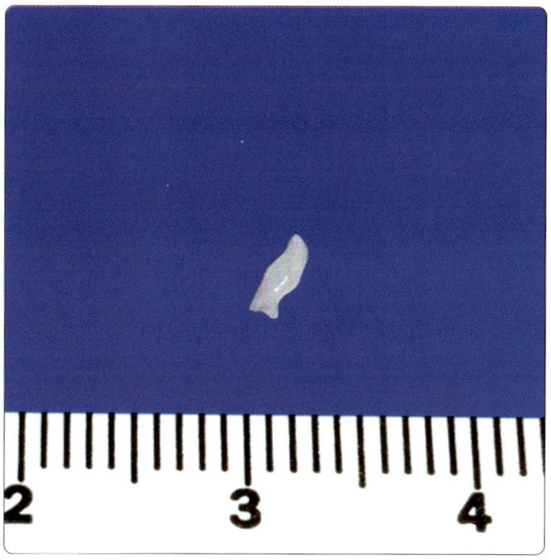

(Left) *The serosal surface of a seromuscular colonic biopsy is shown here lying en face. The specimen should not be embedded in this orientation, as this would make evaluation of innervation of the bowel wall difficult.* **(Right)** *The seromuscular biopsy should be embedded on edge in order to best represent the myenteric plexus on frozen section.*

Seromuscular Colon Biopsy for Frozen Section

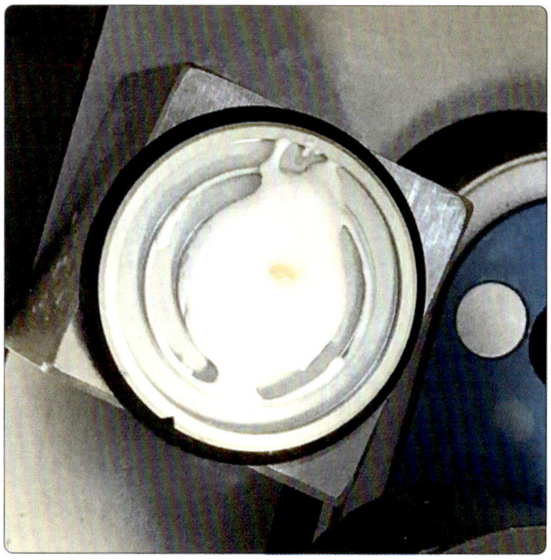

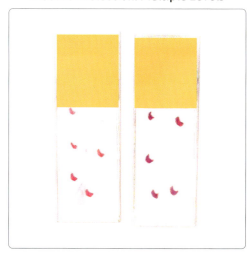

Hirschsprung Disease Pull-Through Specimen

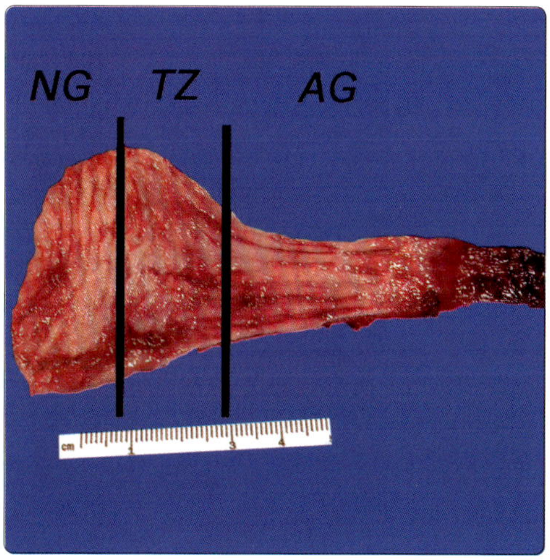

(Left) *The seromuscular biopsy is seen here embedded on edge in OCT gel. The biopsy should represent the entire outer longitudinal layer of the muscularis propria, and at least most of the inner circular layer.* **(Right)** *Colonic pull-through specimen for HD shows the dilated normal ganglionic portion proximally, the aganglionic zone distally, and the angulated transition zone (TZ) between the black lines. Frozen sections taken within the TZ may reveal hypoganglionosis along with hypertrophied nerve fibers.*

Frozen Section Slides for Hirschsprung Disease Evaluation: Multiple Levels

Normal Colon on Frozen Section

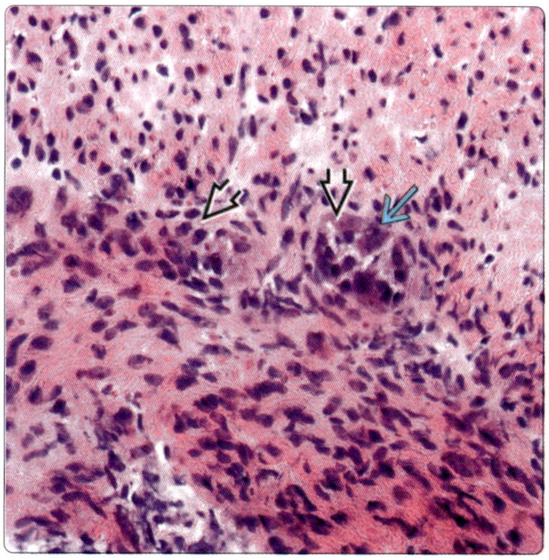

(Left) *Examination of multiple deeper levels of each biopsy specimen is necessary to confidently rule out the presence of ganglion cells on frozen section.* **(Right)** *Frozen section evaluation shows ganglion cells arranged in clusters ⇨. They may be present singly as well. Large, round, eccentric nuclei within eosinophilic cytoplasm alert the observer to their presence. Vague nucleoli can be seen in some of the ganglion cells →.*

SURGICAL/CLINICAL CONSIDERATIONS

Goal of Consultation

- Determine whether proximal and distal margins are free of dysplasia and carcinoma
- Determine whether proximal margin is free of Barrett esophagus

Change in Patient Management

- Additional tissue at proximal or distal margin may be resected

Clinical Setting

- Patients with carcinoma usually present with symptoms related to mass lesion
  - Usually no prior history of esophageal disorder
  - Surgery undertaken with curative intent in most patients
- Majority of lesions are diagnosed by endoscopic biopsy
  - Primary diagnosis optimally made on permanent sections
- Surgery often preceded by neoadjuvant therapy, including chemotherapy and radiation

SPECIMEN EVALUATION

Gross

- Identify esophagus, stomach, and duodenum (if present in complete gastrectomy)
- Examine outer surface for tumor involvement
- Open specimen as close to stapled margin as possible for accurate measurements
  - Ink proximal and distal margins
- Avoid cutting through tumor when opening specimen
  - Location of tumor can generally be determined by palpating interior surface of esophagus prior to opening it
- Identify cancer site
  - Cancers at gastroesophageal junction are usually adenocarcinomas
    - Often associated with Barrett esophagus
      - Barrett esophagus consists of salmon-pink columnar mucosa interspersed within gray-white squamous mucosa
  - Cancers in stomach are usually adenocarcinomas
    - Wide variation in gross appearance: Polypoid fungating masses to ulceroinfiltrative lesions
    - Signet ring cell carcinomas may present with diffusely thickened muscularis propria and normal overlying mucosa ("linitis plastica")
  - Lesions of esophageal or gastric wall are usually leiomyomas or gastrointestinal stromal tumors (GIST)
- After neoadjuvant treatment, there may only be an ulcerated indurated region that represents tumor bed
- Distance of residual cancer or tumor bed to closest proximal and distal margins is measured
  - Tumors can invade beneath normal overlying mucosa for extended distance
    - Margin can appear normal by gross examination
    - Full-thickness sections to include entire wall are necessary for complete evaluation

Frozen Section

- Margin evaluation must include full cross section, including mucosa, submucosa, and muscularis propria
  - Mucosa can sometimes curl over at cut edge of specimen due to retraction of muscularis propria
  - It may be necessary to pull muscularis propria back slightly to get full-thickness section
- Distal (gastric) margin is usually far from carcinoma
- An en face margin can be taken when residual tumor/tumor bed is > 1.0 cm from margin
  - Examines larger portion of margin
  - Distance of tumor from margin cannot be determined
- A perpendicular margin should be taken when residual tumor or tumor bed is < 1.0 cm from margin and when distance to margin may govern additional surgery
  - Surgeon should specify if distance to margin is needed
  - A perpendicular margin samples only 1 small portion of margin

Gastroesophageal Junction Carcinoma

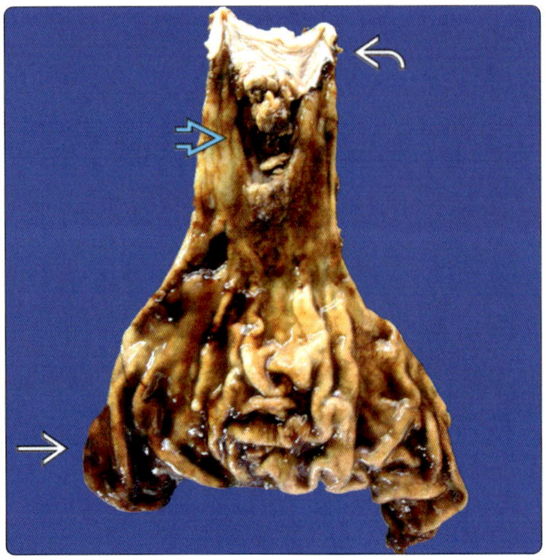

Gastroesophageal Junction Carcinoma

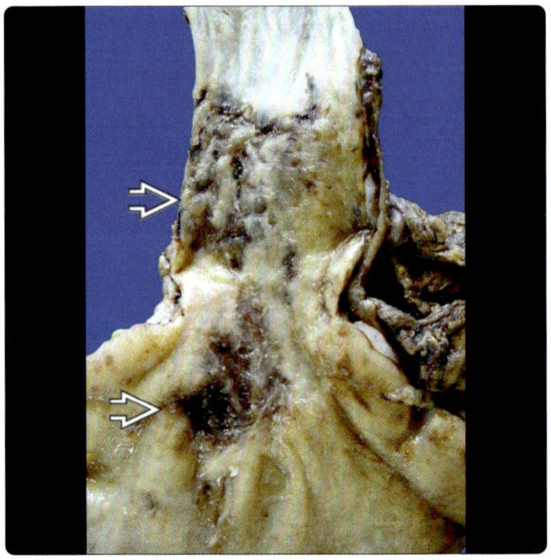

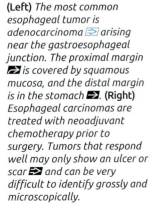

(Left) *The most common esophageal tumor is adenocarcinoma* ⇨ *arising near the gastroesophageal junction. The proximal margin* ➡ *is covered by squamous mucosa, and the distal margin is in the stomach* ➡. **(Right)** *Esophageal carcinomas are treated with neoadjuvant chemotherapy prior to surgery. Tumors that respond well may only show an ulcer or scar* ➡ *and can be very difficult to identify grossly and microscopically.*

- Surgeon should be aware that entire margin has not been examined and that additional sampling on permanent sections could show areas of carcinoma

MOST COMMON DIAGNOSES

Barrett Esophagus

- Normal esophageal squamous mucosa is replaced by metaplastic columnar mucosa
  - Typically appear as tongues of columnar epithelium lining distal esophagus
  - Salmon pink granular columnar mucosa replaces gray-white glistening squamous mucosa
- Neoplastic lesions are grossly visible as nodules or masses or as depressed ulcerated lesions
- Surgeons usually attempt to remove entire Barrett segment at surgery for cancer but may not be feasible in all cases due to length of affected segment

Adenocarcinoma, Tubular Type

- Usually arise in distal esophagus in background of Barrett esophagus
- Gland-forming tumors with variable grades of differentiation

Adenocarcinoma, Signet Ring Cell Type

- Signet ring cell carcinomas are more common in stomach
- Involvement can be difficult to detect grossly and on frozen section
- There are useful features to distinguish signet ring cells from histiocytes and lymphoid cells
  - Clustering of tumor cells
  - Cytoplasmic mucin vacuoles
  - Nuclear hyperchromasia

Squamous Cell Carcinoma

- Usually affect midproximal esophagus
- May be exophytic, ulcerating, or present as stricture
- Surgery preceded by preoperative radiation therapy in most cases
  - Radiation atypia may be difficult to distinguish from dysplasia
- Esophageal margin should be evaluated for dysplasia and invasive carcinoma
  - Some carcinomas are multifocal

Leiomyoma and Gastrointestinal Stromal Tumor

- Incidental leiomyomas and GIST are common in esophagogastrectomy specimens
  - It is not necessary to distinguish between these 2 lesions on frozen section
- Well-circumscribed, tan-gray masses
  - Spindle or epithelioid cells
- Usually deep seated in muscularis
- Margins can be evaluated grossly

Granular Cell Tumor

- Located in submucosa or muscularis propria
  - Borders can be circumscribed or irregular
- Abundant granular pink cytoplasm
- Only rare tumors (< 5%) behave in malignant fashion
  - May have necrosis, spindle cell pattern, nuclear atypia, increased mitoses, and usually large size (> 5 cm)
- Overlying mucosa is intact
  - Pseudoepitheliomatous hyperplasia overlying granular cell tumor can mimic squamous cell carcinoma

REPORTING

Frozen Section

- Margins positive or negative for dysplasia, invasive carcinoma, &/or intestinal metaplasia
- If carcinoma is close to margin, distance from margin is reported

PITFALLS

Carcinoma vs. Treatment-Related Changes

- Many patients are treated with preoperative chemotherapy &/or radiation therapy
- Carcinomas can be difficult to identify
  - Scattered atypical cells in fibrotic tumor bed
  - Mucin pools with scarce or absent tumor cells
- Atypical changes in benign cells can mimic carcinoma
  - Squamous mucosa
    - Radiation atypia appears as large cells with vacuolated cytoplasm
      - Atypia also present in stromal cells
    - Dysplasia shows cells with high nuclear:cytoplasm ratio
  - Endocrine cell clusters
    - Neuroendocrine cells are resistant to treatment and may form small clusters
  - Esophageal ducts and glands
    - Nuclear atypia and squamous metaplasia may mimic cancer invading in wall
  - Stroma
    - Nuclear atypia in fibroblasts
    - Thickened blood vessels
  - Adventitial skeletal muscle
    - Degenerating skeletal muscle may mimic cancer
      - However, cells are generally multinucleated
    - Located in perimuscular adventitial tissue; associated with areas of more recognizable muscle
- Tumor bed at margin
  - Foci of necrosis, calcification, and fibrosis or acellular mucin pools seen in cases with complete response to therapy

False-Negative Margin

- Carcinoma deep in submucosa or muscularis propria can be missed if full-thickness section is not taken

SELECTED REFERENCES

1. Spicer J et al: Diagnostic accuracy and utility of intraoperative microscopic margin analysis of gastric and esophageal adenocarcinoma. Ann Surg Oncol. 21(8):2580-6, 2014
2. Chennat J et al: Advanced pathology under squamous epithelium on initial EMR specimens in patients with Barrett's esophagus and high-grade dysplasia or intramucosal carcinoma: implications for surveillance and endotherapy management. Gastrointest Endosc. 70(3):417-21, 2009
3. Prasad GA et al: Significance of neoplastic involvement of margins obtained by endoscopic mucosal resection in Barrett's esophagus. Am J Gastroenterol. 102(11):2380-6, 2007

Esophageal Adenocarcinoma

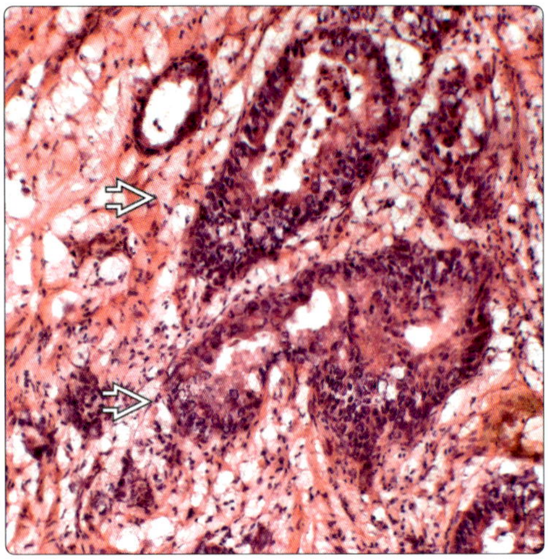

Esophageal Adenocarcinoma

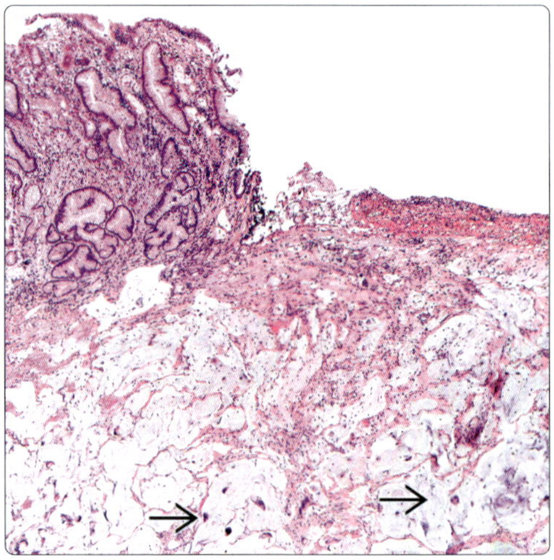

(Left) *The most common type of esophageal adenocarcinoma resembles colonic adenocarcinoma* ➡ *and is well or moderately differentiated. Signet ring cell carcinoma and mucinous carcinoma are less common types. Barrett mucosa is frequently present.* **(Right)** *Esophageal carcinomas are often treated with neoadjuvant chemoradiation therapy. The residual adenocarcinoma may consist of only large mucin pools with scattered viable tumor cells* → *in the tumor bed.*

Squamous Cell Carcinoma

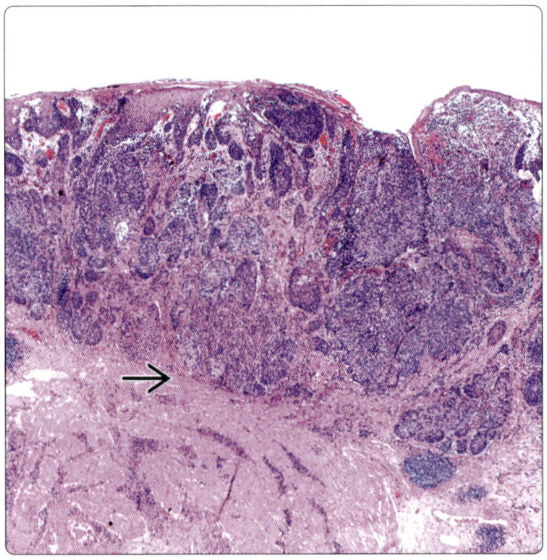

Squamous High-Grade Dysplasia

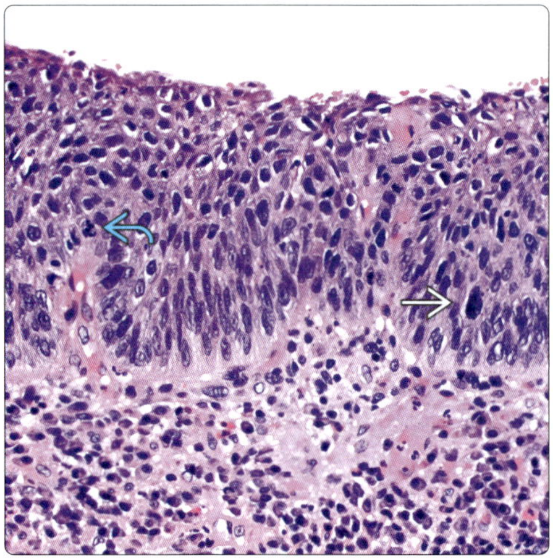

(Left) *Squamous cell carcinomas are the 2nd most common type of esophageal cancer. They occur at any site but are more common in the proximal esophagus. This carcinoma is invasive into the muscularis propria* →*.* **(Right)** *Squamous dysplasia or carcinoma in situ are often associated with squamous cell carcinomas. There is an absence of maturation, high nuclear:cytoplasmic ratio, pleomorphic nuclei* ➡*, and easily identified mitotic figures* ↪*.*

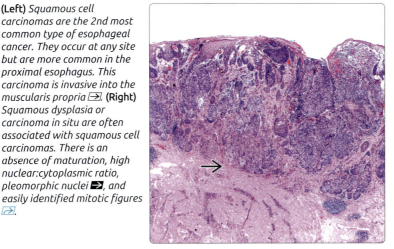

Squamous Cell Carcinoma

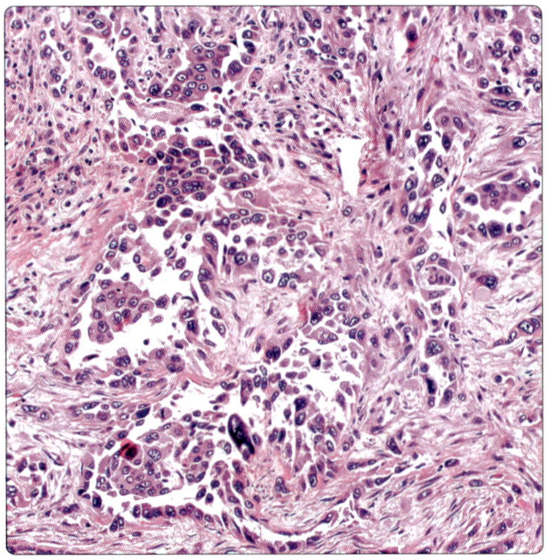

Verrucous Squamous Cell Carcinoma

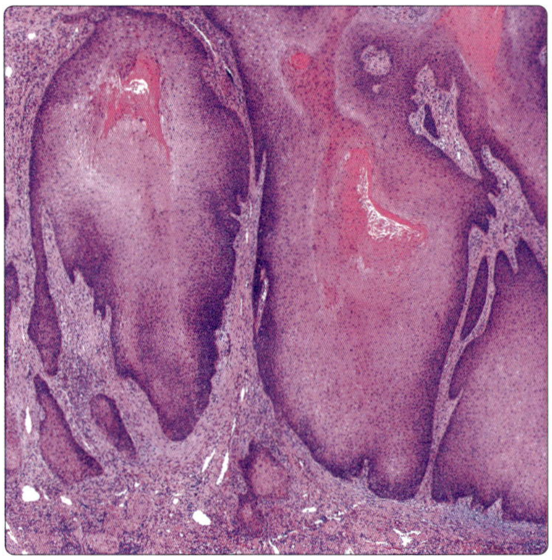

(Left) *Some squamous cell carcinomas show central acantholysis, resulting in a pseudoglandular pattern that may be mistaken for an adenocarcinoma. Keratinized cells with deep eosinophilic cytoplasm are helpful to recognize the cells as squamous.* **(Right)** *Verrucous squamous cell carcinoma is a rare esophageal tumor that forms a wart-like, exophytic mass on endoscopy. It is difficult to diagnose preoperatively, as superficial biopsies may not show atypia. The carcinoma invades along a broad pushing front.*

Signet Ring Cell Carcinoma

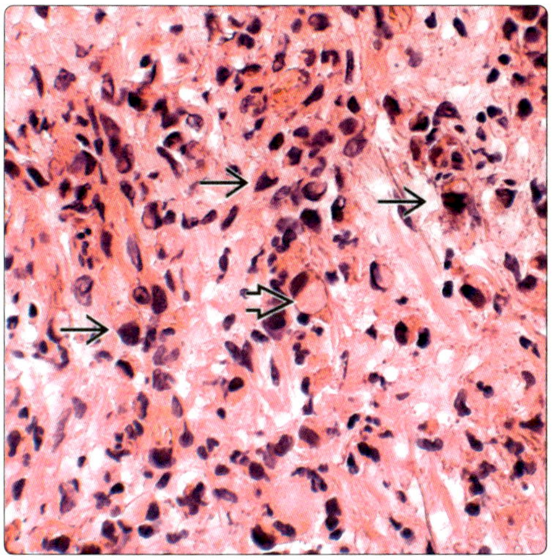

Esophageal Margin

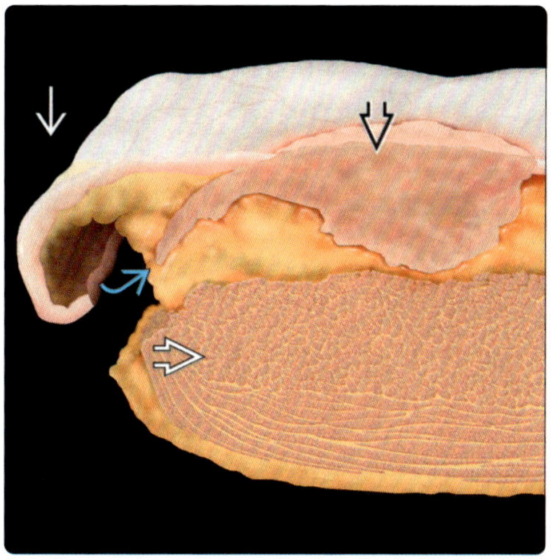

(Left) *Signet ring cells* ➡ *can be difficult to recognize on frozen section due to bland nuclei and single cell infiltration. Clustering of cells, cytoplasmic mucin, and nuclear hyperchromasia* ➡ *are helpful to distinguish them from histiocytes and lymphoid cells.* **(Right)** *The muscularis* ➡ *retracts after being cut, resulting in the squamous mucosa curling over the edge of the proximal margin* ➡*. If only the normal mucosa is taken for frozen section, invasive carcinoma* ➡ *invading in the submucosa* ➡ *can be missed at the margin.*

Signet Ring Cell Carcinoma: Lymph-Vascular Invasion

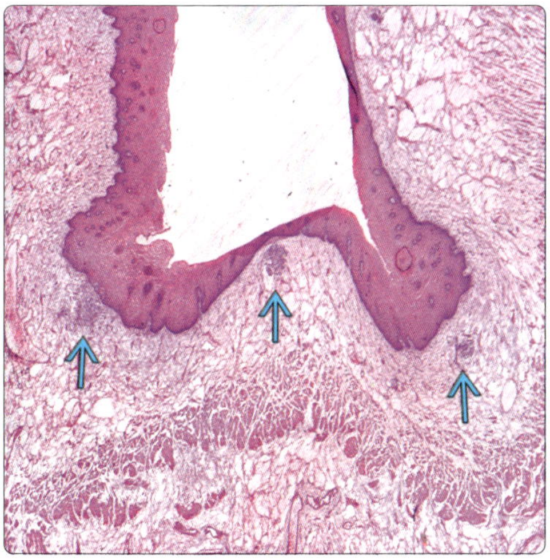

Esophagus: Positive Margin in Submucosa

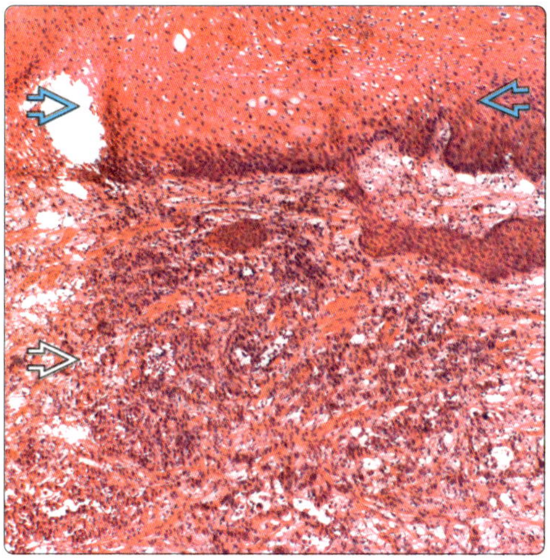

(Left) *The proximal margin of resection may be positive due to extensive lymph-vascular invasion by tumor cells* ➡*. In such cases, systemic dissemination is likely, and taking an additional margin is unlikely to impact patient outcome.* **(Right)** *Invasive carcinoma may be present* ➡ *beneath normal overlying mucosa* ➡*. Full-thickness sections are important to avoid false-negative diagnosis.*

Esophagus: Positive Margin in Submucosa

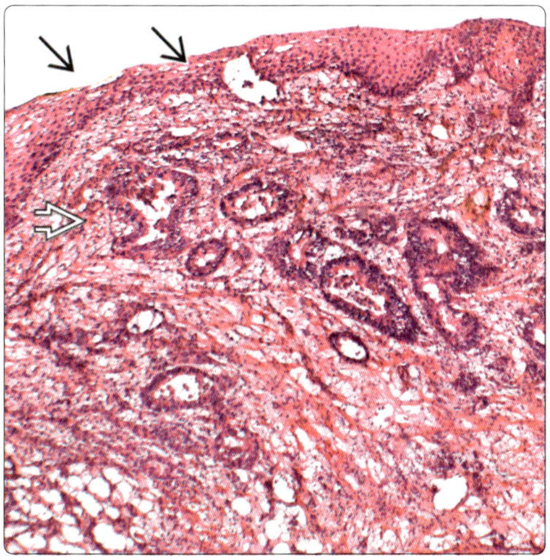

Esophagus: Positive Margin in Muscularis

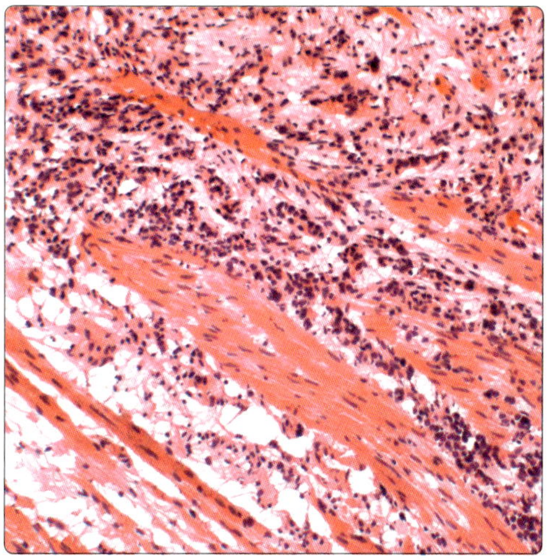

(Left) *The overlying squamous mucosa* ➡ *would appear grossly normal at this margin. However, adenocarcinoma* ➡ *is present invading below the mucosa, and the margin is positive in this en face section.* **(Right)** *Carcinomas can be present at the margin in the muscularis propria. It is important for the margin section to be full thickness and not just include the mucosa and submucosa.*

(Left) *Esophageal carcinomas are often treated with preoperative chemotherapy or radiation therapy. The remaining tumor bed may consist of a subtle area of fibrosis or ulceration* ⇒. *Residual carcinoma at the margin may be difficult to identify.* **(Right)** *A carcinoma with a marked response to chemotherapy often consists of scattered foci of residual tumor cells* ⇒ *in the submucosa. If the tumor bed is present at the margin, it should be reported, as this may not be predictive of a true negative margin.*

Tumor Bed After Neoadjuvant Therapy: Gross Appearance

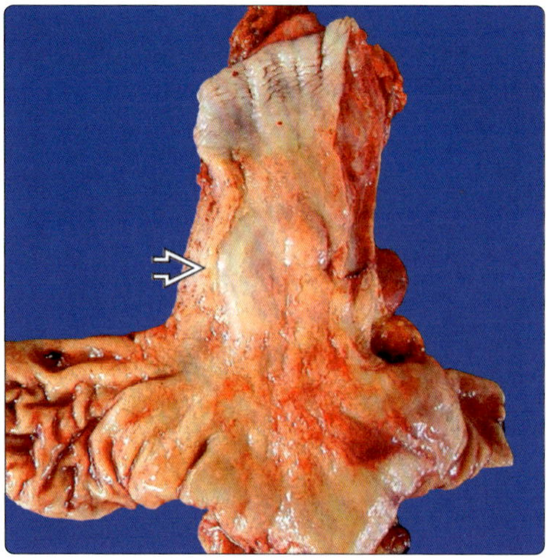

Esophageal Carcinoma After Neoadjuvant Therapy

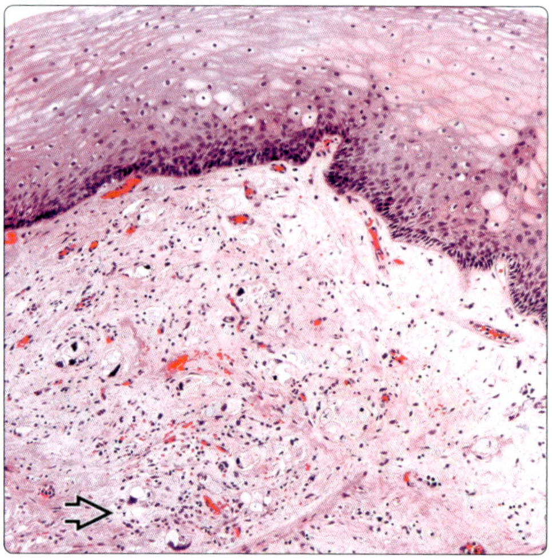

(Left) *Carcinoma after neoadjuvant therapy often shows marked cytoplasmic vacuolation* ↪, *and the cells may be mistaken for macrophages intermingled with other inflammatory cells in the tumor bed. The marked nuclear hyperchromasia* ⇒ *helps in correctly identifying the cells as residual carcinoma.* **(Right)** *Residual carcinoma* ↪ *may be present as scattered cells deep in the muscularis propria* ⇒ *at the proximal margin and can be easily missed if a full-thickness section is not examined carefully.*

Esophageal Carcinoma After Neoadjuvant Therapy

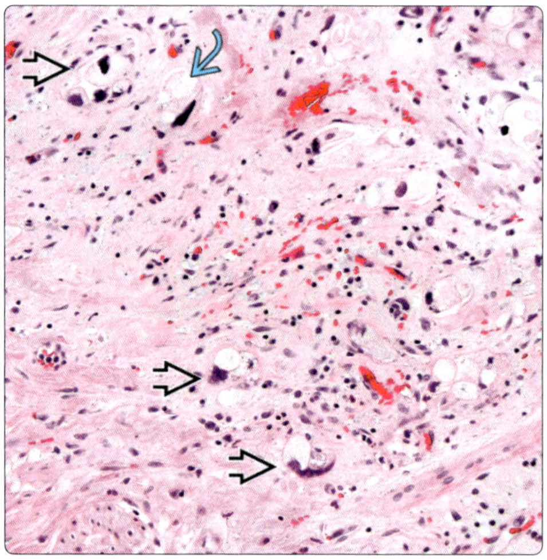

Esophageal Carcinoma After Neoadjuvant Therapy

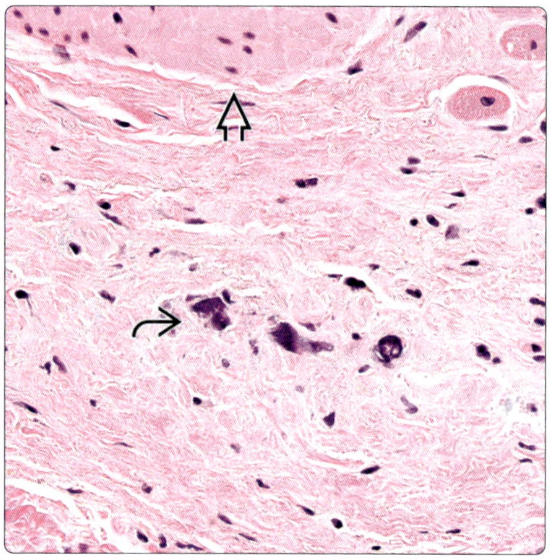

(Left) *Endocrine cells are resistant to chemoradiation effect and persist as clusters* → *in the mucosa at the tumor site. These cells may be mistaken for residual tumor on frozen section.* **(Right)** *Degenerating skeletal muscle* ⇒ *as a result of neoadjuvant treatment can be mistaken for residual tumor. The nuclei migrate to the center of the cells and are hyperchromatic. Clues to identifying these cells as muscle cells are the presence of multiple nuclei and location adjacent to normal muscle* →*.*

Neoadjuvant Therapy: Endocrine Cell Clusters

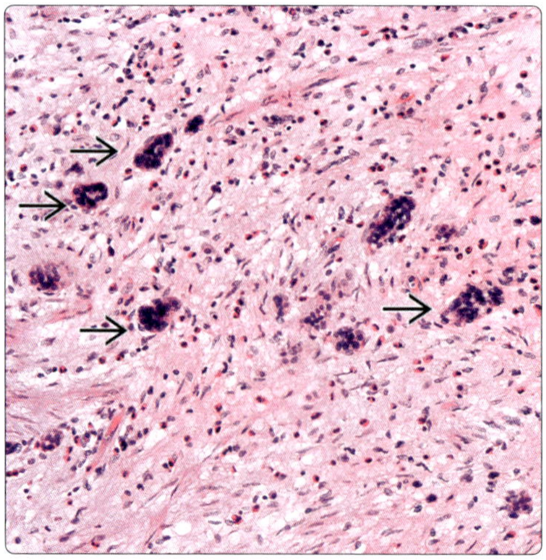

Neoadjuvant Therapy: Degenerating Skeletal Muscle

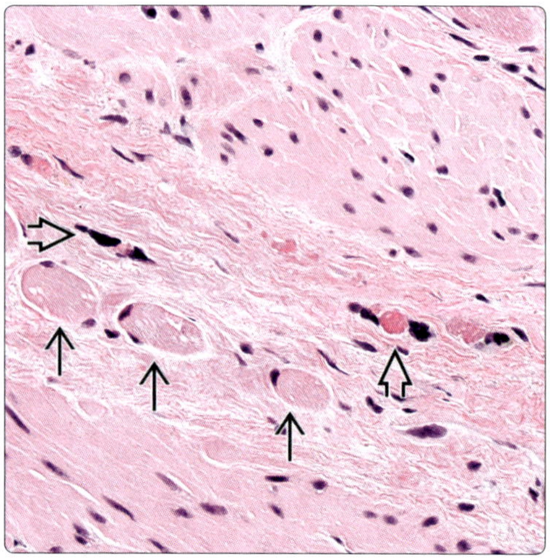

Esophageal Duct

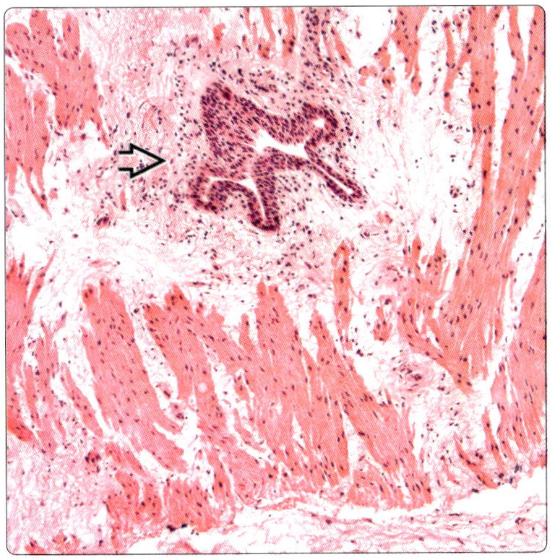

Neoadjuvant Therapy: Esophageal Duct

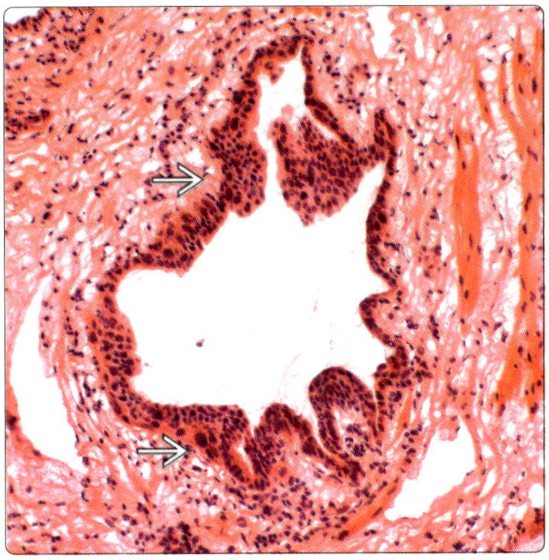

(Left) *A benign normal esophageal duct* ⇨ *is present within the muscularis. The presence of a glandular structure in this location could be mistaken for invasive carcinoma.* **(Right)** *Therapy can cause nuclear atypia* ➡ *and squamous metaplasia in esophageal ducts. These changes may be mistaken for residual carcinoma, particularly when seen in a glandular structure in the wall of the esophagus.*

Barrett Esophagus

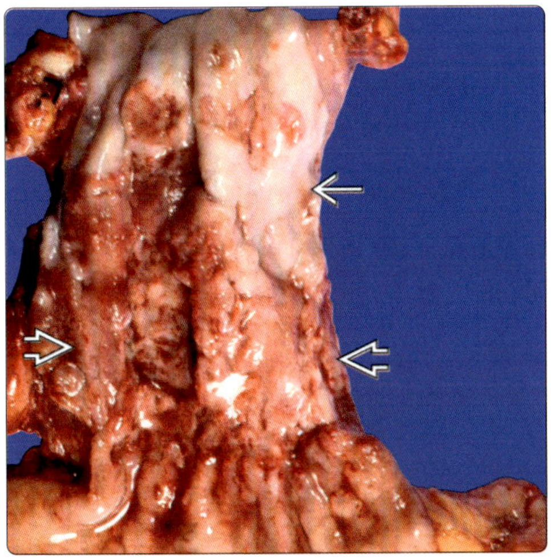

Granular Cell Tumor

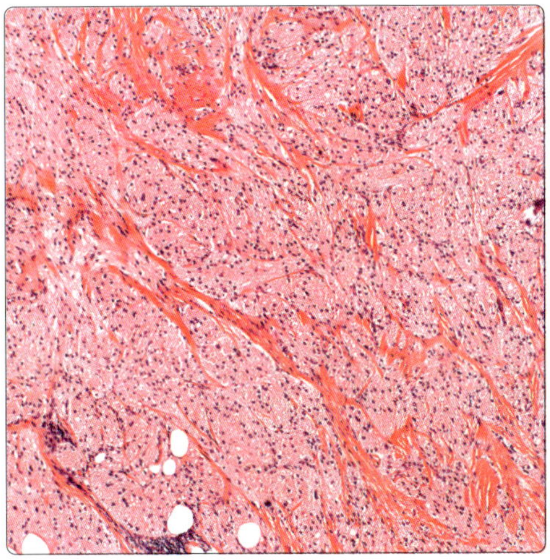

(Left) *The normal pearly gray esophageal squamous mucosa* ➡ *is replaced by pink, granular columnar mucosa* ⇨ *in Barrett esophagus.* **(Right)** *Granular cell tumors show abundant granular eosinophilic cytoplasm and nuclei with open chromatin and prominent nucleoli. Reactive squamous cell changes in the mucosa above a granular cell tumor can mimic invasive squamous cell carcinoma.*

Leiomyoma

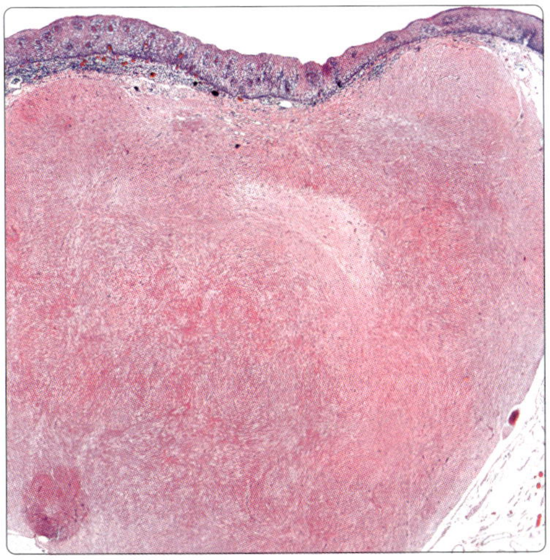

Leiomyoma

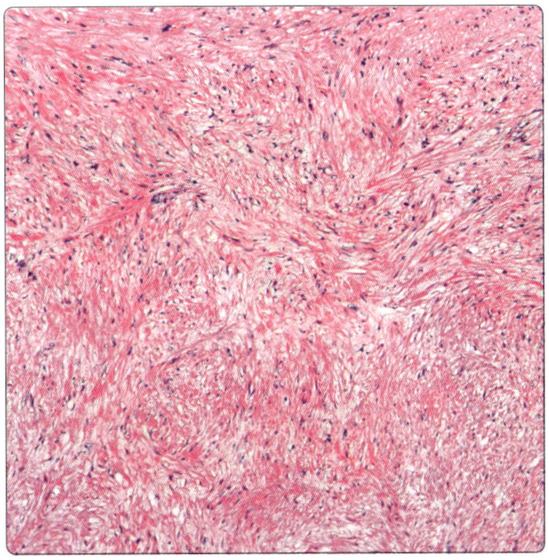

(Left) *Leiomyomas form circumscribed submucosal masses. Gastrointestinal stromal tumor also occurs in the esophagus but is less common. The final classification is not important for intraoperative consultation.* **(Right)** *Leiomyomas consist of fascicles of bland-appearing smooth muscle cells. Nuclear pleomorphism and mitoses should not be seen.*

SURGICAL/CLINICAL CONSIDERATIONS

Goal of Consultation

- Determine if mass-forming lesion of fallopian tube is benign or malignant
- Diagnose suspected tubal pregnancies by identifying products of conception

Change in Patient Management

- Additional biopsies may be taken for staging if carcinoma is present
- If ectopic pregnancy is present, salpingectomy or salpingotomy is performed
  - Additional surgical exploration is not necessary to identify alternative sites

Clinical Setting

- Vast majority of serous carcinomas arise in fimbriae of fallopian tubes
  - Women with *BRCA1* or *BRCA2* or *TP53* (Li-Fraumeni syndrome) germline mutations are at high risk
    - ~ 10% will be diagnosed with occult carcinoma
  - Tubal carcinoma is difficult to diagnose preoperatively
    - Inflammatory conditions are more common than malignancy
- Women with elevated hCG levels, but without documented intrauterine pregnancy, may have ectopic pregnancy
  - Rupture and hemorrhage can be life threatening
  - Majority of cases are diagnosed by ultrasound and managed conservatively
  - In rare cases, clinical evaluation is inconclusive, and intraoperative examination may be helpful

SPECIMEN EVALUATION

Gross

- Describe size (length and diameter) and presence, absence, or obliteration of fimbriated end
  - Tubal carcinomas typically arise within fimbriae
    - Close inspection for adhesions, discoloration, or masses is critical
    - Fusion or loss of fimbriae within adnexal mass is suggestive of serous carcinoma
- Patency of lumen is determined with probe
  - Plastic ring may be present if there has been prior tubal ligation
- Serosal surface is described
  - Normal: Smooth and glistening
  - Adhesions: Rough surface and attached tissue
  - Masses
  - Paratubal cysts
  - Purulent or fibrinous exudates
  - Rupture
- For tubes removed as part of prophylactic salpingectomy
  - If grossly normal or if only cysts are present, fixation without sectioning is recommended
    - Likelihood of diagnosing carcinoma is very small
    - Detection of precursor lesions and small carcinomas may be compromised unless specimen is optimally fixed and processed for permanent sections
  - If solid nodule > 0.5 cm is present and small, representative portion can be sampled, frozen section may be appropriate
    - Frozen section should only be performed if surgeon will perform additional staging procedures if carcinoma is diagnosed
- If mass is present within ampulla or isthmus of tube
  - Make serial cross sections of tube; note any tubal contents
    - Purulent exudate
    - Hemorrhage
    - Placental or fetal tissue with membranes
    - Masses
    - Areas of firmness or discoloration

Frozen Section

- In general, frozen section diagnosis of small (< 5 mm) lesions of tube is contraindicated
- If there is larger solid mass, small portion may be frozen to determine if carcinoma is present

(Left) *The normal fallopian tube is divided into the isthmus (adjacent to the uterus) ➩, infundibulum ➩, ampulla ➩, and fimbriae ➩. The lumen should be patent and the fimbriae thin and delicate.* **(Right)** *The classic gross description of tubal carcinoma is of massive tubal dilation ➩ and fusion of the fimbriae ➩, the so-called sausage tube.*

Normal Fallopian Tube

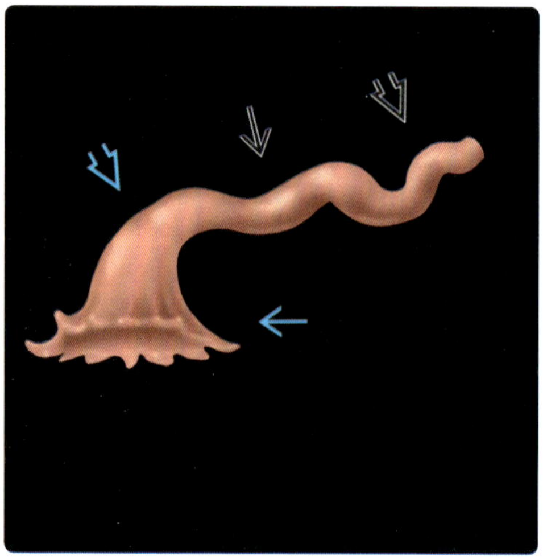

Fallopian Tube Carcinoma

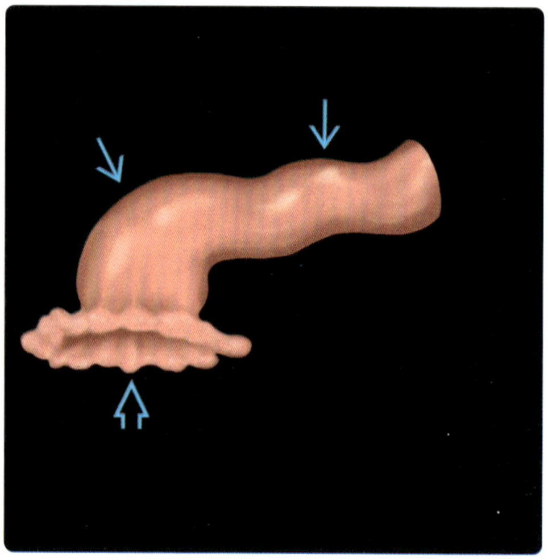

- In absence of mass, frozen section should not be undertaken
  - Lesions should never be entirely frozen
- Tubes without solid gross lesions should be evaluated on permanent sections
- Cysts and grossly normal tissue are highly unlikely to yield sufficient findings for diagnosis of malignancy

- In setting of suspected ectopic pregnancies, areas of hemorrhage and blood clot often contain products of conception if they are not readily evident
  - Frozen section can be helpful to document placental or fetal tissues

MOST COMMON DIAGNOSES

Serous Lesions

- Serous lesions can be in situ or invasive
- **Serous tubal intraepithelial carcinoma (STIC)**
  - In isolation, STIC is unlikely to be identified grossly
    - Lacks invasion into underlying stroma
  - STIC may be seen in areas adjacent to mass-forming invasive carcinoma
    - Supports origin as primary tubal carcinoma vs. carcinoma arising in ovary, peritoneum, or endometrium
  - Identified at low power by irregular epithelial thickness with exfoliation of tumor cells
    - High nuclear:cytoplasmic ratio and loss of cilia
  - Nuclei show marked pleomorphism
    - Enlarged nuclei with prominent nucleoli
    - Loss of nuclear polarity
    - Frequent mitoses
    - Hyperchromasia
    - Apoptotic bodies common
  - Histologic features should recapitulate those seen in invasive serous carcinoma
  - May require supportive immunohistochemical studies for p53 and Ki-67 for diagnosis
- **Invasive serous carcinoma**
  - Grossly may present as fimbrial masses or adhesion to ovary
    - Occasionally may occupy entire tube, resulting in sausage-like gross appearance
  - 90% of fallopian tube carcinomas are serous
    - 3-20% are bilateral
    - Most common in women in their 40s-60s
  - Similar histologic features as STIC but with invasion into underlying stroma
  - Frequently associated with lymph-vascular invasion, which may be identified on frozen sections

Adenomatoid Tumor

- Most common benign tumor of fallopian tube and broad ligament
  - Small, tan-white nodule on serosal surface
    - Frozen section is unnecessary and should be avoided
  - Histologically may be complex
    - Small pseudoglandular spaces
    - Lined by flat to cuboidal cells
      - Occasional pleomorphism can be present
    - Stroma composed of smooth muscle and hyalinized connective tissue

Ectopic Pregnancy

- Most common implantation site for ectopic pregnancy is fallopian tube
  - Unusual sites are ovary, abdomen, cervix, or caesarean section scar
  - Increased risk is associated with endometriosis, pelvic inflammatory disease, and prior surgery
- 87-99% of tubal pregnancies can be diagnosed by transvaginal ultrasound
  - Very rare that ultrasound examination does not document ectopic implantation after positive pregnancy test
  - Termed pregnancy of unknown location (PUL)
- Many women are treated medically with methotrexate
- Surgical treatment can be by salpingotomy or salpingectomy
  - Intraoperative evaluation may be useful for cases with unclear clinical and imaging characteristics
  - Grossly may appear as swollen tube with vascular congestion, hemorrhage, or perforation
  - Presence of fetal villi, gestational sac, implantation site, or embryonic parts is diagnostic
- Areas of hemorrhage and blood clot may yield diagnostic tissue
  - Placental and fetal tissues may not be grossly evident

Infarction

- Edematous, hemorrhagic tube grossly
- Widespread hemorrhagic necrosis commonly present microscopically

Transitional Cell Lesions

- Transitional cell metaplasia
  - Also termed Walthard nests
  - Common benign finding; not proven to be precursor lesion
  - Gross appearance is of multiple small (0.1 to 0.2 cm) nodules on serosal surface near isthmus
    - Frozen section is unnecessary and should be avoided
- Transitional cell carcinoma
  - 10% of primary fallopian tube carcinomas
  - Most common in women in their 40s-50s
  - Increased risk in women with *BRCA1* or *BRCA2* mutations
  - Histologic appearance is similar to urinary tract transitional carcinomas
    - Solid and papillary sheet-like growth
    - High-grade nuclei
    - Frequent mitoses
  - Are thought to represent a histologic variant of serous carcinoma (solid, endometrioid, and transitional-type (SET) tumors)

Inflammatory Conditions

- Can be associated with endometriosis, pelvic inflammatory disease, and chronic endometritis
  - Risk factor for ectopic pregnancy
  - Usually bilateral
  - Some cancers are associated with inflammation and abscess formation

- May be caused by tuberculosis, actinomycosis, coccidioidomycosis, Crohn disease, or sarcoidosis
- Can result in tubal mass &/or distension and thickening of tubal plicae, mimicking carcinoma
- Chronic active salpingitis can result in salpingitis follicularis
    - Fused plicae due to fibrin deposition result in follicle-like structures

Salpingitis Isthmica Nodosa

- Diverticular disease of tubes
    - Surrounded by smooth muscle
    - Only mild inflammation
- Grossly appears as yellow-white nodules near isthmus
    - Frozen section is unnecessary and should be avoided

Mesonephric Remnant of Broad Ligament

- May form smooth nodule in wall of tube
- Composed of small tubules with low columnar to cuboidal cells
    - Lack cilia
- Surrounded by prominent smooth muscle
- May have cystic component
- Frozen section is unnecessary and should be avoided

Leiomyoma

- Can form smooth nodules in wall of fallopian tube
- Formed of bland spindle-shaped smooth muscle cells
- Frozen section is unnecessary and should be avoided

REPORTING

Gross Evaluation

- Grossly normal tubes or tubes with only small cystic or solid nodules (< 5 mm) may be reported as such
    - Further processing and diagnosis should be deferred to permanent sections

Frozen Section

- Report "invasive serous carcinoma, high grade" when serous carcinoma is identified
- STIC is difficult if not impossible to diagnose by frozen section
    - Report "severe tubal atypia" with explanation of the features that are present and defer final diagnosis to permanent sections
- Report "tubal ectopic pregnancy" when identifiable products of conception are present

PITFALLS

Transitional Cell Metaplasia

- May mimic tubal intraepithelial carcinoma due to increased epithelial thickness and increased nuclear density
- Lesions consist of bland cells with streaming nuclei oriented perpendicularly to epithelial base
- Pleomorphism and mitotic activity should be absent

Endometriosis

- Endometrial glands and stroma present in lumen or within tubal wall
- Endometriosis may form mass or areas of extensive hemorrhage mimicking neoplasm or possible ectopic pregnancy

Metastasis

- Metastatic adenocarcinoma (usually colonic, appendiceal, or ovarian) may mimic primary malignancy
    - Mucin production and colonization of epithelium is typically present
- Clinical history of prior malignancy is important for final classification

SELECTED REFERENCES

1. Savelli L et al: Misdiagnosed ectopic pregnancy mimicking adnexal malignancy: a report of two cases. Ultrasound Obstet Gynecol. 41(2):223-5, 2013
2. Vang R et al: Fallopian tube precursors of ovarian low- and high-grade serous neoplasms. Histopathology. 62(1):44-58, 2013
3. Elsokkari I et al: Primary transitional cell carcinoma of the fallopian tube. J Obstet Gynaecol Res. 37(11):1767-71, 2011
4. Rabban JT et al: Correlation of macroscopic and microscopic pathology in risk reducing salpingo-oophorectomy: implications for intraoperative specimen evaluation. Gynecol Oncol. 121(3):466-71, 2011
5. Yener N et al: Xanthogranulomatous salpingitis as a rare pathologic aspect of chronic active pelvic inflammatory disease. Indian J Pathol Microbiol. 54(1):141-3, 2011
6. Kocak M et al: Primary and bilateral tubal carcinoma is associated with long-standing granulomatous inflammation and primary infertility: a case report. J Obstet Gynaecol Res. 36(4):912-5, 2010
7. Nama V et al: Tubal ectopic pregnancy: diagnosis and management. Arch Gynecol Obstet. 279(4):443-53, 2009
8. Rabban JT et al: Multistep level sections to detect occult fallopian tube carcinoma in risk-reducing salpingo-oophorectomies from women with BRCA mutations: implications for defining an optimal specimen dissection protocol. Am J Surg Pathol. 33(12):1878-85, 2009
9. Rabban JT et al: Transitional cell metaplasia of fallopian tube fimbriae: a potential mimic of early tubal carcinoma in risk reduction salpingo-oophorectomies from women With BRCA mutations. Am J Surg Pathol. 33(1):111-9, 2009
10. Callahan MJ et al: Primary fallopian tube malignancies in BRCA-positive women undergoing surgery for ovarian cancer risk reduction. J Clin Oncol. 25(25):3985-90, 2007
11. Verit FF et al: Primary carcinoma of the fallopian tube mimicking tubo-ovarian abscess. Eur J Gynaecol Oncol. 26(2):225-6, 2005

Early Tubal Carcinoma

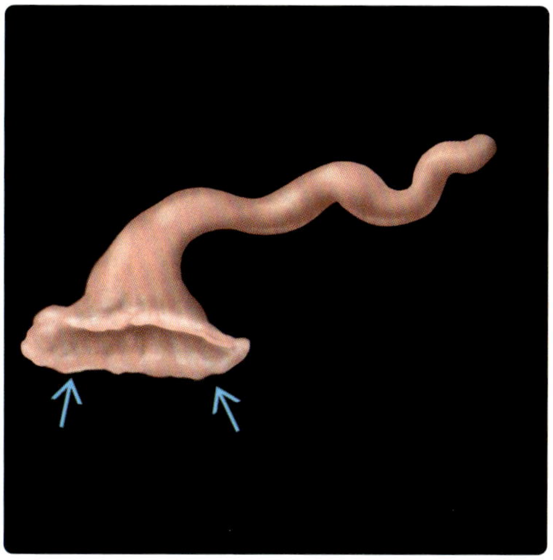

Tubal Intraepithelial Carcinoma

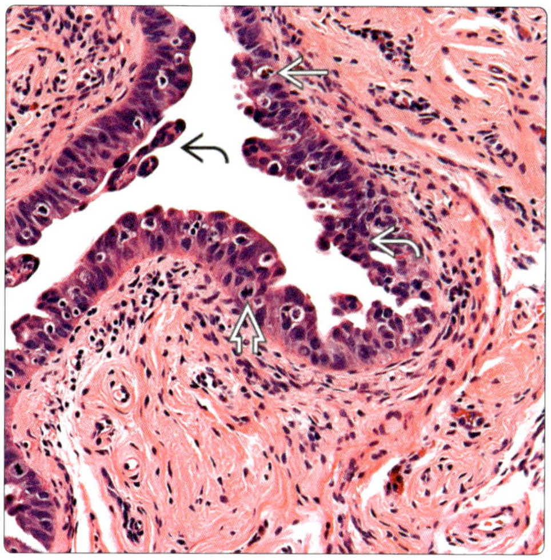

(Left) *Early tubal carcinoma may present as fusion of the fimbriae* ➙ *or as a distinct, yet small, mass arising from the fimbriae.* **(Right)** *Tubal intraepithelial carcinoma displays nuclear crowding, loss of nuclear polarity* ➙*, apoptotic bodies* ➙*, and cellular exfoliation* ➙*. Scattered mitotic figures are identifiable* ➙*. Lesions such as this may be present in grossly normal-appearing fallopian tube fimbriae. This is a diagnosis made best on permanent sections.*

Serous Carcinoma: Gross Appearance

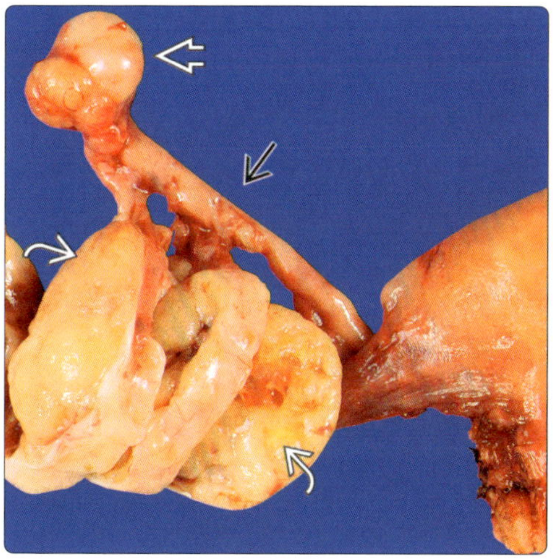

Early Serous Carcinoma

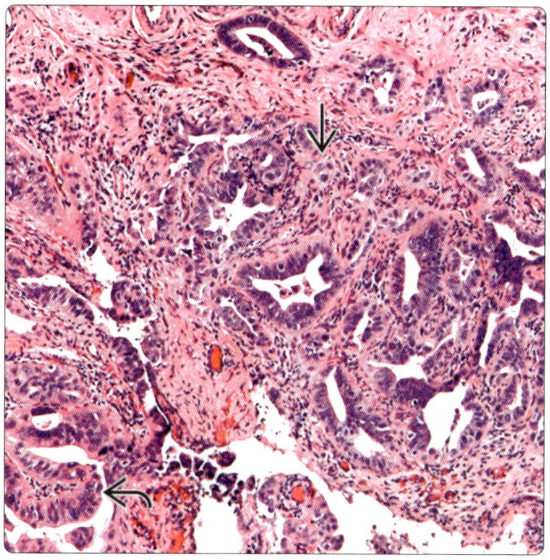

(Left) *This fallopian tube* ➙ *has abnormal fimbrial enlargement and adhesions* ➙*, indicating a possible tubal primary carcinoma. The fimbriae of the tube should be closely examined for gross abnormalities such as this in all surgical resections. In this case, the ovary is enlarged* ➙ *and may also be involved by carcinoma.* **(Right)** *Early serous carcinoma often cannot be appreciated grossly. The presence of focal stromal invasion* ➙ *necessitates the diagnosis of serous carcinoma. Often, a tubal intraepithelial lesion* ➙ *is present.*

Serous Carcinoma

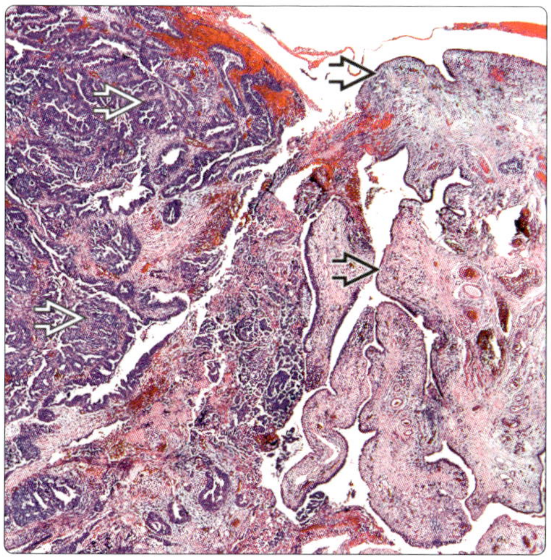

Serous Carcinoma

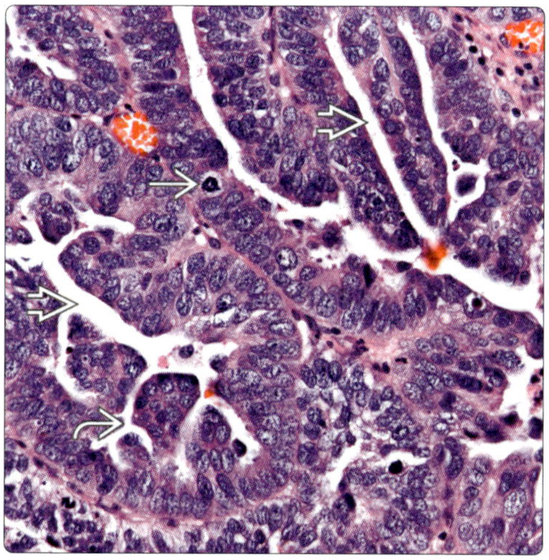

(Left) *Invasive serous carcinoma* ➙ *can be difficult to identify as ovarian or tubal by imaging. In this case, the carcinoma is adjacent to atrophic fallopian tube fimbriae* ➙*.* **(Right)** *High-grade serous carcinoma is characterized by papillary or pseudopapillary structures. Glandular spaces are often slit-like* ➙ *as opposed to round. Epithelial crevasses* ➙ *are often present due to tufting. Numerous mitotic figures* ➙ *are present as well as nuclear pleomorphism.*

(Left) *An ectopic pregnancy can be a medical emergency and is identified by immature placental villi and implantation site within a fallopian tube. Fimbriae underlie the implantation site.* **(Right)** *In the absence of villi and embryonic tissue, the presence of implantation site trophoblasts in the wall of a fallopian tube is sufficient for the diagnosis of an ectopic gestation.*

Tubal Ectopic Pregnancy

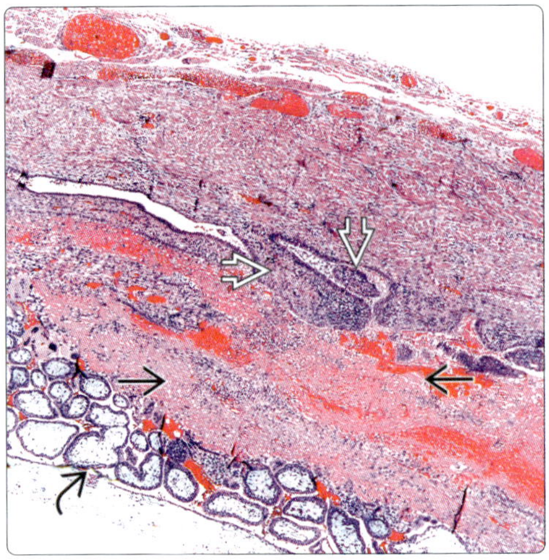

Tubal Ectopic Pregnancy

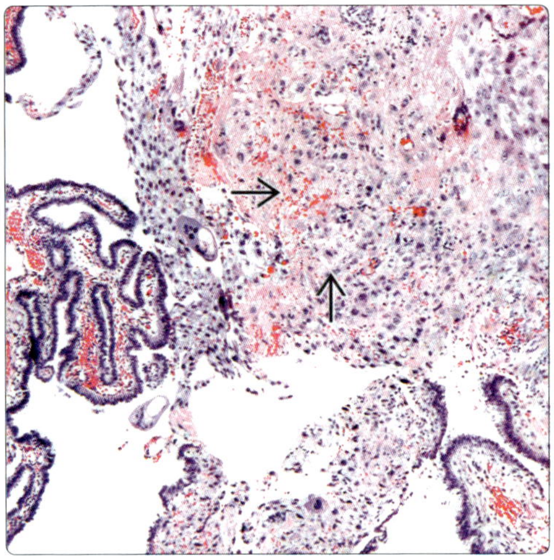

(Left) *Transitional metaplasia of the tubal epithelium, a common benign finding, can cause thickening of the epithelium and may mimic serous intraepithelial carcinoma. The lack of epithelial tufting and tumor cell exfoliation are helpful histologic features in ruling out carcinoma.* **(Right)** *Transitional metaplasia of the tube shows nuclear streaming oriented perpendicular to the epithelial base. Note the conspicuous lack of pleomorphism, loss of nuclear polarity, or mitotic activity.*

Transitional Metaplasia

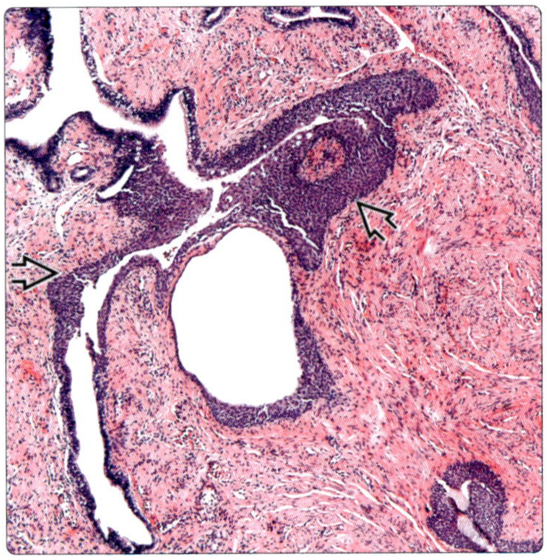

Transitional Metaplasia

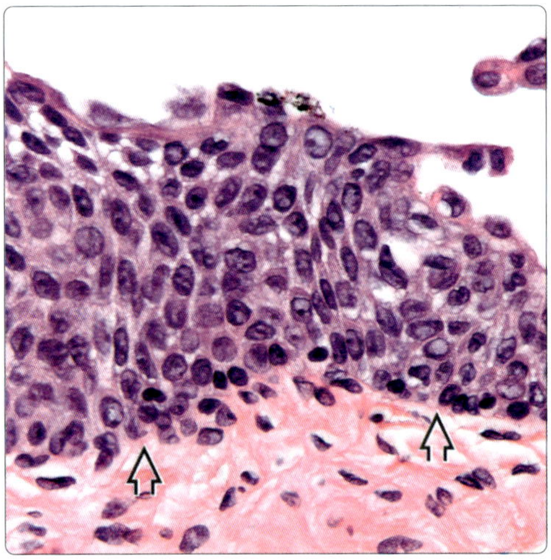

(Left) *Endometrial glands & stroma within the tubal lumen or wall of the tube characterize endometriosis. Abundant hemorrhage is present within the lumen. In this case, the endometrial stroma has extensive pseudodecidual change secondary to treatment with progestins.* **(Right)** *Acute &/or chronic salpingitis often causes thickening of the fallopian tube that may be associated with marked edema, congestion, and fibrin deposition with secondary hydrosalpinx. (From DP: Gynecological.)*

Endometriosis

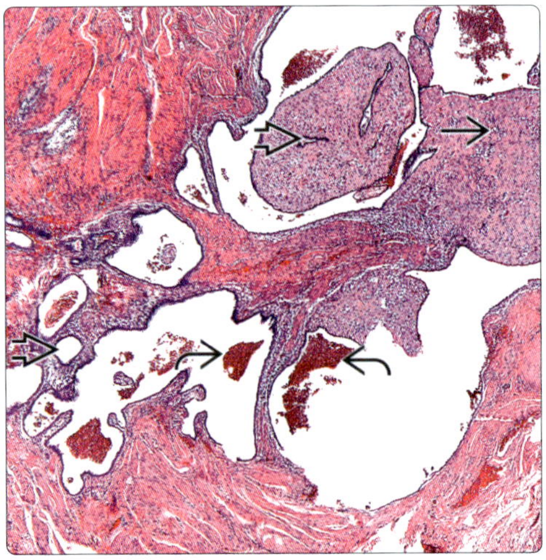

Salpingitis: Gross Appearance

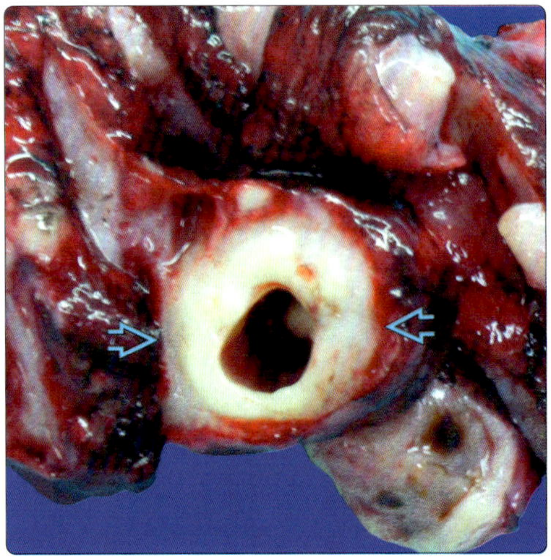

Pseudoxanthomatous Salpingitis

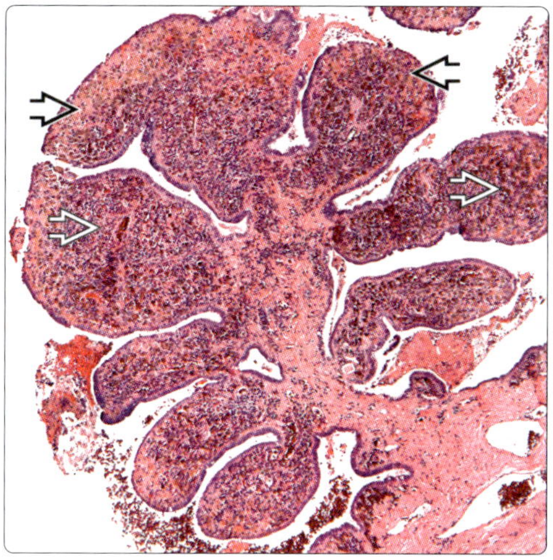

Chronic Salpingitis

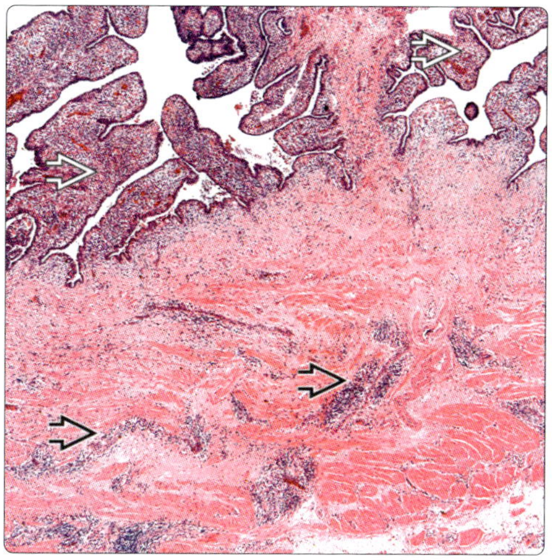

(Left) *Pseudoxanthomatous salpingitis is another cause of tubal wall thickening and edema. Examination of the tube will often yield an intense lymphohistiocytic infiltrate filling the plica ➡ and the wall of the tube. These histiocytes are often full of hemosiderin ➡, which appear brown at low power.* **(Right)** *In chronic salpingitis, aggregates of lymphocytes ➡ and lymphoid follicles may be seen within the wall of the tube and plica ➡. This may cause thickening and dilation and may be concerning for malignancy.*

Mesonephric Remnants, Cysts, and Rests

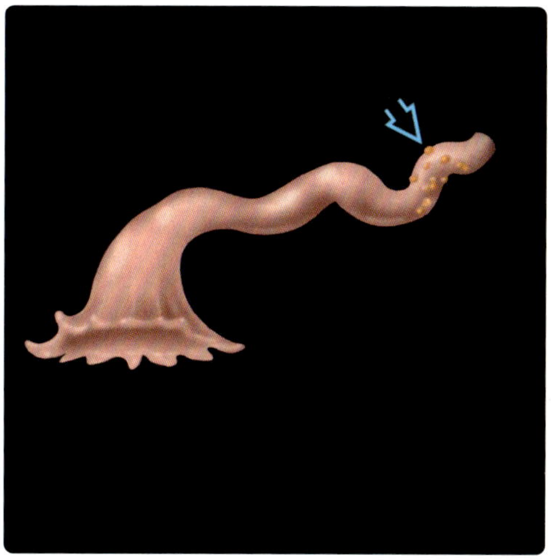

Mesonephric Remnants

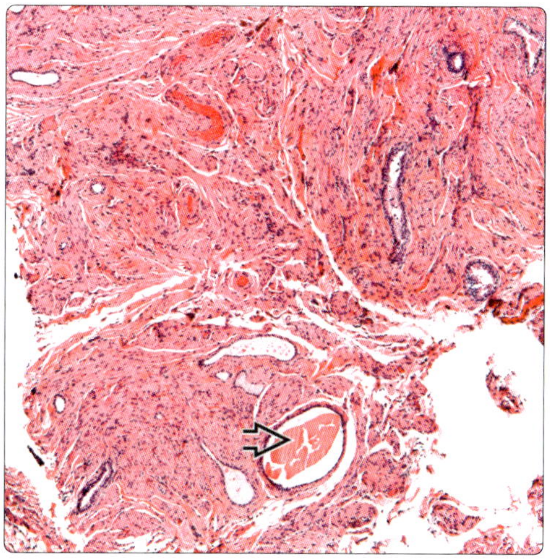

(Left) *Mesonephric remnants that become cystically dilated, small paratubal cysts, and other epithelial rests, such as Walthard rests, may appear as small, clear to yellow nodules ➡ scattered across the serosal surface of the tube.* **(Right)** *Mesonephric remnants may be seen in the paratubal tissue. They are lined by simple cuboidal, nonciliated epithelium. They may become cystic and contain eosinophilic fluid ➡.*

Leiomyoma and Adenomatoid Tumor

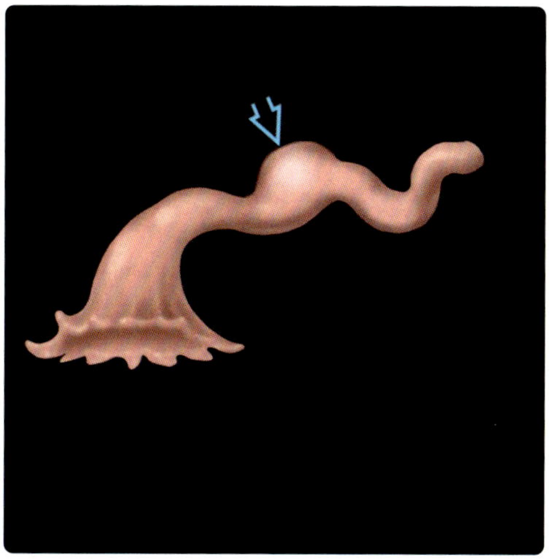

Adenomatoid Tumor

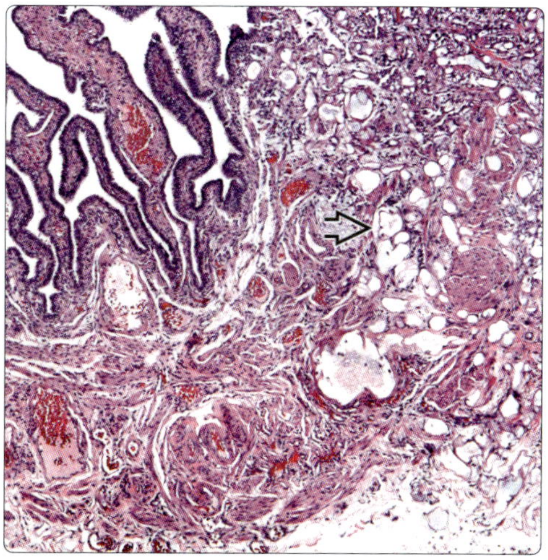

(Left) *Mesenchymal masses, such as adenomatoid tumor (the most common benign tumor of the fallopian tube) and leiomyoma, often present as an eccentric subserosal mass ➡.* **(Right)** *This adenomatoid tumor is adjacent to a tubal lumen. The tumor has small cystic spaces ➡ that may appear gland-like or signet ring-like. The spaces are lined by bland, flat to cuboidal mesothelial cells.*

SURGICAL/CLINICAL CONSIDERATIONS

Goal of Consultation

- Determine if malignancy or dysplasia is present
- Determine if invasive tumor &/or dysplasia has been completely excised

Change in Patient Management

- Malignancies may be excised or treated with radiation therapy
- Multiple biopsies may be used to map extent of tumor &/or dysplasia and determine how much tissue to excise
  - Additional tissue may be resected to achieve tumor-free margins
- In patients with nodal metastases and no known primary tumor, additional biopsies may be obtained if tumor is not identified initially

Clinical Setting

- Presenting symptoms may be mass, ulceration, pain, or difficulty with speech or swallowing
- Some patients present with nodal neck metastases and no known primary
  - Common scenario for oropharyngeal squamous cell carcinoma and nasopharyngeal carcinoma
- Resecting minimal amount of tissue is necessary for optimal functional and cosmetic results
- Residual disease is major determinant of death for patients with head and neck squamous cell carcinomas

SPECIMEN EVALUATION

Gross

- Biopsies for diagnosis are typically small & fragmented
- Resections are often complex
  - If entire resection is sent for margin evaluation, precise orientation is essential
  - Direct consultation with surgeon can be very helpful to identify location of closest margins
  - Differential inking of margins with multiple colors can aid in maintaining orientation
- Margins may be sent as small biopsies from edges of surgical bed (referred to as defect sampling)
  - Mucosal biopsies should be oriented if possible to identify (typically shiny) mucosal surface and minimize tangential sectioning

Frozen Section

- Small biopsies may be completely frozen
- Margins should always be taken perpendicular to actual margin
  - En face margins are not capable of evaluating narrow (1-2 mm) but tumor-free margins
    - Distance to margin cannot be determined and is often clinically important
- Deep margins more often positive than mucosal margins

Cytology

- Touch preps may be performed to evaluate tumors
- Cytology not routinely used for margin evaluation

MOST COMMON DIAGNOSES

Keratinizing (Conventional) Squamous Cell Carcinoma

- Abnormal keratinization (e.g., deep in epithelium), frequent mitoses, necrosis, nuclear pleomorphism and hyperchromasia, &/or desmoplastic stromal response
- Tumors may exhibit differing patterns of invasion
  - Broad pushing front of invasion
    - This pattern is especially challenging in small biopsies and may require presence of adjacent normal tissue to recognize presence of invasion
  - Irregular nests of tumor cells &/or individual infiltrative cells
    - Usually readily recognized

Verrucous Carcinoma

- Extremely well-differentiated variant of squamous cell carcinoma
- Invades as uniform front of invasion with bulbous rete ridges
- Minimal cytologic atypia

(Left) *Squamous cell carcinoma in situ shows full-thickness atypia with loss of normal cellular maturation and irregular cell spacing as well as marked nuclear size variation and hyperchromasia.* **(Right)** *Invasive keratinizing squamous cell carcinoma infiltrates as irregular nests of atypical squamous epithelium with focal areas of keratinization and elicits a loose desmoplastic stromal response.*

Squamous Cell Carcinoma In Situ

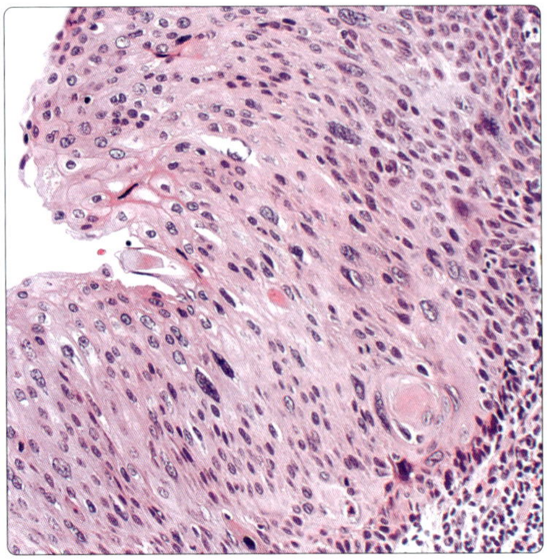

Invasive Squamous Cell Carcinoma

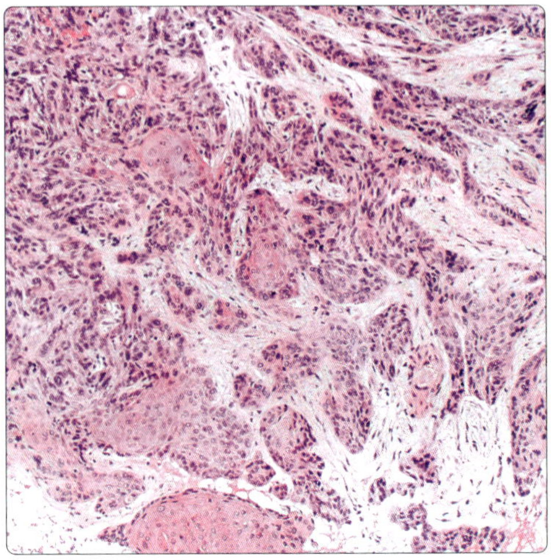

- When strictly defined, only risk of local recurrence
  - Diagnosis should be reserved for excised tumors, as similar features may be seen in areas of conventional squamous cell carcinoma

Basaloid Squamous Cell Carcinoma

- Clinically aggressive variant
- Basaloid tumor cells have scant cytoplasm and high-grade features including necrosis, nuclear hyperchromasia, and frequent mitoses
- Recognition as squamous carcinoma relies on identification of squamous differentiation (keratinization or intercellular bridges) or coexisting component of squamous dysplasia/carcinoma in situ
- Differential diagnosis includes other high-grade small round cell malignancies, especially small cell carcinoma and solid variant adenoid cystic carcinoma
  - Distinction often requires special stains
  - Adequate on frozen section to diagnose as basaloid carcinoma and defer definitive classification

Papillary Squamous Cell Carcinoma

- Associated with high-risk HPV viral types
- In small biopsies, confirmation of invasion may not be possible
- Often represents superficial sampling of bulky, clinically evident malignancy so that definitive confirmation of invasion may not be essential on frozen section

Sarcomatoid (Spindle Cell) Carcinoma

- Recognized by presence of malignant spindle cell proliferation coexisting with conventional squamous cell carcinoma &/or squamous dysplasia
- Differential diagnosis is with melanoma and sarcoma, especially leiomyosarcoma
  - May require special stains, but as many as 50% are negative for epithelial markers
- Behaves similarly to conventional squamous cell carcinoma

Squamous Dysplasia/Squamous Cell Carcinoma In Situ

- Grading and terminology of squamous precursor lesions is controversial
  - There are advocates for 2-tiered (low and high grade) and up to 4-tiered systems (mild, moderate, severe dysplasia, and carcinoma in situ)
    - Reproducibility is poor and diminishes with more grading tiers
- For frozen sections, severe dysplasia/carcinoma in situ at margins will usually prompt additional sampling
- Lesser degrees of dysplasia may not require additional tissue according to surgeon's judgment and clinical circumstances (location, solitary vs. multifocal)
- Diagnostic features include budding of rete ridges, expansion of basal proliferative layer, migration of mitoses into upper cell layers, nuclear hyperchromasia, nuclear size variation, and dyskeratosis

REPORTING

Frozen Section

- Carcinoma (at margin, if applicable, or provide distance to margin if possible)
- Perineural &/or lymph-vascular invasion
- Dysplasia at margin (with grade)

PITFALLS

False-Negative Diagnoses

- Deeper levels in frozen section blocks sometimes reveal cancer missed in initial superficial sections
- Denuded or maloriented blocks may miss dysplasia or make it impossible to assess grade accurately
  - Deeper tissue levels should be attempted to resolve diagnostic uncertainty
  - If necessary, block can be turned 90° to correct orientation
- Sampling error
  - Tissue taken may not include positive margin

False-Positive Diagnoses

- Pseudoinfiltrative growth due to tangential sectioning
  - Deeper levels should be obtained to confirm connection to overlying epithelium
- Duct involvement by severe dysplasia/carcinoma in situ may be mistaken for invasion
  - Uniform distribution, lack of single infiltrative cells, perpendicular orientation to surface epithelium, and connection to surface epithelium aid recognition
- Atypia after radiation therapy may be difficult to distinguish from dysplasia or infiltrating tumor cells
  - Isolated nucleomegaly and cytomegaly with vacuolization of either nucleus or cytoplasm
  - Nuclear:cytoplasmic ratio is preserved
- Necrotizing sialometaplasia creates impression of invasive carcinoma
  - Changes are seen in conjunction with ischemic changes in adjacent tissue, often after prior biopsy
  - Lobulated squamous metaplasia of salivary ducts without marked atypia aids in recognition
    - Benign pattern best appreciated at low power
- Pseudoepitheliomatous hyperplasia
  - Bland nuclear features of pseudoinfiltrative squamous epithelium
  - Especially common with granular cell tumors
    - Essential to look at stroma for diagnostic eosinophilic tumor cells in association with granular cytoplasm
- Candidiasis may cause squamous hyperplasia and reactive epithelial changes that may be mistaken for dysplasia or, rarely, carcinoma
  - Intraepithelial neutrophils are clue to potential presence of fungal organisms
  - If uncertain about presence of dysplasia, diagnosis of squamous atypia may be appropriate with recommendation to rebiopsy if lesion persists after treating infection

SELECTED REFERENCES

1. Amit M et al: Improving the rate of negative margins after surgery for oral cavity squamous cell carcinoma: a prospective randomized controlled study. Head Neck. 38 Suppl 1:E1803-9, 2016
2. Ettl T et al: Positive frozen section margins predict local recurrence in R0-resected squamous cell carcinoma of the head and neck. Oral Oncol. 55:17-23, 2016
3. Olson SM et al: Frozen section analysis of margins for head and neck tumor resections: reduction of sampling errors with a third histologic level. Mod Pathol. 24(5):665-70, 2011

Mild Squamous Dysplasia

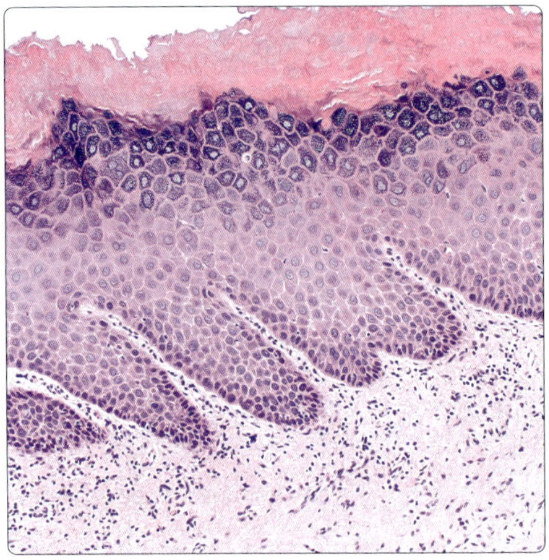

Squamous Cell Carcinoma In Situ

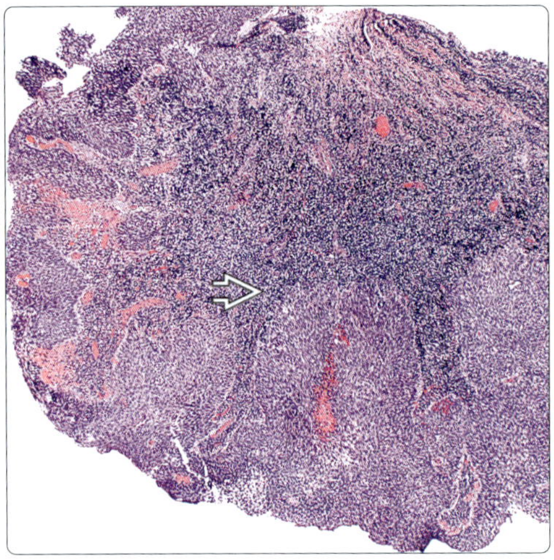

(Left) *Mild dysplasia may be subtle and challenging to distinguish from reactive atypia. The abnormalities are limited to the lower 1/3 of the epithelium with minimal nuclear atypia. Clues include loss of nuclear palisading in the basal proliferative zone and budding of the rete ridges.* **(Right)** *The full-thickness atypia of squamous cell carcinoma in situ is seen along with an area with endophytic growth ➡, concerning for blunt invasion. Assessment is challenging and requires a substantial, well-oriented biopsy to be definitive.*

Squamous Cell Carcinoma In Situ

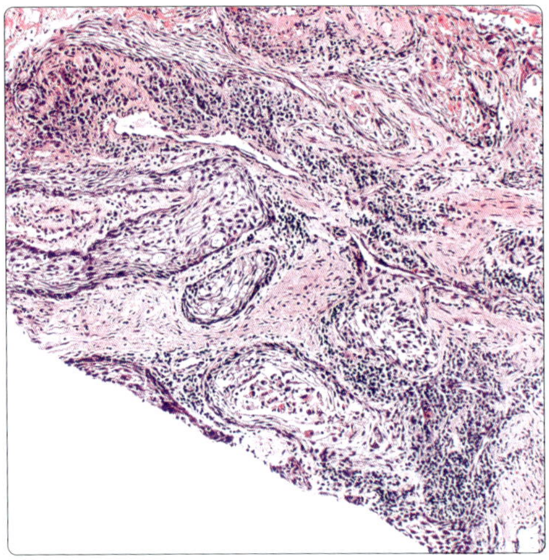

Basaloid Squamous Cell Carcinoma

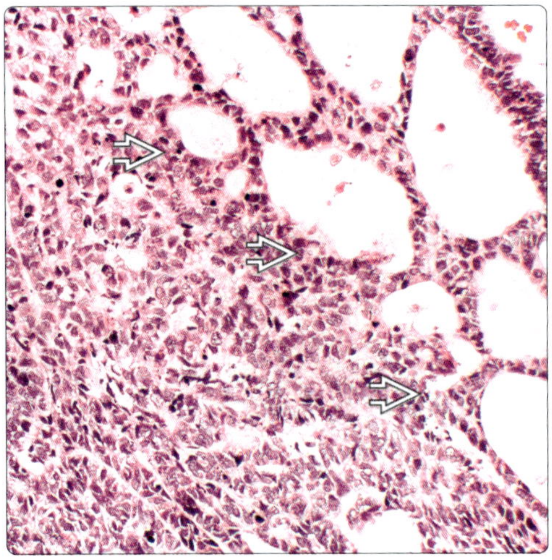

(Left) *Along with squamous cell carcinoma in situ, there are complex anastomosing strands of epithelium that are suggestive of invasion but that ultimately connect with the surface. Caution is needed to avoid misdiagnosing tangential sectioning as invasion.* **(Right)** *This high-grade basaloid carcinoma exhibits adenoid cystic carcinoma-like areas ➡. Recognition as squamous cell carcinoma depends on the identification of a component of conventional squamous cell carcinoma &/or squamous dysplasia.*

Papillary Squamous Cell Carcinoma

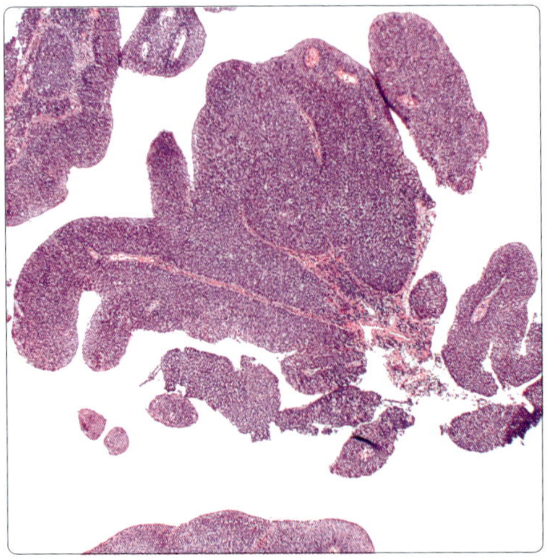

Sarcomatoid (Spindle Cell) Carcinoma

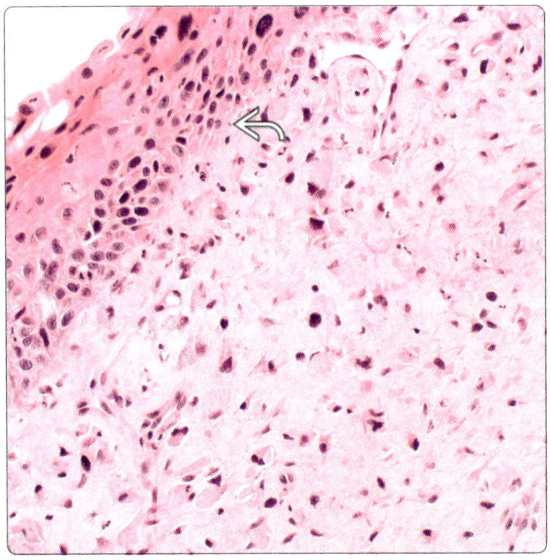

(Left) *Biopsies of papillary squamous cell carcinoma are often composed of superficial exophytic tissue fragments. Fibrovascular cores are lined by basaloid epithelium with full-thickness atypia without maturation. Invasion may be difficult to demonstrate.* **(Right)** *An atypical spindle cell proliferation present within a hyalinized stroma can be recognized as spindle cell carcinoma by associated conventional squamous cell carcinoma or dysplasia ➡.*

Squamous Cell Carcinoma: Perineural Invasion

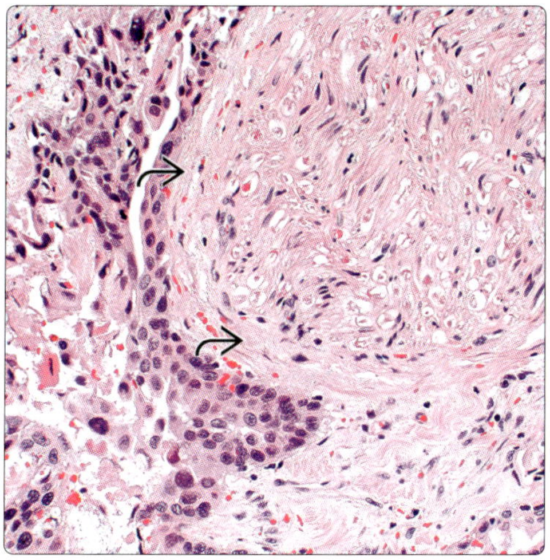

Squamous Cell Carcinoma: Skeletal Muscle Invasion at Deep Margin

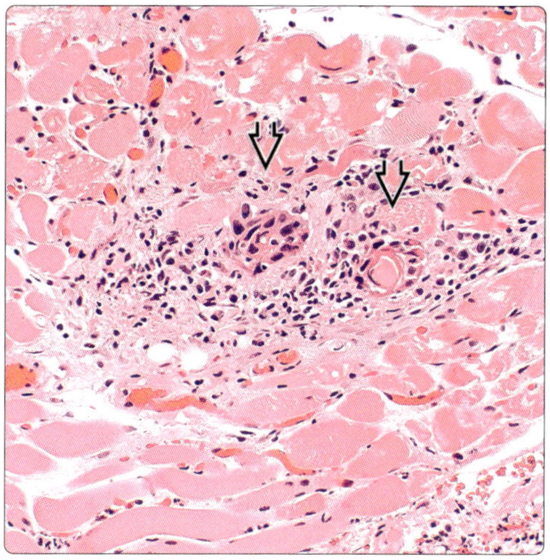

(Left) *Malignant cells from a squamous cell carcinoma abut a large nerve fragment ⇾. Perineural invasion by tumor may require 1 or more additional margins to completely excise the tumor growing along the nerve. This is a common source of residual disease and positive margins.* **(Right)** *Deep soft tissue margins may be involved by foci of squamous cell carcinoma that are discontinuous with the main mass. Such foci can be quite small ⇾, requiring close examination to avoid a false-negative interpretation.*

Necrotizing Sialometaplasia

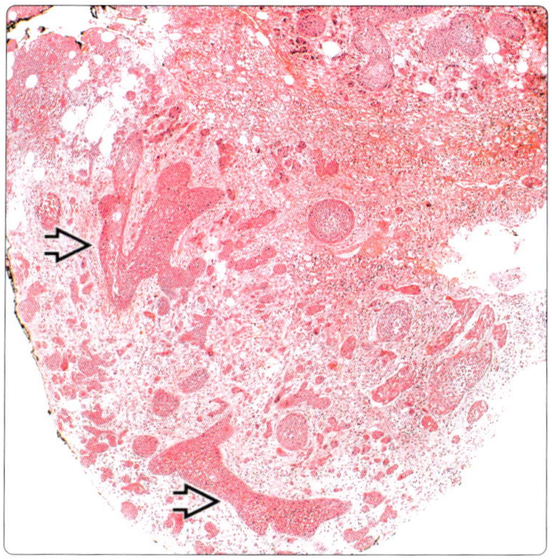

Necrotizing Sialometaplasia

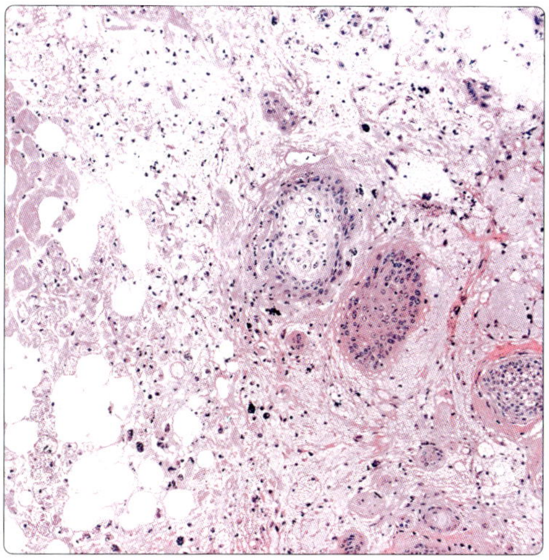

(Left) *Necrotizing sialometaplasia exhibits a pseudoinfiltrative appearance with islands of benign or reactive-appearing squamous epithelium. At low power, the relatively uniform distribution of these islands can be seen as they branch off of salivary ducts undergoing squamous metaplasia ⇾.* **(Right)** *A clue to the diagnosis of necrotizing sialometaplasia is ischemic necrosis in the tissue surrounding the involved salivary gland parenchyma. Enlarged nuclei and mitoses can mimic malignancy.*

Granular Cell Tumor

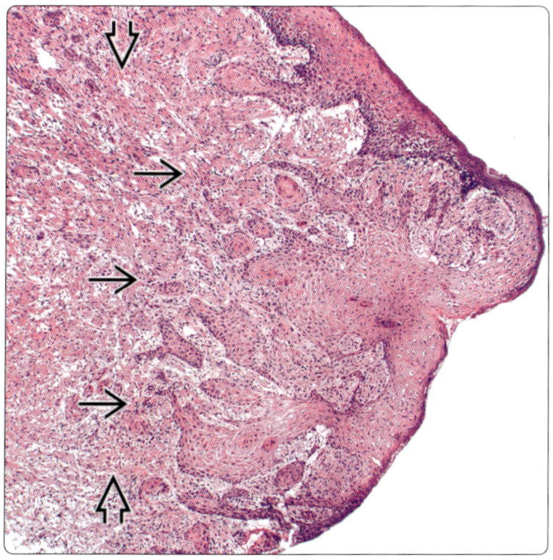

Granular Cell Tumor

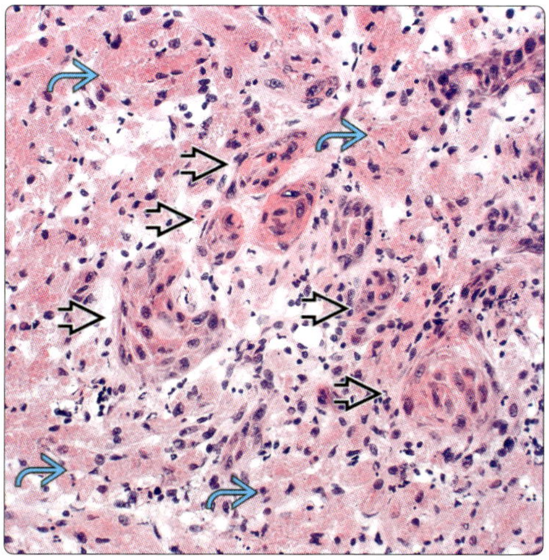

(Left) *Pseudoepitheliomatous hyperplasia ⇾ associated with a granular cell tumor ⇾ is a notorious mimic of infiltrative squamous cell carcinoma. At low power, islands of well-differentiated squamous cells appear to be dropping off from the hyperplastic surface epithelium.* **(Right)** *The cells of this granular cell tumor ⇾, with abundant granular eosinophilic cytoplasm, are surrounded by islands of benign-appearing squamous epithelium ⇾ from overlying pseudoepitheliomatous hyperplasia.*

SURGICAL/CLINICAL CONSIDERATIONS

Goal of Consultation

- Confirm presumed diagnosis of renal cell carcinoma (RCC) in solid renal lesions or of urothelial carcinoma in renal pelvis lesions
- Diagnose cystic renal lesion
- Evaluate parenchymal margin when partial nephrectomy is performed

Change in Patient Management

- If RCC is confirmed, definite surgery (partial or complete nephrectomy) may be performed
- If urothelial carcinoma is confirmed, nephroureterectomy with bladder cuff margin may be performed
- Positive parenchymal margin in partial nephrectomy may result in additional tumor bed resection or performance of complete nephrectomy

Clinical Setting

- Renal masses usually have characteristic findings by imaging
  - Previous core needle biopsies or fine-needle aspirations may not be diagnostic
  - Typically, appropriate management of renal masses is complete surgical excision by radical nephrectomy or partial nephrectomy
- Most common clinically evident renal mass is RCC
  - If mass size requires complete nephrectomy, intraoperative consultation is usually not required
  - Frozen sections may be performed to confirm clinical suspicion of neoplasm in cases with unusual clinical or radiographic findings
- Smaller asymptomatic masses detected by imaging are more likely to be lesions other than carcinoma
- Partial nephrectomy maintains renal function and is preferred in patients with small tumors, impaired renal function, or bilateral tumors
  - Gross examination &/or frozen section of parenchymal margin or frozen section of tumor bed may be performed, particularly in cases where surgeon is uncertain of complete excision of tumor

SPECIMEN EVALUATION

Gross

- **Partial nephrectomy**
  - Consists of portion of kidney, usually with little surrounding nonrenal tissue
    - No major vessels or ureter will be present
  - Cut parenchymal surface is identified
    - Examine surface for any areas with possible tumor involvement
  - Ink parenchymal margin
  - Serially section specimen perpendicular to margin
  - Identify closest approach of tumor to margin
    - If tumor is well defined and rim of normal tissue is present between tumor and margin, gross evaluation is highly predictive of a microscopically negative margin
    - If gross appearance shows possible tumor involvement, tissue may be taken for frozen section
- **Tumor bed biopsies**
  - In some centers, biopsies of cut surface of remaining kidney after partial nephrectomy is performed
  - Tumor bed biopsies consist of small fragments of tissue and are completely frozen
- **Radical nephrectomy**
  - Specimen consists of kidney, ureter, renal vein and artery, perinephric fat, and surrounding Gerota fascia
    - Adrenal gland may or may not be present
    - Distal margins of ureter and vessels are excised and placed in marked cassettes
  - Outer aspect of specimen is examined to identify any areas of tumor involvement
    - Tumor involvement of renal vein is usually identified by preoperative imaging
    - Tumor may be seen extending from hilum into vein

Complete Nephrectomy: Gross Appearance

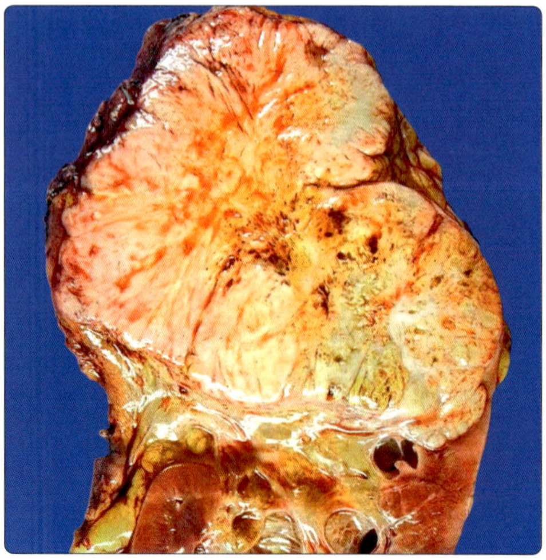

Partial Nephrectomy: Gross Appearance

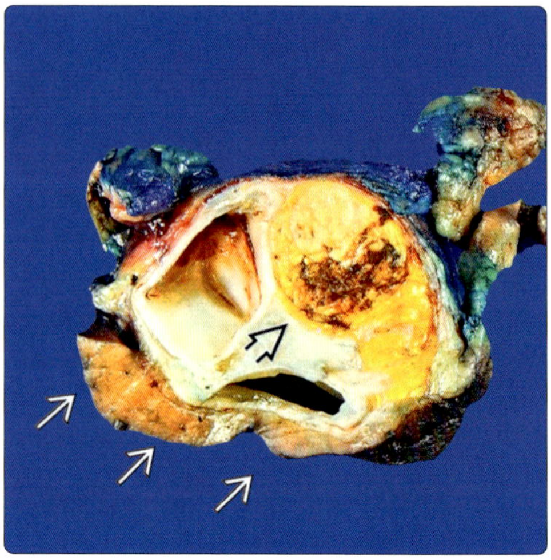

(Left) *A nephrectomy is often performed for malignancies [e.g., this renal cell carcinoma (RCC)] and removes the kidney, ureter, vessels, and sometimes the adrenal. Margins are rarely involved. (Courtesy S. Tickoo, MD.)* **(Right)** *Partial nephrectomy removes the tumor (in this case a clear cell RCC) ⇨ and a rim of normal parenchyma ➡. Gross confirmation of normal tissue at the parenchymal margin can be sufficient without frozen section. (Courtesy S. Tickoo, MD.)*

  - If tumor is identified at margins, differential inking &/or other identification should be utilized to identify these areas for eventual sampling
- Outer portion of specimen is inked
- Probe is placed into ureter
- Incision is made along probe to bisect ureter and plane of section is extended to bisect kidney
  - Allows examination of entire urothelium
- All lesions are identified, including size, number, location, and relationship to margins
  - Many renal tumors can be identified by their gross features
  - Tumor identification may not require frozen section

Frozen Section

- Parenchymal margin of partial nephrectomy can be submitted for frozen section if gross lesion is present
  - If parenchymal margin appears negative by gross examination, frozen sections may not be necessary
- Tumor bed biopsies of partial nephrectomy should be entirely frozen
- Multiple sections of cystic renal lesions and oncocytic lesions may be needed to confirm diagnosis
  - Best accomplished with permanent sections
  - Should only be attempted by frozen section in unusual circumstances in which finding of carcinoma would alter surgical approach

MOST COMMON DIAGNOSES

Clear Cell RCC

- Most common renal tumor
- Well-circumscribed or lobulated golden yellow to red mass with pushing borders
- Gross appearance is often heterogeneous with areas of hemorrhage, necrosis, and cystic degeneration
  - Preoperative renal artery embolization can result in extensive infarction and necrosis
- Gray or tan-white fleshy-appearing areas may represent areas of sarcomatoid differentiation
- Cells have clear to eosinophilic cytoplasm arranged in nests or solid sheets within delicate fibrovascular network
  - Nuclear grade ranges from low to high based on prominence of nucleoli for WHO/ISUP grades 1-3 and nuclear pleomorphism or sarcomatoid or rhabdoid differentiation for WHO/ISUP grade 4
  - Areas with darker eosinophilic cytoplasm are usually higher grade
- RCC with prominent cystic changes may be identified by an inner irregular surface or papillary projection(s)
  - Can be difficult to diagnose on frozen section

Multilocular Cystic Renal Neoplasm of Low Malignant Potential

- Gross appearance is of a multiloculated cystic lesion with no solid nodules
- Histologic examination reveals cysts lined by a layer of cells with clear cytoplasm and low-grade nuclear features and small, nonexpansile clusters of tumor cells within the fibrous septa
- May not be possible to distinguish from clear cell RCC with prominent cystic architecture on frozen section as extensive sampling may be required to exclude solid areas

Clear Cell Tubulopapillary Carcinoma

- Well-circumscribed tumors that are often cystic on gross examination
- Low-grade cells with clear cytoplasm arranged in papillary, branching tubules, or acinar architectures
- Characteristic linear arrangement of nuclei near apical aspect of cells in much of neoplasm

Papillary RCC

- 2nd most common renal neoplasm
- Tumors are often well-circumscribed with fibrous pseudocapsule
- Tumors with hemorrhage or abundant hemosiderin-macrophages appear brown while tumors with abundant foamy histiocytes have tan to yellow color
- Areas with necrosis, hemorrhage, and cystic change are common
- Tumors may have papillary, solid, or trabecular architecture
  - Papillary architecture gives soft friable appearance, which may be mistaken grossly for necrosis
  - Foamy histiocytes may be present within fibrovascular cores
- 2 types
  - Type 1 tumors: Cells with scant amphophilic cytoplasm and low-grade nuclear features
  - Type 2 tumors: Darker eosinophilic cytoplasm, nuclear pseudostratification, and high-nuclear grade

Collecting Duct RCC

- Rare, aggressive neoplasms that are predominantly located within renal medulla but may extend into renal cortex in larger tumors
- Irregular firm gray-white multinodular masses with frequent invasion into renal sinus
  - Hemorrhage, cystic degeneration, and necrosis is common
- Infiltrative with varying tubular, papillary, solid, and cribriform architecture and high-grade nuclear features
- Marked desmoplasia and inflammation is common finding
- Some cases closely resemble high-grade urothelial carcinoma and may be difficult to differentiate on frozen section

Chromophobe RCC

- Well-circumscribed tan to brown homogeneous mass
  - May have central scar, hemorrhage, or necrosis
- Most have solid growth pattern with incomplete fibrovascular septa
  - Nested, alveolar, cystic and other patterns can be present
- Nuclear features
  - Irregular wrinkled nuclei (raisinoid cells) and binucleate cells with prominent perinuclear halos
  - Focal cells may have hyperchromatic, degenerative nuclei
- Cytoplasm
  - Abundant, granular, and pale pink with prominent well-defined cell membranes

- Eosinophilic variant has darkly staining cytoplasm
  - Tend to have fewer perinuclear halos and wrinkled-appearing nuclei
- May be difficult to distinguish from oncocytoma
- Frozen section diagnosis of "oncocytic renal neoplasm" may be preferable unless chromophobe carcinoma can clearly be diagnosed

Oncocytoma

- Well-circumscribed tan to dark brown mass, which can resemble chromophobe RCC grossly
  - Central scar is common
  - No necrosis
- Usually, pattern is of nests of cells in hypocellular stroma
  - Can also form cysts and tubules
  - Sheets of cells, like chromophobe RCC, is less common
  - Small papillae may be only focal finding within cysts or dilated tubules
- Nuclei
  - Round and regular with vesicular chromatin and central nucleoli
  - Lacks perinuclear halos present in chromophobe RCC
  - Foci with pleomorphic, hyperchromatic, degenerative nuclei may be present (more common than in chromophobe RCC)
- Cytoplasm
  - Granular and eosinophilic without distinct cell membranes that are present in chromophobe RCC
  - Clear cells absent or only focally present within area of scar
- Tumor extension into perinephric fat or vascular spaces does not exclude diagnosis of oncocytoma
- Definitive diagnosis may not be possible on frozen section

Angiomyolipoma

- Tumor within perivascular epithelioid cell tumor (PEComa) class of tumors, vast majority are benign
- Usually well circumscribed with gross appearance depending on proportion of adipose tissue, smooth muscle, and blood vessels present
  - Imaging findings may be diagnostic due to admixture of adipose tissue
- Consists of varying proportions of dystrophic blood vessels, smooth muscle, and adipose tissue
  - Blood vessels have thick hyalinized walls with spindle cells radiating outward from vascular wall
  - Smooth muscle appears as spindle cells arranged in fascicles or as epithelioid cells
- Diagnosis can be difficult on frozen section
  - Adipose tissue can be misinterpreted as artifactual clefts on frozen section
  - Tumors with predominant smooth muscle component can resemble smooth muscle neoplasm or sarcomatoid RCC
  - Adipose predominant angiomyolipomas may be difficult to distinguish from well-differentiated liposarcoma
- Multifocal &/or bilateral tumors may be associated with tuberous sclerosis

Urothelial Carcinoma

- May occur as papillary lesion involving renal pelvis or as infiltrative lesion, which involves renal parenchyma
- Histologically similar to urothelial carcinoma of bladder
- Carcinomas invasive into renal parenchyma can be difficult to differentiate from collecting duct carcinoma or other centrally located high-grade RCCs

Malakoplakia

- Most common in patients with immunosuppression due to organ transplant, chemotherapy for malignancy, or diabetes
- Forms small, soft yellow plaques and nodules
- Sheets of eosinophilic histiocytes (von Hansemann cells) with intracytoplasmic targetoid basophilic inclusions (Michaelis-Guttman bodies) and admixed acute and chronic inflammation
  - May occasionally have associated fibrosis or spindled appearance
- Michaelis-Gutmann bodies are pathognomonic and can be identified on frozen sections

Xanthogranulomatous Pyelonephritis

- Associated with urinary tract obstruction and staghorn calculi
- Single or multiple golden yellow lesions, typically with hydronephrosis
- Sheets of foamy histiocytes are associated with mixed inflammatory infiltrate
  - Lack delicate network of fibrovascular septa of clear cell RCC
  - Nuclei of histiocytes are bland

Cystic Lesions

- Renal cysts can be congenital, sporadic, or acquired due to long-term hemodialysis
  - Hemorrhage &/or inflammatory changes can make distinction from solid neoplasms difficult by imaging
  - Lined by single layer of flat or cuboidal bland epithelial cells
- RCC can have extensive necrosis and appear cystic, with gross appearance mimicking hemorrhagic simple cyst
  - All cysts should be carefully examined for mural nodules or papillary projections
  - Multiple sections may be required to locate focus of RCC within cyst wall
- Acquired cystic kidney disease occurs in > 30% of patients with end-stage renal disease
  - 5-10% of patients develop RCC
    - Acquired cystic disease-associated RCC is most common subtype of RCC but other subtypes also occur
  - Extensive sampling may be necessary to diagnose carcinoma and is not commonly requested as part of intraoperative consultation

Mixed Epithelial and Stromal Tumor Family

- Uncommon benign tumors that are most common in perimenopausal women
- Most often identified near renal pelvis but can extend into renal cortex
- Can resemble multilocular cystic renal neoplasm of low malignant potential on imaging and gross examination

- Morphologic spectrum ranges from predominantly cystic tumors (adult cystic nephromas) to tumors with both solid and cystic components (mixed epithelial and stromal tumor (MEST) family)
  - Cysts are lined by single layer of flat, cuboidal, or hobnail epithelium with bland nuclear features
    - Clear cytoplasm, if present, should only be focal
  - Fibrous septa and solid areas are composed of fibrous or ovarian-type stroma or smooth muscle

Papillary Adenomas

- Benign, usually incidental lesions, may be multiple
- Adenomas are nonencapsulated neoplasms < 15 mm in size with papillary &/or tubular architecture and low-grade nuclei
  - Do not have cells resembling those of clear cell or chromophobe carcinomas
  - Can be associated with foamy macrophages or psammoma bodies
- May be difficult to distinguish from low-grade carcinoma when present at parenchymal margin on frozen section
  - Usually located away from main mass
  - Often histologically distinct from main mass

Lymphoma

- Usually occurs as secondary involvement in systemic disease
- Homogeneous gray to white mass involving cortex or medulla, may occur as distinct mass lesion or diffusely involve kidney
- Extensive necrosis may be present, making interpretation of frozen sections difficult
- Most common is large B-cell type

Metastases

- Often prior clinical history of malignancy is present
- May be solitary tumor, mimicking primary renal neoplasm

REPORTING

Gross

- If lesion has gross features of RCC, this finding can be reported
- Gross confirmation of negative parenchymal margin of partial nephrectomy is highly predictive of no residual carcinoma

Frozen Section

- If findings characteristic for specific neoplasm are present, diagnosis may be reported
  - Often, categorization of lesion as benign or malignant provides surgeon with sufficient information
  - Distinguishing renal tumors from urothelial carcinoma, when possible, can alter surgical management
  - In difficult cases, such as cystic lesions or oncocytic neoplasms, deferment to permanent sections may be necessary and appropriate
- For parenchymal margin of partial nephrectomy, presence or absence of tumor at margin should be reported
  - Value of frozen section evaluation in this setting has been questioned
    - Recent studies have suggested positive surgical margin has little impact on risk of local recurrence or overall patient survival
    - Evaluation of tumor bed by surgeon for complete tumor removal has been shown to be accurate predictor of negative margin
    - Studies have shown poor correlation between frozen section diagnosis and final diagnosis
- Tumor bed biopsies may be more difficult to interpret in absence of information about primary lesion and distance from margin
  - Evaluation of partial nephrectomy specimen is preferable

PITFALLS

Crush Artifact

- Crushed benign renal tubules can be difficult to interpret in parenchymal margin sections
- Features supporting benign tubules
  - Absence of nuclear atypia within tubules
  - Presence of glomeruli within surrounding renal parenchyma

Lesions With Foamy Cytoplasm

- Benign lesions containing histiocytes with foamy or eosinophilic cytoplasm may be difficult to distinguish from clear cell RCC on frozen section
  - Xanthogranulomatous pyelonephritis
  - Malakoplakia
  - Fat necrosis

Oncocytic Neoplasms

- Some RCCs, such as chromophobe RCC, can have brightly eosinophilic cytoplasm
  - Can be misdiagnosed as benign oncocytoma with limited sampling on frozen section
- Diagnosis of "oncocytic neoplasm" is preferred unless malignancy can clearly be diagnosed

Cystic Lesions

- Cystic &/or necrotic RCC can be difficult to differentiate from hemorrhagic cysts on frozen section
  - May require multiple sections to locate RCC within cyst wall

Urothelial vs. Collecting Duct Carcinoma

- Invasive urothelial carcinoma and collecting duct carcinoma both appear as infiltrative lesions with desmoplastic reaction

Papillary Adenoma at Margin

- Generally small lesions located away from main tumor
- Usually does not resemble renal tumor

SELECTED REFERENCES

1. Laganosky DD et al: Surgical margins in nephron-sparing surgery for renal cell carcinoma. Curr Urol Rep. 18(1):8, 2017
2. Alemozaffar M et al: The importance of surgical margins in renal cell and urothelial carcinomas. J Surg Oncol. 113(3):316-22, 2016
3. Shen SS et al: Use of frozen section in genitourinary pathology. Pathology. 44(5):427-33, 2012

Contents

(Left) *Clear cell RCC usually forms a golden yellow circumscribed mass with hemorrhage. This tumor has invaded the renal vein, an important prognostic factor that is usually detected on presurgical imaging. (Courtesy S. Tickoo, MD.)* **(Right)** *Frozen section of a grade 1 clear cell RCC shows nests of cells with clear cytoplasm and small nuclei surrounded by a network of fibrovascular septa.*

Clear Cell Renal Cell Carcinoma: Gross Appearance

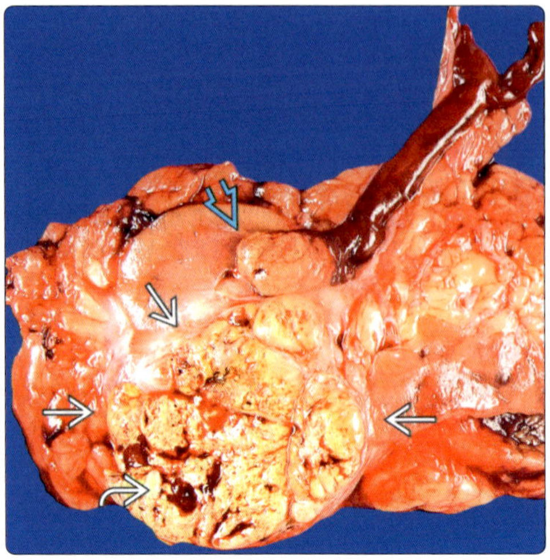

Clear Cell Renal Cell Carcinoma: Grade 1

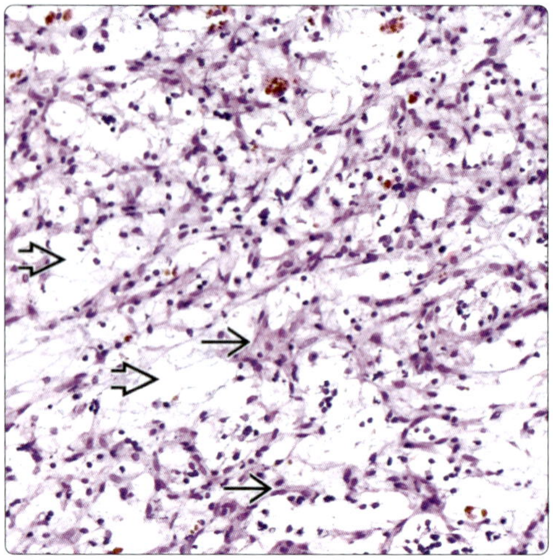

(Left) *Small, hyperchromatic nuclei are typical of a low-grade clear cell RCC. The nuclei may mimic lymphocytes in WHO/ISUP grade 1 lesions.* **(Right)** *Frozen section of a high-grade clear cell RCC (WHO/ISUP grade 3) shows enlarged irregular nuclei with prominent nucleoli. Eosinophilic cytoplasm, rather than clear cytoplasm, is more commonly seen in areas with a higher grade in clear cell RCC.*

Clear Cell Renal Cell Carcinoma: Grade 1

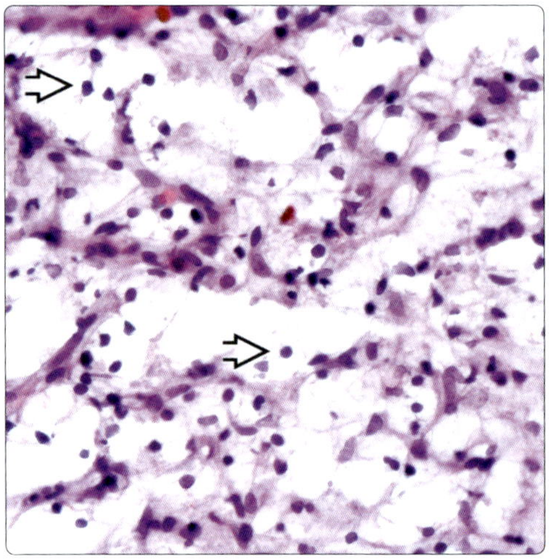

Clear Cell Renal Cell Carcinoma: Grade 3

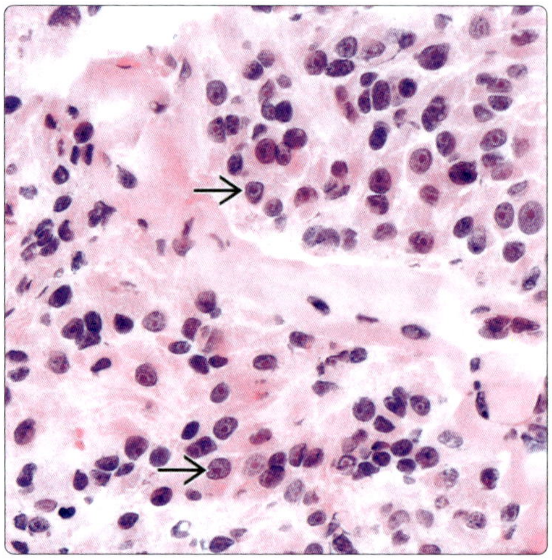

(Left) *The parenchymal margin of a partial nephrectomy often shows changes commonly present in the peritumoral renal parenchyma, such as interstitial fibrosis and chronic inflammation.* **(Right)** *Frozen and crush artifactual changes in the parenchymal margin may obscure the tubular lumina, which may appear worrisome for a neoplastic lesion. The presence of glomeruli as well as the absence of nuclear atypia within the tubular epithelium are helpful in recognizing normal renal tissue.*

Partial Nephrectomy: Parenchymal Margin

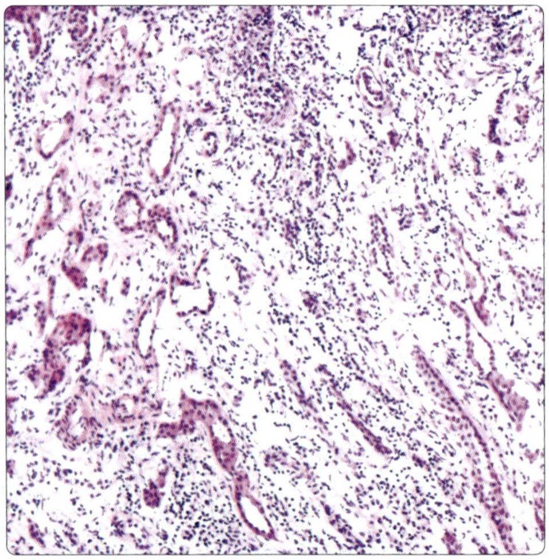

Partial Nephrectomy: Parenchymal Margin

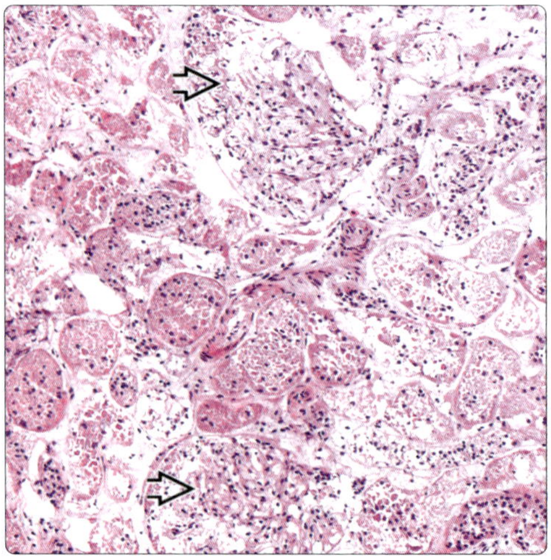

Renal Cell Carcinoma With Necrosis and Hemorrhage

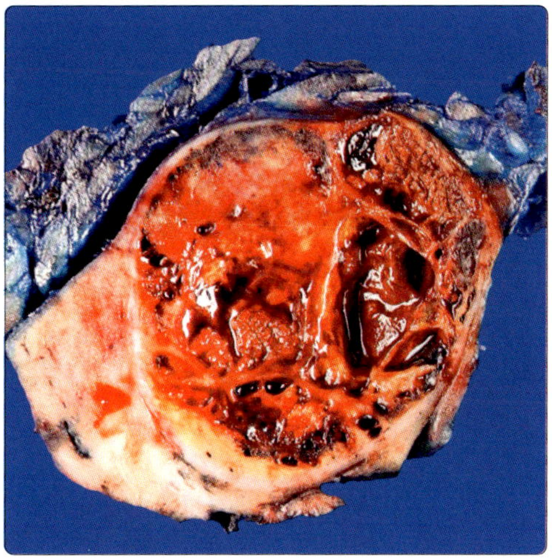

Multilocular Cystic Renal Neoplasm of Low Malignant Potential

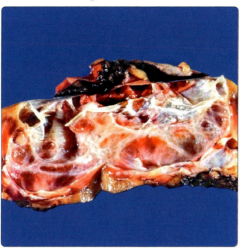

(Left) *Extensive necrosis and hemorrhage can be present in RCC and, at times, grossly mimic a hemorrhagic simple cyst. Multiple histologic sections of the cyst wall may be needed to identify RCC and are best performed on permanent sections. (Courtesy S. Tickoo, MD.)* **(Right)** *Multilocular cystic renal neoplasm of low malignant potential consists of a well-circumscribed multicystic lesion with thin fibrous septations. No solid masses are present within the tumor. (Courtesy S. Tickoo, MD.)*

Clear Cell Renal Cell Carcinoma

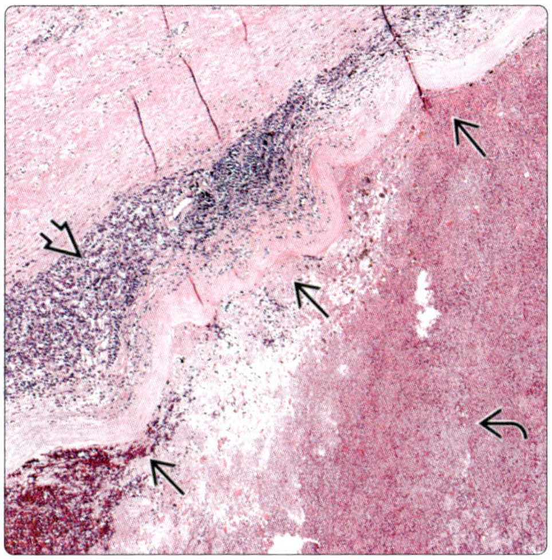

Multilocular Cystic Renal Neoplasm of Low Malignant Potential

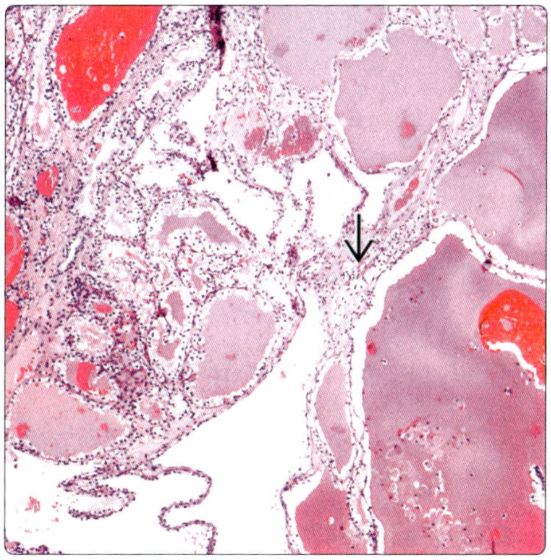

(Left) *This clear cell RCC has extensive central hemorrhage and necrosis ➔ surrounded by a fibrous wall ➔. An area of residual RCC ➔ is present within the fibrous wall.* **(Right)** *Cells with clear cytoplasm line multiple cysts of varying sizes in multilocular cystic renal neoplasm of low malignant potential. A small cluster of tumor cells with clear cytoplasm is present ➔ but no solid masses are formed. (Courtesy S. Tickoo, MD.)*

Clear Cell Renal Cell Carcinoma: Cystic

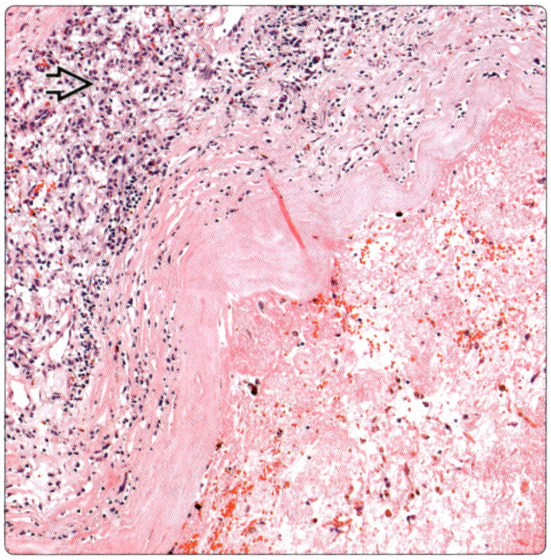

Multilocular Cystic Renal Neoplasm of Low Malignant Potential

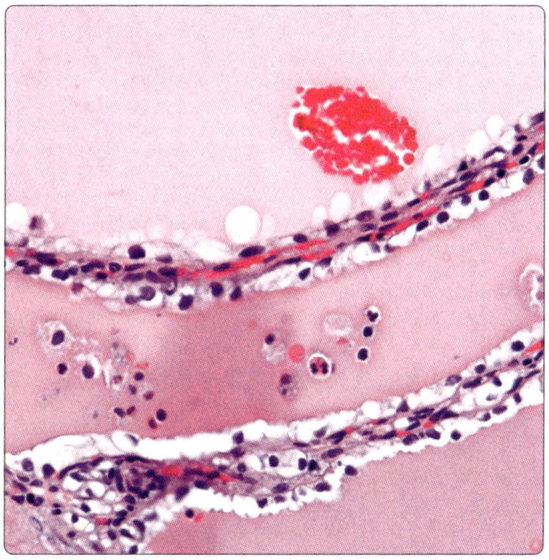

(Left) *A focus of clear cell RCC ➔ is present within the fibrotic wall of this cystically necrotic RCC. Multiple sections of the cyst wall may be necessary before a focus of residual RCC is identified.* **(Right)** *A single layer of cells with clear cytoplasm and low-grade nuclear features (WHO/ISUP grade 1 or 2) is seen lining the cysts. On frozen section, denudation of the cyst-lining cells can make diagnosis difficult and multiple sections may be required. (Courtesy S. Tickoo, MD.)*

(Left) *Papillary RCC is well circumscribed and may have a fibrous pseudocapsule ➡. A brown color can represent areas with hemosiderin, whereas areas with abundant foamy macrophages appear yellow. Areas of hemorrhage, necrosis, and cystic degeneration can be present. (Courtesy S. Tickoo, MD.)* **(Right)** *A fibrous capsule ➡ may be identified on microscopic examination of papillary RCCs, corresponding to the encapsulated appearance seen on gross examination. (Courtesy S. Tickoo, MD.)*

Papillary Renal Cell Carcinoma: Gross Appearance

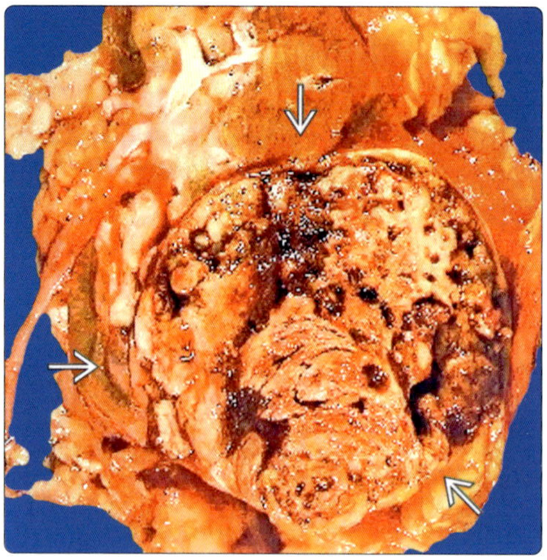

Papillary Renal Cell Carcinoma: Fibrous Capsule

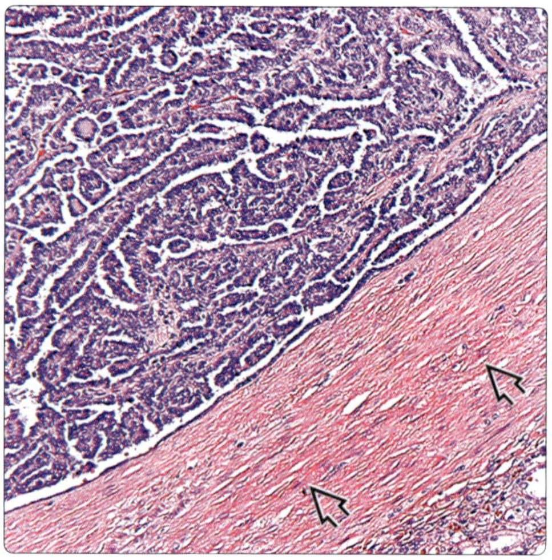

(Left) *A papillary RCC consists of fibrovascular cores lined by cells with abundant, brightly eosinophilic cytoplasm. This gives the tumor a soft texture grossly that can be mistaken for necrosis.* **(Right)** *In some papillary RCCs, abundant foamy macrophages are present within the fibrovascular cores ➡. This can confer a yellow color grossly. The papillary fronds are lined by low-grade nuclei. (Courtesy S. Tickoo, MD.)*

Papillary Renal Cell Carcinoma

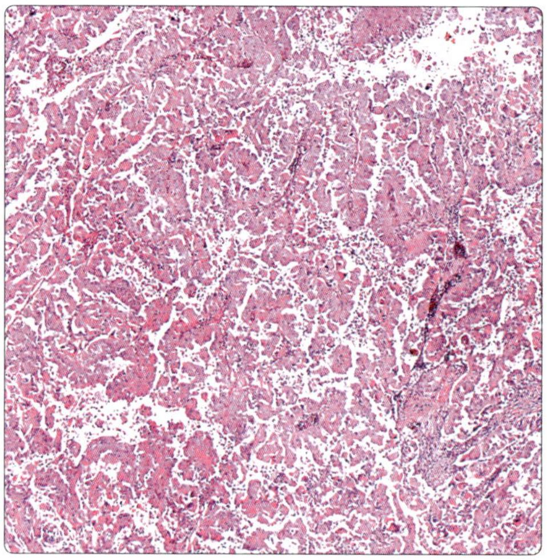

Papillary Renal Cell Carcinoma: Fibrovascular Cores

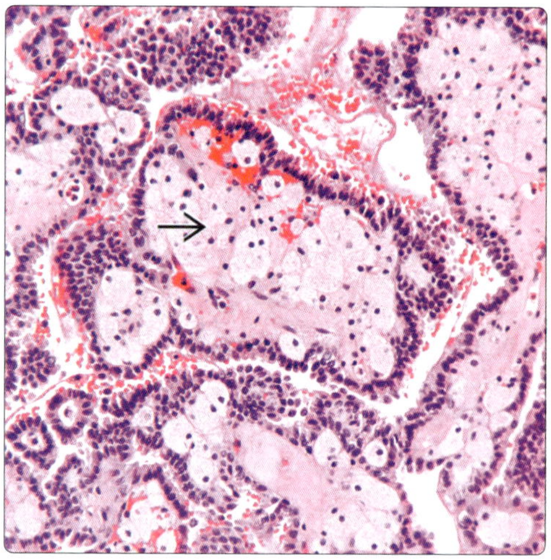

(Left) *Frozen section of a papillary RCC shows cells with scant to moderate amounts of cytoplasm and uniform round nuclei. Papillary RCC, along with clear cell RCCs, are assigned a WHO/ISUP nucleolar grade on permanent sections.* **(Right)** *This papillary RCC has abundant eosinophilic cytoplasm, nuclear stratification, and high-grade nuclear features (WHO/ISUP grade 3).*

Papillary Renal Cell Carcinoma: Nuclear Appearance

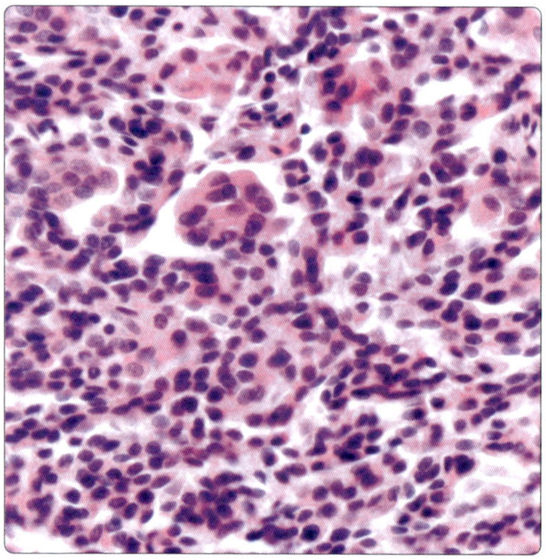

Papillary Renal Cell Carcinoma: High-Grade Nuclei

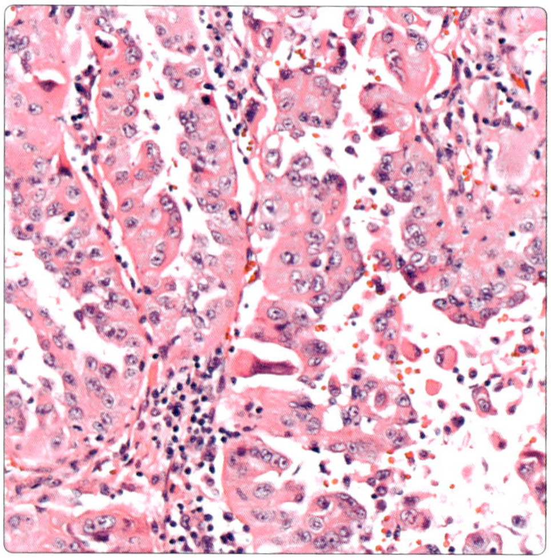

Contents

Chromophobe Renal Cell Carcinoma: Gross Appearance

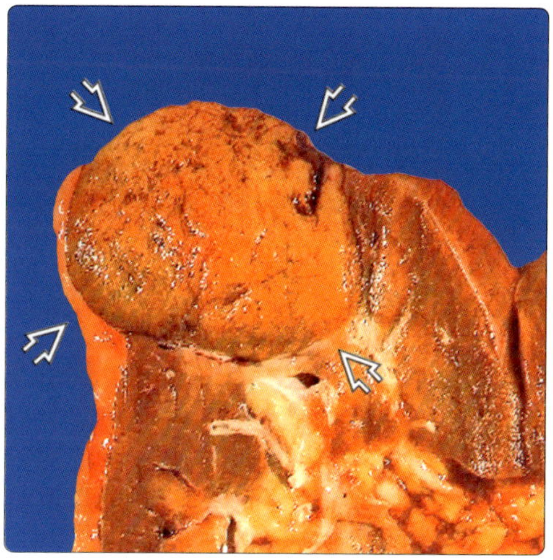

Oncocytoma: Gross Appearance

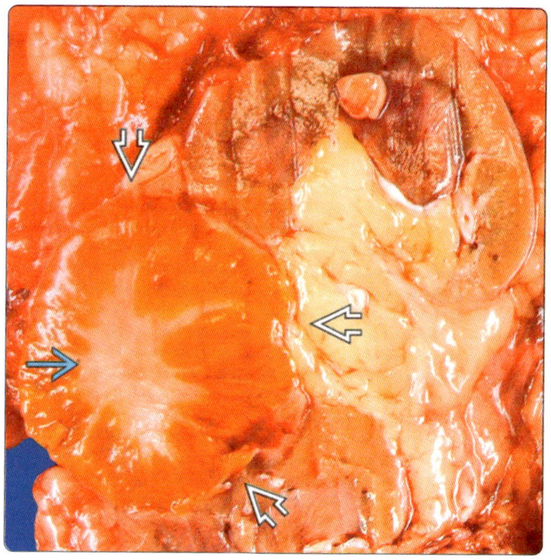

(Left) *Chromophobe RCC forms a well-circumscribed mass with a tan to brown appearance ➔. Although some tumors have a central scar, this feature is more typical of oncocytomas. (Courtesy S. Tickoo, MD.)* **(Right)** *An oncocytoma grows as a well-circumscribed tan-brown tumor ➔. A central scar ➔ is typical but not entirely specific for this tumor type. Some of these tumors reach sizes of up to 12 cm. These tumors can be difficult to distinguish from chromophobe RCC. (Courtesy S. Tickoo, MD.)*

Chromophobe Renal Cell Carcinoma: Nuclear Features

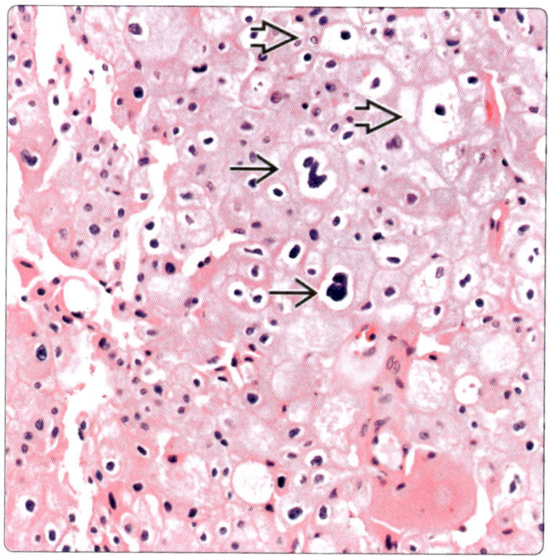

Oncocytoma

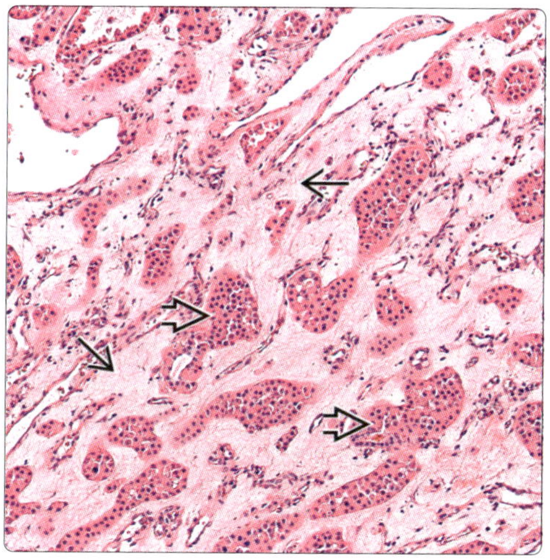

(Left) *Chromophobe RCC usually grows as sheets of cells. The cells often have distinct cell membranes and nuclei with irregular nuclear membranes, giving them a raisinoid appearance ➔. Prominent perinuclear halos ➔ are characteristic and not seen in oncocytomas.* **(Right)** *Oncocytomas typically grow as solid nests of cells with brightly eosinophilic oncocytic cytoplasm ➔ interspersed within a hypocellular stroma ➔. A solid or sheet-like growth pattern is less common.*

Chromophobe Renal Cell Carcinoma

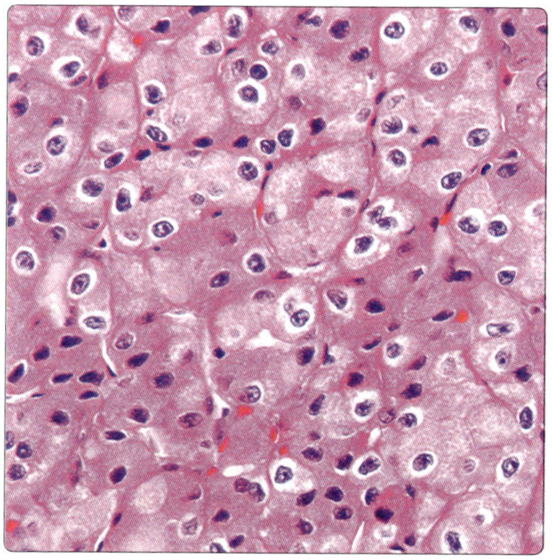

Oncocytoma

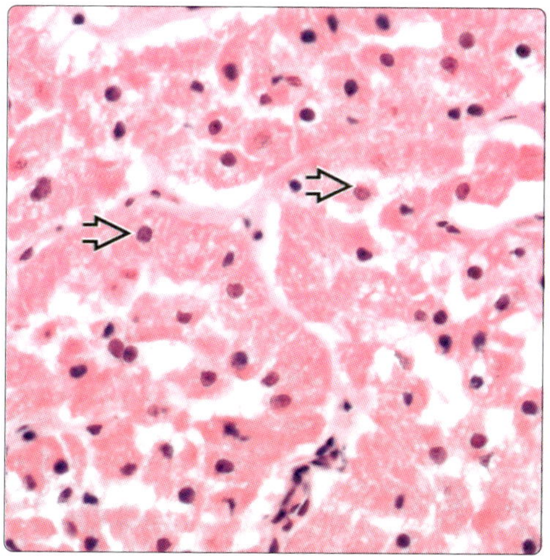

(Left) *The eosinophilic variant of chromophobe RCC has abundant eosinophilic cytoplasm, raisinoid nuclei, and numerous perinuclear halos. (Courtesy S. Tickoo, MD.)* **(Right)** *Cells with abundant granular cytoplasm and round, regular nuclei ➔ are arranged in nests in this frozen section of an oncocytoma. No perinuclear halos or distinct cell membranes are seen. However, distinction from a chromophobe RCC may be difficult on frozen section and "oncocytic neoplasm" may be preferable in this setting.*

Contents

Urothelial Carcinoma: Gross Appearance

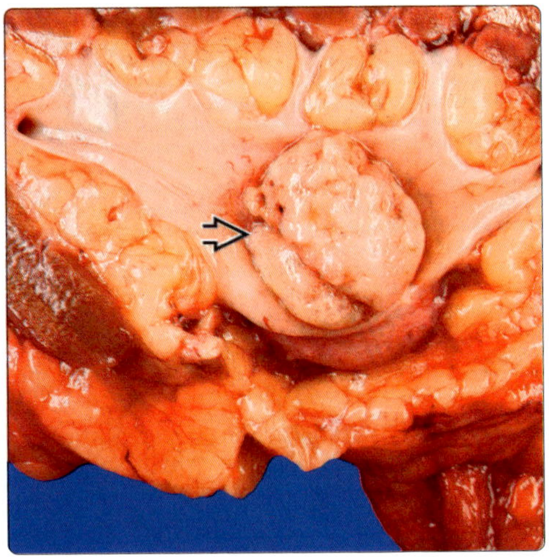

Urothelial Carcinoma: Gross Appearance

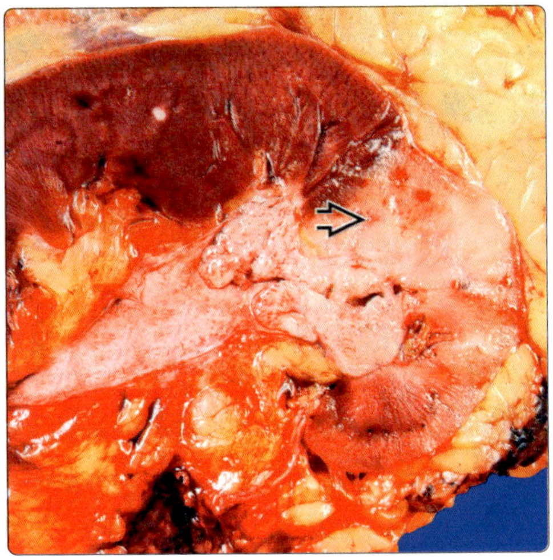

(Left) *This papillary urothelial carcinoma is present in the renal pelvis and has a gross polypoid appearance. The stalk connecting the tumor to the underlying renal pelvis is usually much smaller than the bulging tumor mass. (Courtesy S. Tickoo, MD.)* **(Right)** *This urothelial carcinoma has invaded into the renal parenchyma. These lesions can grossly and microscopically be mistaken for RCC, especially in the absence of an exophytic mass or area of wall thickening in the renal pelvis. (Courtesy S. Tickoo, MD.)*

Papillary Urothelial Carcinoma: High Grade

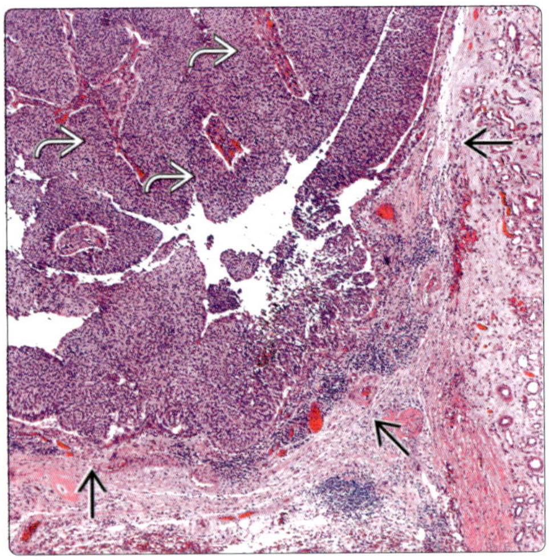

Papillary Urothelial Carcinoma: High Grade

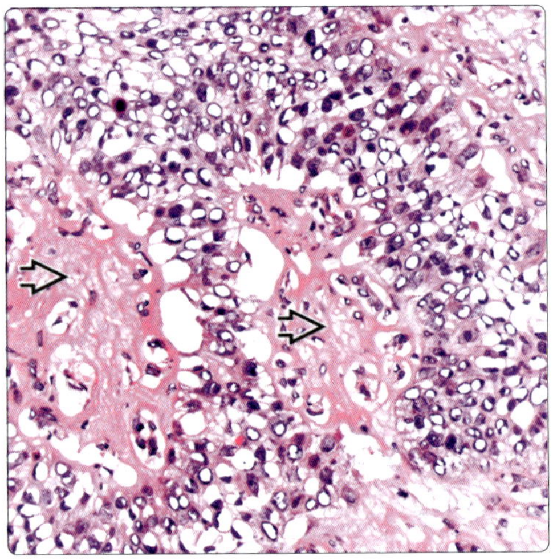

(Left) *This high-grade papillary urothelial carcinoma grows as papillary fronds arising from the urothelium lining the renal pelvis. Invasion into the renal parenchyma can occur from the base of the tumor.* **(Right)** *This high-grade papillary urothelial carcinoma consists of cells with hyperchromasia, pleomorphism, and disorganization lining fibrovascular cores on frozen section. The location and gross appearance of these tumors are helpful in distinguishing them from papillary RCC.*

Papillary Urothelial Carcinoma: High Grade

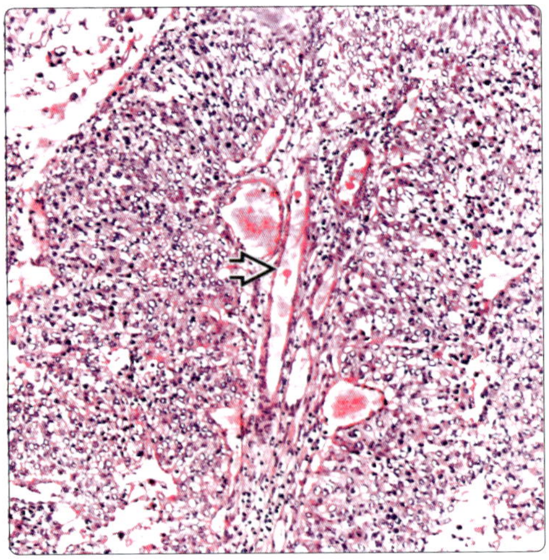

Urothelial Carcinoma: Invasion Into Kidney

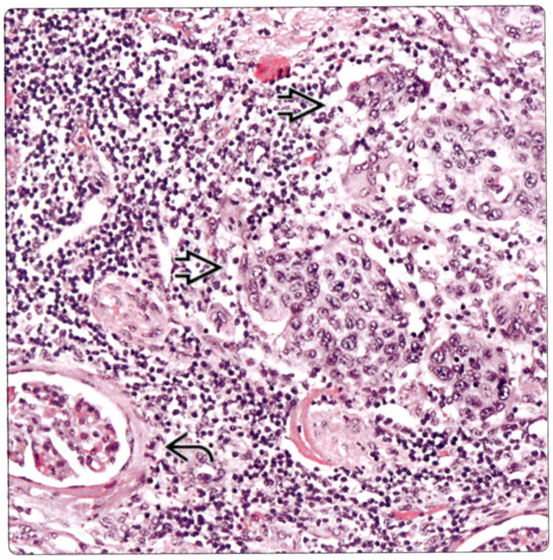

(Left) *A central fibrovascular core is lined by cells showing pleomorphism, disorganization, crowding, and frequent mitotic figures in this high-grade papillary urothelial carcinoma.* **(Right)** *Small nests of invasive urothelial carcinoma are present infiltrating through the renal parenchyma with residual normal glomeruli. Abundant chronic inflammation is present in the surrounding tissue. Differentiation of urothelial carcinoma from high-grade RCC can be difficult. (Courtesy S. Tickoo, MD.)*

Collecting Duct Carcinoma: Gross Appearance

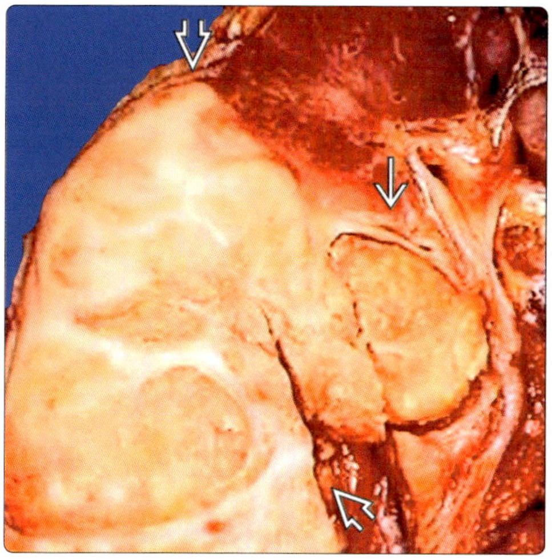

Angiomyolipoma: Gross Appearance

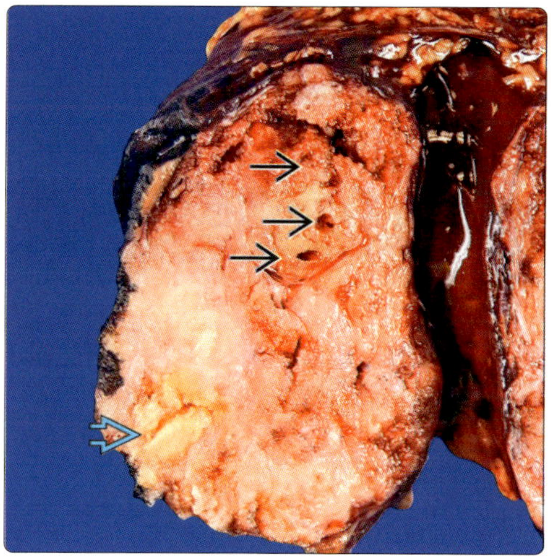

(Left) *This collecting duct carcinoma forms a hard, large, tan to white multinodular mass centered within the medulla of the kidney and extends into the renal cortex. (Courtesy S. Tickoo, MD.)* **(Right)** *Angiomyolipomas (AMLs) form circumscribed masses. The appearance is dependent upon the proportion of fat, smooth muscle, and vascular structures within the tumor. Areas of yellow adipose tissue and blood vessels are present in this tumor. (Courtesy S. Tickoo, MD.)*

Collecting Duct Carcinoma

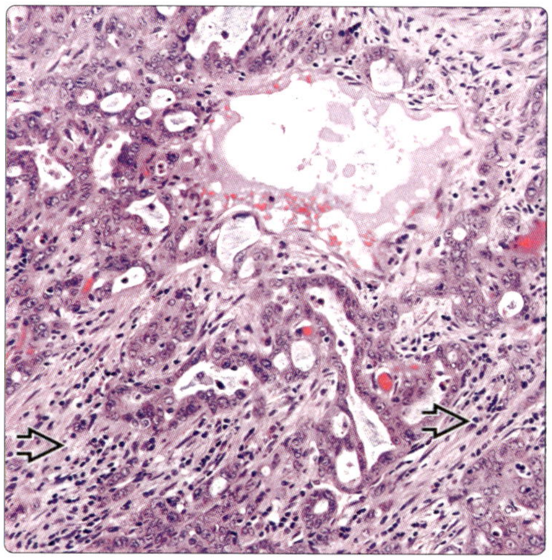

Angiomyolipoma

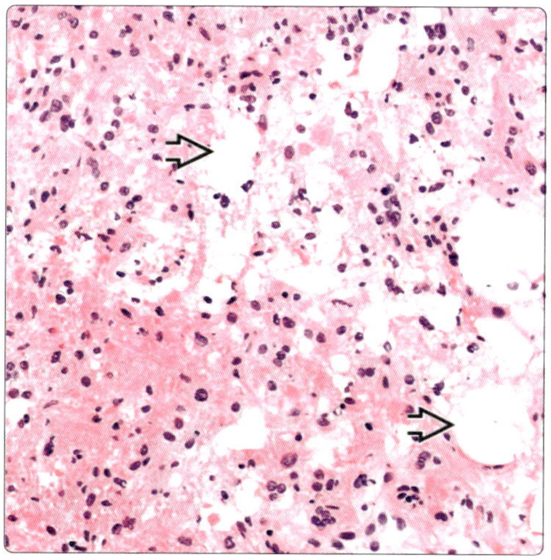

(Left) *Collecting duct carcinoma consists of cells with high-grade cytologic features arranged in tubules and solid nests invading through renal parenchyma. Papillary and cribriform architecture may be present. The stroma is desmoplastic with an inflammatory infiltrate. (Courtesy S. Tickoo, MD.)* **(Right)** *Adipose tissue in AMLs can be mistaken for artifactual clefts on frozen section. Locating areas of fat within a spindle cell proliferation can be helpful in making the correct diagnosis.*

Angiomyolipoma

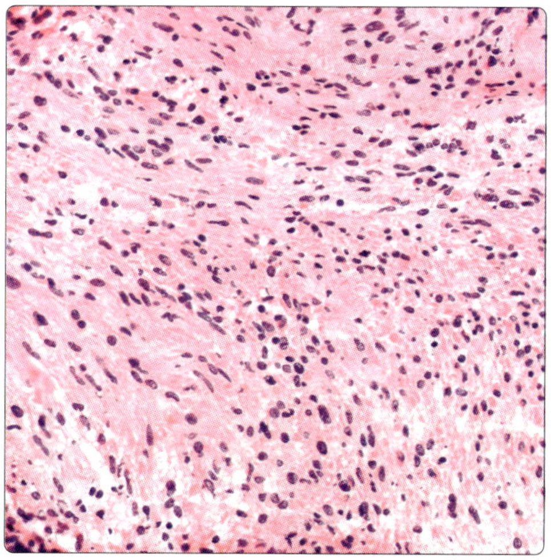

Angiomyolipoma

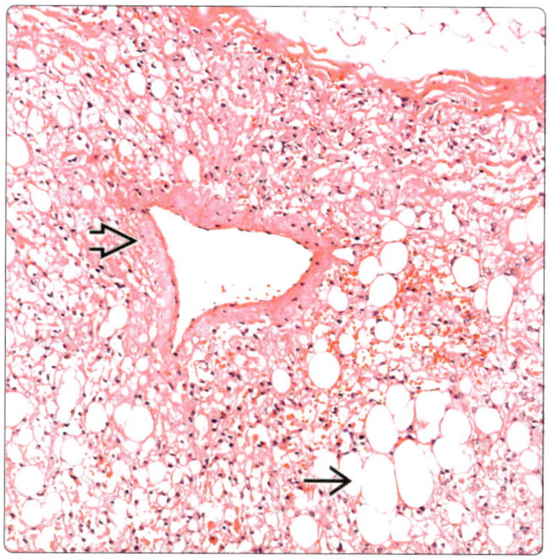

(Left) *Fascicles of spindle cells within angiomyolipomas can be mistaken for sarcomatoid carcinoma. Features characteristic of AMLs, such as fat and dysmorphic vessels with spindle proliferations radiating from the wall, should assist in the diagnosis.* **(Right)** *A thick-walled vessel is present in this permanent section of an AML. The spindle cells often appear to radiate off of the vessel, which is a helpful diagnostic clue. Nests of adipose cells are also present.*

Contents

Xanthogranulomatous Pyelonephritis: Gross Appearance

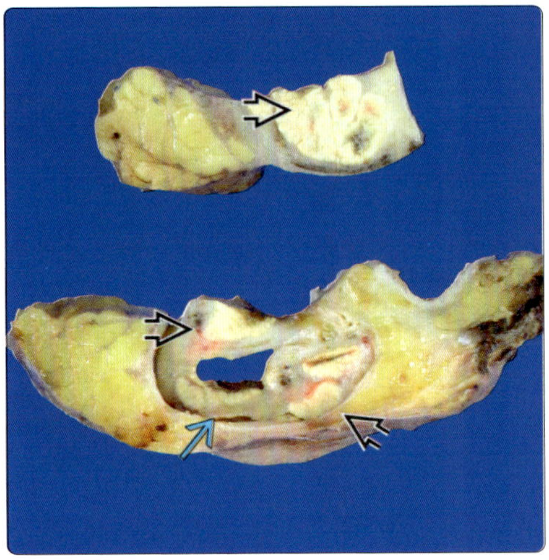

Xanthogranulomatous Pyelonephritis

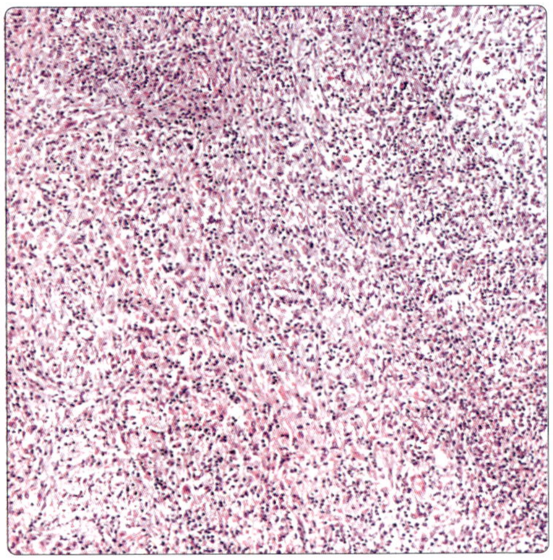

(Left) *Multiple irregular yellow masses ⇨ are present in the renal parenchyma in this case of xanthogranulomatous pyelonephritis. Marked hydronephrosis is present, with only a thin rim of fibrotic-appearing renal parenchyma ⇨.* **(Right)** *Abundant histiocytes with clear to lightly eosinophilic foamy cytoplasm are present in this frozen section of xanthogranulomatous pyelonephritis. Note the absence of delicate fibrovascular septa, which are characteristic of clear cell RCC.*

Xanthogranulomatous Pyelonephritis

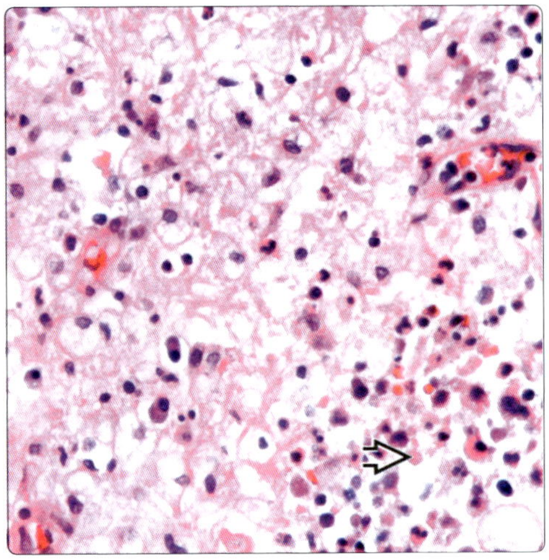

Fat Necrosis

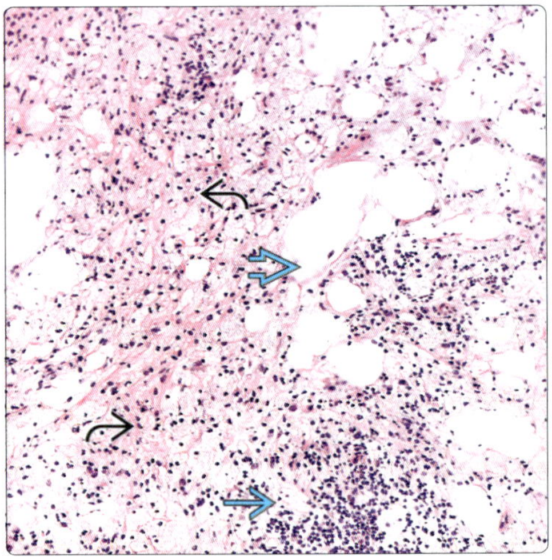

(Left) *A mixed inflammatory infiltrate with microabscess formation ⇨ is present in association with histiocytes with lightly eosinophilic cytoplasm in xanthogranulomatous pyelonephritis.* **(Right)** *The histiocytes with abundant foamy cytoplasm ⇨ in fat necrosis can be mistaken for clear cell RCC on frozen section, especially when evaluating a perinephric mass or a possible metastatic lesion in a patient with a history of RCC. Fat ⇨ and chronic inflammatory infiltrates ⇨ are identified.*

Malakoplakia

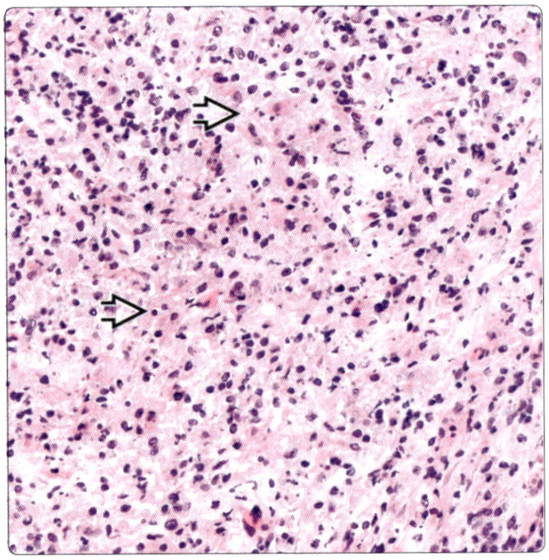

Malakoplakia: Michaelis-Gutmann Bodies

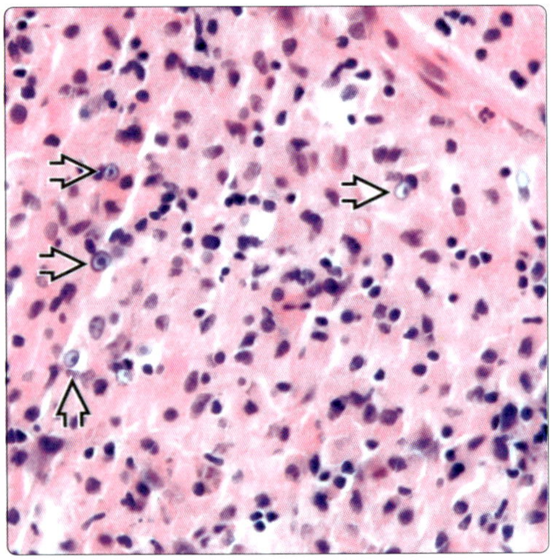

(Left) *Malakoplakia usually occurs in immunocompromised patients and may be seen as soft yellow plaques or nodules. Sheets of histiocytes with eosinophilic cytoplasm ⇨, known as von Hansemann histiocytes, are present in this frozen section. A mixed inflammatory infiltrate is present in the background.* **(Right)** *Numerous basophilic, lamellated targetoid ("owl's eye") Michaelis-Gutmann bodies ⇨ are identified in this permanent section of malakoplakia. These are thought to be mineralized phagosomes.*

Adult Cystic Nephroma: Gross Appearance

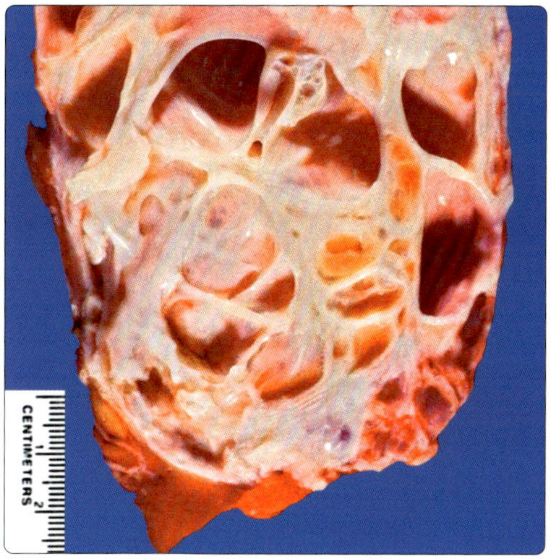

Mixed Epithelial and Stromal Tumor: Gross Appearance

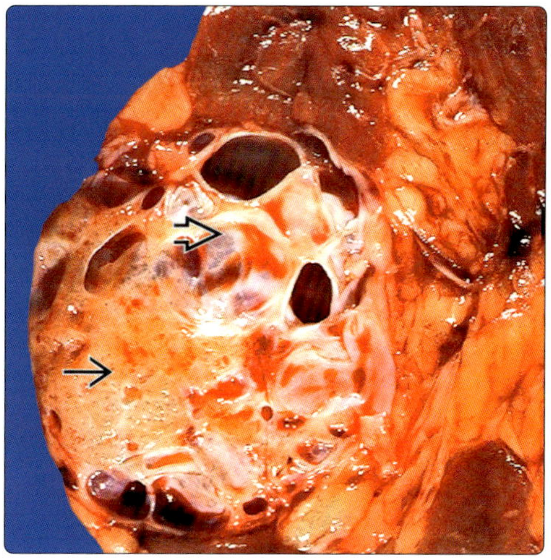

(Left) *Adult cystic nephroma is a predominantly cystic lesion in the mixed epithelial and stromal tumor and may resemble multilocular cystic renal neoplasm of low malignant potential. Both are made of multiple cysts with thin fibrous septations. (Courtesy S. Tickoo, MD.)* **(Right)** *This is a mixed epithelial and stromal tumor composed of areas made of thin-walled cysts ⇨ as well as more solid areas →. (Courtesy S. Tickoo, MD.)*

Mixed Epithelial and Stromal Tumor

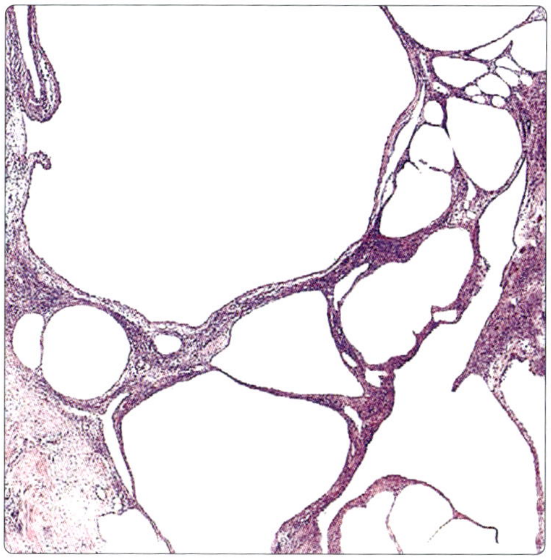

Mixed Epithelial and Stromal Tumor

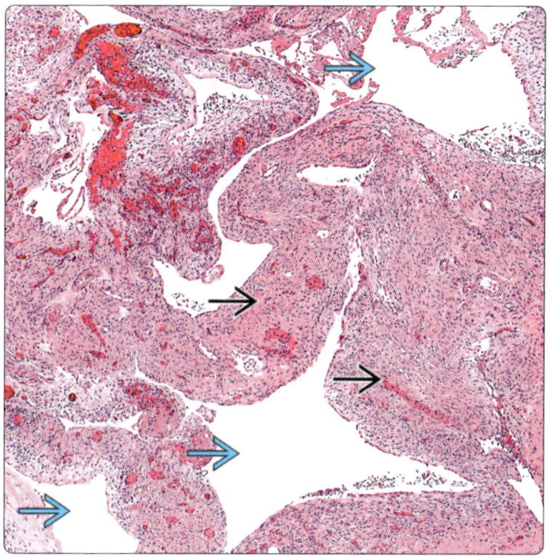

(Left) *Multiple cysts with thin fibrous septations are present in a predominantly cystic mixed epithelial and stromal tumor (MEST) (adult cystic nephroma). The cyst lining often appears flattened, hobnailed, or cuboidal. (Courtesy S. Tickoo, MD.)* **(Right)** *This MEST shows solid components composed of fibrous tissue → in addition to cysts →. The stromal component can consist of dense fibrous tissue, ovarian-type (spindle cell) stroma, &/or smooth muscle.*

Mixed Epithelial and Stromal Tumor

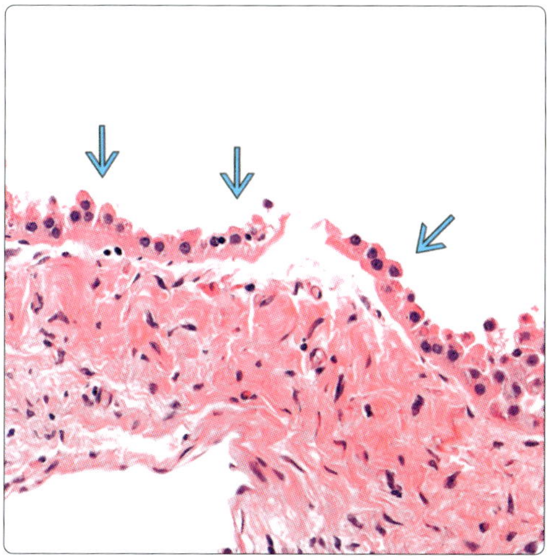

Lymphoma: Gross Appearance

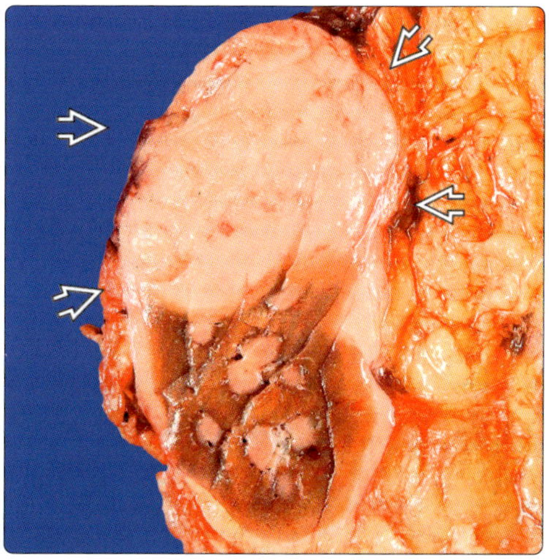

(Left) *A cuboidal epithelial lining → is identified lining a cyst in this MEST. Flattened, hobnailed, and columnar epithelium can also be present in these tumors. Less commonly, urothelial-like and clear cells can be identified lining the cyst walls.* **(Right)** *Lymphomas involving the kidney can form discrete tan/white homogeneous fleshy masses ⇨. The majority are of large B-cell type. Extensive necrosis can make diagnosis difficult on frozen section. (Courtesy S. Tickoo, MD.)*

SURGICAL/CLINICAL CONSIDERATIONS

Goal of Consultation

- Determine if potential donor kidney is suitable for transplantation
- Suitability of kidney depends on following
  - Pathologic features predictive of adequate renal function
    - ~ 40% of kidneys considered for transplantation under expanded criteria are rejected
  - Donor renal disease
    - Patients may not have been evaluated for renal disease prior to death
    - Some donor kidney disease can resolve after transplantation
      - IgA nephropathy most common; IgA deposits present in 10% of donor biopsies
  - Donor neoplastic disease
    - Any suspicious focal lesions are biopsied

Change in Patient Management

- Kidney will not be used for transplantation if determined to be unsuitable

Clinical Setting

- Clinical criteria are used to select kidneys most likely to become functional allografts
  - Standard criteria donors (SCDs)
    - Donors not defined as expanded criteria donors (ECDs)
  - ECDs
    - All donors age > 60 years
    - Donors age 50-60 years and have at least 2 of following
      - Death from cerebrovascular accident, hypertension, or serum creatinine >1.5 mg/dL
    - Donation after cardiac death
- Organ Procurement and Transplantation Network (OPTN) recommends preimplantation biopsies on subset of potential donors
  - Donors with Kidney Donor Profile Index (KDPI) of > 85%
    - Derived from 10 donor factors: Age, height, weight, ethnicity, history of diabetes or hypertension, cause of death, serum creatinine, hepatitis C virus, and donor after cardiac death status
  - By request of surgeon

Kidney Acceptance Criteria

- Clinical features of donor and potential recipient and pathologic findings of donor kidney are taken into consideration
  - No absolute cutoff has been established for any pathologic criteria
  - Double transplants are possible if there is concern about renal function

SPECIMEN EVALUATION

Gross

- Usually small wedge biopsies but can be needle biopsy
- Tissue should be gently blotted to remove excess fluid

Frozen Section

- Entire specimen is used for frozen section
- If capsule can be identified, specimen should be oriented so that sections are perpendicular to capsule

Reliability

- Renal specialist pathologist versus on-call general pathologist
  - 1 study found evaluation of donor biopsies by renal pathologist was correlated with 1-year graft function and death-censored graft survival
    - Evaluation by on-call pathologists, however, had no correlation with graft outcome
  - Training of on-call pathologists is recommended if renal pathologist is not available
  - If no renal pathologist is available on site, whole slide imaging with remote interpretation by renal pathologist may be option in some centers
- Reproducibility
  - Good to fair reproducibility among pathologists for some features

(Left) *This donor kidney biopsy appears edematous and the glomeruli appear hypercellular ➡. These are common artifacts of frozen sections. The percentage of globally sclerotic glomeruli ➡ is routinely reported.* **(Right)** *Frozen section artifacts are not seen in formalin-fixed permanent sections stained with PAS. This glomerulus has normal cellularity. There is mild intimal hyalinosis of an arteriole ➡.*

Donor Biopsy: Frozen Section

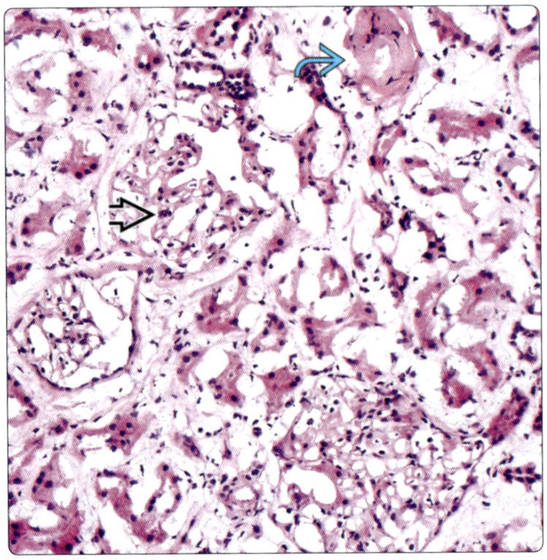

Donor Biopsy: Permanent Section

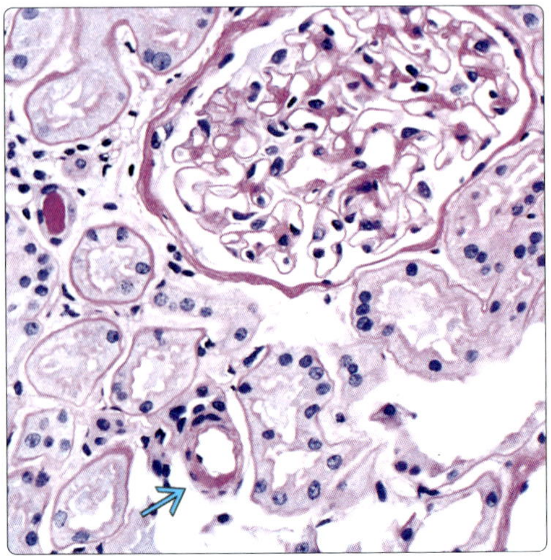

- Number of viable and globally sclerotic glomeruli, percentage of global glomerulosclerosis, interstitial fibrosis, and arteriosclerosis
- Poor reproducibility for arteriolar hyalinosis on frozen sections
  - Significant discrepancy from reproducibility on permanent sections
- Acute tubular injury shows poor reproducibility on frozen and permanent sections

EVALUATION OF DONOR BIOPSY

Sample Adequacy

- Size
  - Wedge biopsy 10 mm long x 5 mm wide x 5 mm deep
- Structures present
  - At least 25 glomeruli should be present, including glomeruli from deep cortex
  - At least 2 arteries should be present

Histologic Features

- Chronic changes
  - Present in many biopsies
  - Usually increase with donor age
- Glomerulosclerosis
  - Glomerulus is replaced by solid eosinophilic fibrosis
  - Percentage of globally sclerotic glomeruli important (global glomerulosclerosis)
    - > 20% is associated with higher incidence of delayed graft function (DGF) requiring transient dialysis and higher creatinine (Cr) at 3-24 months
      - Variable effect on graft survival
  - No absolute cutoff point for percent of global glomerulosclerosis has been determined
  - Sclerotic glomeruli are predominately in subcapsular cortex in arteriosclerosis and often overestimated in wedge biopsies
  - Strong correlation with age
- Arteriosclerosis
  - Moderate arteriosclerosis (> 25% luminal narrowing) is predictor of worse graft outcome (graft loss, DGF, higher Cr)
- Interstitial fibrosis and tubular atrophy
  - Not consistently predictive of graft function
- Thrombi in glomeruli and arteries
  - Head trauma in donor can precipitate thrombotic microangiopathy
  - Even with glomerular thrombi, good outcome is possible
  - Reporting percentage of glomeruli with thrombi may not represent extent of thrombi in graft
    - Percentage of glomerular area involved by thrombi (segmental versus diffuse) may convey better extent of thrombosis, but this has not been well studied
  - Cholesterol emboli may be contraindication to transplantation
- Other features
  - Renal infarct: May be associated with vascular changes
  - Tumors
    - Patients may have unsuspected neoplasms
    - Angiomyolipoma is most common benign renal tumor (0.1-0.2% of population)
      - Involved kidneys have been used successfully for transplantation
      - May be contraindication to transplantation in some settings
    - Small well-differentiated renal cell carcinomas may be resected and kidney used for transplantation
  - Mesangial nodules
    - Often associated with diabetes
  - Pigmented casts in tubules
    - Myoglobin casts associated with rhabdomyolysis
      - May not be contradiction to transplantation
  - Interstitial inflammation
    - Lymphocytic infiltrates are common finding
      - Very rarely due to lymphoma or leukemia
    - Granulomatous inflammation may be contraindication for transplantation

Maryland Aggregate Pathology Index (MAPI)

- Subset (~ 12%) of kidneys from donors unsuitable by clinical criteria have normal histologic features
- MAPI can be used to predict likelihood of graft survival at 5 years based on pathologic features
- Aggregate score is predictive of graft survival
  - Scores 0-7: 90%
  - Scores 8-11: 63%
  - Scores 12-15: 53%
- 5 histologic features are evaluated, and points for each are added to create score
  - Global glomerulosclerosis
    - If ≥ 15%: 2 points
  - Wall:lumen ratio of interlobular arteries (width of wall at 2 points/diameter of lumen)
    - If ≥ 0.5: 2 points
  - Periglomerular fibrosis (thickening, wrinkling, and reduplication of Bowman capsule)
    - If present: 4 points
  - Arteriolar hyalinosis (amorphous, homogeneous eosinophilic deposits in walls of arterioles)
    - If present: 4 points
  - Scar (focus of sclerosis and renal parenchymal fibrosis and atrophy involving at least 10 tubules)
    - If present: 3 points

REPORTING

Donor Biopsy

- Site and type of specimen (wedge or needle core biopsy)
- Number of glomeruli, number of globally sclerotic glomeruli, percentage of global glomerulosclerosis
- Number of arteries (not arterioles)
- Histologic features (graded as none, mild, moderate, or severe)
  - Interstitial fibrosis, tubular atrophy, interstitial inflammation, arterial intimal fibrosis, glomerular thrombi
- Any other notable feature (e.g., nodular glomerulosclerosis, focal segmental glomerulosclerosis, tumor)

PITFALLS

Wedge Biopsies

- Sclerotic glomeruli overestimated in wedge biopsies

Donor Biopsy Reporting and Scoring Sheet

Features	Notes
Type of specimen	Wedge biopsy, core needle biopsy
Number of glomeruli	Number of unique glomeruli that are available for evaluation are counted
Number of globally sclerosed glomeruli	Periglomerular sclerosis and focal glomerulosclerosis are included under other findings
Percentage of global glomerulosclerosis	Number of globally sclerosed glomeruli over number of total glomeruli
Number of arteries (not arterioles)	Artery defined as vessel with internal elastic lamina, or diameter > 1/3 diameter of typical glomerulus, or vessel with 3 or more layers of smooth muscle

Following Findings Are Scored

Score	None	Mild	Moderate	Severe
Interstitial fibrosis	None (< 5% cortex)	Mild (6-25%)	Moderate (26-50%)	Severe (> 50% of cortex involved)
Tubular atrophy	None (0% cortex)	Mild (< 25%)	Moderate (26-50%)	Severe (> 50% of cortical tubules involved)
Interstitial inflammation	None (< 10% cortex)	Mild (10-25%)	Moderate (26-50%)	Severe (> 50% of cortex involved)
Arterial intimal fibrosis (arteriosclerosis)	None (0% luminal narrowing)	Mild (< 25%)	Moderate (26-50%)	Severe (> 50% vascular narrowing)
Arteriolar hyalinosis (hyaline restricted to subendothelial layer)	None	Mild (at least 1 arteriole)	Moderate (> 1 arteriole)	Severe (circumferential, multiple arterioles)
Glomerular thrombi	None	Mild (< 10% of capillaries occluded in most severely affected glomerulus)	Moderate (10-25% capillaries occluded)	Severe (> 25% capillaries occluded)
Acute tubular injury or necrosis	None	Mild (epithelial flattening, tubule dilation, nuclear dropout, loss of brush border)	Moderate (focal coagulative type necrosis)	Severe (infarction)
Other notable findings				
Findings	Focal segmental glomerulosclerosis	Nodular glomerulosclerosis	Tumor	Others

Liapis H et al: Banff histopathological consensus criteria for preimplantation kidney biopsies. Am J Transplant. 17(1):140-150, 2017

- Superficial biopsy may overrepresent globally sclerotic glomeruli, which tend to be subcapsular in patients with arteriosclerosis
- Arteries may be absent

Superficial Biopsy

- Superficial biopsy may only have capsule present

Frozen Section Artifacts

- Glomeruli
  - Glomeruli appear hypercellular
- Interstitium
  - Retraction of epithelial elements can resemble interstitial edema
  - Edema can resemble fibrosis
- Tubules
  - Tubules appear retracted
    - Can be misinterpreted as atrophy or injury
  - Difficult to appreciate acute tubular injury
- Red cell casts lyse on freezing

Specimen Handling

- Cold ischemic time must be minimized
- Biopsies should be kept moist in appropriate preservative
  - Prolonged time in saline can produce artifacts
  - Desiccation can alter appearance

SELECTED REFERENCES

1. Liapis H et al: Banff histopathological consensus criteria for preimplantation kidney biopsies. Am J Transplant. 17(1):140-150, 2017
2. Azancot MA et al: The reproducibility and predictive value on outcome of renal biopsies from expanded criteria donors. Kidney Int. 85(5):1161-8, 2014
3. Haas M: Donor kidney biopsies: pathology matters, and so does the pathologist. Kidney Int. 85(5):1016-9, 2014

Donor Biopsy: Frozen Section

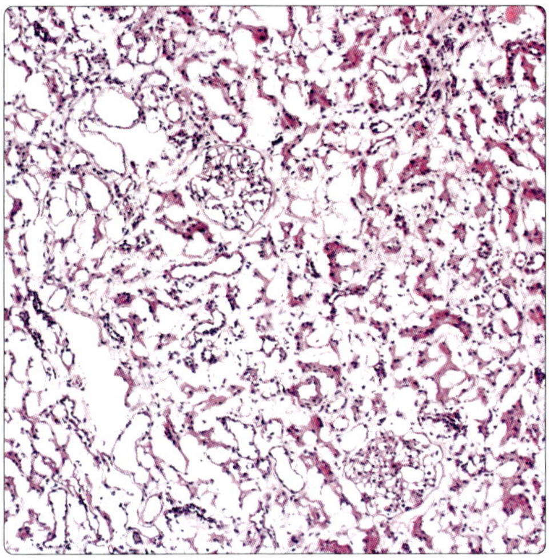

Donor Biopsy: Wedge biopsy

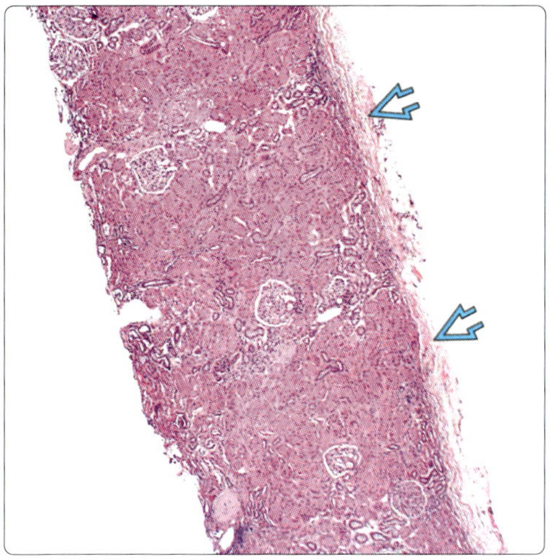

(Left) *This frozen section of a donor biopsy shows apparent interstitial edema, likely the "normal" state of the kidney before dehydration during processing. The tubular morphology is uninterpretable. The evaluation of features predictive of graft function is challenging in specimens with this degree of artifact.* **(Right)** *Most donor biopsies are wedge, instead of needle, biopsies, and sample subcapsular tissue (capsule ⇨). This is a reason why intermediate-sized arteries are not often sampled.*

Donor Biopsy: Glomerular Thrombi

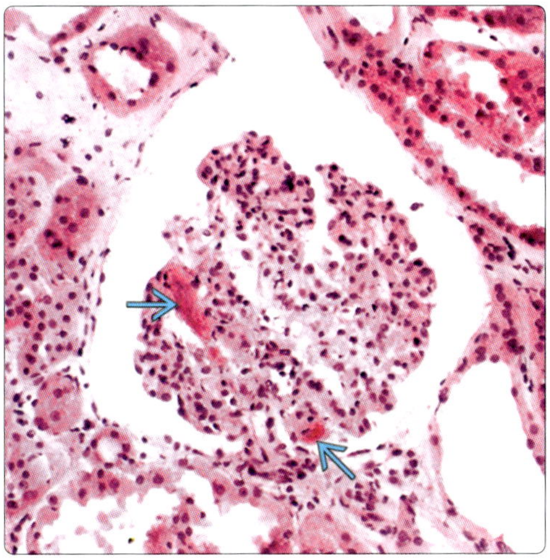

Donor Biopsy: Glomerular Thrombi

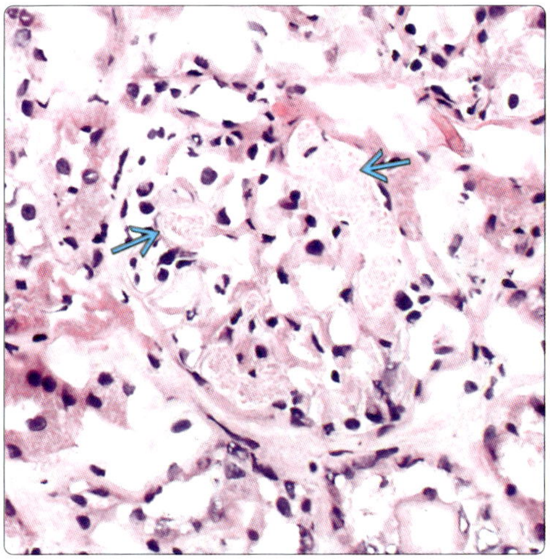

(Left) *This frozen section of a donor biopsy shows fibrin thrombi → in 2 capillary loops. These can be easily overlooked, especially if they are focal. Thrombi are common in donors who died from stroke or head injury. Scattered thrombi do not contraindicate use of the kidney for transplantation.* **(Right)** *Thrombi → in a glomerulus of a donor biopsy can appear pale on some H&E-stained sections, instead of darkly eosinophilic. This can make detection of thrombi difficult.*

Donor Biopsy: Arteriosclerosis

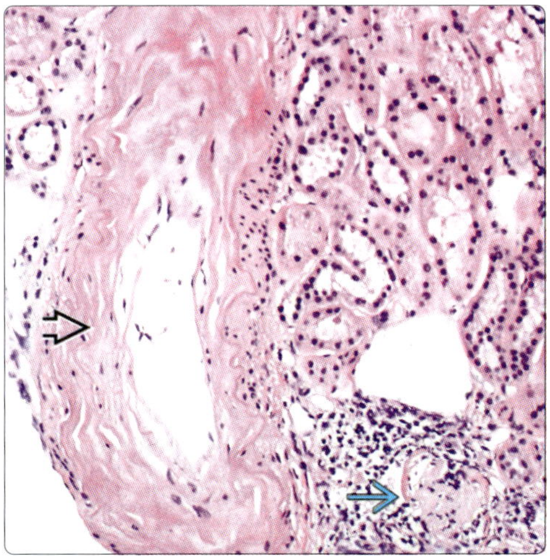

Donor Biopsy: Diffuse Global Glomerulosclerosis

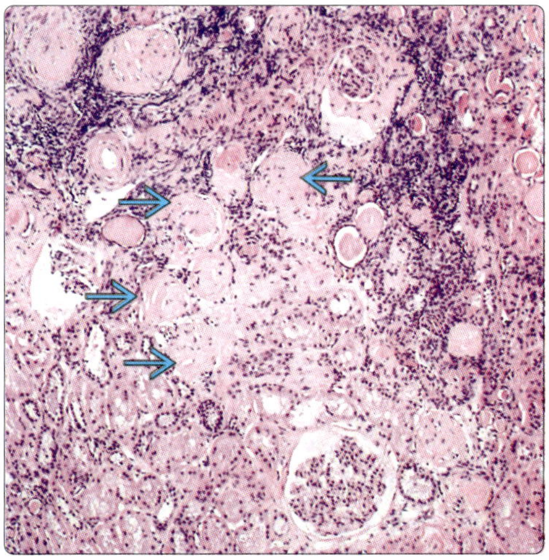

(Left) *A biopsy from a potential donor kidney shows severe arteriosclerosis ⇨. This size artery is not always present in wedge biopsies. A globally sclerotic glomerulus is also seen →.* **(Right)** *This donor kidney biopsy shows > 80% globally sclerotic glomeruli →. The biopsy is not from a subcapsular scar. Both the right and left kidneys showed the same finding. This finding is a reason for rejecting kidneys for transplantation.*

Contents

(Left) *This donor biopsy shows mild arteriolar hyalinosis, which is difficult to recognize on frozen section. The corresponding permanent section showed diffuse diabetic glomerulosclerosis.* **(Right)** *The permanent section of a donor biopsy shows mild to moderate mesangial matrix expansion, readily recognized on a PAS-stained section. There is also arteriolar hyalinosis.*

Donor Biopsy: Diabetic Donor

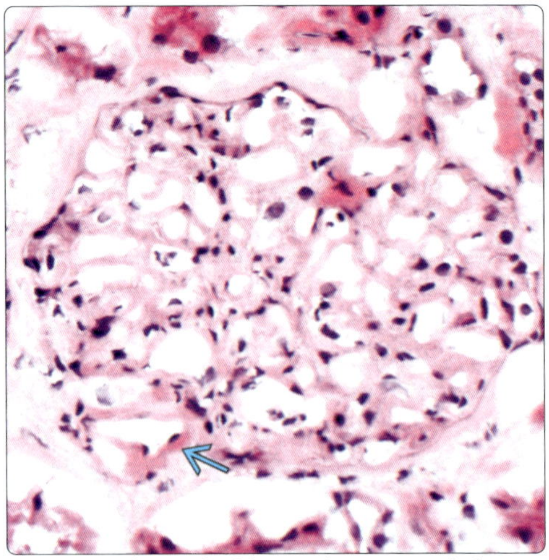

Donor Biopsy: Diffuse Diabetic Glomerulosclerosis

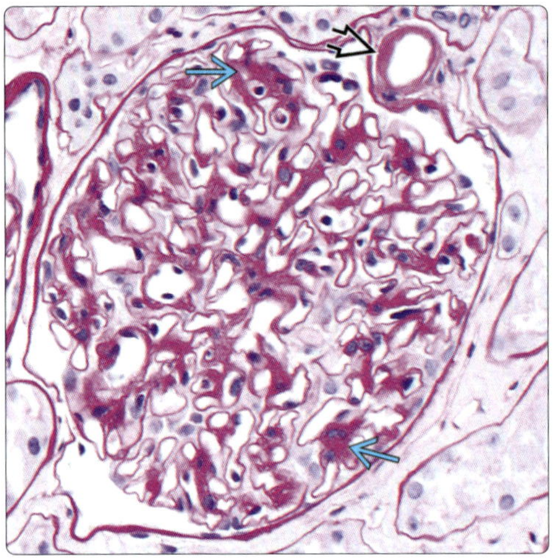

(Left) *This biopsy taken 17 days after transplantation of the kidney shows prominent nodular diabetic glomerulopathy. Both the donor and the recipient were diabetic. The nodules were not apparent in a donor frozen section, even in retrospect. The graft was eventually lost. Donation to a nondiabetic recipient might have been more salutary.* **(Right)** *This kidney shows severe tubular injury with granular eosinophilic casts positive for myoglobin. The cause of death of the donor was trauma.*

Transplanted Kidney Biopsy: Nodular Glomerulosclerosis not Apparent on Frozen Section

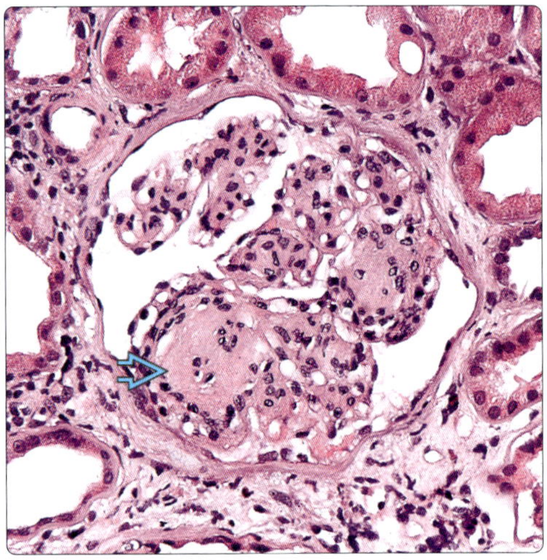

Donor Biopsy: Myoglobin Casts

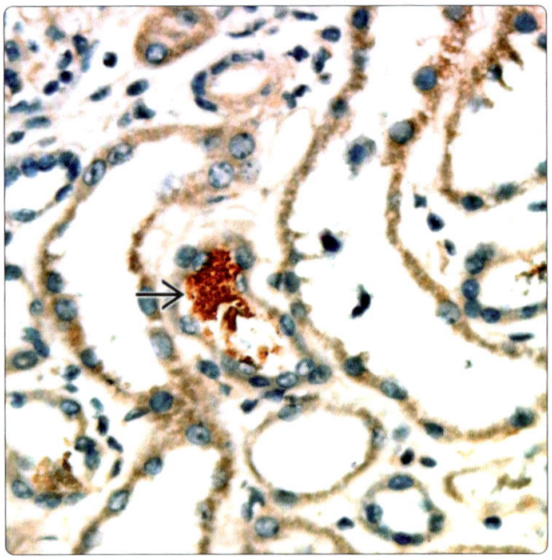

(Left) *Immunofluorescence of a living donor kidney shows IgA deposits in the mesangium. The donor had no evidence of glomerular disease. This may be an incidental finding in donor biopsies. IgA deposits resolve with time in the recipient after donation.* **(Right)** *Immunofluorescence of a biopsy taken 3 months after transplant of a living donor kidney that previously showed prominent IgA deposits in the mesangium now shows loss of the mesangial IgA deposits. The recipient had no clinical evidence of glomerular disease.*

Donor Kidney: Incidental IgA Deposits

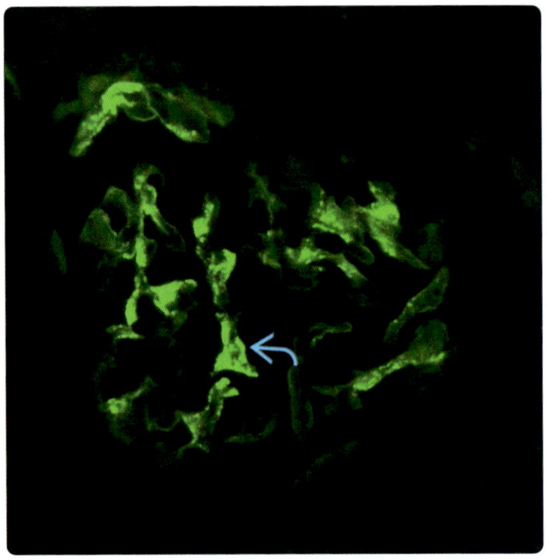

Transplanted Kidney Biopsy: Resolving IgA Deposits Post Transplant

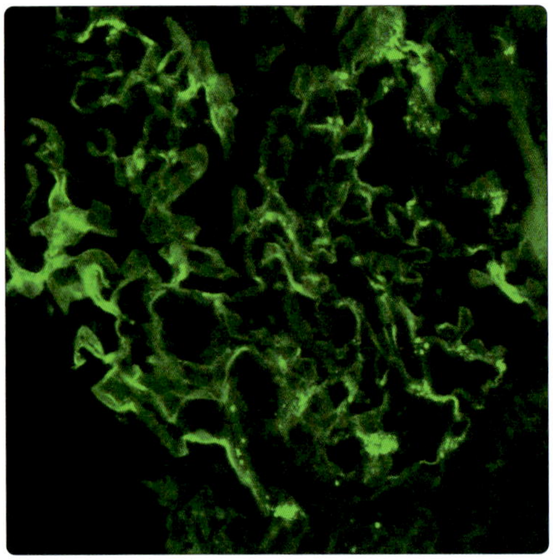

Donor Biopsy: Arteriolar Hyalinosis

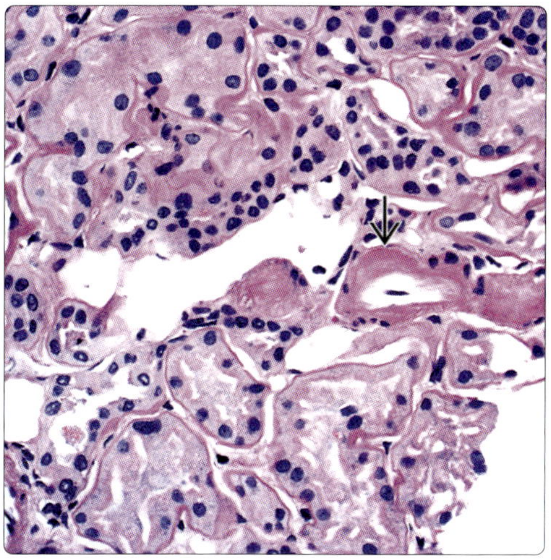

Donor Biopsy: Nodular Arteriolar Hyalinosis

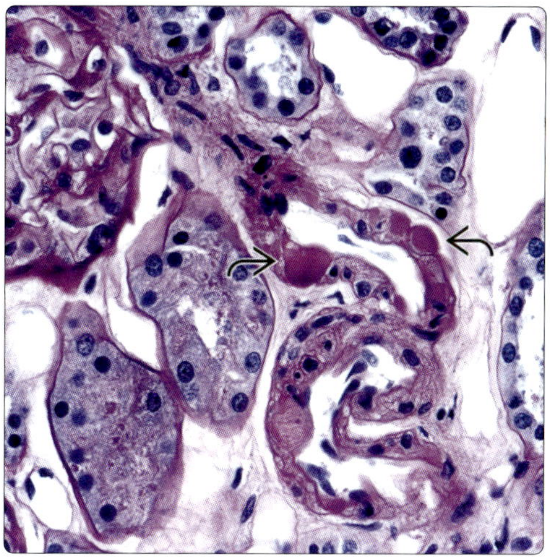

(Left) *Intimal arteriolar hyalinosis → is a feature difficult to identify on a frozen section. This feature is more obvious on this permanent section stained with periodic acid-Schiff.* **(Right)** *Nodular peripheral arteriolar hyalinosis → in a donor biopsy looks exactly like the hyalinosis commonly found in chronic calcineurin inhibitor (CNI) toxicity and was once thought to be specific for CNI. This feature, however, is also uncommonly seen in the absence of CNI administration.*

Donor Biopsy: Permanent Section

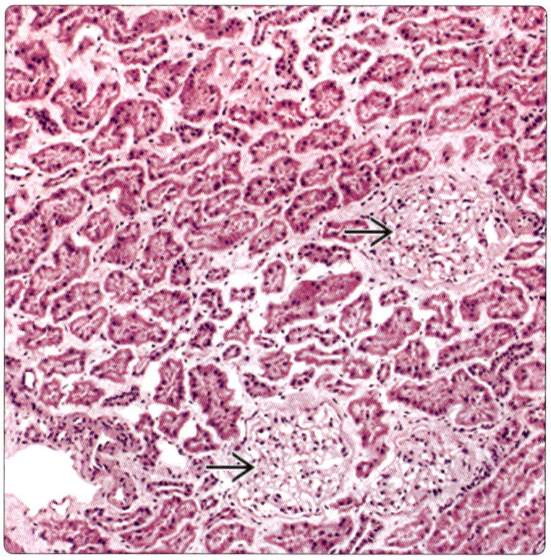

Donor Wedge Biopsy: Frozen Section with Wrinkles

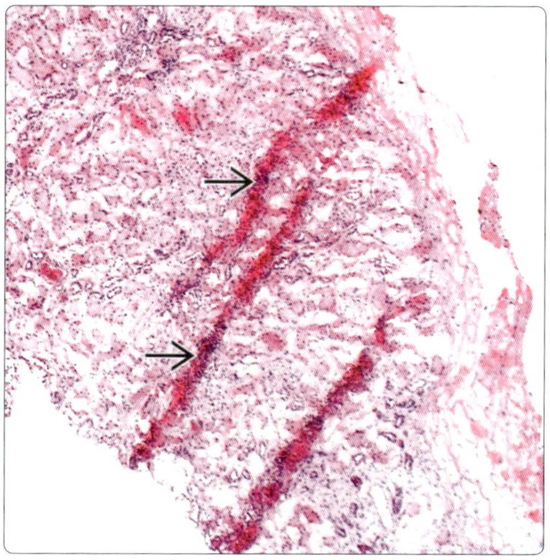

(Left) *The appearance of kidney parenchyma can be different on frozen section and subsequent permanent section. This biopsy looked markedly edematous on frozen section and the glomeruli appeared hypercellular. On permanent section, there is only focal, fine interstitial edema and normal-appearing glomeruli →.* **(Right)** *Frozen sections are more likely than permanent sections to show wrinkles → and folds, which can make interpretation more difficult. Additional sections without artifacts should be prepared.*

Donor Biopsy: Pediatric Patient

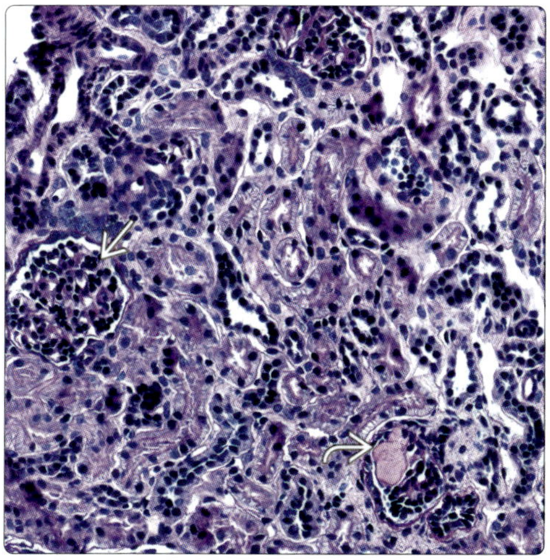

Donor Biopsy: Angiomyolipoma

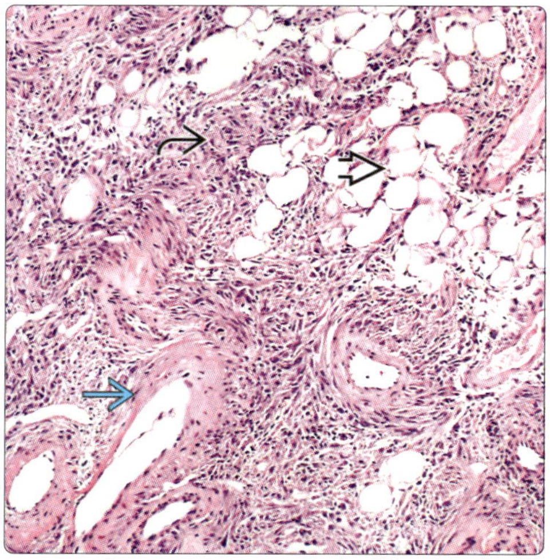

(Left) *A donor kidney biopsy from a child shows immature glomeruli → with crowded podocytes and 1 glomerulus with focal segmental glomerulosclerosis →, probably developmental.* **(Right)** *Unsuspected neoplasms may be found in donor kidneys. This biopsy revealed an angiomyolipoma. The vascular →, smooth muscle →, and adipose tissue → elements characteristic of this tumor are seen.*

SURGICAL/CLINICAL CONSIDERATION

Goal of Consultation

- Determine if renal needle biopsy is adequate for final diagnosis
- Allocate tissue for special studies
  - Light microscopy (LM)
  - Immunofluorescence (IF)
  - Electron microscopy (EM)
  - Other studies depending on clinical situation
    - Culture for organisms
    - Tissue for molecular studies (e.g., tissue saved in fixatives such as RNAlater for RNA isolation)

Change in Patient Management

- If specimen is deemed inadequate, additional needle biopsies will be taken

Clinical Setting

- Medical renal biopsy
  - Generally performed for abnormal renal function or for urinary abnormalities
    - Should include renal cortex with glomeruli
    - Typically require IF and EM studies for final diagnosis
  - Also performed to evaluate renal allografts
    - Allograft biopsies also benefit from IF and sometimes EM studies
    - Some centers perform surveillance (protocol) allograft biopsies at predetermined time points after transplant
    - Surveillance biopsies are evaluated for subclinical rejection, viral infection, recurrent disease, etc.
- Biopsies are usually performed under ultrasound guidance or CT guidance
  - Percutaneous (needle) biopsy
    - Ultrasound-guided, automated gun with 16-gauge to 18-gauge needle is usual
    - 3 biopsy passes provide adequate sample in 84% of cases in native and transplant biopsies (by Banff adequacy criteria)
    - Compared to 18-gauge needle biopsies, 16-gauge needle biopsies provide more glomeruli & higher percentage of adequate biopsies with fewer passes
  - Transjugular renal biopsy may be performed in patients at high risk for bleeding (coagulopathy or thrombocytopenia)
    - Typically yields smaller sample than percutaneous biopsy but sufficient for diagnosis in > 90% of cases
- Generally regarded as safe outpatient procedure
  - Hematuria may occur
    - Postbiopsy microscopic hematuria is usual
    - Gross hematuria in ~ 3.5%
  - Other complications in 1-3% (varies with technique)
    - Higher risk of bleeding with 14-gauge needle biopsy
      - 16-gauge and 18-gauge needle biopsies have lower risk of bleeding
    - Perirenal hematoma ~ 2.5%
    - Bleeding requiring transfusion ~ 0.9%
    - Hemorrhage requiring nephrectomy ~ 0.01%
    - Death ~ 0.02% (2 of 8,971 patients in metaanalysis)
  - Intrarenal arteriovenous fistulas in ~ 7% of allograft biopsies
    - Usually resolve
    - No apparent effect on renal function
  - Page kidney (described by Dr. Irwin Page)
    - Most commonly due to trauma, but rare cases occur due to bleeding after kidney biopsy
    - Compression of kidney by accumulation of blood in perinephric or subcapsular space
    - Usually manifests with renin-dependent reactive hypertension due to renal ischemia
      - Occasionally presents with renal insufficiency

Quality Improvement

- On-site adequacy assessment and adequacy statement in renal biopsy report may improve renal biopsy adequacy
- In 1 study
  - 22% of biopsies without on-site evaluation were considered inadequate

Fresh Renal Biopsy: Gross Examination

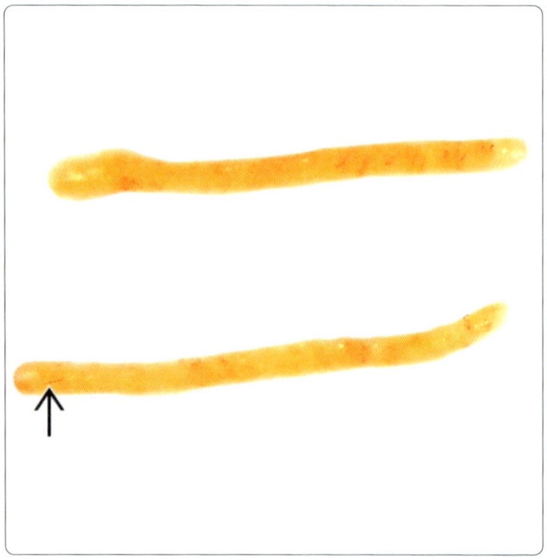

Fixed Renal Biopsy: Gross Examination

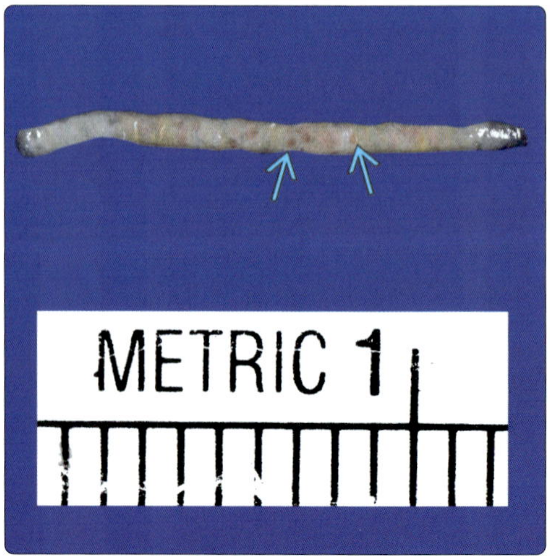

(Left) *Renal 16-gauge cores are typically 1 mm in diameter x 10-20 mm long (these are ~ 13 mm). Glomeruli are pale or congested bulges; red cell casts are brown streaks ➔ or dots. (Courtesy C. Swetts, MD.)* **(Right)** *A kidney transplant biopsy from a briefly formalin-fixed sample shows glomeruli ➔ that are rounded and darker tan than surrounding tissue.*

- Only ~ 6% of biopsies with on-site evaluation were considered inadequate

SPECIMEN EVALUATION

Gross

- Biopsies must only be touched by forceps free of fixatives
  - Minute amounts of formalin can alter antigenicity of tissue used for IF
  - Glutaraldehyde contamination can complicate interpretation by LM and IF
- Needle biopsies are best examined under stereomicroscopy (dissecting microscope)
  - If dissecting microscope is not available, renal biopsies can be examined using magnifying glass
- For evaluation of allografts, ≥ 10 glomeruli and 2 arteries must be present (Banff criteria)
  - Glomeruli are pink to red nodules ("raspberries") in pale-tan background on examination of fresh tissue
    - Formalin or glutaraldehyde fixation alters appearance; glomeruli appear slightly more tan on tan background
    - Glomeruli difficult to identify on tissue preserved in IF transport medium (Zeus)
      - Tissue appears white and opaque

Allocation of Tissue

- In majority of cases, tissue is saved for LM, IF, and EM
  - Appropriate allocation of tissue depends on several factors
    - Clinical differential diagnosis
    - Focality of expected disease
    - Amount of tissue available
- LM
  - Tissue is fixed in formalin
  - Standard histochemical stains are H&E, PAS, Jones-methenamine silver, and trichrome
  - Additional stains ordered depending on clinical setting and LM appearance
- IF
  - Cortex and medulla are placed in Zeus transport solution (Michel solution)
  - Standard immunohistochemical studies are IgA, IgG, IgM, kappa, lambda, C3, C1q, albumin, and fibrin
    - C4d is added for allograft biopsies to evaluate for antibody-mediated rejection
  - If no glomeruli are present in tissue submitted in Zeus medium, IF staining may still be contributory
    - Detection of monoclonal immunoglobulin deposition disease, light-chain cast nephropathy, light-chain (AL) or heavy-chain (AH) amyloidosis, etc.
    - C4d staining of peritubular capillaries for transplant biopsies (C4d may also be performed by immunoperoxidase staining)
  - If no glomeruli present in frozen IF tissue, IF can be performed on pronase-digested paraffin sections
    - Pronase-digested paraffin IF less sensitive than routine IF on frozen tissue
- EM
  - Tissue with few glomeruli are saved in Karnovsky glutaraldehyde/paraformaldehyde fixative
  - If limited tissue, tissue processed for LM can be deparaffinized for EM
    - This technique shows some artifacts that can inhibit interpretation
    - Artifactual glomerular basement membrane thinning does not allow for diagnosis of thin glomerular basement membrane nephropathy on deparaffinized samples
    - Loss of cellular detail
    - Podocyte foot processes and endothelial cells may not be evaluable
    - Histology technician may cut fewer sections to save tissue for potential EM studies on deparaffinized tissue

Frozen Section

- In general, tissue should be allocated for special studies and should not be frozen for histologic examination

REPORTING

Gross

- Reports should include
  - Fixative or transport media in which specimens were received
  - Specimen measurements
  - Adequacy of sample
  - Allocation of tissue

PITFALLS

Evaluation of Number of Glomeruli

- In limited samples, arteries may look like glomeruli
  - Helpful to look for at least 2 glomeruli near each other
- Very small ischemic glomeruli may not be apparent grossly, even under dissection microscope

SELECTED REFERENCES

1. Chunduri S et al: Adequacy and complication rates with 14- vs. 16-gauge automated needles in percutaneous renal biopsy of native kidneys. Semin Dial. 28(2):E11-4, 2015
2. Geldenhuys L et al: Percutaneous native renal biopsy adequacy: a successful interdepartmental quality improvement activity. Can J Kidney Health Dis. 2:8, 2015
3. Gilani SM et al: Role of on-site microscopic evaluation of kidney biopsy for adequacy and allocation of glomeruli: comparison of renal biopsies with and without on-site microscopic evaluation. Pathologica. 105(6):342-5, 2013
4. Goldstein MA et al: Nonfocal renal biopsies: adequacy and factors affecting a successful outcome. J Comput Assist Tomogr. 37(2):176-82, 2013
5. Mai J et al: Is bigger better? A retrospective analysis of native renal biopsies with 16 Gauge versus 18 Gauge automatic needles. Nephrology (Carlton). 18(7):525-30, 2013
6. Corapi KM et al: Bleeding complications of native kidney biopsy: a systematic review and meta-analysis. Am J Kidney Dis. 60(1):62-73, 2012
7. Kurban G et al: Needle core biopsies provide ample material for genomic and proteomic studies of kidney cancer: observations on DNA, RNA, protein extractions and VHL mutation detection. Pathol Res Pract. 208(1):22-31, 2012
8. Sis B et al: Banff '09 meeting report: antibody mediated graft deterioration and implementation of Banff working groups. Am J Transplant. 10(3):464-71, 2010
9. Kamar N et al: Acute Page kidney after a kidney allograft biopsy: successful outcome from observation and medical treatment. Transplantation. 87(3):453-4, 2009
10. Misra S et al: Safety and diagnostic yield of transjugular renal biopsy. J Vasc Interv Radiol. 19(4):546-51, 2008

(Left) *The kidney is often biopsied percutaneously under ultrasound or CT guidance using a posterior approach.* **(Right)** *This sagittal image of the left kidney was obtained during an ultrasound-guided biopsy. The image shows a core biopsy needle that has been introduced into the cortex of the lower renal pole using real-time guidance. The needle trajectory is directed away from the renal hilum to reduce the risk of injury to hilar vessels and the urinary collecting system.*

Renal Biopsy Procedure

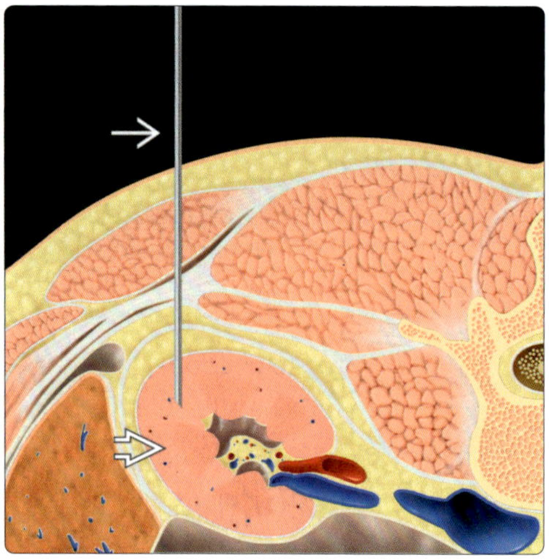

Renal Biopsy Under Ultrasound Guidance

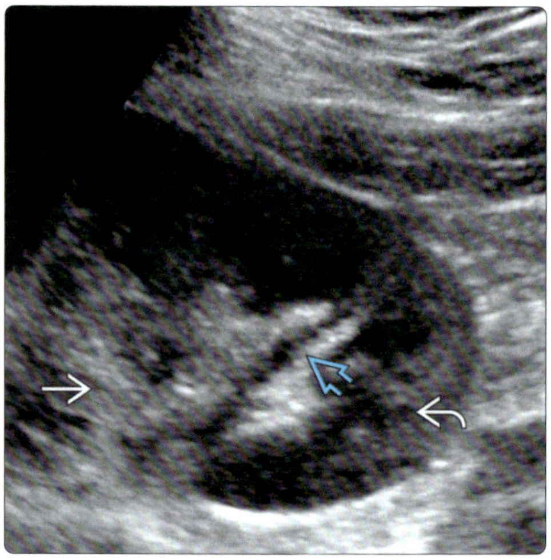

(Left) *A 39-year-old man underwent percutaneous kidney biopsy for chronic renal failure. He subsequently developed hypertension (180s/100s) and renal failure. A CT scan showed a subcapsular hematoma, that resulted in decreased renal perfusion (acute Page kidney).* **(Right)** *An ultrasound image shows an AV fistula at a recent biopsy site in the lower pole of a renal transplant. Doppler waveform at the fistula shows typical high-velocity, low-resistance blood flow. (Courtesy T. Atwell, MD.)*

Renal Biopsy: Acute Page Kidney Complication

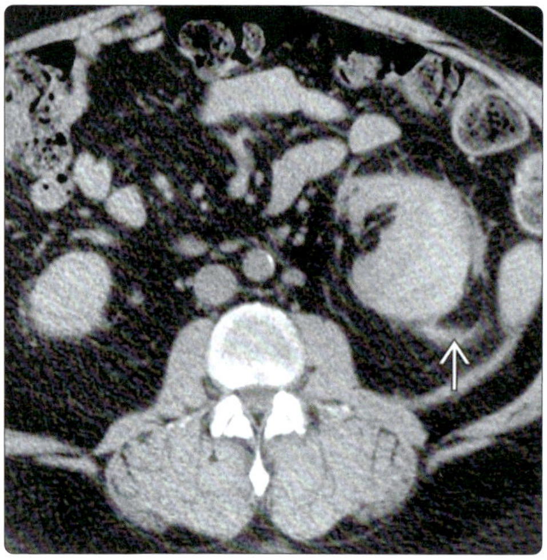

Renal Biopsy: Arteriovenous Fistula Complication

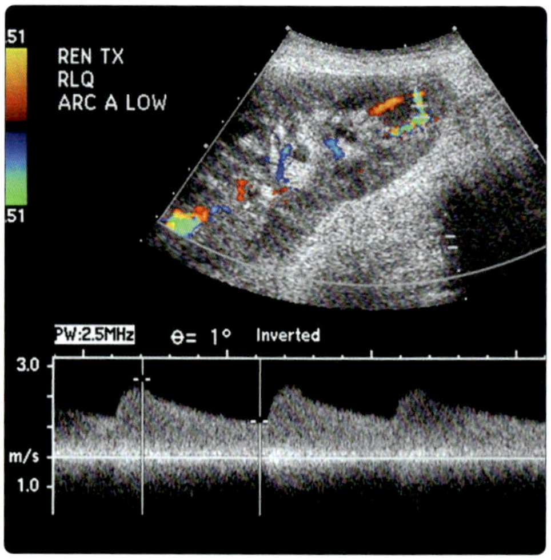

(Left) *An adequate sample is essential to detect focal lesions. This is a case of focal necrotizing and crescentic glomerulonephritis that is pauciimmune. Only 2 glomeruli show cellular crescents, whereas the other glomeruli look normal.* **(Right)** *An abdominal CT scan shows a moderate-sized left retroperitoneal perinephric hematoma following a percutaneous kidney biopsy. An acute bleed tracked along the left pericolic gutter and psoas muscle.*

Renal Biopsy: Disease With Focal Lesions

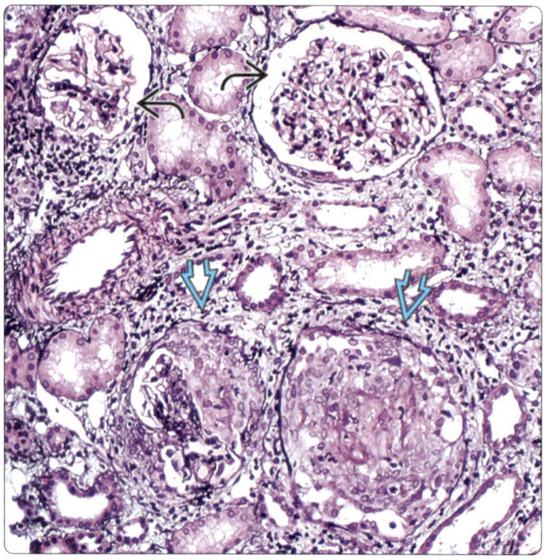

Renal Biopsy: Perinephric Hematoma Complication

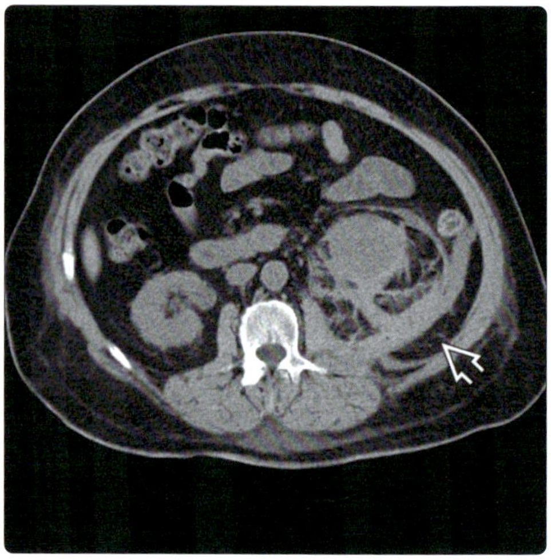

Renal Biopsy: Diffuse Disease

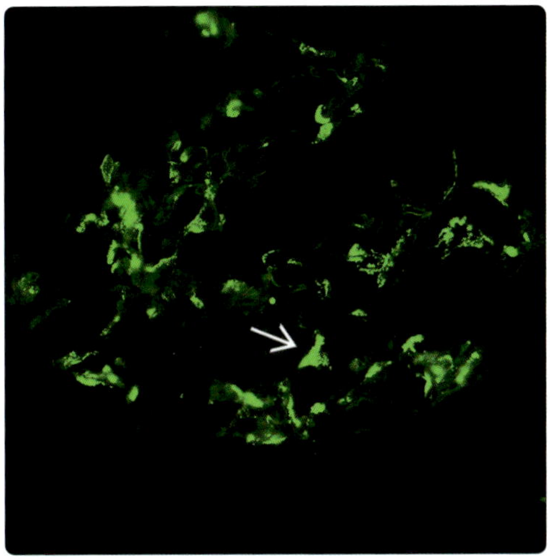

Renal Biopsy: Focal Disease

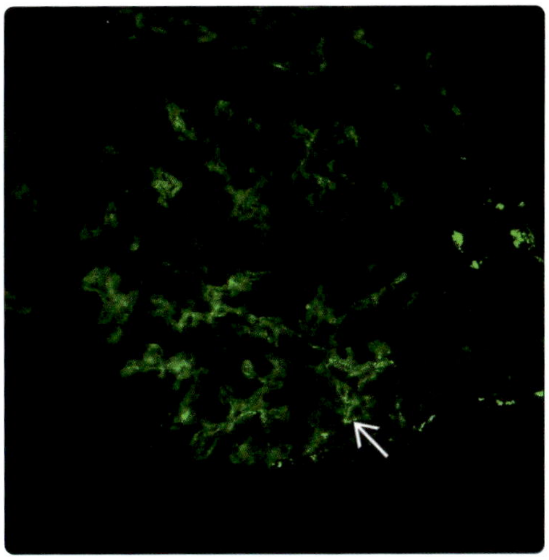

(Left) *Immunofluorescence staining for IgA is diffuse in IgA nephropathy, so even 1 glomerulus present in IF tissue should be sufficient to make a diagnosis of IgA nephropathy with correlating features by light microscopy and EM. This image shows granular mesangial staining for IgA* ➡. **(Right)** *Immunofluorescence staining in cryoglobulinemic glomerulonephritis can be variable between glomeruli. In this glomerulus, there is only trace segmental staining for C3* ➡. *A larger IF sample would be helpful to support this diagnosis.*

Renal Biopsy: Limited Tissue Sample

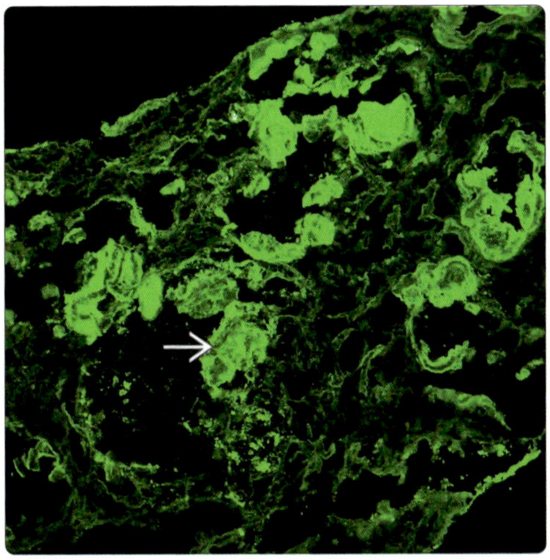

Renal Biopsy: Value of Tissue for Electron Microscopy

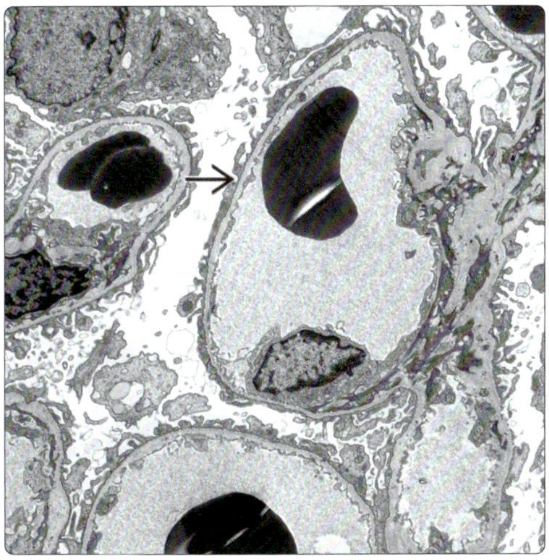

(Left) *Immunofluorescence staining can be contributory for some diseases, even in biopsies without glomeruli. This patient with acute renal failure had cast nephropathy with casts* ➡ *that stain for λ- but not κ-light chain.* **(Right)** *A woman underwent biopsy for a history of longstanding microscopic hematuria. By light microscopy and IF the glomeruli were normal. EM shows thin glioblastomas GBMs* ➡ *(mean: 240 nm). This diagnosis of thin GBM nephropathy cannot be made by EM on deparaffinized tissue due to thinning artifact.*

Renal Biopsy: Allograft Sampling for Rejection

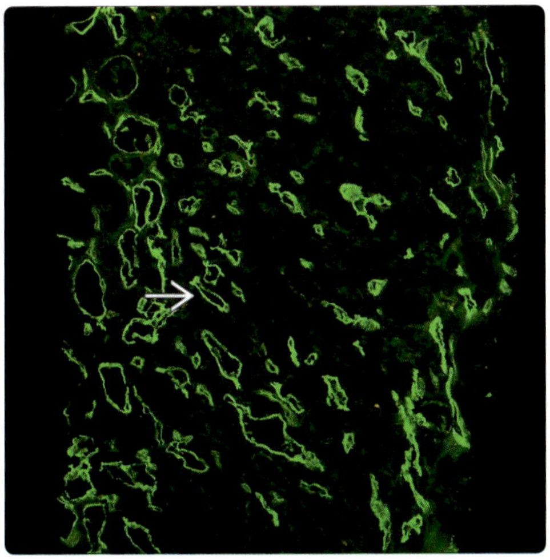

Renal Biopsy: Value of Tissue for Electron Microscopy

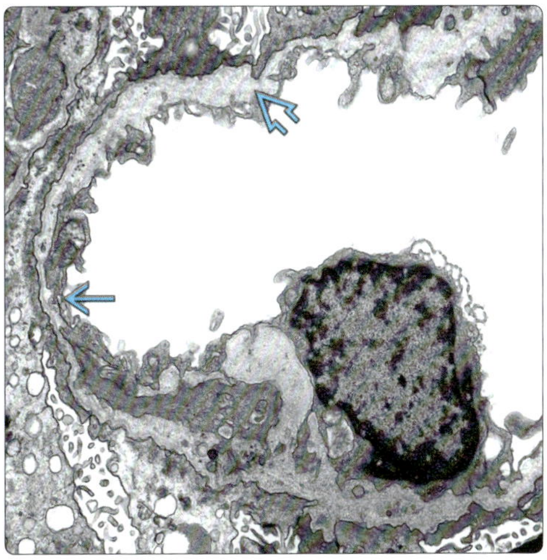

(Left) *C4d staining to evaluate humoral rejection can be interpreted on specimens with medulla and without glomeruli. In this case, there is diffuse bright peritubular capillary staining for C4d* ➡. **(Right)** *This biopsy is from a 13-year-old boy with a history of hematuria, mild proteinuria, and hearing loss. By EM, there is marked basement membrane thinning* ➡ *with lamellations or "basketweaving"* ➡. *The diagnosis of Alport syndrome is best made on tissue fixed in glutaraldehyde rather than on deparaffinized tissue.*

SURGICAL/CLINICAL CONSIDERATIONS

Goals of Consultation

- Provide preliminary frozen section (FS) differential diagnosis of tumor in nephrectomy specimens
  - Differentiate between benign vs. malignant tumors
  - Differentiate between Wilms vs. other tumor types
  - FS to provide definitive final diagnosis should be avoided
- Allocate tissue for special studies
- Evaluate margins
  - Evaluation of vascular and ureteral margins by FS is usually not needed for pediatric renal tumors
  - Parenchymal resection margin may be evaluated in the case of nephron-sparing surgery
- Determine specimen adequacy of core needle biopsy specimens

Change in Patient Management

- FS findings may rule in or out more aggressive tumor types
  - Central vascular access will be placed if adjuvant chemotherapy indicated
  - Diagnosis of renal cell carcinoma (RCC) in older children may result in more aggressive lymph node dissection
- FS findings may influence allocation of tissue for special studies
  - May ensure viable, adequate tissue for treatment protocols

Clinical Setting

- Renal tumors are rare in children
  - Only ~ 600 cases per year in USA
  - 80% are Wilms tumor
    - Other tumor types include: Congenital mesoblastic nephroma (CMN), RCC, angiomyolipoma
- Role of imaging
  - MR is valuable in distinguishing Wilms tumor from nephrogenic rests (NRs) and nephroblastomatosis
- Role of biopsy in evaluation of pediatric renal tumors
  - In majority of cases, biopsy prior to chemotherapy is not necessary and is discouraged
  - Indications for pediatric renal tumor biopsy with possible FS
    - Unusual clinical features
      - Age > 8 years to rule out non-Wilms tumor
      - Atypical imaging findings
    - **Biopsies should be avoided when possible**
      - **Tumor spill due to biopsy upstages malignant tumors to stage III**
      - **Increases risk of recurrence**
- Bilateral Wilms renal tumors (BWT)
  - 5-10% of pediatric renal tumors are bilateral with some exceptions
    - Congenital mesoblastic nephroma is unilateral
    - Bilateral clear cell sarcomas and rhabdoid tumors of kidney are rare
  - Prevalence of BWT is higher in predisposition syndromes, such as **W**ilms tumor, **a**niridia, **g**enitourinary anomalies, **r**etardation/**B**eckwith-**W**iedemann **s**yndrome (WAGR/BWS)
    - Up to 22% of BWT patients have predisposition syndrome
  - Initial pretreatment biopsies for BWT are now controversial
    - Difficult to distinguish Wilms from NRs histologically
    - Biopsy may miss anaplasia
    - Tumor spillage due to biopsy will upstage tumor
  - Indications for biopsy in BWT with possible FS
    - Patient > 10 years old to rule out non-Wilms tumor
      - But biopsy may not rule out anaplasia
    - Atypical imaging
    - If biopsy indicated, important to biopsy both kidneys
      - In 20% of cases, pathology is not same bilaterally
  - Radiologic correlation is important to evaluate for NRs and nephroblastomatosis
    - MR more widely used in evaluation of bilateral tumors

SPECIMEN EVALUATION

Gross

- **Nephrectomy specimen**

Wilms Tumor: CT Appearance

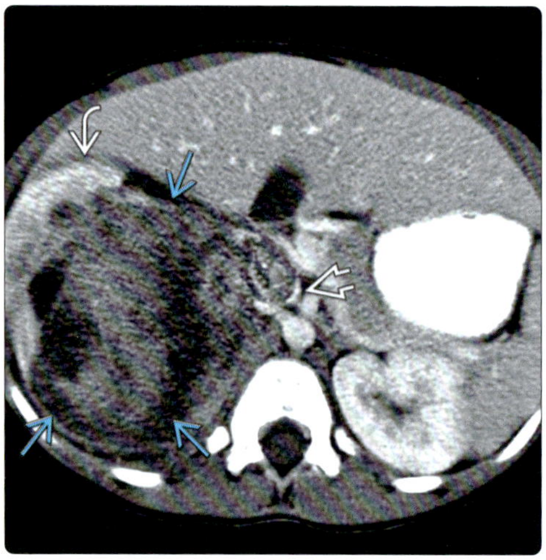

Wilms Tumor: Triphasic

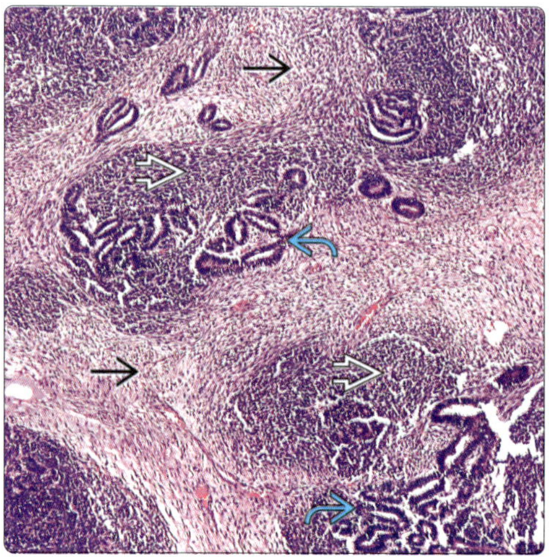

(Left) *Wilms tumor is the most common pediatric renal tumor, seen here on CT as a partially enhancing mass ➔ within the kidney ➔. A tumor thrombus in the inferior vena cava is surrounded by a crescent of contrast ➔.* **(Right)** *Triphasic Wilms tumor is composed of an epithelial component ➔, a mesenchymal component ➔, and blastema ➔. This same histologic appearance may be seen in hyperplastic nephrogenic rests (NRs).*

- Ureter and renal vessels are identified
    - Renal vein is examined for tumor thrombus
        - Vein may retract, resulting in tumor thrombus protruding from lumen
        - Not considered positive margin if thrombus has not been transected and vascular wall at margin is not invaded
- Presence of adrenal gland determined
    - May or may not be present
- External surface of kidney is inspected for possible tumor involvement
    - Important to determine and record whether or not capsule is grossly intact
- Intact specimen is photographed
- Kidney is weighed
    - Weight may serve as eligibility factor in clinical trials
- Distal margins of ureter and vessels are removed and placed in marked cassette
- **Capsule is inked prior to bisecting kidney**
    - Best 1st cut should pass through midline of kidney in coronal plane
- All lesions are identified and described
    - Location: Hilum, parenchyma
        - Involvement of renal sinus, renal vein, ureter
    - Size, number, color, and border
    - Cysts, necrosis, hemorrhage
- Tumors are allocated for special studies
    - Children's Oncology Group protocol for tissue allocation
        - Same for all pediatric renal tumors
    - Frozen tissue
        - ≥ 1 g snap-frozen in liquid nitrogen or cold isopentane in 2 or more vials
        - Tumor and nontumor tissue frozen
        - NRs may also be frozen
    - Other ancillary studies
        - Cytogenetics, touch preparations, flow cytometry, electron microscopy
- Specimen is refrigerated in formalin overnight prior to taking permanent sections
    - This renders specimen much less friable and easier to section
        - Retains color as seen in fresh state

Frozen Section

- **Nephrectomy**: Representative section of tumor is frozen
- **Needle Biopsy**: 1 core is frozen

MOST COMMON DIAGNOSES

Wilms Tumor

- Synonymous with nephroblastoma
- Most common pediatric renal tumor (~ 80%)
- Peak incidence: 2-4 years of age
    - Uncommon < 6 months of age
- MR appearance: Solitary spherical mass that compresses surrounding renal parenchyma
    - 7% multicentric
- Gross appearance: Well-circumscribed lobulated mass with variegated appearance
    - Extensive necrosis and hemorrhage are common
    - May be cystic
- Microscopic appearance: May be triphasic, biphasic, or monophasic
    - Varying amounts of each component can mimic many other tumors
- Differential diagnosis for triphasic Wilms tumor
    - NRs and nephroblastomatosis
        - 1/3 of kidneys with Wilms tumor also have NRs
- Differential diagnosis for blastemal-predominant Wilms tumor
    - NRs, nephroblastomatosis
    - Renal neuroblastoma
    - Renal primitive neuroectodermal tumor
    - Renal lymphoma
    - Cellular variant of CMN
- Differential diagnosis for stromal-predominant Wilms tumor
    - Classic variant of CMN
    - Angiomyolipoma
- Differential diagnosis for epithelial-predominant Wilms tumor
    - Metanephric adenoma
    - Papillary RCC
- Differential diagnosis for teratoid Wilms tumor
    - Renal teratoma, immature

Nephrogenic Rests and Nephroblastomatosis

- Increases risk of development of metachronous bilateral tumors
    - Present in up to 90% of synchronous bilateral Wilms tumors
    - Present in in up to 94% of metachronous bilateral Wilms tumors
- May be indistinguishable from Wilms tumor histologically if entire NR is not sampled
- MR appearance of NRs: Ovoid, oblong, or lenticular mass or masses
    - Perilobar NRs are subcapsular and usually take shape of renal capsule
    - Intralobar NRs can be irregular in shape
    - Often multiple
- Gross appearance of NRs: Pale masses near cortex
- MR appearance of diffuse perilobar nephroblastomatosis: Masses expand cortex, forming cortical rind that preserves cortical shape
- Developmental stages of NRs
    - Dormant/incipient
    - Sclerosing/regressing
    - Obsolescent
    - Hyperplastic

Congenital Mesoblastic Nephroma (CMN)

- Presents congenitally or within 1st year of life
- Unilateral tumor arising in central portion of kidney
- Classic variant
    - Composed of intersecting spindle cell fascicles reminiscent of fibromatosis
    - No consistent translocation identified
- Cellular variant
    - Composed of plump spindle cells

Clear Cell Sarcoma of Kidney

- Mean age at diagnosis: 3 years
- Wide array of histologic variants
  - Classic variant: Clear cells arranged within delicate fibrovascular network

Rhabdoid Tumor

- Mean age at diagnosis: ~ 17 months
  - > 90% diagnosed by 3 years of age
- Sheets of large cells
  - Large round nuclei with prominent nucleoli
  - Abundant eosinophilic cytoplasm
  - Cytoplasmic eosinophilic perinuclear inclusions

Primitive Neuroectodermal Tumor

- Most common in adolescents and young adults
- Sheets of small, round, blue cells
- Rosetting may be seen to varying degrees

Lymphoma

- Rare in kidney
- Sheets of small, round, blue cells
- Flow cytometry, cytogenetics, and immunoperoxidase studies are helpful to achieve final diagnosis

Angiomyolipoma

- Associated with tuberous sclerosis complex
- Admixture of smooth muscle, vessels, and adipose tissue in varying proportions

Renal Cell Carcinoma (RCC) in Pediatric Patients

- Account for < 5% of new pediatric renal tumors
  - More common than clear cell sarcoma of kidney and renal rhabdoid tumor
- Average age at presentation: 9-10 years
- **Adult-type renal clear cell carcinoma**
  - Very rare in absence of underlying genetic condition
    - Tuberous sclerosis complex, von Hippel-Lindau disease
- **Renal tumors with Xp11.2 translocation**
  - Outnumber conventional RCCs in children
  - Most have tubulopapillary configuration histologically
- **Papillary RCC**
  - 2nd most common type in children
  - Differential diagnosis
    - Differentiated epithelial Wilms tumor
    - Metanephric adenoma
- **Renal medullary carcinoma**
  - Rare, aggressive carcinoma with mean survival of 4 months
  - Associated with sickle cell anemia

REPORTING

Frozen Section

- Triphasic small round blue cell tumor
  - Report "triphasic renal tumor consistent with Wilms tumor versus nephrogenic rest"
- Biphasic or monophasic small round blue cell tumor
  - Report "small round blue cell tumor, differential diagnosis includes pediatric renal tumor versus nephrogenic"
- Stromal-predominant tumor
  - Report "renal tumor with smooth muscle/skeletal muscle/mesenchymal/cartilaginous (etc.) differentiation"
    - Differential diagnosis depends on histologic findings

Reliability

- Correlation of FS and permanent diagnosis
  - Literature reports diagnostic accuracy between 78-98% in pediatric solid tumors
    - 89% correlation reported in distinguishing Wilms vs. non-Wilms
    - 94% correlation reported in distinguishing benign from malignant tumors

PITFALLS

Nephrogenic Rests vs. Wilms Tumor

- Can be histologically indistinguishable on biopsy specimens
- Radiographic studies are helpful in making distinction
- **Communication with surgeon is important to avoid unnecessary nephrectomy**
- Wilms tumor
  - Spherical
  - Peritumoral capsule histologically
- NRs
  - Oblong or irregular shape
  - More likely to be multiple
  - Nonencapsulated histologically
  - Perilobar rests usually take shape of cortex
  - Intralobar rests are often admixed with renal tissue and not well circumscribed
  - Psammoma bodies more likely to be present
- Diffuse hyperplastic perilobar nephroblastomatosis
  - Presents as thickened cortical rind that preserves cortical shape

Treatment Effect

- Residual differentiated Wilms tumor cells are commonly found in postchemotherapy surgical specimens
  - Mature, quiescent-appearing tubules are considered to be regressive changes

Sampling Error

- FSs and core needle biopsies can miss diagnostic areas

Improper Utilization of Frozen Section

- FS should not be used for
  - Definitive diagnosis of histologic tumor type
  - Determination of Wilms tumor vs. NR/nephroblastomatosis
  - Diagnosis of anaplasia
- Best to defer diagnosis to permanent sections

SELECTED REFERENCES

1. Carrasco A Jr et al: Reliability of intraoperative frozen section for the diagnosis of renal tumors suspicious for malignancy in children and adolescents. Pediatr Blood Cancer. 64(8), 2017
2. Millar AJ et al: Management of bilateral Wilms tumours. Pediatr Surg Int. 33(4):461-469, 2017
3. Irtan S et al: Wilms tumor: "State-of-the-art" update, 2016. Semin Pediatr Surg. 25(5):250-256, 2016
4. Perlman EJ: Pediatric renal tumors: practical updates for the pathologist. Pediatr Dev Pathol. 8(3):320-38, 2005

Wilms Tumor and Nephrogenic Rests: MR Appearance

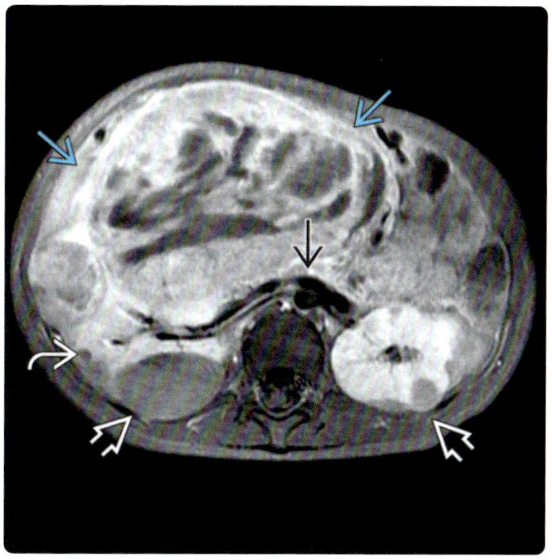

Wilms Tumor and Nephrogenic Rests: Gross Appearance

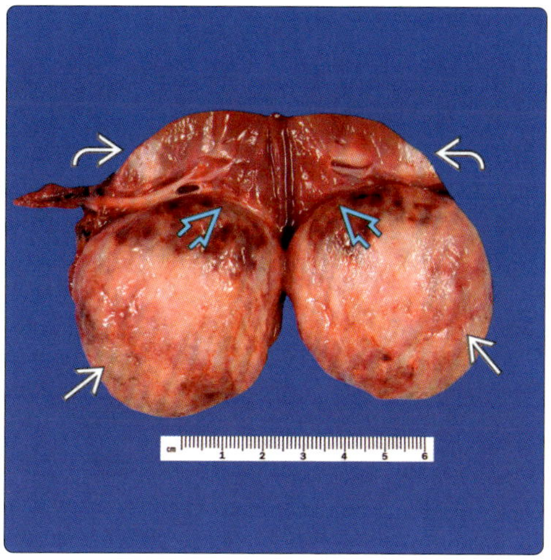

(Left) *Axial T1WI C+ MR shows a large Wilms tumor growing anteriorly from the right kidney. NRs form oblong nonenhancing masses along the capsules of both kidneys. The renal veins and the inferior vena cava are compressed but patent.* **(Right)** *Bivalved kidney reveals a spherical tan-pink Wilms tumor compressing the adjacent residual renal parenchyma. A tan perilobar NR is present in a subcortical location.*

Nephroblastomatosis: CT Appearance

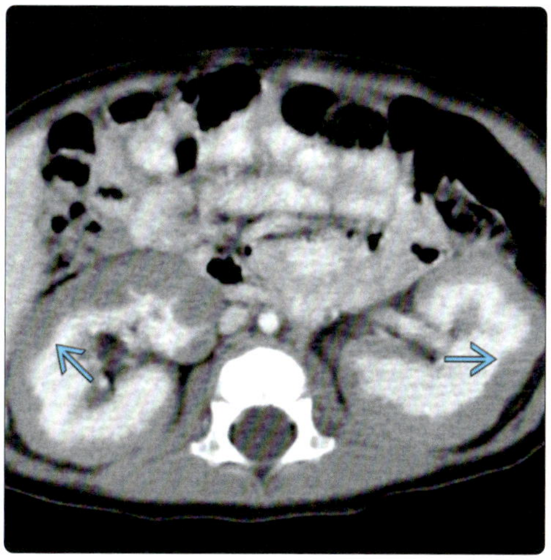

Nephroblastomatosis: Gross Appearance

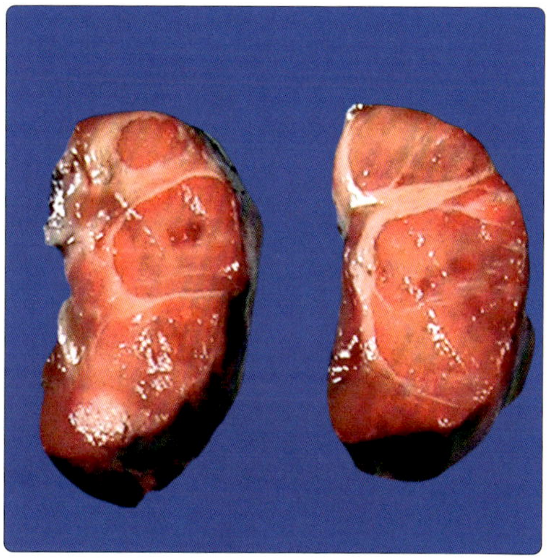

(Left) *Axial CECT of the abdomen shows a rind of homogeneous hypodense tissue surrounding both kidneys. Nephroblastomatosis characteristically has a homogeneous appearance and does not enhance compared with the remainder of the renal parenchyma.* **(Right)** *Serial sections of a partial nephrectomy specimen from a patient with bilateral diffuse hyperplastic perilobular nephroblastomatosis demonstrate an expanded cortex containing nephrogenic tissue. The cortex is expanded but maintains its shape.*

Wilms Tumor

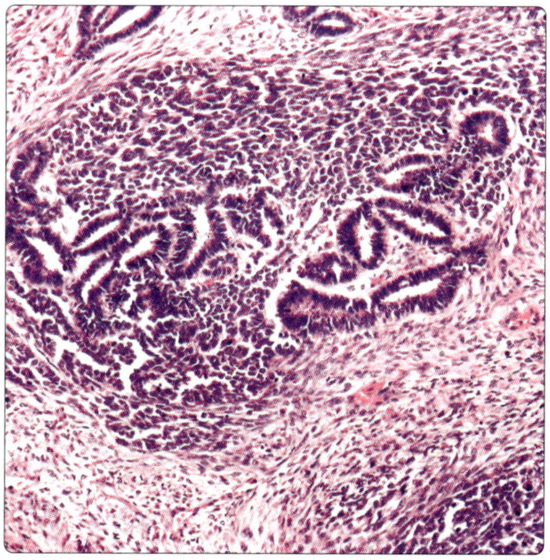

Nephroblastomatosis: Triphasic

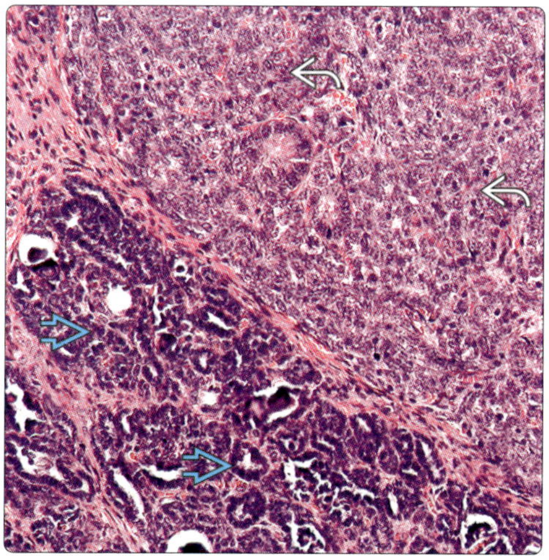

(Left) *Wilms tumor can be histologically indistinguishable from nephroblastomatosis or hyperplastic NRs. The appearance by imaging and on gross examination can be helpful in making this distinction.* **(Right)** *Triphasic nephroblastomatosis may be treated with nephron-sparing surgery or chemotherapy. Although the tubules and blastema appear quiescent, the hyperplastic focus on the right contains cells cytologically similar to Wilms tumor.*

(Left) *Tubular structures are seen in this frozen section of a pediatric renal tumor nephrectomy specimen, placing Wilms tumor high on the preliminary differential diagnosis. The nature of the stromal tissue is difficult to discern on frozen section.* (Right) *Renal biopsy from a child with bilateral tumors reveals a triphasic primitive tumor. Although these features are consistent with Wilms tumor, it is difficult to exclude a NR histologically. Radiographic correlation is useful in this evaluation.*

Wilms Tumor: Frozen Section

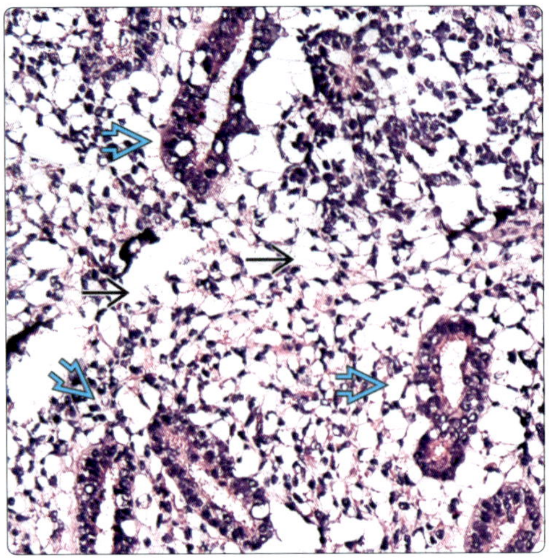

Renal Core Needle Biopsy

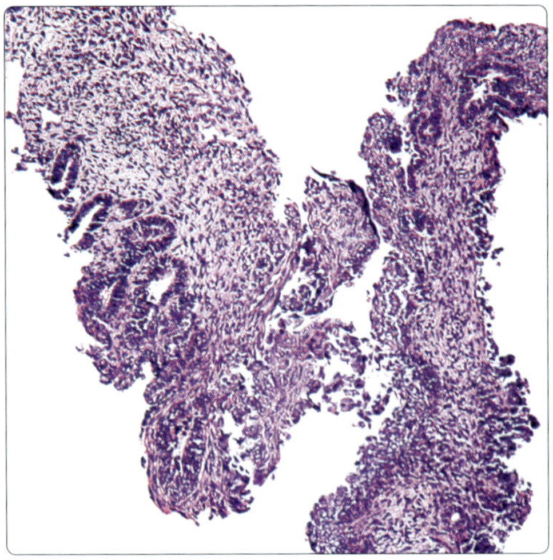

(Left) *A small Wilms tumor is spherical and compresses the surrounding renal parenchyma in this bivalved specimen. A fibrous pseudocapsule encases the tumor.* (Right) *Perilobar NRs are oblong or lenticular and follow the cortical contour. They are well circumscribed but unencapsulated. Intralobar NRs are irregularly shaped. Wilms tumors are spherical, can result in cortical bulging, and are surrounded by a pseudocapsule. Nephroblastomatosis expands the cortex with a cortical rind that preserves renal shape.*

Wilms Tumor: Gross Appearance

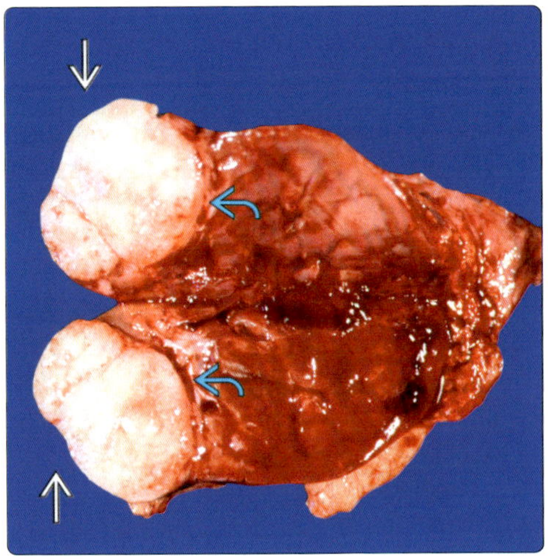

Nephrogenic Rests vs. Wilms vs. Nephroblastomatosis

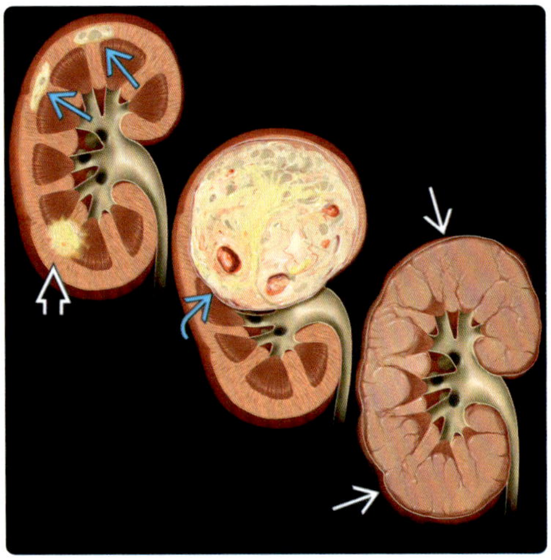

(Left) *Sclerosing NRs are seen in a perilobar (subcapsular) location. Perilobar NRs, unlike Wilms tumor, often have an elongate shape that follows the cortical contour. Also, unlike Wilms tumor, both perilobar and intralobar NRs are unencapsulated.* (Right) *NR after chemotherapy consists of cells with small, quiescent-appearing nuclei forming sheets and tubular structures with psammoma bodies within a collagenous background.*

Nephrogenic Rests: Sclerosing

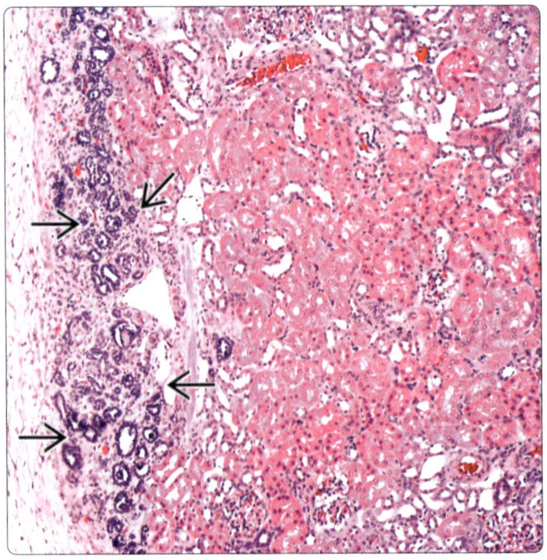

Wilms Tumor: Nephrogenic Rests and Treatment Effect

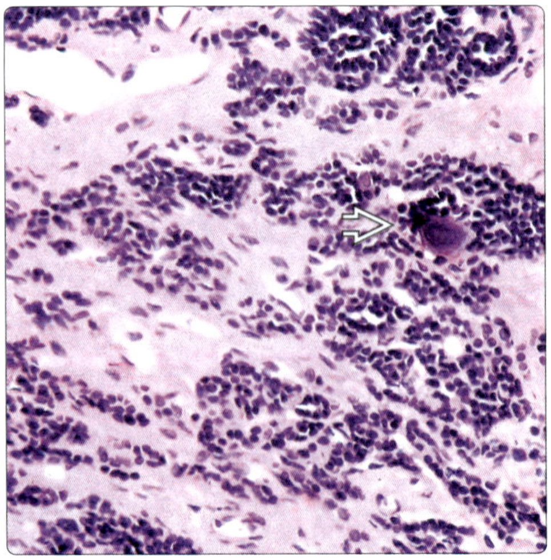

Wilms Tumor: Blastema

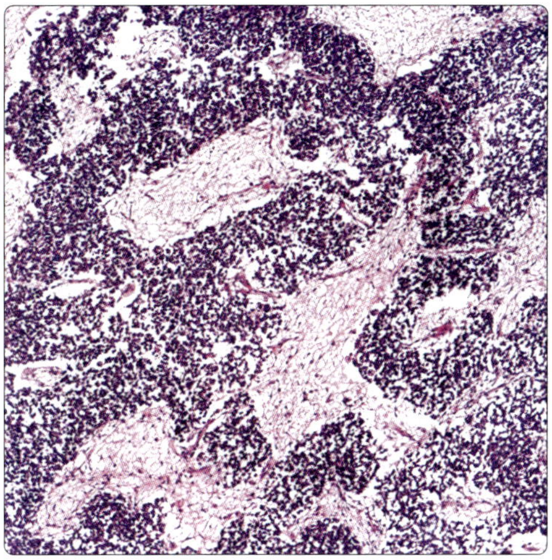

Wilms Tumor: Anaplasia

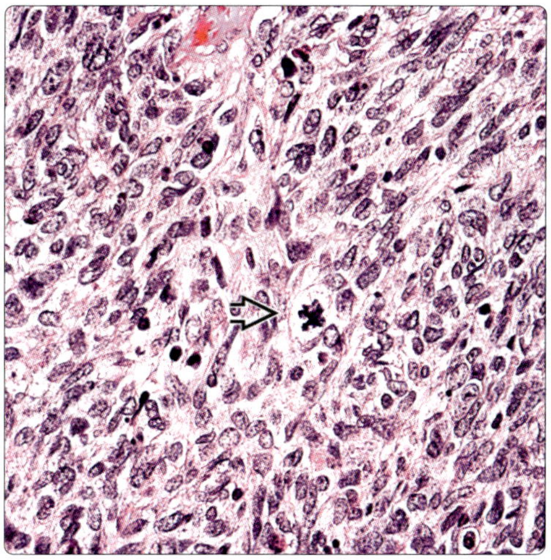

(Left) *Frozen sections are sometimes performed on pediatric renal tumors to establish a differential diagnosis to aid in tissue procurement. This permanent section of a frozen section of a biphasic Wilms tumor shows blastema arranged in a serpentine pattern, which is highly characteristic.* **(Right)** *Anaplasia in Wilms tumor should be evaluated on permanent sections rather than on frozen sections. Anaplasia is composed of large, hyperchromatic nuclei and large, hyperdiploid mitotic figures* ⇨.

Wilms Tumor: Cartilaginous Differentiation

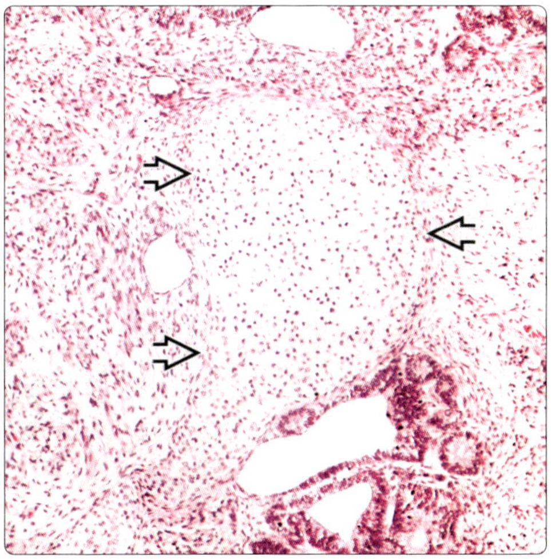

Wilms Tumor: Skeletal Muscle Differentiation

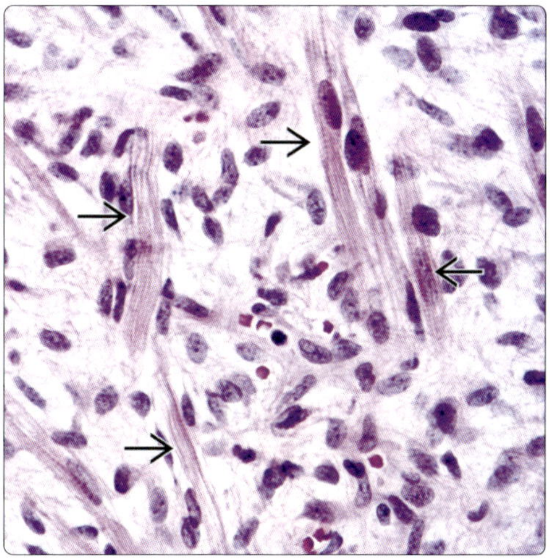

(Left) *The mesenchymal component of Wilms tumor can include striated muscle, cartilage, bone, adipose tissue, and fibrous tissue. This tumor shows cartilaginous differentiation* ⇨. **(Right)** *The mesenchymal component of Wilms tumors can be highly variable and demonstrate heterologous differentiation, such as striated skeletal muscle* → *or smooth muscle. Rhabdomyoid differentiation can be present and, in some cases, is malignant (termed "rhabdomyosarcomatous Wilms tumor").*

Primitive Neuroectodermal Tumor

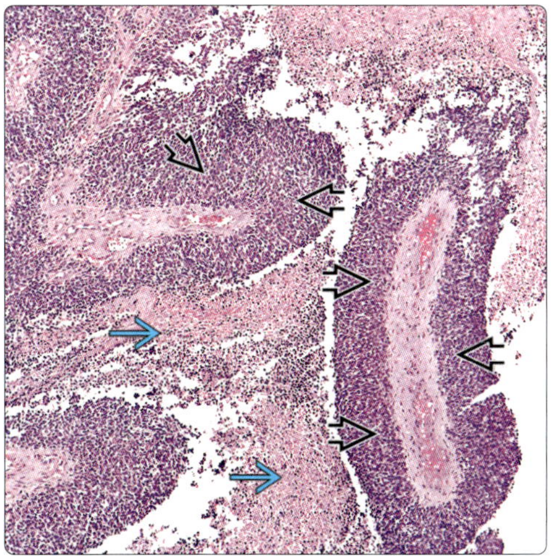

Primitive Neuroectodermal Tumor

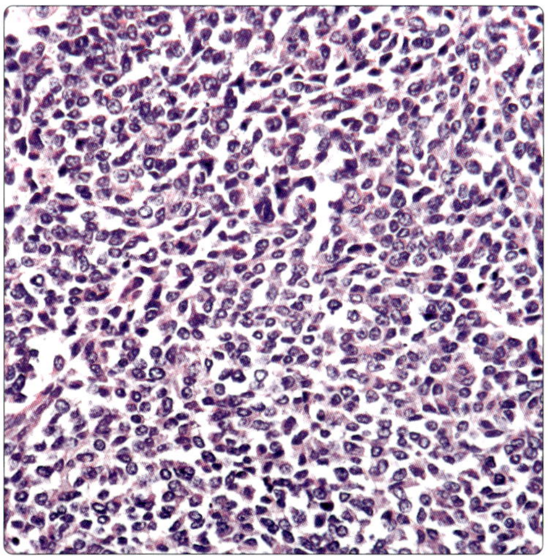

(Left) *This case of renal PNET in a teenager shows sheets of small round blue cells demonstrating geographic necrosis* → *with perivascular sparing* ⇨. *This is a common finding in PNET.* **(Right)** *Renal PNET is composed of sheets of small round blue cells and may be difficult to distinguish from a monophasic Wilms tumor on frozen section. Additional studies needed for final diagnosis include CD99, which shows membranous positivity, and cytogenetics or FISH, identifying the EWS-FLI1 translocation.*

(Left) *Congenital mesoblastic nephroma is the most common renal tumor in infants. It tends to arise centrally. The classic variant has a distinct gross appearance showing a pale-tan, thick, trabeculated, and whorled fibrous surface. The tumor-kidney interface is indistinct ➡. Necrosis and cysts are more common in the cellular variant.* **(Right)** *The classic variant of congenital mesoblastic nephroma consists of spindle cells arranged in long intersecting fascicles and resembles fibromatosis. Entrapped renal parenchyma ↪ is seen.*

Congenital Mesoblastic Nephroma, Classic: Gross Appearance

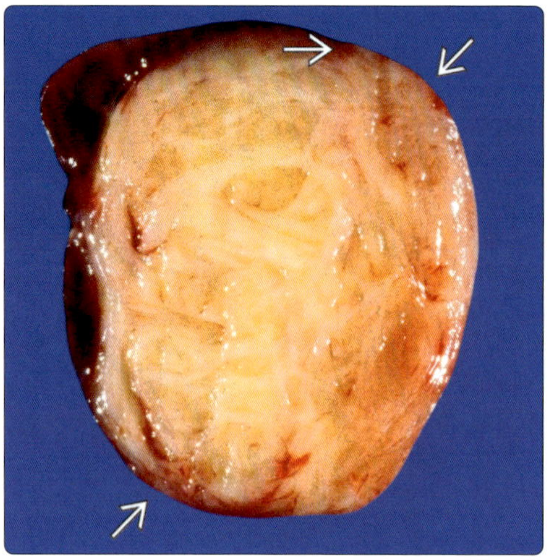

Congenital Mesoblastic Nephroma, Classic

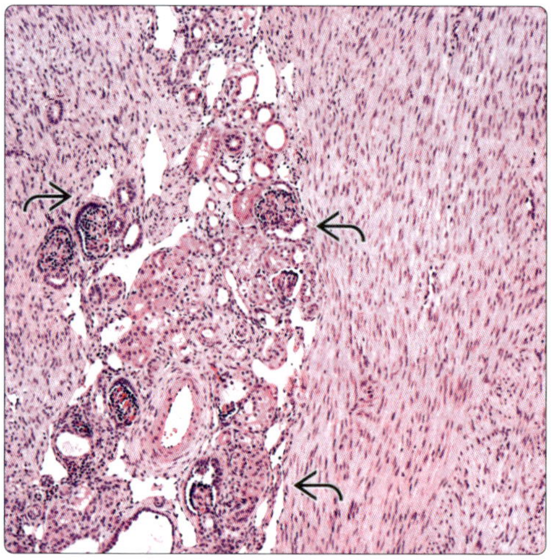

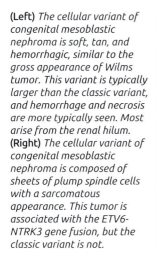

(Left) *The cellular variant of congenital mesoblastic nephroma is soft, tan, and hemorrhagic, similar to the gross appearance of Wilms tumor. This variant is typically larger than the classic variant, and hemorrhage and necrosis are more typically seen. Most arise from the renal hilum.* **(Right)** *The cellular variant of congenital mesoblastic nephroma is composed of sheets of plump spindle cells with a sarcomatous appearance. This tumor is associated with the ETV6-NTRK3 gene fusion, but the classic variant is not.*

Congenital Mesoblastic Nephroma, Cellular: Gross Appearance

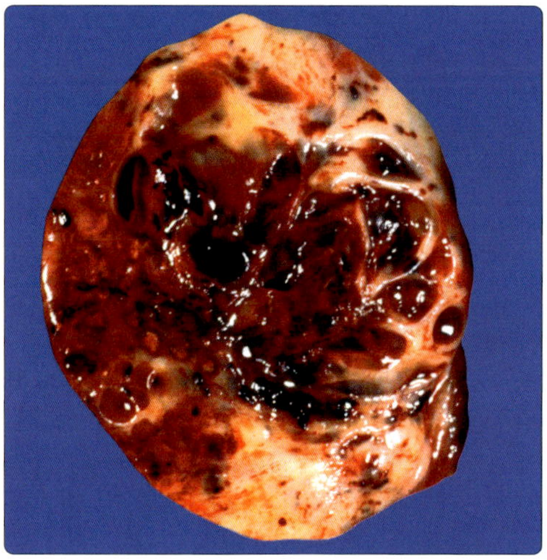

Congenital Mesoblastic Nephroma, Cellular

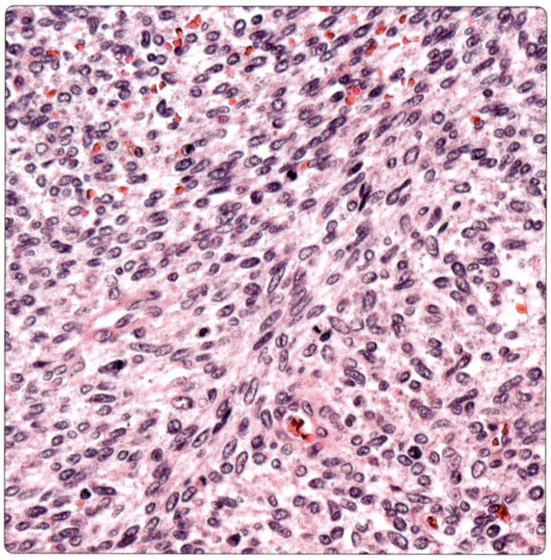

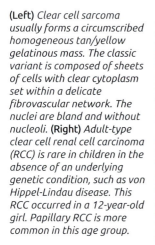

(Left) *Clear cell sarcoma usually forms a circumscribed homogeneous tan/yellow gelatinous mass. The classic variant is composed of sheets of cells with clear cytoplasm set within a delicate fibrovascular network. The nuclei are bland and without nucleoli.* **(Right)** *Adult-type clear cell renal cell carcinoma (RCC) is rare in children in the absence of an underlying genetic condition, such as von Hippel-Lindau disease. This RCC occurred in a 12-year-old girl. Papillary RCC is more common in this age group.*

Clear Cell Sarcoma of Kidney

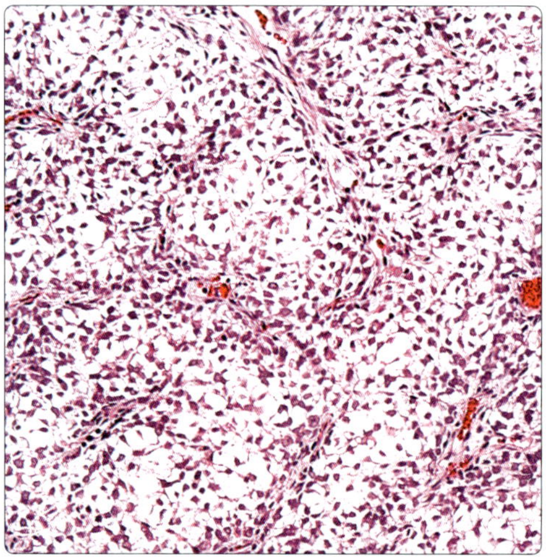

Renal Cell Carcinoma: Clear Cell Type

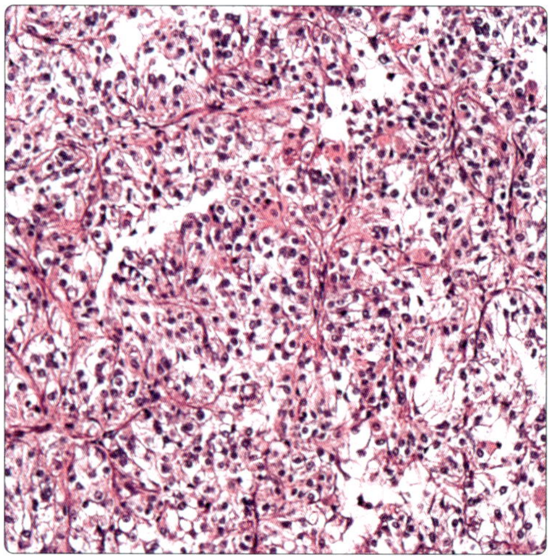

Renal Cell Carcinoma: Medullary Type

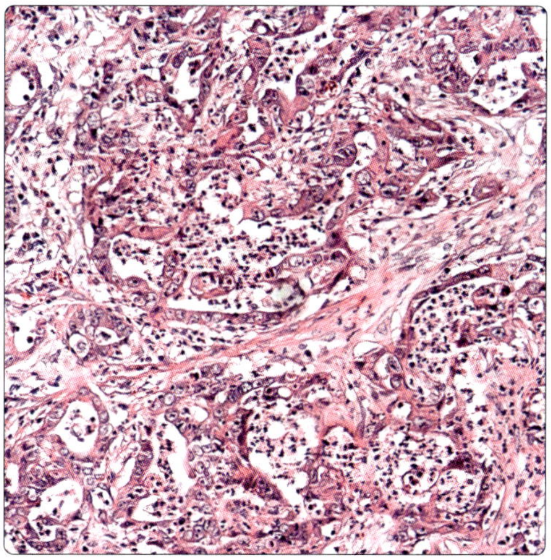

Renal Teratoma

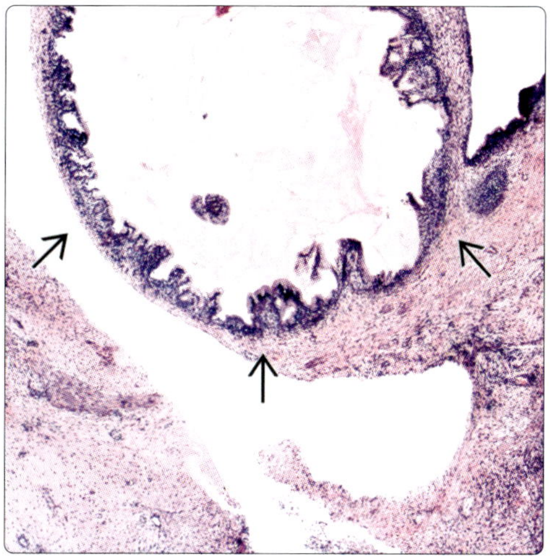

(Left) *Medullary RCC is a rare, aggressive tumor with a predilection for patients with sickle cell hemoglobinopathy. Irregular glands with highly atypical nuclei and associated acute inflammation with necrosis are characteristic.* **(Right)** *Most pediatric renal tumors diagnosed as immature teratomas may actually be teratoid Wilms tumors. The presence of mature organoid differentiation, such as this gastric-type structure lined by gastric epithelium and surrounded by muscularis ⇒, is diagnostic of a teratoma.*

Angiomyolipoma

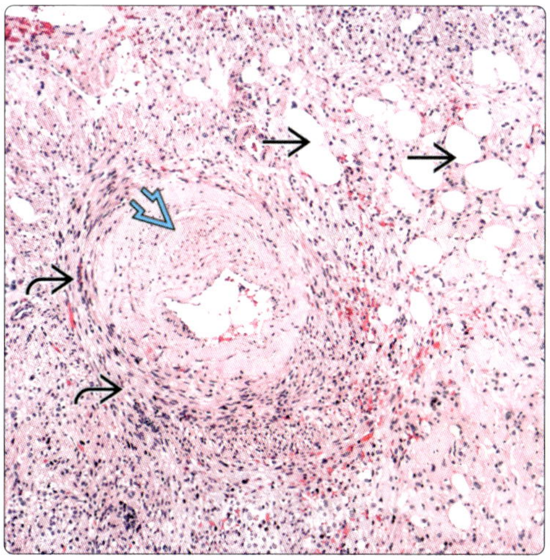

Angiomyolipoma: Renal Biopsy

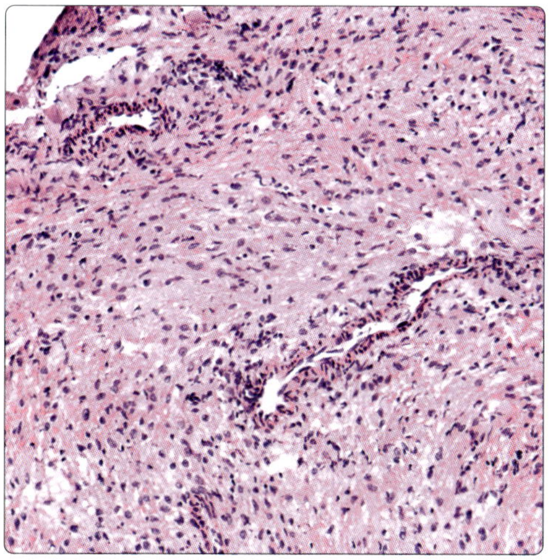

(Left) *The radiologic appearance of angiomyolipoma is often diagnostic due to the admixture of tissue types. These tumors consist of smooth muscle ⇒, blood vessels ⇒, and adipose tissue ⇒.* **(Right)** *Frozen section from a child with bilateral renal tumors shows smooth muscle differentiation and muscular vessels. These features, in conjunction with the radiographic impression and history of tuberous sclerosis, make angiomyolipoma the favored diagnosis.*

Rhabdoid Tumor

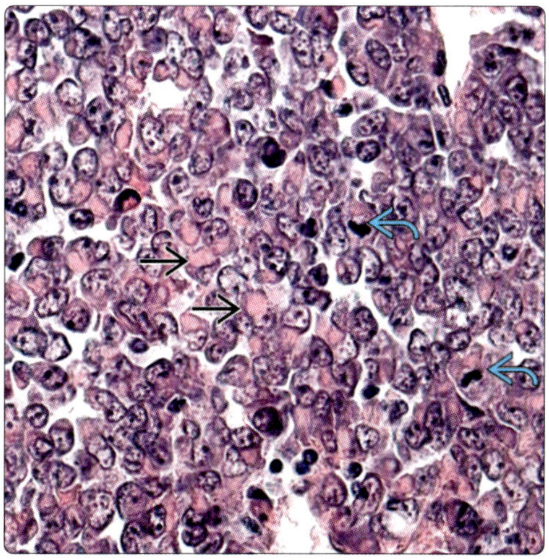

Rhabdoid Tumor: Frozen Section

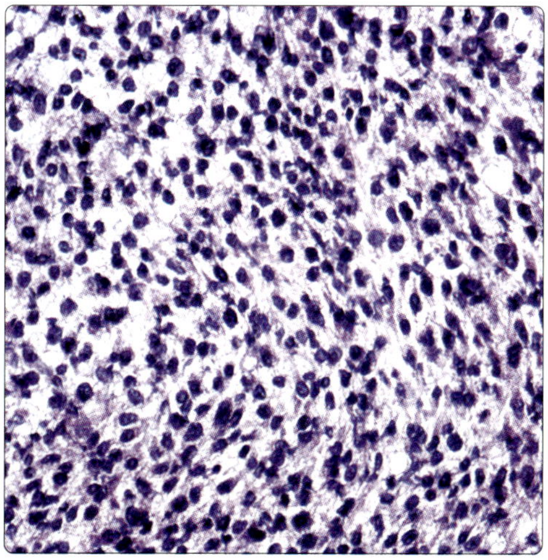

(Left) *Renal malignant rhabdoid tumors are composed of sheets of large cells with large, round eccentric nuclei with prominent nucleoli and eosinophilic cytoplasmic inclusions ⇒. Mitotic rate is high ⇒.* **(Right)** *Typical nuclear and cytoplasmic features are not evident in this frozen section of a renal malignant rhabdoid tumor. Definitive diagnosis is best deferred to permanent sections.*

Contents

SURGICAL/CLINICAL CONSIDERATIONS

Goal of Consultation

- Determine if malignancy or dysplasia are present
- Determine if margins are free of carcinoma or dysplasia

Change in Patient Management

- Carcinoma may be excised or treated with radiation therapy if margins are positive
- Multiple biopsies may be used to map extent of tumor and determine how much tissue to resect
- Additional tissue may be taken at areas of margin involvement to obtain clear margins

Clinical Setting

- Smoking and alcohol use are major risk factors for conventional squamous cell carcinoma
  - No correlation between high-risk HPV and morphology in larynx
- Patients with advanced carcinoma, airway compromise, or recurrent carcinoma may undergo total laryngectomy
- Patients with limited involvement or in situ carcinoma may be treated with partial laryngectomy

SPECIMEN EVALUATION

Gross

- Biopsies often small and fragmented
- Total laryngectomy
  - Superior mucosal margins are margins most likely to be positive for carcinoma
    - Anterior/lateral soft tissue margins may be involved if tumor is advanced
  - Specimen may contain pharyngeal or thyroid tissue
- Partial laryngectomy
  - Orientation by surgeon may be necessary
- Margins may be submitted separately as small specimens by surgeon

Frozen Section

- Small biopsies and separate margins may be completely frozen
- If mucosa can be identified, specimen should be embedded perpendicularly to allow for assessment of invasion
- Margins should always be taken as perpendicular sections
  - En face margins are not capable of evaluating narrow (1-2 mm) but tumor-free margins

MOST COMMON DIAGNOSES

Conventional Squamous Cell Carcinoma

- Most common; typically keratinizing and graded according to degree of differentiation
- May exhibit different patterns of invasion
  - Broad pushing front of invasion
    - Challenging to assess in small biopsies and may require presence of adjacent normal tissue to recognize presence of invasion
  - Irregular nests &/or individual infiltrative cells
    - Usually easy to recognize in small biopsies
- Abnormal keratinization, frequent mitoses, necrosis, nuclear pleomorphism and hyperchromasia, &/or desmoplastic stromal response may be appreciated

Verrucous Carcinoma

- Well-differentiated variant with minimal cytologic atypia
- Uniform front of invasion with bulbous rete ridges
- When strictly defined, only poses risk of local recurrence
- Diagnosis should be reserved for excised tumors, as similar foci may be seen in conventional squamous cell carcinoma

Basaloid Squamous Cell Carcinoma

- Clinically aggressive variant recognized in larynx
- More common in supraglottis and piriform sinus
- Basaloid tumor cells have scant cytoplasm and high-grade features including necrosis and frequent mitoses
- Foci of keratinizing squamous cell carcinoma may be seen
- Must be distinguished from oropharyngeal HPV-associated squamous cell carcinoma, which has favorable prognosis
  - Oropharyngeal carcinomas can extend to larynx

Invasive Squamous Cell Carcinoma

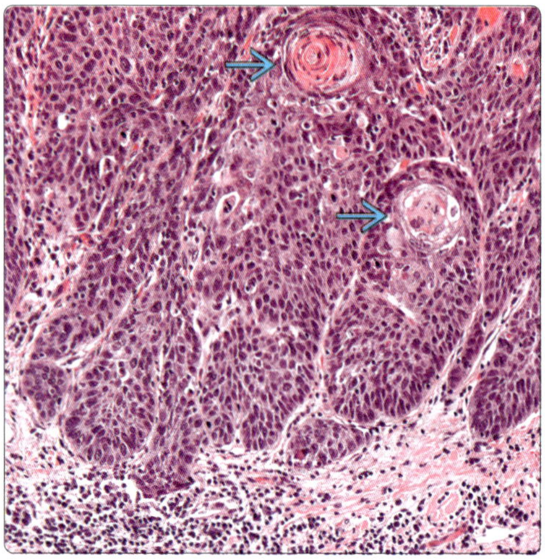

Verrucous Carcinoma

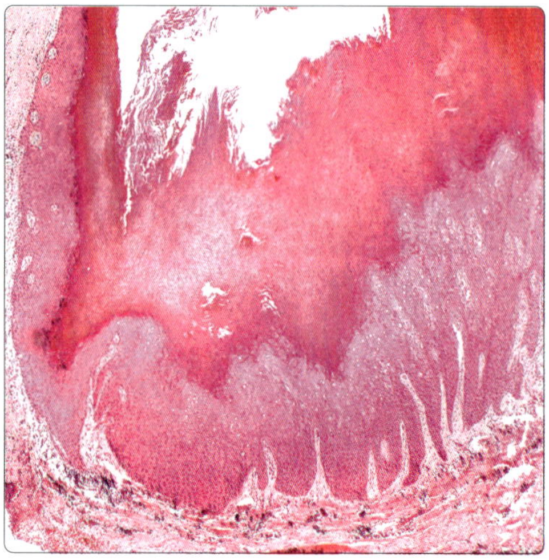

(Left) *Invasive keratinizing squamous cell carcinoma is the most common laryngeal malignancy and is characterized by irregular infiltrating nests of atypical squamous cells with focal areas of keratinization* ➡*. A desmoplastic stromal response is often present.* **(Right)** *Verrucous carcinoma invades as a broad, uniform pushing front. This is a difficult pattern of invasion to recognize in small biopsies. The diagnosis should be reserved for completely excised tumors.*

- Other high-grade round cell malignancies, especially small cell carcinoma, must be considered
  - Distinction often requires special stains
  - Adequate on frozen section to diagnose as basaloid neoplasm/malignancy and defer to permanent sections

Papillary Squamous Cell Carcinoma

- Exophytic, fibrovascular cores lined by malignant squamous epithelium (keratinizing or nonkeratinizing)

Sarcomatoid (Spindle Cell) Carcinoma

- Malignant spindle cell proliferation coexisting with conventional squamous cell carcinoma &/or dysplasia
- In absence of dysplasia or carcinoma in situ, preliminary diagnosis of atypical spindle cell neoplasm sufficient
- Final diagnosis needs to be deferred for immunohistochemical studies (keratins, p63) to differentiate from reactive stromal proliferations (e.g., contact ulcer) and sarcoma

Squamous Dysplasia and Carcinoma In Situ

- High-grade dysplasia or carcinoma in situ will usually prompt excision of lesion or partial laryngectomy
  - Grading controversial
  - Conventionally graded as mild (involving lower 1/3 of epithelium), moderate (up to 2/3 of epithelium), and severe (> 2/3 of epithelium)
  - Recent proposal by 2017 WHO for 2-tier system of low grade and high grade (encompassing moderate and severe dysplasia and carcinoma in situ)
- Carcinoma in situ shows features of conventional squamous cell carcinoma but without invasion

Neuroendocrine Tumors

- Classified as well, moderately, and poorly differentiated
  - Distinction between well- and moderately differentiated tumors deferred to resection
- **Well-differentiated neuroendocrine carcinoma (typical carcinoid)**
  - Organoid growth pattern with nests, trabeculae, cords, or sheets; may form rosettes
  - Pale, eosinophilic or clear cells with stippled salt-and-pepper chromatin and minimal nuclear atypia
  - Mitotic index < 2 per 10 HPF
- **Moderately differentiated neuroendocrine carcinoma (atypical carcinoid)**
  - Morphologically similar to well-differentiated tumors but may show more nuclear atypia
  - Mitotic index 2-10 per 10 HPF
- **Poorly differentiated neuroendocrine carcinoma**
  - Classified as large cell or small cell carcinoma
  - Mitotic index > 10 per 10 HPF
- Immunohistochemistry (positive for neuroendocrine markers and keratin) and clinical correlation (e.g., serum calcitonin) may be necessary to differentiate from paraganglioma and medullary thyroid carcinoma

Radiation Atypia

- May be seen for prolonged time periods after radiation
- Isolated cells with nucleomegaly and cytomegaly with vacuolization of either nucleus or cytoplasm
  - Malignancies typically show atypia throughout lesion
- Nuclear:cytoplasmic ratio preserved

Squamous Papilloma and Respiratory Papillomatosis

- Majority related to low-risk HPV (6 or 11)
- Malignant transformation rare (1-4%), except for history of prior irradiation
- Papillary lesion lined by bland squamous epithelium
  - Mitoses usually limited to basal layer
- Koilocytes may be seen
- Distinguished from papillary squamous cell carcinoma by lack of full-thickness atypia and pleomorphism

REPORTING

Frozen Section

- Invasive or in situ carcinoma (at margin, if applicable, or provide distance to margin if possible)

PITFALLS

Pseudoepitheliomatous Hyperplasia

- Bland nuclear features with pseudoinfiltrative pattern
- Especially common overlying granular cell tumor
  - Essential to look in stroma for diagnostic epithelioid tumor cells with granular eosinophilic cytoplasm

Candidiasis

- May cause squamous hyperplasia and reactive epithelial changes that can be mistaken for dysplasia or carcinoma
- Intraepithelial neutrophils clue to potential presence of fungi
- If uncertain about dysplasia, diagnosis of squamous atypia may be appropriate with recommendation to rebiopsy if lesion persists after treating infection

Reactive Transitional/Metaplastic Epithelium

- Often seen in vocal cord region at transition between squamous and respiratory epithelium
- Can show reactive atypia without obvious maturation, especially in setting of inflammation or prior treatment
  - May create difficulties in distinction from high-grade dysplasia or carcinoma in situ
- May show occasional mitotic figures but usually lacks marked nuclear size variability and irregularity

Laryngeal Polyp (Vocal Cord Polyp or Nodule)

- Arises secondary to repeated trauma (e.g. intubation, vocal abuse)
- Squamous epithelium may show reactive atypia and pseudoinvasive pattern, mimicking dysplasia or carcinoma
- Deeper levels may demonstrate continuity between squamous nests and surface
- Presence of typical stromal changes (hyaline, myxoid, edematous, vascular) may aid in distinction

SELECTED REFERENCES

1. Du E et al: Refining the utility and role of frozen section in head and neck squamous cell carcinoma resection. Laryngoscope. 126(8):1768-75, 2016
2. Kao HL et al: Head and neck large cell neuroendocrine carcinoma should be separated from atypical carcinoid on the basis of different clinical features, overall survival, and pathogenesis. Am J Surg Pathol. 36(2):185-92, 2012
3. Lewis JS Jr et al: Transcriptionally-active high-risk human papillomavirus is rare in oral cavity and laryngeal/hypopharyngeal squamous cell carcinomas--a tissue microarray study utilizing E6/E7 mRNA in situ hybridization. Histopathology. 60(6):982-91, 2012

(Left) *In the setting of candidiasis, squamous epithelium can show reactive changes including hyperplasia, parakeratosis, and mitotic activity near the basal layer* ➔*. Although the features may be worrisome for dysplasia, the presence of intraepithelial neutrophils* ⇨ *is a clue to the potential presence of fungal hyphae.* **(Right)** *Fungal forms can be found in the parakeratotic layer and may be visible on H&E* ⇨ *or with PAS stain with diastase digestion. Note the characteristic pseudohyphae of Candida species.*

Squamous Hyperplasia in Candidiasis

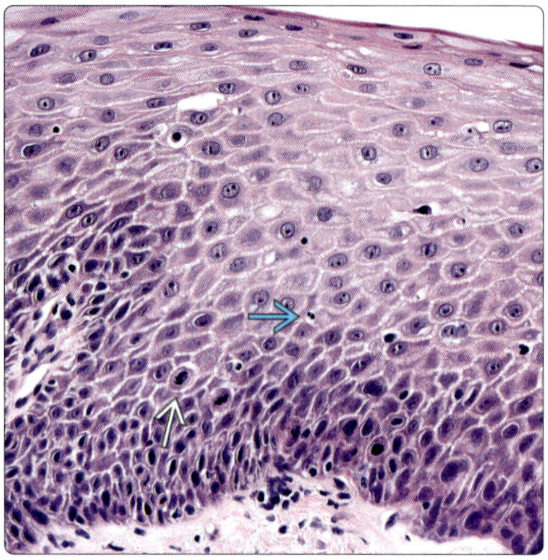

Candidiasis

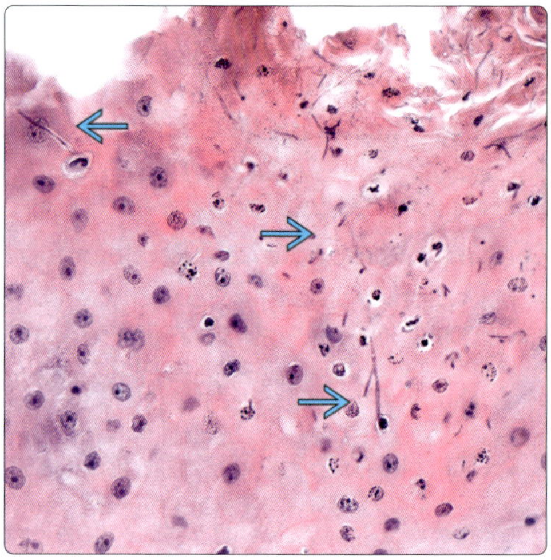

(Left) *Vocal cord polyps are common lesions that are identifiable by characteristic stromal changes. In this example, there is marked stromal myxoid change. The overlying epithelium shows normal maturation without atypia.* **(Right)** *This vocal cord polyp has extensive hyaline-vascular stromal change. The paucicellular hyaline material may prompt concern for amyloid deposition, but special stains are invariably negative. The overlying epithelium may show reactive changes in some cases.*

Vocal Cord Polyp

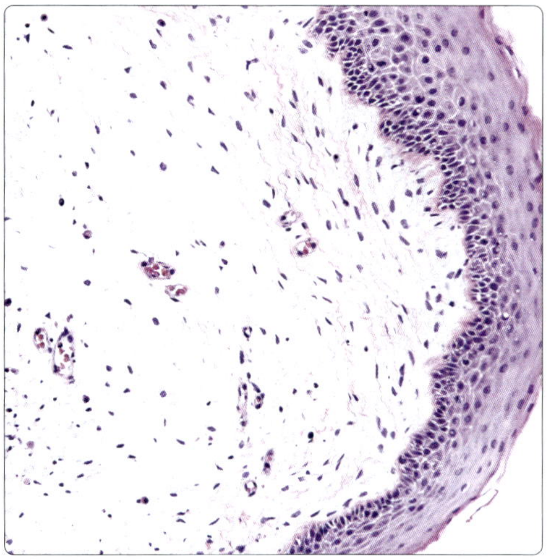

Vocal Cord Polyp

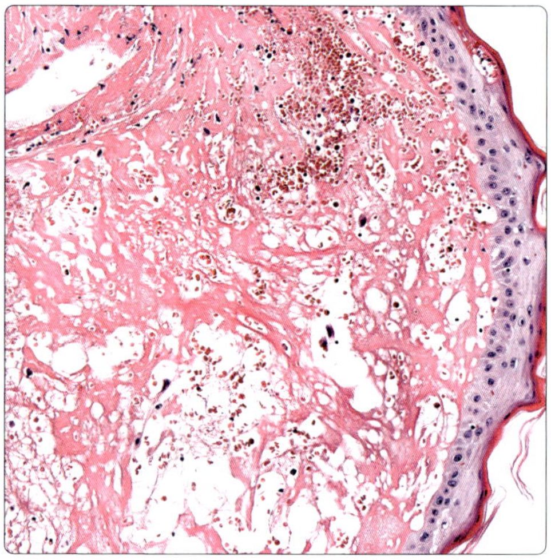

(Left) *Tangential sectioning can give the false impression of invasion in a vocal cord polyp. Deeper levels can be helpful to show that the bland pseudoinfiltrative epithelium* ⇨ *connects to the surface epithelium as more of the lesion is seen.* **(Right)** *Patients receiving radiation therapy for squamous cell carcinoma may develop laryngeal ulcers. This ulcer has islands of squamous epithelium in stroma* ⇨*, creating an impression of invasion. Note, however, the uniform distribution and lack of atypia in these epithelial islands.*

Vocal Cord Polyp

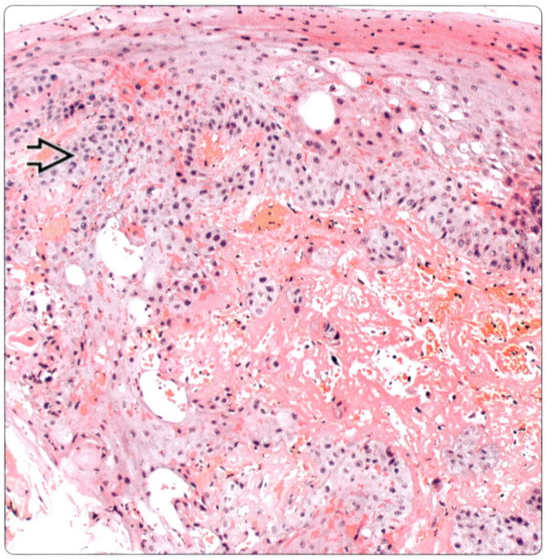

Postradiation Ulcer

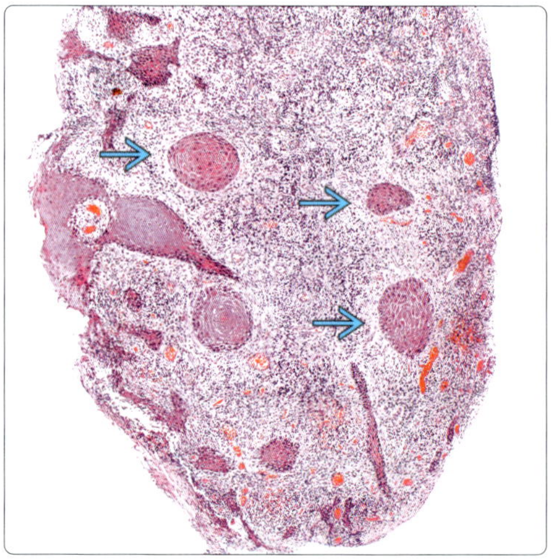

Contents

Neuroendocrine Carcinoma

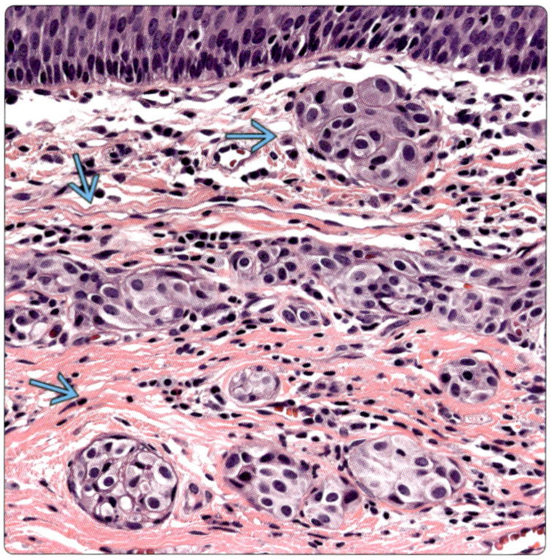

Squamous Cell Carcinoma In Situ

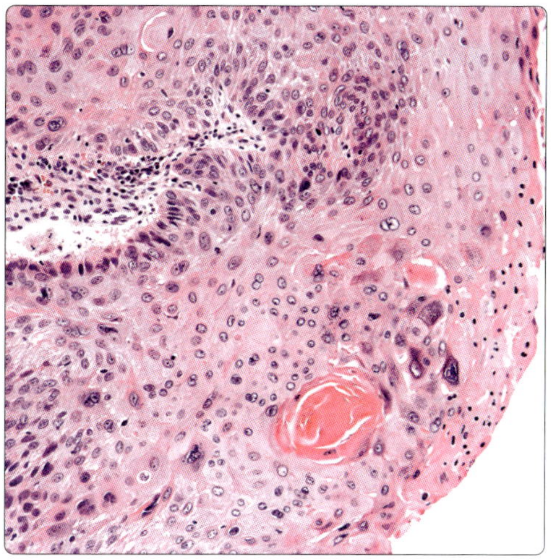

(Left) *Neuroendocrine carcinomas infiltrate as cords and nests of cells with round nuclei and dispersed chromatin →. The diagnosis of moderately differentiated neuroendocrine carcinoma is deferred to permanent section as a mitotic count is required for classification. Ancillary studies should be performed to exclude mimics.* **(Right)** *Squamous cell carcinoma in situ in small and tangentially oriented biopsies can be challenging to assess for invasion and may require deeper levels. Note the lack of maturation.*

Squamous Papilloma

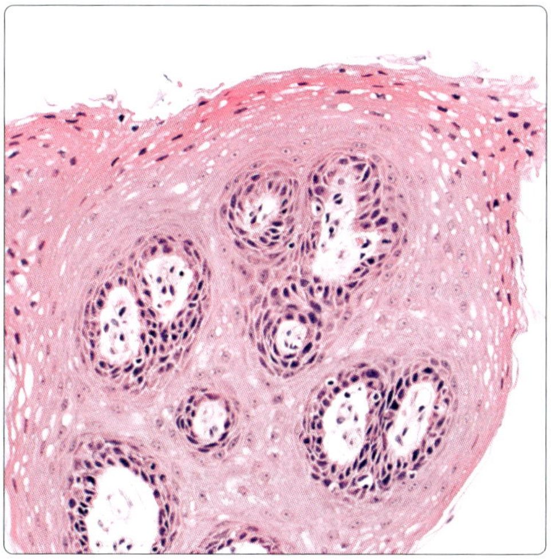

Postintubation Ulcer (Contact Ulcer)

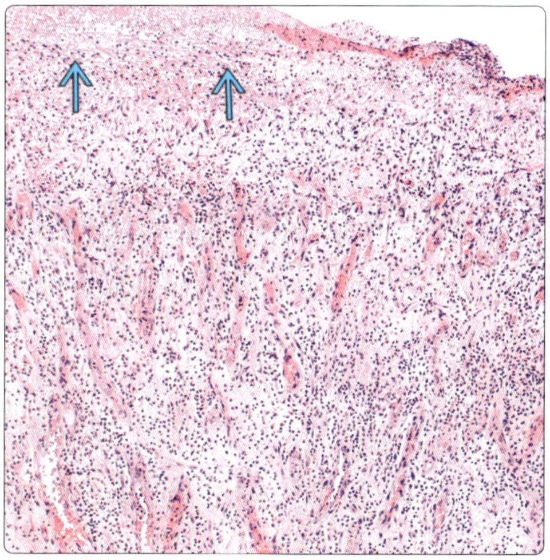

(Left) *Squamous papillomas are exophytic with fibrovascular cores lined by bland squamous epithelium. Many are associated with low-risk HPV.* **(Right)** *Postintubation contact ulcer shows abundant granulation tissue with uniformly distributed blood vessels arranged perpendicularly to the surface. These polypoid lesions on vocal cord may be concerning for malignancy. Note abundant surface fibrin deposition →, inflammation, and vascular proliferation. Contact ulcers from vocal abuse show similar findings.*

Granular Cell Tumor

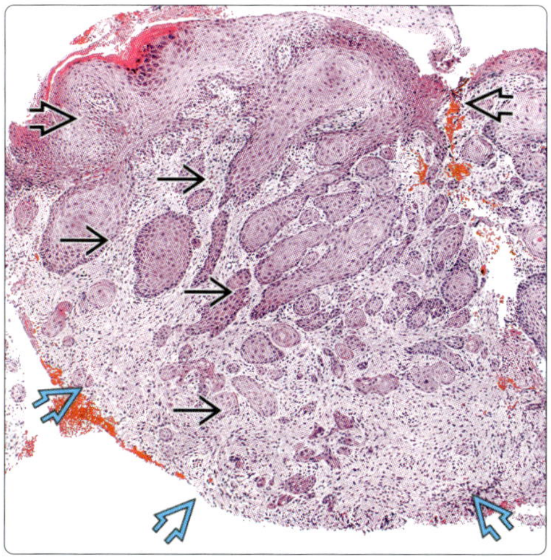

Granular Cell Tumor

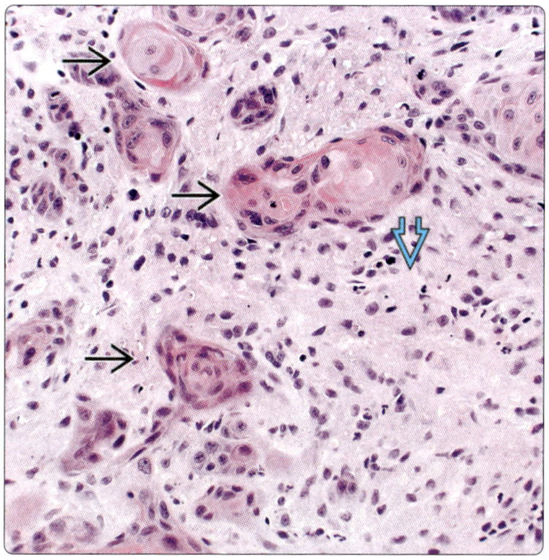

(Left) *Pseudoepitheliomatous hyperplasia ⇒ overlying a granular cell tumor ⇒ is a notorious mimic of infiltrative squamous cell carcinoma. Islands of well-differentiated squamous cells → appear to be dropping off from the hyperplastic surface epithelium.* **(Right)** *The cells of a granular cell tumor ⇒ should be sought at the base of an area of pseudoepitheliomatous hyperplasia. The cells are present surrounding islands of benign-appearing squamous epithelium →.*

SURGICAL/CLINICAL CONSIDERATIONS

Goal of Consultation

- Diagnosis of incidental small, white, subcapsular liver mass discovered during surgery

Change in Patient Management

- If lesion is malignant, surgery may be aborted or completed with palliative intent only

Clinical Setting

- Lesion on surface of liver may be seen preoperatively by imaging, at time of surgery, or during staging laparoscopy

SPECIMEN EVALUATION

Gross

- Specimen is usually small excisional biopsy that cannot be oriented

Frozen Section

- Entire specimen is generally frozen

MOST COMMON DIAGNOSES

Bile Duct Hamartoma (von Meyenburg Complex)

- Often multiple and generally small (< 0.5 cm)
- Circumscribed proliferation of ectatic well-formed ducts
  - Often with intraluminal bile
  - In loose or sclerotic stroma
  - Lined by cuboidal cells without atypia, mitoses, or architectural atypia

Bile Duct Adenoma (Peribiliary Gland Hamartoma)

- Usually solitary, small (< 1 cm), but can be large (4 cm)
- Circumscribed proliferation of small tubules with compressed lumina in fibrous stroma
  - Lined by cuboidal cells without atypia or mitoses
  - Tubules may show closely packed back-to-back architecture
  - Can have mucinous metaplasia or neuroendocrine appearance

Metastatic Carcinoma

- Moderately and poorly differentiated adenocarcinomas are easily diagnosed based on cytologic atypia
- Diagnosis of metastatic well-differentiated adenocarcinoma can be challenging
  - Greater nuclear enlargement and nucleolar prominence in well-differentiated carcinoma compared with benign bile duct lesions
  - Intraluminal necrosis favors metastatic carcinoma

Inflammatory Changes

- Hyalinized nodule may be due to granulomas from prior infection or current infection

Hemangioma

- Infarcted or sclerosed hemangioma may also mimic metastatic carcinoma on intraoperative examination

Cystic Lesions

- Benign biliary or mesothelial cysts may also mimic metastatic carcinoma on diagnostic laparoscopy

REPORTING

Frozen Section

- If benign, report as benign glandular proliferation, diagnostic features of malignancy not seen
- If malignant, report as metastatic carcinoma

PITFALLS

False-Positive Diagnosis

- Bile duct adenoma is most common liver lesion mistaken for adenocarcinoma or cholangiocarcinoma

SELECTED REFERENCES

1. Aishima S et al: Bile duct adenoma and von Meyenburg complex-like duct arising in hepatitis and cirrhosis: pathogenesis and histological characteristics. Pathol Int. 64(11):551-9, 2014

Bile Duct Hamartomas of Liver Capsule: Gross Appearance

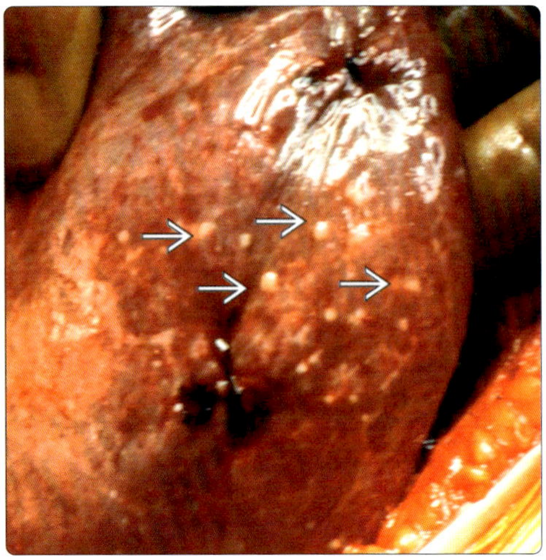

Metastatic Carcinoma to Liver: Gross Appearance

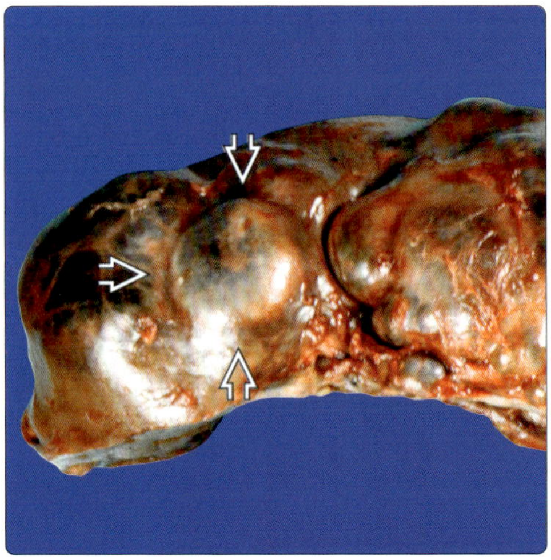

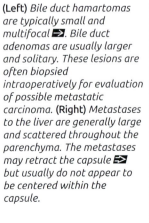

(Left) *Bile duct hamartomas are typically small and multifocal ➡. Bile duct adenomas are usually larger and solitary. These lesions are often biopsied intraoperatively for evaluation of possible metastatic carcinoma.* **(Right)** *Metastases to the liver are generally large and scattered throughout the parenchyma. The metastases may retract the capsule ➡ but usually do not appear to be centered within the capsule.*

Bile Duct Hamartoma

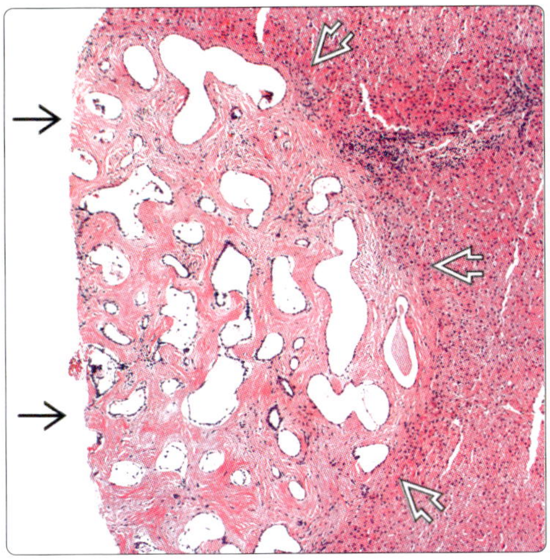

Metastatic Carcinoma

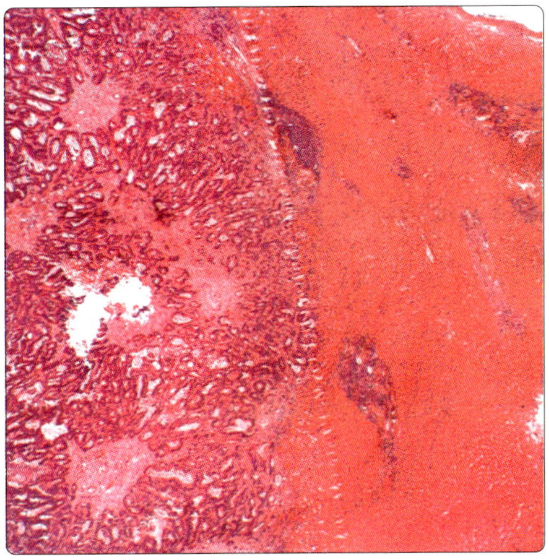

(Left) *Bile duct hamartomas form small, white, well-circumscribed ➡ nodules on the surface of the liver ⇨. Dilated tubules lined with low cuboidal cells are present within a densely fibrotic stroma. The tubules are clearly delineated and do not form complex anastomosing patterns, as would be present in many cases of carcinoma.* **(Right)** *Small metastases to the liver can occasionally form small nodules on the surface of the liver that mimic bile duct adenomas and hamartomas.*

Bile Duct Adenoma

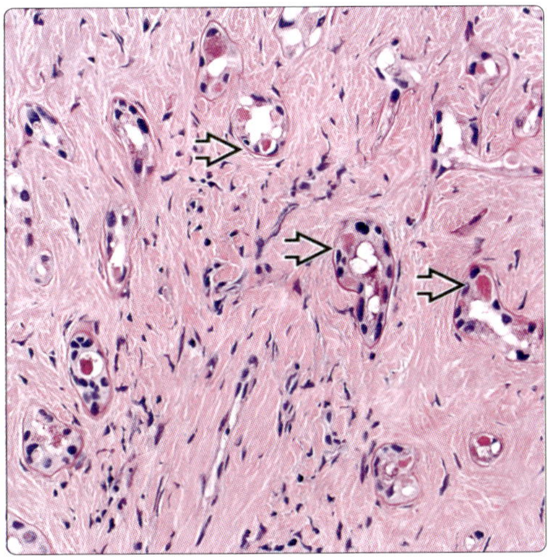

Metastatic Adenocarcinoma

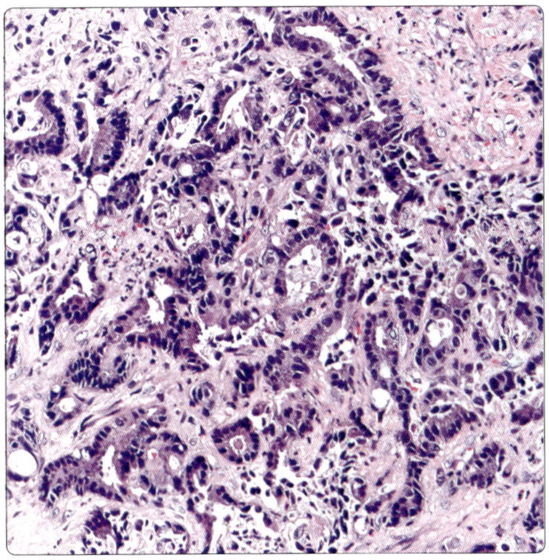

(Left) *Bile duct adenomas grow as small, angulated, tubular structures with small lumina. These tumors may show mucinous metaplasia with intracytoplasmic mucin ⇨. This feature can make distinction from metastatic adenocarcinoma challenging in some cases.* **(Right)** *Metastatic carcinomas often have a complex pattern of small anastomosing glands rather than distinct separate tubules. The nuclear changes (enlargement and hyperchromasia) are helpful in confirming malignancy.*

Bile Duct Adenoma

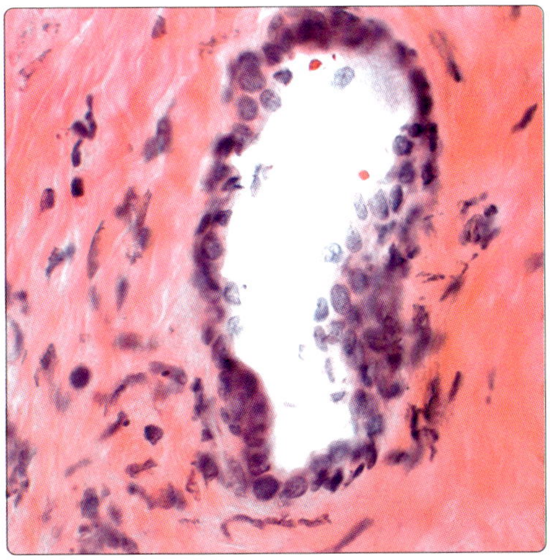

Metastatic Adenocarcinoma

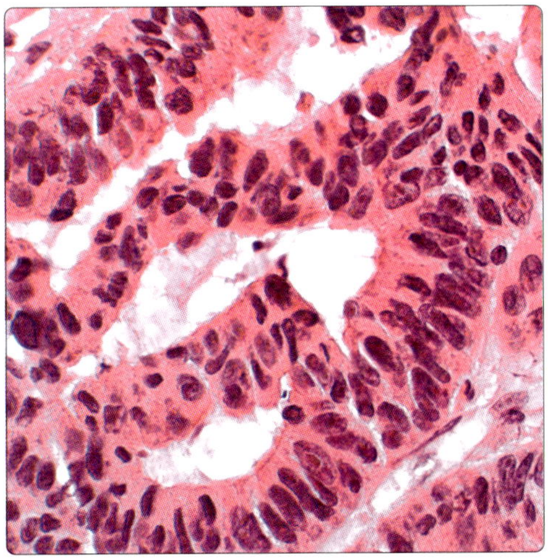

(Left) *The nuclei in this tubule from a bile duct adenoma appear slightly enlarged and stacked due to freezing of artifact, thickness of section, and tangential sectioning. Additional sections may be necessary to avoid an overdiagnosis of malignancy.* **(Right)** *Metastatic adenocarcinoma usually has a complex glandular pattern rather than forming individual glandular spaces. This colonic adenocarcinoma has characteristic tall columnar cells.*

SURGICAL/CLINICAL CONSIDERATIONS

Goal of Consultation

- Evaluation of donor liver prior to transplantation

Change in Patient Management

- Pathologic findings are used to decide whether or not liver is suitable for transplantation
  - Livers with high risk of allograft failure will not be used for transplantation

Clinical Setting

- Criteria for acceptance have been expanded to include organs at greater risk of reduced function or graft failure
  - There is a shortage of livers, resulting in patient mortality while waiting for an available organ
- The following features are no longer used to automatically exclude a liver from consideration
  - Age (> 60 years), viral hepatitis, steatosis, alcohol abuse, acute infection, hypotension, hypoxemia, cardiovascular disease, donation after cardiac death, chronic renal failure
- Appearance of liver capsule can be evaluated by surgeon
  - Sharp edges correlate with absence of steatosis, and rounded edges correlate with presence of steatosis
  - However, appearance at surgery underestimates amount of steatosis
- Histologic evaluation of liver is helpful to predict organs at greatest risk
  - Degree of macrovesicular steatosis is the most useful criteria for accepting or rejecting a graft

SPECIMEN EVALUATION

Gross

- Either wedge biopsy (≥ 1.5 cm^2) or cutting needle biopsy (≥ 2 cm in length) from anterior-inferior edge of liver is performed
  - If gross mass lesion is present, separate biopsy of noninvolved liver is also evaluated
  - Needle biopsy is preferred for evaluating fibrosis
    - Subcapsular liver sampled in wedge biopsy often has thick trabeculae that may be mistaken for advanced fibrosis
- Biopsy should be processed as quickly as possible
  - Fat is diminished after even a few minutes of exposure to air
  - Saline can cause distortion (chromatin clumping and edema of extracellular spaces)
- Specimens are ideally received and evaluated immediately after biopsy

Frozen Section

- Tissue should be gently blotted dry to reduce ice crystal artifact
  - However, excessive blotting can remove fat from specimen
- Entire specimen is frozen

FEATURES TO BE EVALUATED

Macrovesicular Steatosis

- Single, dominant, lipid vacuole displacing nucleus to periphery of cell
- Usually centrilobular
- Severity is graded
  - Mild: < 30% of hepatocytes
  - Moderate: 30-60% of hepatocytes
    - Increased risk of complications
    - Liver may be accepted for transplant in some settings
  - Severe: > 60% of hepatocytes
    - Absolute contraindication for transplantation due to high risk of graft malfunction

Microvesicular Steatosis

- Numerous small lipid droplets that do not cause displacement of nucleus to periphery of cell
  - Nucleus is located in center of cell
- Graded in same manner as macrovesicular steatosis
- Minimal effect on graft function
  - Common finding
- Often seen in cases of macrovesicular steatosis

Normal Liver

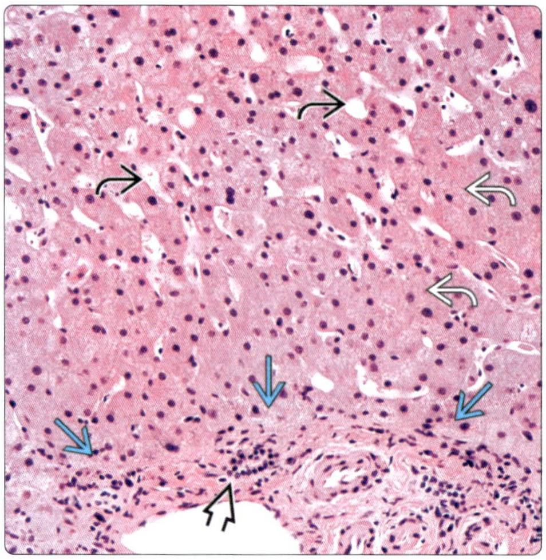

Normal Liver

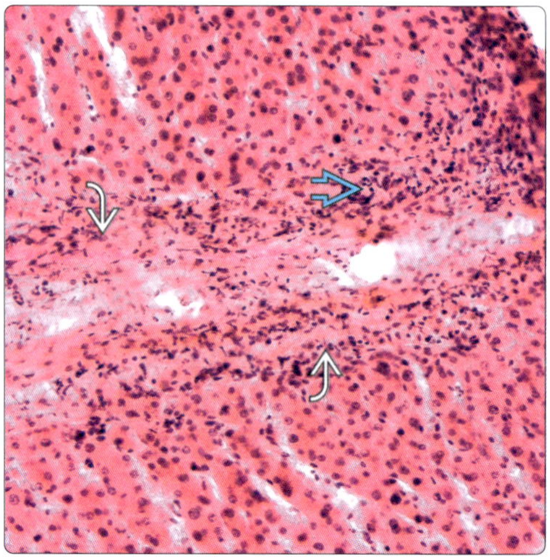

(Left) *Each component of the liver parenchyma is evaluated systematically: Portal tracts with duct ⇒, artery and vein, portal-lobular interface ⇒, hepatocytes ⇒, and sinusoids ⇒.* **(Right)** *The degree of inflammation ⇒ in portal tracts may be overestimated and the portal-lobular interface may appear blurred ⇒ on frozen sections, which are usually thicker than standard paraffin sections.*

Fibrosis

- Portal and periportal fibrosis may be difficult to evaluate on frozen sections
  - Fibrous capsule of liver and subcapsular areas of fibrosis should be distinguished from significant fibrosis
  - Wedge biopsies can be difficult to evaluate for fibrosis
- Bridging fibrosis is easily detected
- Nodularity of liver and bridging fibrosis are indicative of cirrhosis and are contraindication to transplantation

Necrosis

- Apoptotic hepatocytes (acidophil bodies)
- Centrilobular necrosis
- Reported as
  - Focal (< 10%) or extensive (≥ 10%)
  - Mild or severe

Mass Lesions

- Benign lesions are not contraindication for transplantation
  - Capsular nodule or nodules
    - Bile duct adenoma (peribiliary gland hamartoma)
    - Bile duct hamartoma (von Meyenburg complex)
  - Focal nodular hyperplasia
  - Hepatocellular adenoma
    - May be difficult or impossible to distinguish from well-differentiated hepatocellular carcinoma on frozen section
- Biopsy away from mass should also be evaluated
- Malignancy
  - Diagnosis of hepatocellular carcinoma, metastatic carcinoma, or other malignancy is absolute contraindication for transplantation

Portal Inflammation

- Mild chronic inflammation of portal triad is common in hospitalized patients
  - Not contraindication for transplantation
- Severe lymphoplasmacytic portal infiltrate with interface hepatitis (piecemeal necrosis) should raise possibility of viral hepatitis
- Reported as mild, moderate/severe

Iron Deposition

- **Hepatocellular siderosis**
  - Coarse, dark brown granular pigment in periportal hepatocytes; graded semiquantitatively from 1-4+
  - Grades > 2 may be contraindication for transplantation
    - Organs from patients with hereditary hemochromatosis or secondary iron overload can be used if fibrosis is not advanced
- **Kupffer cell siderosis**
  - Common finding; typically mild, cannot be detected easily on frozen section

Other Pigments

- Lipofuscin (very fine brown granules in centrilobular hepatocytes)
  - Increased with age and can be extensive
  - Not contraindication to transplantation
- Bile (green to gold/brown granules) in perivenular hepatocytes or within canaliculi
  - Not contraindication to transplantation

Granulomas

- Nonnecrotizing fibrotic granulomas may be residue of prior infection (e.g., histoplasmosis)
  - Not contraindication to transplantation
- Necrotizing granulomas may indicate current infection and lead to rejection of organ for transplant

Congestion

- Dilated sinusoids alone are a nonspecific finding
- Atrophy of perivenular hepatocytes and sinusoidal dilatation often consequence of terminal ischemic injury

Duct Damage

- Seen in primary biliary disorders, such as primary biliary cirrhosis and primary sclerosing cholangitis
- Ductular proliferation is also indirect evidence of duct damage

Thrombi

- Rarely seen in central or portal veins

REPORTING

Frozen Section

- Features reported
  - Steatosis: Presence or absence and percentage of hepatocytes affected
    - Minimal or mild (up to 30% of hepatocytes) may be acceptable for transplantation
    - Severe (> 60%) is associated with nonfunctioning graft
  - Extent of inflammation &/or hepatocyte necrosis
    - Mild focal necrosis may occur during harvesting of organ
    - Severe or extensive necrosis is associated with graft failure
  - Fibrosis: Presence or absence
  - Alcohol-induced injury: Associated with compromise of graft weeks to years after transplantation
    - Fibrosis
    - Moderate to severe fatty change
    - Marked hepatocytic necrosis ± cholestasis
    - Mallory hyaline/ballooning degeneration
- Biopsies consisting entirely or predominantly of capsule are inadequate for evaluation
  - Additional biopsy should be requested
- Representative slides should be retained by recipient institution to aid in evaluating graft after transplantation

PITFALLS

Superficial Biopsy

- Very superficial biopsy may only sample capsule
  - Glisson capsule can penetrate into parenchyma for 0.5 cm or more
- If cause of death was trauma, there may be peripheral hemorrhage and inflammation
- Deeper biopsy &/or needle biopsy should be requested

Lipofuscin

- Can be normal finding in older patients in a centrilobular location
- Can be mistaken for cholestasis

Contents

Criteria for Liver Transplantation Based on Frozen Section Features

Finding	Acceptable for Transplantation	Unacceptable for Transplantation
Steatosis, macrovesicular	< 10% of hepatocytes involved	≥ 30% of hepatocytes involved
Steatosis, microvesicular	Any type	Not applicable
Viral hepatitis	In positive recipients: Grade < 2 Batts and Ludwig; grade < 5 modified histological activity index (mHAI) (Ishak/Knodell)	In all recipients: Grade ≥ 2 Batts and Ludwig; grade ≥ 5 mHAI (Ishak/Knodell)
Fibrosis	Stage < 2 Batts and Ludwig or mHAI (Ishak/Knodell)	Stage ≥ 2 Batts and Ludwig or mHAI (Ishak/Knodell)
Granulomas	"Burned-out" or fibrotic/calcified granulomas	Active granulomas, caseating or noncaseating
Nonspecific portal inflammation	Mild	> Mild (particularly if viral hepatitis status of donor is unknown)
Necrosis	< 10% of liver area	≥ 10% of liver area
Malignancy	No	Yes

Batts and Ludwig inflammation grades are 0 (no activity), 1 (minimal), 2 (mild), 3 (moderate), 4 (severe), and fibrosis stages are 0 (none), 1 (portal fibrosis), 2 (periportal fibrosis), 3 (septal fibrosis), and 4 (cirrhosis).

Batts KP et al: Chronic hepatitis. An update on terminology and reporting. Am J Surg Pathol. 19(12):1409-17, 1995.

Modified Histological Activity Index Grading (Ishak/Knodell)

Category	Score	Category	Score
Periportal or periseptal interface hepatitis (piecemeal necrosis)		**Confluent necrosis**	
Absent	0	Absent	0
Mild (focal, few portal areas)	1	Focal confluent necrosis	1
Mild/moderate (focal, most portal areas)	2	Zone 3 necrosis in some areas	2
Moderate (continuous around < 50% of tracts or septa)	3	Zone 3 necrosis in most areas	3
Severe (continuous around > 50% of tracts or septa)	4	Zone 3 necrosis and occasional portal-central (P-C) bridging	4
		Zone 3 necrosis and multiple P-C bridging	5
		Panacinar or multiacinar necrosis	6
Focal (spotty) lytic necrosis, apoptosis, and focal inflammation*		**Portal inflammation**	
Absent	0	None	0
≤ 1 focus per 10x objective	1	Mild, some or all portal areas	1
2-4 foci per 10x objective	2	Moderate, some or all portal areas	2
5-10 foci per 10x objective	3	Moderate/marked all portal areas	3
> 10 foci per 10x objective	4	Marked, all portal areas	4

**The score for each of the categories is added for a total score from 0-18.*

Ishak K et al: Histological grading and staging of chronic hepatitis. J Hepatol. 22(6):696-9, 1995.

- Can be mistaken for iron deposits (should be in periportal location)

Air-Dried Specimens

- Diminishes amount of fat present

Specimens in Saline

- Can make evaluation of necrosis difficult
  - May cause clumping of cytoplasm and extracellular fluid
- Ice crystal artifact can create clear spaces that mimic fat droplets and lead to overestimation of steatosis
  - Staining quality will be poor in hepatocytes
  - Artifact is present throughout tissue

Gauze or Towel

- Can cause fat to diffuse out of tissue and result in underestimate of steatosis
- May create artifactual holes in tissue

SELECTED REFERENCES

1. Flechtenmacher C et al: Donor liver histology–a valuable tool in graft selection. Langenbecks Arch Surg. 400(5):551-7, 2015
2. Hołówko W et al: Reliability of frozen section in the assessment of allograft steatosis in liver transplantation. Transplant Proc. 46(8):2755-7, 2014
3. Melin C et al: Approach to intraoperative consultation for donor liver biopsies. Arch Pathol Lab Med. 137(2):270-4, 2013
4. Transplant Pathology Internet Services: Liver. http://tpis.upmc.com/changebody.cfm?url=/tpis/liver/LDonorFS.jsp. Reviewed December 3, 2013. Accessed December 3, 2013.

Macrovesicular Steatosis: Mild (< 30%)

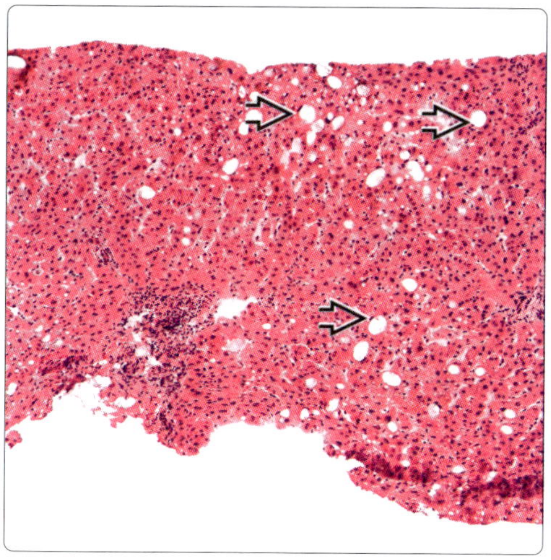

Macrovesicular and Microvesicular Steatosis

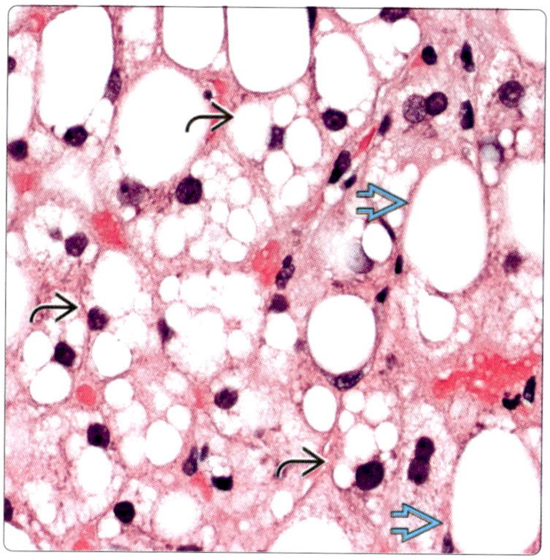

(Left) *The extent of macrovesicular steatosis is the strongest predictive factor for graft failure. This biopsy shows mild macrovesicular steatosis ⇨ involving < 30% of the biopsy.* **(Right)** *In macrovesicular steatosis, a single fat vacuole displaces the nucleus to the periphery ⇨. In microvesicular steatosis, there are multiple small vacuoles, and the nucleus is located centrally ↗.*

Macrovesicular Steatosis: Moderate (30-50%)

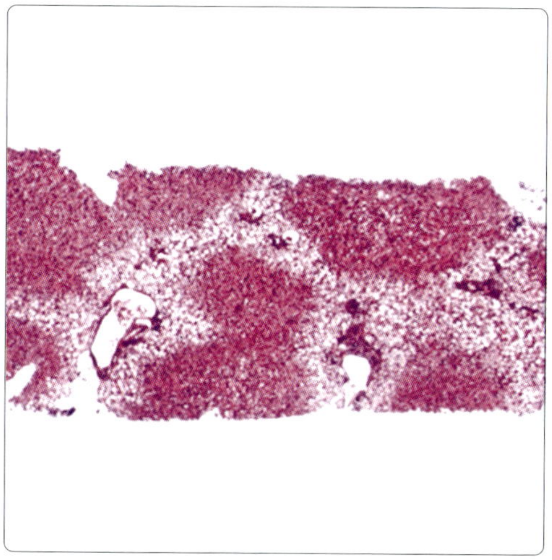

Microvesicular Steatosis

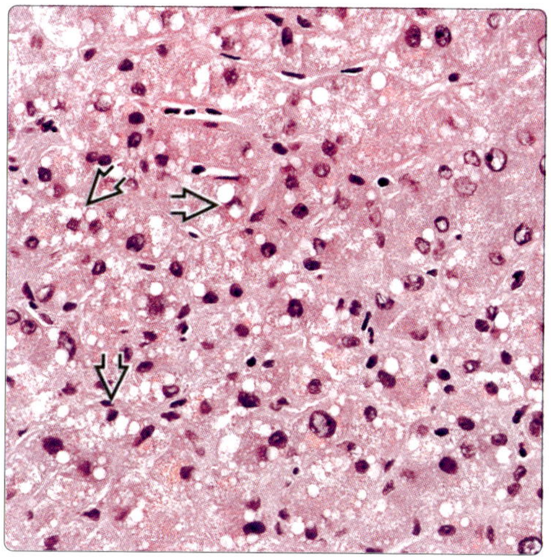

(Left) *This macrovesicular steatosis has a periportal distribution and approaches the 30% cut-off. The quantity of steatosis is more important than the distribution.* **(Right)** *Microvesicular steatosis is a common finding and is graded in the same manner as macrovesicular steatosis. However, this finding is not as important in predicting graft function. Multiple small vacuoles with a central nucleus ⇨ are seen.*

Macrovesicular Steatosis: Severe (> 60%)

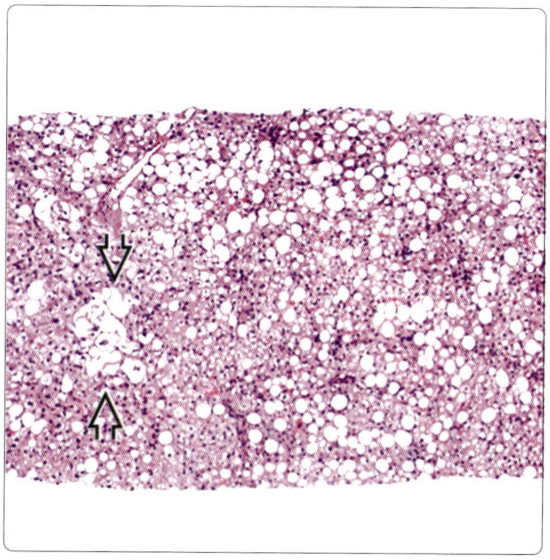

Mallory Hyaline

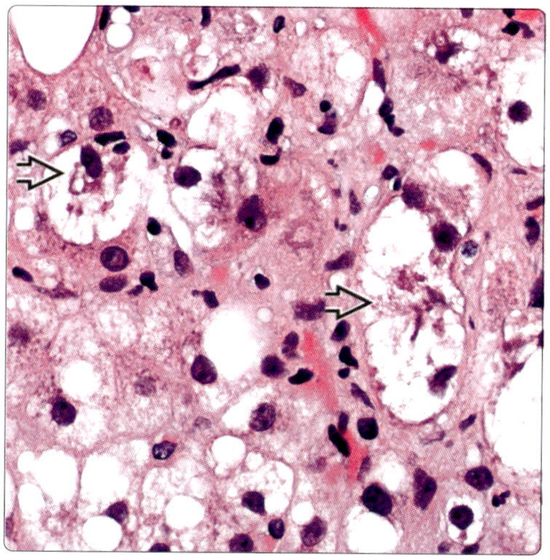

(Left) *In this biopsy, severe macrovesicular steatosis diffusely involves the majority of the liver parenchyma. Foci of ballooning degeneration ⇨ are apparent, even at low magnification.* **(Right)** *Mallory hyaline ⇨ is observed as ropy, intracytoplasmic inclusions, typically in a perinuclear location. The presence of Mallory hyaline is not etiologically specific but is most commonly seen in the setting of a toxic/metabolic steatohepatitis.*

(Left) *There is mild sinusoidal dilatation in the centrilobular zone. This is a nonspecific finding and is not clinically significant. A portal tract is present.* **(Right)** *Mild sinusoidal dilatation diffusely involves the centrilobular and midzonal sections surrounding the central vein in this biopsy. Centrilobular congestion is only clinically important if seen in conjunction with atrophy of perivenular hepatocytes due to terminal ischemic injury.*

Congestion: Centrilobular

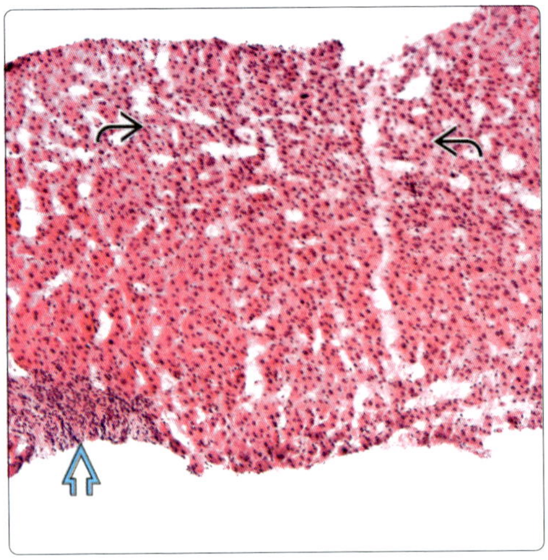

Congestion: Centrilobular/Midzonal

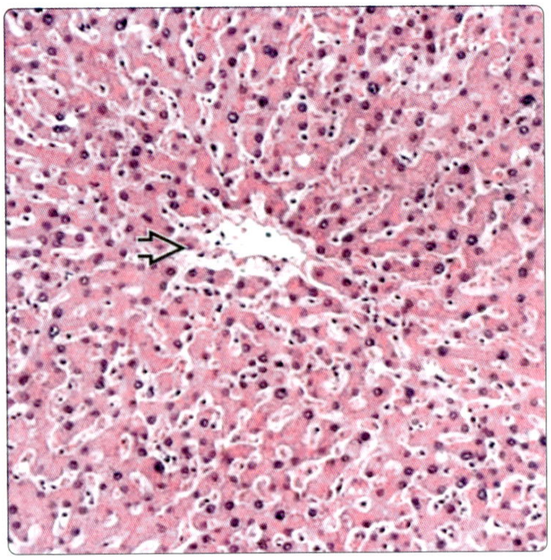

(Left) *Centrilobular congestion is present with thinned-out hepatic cords, consistent with atrophy. The central vein at the top of the image helps in determining the predominant zone of hepatic damage.* **(Right)** *Hepatocytic damage and dropout and perivenular hemorrhage are present in this liver biopsy. Mild focal necrosis can be seen during the harvesting of the graft.*

Congestion: Centrilobular

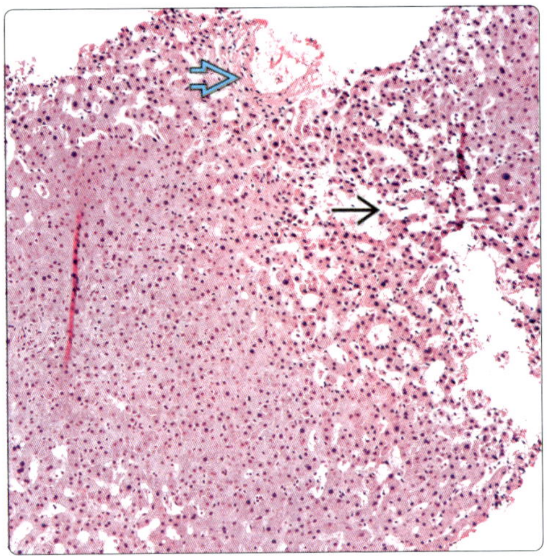

Perivenular Hemorrhage and Necrosis

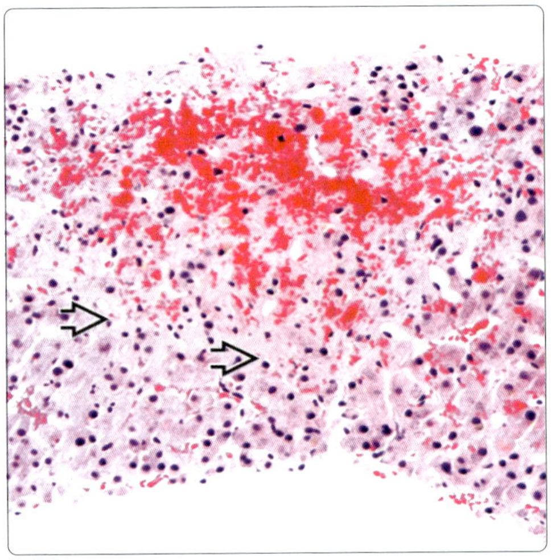

(Left) *In cholestasis, the green to golden granules of bile may be seen in intracellular or canalicular locations. Feathery degeneration of hepatocytes is typical of cholestatic hepatocellular injury.* **(Right)** *Lipofuscin is composed of fine yellow/brown granules. A perivenular distribution is common and should not be mistaken for increased intracellular iron deposition or cholestasis.*

Cholestasis

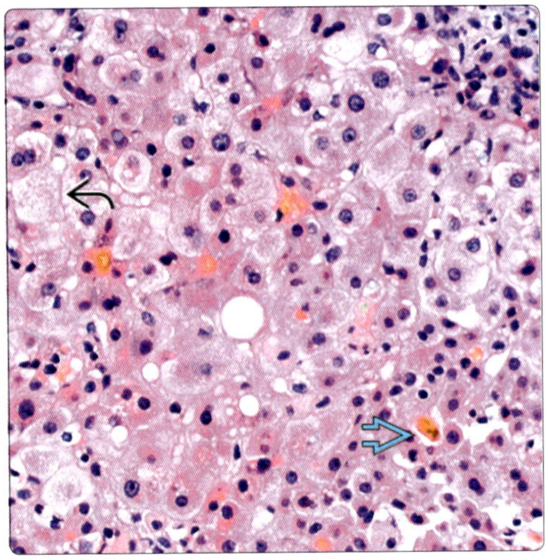

Lipofuscin: Perivenular

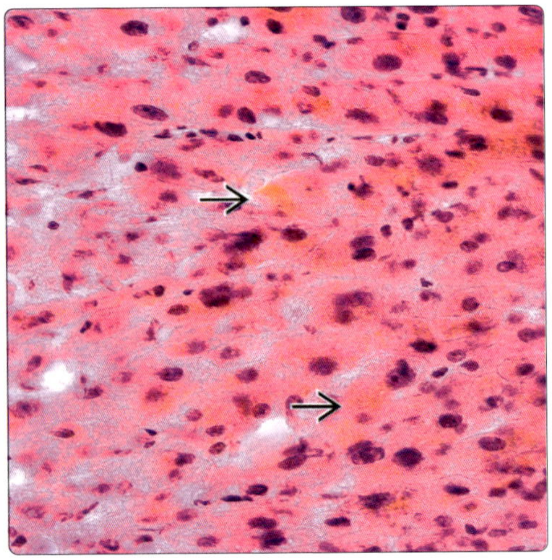

Sinusoidal Inflammation: Mild

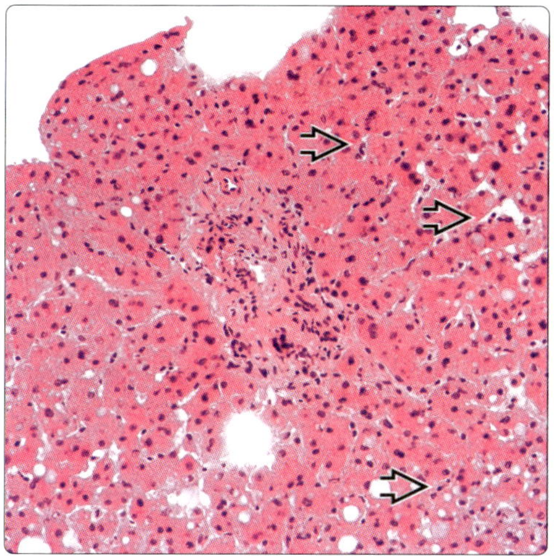

Portal Inflammation: Mild

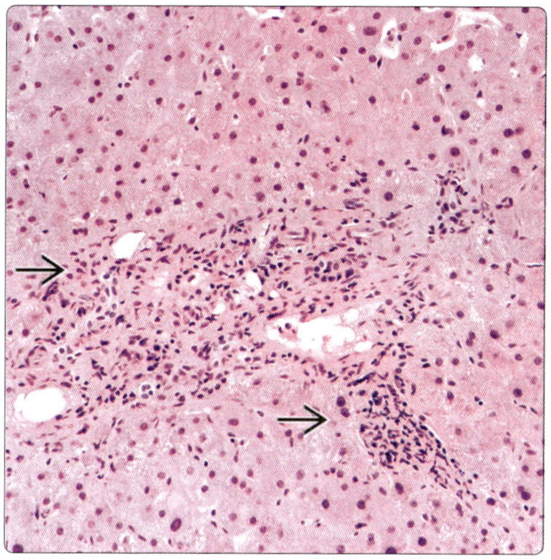

(Left) *Inflammation in the liver parenchyma may be portal, sinusoidal, or lobular. Portal inflammation is typical of viral hepatitis. In this biopsy, portal inflammation is minimal, but the parenchyma shows mild sinusoidal mononuclear cell infiltration.* **(Right)** *Mild portal inflammation is etiologically nonspecific and does not have any impact on the acceptability of a liver for transplantation. Mild portal and periportal fibrosis is also present in this case.*

Portal/Periportal Inflammation

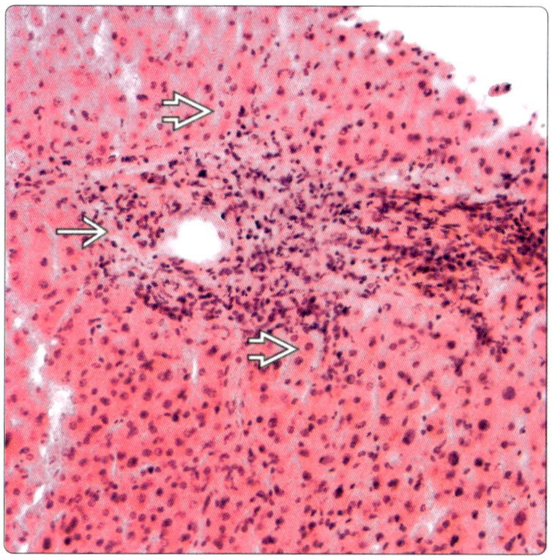

Portal Inflammation: Moderate

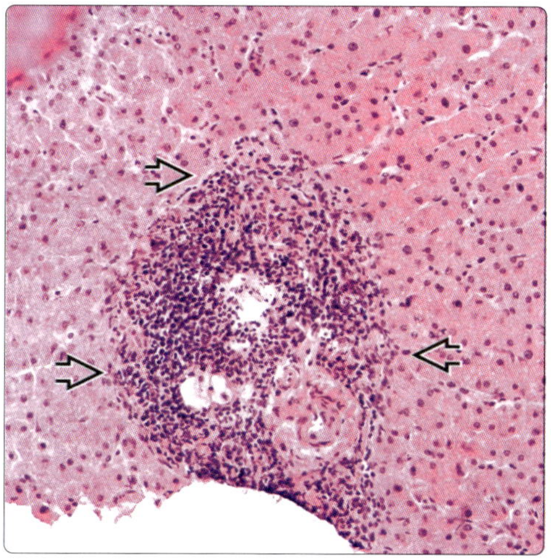

(Left) *A moderate portal mononuclear cell infiltration is present. There is also some piecemeal necrosis where the inflammatory cells spill over from the portal tracts into adjacent hepatic parenchyma.* **(Right)** *Piecemeal necrosis (also known as interface hepatitis) involves almost the entire circumference of this portal tract. This degree of inflammatory infiltrate and hepatocellular injury should raise suspicion for an underlying viral hepatitis.*

Portal Inflammation: Severe

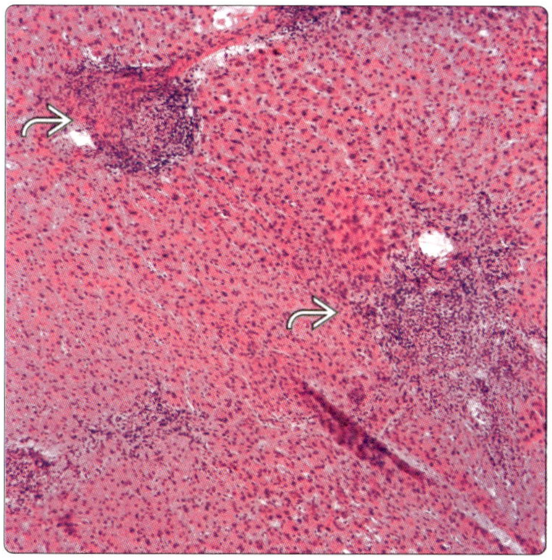

Cytomegalovirus Hepatitis

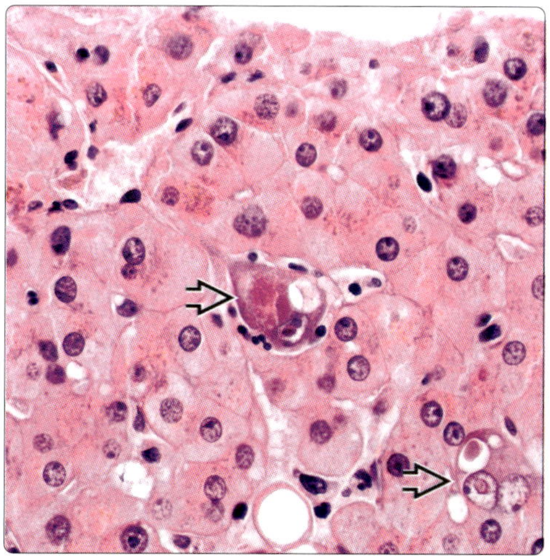

(Left) *The likelihood of viral hepatitis increases if most or all portal tracts show a moderate to severe degree of mononuclear inflammation, as seen in this liver from a patient with HCV viral hepatitis. Livers with HCV may be transplanted into HCV-positive patients.* **(Right)** *Inflammation may be mild or absent in cases of cytomegalovirus (CMV) hepatitis. The diagnosis rests on demonstration of typical "owl's-eye" inclusions within hepatocytes. Livers with CMV can be transplanted into CMV-positive recipients.*

SURGICAL/CLINICAL CONSIDERATIONS

Goal of Consultation

- Evaluation of margins
- Determine whether liver mass is benign or malignant, if possible

Change in Patient Management

- If lesion is benign, wide margin of resection is unnecessary
- If malignant lesion is present at margin, additional tissue is removed, if surgically feasible
- Primary resection, such as Whipple procedure, is not performed if hepatic metastasis is confirmed

Clinical Setting

- Liver lesions are usually diagnosed by core needle biopsy or fine-needle aspiration prior to surgery
- Patients may benefit from resection of
  - Hepatocellular adenoma
  - Focal nodular hyperplasia if increasing in size
  - Hepatocellular carcinoma
  - Intrahepatic cholangiocarcinoma
  - Metastases to liver
    - Oligometastatic carcinomas (colon carcinoma most common primary site)
    - Neuroendocrine tumors
- Malignant lesions are resected with margin of at least 1 cm, if possible
- Superficial or capsular liver mass may be detected during operation for another reason
  - Surgeon may request intraoperative evaluation to guide surgery and for staging

SPECIMEN EVALUATION

Gross

- Measure specimen in 3 dimensions
- Cut parenchymal margin (without capsule) of liver is identified
  - Evaluate surface for any areas grossly suspicious for tumor involvement
- Ink margin
  - Liver capsule is not margin and should not be inked
- Thinly slice specimen perpendicular to margin
  - Identify all mass lesions
  - Number of metastatic foci found in resection has clinical and prognostic relevance
    - Correlation with number of lesions seen on imaging is necessary to ensure surgeon removed all foci of tumor
    - Slices must be 4-5 mm thick to detect small metastatic foci
- Measure closest distance to margin
- Only fibrotic tumor bed may be visible in posttreatment resections

Frozen Section

- If there is grossly suspicious area for margin involvement, perpendicular frozen section is evaluated

MOST COMMON DIAGNOSES

Metastatic Carcinoma

- Most common diagnosis (~ 25% of total, ~ 75% of malignant diagnoses)
- Multiple hard white masses
  - Often have central necrosis

Hepatocellular Carcinoma

- 2nd most common diagnosis (~ 25% of malignant diagnoses)
- May present as solitary mass, dominant mass with satellite nodules, or rarely, in diffusely infiltrative pattern
  - Variegated yellow-white appearance with necrosis and hemorrhage in larger lesions
- Surrounding liver is usually cirrhotic
  - Nodule within nodule may be area of carcinoma with dominant nodule or carcinoma arising in dysplastic nodule
- Tumor cells closely resemble normal hepatocytes when well differentiated

Metastatic Carcinoma to Liver: Gross Appearance

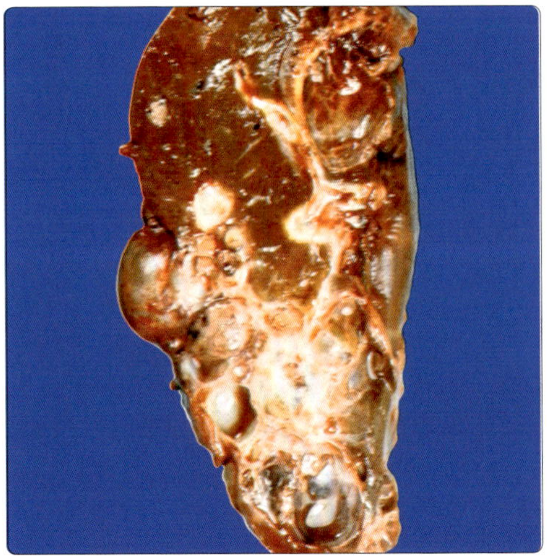

Metastatic Colon Carcinoma to Liver

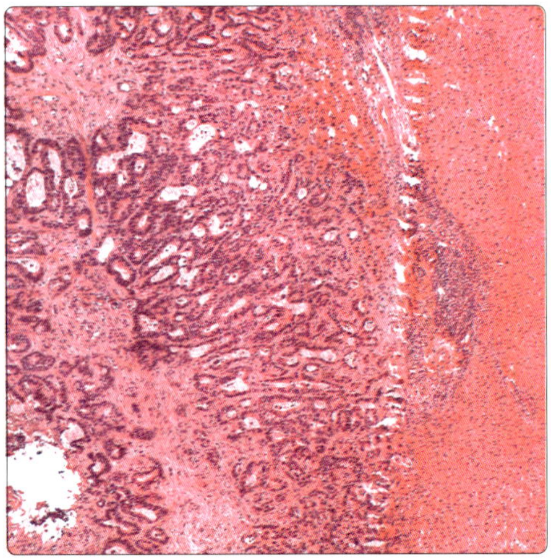

(Left) *Surgeons often request intraoperative evaluation of the hepatic margin to ensure complete resection of metastatic tumors. Colon carcinoma and intestinal carcinoids are examples of common tumors with a propensity for liver metastasis.* **(Right)** *Metastatic colon carcinoma shows glands lined by tall columnar cells with dirty intraluminal necrosis. Resections performed after chemotherapy may only show necrosis ± calcifications. Surgeons attempt to obtain negative margins when possible.*

- Large polygonal cells with large nucleus, prominent nucleolus, and abundant cytoplasm
  - Canalicular bile may be present and support origin in liver
  - Thickened trabeculae with > 2 cells
  - Absent portal tracts
- Poorly differentiated carcinomas are more easily recognized as malignant, but distinction of hepatocellular from cholangiocarcinoma may be difficult
- Fibrolamellar variant
  - Occurs in young patients; no cirrhosis in background
  - Lamellar collagen bands surround tumor nests
  - Tumor cells show cytoplasmic inclusions and prominent cherry red nucleoli

Cholangiocarcinoma

- Most carcinomas are advanced at time of diagnosis
- Large, gray-white, hard, irregular masses
- Cholangiocarcinoma cannot be distinguished from metastatic adenocarcinoma on frozen section

Bile Duct Adenoma/Hamartoma

- Form small (< 1 cm) to large (up to 4 cm) white circumscribed nodules on liver capsule
- Often biopsied during abdominal surgery to exclude metastasis
- Circumscribed borders
- Well-formed small tubules, variable collagen
  - Bile may be present in hamartomas
- Minimal nuclear atypia, may show cytoplasmic globules

Hepatocellular Adenoma

- Majority occur in young women
  - Resected due to risk of rupture and hemorrhage
- Solitary encapsulated mass with homogeneous appearance that resembles surrounding liver
  - Can be very large (up to 30 cm)
- Consists of normal-appearing hepatocytes in trabeculae that are 1-2 cells thick
  - Macrovesicular steatosis common
  - Lacks portal tracts (with exception of inflammatory variant)
  - Uniform cell population without mitotic activity
- May be difficult to distinguish from well-differentiated hepatocellular carcinoma on frozen section
  - Trabecular thickness, pseudoglandular formation, and high-grade nuclear atypia are helpful features to suggest carcinoma
- Surrounding liver is normal in appearance
  - Carcinomas often associated with cirrhosis
- Gross evaluation of margin is sufficient

Focal Nodular Hyperplasia

- Usually solitary gray-white unencapsulated mass located beneath liver capsule
  - Resected when large and symptomatic
- Majority are < 5 cm
- There is characteristic central fibrotic area with broad strands radiating out in stellate pattern
  - May be absent in small lesions
  - Fibrous septa may have abnormal arteries with intimal proliferation and muscular hypertrophy
  - Proliferation of small bile ducts at edge of fibrous septa
- Parenchyma within lesion is nodular
  - Pattern looks cirrhotic
    - Important to note that entire liver is not cirrhotic

Hemangioma

- Usually diagnosed by imaging
  - May undergo preoperative embolization to reduce hemorrhage
- Gross removal of lesion is sufficient

Mucinous Cystic Neoplasm (Biliary Cystadenoma)

- Females 20-70 years of age
- Unilocular or multilocular
- Cysts lined by pancreaticobiliary or mucinous epithelium with adjacent ovarian-type stroma

Pediatric Tumors

- Rare
  - Tissue for ancillary studies should be considered (electron microscopy, cytogenetic studies, snap frozen for molecular studies)
- Some tumors that occur in adults also occur in children
  - Hepatocellular carcinoma, focal nodular hyperplasia, hepatocellular adenoma
- **Hepatoblastoma**
  - Large circumscribed mass with variegated appearance, including cysts, necrosis, and hemorrhage
- **Mesenchymal hamartoma**
  - Large circumscribed mass with multiple cystic spaces filled with fluid
    - Solid areas may fibrotic, myxoid, with entrapped foci of normal liver
- **Embryonal (undifferentiated) sarcoma**
  - Circumscribed soft tumor with solid and cystic appearance

REPORTING

Frozen Section

- Margins are reported as positive or negative
  - Distance to margin for hepatocellular carcinomas should be reported
- Definitive diagnosis may not be possible on frozen section
  - Preliminary diagnosis of hepatocellular tumor or metastatic carcinoma, for example, is usually sufficient for intraoperative management

PITFALLS

Bile Duct Adenoma/Hamartoma vs. Metastasis

- Small size, circumscribed borders, and bland cytologic features favor benign lesion
- Tall columnar cells, dirty necrosis, solid nests of cells, and desmoplastic stroma favor metastatic carcinoma

SELECTED REFERENCES

1. Bhutiani N et al: Impact of surgical margin clearance for resection of secondary hepatic malignancies. J Surg Oncol. 113(3):289-95, 2016
2. Lafaro K et al: The importance of surgical margins in primary malignancies of the liver. J Surg Oncol. 113(3):296-303, 2016
3. Rakha E et al: Accuracy of frozen section in the diagnosis of liver mass lesions. J Clin Pathol. 59(4):352-4, 2006

(Left) *Malignant hepatocellular lesions show a variegated appearance with hemorrhage and necrosis ➡. This hepatocellular carcinoma (HCC) is unusual in that it is arising in a noncirrhotic background ⇨.* **(Right)** *Well-differentiated HCC can be difficult to distinguish from adenoma on frozen section. In this case, definite thickening of hepatic cord architecture is not seen. The final classification is best deferred to permanent sections.*

Hepatocellular Carcinoma: Gross Appearance

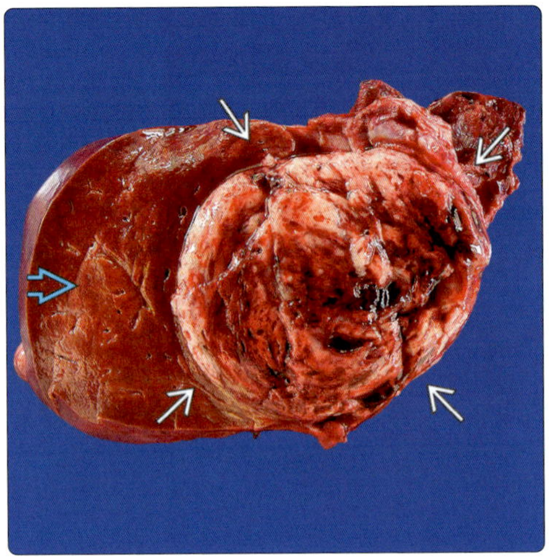

Hepatocellular Carcinoma

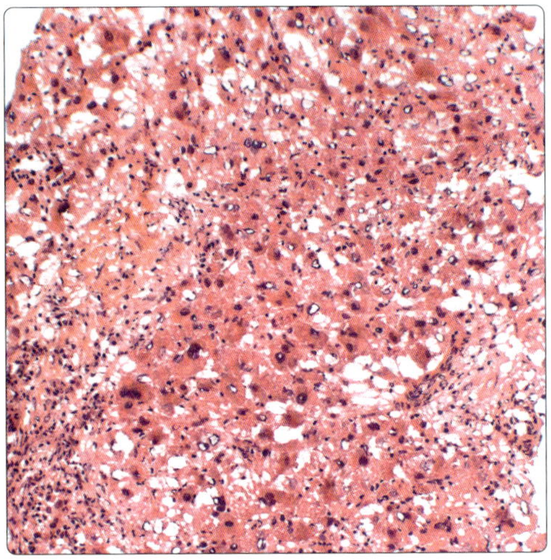

(Left) *The margin of a liver resection typically shows cautery artifact, and this can make evaluation very difficult. It is always important to correlate the gross appearance of the lesion and margin with the microscopic findings on frozen section. This HCC was present at the inked resection margin grossly and was confirmed microscopically ➡.* **(Right)** *This margin ⇨ of a liver resection for HCC consists of normal tissue with 1-2 cells thick hepatic cords and several portal triads ⇨.*

Hepatocellular Carcinoma: Positive Margin

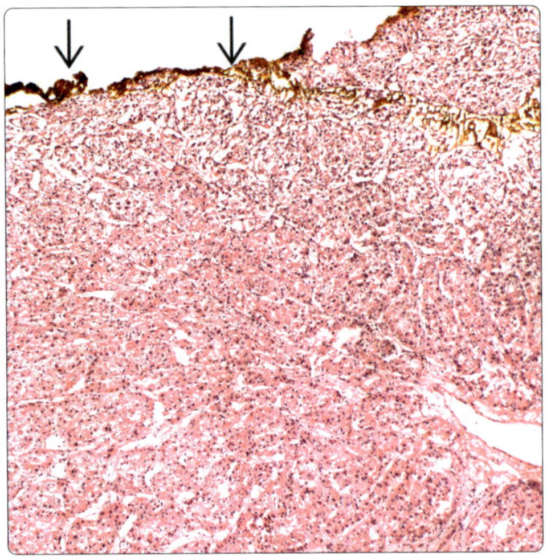

Liver Resection: Negative Margin

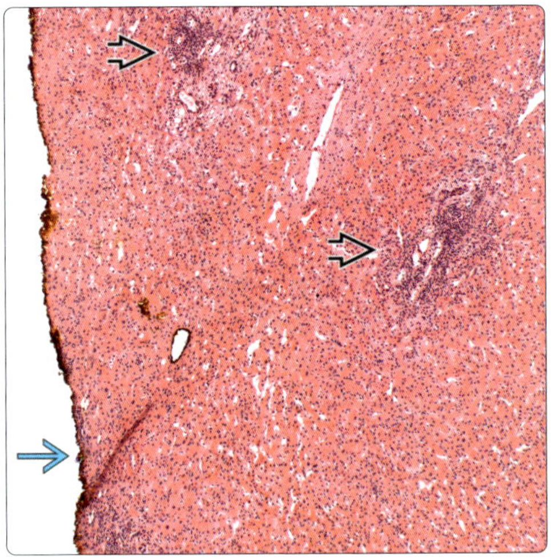

(Left) *Nonneoplastic liver is best recognized on frozen sections by the presence of portal tracts. Portal structures are absent in HCC and hepatic adenomas with the exception of inflammatory hepatic adenomas. A thickened cord architecture is helpful in making a diagnosis of HCC.* **(Right)** *Fibrolamellar HCC occurs in young patients without cirrhosis. Tumor cells with prominent nucleoli and cytoplasmic inclusions grow in nests surrounded by dense collagen bundles in parallel lamellae.*

Hepatocellular Carcinoma

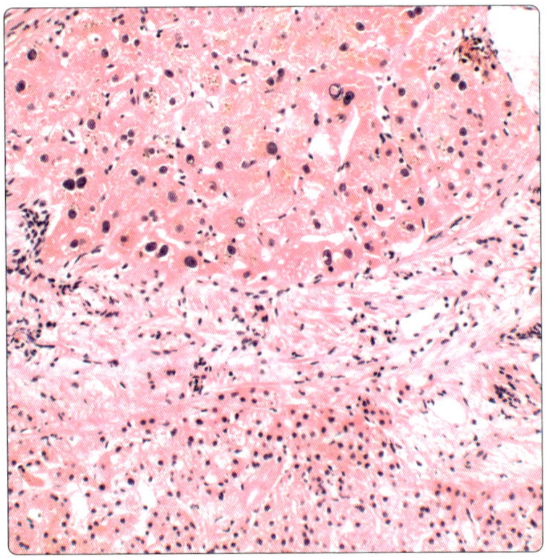

Fibrolamellar Carcinoma

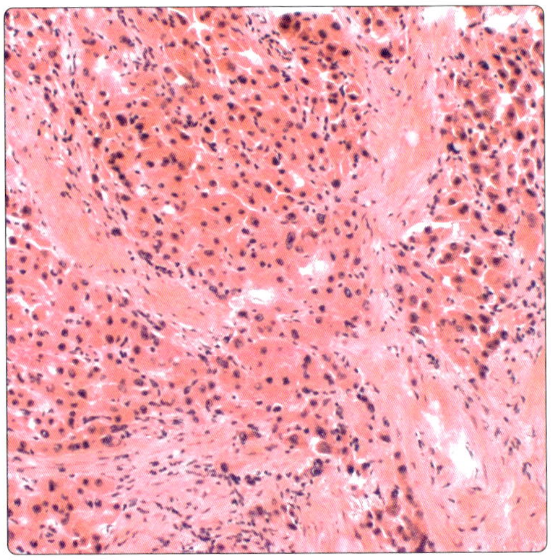

Focal Nodular Hyperplasia: Gross Appearance

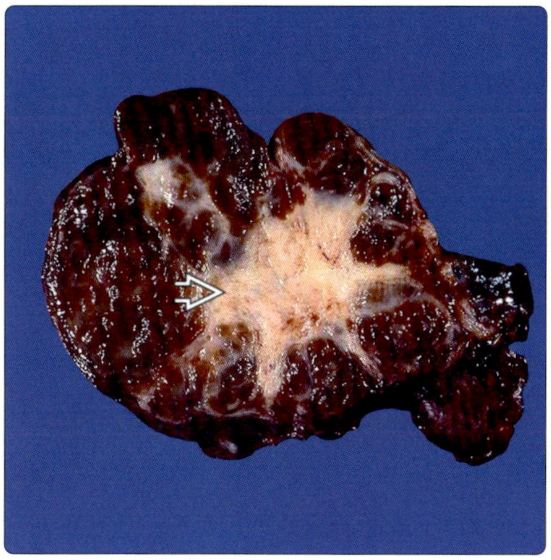

Focal Nodular Hyperplasia

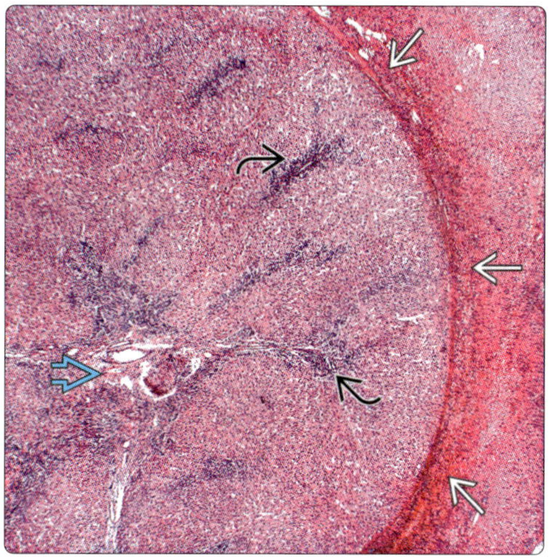

(Left) *Focal nodular hyperplasia appears as a circumscribed mass with a characteristic central scar that radiates out in a stellate configuration. The remainder of the cut surface of the lesion resembles normal liver parenchyma or appears nodular.* **(Right)** *Focal nodular hyperplasia has a well-demarcated border. Delicate fibrous septa radiate out from the central scar and show marked ductular proliferation and abnormal blood vessels.*

Hepatocellular Adenoma: Gross Appearance

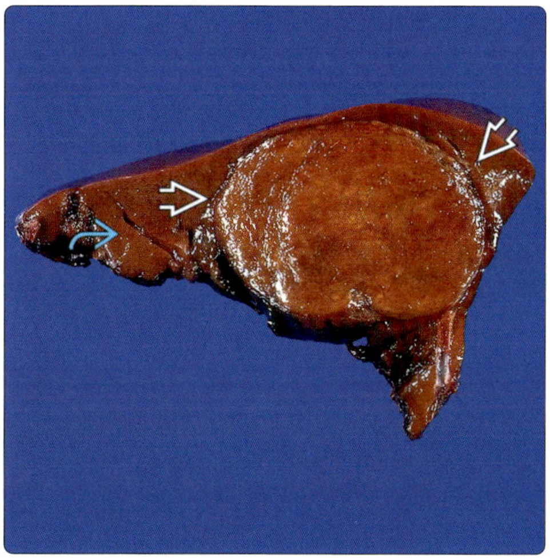

Hepatocellular Adenoma

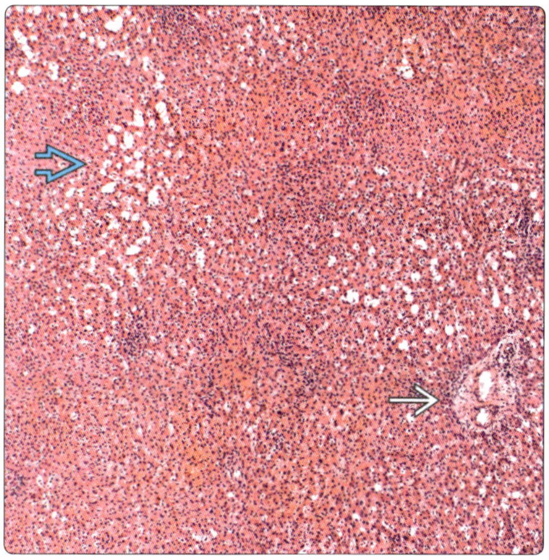

(Left) *Hepatocellular adenomas are well-circumscribed tumors with a homogeneous smooth cut surface that resembles adjacent nonneoplastic liver parenchyma.* **(Right)** *Hepatic adenomas usually do not have portal tracts. However, the inflammatory (formerly known as telangiectatic) variant may have portal tract-like structures with a lymphoid infiltrate. The sinusoids may be markedly dilated in a subset of cases.*

Mucinous Cystic Neoplasm: Gross Appearance

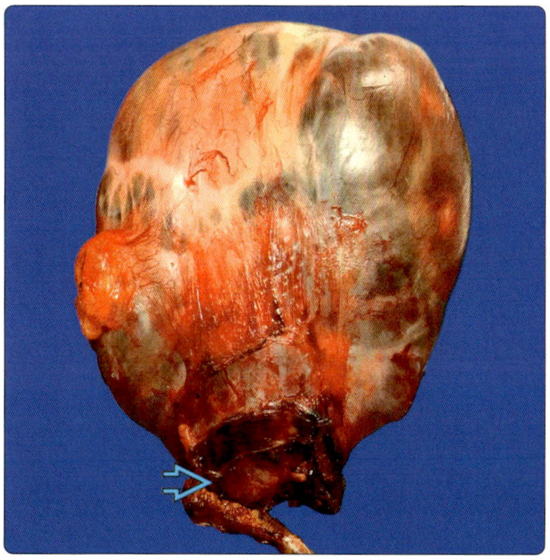

Sclerosed Hemangioma

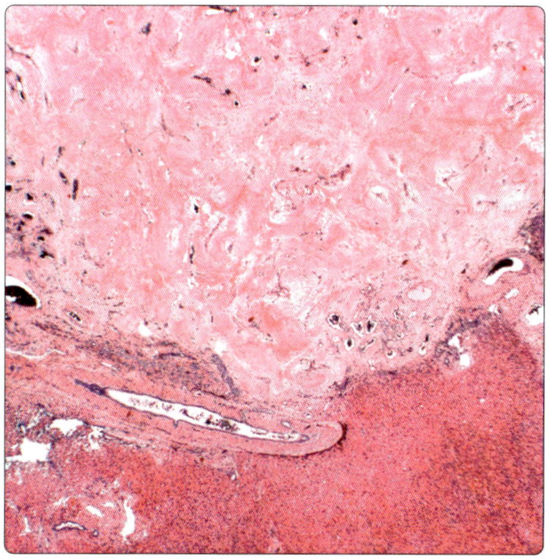

(Left) *Mucinous cystic neoplasms of the liver (also known as biliary cystadenomas) are unilocular or multilocular cystic lesions with a pancreaticobiliary or mucinous lining epithelium rimmed by ovarian-type stroma. The resection margin is seen as a cut surface.* **(Right)** *Hemangiomas are the most common primary hepatic tumor and may undergo infarction and hyalinization. This sclerosed hemangioma is composed of thick-walled vessels widely separated by abundant collagen.*

SURGICAL/CLINICAL CONSIDERATIONS

Goal of Consultation

- To identify and diagnose difficult-to-image lung lesions in wedge resections that require T bar placement to ensure removal by surgeon

Change in Patient Management

- If malignancy is identified, surgeon may elect to perform lobectomy &/or sample lymph nodes
- More limited surgery may be considered for adenocarcinoma in situ (AIS) or minimally invasive adenocarcinoma (MIA)
  - However, definitive diagnosis of AIS or MIA requires evaluation of entire lesion on permanent sections
    - Decision to alter surgical approach requires clinical judgment based on constellation of features
- If lesion cannot be identified in specimen, possibility that lesion was not removed must be considered

Clinical Setting

- Asymptomatic lung lesions may be detected when patients undergo lung cancer screening
  - United States Preventative Services Task Force has issued recommendations for screening
    - Annual low-dose computed tomography (CT) is recommended for individuals between ages of 55-80 with 30-year history of smoking who currently smoke or have quit smoking within last 15 years
- Incidental lung lesions may also be detected when patients undergo CT examination for other reasons
- Lung imaging by CT can detect small lesions (< 2 cm) and lesions of low density (ground-glass opacities)
  - Lesions that require excision include
    - Lesions increasing in size
    - Solid or partially solid masses
  - ~ 75% are carcinoma and 25% benign lesions
  - Diagnosis of small lesions and ground-glass opacities by needle biopsy can be difficult
    - Ground-glass opacity consists of area of increased hazy density with preserved bronchial and vascular markings
      - May be due to thickened alveolar septa or partial filling of air spaces with cells, fluid, or debris
      - Adequate sampling for definitive diagnosis is difficult
    - Small lesions can be difficult to target precisely
- Clinical decision may be made to perform limited lung surgery
  - Imaging shows lesion of low risk for invasive carcinoma
  - Diagnosis is expected to be AIS or MIA
    - 100% survival with excision only
      - Lymph nodes are not involved
    - Surgeon must be aware that AIS and MIA can only be diagnosed after complete evaluation of specimen on permanent sections
  - Patient has limited lung capacity or other comorbidity
  - Contralateral lung surgery is planned
  - Patient preference
- Small masses and ground-glass opacities may be difficult or impossible to identify in patient during operation
  - In open resections, surgeon may not be able to detect lesion by palpation with confidence
  - In image-guided video-assisted thoracoscopic surgery (iVATS), lung is not accessible for palpation
- Multiple methods have been developed to help surgeon identify lesion
  - Intraoperative ultrasound
  - Percutaneous injection of dye
  - Image-guided placement of wires, hooks, or T bars
- T bars are placed under CT guidance immediately prior to operation
  - 1 T bar may be placed to mark location of single lesion
  - 2 T bars may be placed to either mark 2 separate lesions or to bracket area of increased density
  - Shape of bar aids in anchoring wire in tissue
- Patient is transferred to operating room, and surgeon performs wedge resection to remove T bar and surrounding lung tissue

Lung Imaging

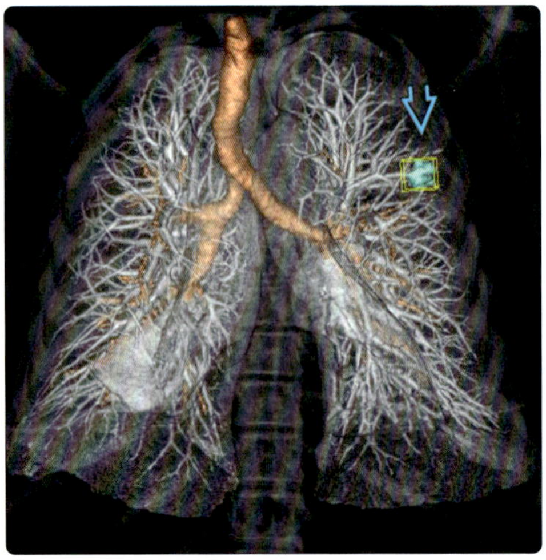

CT Scan: Ground-Glass Opacity

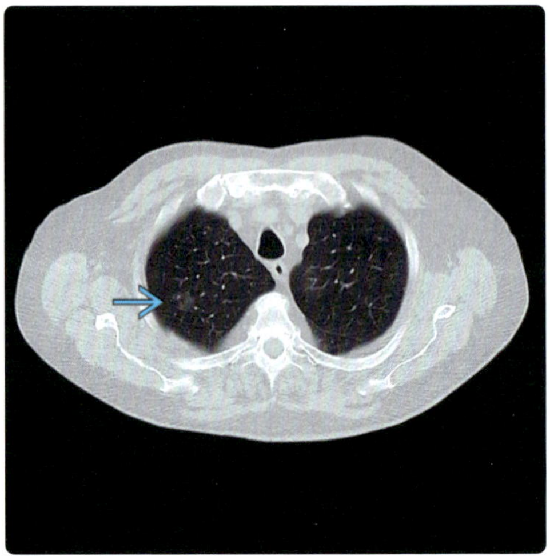

(Left) *CT scans can detect small (< 2 cm) lung lesions ➡ as well as lesions of low density (ground-glass opacities). Over 1/2 of these lesions are malignant. Lung-preserving surgery can be challenging as these lesions are often difficult to identify intraoperatively by the surgeon. (Courtesy R. Gill, MD.)* **(Right)** *CT scan shows a ground-glass opacity ➡ in the lung that increased in size over time. A lesion increasing in size is suspicious for malignancy. This is an indication for excision. (Courtesy R. Gill, MD.)*

- Radiograph of specimen is performed

SPECIMEN EVALUATION

Specimen Radiograph

- Specimen is imaged by CT
  - Image can document presence of T-bar
  - Lesion may not be seen due to collapse of surrounding lung tissue

Gross

- Protruding wire with T bar is identified
- Intact specimen is gently palpated (so as to not dislodge T bar) to attempt to identify lesion
  - If lesion can be palpated, location is noted within specimen with respect to T bar
  - Pleura adjacent to mass is inspected to determine if lesion involves pleura or if pleura is freely mobile over lesion
- If palpable mass is identified, specimen is incised through mass
  - Entire mass should be serially sectioned
    - Carcinomas can be associated with fibrotic scars
    - Presence of firm mass adjacent to scar is suggestive of carcinoma
      - All areas grossly suspicious for carcinoma should be evaluated by frozen section
  - Size of mass and relationship to margin and pleura are noted
  - Representative section(s) of mass and closest margin are taken for frozen section
- If palpable mass is not identified, specimen is serially sectioned and each section carefully examined for visible lesions and gently palpated
  - Lesion may be subtle area of slightly increased firmness, paler in color than surrounding lung parenchyma
- There are 2 methods to evaluate margin
  - Standard method is to cut away staple line and remove as little lung tissue with staples as possible
    - Exposed lung parenchyma is inked to mark parenchymal margin
    - Margin is taken as perpendicular section, including inked tissue edge in area closest to lesion
  - If lesion is close to staple line, and lung preserving surgery is goal, tissue section containing both lesion and tissue with staples may be taken for frozen section
    - This method can only be used with stapling devices that do not result in interlocked staples
    - Exposed lung parenchyma at edge of staple line is inked
    - Specimen is serially sectioned, and site closest to lesion identified
    - Section is taken perpendicular to margin
      - Scissors are used to cut through staple line
    - Tissue is mounted with staples closest to blade
    - As block is faced, staples will become evident by grating against cryostat blade and creating tears in tissue
    - Block on chuck is removed from cryostat
    - Staples are removed from tissue with forceps
    - Block on chuck is replaced in cryostat
      - Surface of tissue is covered with embedding medium to refreeze tissue
    - Blade is replaced
    - Deeper sections showing lesion and margin are taken
    - This method allows evaluation of true tissue margin, which is present in tissue that was stapled

Frozen Section

- Representative section of lesion is taken for frozen section
- If carcinoma is identified, closest margin should be examined by frozen section unless lobectomy is planned

MOST COMMON DIAGNOSES

Adenocarcinoma In Situ

- Lesions classified as AIS have excellent prognosis
  - 100% disease-specific survival
  - No nodal involvement
- Definitive diagnosis of AIS can only be made after entire lesion is examined on permanent sections
- Gross appearance is typically subtle area of increased density with paler color compared to surrounding lung parenchyma
- Classification as AIS requires
  - Solitary lesion
  - Size ≤ 3 cm
  - Pure lepidic pattern
    - Alveolar walls should be thin or expanded by lymphocytic infiltrate
  - Not mucinous in type, or only rarely
  - No vascular or pleural involvement
  - No necrosis
  - No spread through air spaces
    - Defined as tumor cells within air spaces beyond edge of main tumor as determined by gross examination or at low power
    - Tumor cells must be distinguished from alveolar macrophages
    - Can be very difficult to distinguish from artifactual displacement of tumor cells
- AIS is distinguished from reactive atypia by nuclear features
  - Variation in size (~ 60% of cases)
  - Atypical enlarged and irregular nuclei (~ 80% of cases)
  - Prominent macronucleoli (< 10% of cases)
  - Atypical mitoses (~ 25% of cases)
- Inflammatory changes, such as granulomatous inflammation, acute inflammation, &/or organizing pneumonia would be more likely to be associated with reactive atypia
- Atelectasis after excision may cause lepidic pattern of AIS to mimic adenocarcinoma associated with desmoplastic response

Minimally Invasive Adenocarcinoma (MIA)

- Some lesions that would otherwise fulfill criteria for AIS have small (< 0.5 cm) foci of invasion
- Definitive diagnosis of MIA can only be made after complete evaluation of lesion on permanent sections

Invasive Carcinoma

- Malignant lesions that do not fulfill criteria for AIS or MIA would be classified as adenocarcinoma or other types of carcinoma
  - Multiple growth patterns are often present
- These lesions would typically undergo complete lobar excision and sampling of regional lymph nodes

Atypical Adenomatous Hyperplasia

- Defined as small (≤ 0.5 cm) lesion
  - Generally seen as incidental finding, often adjacent to carcinoma
  - It is highly unlikely that atypical adenomatous hyperplasia would be detected by imaging
- Cells lining alveoli are cuboidal with hyperchromatic and variably atypical nuclei
  - Cell population is distinct from cells lining adjacent uninvolved alveoli

Metastatic Carcinoma

- Solitary lung masses in patients with history of malignancy may be metastasis or new primary lung cancer
- Comparison to patient's prior tumor is of value

Chondroid Hamartoma

- May present as ground-glass nodule on imaging
- Grossly, hamartomas form well-circumscribed masses with white to blue-gray glassy appearance
- Tumor consists of bland cartilage
  - Adjacent hamartomatous areas of adipose tissue, fibrous tissue, &/or muscle may correlate with ground-glass appearance

Inflammatory Changes

- Many types of inflammatory lung disease can cause ground-glass opacities
- Reactive pneumocytes must be distinguished from neoplastic tumor cells
  - Cuboidal to hobnail in shape
  - Nuclear atypia can be marked
  - Changes are usually diffuse with no clear demarcation of discrete lesion
    - Interface between lepidic pattern carcinoma and surrounding benign lung parenchyma is usually easily discerned
      - Sections that include both lesion and surrounding lung tissue are helpful
  - Surrounding tissue should include changes associated with reactive hyperplasia
    - Inflammation, fibrosis, acute lung injury, granulomas

Infection

- Many types of infections can cause ground-glass opacities
  - Cytomegalovirus pneumonia, herpes simplex virus pneumonia, pneumocystis pneumonia, *Aspergillus* infection
- If infection is suspected, tissue should be taken for appropriate cultures

REPORTING

Gross Findings

- Presence or absence of lesion at site of T bar(s) is documented

Frozen Section

- Results of frozen section are reported
  - In general, diagnosis of malignant or not malignant is sufficient
  - If patient has history of malignancy, opinion as to likelihood lesion is metastasis may be helpful
- It is helpful to include if findings would be consistent with AIS or MIA or if these diagnoses are excluded
  - However, surgeon should be aware that final classification requires microscopic evaluation of entire lesion on permanent sections

PITFALLS

Overdiagnosis of Invasive Carcinoma

- Benign changes can mimic malignancy on frozen section
  - Squamous metaplasia, bronchial metaplasia, reactive pneumocyte hyperplasia
  - Extensive background inflammation and fibrosis can make distinction of reactive changes from carcinoma difficult
- Carcinoma should show features of nuclear atypia and variation in cell size
  - There should be sharp change in cytologic appearance at border with normal lung parenchyma
- Collapse of alveoli in specimens can create patterns that mimic invasion
- Diagnosis of carcinoma should only be made when diagnosis is certain

Underdiagnosis of Invasive Carcinoma

- Final diagnosis of AIS or MIA requires complete microscopic evaluation of lesion
  - Frozen section only evaluates portion of specimen

SELECTED REFERENCES

1. He P et al: Diagnosis of lung adenocarcinoma in situ and minimally invasive adenocarcinoma from intraoperative frozen sections: an analysis of 136 cases. J Clin Pathol. 69(12):1076-1080, 2016
2. Liu S et al: Precise diagnosis of intraoperative frozen section is an effective method to guide resection strategy for peripheral small-sized lung adenocarcinoma. J Clin Oncol. 34(4):307-13, 2016
3. Gill RR et al: Image-guided video assisted thoracoscopic surgery (iVATS) - phase I-II clinical trial. J Surg Oncol. 112(1):18-25, 2015
4. Hsu HH et al: Localization of nonpalpable pulmonary nodules using CT-guided needle puncture. World J Surg Oncol. 13:248, 2015
5. Trejo Bittar HE et al: Accuracy of the IASLC/ATS/ERS histological subtyping of stage I lung adenocarcinoma on intraoperative frozen sections. Mod Pathol. 28(8):1058-63, 2015

T Bar Placement Under CT Guidance

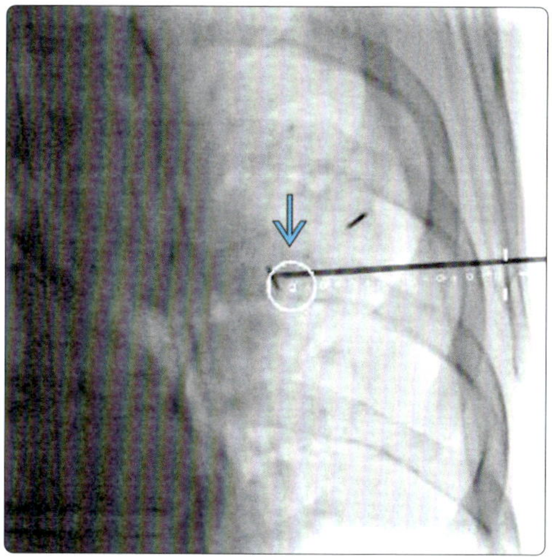

CT Scan: Specimen Image

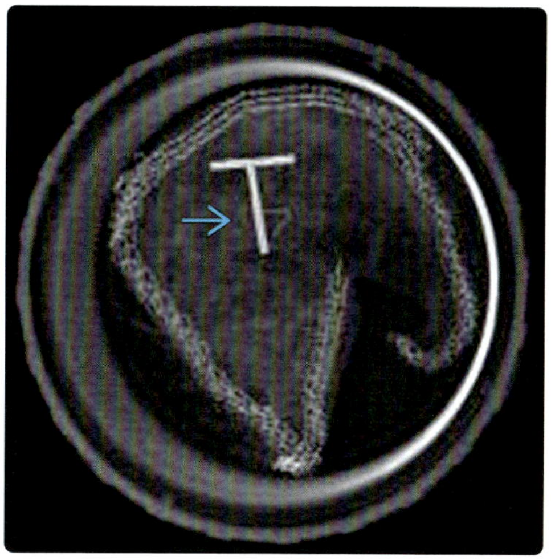

(Left) *If a small mass or ground-glass opacity will be difficult to identify intraoperatively, the lesion can be marked to assist the surgeon. Immediately prior to surgery, a radiologist percutaneously places a T bar at the site of the lung lesion . (Courtesy R. Gill, MD.)* **(Right)** *Specimen CT shows the T bar . The lung parenchyma collapses after excision, and this generally precludes the ability to identify the lesion. In this case, the targeted ground-glass opacity cannot be seen. (Courtesy R. Gill, MD.)*

Lung iVATS Resection: Gross Evaluation

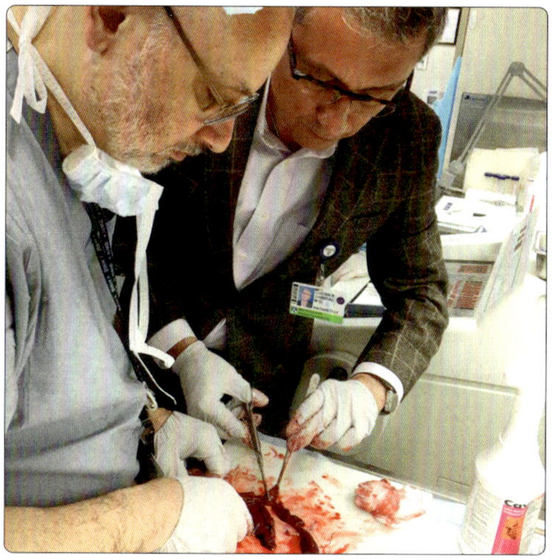

Lung iVATS Resection: Intact Specimen

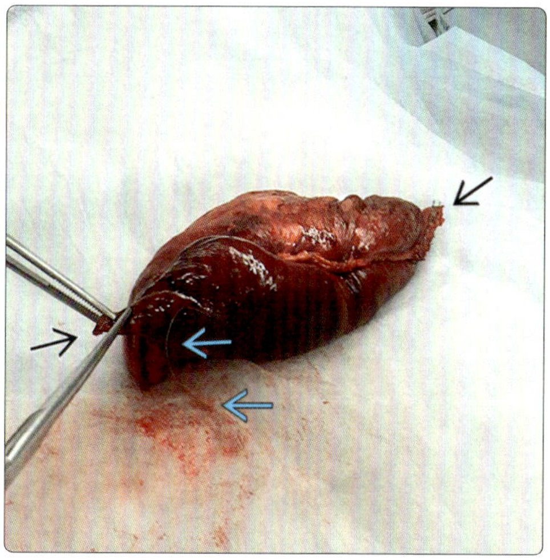

(Left) *Lung excisions using T bars to localize a small or subtle lesion can be difficult to evaluate. It is often very important for the surgeon and pathologist to collaborate to identify the lesion. (Courtesy R. Bueno, MD and L. Chirieac, MD.)* **(Right)** *The wire from the T bar protrudes from the specimen . The staple line is identified. The specimen radiograph may be used to help identify the likely location of the tip of the T bar within the specimen.*

Lung iVATS Resection: Palpation of Intact Specimen

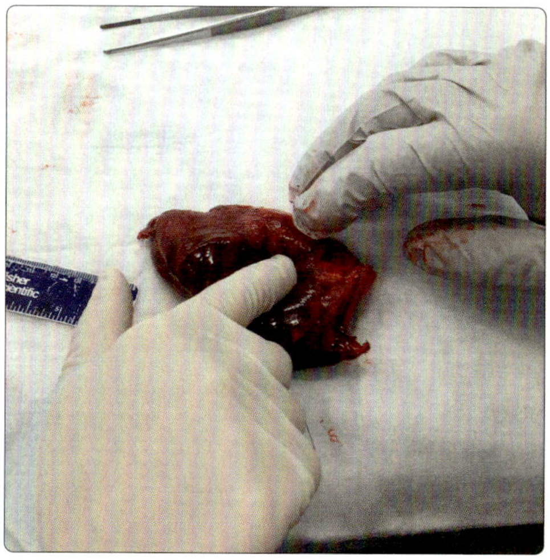

Lung iVATS Resection: Serial Sections

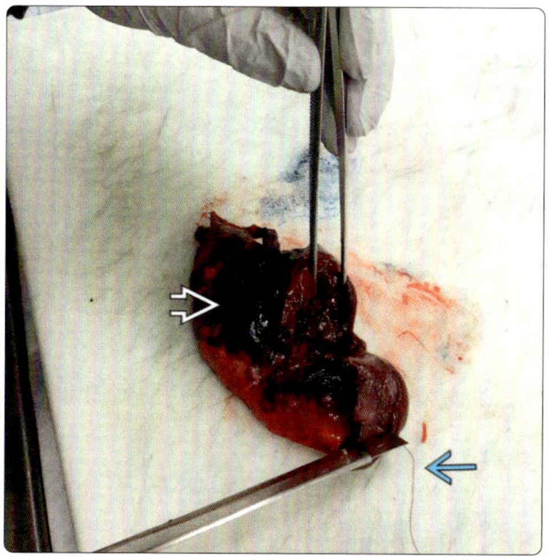

(Left) *The intact specimen is carefully palpated to determine if a mass can be identified. However, the majority of the lesions will be too small or too diffuse to be palpable prior to sectioning.* **(Right)** *The lung parenchyma exposed after removing the staple line has been inked black to mark the margin . The specimen is thinly sectioned starting near the wire of the T bar . Each section is examined for visual evidence of a lesion.*

Lung iVATS Resection: Serial Sections

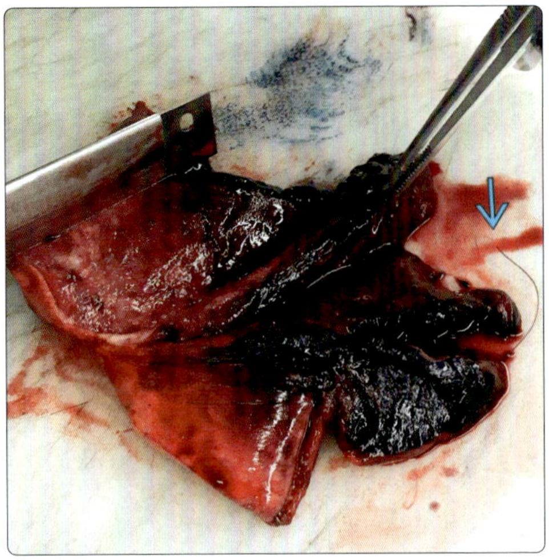

Well-Differentiated Adenocarcinoma: Gross Appearance

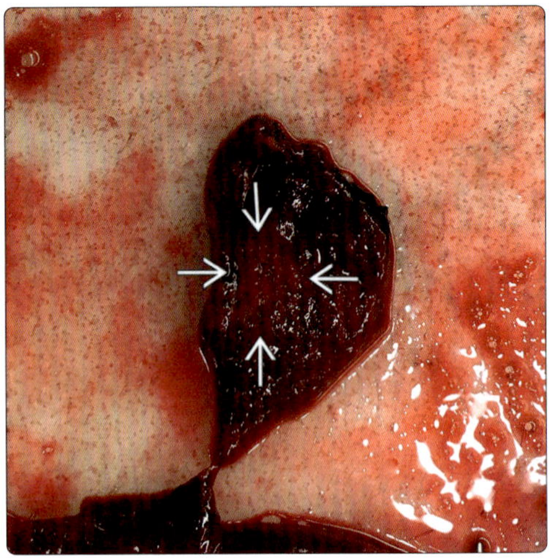

(Left) *This lung wedge resection has been thinly sectioned. The T bar wire is left in place to help identify the likely site of the lesion. A lesion was not evident by visual inspection in this specimen.* **(Right)** *This 1.1-cm well-differentiated mucinous adenocarcinoma has a predominantly lepidic pattern and formed a ground-glass opacity by imaging. The carcinoma was difficult to identify grossly, as it is only slightly paler than the surrounding lung parenchyma and only slightly firmer to palpation.*

Moderately Differentiated Adenocarcinoma: Gross Appearance

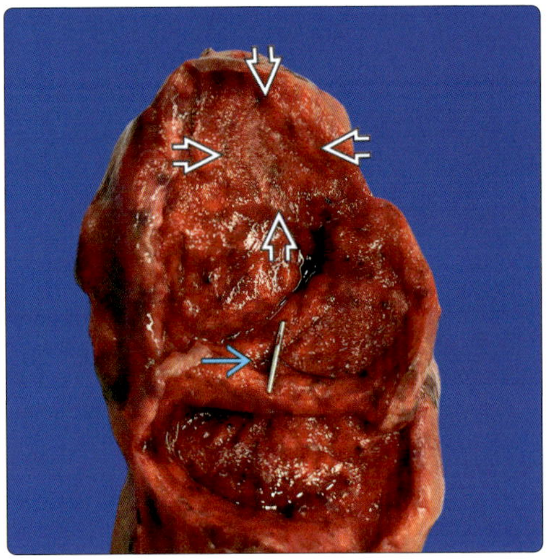

Metastatic Melanoma: Gross Appearance

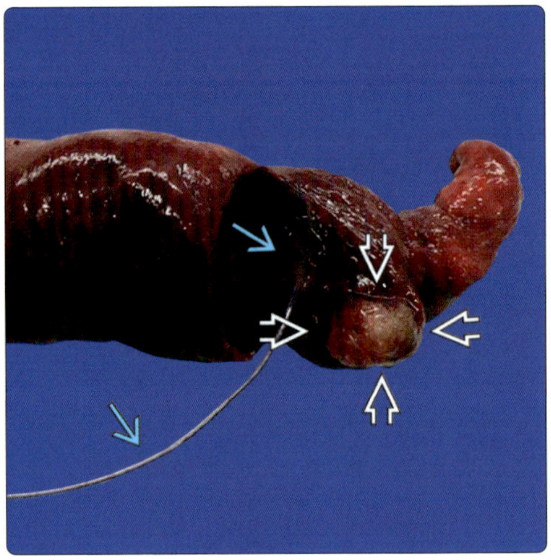

(Left) *This 1.3-cm moderately differentiated carcinoma with a lepidic pattern presented clinically as a ground-glass opacity increasing in size. A T bar was used to localize the lesion. The lesion is very difficult to identify grossly, as it was only marginally firmer than the surrounding lung parenchyma.* **(Right)** *This 0.7-cm metastasis from a known melanoma forms a grossly evident mass adjacent to the T bar. A T bar was used due to the small size of the lesion.*

Lung Lesion: Frozen Section

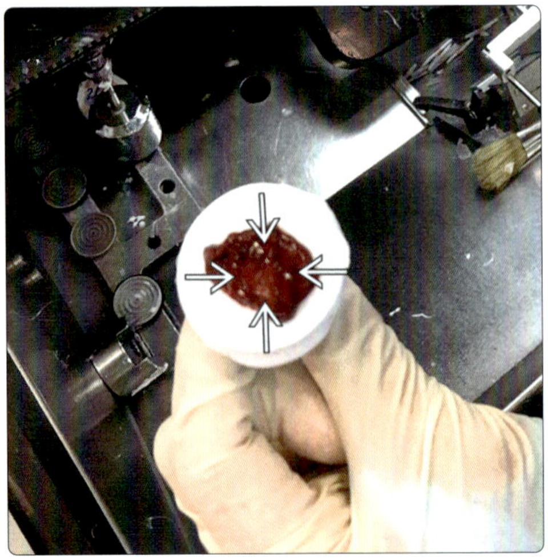

Lung Lesion: Frozen Section

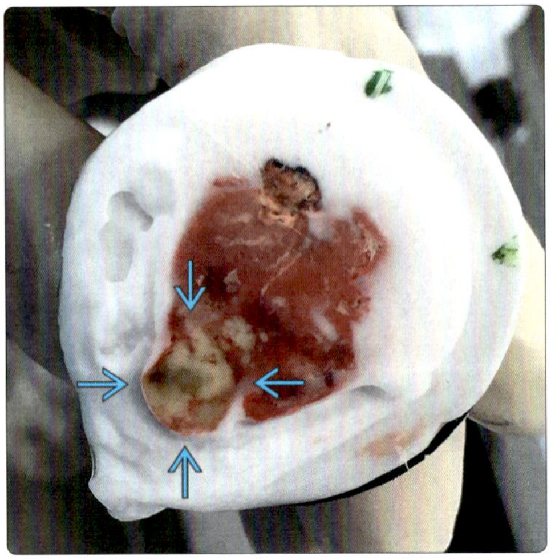

(Left) *A frozen section of the grossly identified lesion is essential to document that the targeted lesion has been removed and to determine if the lesion is benign or malignant.* **(Right)** *A solid mass that is readily identifiable grossly is more likely to be an invasive adenocarcinoma and less likely to be adenocarcinoma in situ, minimally invasive adenocarcinoma, or benign inflammatory changes. The microscopic findings should always be correlated with the gross appearance.*

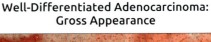

Well-Differentiated Adenocarcinoma: Frozen Section

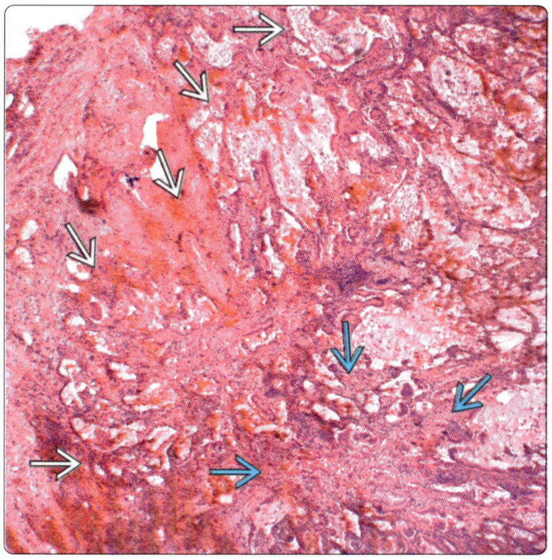

Well-Differentiated Adenocarcinoma: Frozen Section

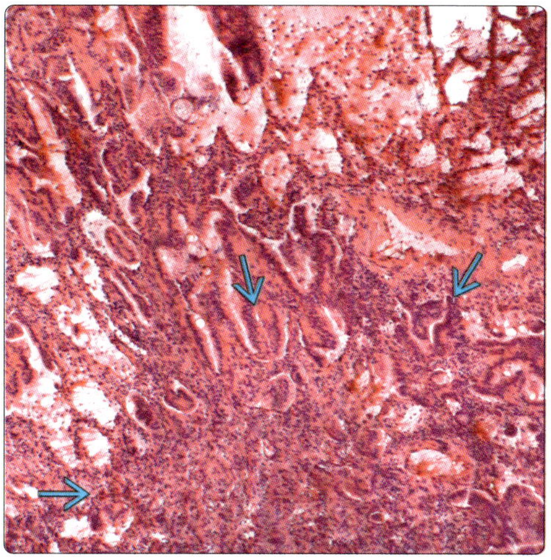

(Left) *Invasive adenocarcinomas usually form palpable masses due to a desmoplastic response associated with clearly malignant infiltrating glands, as seen in the center of this cancer ⇨. The lepidic pattern at the periphery of this carcinoma ➡ is typically more difficult to appreciate grossly.* **(Right)** *Invasive adenocarcinomas are usually easily recognized on frozen section, as they form a solid mass of malignant gland-forming tumor cells associated with a desmoplastic response ⇨.*

Mucinous Adenocarcinoma: Lepidic Pattern

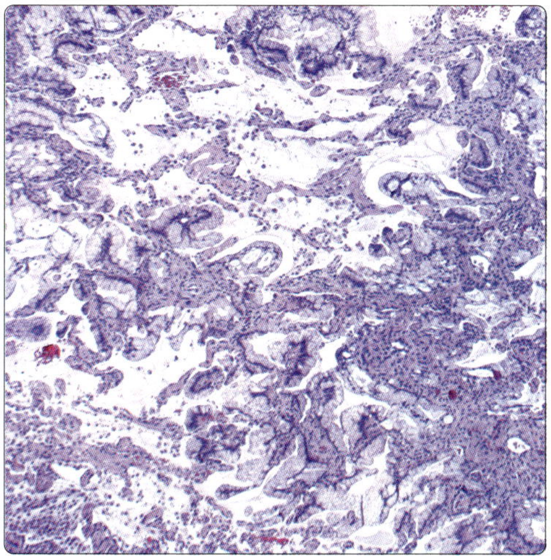

Mucinous Adenocarcinoma

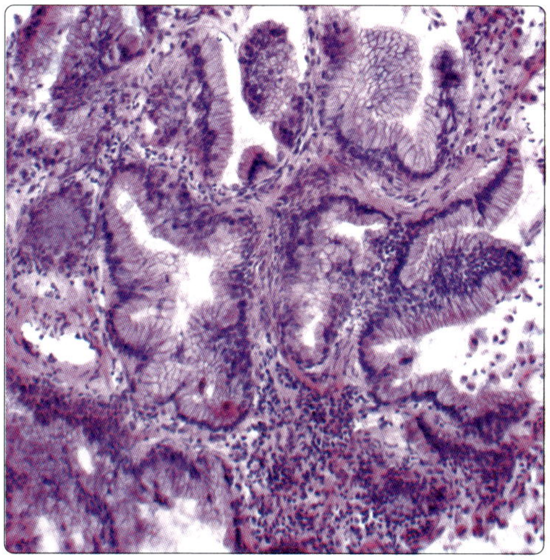

(Left) *Mucinous adenocarcinomas can have a lepidic growth pattern. These cancers are typically only slightly firmer than normal lung parenchyma to palpation. Mucin may be grossly apparent.* **(Right)** *Mucinous adenocarcinomas are usually easily recognized on frozen section as the cells do not resemble normal pneumocytes. The tumor consists of tall columnar cells with abundant mucin in the cytoplasm.*

Adenocarcinoma: Lepidic Pattern

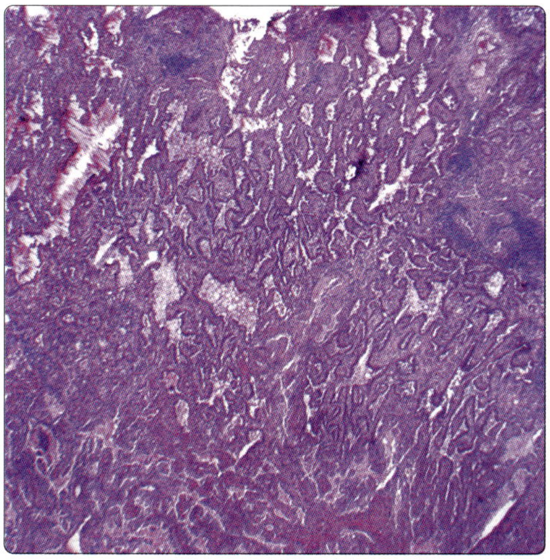

Adenocarcinoma: Lepidic Pattern

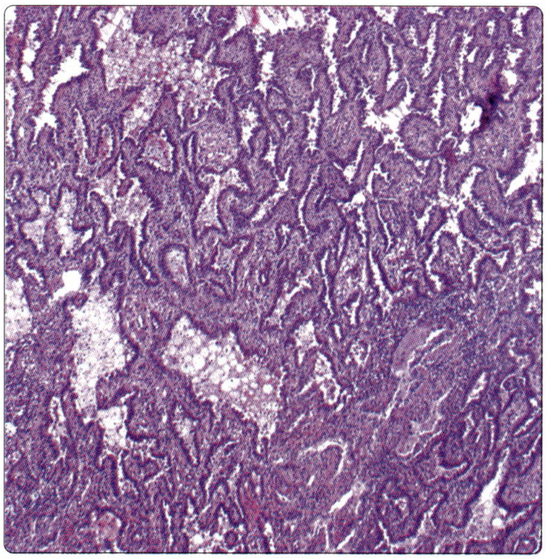

(Left) *An adenocarcinoma with a lepidic pattern does not have the desmoplasia associated with frankly invasive carcinomas. These cancers can form areas of only slightly increased density by palpation and blend into the surrounding breast parenchyma.* **(Right)** *The lepidic pattern of an adenocarcinoma resembles normal lung parenchyma. The septa may be thin, slightly thickened, &/or involved by a lymphocytic infiltrate.*

Adenocarcinoma: Lepidic Pattern

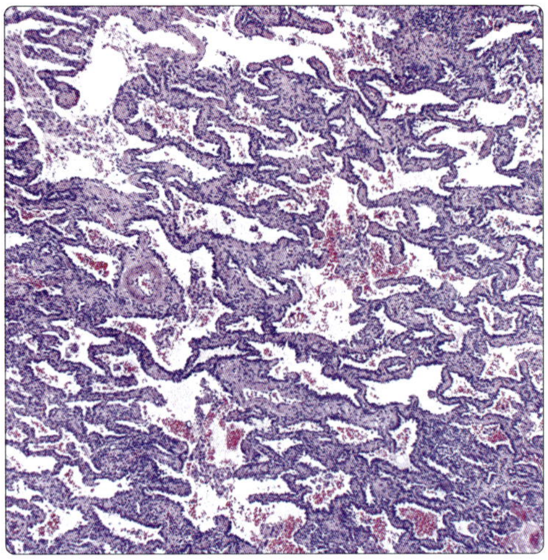

Adenocarcinoma: Lepidic Pattern, Cytologic Features

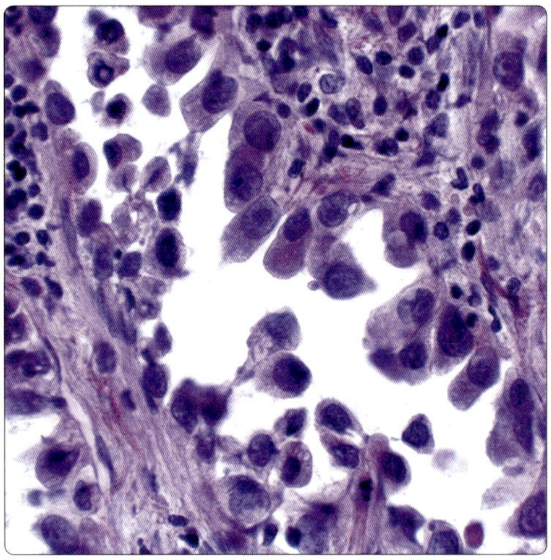

(Left) *The tumor cells of a lepidic-pattern adenocarcinoma are bland and typically lack nucleoli and mitoses. They are more difficult to distinguish from normal or reactive pneumocytes as compared to mucinous carcinomas.* **(Right)** *The cells of adenocarcinomas can have atypical enlarged and irregular nuclei with prominent nucleoli. Mitotic figures may be present. Carcinomas are sharply demarcated from the surrounding benign lung parenchyma, whereas reactive changes are diffusely present.*

Minimally Invasive Adenocarcinoma: Focal Invasion

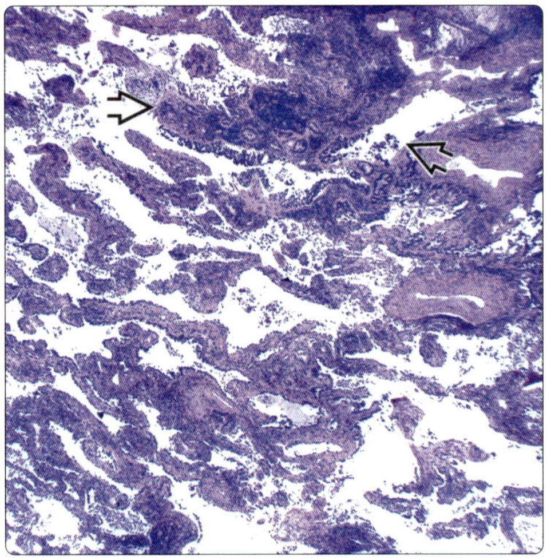

Minimally Invasive Adenocarcinoma

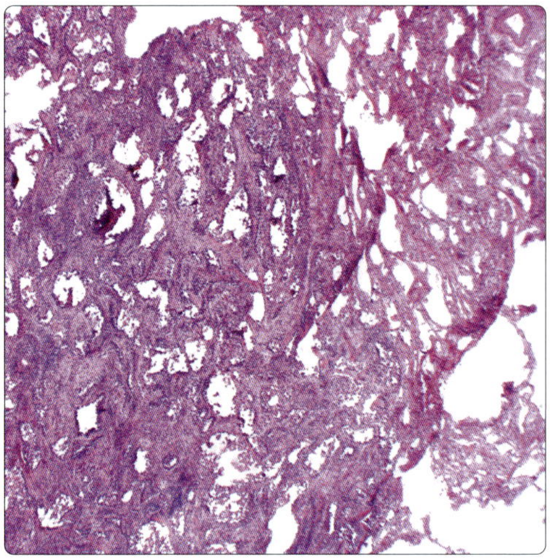

(Left) *Minimally invasive adenocarcinoma can be difficult or impossible to distinguish from adenocarcinoma in situ on frozen section, as the areas of invasion, by definition, are very small ⇨.* **(Right)** *Minimally invasive adenocarcinoma always has to be a provisional diagnosis on frozen section, as the extent of invasion cannot be determined with certainty until the entire specimen has been examined. A decision to limit surgery must also be based on clinical considerations.*

Minimally Invasive Adenocarcinoma: Macrophages in Air Spaces

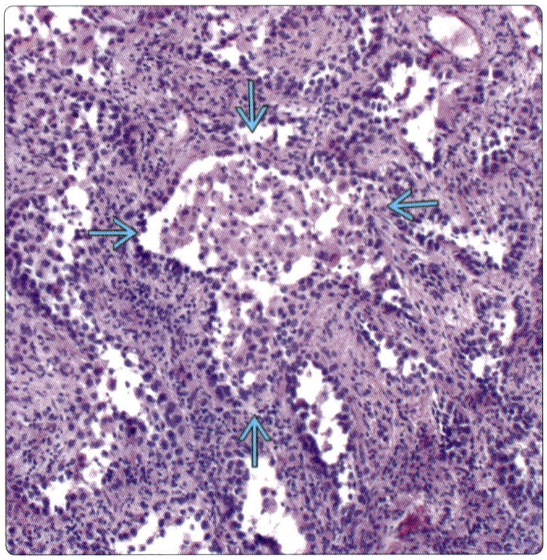

Minimally Invasive Adenocarcinoma: Cytologic Features

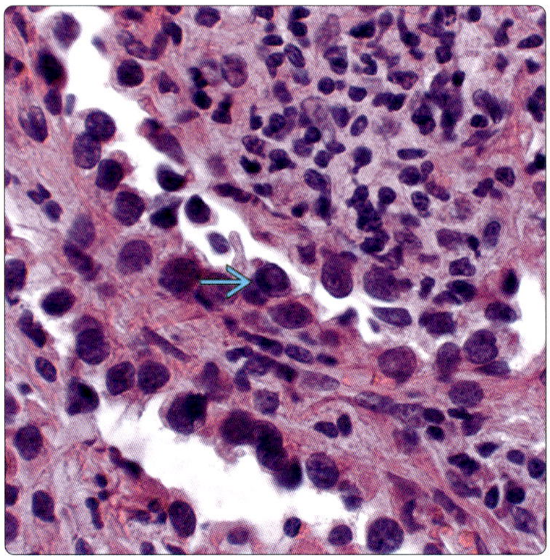

(Left) *Macrophages in airspaces → usually have foamy abundant cytoplasm and contain pigment. They should be distinguished from tumor cells in air spaces, which should not be seen in adenocarcinoma in situ.* **(Right)** *The tumor cells of a minimally invasive carcinoma can be variable in cell size and have prominent nucleoli. Nuclear pseudoinclusions → may be present in carcinomas but can also be present in reactive atypia.*

Atypical Adenomatous Hyperplasia

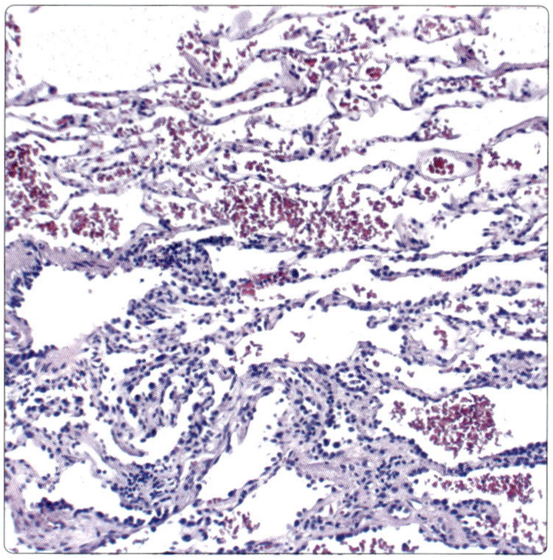

Atypical Adenomatous Hyperplasia: Cytologic Features

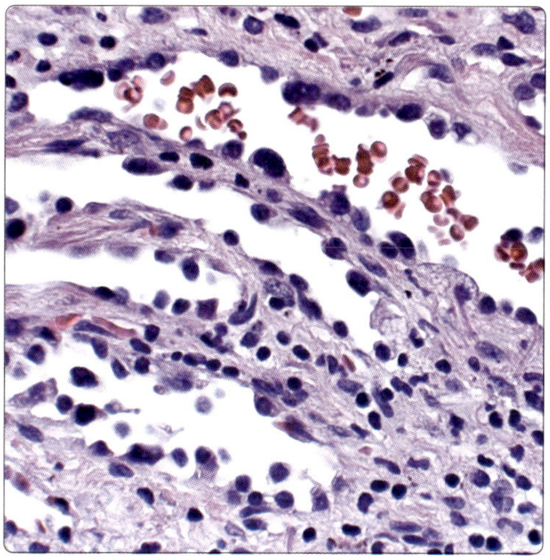

(Left) *Atypical adenomatous hyperplasia is typically an incidental finding, measuring ≤ 0.5 cm. It may cause problems in interpretation when present in the same specimen with a well-differentiated invasive adenocarcinoma with a lepidic pattern.* **(Right)** *The cells of atypical adenomatous hyperplasia are cuboidal with hyperchromatic nuclei. There is usually a distinct change in appearance at the interface with the adjacent normal lung parenchyma.*

Atypical Adenomatous Hyperplasia: Margin

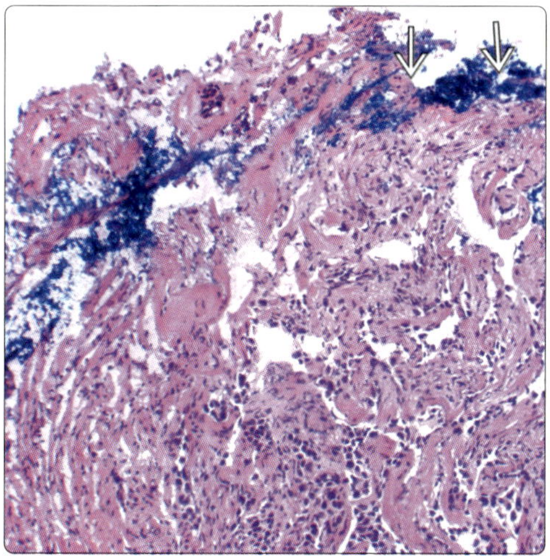

Tumor Cells in Alveolar Spaces

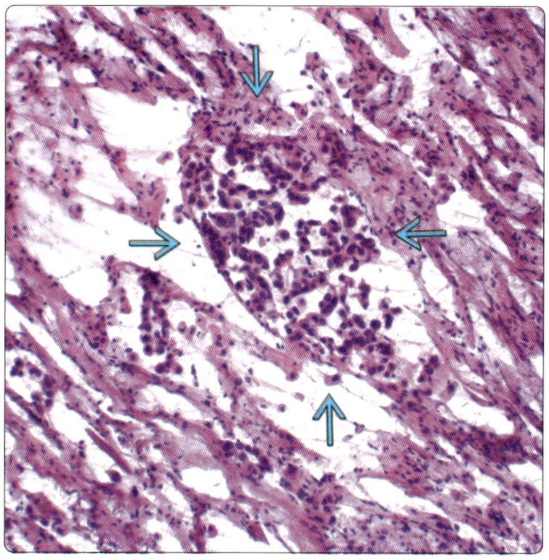

(Left) *Atypical adenomatous hyperplasia is present at the inked margin ➔. In this frozen section, it was not possible to be sure that this was not a portion of the patient's well-differentiated carcinoma. Additional tissue was taken to ensure the margin was free of carcinoma.* **(Right)** *Tumor cells in alveolar spaces ➔ should be distinguished from histiocytes. This finding can be associated with carcinomas but should not be seen in adenocarcinoma in situ. However, artifactual displacement of tumor cells can mimic this finding.*

Organizing Pneumonia

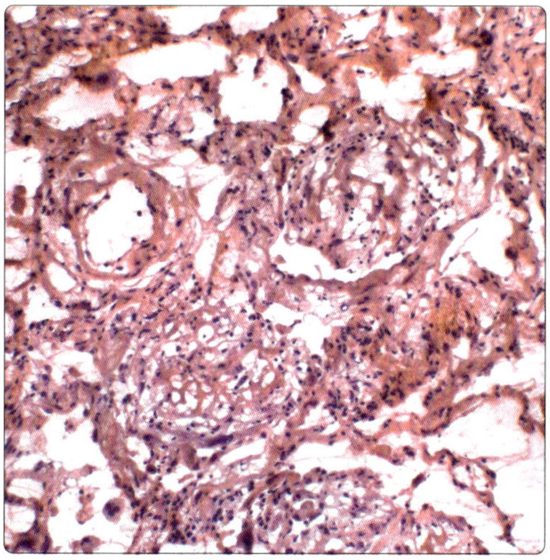

Chondroid Hamartoma

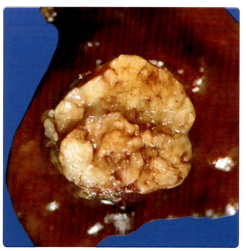

(Left) *Focal areas of pneumonia can form ground-glass opacities. On frozen section, areas of organization should not be mistaken for desmoplasia. Reactive changes in pneumocytes are usually present throughout the specimen. A sharp demarcation from the surrounding lung parenchyma is not seen.* **(Right)** *Benign neoplasms can form ground-glass nodules. Although a chondroid hamartoma forms a solid mass, adjacent hamartomatous changes can include air spaces.*

SURGICAL/CLINICAL CONSIDERATIONS

Goal of Consultation

- Determine if malignancy is present at margin
  - Type of margin depends on type of specimen
    - Bronchial margin: Lobectomy or pneumonectomy
    - Parenchymal margin: Wedge resection and possibly lobectomy
    - Chest wall margin: Lung resection in continuity with adjacent ribs and chest wall
      - Performed in cases in which carcinoma invades from lung into chest wall
      - Many patients will have received preoperative therapy due to extent of tumor

Change in Patient Management

- Additional tissue may be resected to achieve tumor-free margin
- Results may allow further intraoperative staging of patient
- Residual carcinoma at margins may be poor prognostic factor
  - Patients may receive additional therapy

Clinical Setting

- Patient has diagnosis of lung tumor, either made prior to surgery or intraoperatively
  - Complete resection with negative margins may be curative in some patients
  - Residual tumor at bronchial margin may compromise anastomosis
  - Some patients may benefit from tumor debulking if complete resection of margins is not possible

SPECIMEN EVALUATION

Gross

- Bronchial margin
  - Identify bronchus protruding from specimen
  - Determine and record distance from tumor to margin
    - Adenocarcinomas can infiltrate 2 cm from main lesion to margin
    - Squamous cell carcinomas can infiltrate 1.5 cm from main lesion to margin
    - Carcinomas > 3 cm away are rarely present at margin
- Parenchymal margin
  - Large resections &/or tumor not close to staple line
    - Trim staple line as close as possible to staples
    - Ink lung parenchyma revealed by opening of staple line
    - Section specimen and determine closest approach of carcinoma to margin
    - Perpendicular section of margin closest to tumor is taken for frozen section
  - Small resection &/or tumor very close to staple line
    - Surgeons may try to minimize amount of tissue removed for patients with limited lung capacity
    - There is ~ 2 to 3 mm of lung tissue within staple line
      - True margin is at edge of staple line
      - Removing staples from specimen results in excessive tearing of tissue, which will then not be suitable for microscopic evaluation
    - In selected cases, tissue within staple line may be examined by frozen section
      - Outer edge of staple line is inked
      - Lung tissue is serially sectioned up to staple line
      - Closest approach of tumor to staple line is identified
      - Staple line is cut with scissors in order to remove block of tissue for freezing
      - Tissue is less likely to tear during removal of staples when it is frozen and stabilized in embedding medium
- Chest wall margin
  - Identify and ink true soft tissue margin(s)
  - If ribs are removed, and carcinoma invades into ribs, the cut section of the ribs are also margins
    - Bone margins are usually not evaluated intraoperatively but can be identified on permanent sections

Bronchial Margin

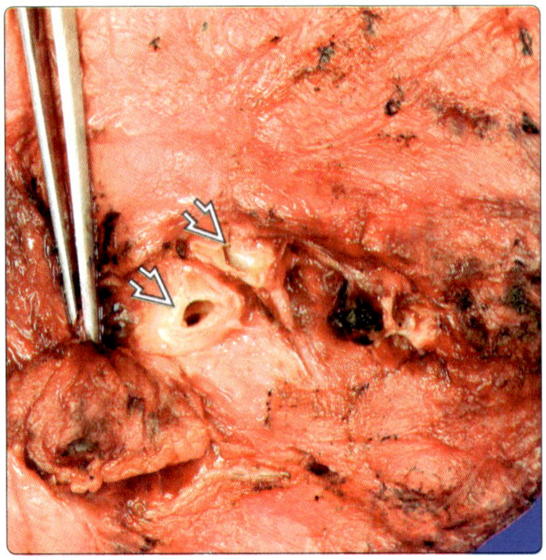

Bronchial Margin

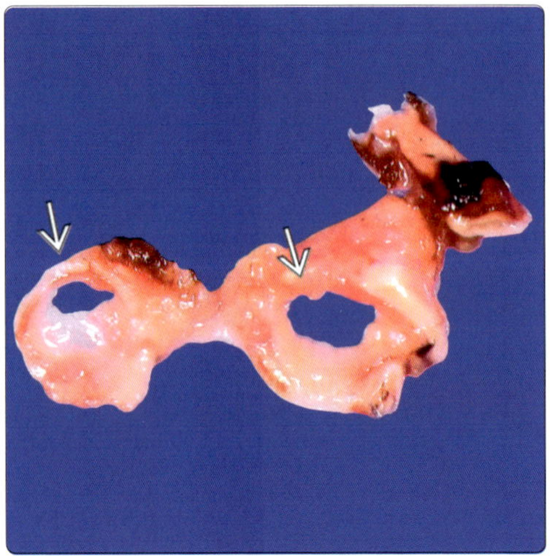

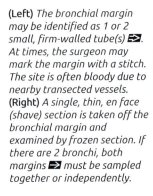

(Left) *The bronchial margin may be identified as 1 or 2 small, firm-walled tube(s) ➡. At times, the surgeon may mark the margin with a stitch. The site is often bloody due to nearby transected vessels.* **(Right)** *A single, thin, en face (shave) section is taken off the bronchial margin and examined by frozen section. If there are 2 bronchi, both margins ➡ must be sampled together or independently.*

- If bone involvement is suspected clinically or on gross examination, it may be possible to use cytologic preparations from marrow portion of the rib margins

Frozen Section

- **Bronchial margin**
  - En face (shave) section of entire (circumferential) bronchial ring is taken
    - If > 1 bronchus is present, sample all bronchi
    - If large, bronchial ring may be bisected &/or > 1 frozen section block prepared
  - Avoid including adjacent lung parenchyma and peribronchial lymph nodes
  - Embed with true margin face up such that true margin is 1st frozen section
- **Parenchymal margin**
  - Margin section below staple line
    - Perpendicular section at site closest to tumor is used for frozen section
  - Margin section with staple line
    - Tissue is mounted on chuck such that blade passes 1st through edge with staples
    - Block is faced until blade hits staple or staple can be seen
      - Staple(s) grate against blade
      - Staples cause tears in section
    - Chuck is removed from cryostat
    - Forceps are used to pull staple (or staples) from block
      - This must not be attempted while chuck is in cryostat
      - It would be dangerous to work near cryostat blade
    - Staples can only be removed if they are not interlocking
      - If surgeons request this technique, they must use correct type of staple
    - Surface of block is recovered with embedding medium and briefly placed in cryostat to refreeze surface
    - Chuck is replaced in cryostat in same orientation
    - Different area of blade or new blade is used
    - Sections are then cut from block
      - Tissue at staple line appears pinched and compressed
      - Oval holes in tissue identify site of staples
      - Typically 2-3 additional mm of tissue at margin can be evaluated
- **Chest wall margin**
  - Perpendicular section at site closest to tumor is taken for frozen section
  - Transected ribs cannot be evaluated by frozen section and must be decalcified and evaluated on permanent section

Cytology

- Touch preps are usually not performed on lung margins
- General cytologic features of benign and malignant cells apply
- Not recommended for bronchial margins as location of tumor cannot be determined

MOST COMMON DIAGNOSES

Margin Negative for Malignancy

- By far most common diagnosis in bronchial and lung margins
  - > 95% of bronchial margins are free of carcinoma
- Parenchymal margins are almost never positive if lung tumor is palpable

Invasive Carcinoma Present at Margin

- **Bronchial margin**
  - Carcinomas of salivary-gland like origin (e.g., adenoid cystic carcinoma, mucoepidermoid carcinoma) are uncommon but have higher rates of positive margins
  - Squamous cell carcinoma or small cell carcinoma are rarely at bronchial margin
  - Positive bronchial margin is unusual in adenocarcinoma due to its typical peripheral location
- **Parenchymal margin**
  - May be close or positive for carcinoma if tumor is difficult for surgeon to palpate
    - Lepidic pattern lesions are often only slightly firm, and edges are difficult to identify
    - Some lepidic pattern adenocarcinomas are multifocal
  - Significance of dispersed tumor cells in airspaces is unclear
    - It is difficult to distinguish artifactual displacement from tumor spread
- Chest wall margin
  - Majority of these cancers will have been treated with chemotherapy ± radiation therapy prior to surgery
  - Carcinomas can be very difficult to identify after treatment
    - Often consist of small foci of tumor scattered over fibrotic tumor bed
    - May not form grossly evident mass
  - Atypia in normal cells can mimic malignancy

Squamous Cell Carcinoma In Situ of Bronchus

- In situ carcinoma may not be indication for resection
  - However, stromal invasion must be excluded as this would be reason for resecting additional bronchus

Carcinoma in Lymphatics

- Tumor in lymphatics is generally not indication for additional surgery
  - It is always important to document that stromal invasion is not present

Carcinoid Tumor

- Endobronchial location is common site
  - Tumor can invade below normal bronchial mucosa
- These tumors are vascular and may be bloody upon sectioning

Lymphoma

- Lymphoma may be present at bronchial margin
  - May not be indication for additional surgery unless there is extensive involvement and anastomosis may be compromised

REPORTING

Frozen Section

- Bronchial margin
  - If tumor is present, report its specific location
    - Invasive carcinoma within or beyond cartilage ring of bronchus
    - Carcinoma in situ in bronchial mucosa
    - Carcinoma in lymph-vascular spaces
    - Metastatic carcinoma in peribronchial lymph node
    - Carcinoma in peribronchial lung tissue (not present at margin)
  - Invasive carcinoma within bronchial ring is only definitive indication for additional margin resection
- Parenchymal margin
  - Report if carcinoma is present at margin
    - Dispersed tumor cells in air spaces are not usually considered to be positive margin
  - "Spread through air spaces" (STAS) has been reported to be risk factor for recurrence when found in wedge resections
    - Solid nests, micropapillary clusters, and single cells are seen in air spaces beyond edge of carcinoma
    - Significance of this finding at or close to margin is not yet clear
    - This finding is difficult to distinguish from artifactual displacement of tumor
- Chest wall margin
  - Report if carcinoma is present at margin
  - If there has been presurgical treatment, it may be difficult to distinguish residual carcinoma from treatment effects

Reliability

- False-positive diagnoses occur in ~ 2% of cases
  - Usually due to misdiagnosing small atypical foci that are not well visualized as carcinoma
    - May be helpful to prepare deeper levels of frozen section
- False-negative diagnoses occur in ~ 2% of cases
  - Failure to see entire bronchial margin
    - Full-circumferential margin must be evaluated
  - Isolated tumor nests or cells hidden by tissue section fold or disrupted by ice crystal artifact may be missed

PITFALLS

Carcinoma In Situ vs. Squamous Metaplasia or Reserve Cell Hyperplasia

- Cytologic atypia and loss of polarity are generally more prominent in carcinoma in situ

Failure to Report Location of Carcinoma in Bronchial Margin

- Reporting margin "positive for carcinoma" is not sufficient
- Location of carcinoma may determine whether or not additional tissue should be taken

Carcinoid Tumor

- Can undermine normal bronchial mucosa and be difficult to identify at margin

Small Cell Carcinoma vs. Peribronchial Lymph Node

- Cells of small cell carcinoma have larger nuclei and often show nuclear molding and tumor necrosis
- Normal organized lymph node architecture (e.g., cortex) is not present

Invasive Carcinoma vs. Radiation-Induced Vascular Changes

- Radiation can lead to significant "smudgy" nuclear atypia in endothelial and stromal cells
- Nest/cohesive architecture typical of carcinomas is usually absent

Invasive Carcinoma vs. Submucosal Glands With Radiation Atypia

- Submucosal glands with radiation changes retain lobular arrangement and demonstrate "smudgy" nuclear atypia

Spread Through Air Spaces vs. Alveolar Macrophages

- Tumor cells in air spaces should resemble carcinoma and have atypical nuclei with nucleoli
  - Cells frequently form solid nests or micropapillary structures
  - STAS is most commonly seen in association with carcinomas with following features: High-grade morphology, micropapillary and solid patterns, and lymph-vascular invasion
- Alveolar macrophages typically have abundant foamy cytoplasm and often have pigment granules
  - Nuclei are small and uniform and often have folds

Spread Through Air Spaces vs. Artifactual Displacement

- Tumor cells can be dislodged during handling of specimen
  - In this circumstance, numerous clusters of tumor cells are often randomly distributed over tissue section and at edges of section
    - STAS is confined to 1- to 3-mm zone beyond edge of tumor in majority of cases (~ 75%)
  - Tumor cells can be dislodged from alveolar walls and be present as linear strips of tissue

SELECTED REFERENCES

1. Borczuk AC: Challenges of frozen section in thoracic pathology: lepidic lesions, limited resections, and margins. Arch Pathol Lab Med. 141(7):932-939, 2016
2. Collaud S et al: Survival according to the site of bronchial microscopic residual disease after lung resection for non-small cell lung cancer. J Thorac Cardiovasc Surg. 137(3):622-6, 2009
3. Butnor KJ: Avoiding underdiagnosis, overdiagnosis, and misdiagnosis of lung carcinoma. Arch Pathol Lab Med. 132(7):1118-32, 2008
4. Wind J et al: Residual disease at the bronchial stump after curative resection for lung cancer. Eur J Cardiothorac Surg. 32(1):29-34, 2007
5. Thunnissen FB et al: Implications of frozen section analyses from bronchial resection margins in NSCLC. Histopathology. 47(6):638-40, 2005
6. Maygarden SJ et al: Bronchial margins in lung cancer resection specimens: utility of frozen section and gross evaluation. Mod Pathol. 17(9):1080-6, 2004
7. Passlick B et al: Significance of lymphangiosis carcinomatosa at the bronchial resection margin in patients with non-small cell lung cancer. Ann Thorac Surg. 72(4):1160-4, 2001

Bronchial Margin: Microanatomy

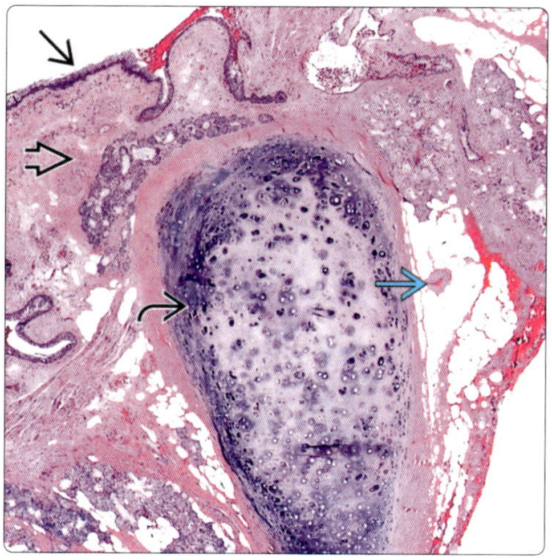

Normal Bronchial Epithelium

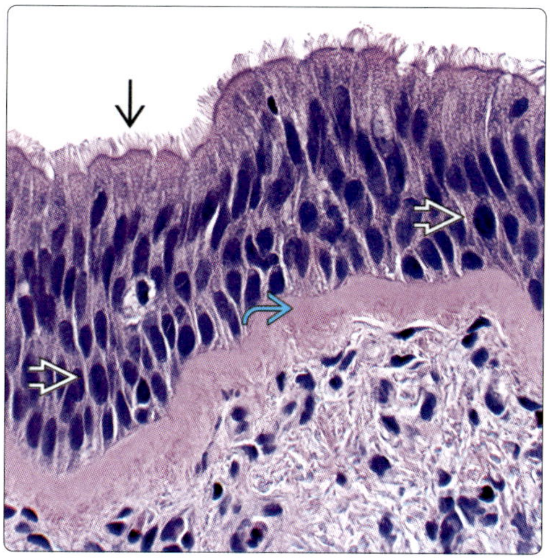

(Left) *At low power, the microanatomical structures of a bronchus include the surface respiratory epithelium ➡, submucosa containing seromucous glands ➡, hyaline cartilage rings ➡, and peribronchial fat ➡. Lymphatics are present within the bronchial wall.* **(Right)** *Normal bronchial mucosa consists of ciliated ➡ pseudostratified (respiratory) epithelium anchored to the underlying submucosa by the basement membrane ➡. Reserve cells ➡ are present above the basement membrane.*

Reserve Cell Hyperplasia

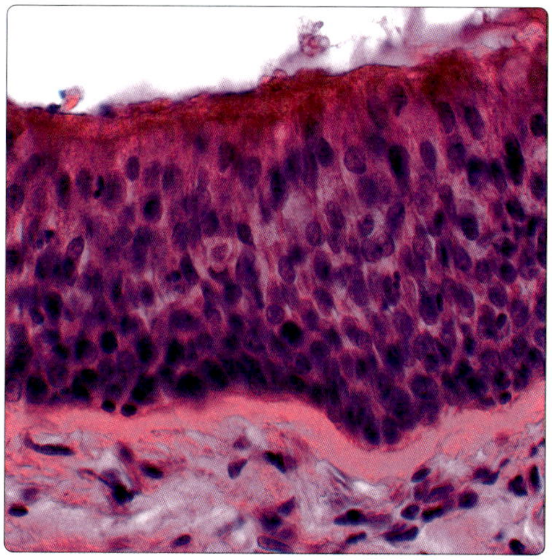

Squamous Dysplasia

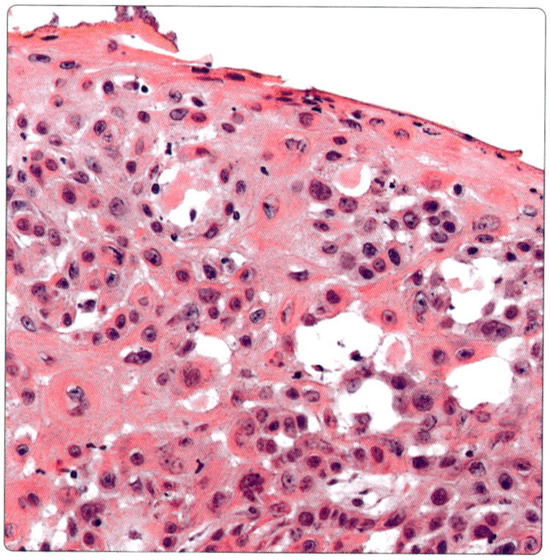

(Left) *This area of reserve cell hyperplasia was misinterpreted as severe dysplasia on frozen section. The thickness of the section contributes to the impression of nuclear hyperchromasia and atypia. However, the cells in reserve cell hyperplasia are small, monomorphic, and tightly packed.* **(Right)** *In squamous dysplasia, the cells are generally larger and show more pronounced nuclear atypia and pleomorphism than in reserve cell hyperplasia. Loss of maturational polarity distinguishes dysplasia from squamous metaplasia.*

Bronchial Margin: False-Negative Interpretation

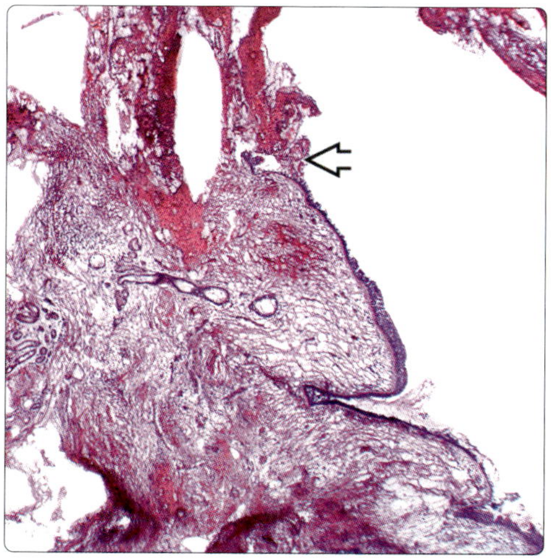

Bronchial Margin: Positive for Carcinoma

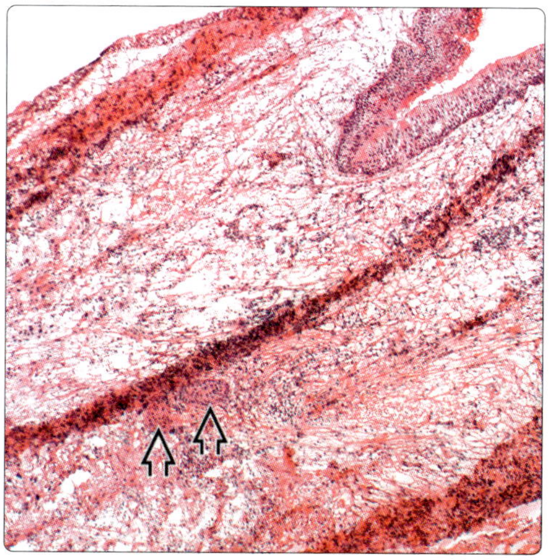

(Left) *Carcinoma at the bronchial margin was missed in this frozen section. The bronchial mucosa and wall end abruptly ➡, indicating that a complete cross section is not present on the slide. If additional sections had been cut, the carcinoma would have been seen in the area of the bronchus missing on this level.* **(Right)** *There are scattered invasive tumor cells ➡ in the submucosal tissue in this frozen section of the bronchial margin. Interpretation is made more difficult due to the ice crystal artifact and folding of the tissue.*

Bronchial Margin: Positive for Carcinoid Tumor

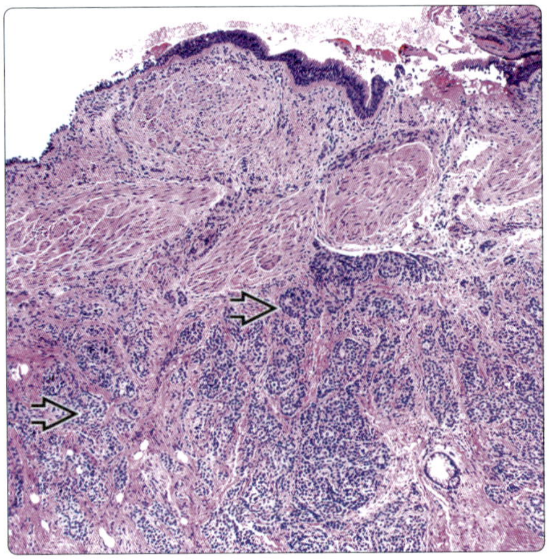

Bronchial Margin: Lymph-Vascular Involvement

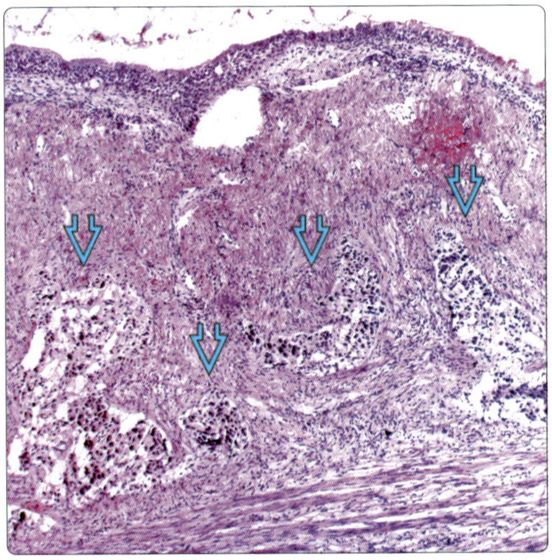

(Left) *Grossly, a carcinoid tumor was located only 2 mm from the bronchial margin. On frozen section, the tumor clearly involves the submucosal stroma at the resection margin within the cartilage ring.* **(Right)** *Carcinoma is present in multiple lymphatics at the bronchial margin. It is very important to report the location of the carcinoma. Although this is a poor prognostic factor, it may not indicate additional surgery as it is not possible to completely resect an intravascular tumor.*

Small Cell Carcinoma

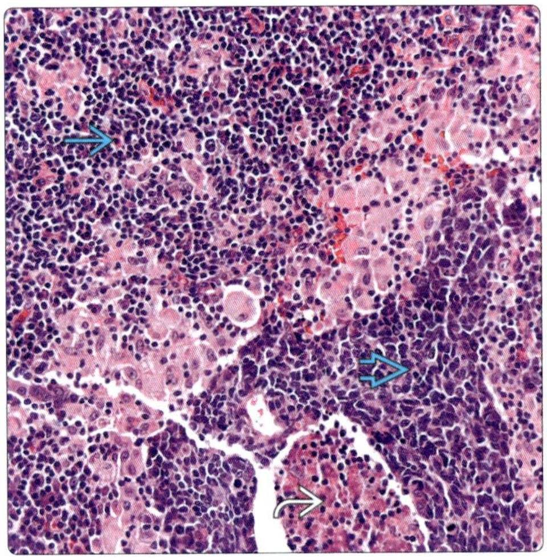

Parenchymal Margin: Staples

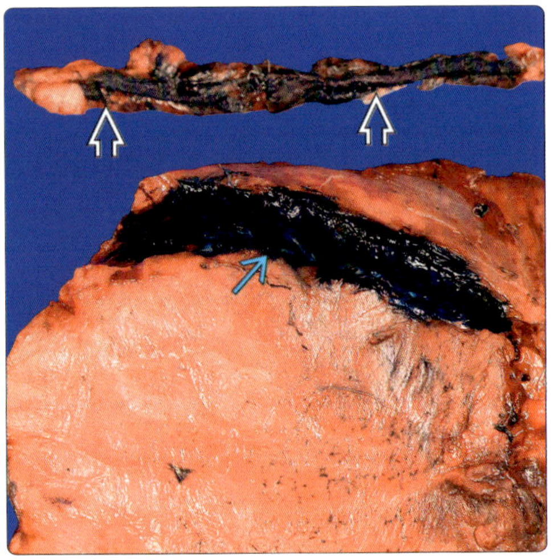

(Left) *Small cell carcinoma can be easily mistaken for benign lymphocytes or a portion of a hilar lymph node at the bronchial margin. Clues to the correct identification may include tumor necrosis &/or larger cells with nuclear molding.* **(Right)** *If a stapled parenchymal margin is to be evaluated, the staple line can 1st be carefully dissected off the specimen. The exposed lung parenchyma at the margin is inked. Parenchymal margins may be present on a wedge biopsy or a lobectomy.*

Parenchymal Margin: Section

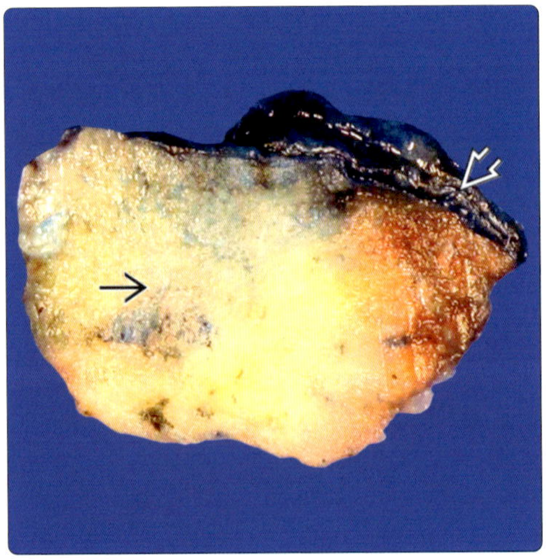

Parenchymal Margin: Squamous Cell Carcinoma

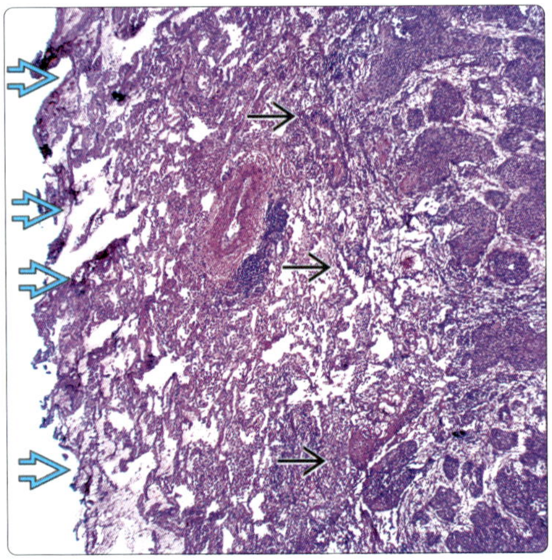

(Left) *If a tumor is grossly identified near the parenchymal margin, 1 perpendicular section demonstrating the closest margin to the tumor is ideal. Any representative section of the margin will suffice if the tumor is located farther away.* **(Right)** *This squamous cell carcinoma is close to but not at the parenchymal margin, which has been marked with blue ink. It is important to ensure that the tumor and margin section is a full face cut and that there is no tissue missing from the center.*

Lung Wedge Resection: Margin

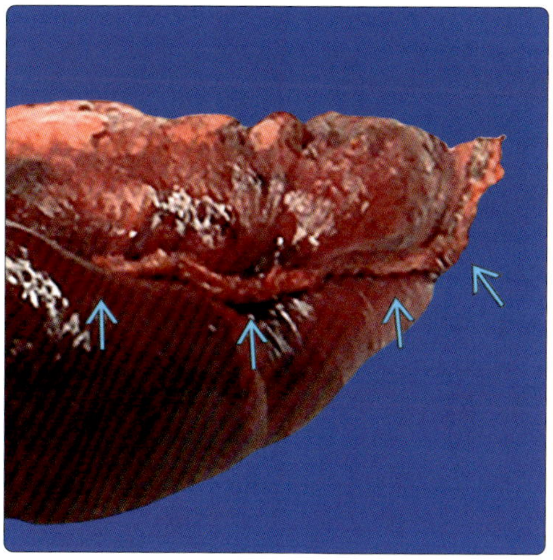

Frozen Block With Staple Line

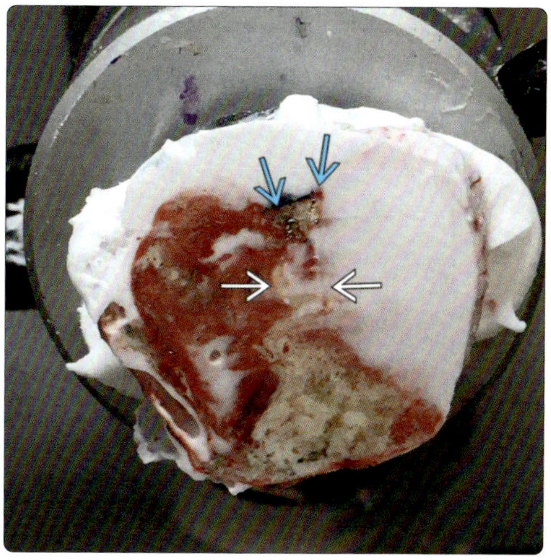

(Left) *The true margin of a lung wedge resection is the tissue containing staples* →*. The staples cannot be removed from the gross specimen, as the tissue would become too shredded to be interpretable. However, once a thin section of tissue is frozen in a block, it is possible to remove 1 or 2 staples while the tissue is stabilized.* **(Right)** *Perpendicular section of the margin containing staples is cut on the cryostat until the staples are seen at the surface of the block* →*. Note that the staples cause tears in the subjacent tissue* ➡*.*

Frozen Block: Removing Staples

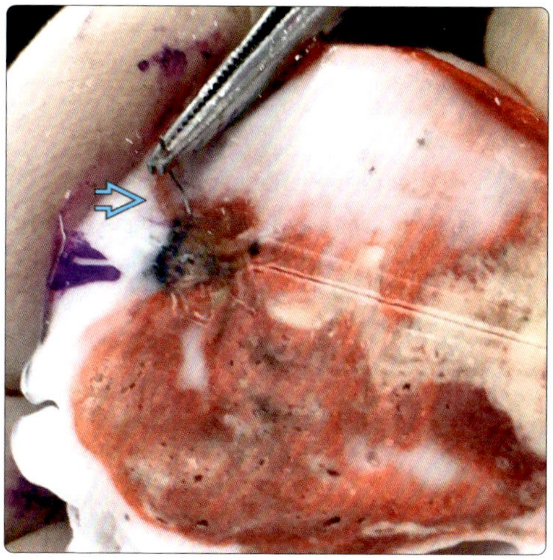

Squamous Cell Carcinoma: True Margin Negative

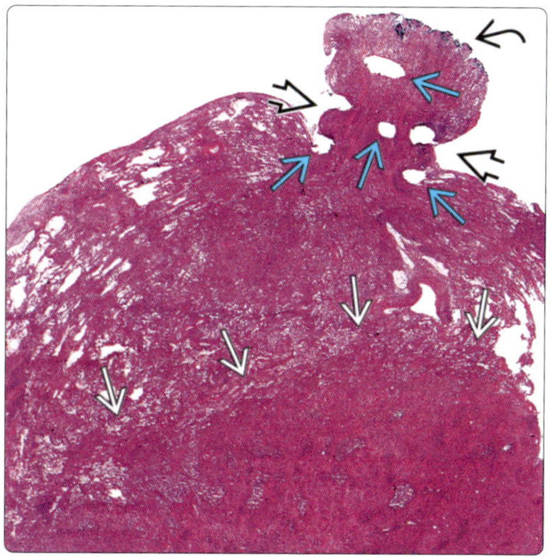

(Left) *After the frozen block is sectioned until the staples are visible, the chuck is removed from the cryostat. A forceps is used to remove the staples* ⇨*. Because the tissue is frozen and stabilized, minimal tissue tearing results from this procedure.* **(Right)** *The tissue at the staple line is pinched, forming a narrow neck* ⇨*. The former location of the staples is marked by oval holes* →*. The true margin is the inked tissue beyond the staple line* ↶*. This squamous cell carcinoma* ➡ *is not present at the true margin or the "margin" below the staples.*

Adenocarcinoma: True Margin Positive

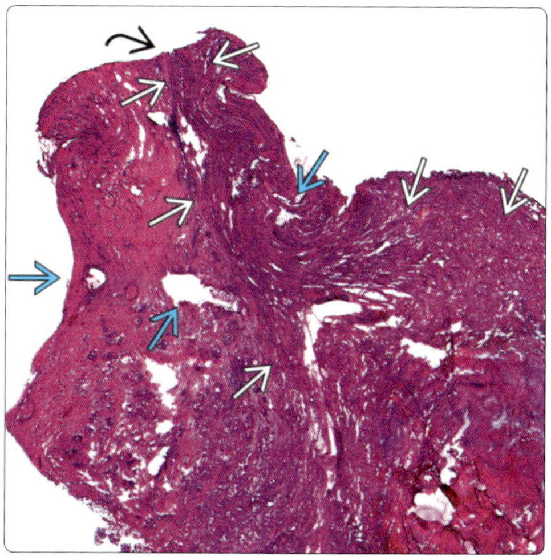

Adenocarcinoma: True Margin Negative

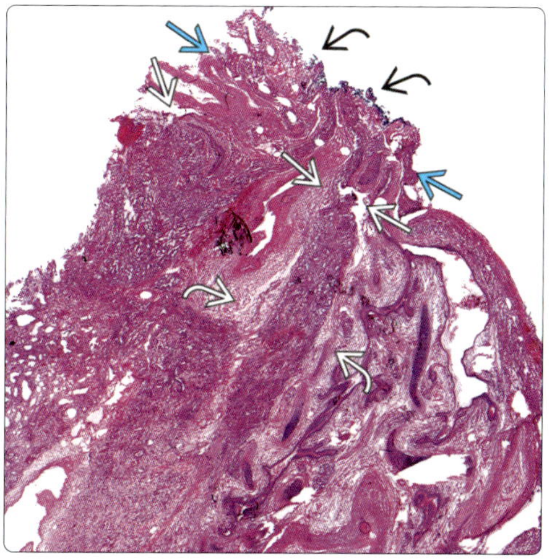

(Left) *This adenocarcinoma* ➡ *is present at the true inked margin beyond the staple line* ↷*, which is identified by oval holes in the tissue* →*.* **(Right)** *This adenocarcinoma* ➡ *is present at the "margin"* ➡ *if the staple line (identified by a series of holes* →*) had been removed. However, the true inked margin beyond the staples is free of carcinoma* ↷*.*

SURGICAL/CLINICAL CONSIDERATIONS

Goal of Consultation

- Provide preliminary diagnosis for patients with diffuse lung disease and aid in allocation of tissue for special studies

Change in Patient Management

- Preliminary diagnosis can help guide immediate management (inflammatory vs. infection vs. neoplasm)

Clinical Setting

- Majority of patients are critically ill; clinical differential diagnosis includes variety of neoplastic, infectious, or inflammatory causes

SPECIMEN EVALUATION

Gross

- Specimen is serially sectioned and examined thoroughly to exclude any focal or mass lesions
- Specimen kept sterile in case tissue needs to be taken for cultures or other special studies (1 cm^3 is minimal amount of tissue for testing)
  - Bacterial, viral, and fungal cultures should be considered if infection under consideration

Frozen Section

- Representative section of tissue is frozen

MOST COMMON DIAGNOSES

Bronchopneumonia/Abscess

- Tissue may need to be taken for culture if not already done so clinically

Granulomatous Inflammation

- Necrotizing granulomas favor infection, and diagnostic findings (e.g., fungal yeast or hyphae) should be mentioned, if present
- Numerous confluent, well-formed, nonnecrotizing granulomas in lymphangitic distribution suggest sarcoidosis
- Rare, poorly formed interstitial granulomas or histiocyte aggregates may suggest hypersensitivity pneumonitis
- Confluent (geographic) zones of necrosis with scattered multinucleated giant cells and **without** well-formed granulomas may suggest granulomatosis with polyangiitis (Wegener granulomatosis)

Viral Infection

- Must demonstrate viral inclusions
  - Often in background of necrotizing pneumonitis or diffuse alveolar damage
  - Prominent nucleoli in reactive pneumocytes can mimic inclusions but lack peripheral halo

Interstitial Lung Disease

- If ILD is suspected on frozen section, final diagnosis should be deferred to permanent sections for thorough sampling

REPORTING

Frozen Section

- Description of histologic findings is generally sufficient (e.g., nonnecrotizing granulomatous inflammation, patchy interstitial fibrosis)
- Absence of neoplasm should be noted
- Most nonneoplastic entities will require evaluation of permanent sections, thus final diagnosis is often deferred

PITFALLS

Failure to Identify Malignant Process

- Dense inflammatory infiltrates can obscure malignant cells

Reactive Pneumocytes in Diffuse Alveolar Damage

- Can simulate carcinoma infiltrating interstitium

Squamous Metaplasia of Bronchioles

- Can mimic squamous cell carcinoma
- Often seen in association with mechanical ventilation

SELECTED REFERENCES

1. Sienko A et al: Frozen section of lung specimens. Arch Pathol Lab Med. 129(12):1602-9, 2005
2. Renshaw AA: The relative sensitivity of special stains and culture in open lung biopsies. Am J Clin Pathol. 102(6):736-40, 1994

Wedge Biopsy of Lung

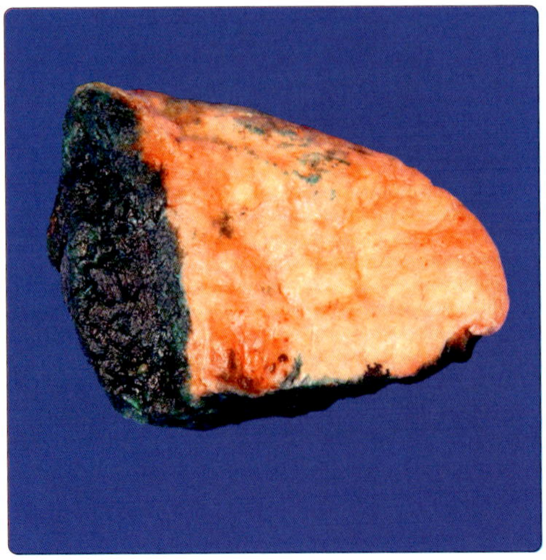

Lung Wedge Biopsy: Sectioning

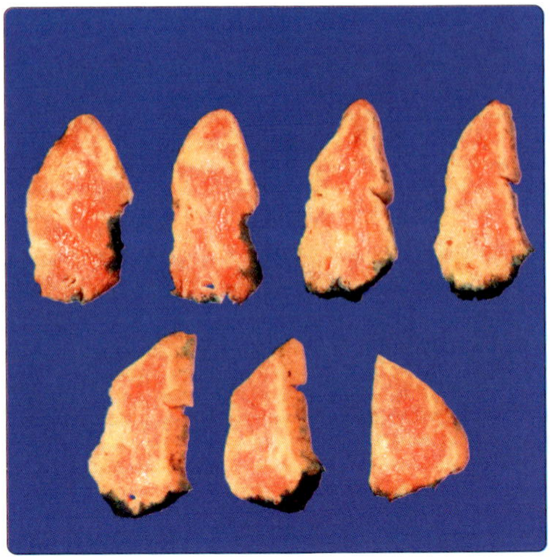

(Left) *Tissue procured to diagnose nonneoplastic lung disease is generally taken as a wedge-shaped fragment from the periphery of 1 or multiple lobes. Staples in the margin, if present, must be removed. Margins are inked in case malignancy is found.* **(Right)** *A lung wedge biopsy is serially sectioned in parallel to the long axis of the specimen and examined for any focal lesions. A representative section may be submitted for frozen section evaluation.*

Acute Bronchopneumonia

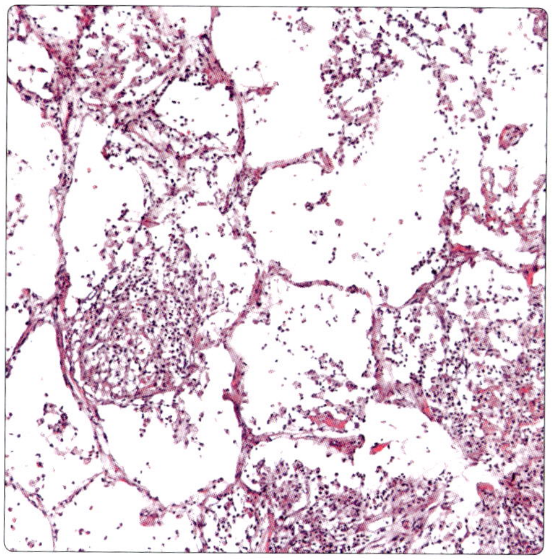

Acute Bronchopneumonia

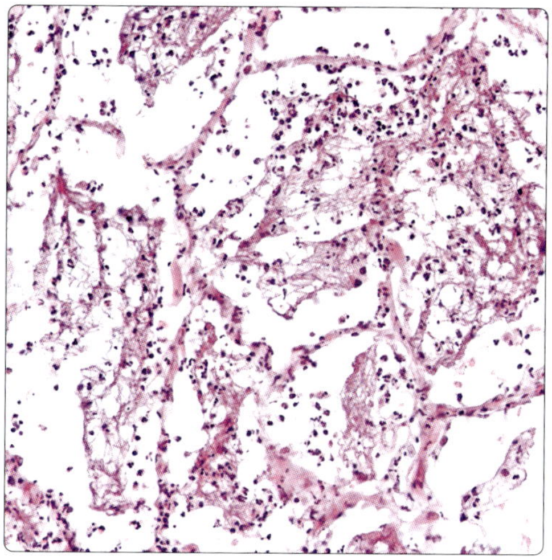

(Left) *Acute bronchopneumonia is characterized by predominantly acute inflammatory cells (neutrophils) within the alveolar spaces &/or lumina of bronchioles. This finding can be diffuse, patchy, or somewhat focal. The infiltrate may also be associated with food particles in cases of aspiration pneumonia.* **(Right)** *The neutrophilic infiltrate may be associated with bacterial clusters, fungal elements, or food material depending on the etiology. Tissue should always be sent for culture.*

Viral Infection

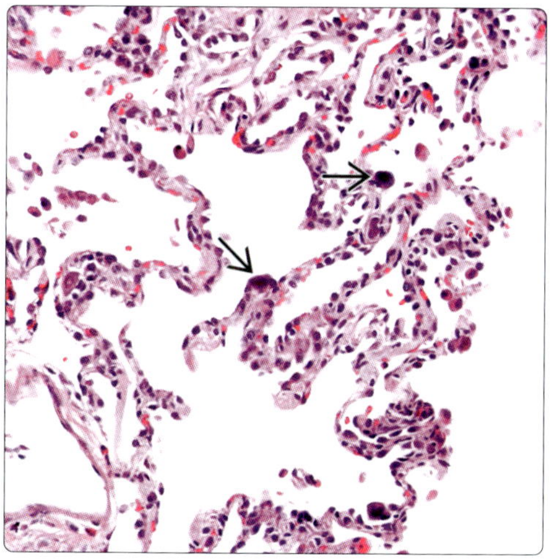

Cytomegalovirus Pneumonitis

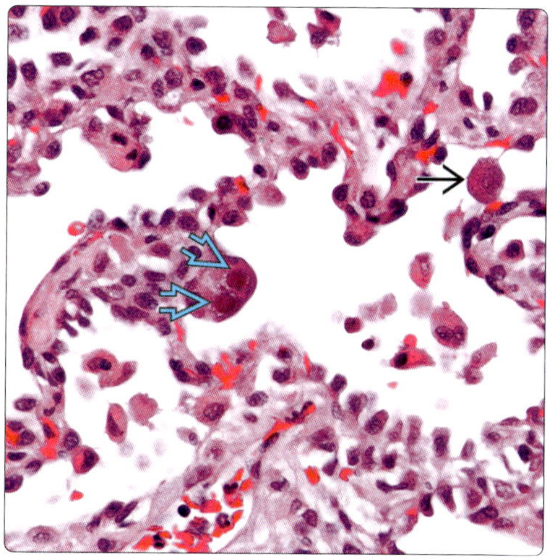

(Left) *A diagnostic finding in certain viral infections is the presence of nuclear &/or cytoplasmic inclusions. These inclusions → vary in size but most stain darkly, allowing for identification at low magnification. The background lung may show necrosis, pneumonitis, or diffuse alveolar damage.* **(Right)** *This image shows 2 nuclear owl's eye inclusions → with peripheral clear halo and 1 eosinophilic granular cytoplasmic inclusion → characteristic of cytomegalovirus infection.*

Granulomatous Inflammation

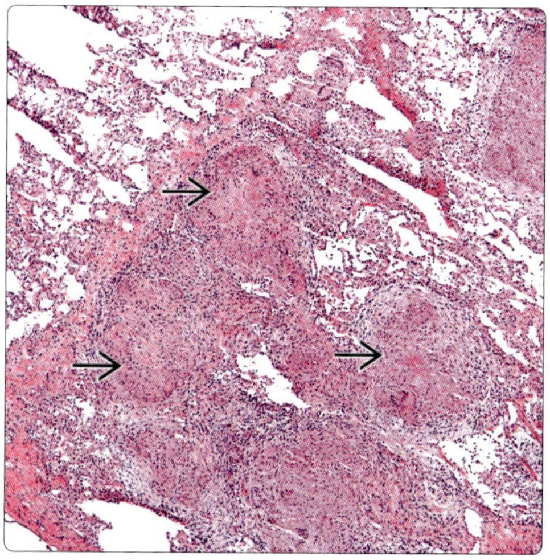

Necrotizing Granulomas

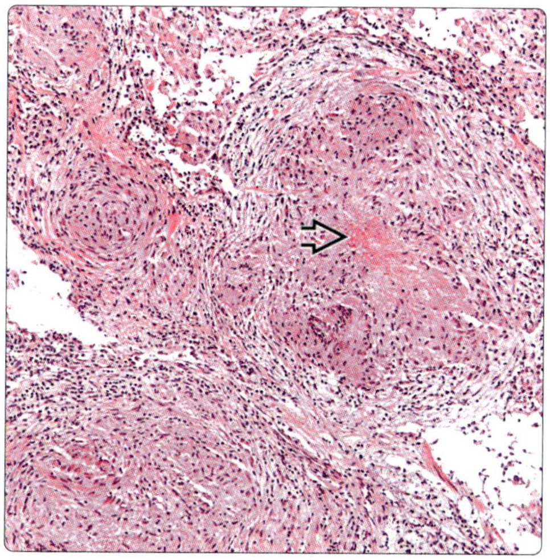

(Left) *Nodular, granulomatous inflammation → in the lung typically raises a differential diagnosis that includes infection (most common), sarcoidosis, aspiration, and foreign body reaction. It can also clinically and grossly mimic a neoplasm.* **(Right)** *Well-formed granulomas with central necrosis (caseation) → strongly favor infection (particularly fungal or mycobacterial), whereas nonnecrotizing, confluent granulomas suggest sarcoidosis. Identification of foreign material supports aspiration.*

(Left) *Sometimes pulmonary granulomas are less well defined and more poorly formed and may even mimic an inflammatory or fibrosing interstitial lung disease. These cases can be challenging, but careful examination will usually turn up the characteristic multinucleated giant cells* ⇨ *seen in most of these lesions.* (Right) *This particular case showed several encapsulated yeast forms* ⇨ *within the multinucleated giant cells. A diagnosis of Cryptococcus infection was rendered.*

Loose Granulomas

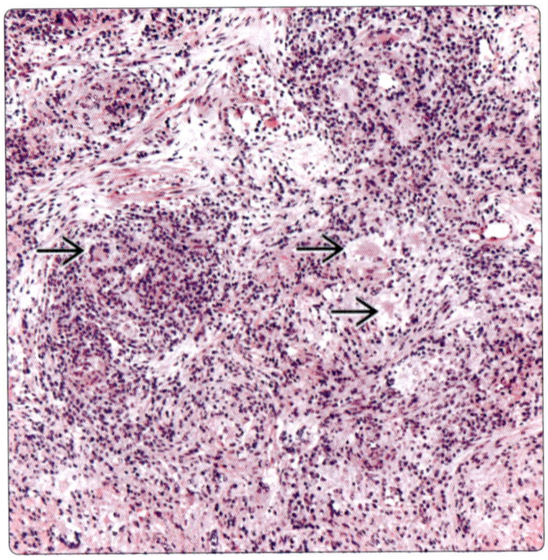

Cryptococcus Infection

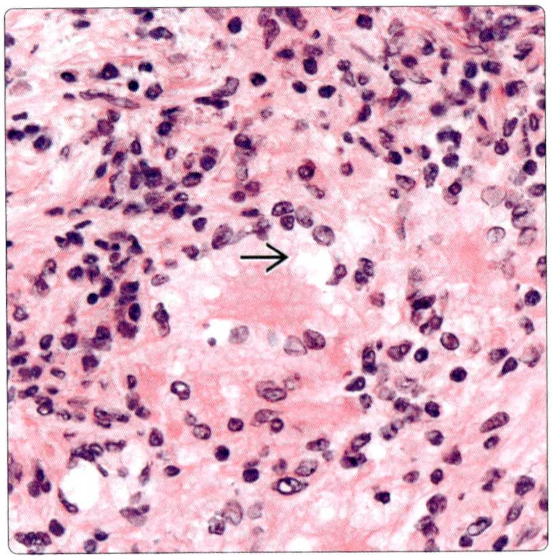

(Left) *Some fungal or mycobacterial infections present as a diffuse intra- and extraalveolar infiltrate of large, foamy macrophages* ⇨*. In this setting, diagnostic features, such as fungal yeast forms, are usually easier to detect than in cases predominantly demonstrating granulomas.* (Right) *Upon high magnification, numerous glassy, circular yeast forms* ⇨ *can be identified within the foamy histiocytes. The morphology suggested Cryptococcus, which was confirmed by culture.*

Foamy Histiocytic Infiltrate

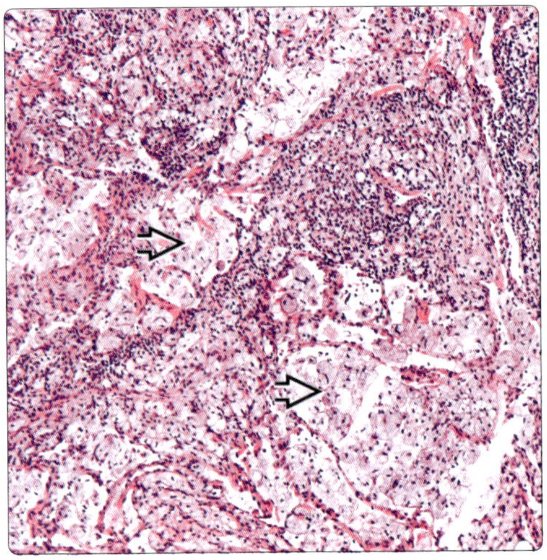

Fungal Infection

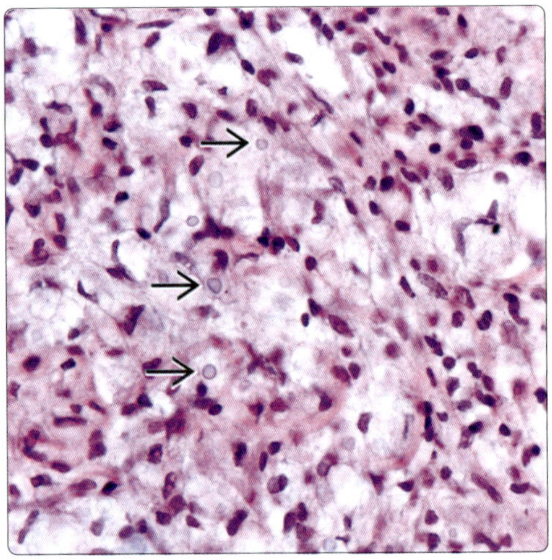

(Left) *Organizing pneumonia* ⇨ *is a relatively common finding in both neoplastic and nonneoplastic lung specimens. In general, this finding is very nonspecific and may indicate 1 of several etiologies, including infection, adverse drug effect, various interstitial lung diseases, and cryptogenic organizing pneumonia, among others.* (Right) *Organizing pneumonia* ⇨ *is identified as irregular "plugs" of loose, myxoid fibroblastic tissue within the alveoli &/or bronchioles.*

Organizing Pneumonia

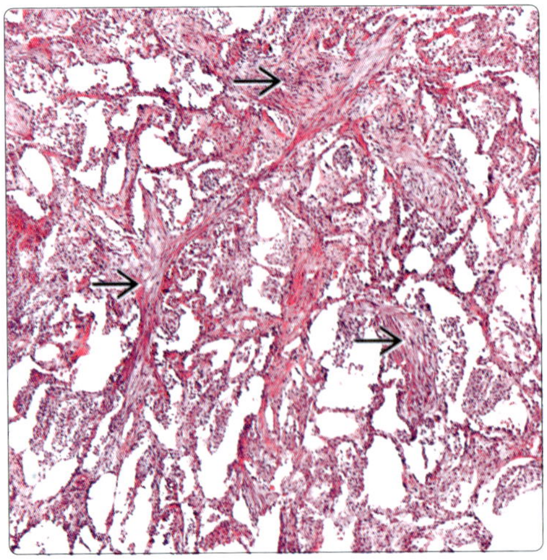

Organizing Pneumonia

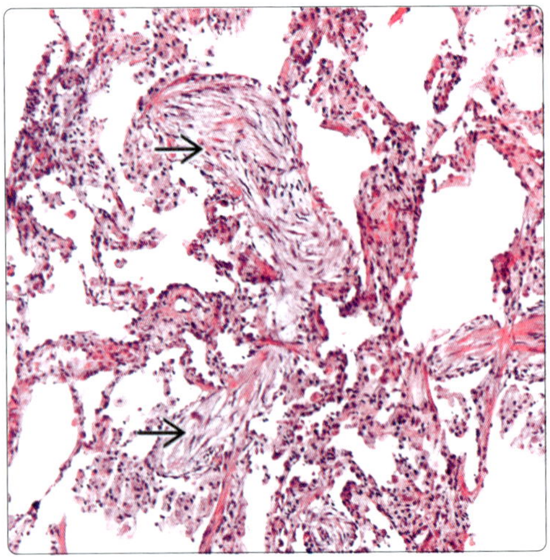

Diffuse Interstitial Fibrosis

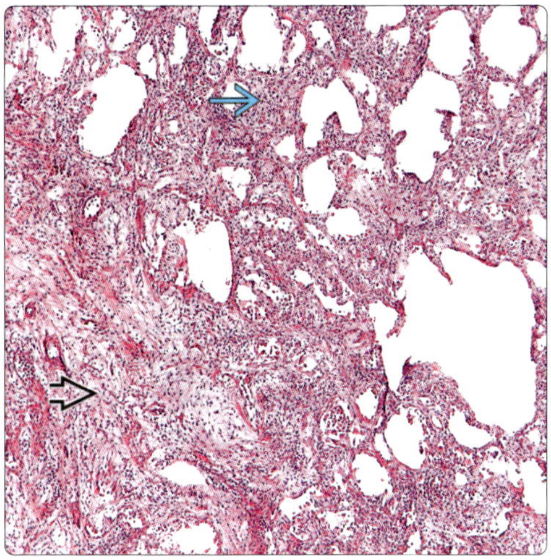

Hypersensitivity Pneumonia

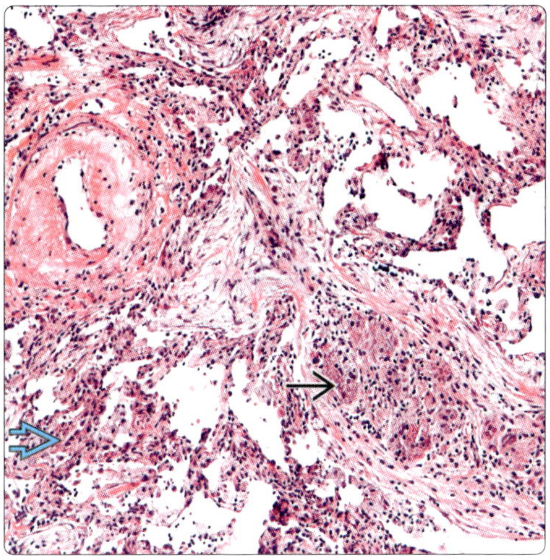

(Left) *The presence of diffuse or patchy interstitial fibrosis may indicate the presence of an interstitial lung disease, such as usual interstitial pneumonia; however, a localized scar is also a consideration. These specimens are best deferred to the permanent sections for diagnosis.* **(Right)** *Hypersensitivity pneumonia may be suggested if the classic findings of loose interstitial histiocytic aggregates and a chronic interstitial inflammatory infiltrate are present in frozen section.*

Diffuse Alveolar Damage

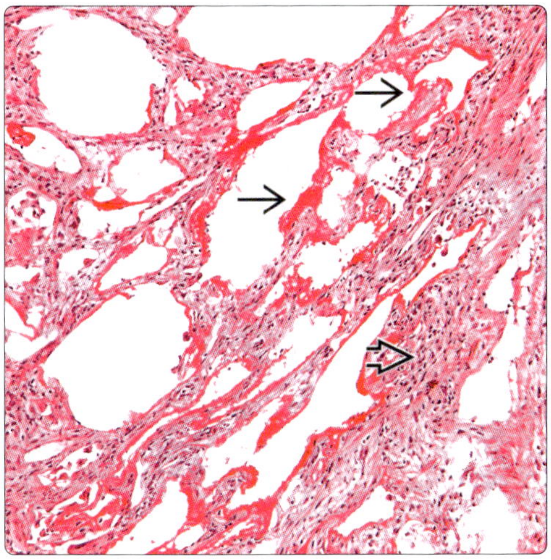

Diffuse Alveolar Damage: Reactive Pneumocytes

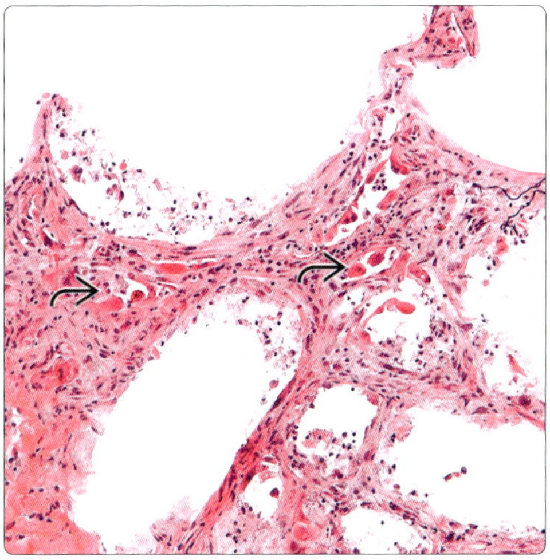

(Left) *The presence of hyaline membranes is diagnostic of diffuse alveolar damage. Other classic findings include interstitial widening with marked edema and prominent, reactive pneumocytes. In this setting, viral inclusions or other diagnostic clues of infection may be present.* **(Right)** *Reactive pneumocytes in diffuse alveolar damage can be alarmingly large and eosinophilic and may mimic an invasive carcinoma. However, the overall clinical and morphologic context is often incompatible with malignancy.*

Lipoid Pneumonia

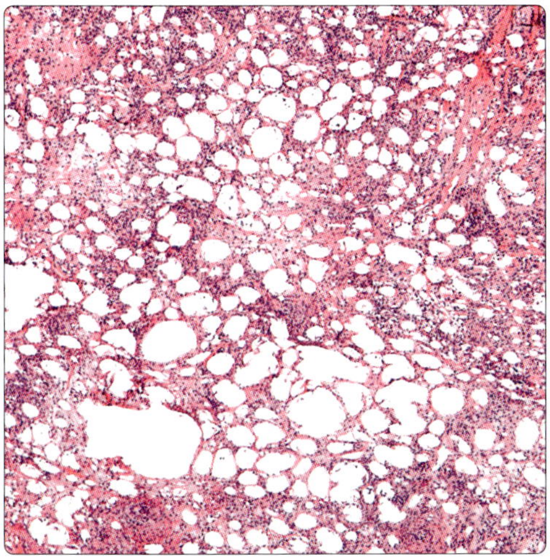

Lipoid Pneumonia

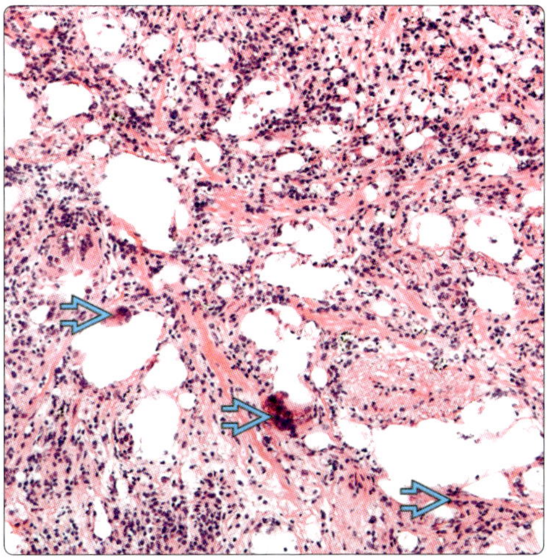

(Left) *Exogenous lipoid pneumonia is an unusual event caused by an aspiration of some form of ingested oil (usually mineral oil). The subsequent tissue reaction involves foreign body giant cells, histiocytes, and fibrosis and creates a nodular, Swiss cheese morphologic appearance.* **(Right)** *Although the oil often washes/processes out of the tissue, the clear spaces left behind are typically surrounded by foamy histiocytes and multinucleated giant cells. Necrosis is not typically identified.*

Contents

SURGICAL/CLINICAL CONSIDERATIONS

Goal of Consultation

- Provide or confirm diagnosis of lung mass
- If malignant, margin of specimen should be evaluated

Change in Patient Management

- If diagnosis of malignancy is made, additional surgery may be performed to achieve tumor-free margins &/or stage tumor
- Subtyping adenocarcinoma (e.g., acinar, papillary) not necessary at time of frozen section

Clinical Setting

- Lung masses may be detected due to symptoms, by screening, or as incidental findings
  - Lung masses causing symptoms are usually larger masses (> 2 cm)
    - Generally diagnosed prior to surgery through transbronchial or CT-guided biopsy and do not necessarily require confirmation
  - Screening using low-dose computed tomography (CT) has been recommended by United States Preventative Services Task Force for persons between ages 55-80 with 30-year history of smoking who currently smoke or have quit smoking within last 15 years
    - These lesions are commonly small masses (< 2 cm) or ground-glass opacities (lesions of low density)
    - Excision is often necessary for diagnosis
      - ~ 70% primary lung malignancies, ~ 10% metastases, and ~ 20% nonmalignant lesions
    - Malignancies in this setting are more likely to be adenocarcinoma in situ (AIS), minimally invasive adenocarcinoma (MIA), or adenocarcinomas with lepidic pattern
  - Incidental lung masses may be detected on CT scans performed for other reasons

SPECIMEN EVALUATION

Gross

- Masses may be excised by wedge resection, lobectomy, or pneumonectomy
- Pleural surface should be carefully inspected
  - Adhesions: May be associated with inflammatory changes or invasion of tumor through pleura
  - Puckering: Usually due to retraction by carcinoma that has invaded into, but not through, pleura
    - Pleural invasion is used for staging and is important prognostic factor
  - Lymphangitic spread: White color of pleural lymphatics indicating extensive lymph-vascular invasion
- Specimen is palpated to identify site of all masses and relationship to any pleural changes
  - Pleura will not move freely over carcinomas that have invaded into pleura
- Specimen is completely serially sectioned to reveal any palpated mass and smaller &/or less firm masses
  - Any areas of possible pleural involvement should be preserved for later evaluation by permanent sections
- Size and location of all masses are recorded
- Distance of lesions to parenchymal margins and bronchial margins is recorded

Frozen Section

- Representative section of mass is frozen
- If lesion has "cheesy" or necrotic surface, touch preps may be indicated in lieu of frozen sections to avoid potential contamination of cryostat with infectious organism (e.g., *Mycobacterium tuberculosis*)
- If surgical margin is nearby, 1 section may be able to demonstrate both mass and margin

Cytology

- Touch preps of cut surface of mass lesion may be helpful if conservation of tumor tissue for permanent section is necessary or if infectious granulomatous disease is possible
  - Suspicion for lymphoma generally requires fresh tissue sent for additional ancillary testing (e.g., flow cytometry)

Invasive Adenocarcinoma

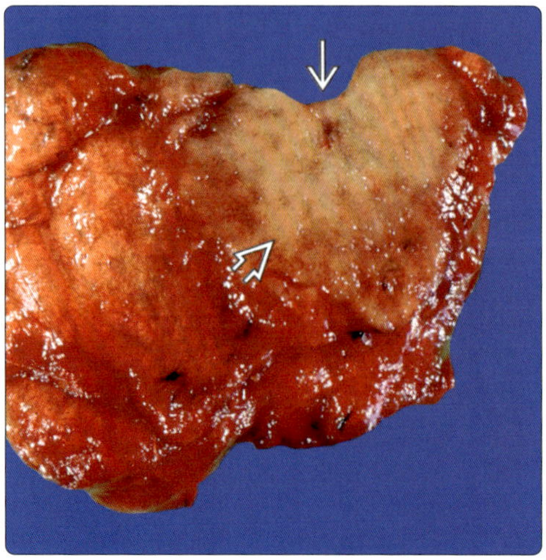

Invasive Adenocarcinoma

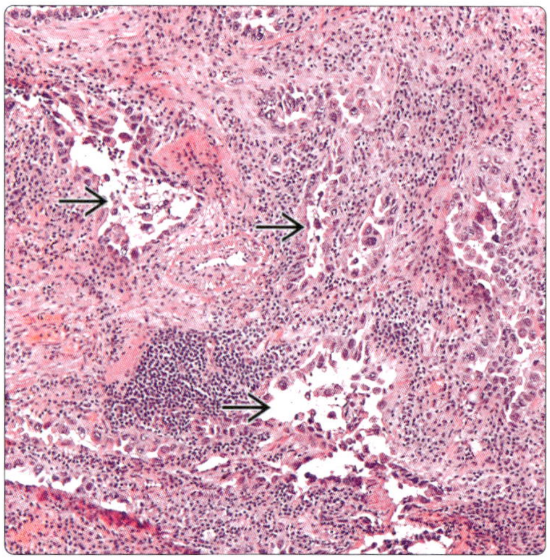

(Left) *Pulmonary adenocarcinoma ➡ is most often seen in a peripheral location and may show "puckering" ➡ or indentation of the pleural surface if the visceral pleura is involved. (Courtesy G. Gray, MD.)* **(Right)** *The majority of cases of well- to moderately differentiated invasive adenocarcinoma characteristically demonstrate obvious gland formation ➡, distinguishing this type of cancer from squamous cell carcinoma.*

- Presence of granulomas on touch prep from small necrotic mass suggests infectious etiology, and subsequent frozen section may not be indicated

MOST COMMON DIAGNOSES

Adenocarcinoma: Conventional/Nonlepidic Pattern

- Most common diagnosis
- Generally presents as solid, discrete mass
- Morphology (glandular vs. solid) depends heavily on degree of differentiation
- Desmoplastic stroma or extensive chronic inflammatory response is often seen

Adenocarcinoma: Lepidic Pattern

- Grossly forms ill-defined, firmer area of lung parenchyma
  - Multiple lesions may be present
  - Lymphomas and focal pneumonia can have similar gross appearance
- Histologic appearance resembles normal lung parenchyma with alveolar walls lined by atypical cells

Adenocarcinoma In Situ (AIS) and Minimally Invasive Adenocarcinoma (MIA)

- AIS and MIA are unlikely to form mass by imaging and are more likely to present as ground-glass opacity
  - Excellent prognosis
  - May be treated with limited (sublobar) excision and no sampling of lymph nodes
  - Decision by surgeon to perform more limited surgery should include consideration of imaging and patient features
    - AIS and MIA can only be diagnosed with certainty after complete evaluation of lesion on permanent sections
    - It is helpful for pathologist to clearly indicate when AIS and MIA are excluded by frozen section
- Classification as AIS requires
  - Solitary lesion measuring < 3 cm
  - Pure lepidic growth pattern
  - No invasion
  - Lacks tumor necrosis and invasion of vessels or pleura
  - Lacks intraalveolar tumor spread
    - However, it is difficult to distinguish this finding from artifactual displacement of tumor cells
- MIA is used for lesions that would otherwise qualify for AIS but have small (< 0.5 cm) areas of invasion
  - In setting of multiple small invasive foci, total percentages of invasive foci can be summed and multiplied by overall tumor diameter
    - Example: 10% invasive component in 2-cm tumor = 2 x 0.1 = 0.2 cm estimated size of invasion

Squamous Cell Carcinoma

- More likely to be centrally located than adenocarcinomas
- May have gritty cut surface depending on amount of keratin production by tumor

Small Cell Carcinoma

- Rarely resected as many have metastasized at time of diagnosis

Non-Small Cell Carcinoma, Not Further Classified

- Acceptable diagnosis in setting of poorly differentiated large cell carcinoma for which thorough sampling &/or immunohistochemistry is necessary for precise classification

Metastatic Carcinoma/Sarcoma

- Previous documented history of malignancy (e.g., colonic adenocarcinoma, osteosarcoma) is invaluable
- Metastatic disease to lung is more likely to present as multiple nodules rather than as single nodule
- Distinction between primary malignancy and metastasis may not always be possible at time of frozen section

Carcinoid

- Most cases occur centrally, especially in endobronchial location
  - Often bilobed with endobronchial component and component in bronchial wall
- Patients are generally younger than typical patient with lung carcinoma

Chondroid Hamartoma

- Generally small and well circumscribed
- Typically demonstrates blue-gray, glassy cut surface due to cartilaginous composition

Granuloma

- Usually small (< 1 cm) and round; may be multiple
- Cut surface varies from soft/necrotic to solid/firm to bony/rock hard
- Granulomas with necrotic/"cheesy" cut surface are more likely to contain fungi (e.g., *Histoplasma*) or mycobacteria, among other organisms
- Tissue should be kept sterile and sent for cultures
  - Frozen sections should be avoided to minimize exposure of personnel to infectious agents and contamination of cryostat

Other Nonneoplastic Inflammatory Changes

- Entities known to present with nodularities include abscess, organizing pneumonia (round pneumonia), granulomatosis with polyangiitis (formerly termed Wegener granulomatosis), and hypersensitivity pneumonitis

Atypical Adenomatous Hyperplasia

- Incidental finding that should not create grossly identifiable mass lesion
- Size: < 5 mm
- May be difficult to distinguish from lepidic pattern adenocarcinoma if present at margin

Lymphoma

- Most common are extranodal marginal zone lymphoma (lymphoma of mucosa-associated lymphoid tissue) and diffuse large B-cell lymphoma
- Tissue should be taken for special studies (e.g., special fixatives, frozen tissue, tissue for flow cytometry)

Intraparenchymal Lymph Node

- Often located near pleura and grossly black due to anthracotic pigment

Lepidic-Pattern Adenocarcinoma vs. Reactive Atypia

Feature	Lepidic-Pattern Adenocarcinoma	Reactive Atypia of Type 2 Pneumocytes
Fibrosis associated with cells	Limited to area of atypical cells	Often > area of atypical cells
Cell types present	1 cell type	Mix of > 1 type
Nuclear inclusions	Frequent, often large	Rare, usually small
Cilia	Absent	May be present
Interface with normal lung	Usually abrupt	Usually single row of cells
Growth pattern	Lepidic but may have projecting tufts or buds; aerogenous spread may be seen	Usually single row of cells
Atypical mitoses	Present in ~ 25%	Absent

Differential Diagnosis of Tumors With Solid Pattern

Feature	Carcinoid	Squamous Cell Carcinoma	Breast Metastasis	Lymphoma
Central location	80-90%	90%	10%	10%
Hyaline stroma > 25%	90%	0%	55	10%
Organoid pattern	70%	0%	5%	20% (fills alveolae)
Salt and pepper chromatin	60%	0%	0%	40%
Nuclear pleomorphism	40%	90%	95%	60%
Irregular nuclear membrane	30%	95%	95%	75%
Mitoses > 5/10 HPF	10%	90%	100%	20%
Spindle cells	May be present (peripheral location)	Often present	Rarely present	Absent

REPORTING

Frozen Section

- Diagnosis of malignant or benign lesion is usually sufficient for intraoperative management
  - Subtypes of carcinoma are not critical intraoperatively
  - If patient has known primary carcinoma elsewhere, surgeon may want opinion as to whether lesion is likely metastasis or primary carcinoma
    - Distinction may not be possible on frozen section
- Some surgeons may want pathologist to distinguish between frank invasive carcinoma, AIS, and MIA
  - Surgeon should be aware that AIS and MIA can only be definitively diagnosed on permanent sections

PITFALLS

Lepidic Pattern Adenocarcinoma vs. Nonneoplastic Inflammatory Changes

- Atelectasis of lung parenchyma after excision combined with reactive atypia can mimic invasive adenocarcinoma
- Primary distinction is made by more pronounced nuclear atypia in adenocarcinomas
  - There is usually clear interface between carcinomas and adjacent normal lung parenchyma, whereas reactive atypia is more diffuse
  - Adenocarcinoma is more likely to show nuclear inclusions
- Carcinomas generally have thicker septal walls

Metastatic Carcinoma vs. Primary Lung Carcinoma

- Important to know history of any prior malignant tumors and histologic type
- May not be possible to make this distinction on frozen section

Lymphoma vs. Intraparenchymal Lymph Node

- Lymphoma generally is larger with irregular border and lacks tan, fleshy cut surface of lymph node
- Histologic architectural hallmarks of lymph node (capsule, subcapsular sinus, etc.) should be sought if tissue is frozen
- Pure cytologic evaluation (i.e., touch prep only) may be of limited use depending on grade of lymphoma

Necrotic Malignancy vs. Necrotic Granuloma

- Distinction can be challenging if lesion is totally necrotic
- Malignancies (both primary and metastatic) are generally larger than infectious lesions
- Granuloma formation on touch prep or frozen section suggests infectious origin, but rare exceptions exist
- Tissue should be taken for cultures if infectious process is suspected

SELECTED REFERENCES

1. Borczuk AC: Challenges of frozen section in thoracic pathology: lepidic lesions, limited resections, and margins. Arch Pathol Lab Med. 141(7):932-939, 2016
2. He P et al: Diagnosis of lung adenocarcinoma in situ and minimally invasive adenocarcinoma from intraoperative frozen sections: an analysis of 136 cases. J Clin Pathol. 69(12):1076-1080, 2016
3. Trejo Bittar HE et al: Accuracy of the IASLC/ATS/ERS histological subtyping of stage I lung adenocarcinoma on intraoperative frozen sections. Mod Pathol. 28(8):1058-63, 2015

Adenocarcinoma, Lepidic Pattern: Gross Appearance

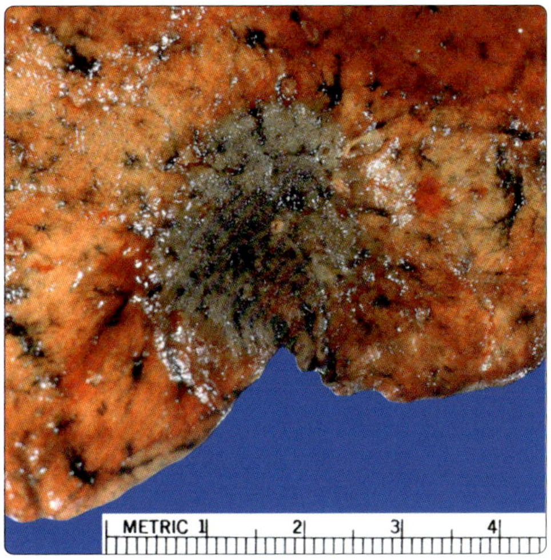

Adenocarcinoma, Lepidic Pattern

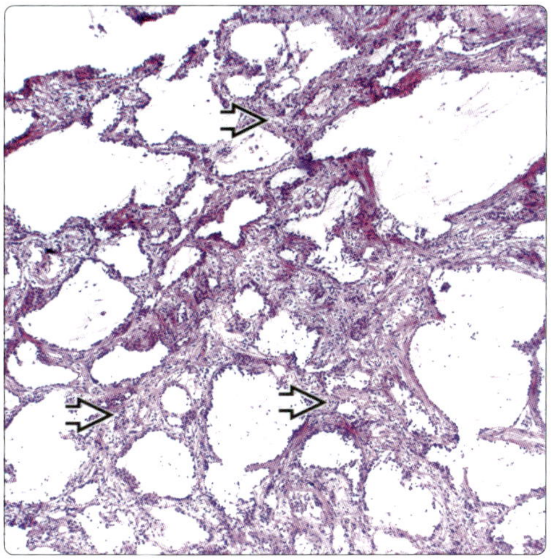

(Left) *Adenocarcinomas with a pure lepidic pattern (formerly bronchioloalveolar type) are often less discrete grossly than overtly invasive adenocarcinomas and may be easily overlooked or confused with round pneumonia (a coin lesion). (Courtesy G. Gray, MD.)* **(Right)** *Lepidic-pattern adenocarcinomas have thickened interstitial septa ⇨; however, thickened walls can also be seen in reactive and inflammatory conditions. The diagnosis of carcinoma is predominantly based on the evaluation of the tumor cells.*

Adenocarcinoma, Lepidic Pattern: Cytologic Features

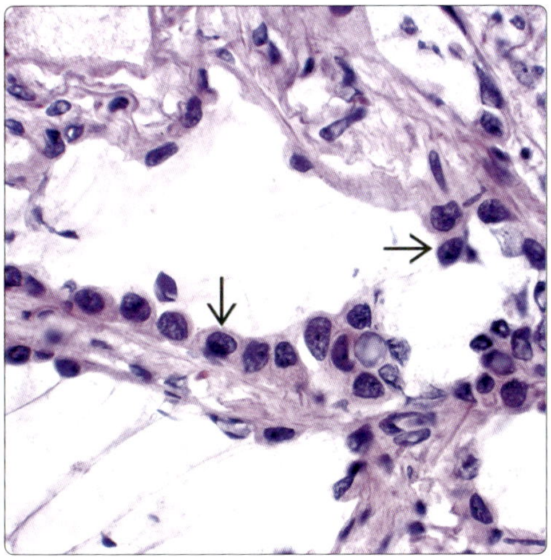

Adenocarcinoma, Lepidic Pattern: Nuclear Inclusions

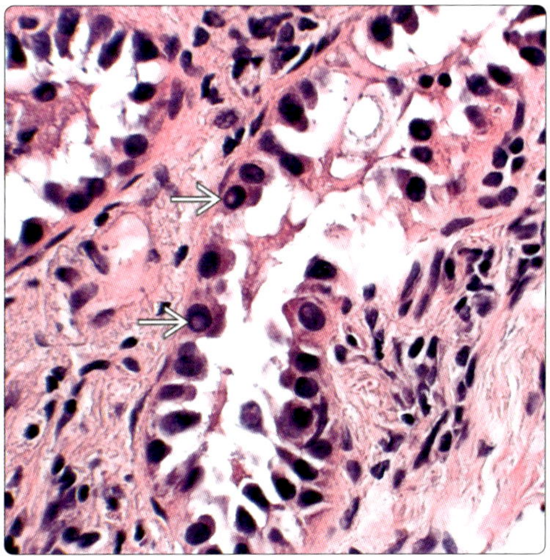

(Left) *In contrast to reactive nonneoplastic conditions, the nuclei → in lepidic-pattern adenocarcinomas are larger, often more hyperchromatic, and variable in size.* **(Right)** *Nuclear inclusions ➡ are commonly seen in lepidic-pattern adenocarcinoma (shown) but are less common and more inconspicuous in reactive atypia. Inclusions are cytoplasmic invaginations and should be round and of the same color as the cytoplasm. Inclusions must be distinguished from nuclei with chromatin clearing due to freezing artifact.*

Mucinous Adenocarcinoma, Lepidic Pattern

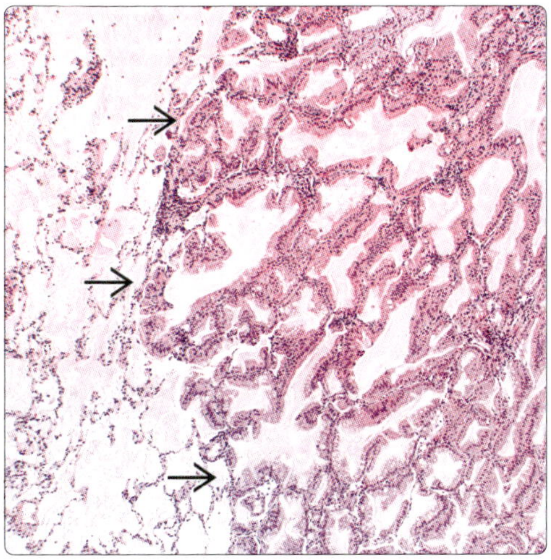

Mucinous Adenocarcinoma, Lepidic Pattern

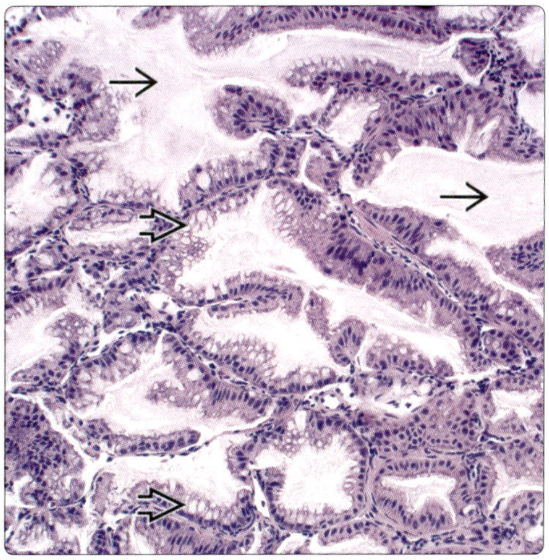

(Left) *Mucinous adenocarcinomas with a lepidic pattern are more easily recognized than their nonmucinous (serous) counterparts because the interface between tumor and normal lung is very well demarcated →. Reactive atypia is not typically associated with mucin production.* **(Right)** *The cells of a lepidic-pattern mucinous adenocarcinoma are always tall/columnar and contain abundant apical mucin ⇨. Extracellular mucin → within alveolar spaces is common and also may be abundant.*

(Left) *Pulmonary squamous cell carcinoma* → *is often a large tumor and generally arises in a central location, as evidenced grossly and microscopically by its proximity to, or involvement with, a bronchus (i.e., of bronchogenic origin)* ➡*. (Courtesy G. Gray, MD.)* **(Right)** *Squamous cell carcinoma may have a gritty or grainy cut surface* ⇨*, depending on the amount of keratin produced. Note the direct involvement of the tumor with the adjacent bronchus* ➡*. (Courtesy G. Gray, MD.)*

Squamous Cell Carcinoma: Gross Appearance

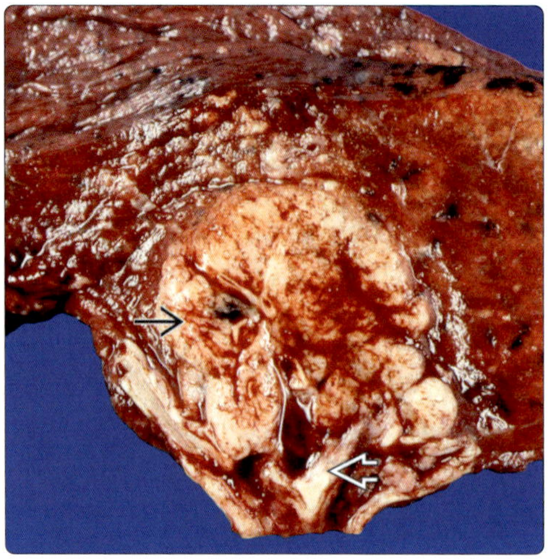

Squamous Cell Carcinoma: Gross Appearance

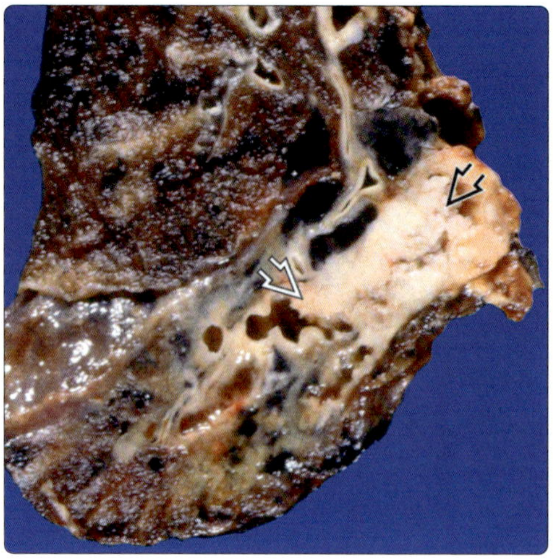

(Left) *Squamous cell carcinoma characteristically shows irregular nests of eosinophilic cells within a desmoplastic stroma. Glandular lumen formation is not present. Necrosis is often prominent.* **(Right)** *The majority of squamous cell carcinomas are composed of eosinophilic tumor cells* →*. However, the cells of the basaloid variant of squamous cell carcinoma are smaller and may mimic small cell carcinoma. Depending on the degree of differentiation, keratin production may be abundant or absent.*

Squamous Cell Carcinoma: Nests and Desmoplastic Stroma

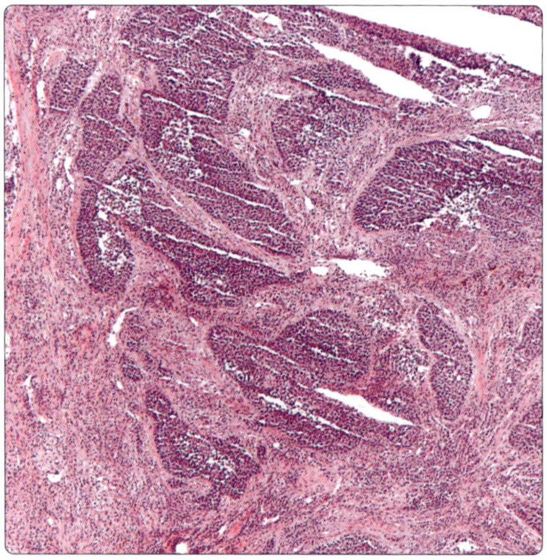

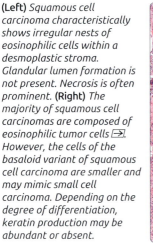

Squamous Cell Carcinoma: Cytologic Features

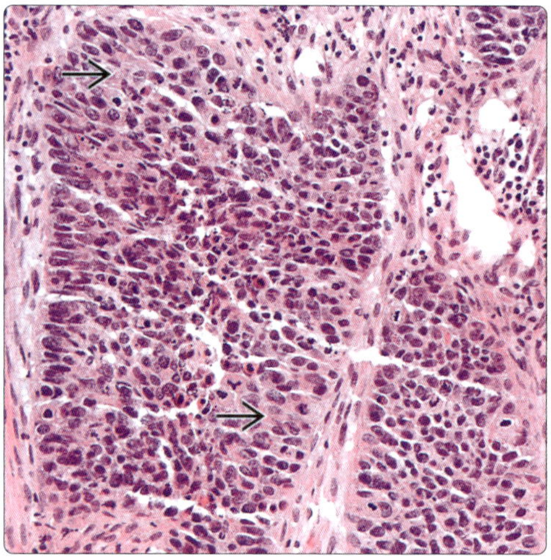

(Left) *Small cell carcinoma* → *generally has a white fleshy surface and is usually located centrally. Note the hilar lymph node involvement* ➡*. These tumors are not typically resected because many have metastasized at the time of diagnosis. (Courtesy G. Gray, MD.)* **(Right)** *Small cell carcinoma is composed of nests and sheets of small cells, and necrosis is common. Importantly, some cases may show peripheral nuclear palisading* →*, leading to confusion with basaloid squamous cell carcinoma.*

Small Cell Carcinoma: Gross Appearance

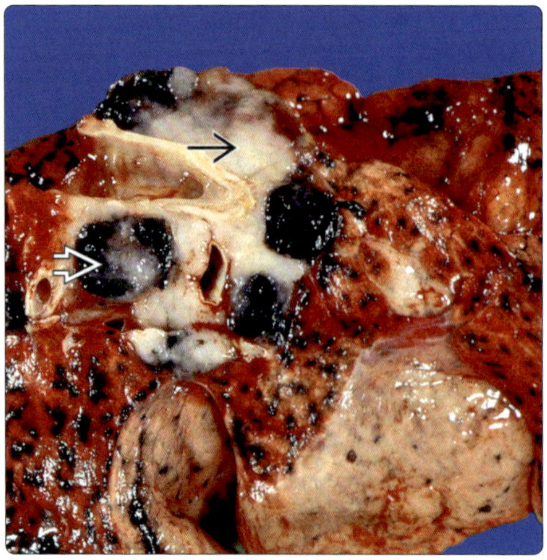

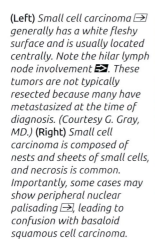

Small Cell Carcinoma: Morphology

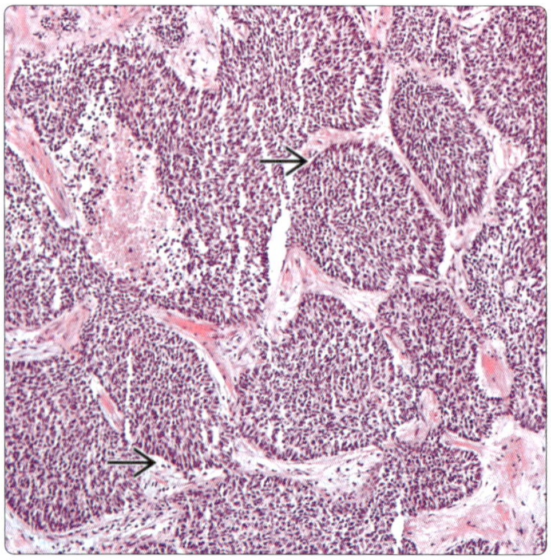

Small Cell Carcinoma: Abundant Mitoses

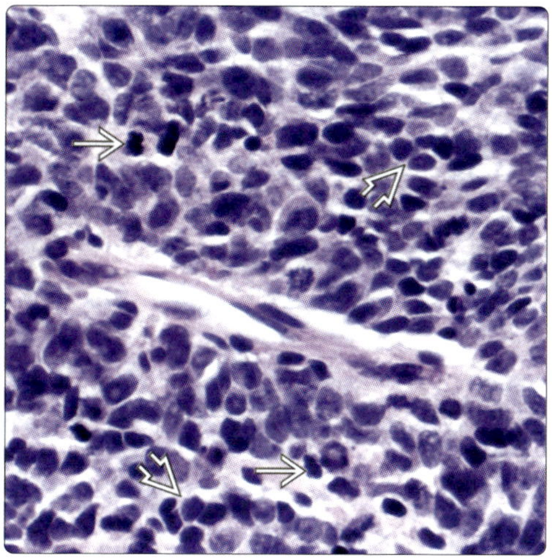

Small Cell Carcinoma: Crush Artifact

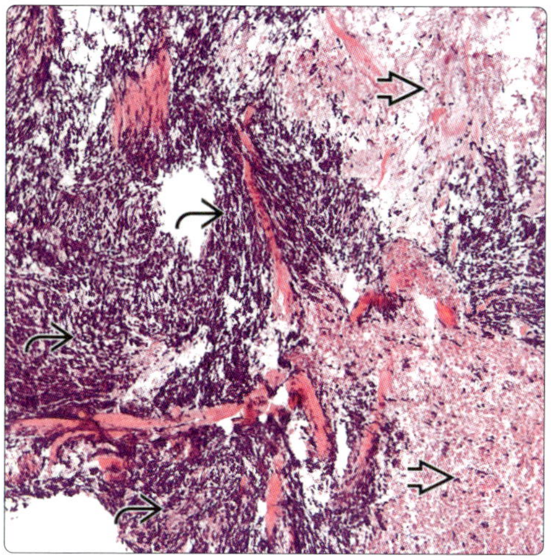

(Left) *Helpful clues to the diagnosis of small cell carcinoma include numerous dark, overlapping, small to medium-sized nuclei, abundant mitoses* ➡*, scant cytoplasm, and nuclear molding* ➡. **(Right)** *The cells of small cell carcinoma are very fragile and easily disrupted. As a result, they often show marked crush artifact* ↪ *and may be difficult to distinguish from benign lymphoid tissue. Other less disrupted areas are usually more likely to be diagnostic. Note the prominent necrosis* ⇨*.*

Carcinoid Tumor: Gross Appearance

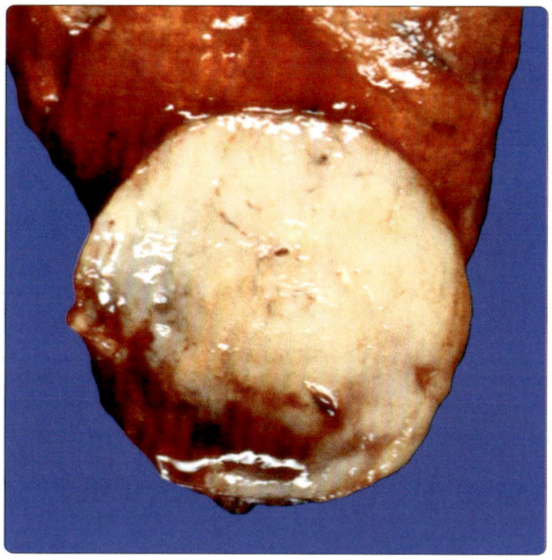

Endobronchial Carcinoid Tumor: Gross Appearance

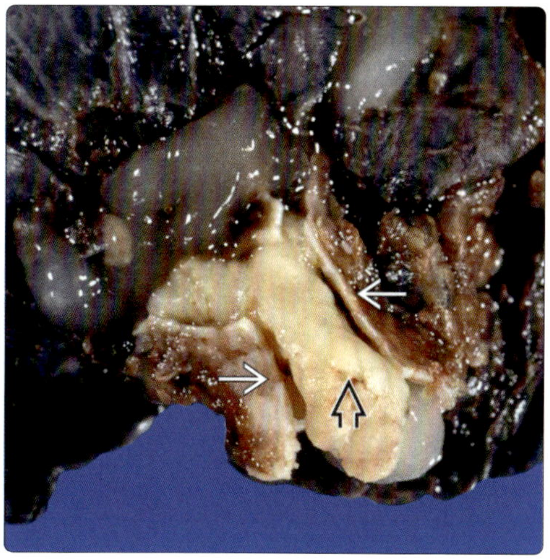

(Left) *Carcinoid tumors are generally well-circumscribed neoplasms and often have a yellow or white-yellow, glistening cut surface. They can be located centrally or peripherally. (Courtesy G. Gray, MD.)* **(Right)** *Some carcinoid tumors arise in an endobronchial location and may extend into the bronchial lumen as a polypoid growth* ⇧ *between the bronchial walls* ➡*. Obstruction may produce symptoms. Some tumors may be mistaken for congealed mucin. (Courtesy G. Gray, MD.)*

Carcinoid Tumor: Morphology

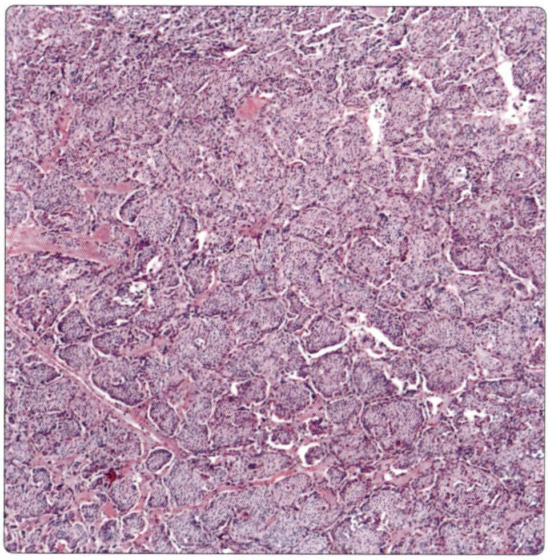

Carcinoid Tumor: Cytologic Features

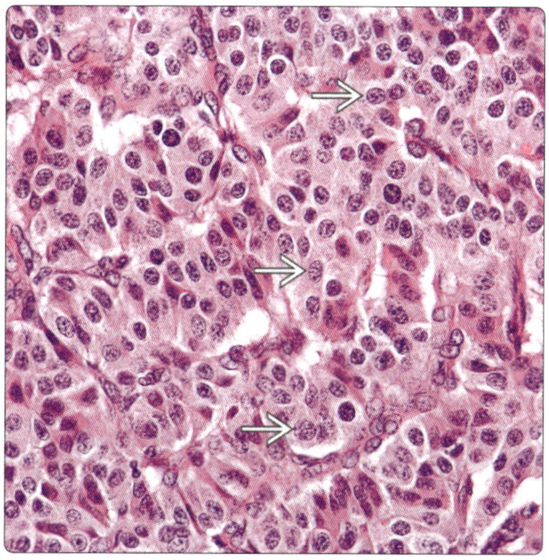

(Left) *Most carcinoid tumors display a prominent nested growth pattern that somewhat resembles a poorly differentiated carcinoma. However, necrosis and mitoses are generally absent. A capillary vascular network between the nests is typically present. Trabecular/corded or acinar growth patterns may also be present in these tumors, helping with identification.* **(Right)** *Carcinoid tumor nuclei usually demonstrate a uniform speckled or salt and pepper chromatin pattern* ➡ *that is diagnostically useful.*

(Left) *Metastatic disease to the lungs is more likely to present as multiple discrete nodules ➔ of varying sizes instead of 1 dominant mass. Multiple lobes of the lung are also more likely to be involved and suggest metastases. (Courtesy G. Gray, MD.)* (Right) *Although it can be very challenging to distinguish a primary lung carcinoma from a metastasis, some clues can usually be identified. Note the tall columnar cells, dirty necrosis ⇒, and the overall confluence of this metastatic colonic adenocarcinoma.*

Metastases to Lung: Gross Appearance

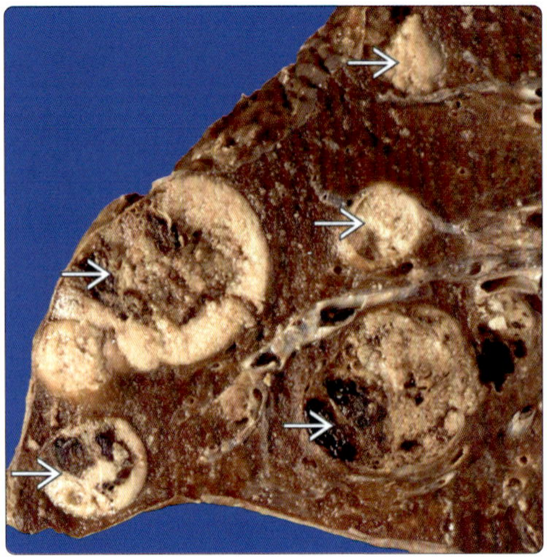

Metastatic Colon Carcinoma

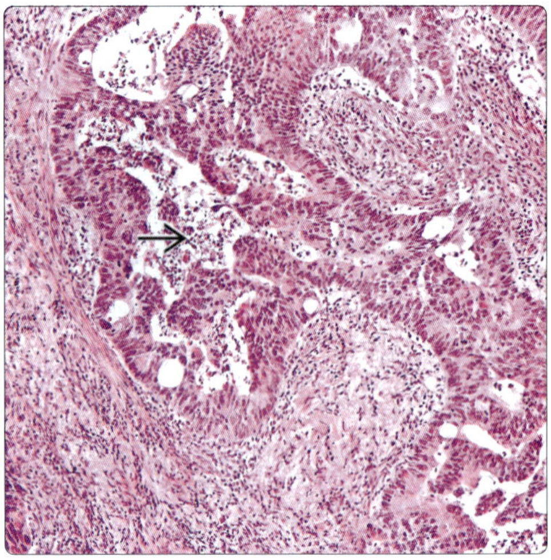

(Left) *In cases of metastatic melanoma, the presence of grossly identifiable dark pigment ➔ is a helpful clue to the diagnosis, if present. (Courtesy G. Gray, MD.)* (Right) *Melanomas, both primary and metastatic, can be difficult to distinguish from carcinoma on frozen section. A documented history of prior melanoma is always helpful to support metastatic disease, but the presence of brown melanin pigment ⇒ may suggest the diagnosis as well.*

Metastatic Melanoma: Gross Appearance

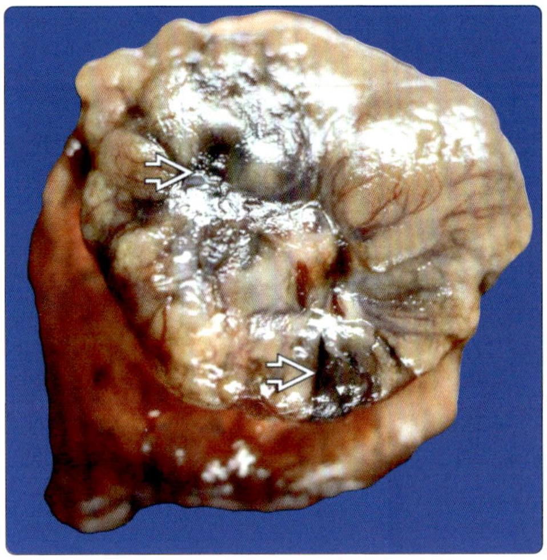

Metastatic Melanoma: Melanin Pigment

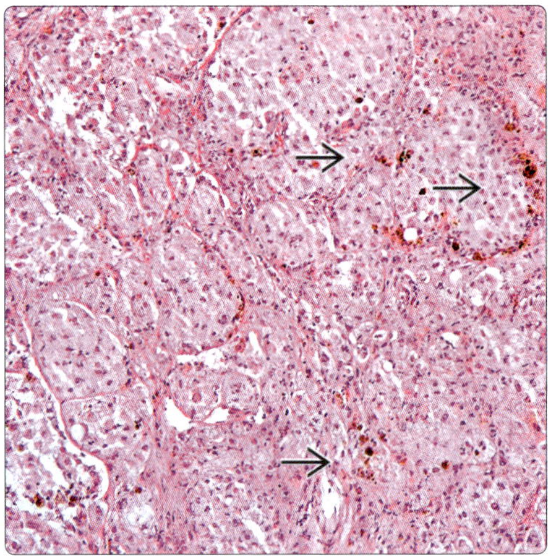

(Left) *Cytologic techniques may be preferred over frozen section in some clinical circumstances (e.g., multiple lung masses in a patient with a history of widely metastatic breast cancer). This touch prep shows metastatic breast carcinoma ⇒ to the lung.* (Right) *Pulmonary hamartoma generally presents as a small, very well-circumscribed lesion. It is composed mainly of benign cartilage and will have a white-gray, glassy &/or focally myxoid cut surface. (Courtesy G. Gray, MD.)*

Metastatic Breast Carcinoma: Touch Prep

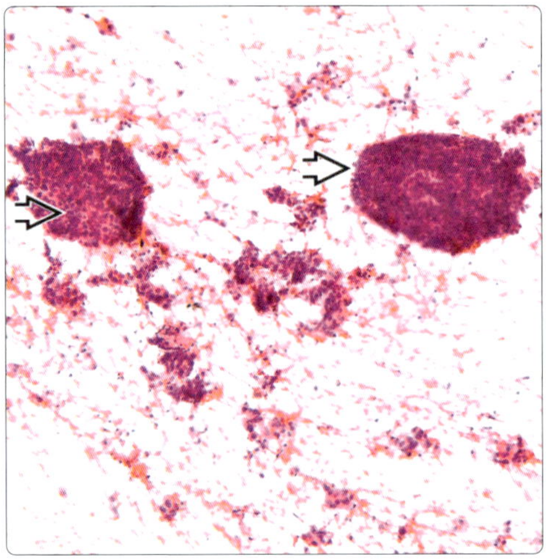

Chondroid Hamartoma: Gross Appearance

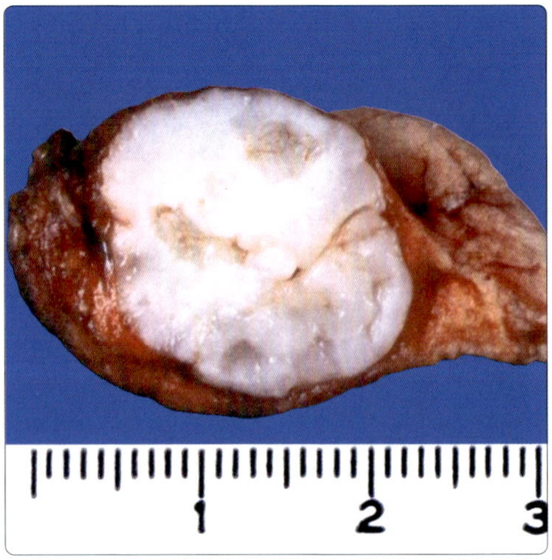

Chondroid Hamartoma: Hyaline Cartilage

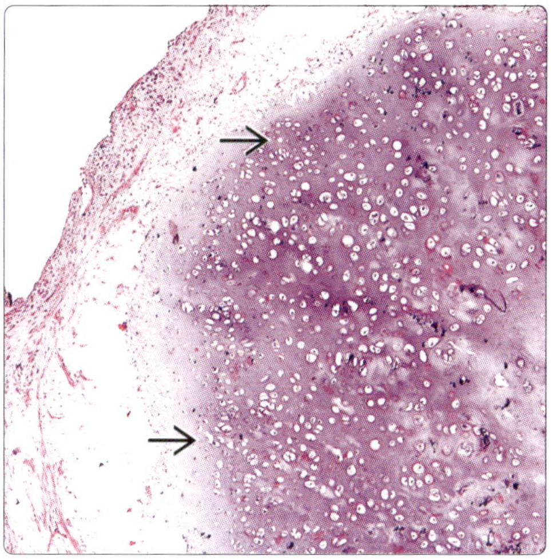

Chondroid Hamartoma: Fat, Fibrous Tissue, and Respiratory Epithelium

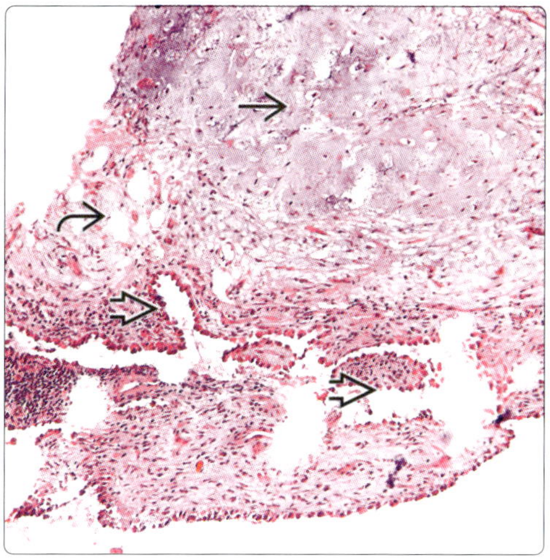

(Left) *The main finding in a pulmonary hamartoma is a lobulated, well-circumscribed proliferation of bland cartilage ➔. A metastatic chondrosarcoma is always in the differential diagnosis. However, in this latter case, the cartilage is generally cytologically malignant, and the patient almost always has a previous history.* **(Right)** *Adjacent foci of fat ➚, fibrous tissue, &/or muscle with an overlying nonneoplastic respiratory epithelium ⇨ are typically present, in addition to cartilage ➔ in pulmonary hamartomas.*

Granuloma: Gross Appearance

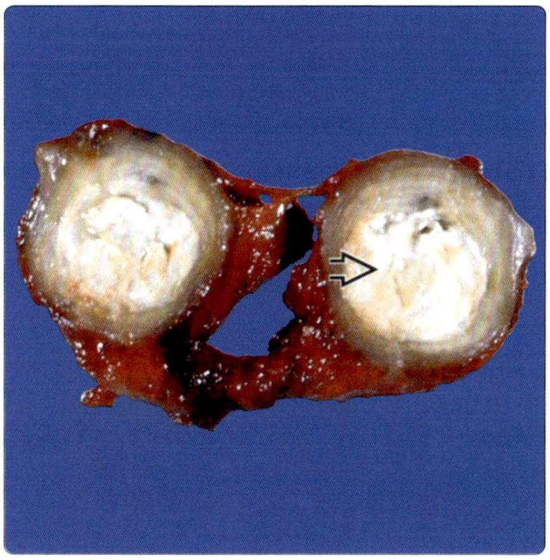

Infectious Granuloma

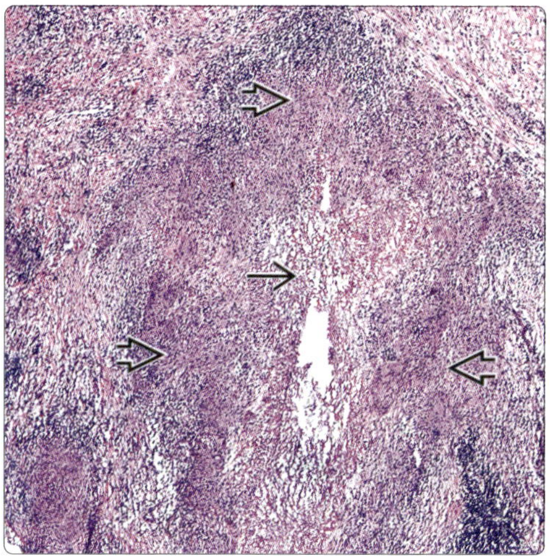

(Left) *It is not uncommon for a limited peripheral wedge biopsy to be taken to evaluate a small nodule in a patient with a large mass elsewhere. Granulomas are usually small and well circumscribed, and they may have a fibrous, bony, or "cheesy" necrotic ⇨ cut surface. Touch preps are recommended for initial intraoperative evaluation of necrotic lesions. (Courtesy G. Gray, MD.)* **(Right)** *A typical infectious granuloma is shown with a rim of epithelioid histiocytes ⇨ and giant cells as well as central necrosis ➔.*

Lymphoma: Gross Appearance

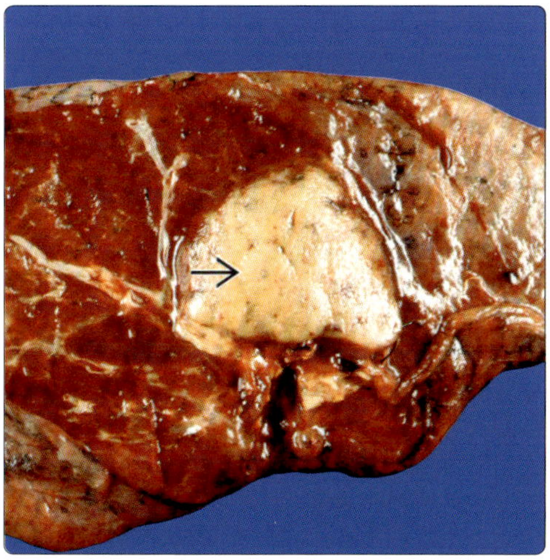

Lymphoma: Touch Prep

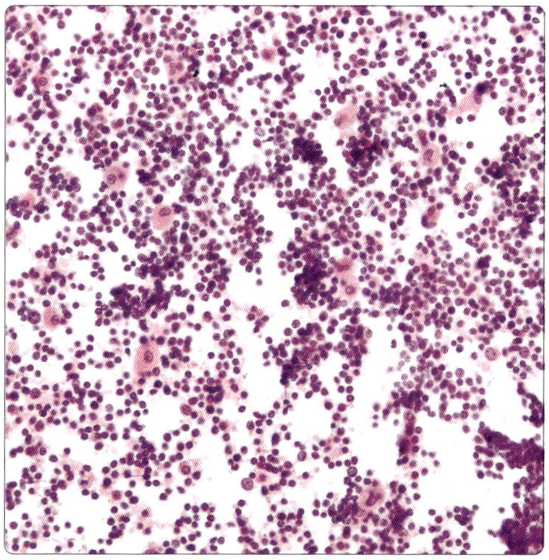

(Left) *Lymphomas of the lung may demonstrate a variety of gross appearances, from nodularity ➔ to apparent consolidation associated with bronchovascular structures. If a diagnosis of lymphoma is suspected, it is important to collect fresh tissue for additional ancillary testing. (Courtesy G. Gray, MD.)* **(Right)** *Touch prep of a lymphoma will generally show dyscohesive sheets of variably atypical lymphoid cells and should trigger further diagnostic work-up (i.e., flow cytometry, cytogenetics, etc.).*

Contents

SURGICAL/CLINICAL CONSIDERATIONS

Goal of Consultation

- Patients with breast cancer
  - Determine if macrometastatic (≥ 2 mm) carcinoma present in sentinel lymph node(s)
    - Metastases < 2 mm may or may not be detected but should be reported if identified
- Patients with axillary adenopathy
  - Determine cause of adenopathy

Change in Patient Management

- If metastasis present in sentinel lymph node, additional lymph nodes may be excised
  - If no additional surgery planned, there is no need for intraoperative evaluation of lymph nodes
- If lymphoma or infectious disease detected, tissue can be taken for ancillary studies

Clinical Setting

- **Patients with breast cancer**
  - In past, decisions concerning systemic therapy for breast cancer relied heavily on nodal status
  - Currently, biologic type of breast cancer more commonly used for these decisions
  - Nodal status predictive of survival but not response to therapy
  - Recent clinical trials (ACOSOG Z0011 and IBCSG 23-01) showed no significant survival benefit to completion axillary dissection in early-stage breast cancer patients with 1-2 positive sentinel lymph nodes
    - As a result, there has been a significant decline in frozen-section diagnosis of sentinel lymph nodes
    - Intraoperative sentinel lymph node evaluation still utilized in patients who would not fit Z0011 inclusion criteria, including those undergoing neoadjuvant chemotherapy
- **Patients with axillary adenopathy**
  - Axillary lymph nodes may be enlarged due to reactive changes, infection, or malignancy
  - Excision of axillary node may be performed for intraoperative diagnosis
    - In many cases, fine-needle aspiration or core needle biopsy are used for this purpose

SPECIMEN EVALUATION

Gross

- All nodes carefully are bluntly dissected from specimen and counted
  - Number of nodes present and number with metastases used to determine need for additional surgery
  - If each node inked different color, slices from multiple nodes can be frozen in same block
    - Important to be able to count number of nodes with metastasis
  - All fat should be trimmed away from nodes
- If gradient of blue dye is present, metastasis is most likely at blue-stained pole
- Each node thinly sliced at 2-mm intervals
- If node grossly suspicious for lymphoma or granulomatous disease, preservation of nonfrozen tissue helpful for ancillary studies
  - Flow cytometry, frozen tissue (molecular studies), and hematopathology fixatives for suspected lymphoma
  - Cultures for granulomatous disease
- Radioactive nodes detected with usual techniques employed do not expose pathology personnel to dangerous levels of radiation
  - Special protective equipment not required
  - Special storage or disposal of tissue or equipment not necessary
  - If new or nonstandard technique utilized, levels of radiation and resulting risk should be assessed
  - Handling procedures should be approved by institutional radiation safety office

Frozen Section

- If grossly evident metastasis, only 1 representative section need be frozen

Lymph Node: Anatomy

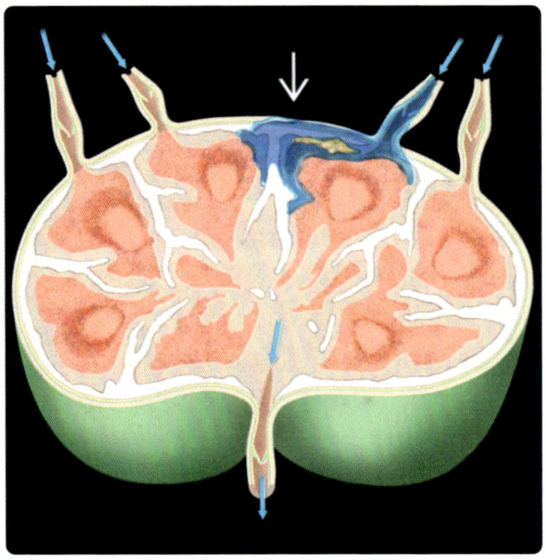

Lymph Node Metastasis: Gross Appearance

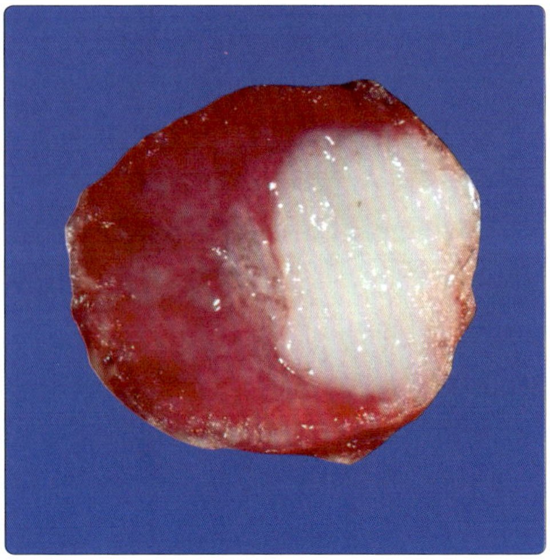

(Left) *Afferent lymphatics, and metastases, enter the node in a central plane. Bisection of the node in this plane is most likely to reveal metastasis. A metastasis is most likely to be near the dye ➡ used for sentinel node detection.* **(Right)** *Metastatic carcinoma usually forms a firm, white mass that replaces the normal brown to red nodal tissue. Smaller metastases, or diffusely infiltrative metastases, may not be grossly visible.*

- Scrape or touch preparation can also be used to document grossly positive lymph node
- If purpose is to detect breast cancer metastasis, all slices of all grossly normal nodes are frozen
  - At least 1 H&E slide including complete cross section of all slices evaluated
- If purpose is to establish diagnosis to explain adenopathy, only one representative section should be frozen
  - Cytologic preparations should be used, when feasible, to preserve tissue for possible ancillary studies

Cytology

- Each cut surface scraped with curved scalpel blade or glass slide and smeared on another slide
- Each node should be separately evaluated
- Useful when either infection or lymphoma suspected
  - Touch imprints, rather than scrape preparations, may be more helpful for lymphoma

Molecular Methods

- One-step nucleic acid amplification (OSNA) currently available assay based on amplification of cytokeratin 19 mRNA
- Proposed as alternative to frozen section
- Although it enables detection of minimal tumor in lymph nodes, clinical utility questionable
  - Cannot reliably determine size of metastasis or extranodal extension
  - Cannot detect cytokeratin 19 (-) carcinomas nor diseases other than carcinoma

MOST COMMON DIAGNOSES

Metastatic Breast Carcinoma

- Most common carcinoma found in axillary nodes of women
  - Metastases from skin cancers next most likely primary site
- Ductal and lobular carcinoma most common types
  - Metastatic tumor almost always resembles primary
    - Preoperative review of slides or reports can be very helpful for correlation
    - If metastatic tumor and primary dissimilar, consider alternative diagnoses (e.g., benign inclusions or metastases from other sites)
  - Metastatic grade I and II lobular carcinomas can be very difficult to identify in nodes
- Metastases may be focal
  - Usually present adjacent to peripheral subcapsular sinus
  - Rare metastases present in center of node
- Sentinel nodes may be sampled after neoadjuvant therapy
  - Metastases that have responded to treatment leave fibrotic tumor bed in 2/3 of cases
    - Useful to report presence of fibrosis consistent with tumor bed when present
  - However, in 1/3 of cases, lymph node with prior metastasis will look completely normal
  - Response to treatment can vary from node to node
  - Residual metastatic carcinoma may be present as scattered foci over tumor bed and difficult to detect on frozen section
    - Cells may have markedly enlarged pleomorphic nuclei and abundant cytoplasm, suggesting that cells may not be viable
      - Viability cannot be determined with certainty based on morphology
      - Any residual tumor cells should be reported

Lymphoma

- Can present as axillary adenopathy
  - Would be unusual and unexpected finding in axillary nodes of woman with breast cancer
  - Women with known low-grade lymphoma/chronic lymphocytic leukemia may have nodal involvement
- Cytologic preparations helpful to reveal morphology and dyscohesive nature of cells
- If sufficient tissue available, tissue should be saved for ancillary studies
  - Frozen tissue (DNA analysis)
  - Flow cytometry
  - Fixatives for hematopathology
    - If Hodgkin lymphoma or diagnoses other than lymphoma are possible, tissue should also be fixed in formalin

Melanoma

- Tumor cells usually appear dyscohesive with markedly pleomorphic nuclei
- Tumors pigmented grossly or microscopically easy to identify
  - However, many metastatic melanomas do not exhibit obvious melanin production
- Patients usually have well-known history of melanoma
  - In rare cases, metastatic melanoma to breast can be mistaken for primary breast carcinoma

Sarcoidosis

- Rarely involves axillary lymph nodes
- Node occupied by confluent noncaseating granulomas
- Infection should be excluded by sending tissue for culture

Benign Epithelial Inclusions

- Ectopic breast tissue or rarely endosalpingiosis may be present as well-formed tubules within node
  - Breast epithelium may show apocrine or squamous metaplasia
  - Breast stroma may or may not be present
  - Endosalpingiosis may contain ciliated cells
- Benign inclusions very rare compared to metastatic well-differentiated breast carcinoma

Silicone

- Can seep out of implants ("bleed") or be released when implant ruptured
- Can be transferred to regional lymph nodes
- Silicone granulomas can be very hard and gritty when cut
  - Gross appearance and texture can closely mimic metastatic carcinoma
- Histiocytes that have taken up silicone may resemble adipocytes or lipoblasts
- Silicone and metastatic carcinoma can be present in same lymph node

Nevus Cell Nests

- Capsular nevus cell rests are small clusters of melanocytic cells present in ~ 5% of lymph nodes
- Consist of short spindle cells with bland nuclei with dispersed chromatin, sometimes associated with melanin
  - Usually morphologically distinct from breast carcinoma
- Generally present within capsule
  - Less commonly involve septa and are present within node

PITFALLS

False-Negative Diagnoses

- **Failure to examine entire node**
  - If not all slices frozen, macrometastases can be missed in ~ 30% of cases
  - Tissue should never be taken from negative nodes in a way that would interfere with detecting all macrometastases
    - Includes tissue taken for alternative techniques such as OSNA
- **Metastatic lobular carcinoma**
  - Can be very difficult to detect in frozen sections or cytologic preparations
    - Single cell infiltrative pattern
    - Scattered throughout node rather than predominantly in peripheral sinuses
  - Tumor cells can resemble normal cells in lymph nodes
    - Grade I carcinomas resemble lymphocytes
    - Grade II carcinomas resemble histiocytes
    - Grade III carcinomas have nuclear pleomorphism and are generally easily recognizable
  - Signet ring cells with mucin vacuoles helpful to recognize tumor cells
    - However, signet ring cells not always present
  - Immunoperoxidase studies for keratin on permanent sections necessary in some cases for final diagnosis
- **Small or unusually located metastases**
  - Metastases < 2 mm may not be present on frozen section or cytologic preparation
    - Micrometastases usually not indication for additional nodal dissection
  - Metastases located in center of node can easily be missed
- **Prior neoadjuvant therapy**
  - Cells may resemble histiocytes and be sparsely distributed
  - Fibrotic stroma extending beyond area of tumor cells is clue to prior treatment
- **Artifacts from surgery and tissue preparation**
  - Ice crystal artifact, tissue folding, and poor staining can compromise ability to recognize metastases
    - Careful attention to trimming away fat and quickly freezing thin slices of tissue should minimize artifacts
    - New slides should be prepared when necessary
  - Cautery from surgery can cause smudging and elongation of nuclei
    - In some cases, definitive diagnosis cannot be made

False-Positive Diagnoses

- **Overestimate extent of disease on cytology**
  - Cytology preparations sensitive but do not assess size of metastasis
  - May correctly detect isolated tumor cells in absence of gross lesion
  - Essential to correlate with gross examination and report gross findings to surgeon
- **Benign breast epithelial inclusions**
  - Metastases should resemble primary carcinoma
    - If metastases appear more differentiated than primary carcinoma, benign inclusions should be considered
- **High endothelial venules**
  - Can resemble tubules when close to capsule
  - Erythrocytes in lumens help identify structure as a blood vessel
- **Germinal centers**
  - Germinal centers near capsule can be mistaken for metastatic carcinoma
  - Large lymphocytes may resemble tumor cells
    - Mitotic figures may be present and may raise concern for carcinoma
  - Germinal centers will include variety of cell types, including tingible body macrophages
    - Comparison to other germinal centers in node can be helpful
- **Giant cells and histiocytes**
  - Giant cells and hemosiderin-laden macrophages may be present in nodes due to prior surgery or implants
  - May obscure small foci of metastatic carcinoma
- **Benign transport**
  - Small clusters of epithelial cells can be seen in lymph nodes after core needle biopsy or surgery for benign or malignant disease
    - Most commonly seen with papillary lesions
    - Immunohistochemical studies can confirm presence of myoepithelial cells in some cases
  - Presence of giant cells and hemosiderin-laden macrophages suggested as evidence for benign transport rather than true metastasis
  - Should not be diagnosed in setting of invasive carcinoma
- **Megakaryocytes**
  - Rarely present in lymph nodes
  - Cells have abundant cytoplasm and large, lobated nuclei with stringy chromatin
    - Cells sparse in number

SELECTED REFERENCES

1. Maguire A et al: Sentinel lymph nodes for breast carcinoma: a paradigm shift. Arch Pathol Lab Med. 140(8):791-8, 2016
2. Fellegara G et al: Benign epithelial inclusions in axillary lymph nodes: report of 18 cases and review of the literature. Am J Surg Pathol. 35(8):1123-33, 2011
3. Weaver DL: Pathology evaluation of sentinel lymph nodes in breast cancer: protocol recommendations and rationale. Mod Pathol. 23 Suppl 2:S26-32, 2010

Lymph Node Sampling

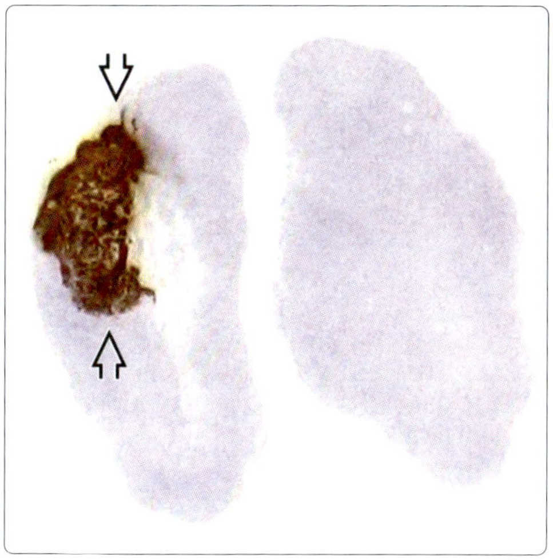

Metastatic Carcinoma: Central Location

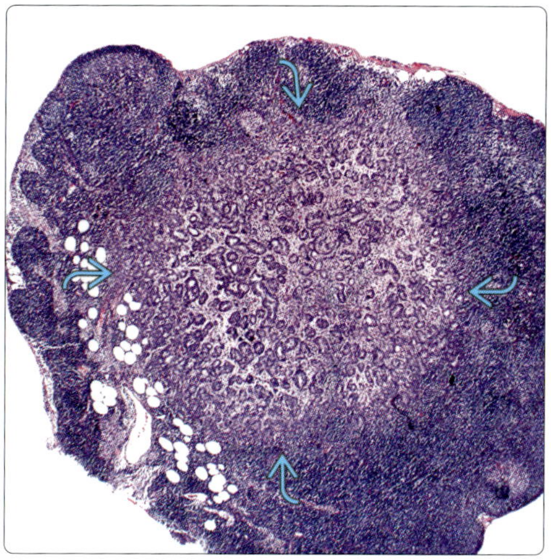

(Left) *Macrometastases are present in only 1/2 of a bisected lymph node in ~ 30% of cases. Therefore, all slices of a grossly negative node must be examined by frozen section or all slices must be sampled for cytology.* **(Right)** *Metastatic carcinoma enters via the afferent lymphatics and is most commonly located in the peripheral sinus adjacent to the capsule. However, occasional metastases are centrally located. The entire surface of the lymph node must be examined.*

Metastatic Carcinoma: Focal Involvement

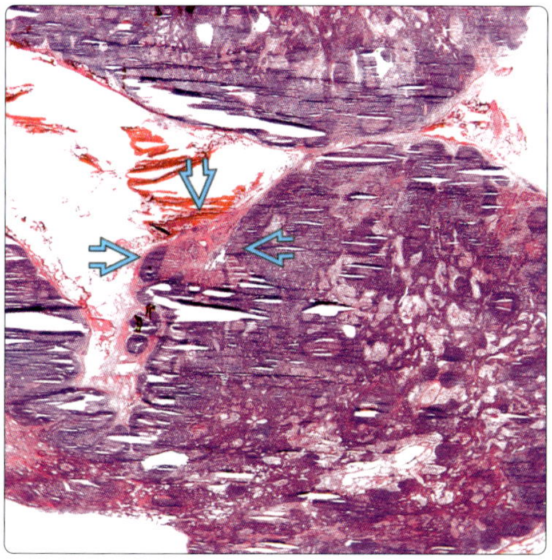

Metastatic Carcinoma: Touch Preparation

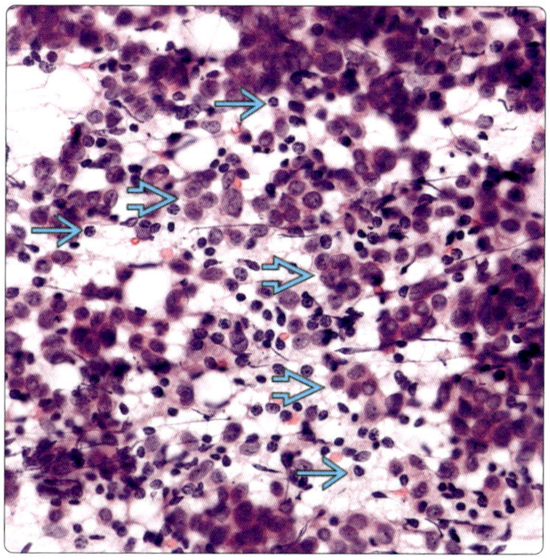

(Left) *Focal involvement of a node by a small metastasis can be difficult to detect. Careful thin sectioning and examination of all slices is important in order to not miss small metastases in large lymph nodes.* **(Right)** *Cytologic preparations are highly suited to documenting metastases in grossly positive lymph nodes. A dual population of neoplastic epithelial cells with large, eccentric atypical nuclei and moderate, dense, eosinophilic cytoplasm, are present in a background of small, mature lymphocytes.*

Lymph Nodes: Inking

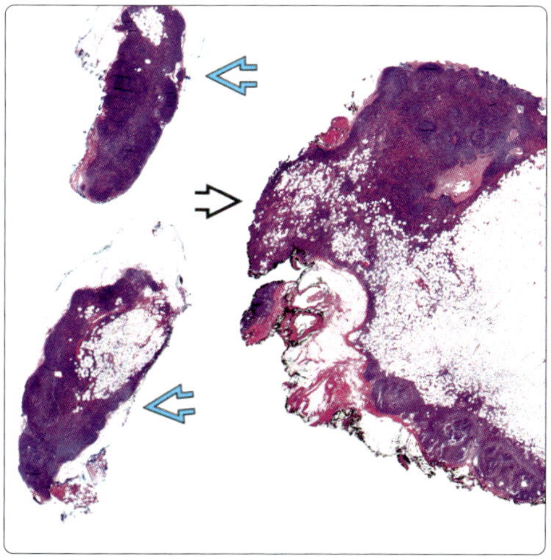

Metastatic Lobular Carcinoma

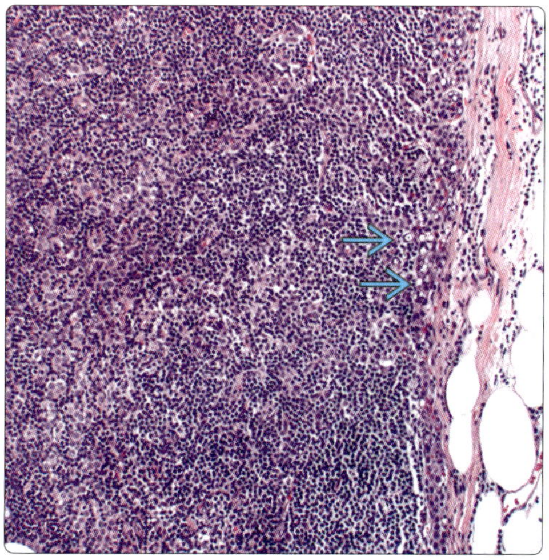

(Left) *The number of positive nodes is an important prognostic factor. This small node has been inked blue and bisected to distinguish it from a 2nd black-inked node. Inking is helpful when multiple small nodes need to be examined.* **(Right)** *Metastatic lobular carcinoma can be very difficult to recognize on frozen section due to the diffuse single cell pattern of infiltration. The cells can closely resemble large lymphocytes or histiocytes. In this case, a few cells with mucin vacuoles help identify the metastasis.*

Lymph Node: Neoadjuvant Therapy

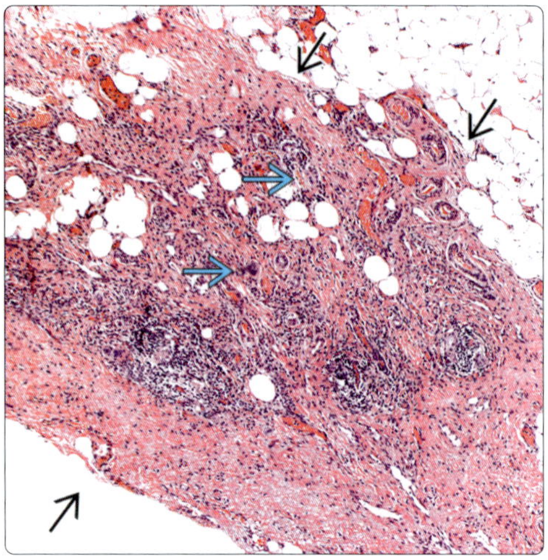

Lymph Node: Neoadjuvant Therapy

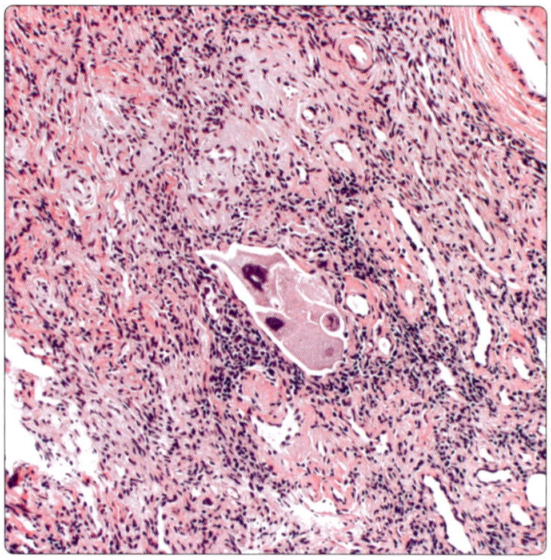

(Left) *A sentinel lymph node may be evaluated after neoadjuvant therapy. Metastases with a marked response to treatment may leave a fibrous scar in the node →. The residual tumor cells can be dispersed and in small clusters →.* **(Right)** *The residual tumor cells after neoadjuvant therapy sometimes show morphological changes, including pleomorphic nuclei and abundant eosinophilic cytoplasm. Although these cells may not be viable, this is not a distinction that can be made on frozen section.*

Small Cell Lymphoma

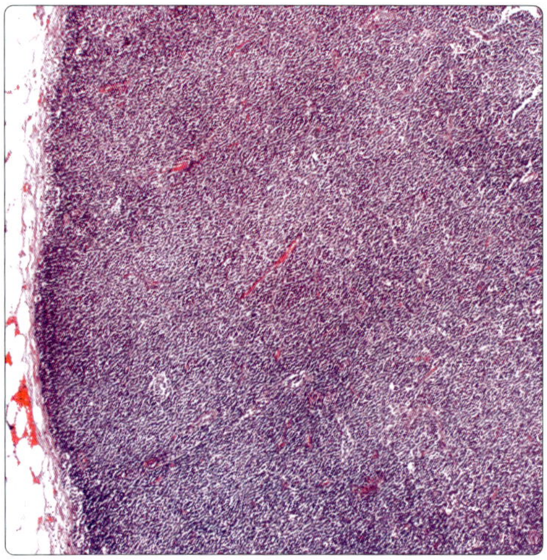

Diffuse Large B-Cell Lymphoma

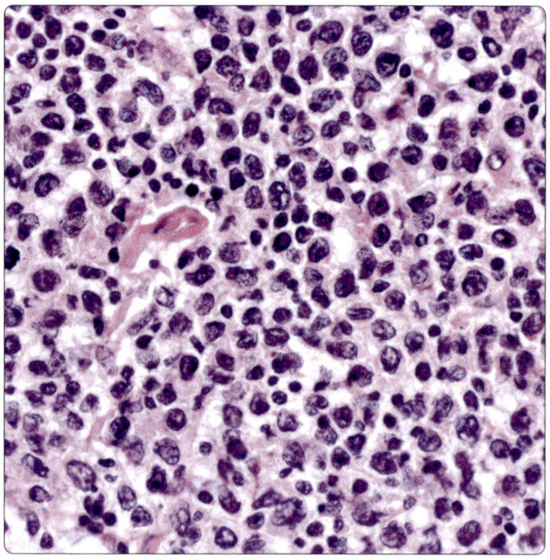

(Left) *Lymphomas can be unexpected findings in nodes evaluated for metastatic carcinoma. Clues to involvement are the effacement of normal architecture and the absence of germinal centers. The peripheral sinuses are obliterated, resulting in a rounded rather than lobulated contour.* **(Right)** *Large cell lymphomas are usually easily identifiable as a malignant tumor. However, it may not be possible to distinguish them from metastatic high-grade lobular carcinoma or melanoma on frozen section.*

Hodgkin Lymphoma

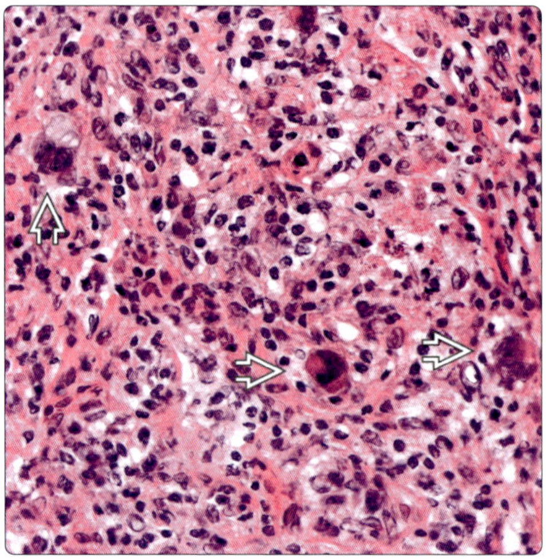

Metastatic Melanoma

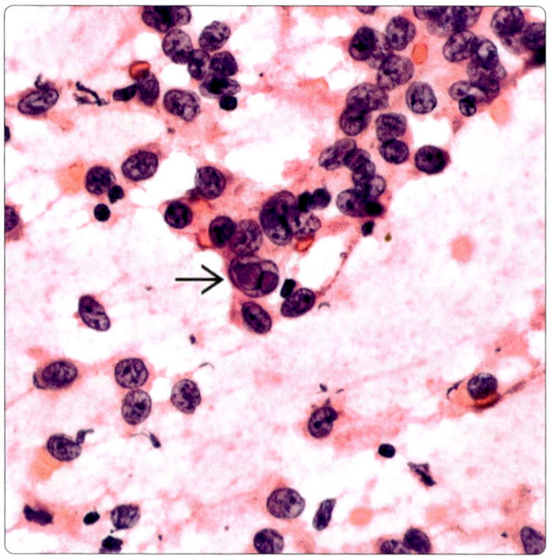

(Left) *Hodgkin lymphoma may present as axillary adenopathy. This example of classic Hodgkin lymphoma shows bi- and multilobed Hodgkin cells → in a background of nonneoplastic lymphocytes. However, diagnostic cells can be scant on frozen section.* **(Right)** *Metastatic melanoma to an axillary lymph node may arise from an upper trunk primary, but in some cases the primary may be unknown. This cytologic scrape preparation shows atypical epithelioid cells with characteristic intranuclear inclusions →.*

Mimic of Metastasis: Blood Vessels

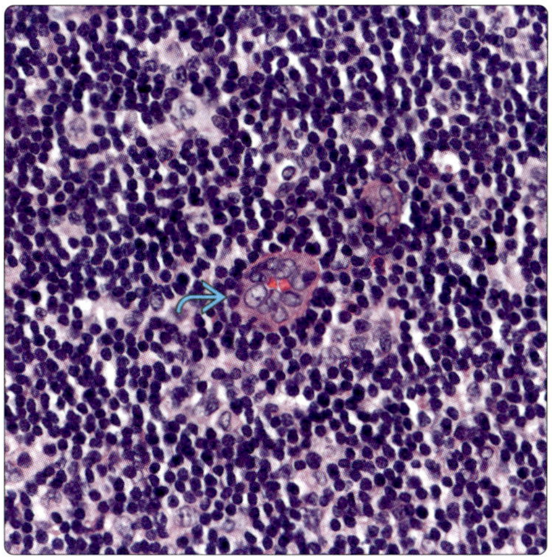

Mimic of Metastasis: Histiocytes

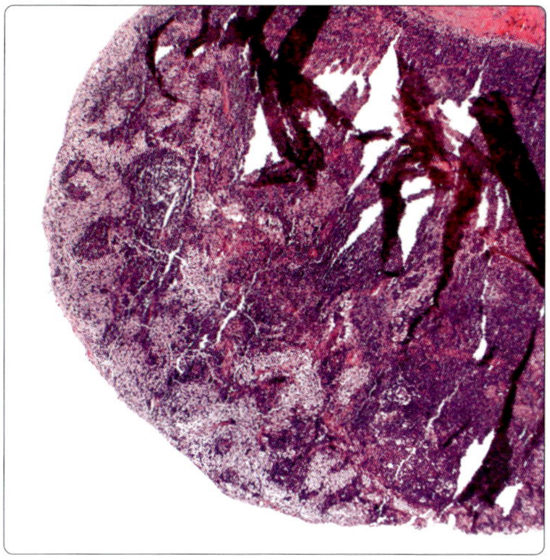

(Left) *Rounded capillaries lined by plump endothelial cells* *can resemble the tubules of adenocarcinoma on frozen section. The presence of luminal erythrocytes demonstrate that the structure is a blood vessel.* **(Right)** *Abundant histiocytes in a subcapsular location can resemble metastatic carcinoma at low power. However, the cells will generally be easily recognizable as histiocytes when more closely examined.*

Mimic of Metastasis: Histiocytes

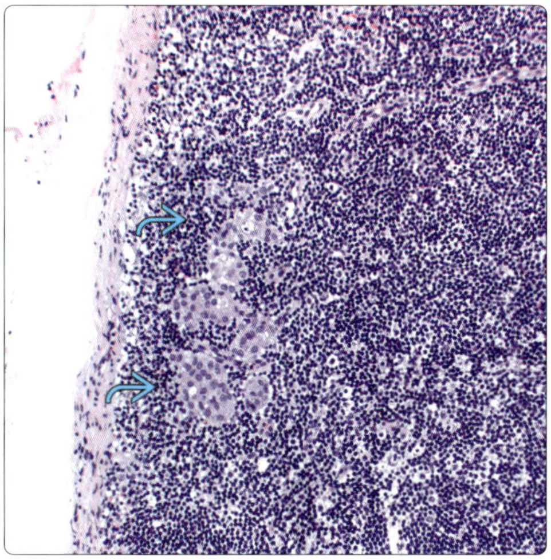

Mimic of Metastasis: Giant Cells

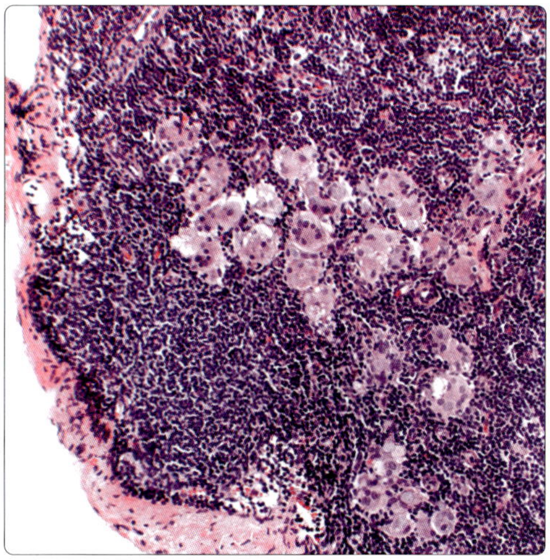

(Left) *Histiocytes* *can occasionally aggregate or cluster in peripheral sinuses such that they mimic metastatic carcinoma. The abundant cytoplasm, often with hemosiderin, is helpful in recognizing the cells as benign.* **(Right)** *Prior biopsy procedures or breast implants may result in a giant cell response in lymph nodes. Multinucleated giant cells with abundant cytoplasm are generally easily distinguished from carcinoma.*

Mimic of Metastasis: Germinal Center

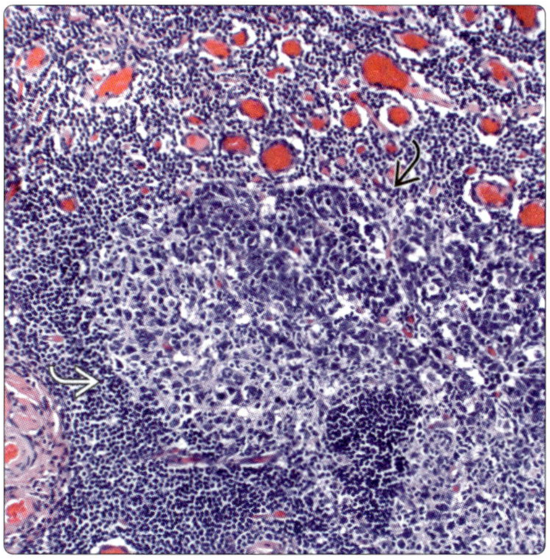

Metastatic Carcinoma Resembling Germinal Center

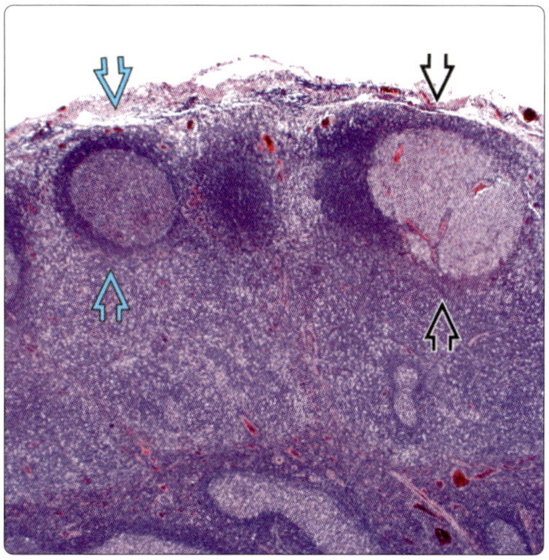

(Left) *This germinal center is located near the periphery of a lymph node and was mistaken for a metastatic carcinoma due to the presence of large lymphocytes and mitoses. The normal light* *and dark* *zones are present. Tingible body macrophages are an important clue.* **(Right)** *This metastatic carcinoma* *could be mistaken for a germinal center* *due to its location and rounded shape.*

(Left) *Benign inclusions often have the appearance of well-formed tubules. Endosalpingiosis can occur in axillary lymph nodes. These glands do not have myoepithelial cells but may have cilia. Immunoperoxidase studies may be necessary to document that they are not metastatic carcinoma.* **(Right)** *Some benign epithelial inclusions have a myoepithelial layer* ➔*, and some are associated with surrounding breast-like stroma. These inclusions are very rare compared to metastatic carcinoma.*

Mimic of Metastasis: Endosalpingiosis

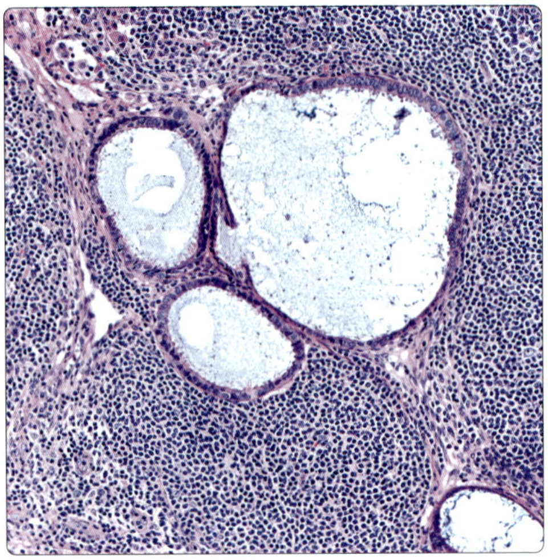

Mimic of Metastasis: Benign Epithelial Inclusion

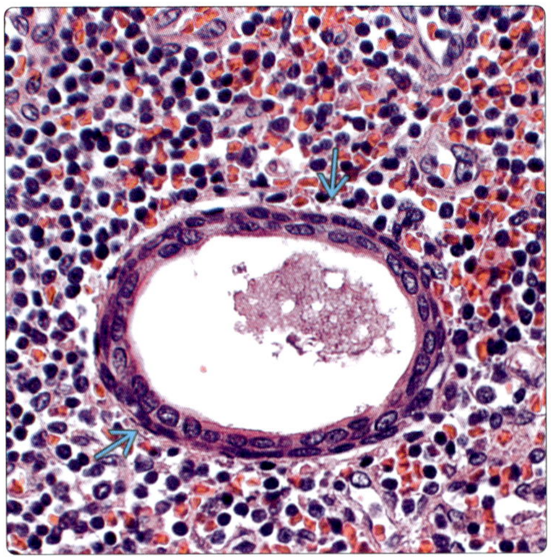

(Left) *Megakaryocytes are occasionally present in nodes* ➔*. They are distinguished from carcinoma by large, convoluted nuclei with smudgy cytoplasm and abundant cytoplasm.* **(Right)** *Nevus cell nests are typically seen in the capsule of lymph nodes. This frozen section shows the characteristic grouped cell arrangement, intracapsular location, and bland uniform nuclei in fibrous stroma. The cells are larger than lymphocytes.*

Mimic of Metastasis: Megakaryocytes

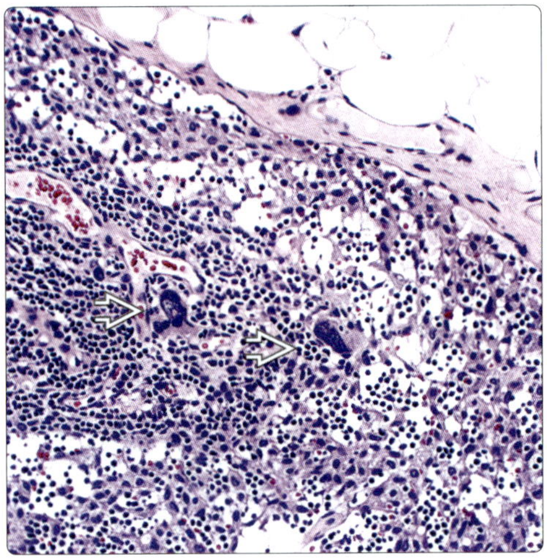

Capsular Nevus Cell Nest

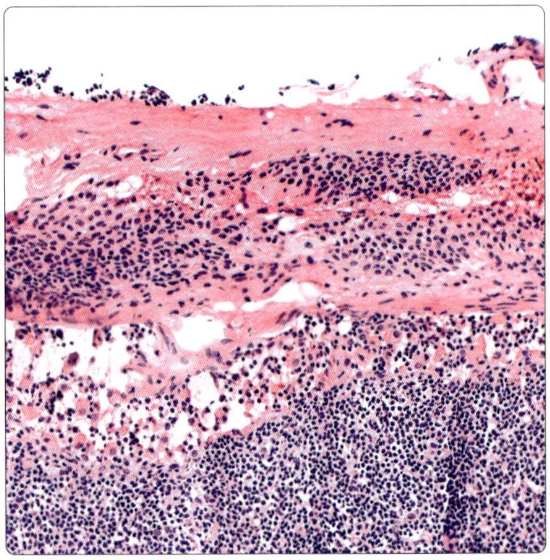

(Left) *A nodal melanocytic nevus is comprised of uniform ovoid cells, some with nuclear grooves, and focal melanin pigment.* **(Right)** *This nevus cell nest* ➔ *is present within a lymph node rather than the usual location in the capsule. In this unusual location, the cells could be mistaken for a metastasis if not recognized as neval cells.*

Capsular Nevus Cell Nest

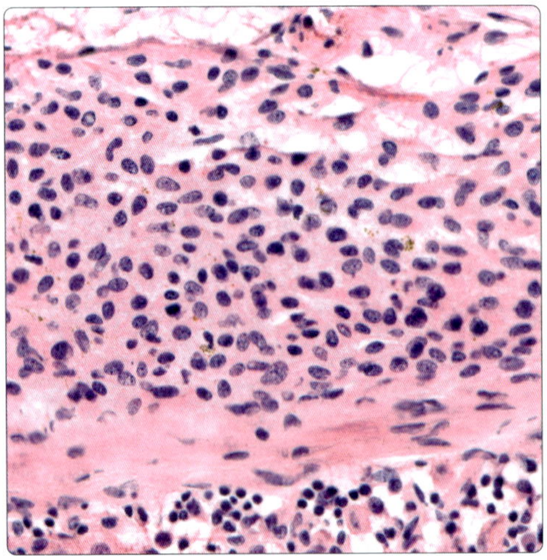

Nevus Cell Nest in Septa of Lymph Node

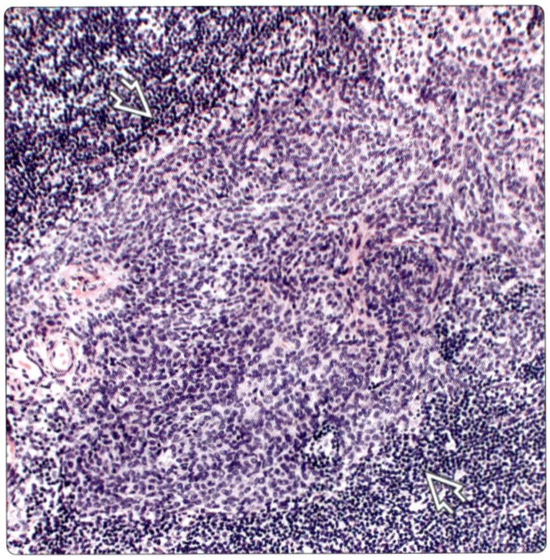

Sarcoidosis

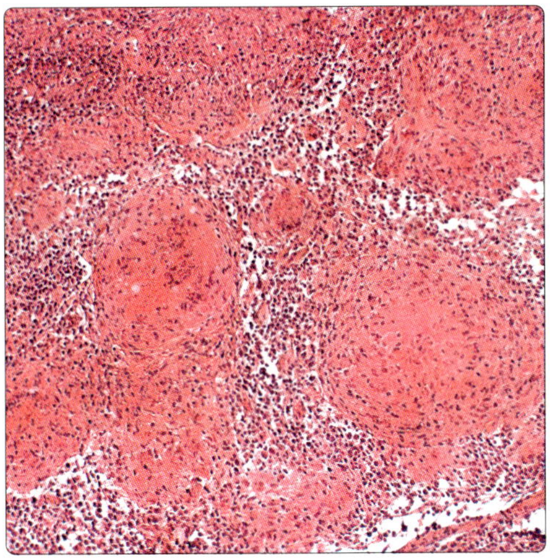

Silicone Reaction

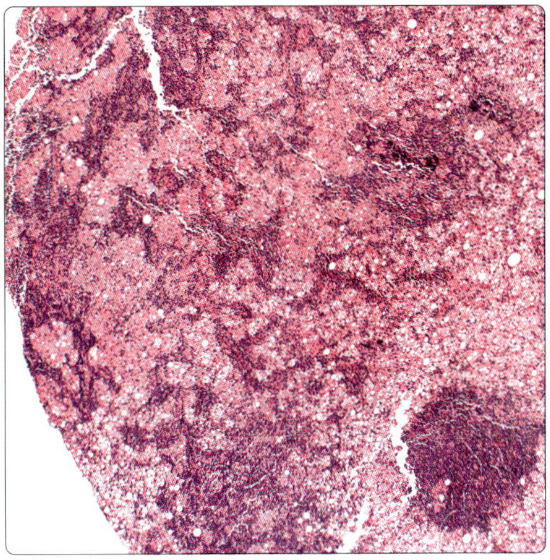

(Left) *Sarcoidosis is a rare finding in an axillary node. Noncaseating granulomas are typical. Infectious etiologies as well as Hodgkin lymphoma associated with granulomas should be considered.* **(Right)** *Silicone granulomas in a node can be hard and gritty when sectioned, mimicking carcinoma on gross examination. The silicone originates in a breast implant that may have ruptured. Metastatic carcinoma can be present in areas of silicone.*

Psammoma Body

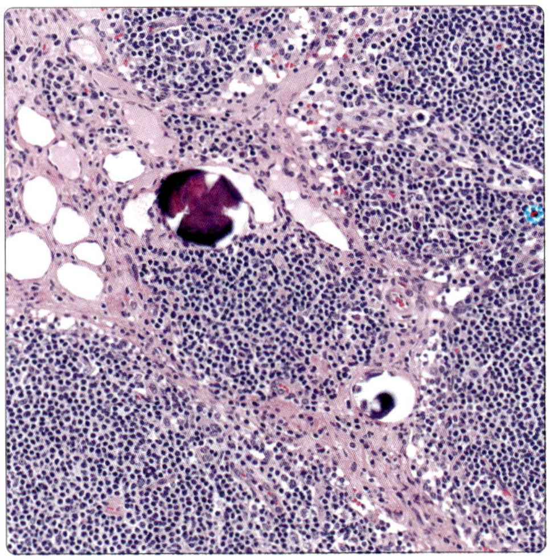

Lymph Node: Folding of Section

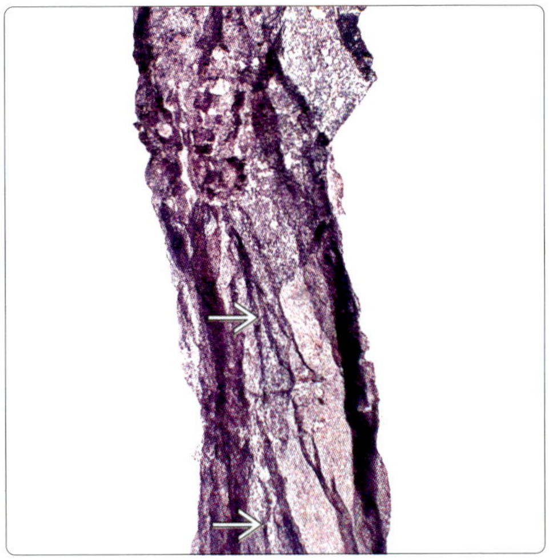

(Left) *Calcifications in axillary nodes may be associated with metastatic breast cancer, metastatic ovarian cancer, or endosalpingiosis. Papillary thyroid cancer would be very unusual at this site.* **(Right)** *This metastasis ➔ is difficult to detect due to the marked folding of the tissue. Additional slides should be prepared for optimal evaluation.*

Cautery Artifact

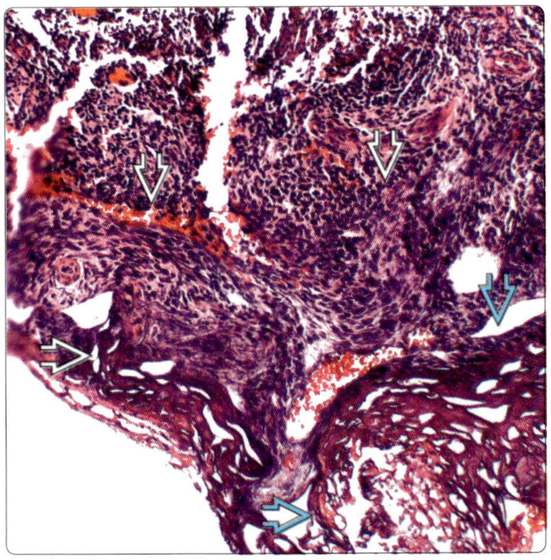

Lymph Node: Uneven Staining

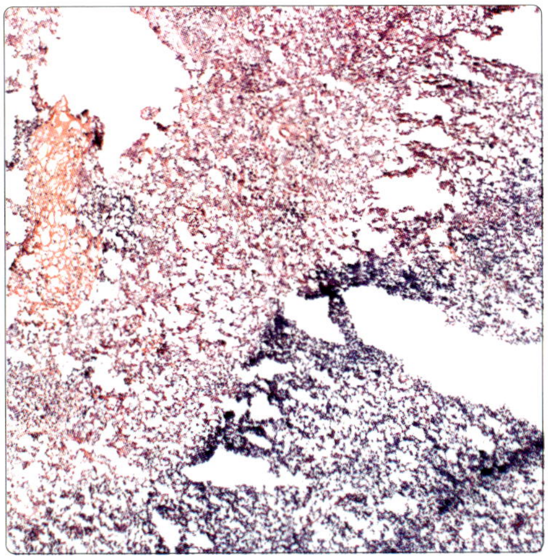

(Left) *Cautery artifact from the removal of a node can cause coagulative necrosis ➔ and elongation of cells ➔, precluding optimal evaluation of a lymph node. These changes could be misinterpreted as metastatic carcinoma or obscure detection of a metastasis.* **(Right)** *The metastasis in this lymph node is more difficult to detect due to the marked ice crystal artifact and uneven staining.*

Contents

SURGICAL/CLINICAL CONSIDERATIONS

Goal of Consultation

- Evaluate peritoneal or inguinal lymph nodes for staging of known carcinoma or to evaluate lymphadenopathy

Change in Patient Management

- Planned surgical procedure for curative intent may be modified or cancelled if metastatic carcinoma is found

Clinical Setting

- Enlarged nodes may be detected during surgery for benign condition
  - If malignant, additional surgical exploration and biopsies may be performed to detect primary carcinoma
- Nodes may be sampled for staging of known carcinomas of abdominal cavity prior to definitive surgery
- For some neoplasms, surgical approach will be altered if metastatic malignancy is detected
  - Pancreatic carcinoma: Pancreatectomy would not be performed
  - Prostate carcinoma: Prostatectomy may not be performed
    - Lymph nodes are no longer commonly evaluated intraoperatively
    - Preoperative serum prostate specific antigen and imaging studies can detect most cases of metastatic carcinoma
- For other neoplasms, surgical treatment is indicated even if metastatic malignancy is present but in some cases may be modified
  - Colon carcinoma: Resection would be performed to relieve/prevent obstruction and control bleeding
  - Ovarian carcinoma: Debulking (cytoreduction) may be performed, depending on size of tumor deposits
- For many neoplasms, extent of surgical treatment may be modified based on presence or absence of metastasis on frozen section
  - Germ cell tumors: Debulking of gross metastatic disease is generally performed
    - Extent of dissection may be greater if frozen section shows viable tumor after treatment
  - Vulvar carcinoma: Absence of tumor in sentinel Cloquet node (superior most deep inguinal node) may indicate lack of need for extensive inguinal dissection
  - Malignant melanoma: Absence of tumor in sentinel Cloquet node may indicate lack of need for extensive inguinal dissection
  - Radical cystectomy for urothelial carcinoma: More extensive nodal dissection may be indicated when frozen sections show metastases in true pelvis
  - Gastric cancer: Some studies indicate more limited surgery may be permissible in patients with negative sentinel lymph nodes, evaluated on intraoperative frozen section
  - Renal cell carcinoma: Absence of tumor in clinically enlarged retroperitoneal lymph nodes may obviate need for more extended node dissection
  - Penile carcinoma: If metastatic tumor is found on frozen section, modified bilateral inguinal lymph node dissection may be converted to classic ilioinguinal lymph node dissection
  - Cervical carcinoma
    - Abdominal radical trachelectomy (rather than radical hysterectomy) has been used to treat patients with frozen section-negative sentinel lymph nodes
    - Positive lymph nodes may precipitate truncated procedure, and addition of neoadjuvant therapy prior to definitive surgery
- For other neoplasms, specific diagnosis can modify how tissue is allocated for special studies
  - Lymphoma: Submission of tissue in special fixatives and for flow cytometry

SPECIMEN EVALUATION

Gross

- Specimen usually consists of excision of nodule presumed grossly to be lymph node
- If surrounded by adipose tissue, nodule should be separated by palpation and dissection

Metastatic Colonic Adenocarcinoma

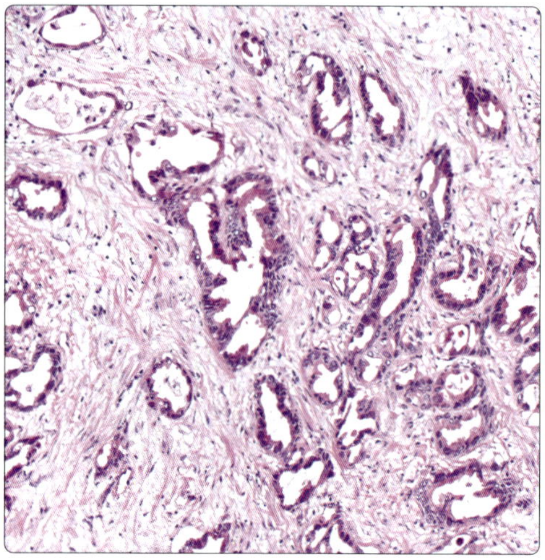

Metastatic Cholangiocarcinoma

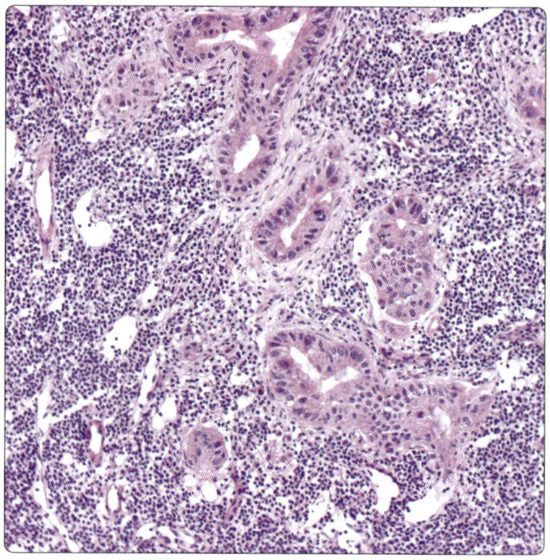

(Left) *Metastases should resemble the primary carcinoma. These irregularly sized and shaped glands comprised of atypical columnar cells elicit a striking desmoplastic reaction, similar to that seen in primary colonic adenocarcinoma.* **(Right)** *The morphology of this metastatic adenocarcinoma is relatively nonspecific, and could be consistent with any pancreaticobiliary site. In this case, the patient had a history of cholangiocarcinoma.*

  - Size and contours (e.g., smooth or irregular) of nodule are recorded
- Nodule is serially sectioned
  - Focal firm white areas are typical of metastatic carcinoma
  - Diffusely enlarged node with fleshy surface is most likely lymphoma
  - Hard, calcified, difficult to cut nodule is most likely infarcted epiploic appendage
  - Mottled nodes with focal necrosis may be involved by infectious process

Frozen Section

- If patient has known carcinoma and biopsy is performed for staging prior to performing surgery, it is preferable to submit entire node for frozen section
  - If only portion of node is frozen, small metastasis can be missed
- If patient does not have known carcinoma, specimen should be sampled such that diagnosis will be possible on permanent sections &/or with ancillary studies
  - Nonfrozen tissue for ancillary studies may be helpful
  - Cytologic preparations are preferred if infection or lymphoma are suspected

Cytology

- Scrape or touch preparations can be made from cut surface(s) of node
- If cytologic preparations do not provide diagnosis, portion of node may be frozen

MOST COMMON DIAGNOSES

Metastatic Malignancy

- Typically, histomorphology resembles that of primary tumor
  - Location and histologic type of known or suspected primary carcinoma is essential information
  - This information will often be known through preoperative records review, or if specimen is submitted as part of sentinel lymph node protocol
- If suspected metastasis does not resemble primary, consider other diagnoses
- Some tumors may elicit obscuring inflammatory responses
  - Granulomatous response: Seminoma, Hodgkin disease, rarely adenocarcinoma
- When there is known neoplasm, most likely to be involved nodes are typically sampled (sentinel or nonsentinel lymph nodes)
  - Cloquet node (deep inguinal node)
    - Vulvar squamous cell carcinoma
    - Malignant melanoma of lower extremity
  - Pelvic lymph nodes
    - Adenocarcinoma of prostate (men)
    - Squamous cell carcinoma of cervix (women)
    - Urothelial carcinoma of bladder
    - Adenocarcinoma of endometrium
  - Paraaortic lymph nodes
    - Pancreatic head adenocarcinoma
    - Germ cell malignancies of testis
    - Adenocarcinoma of endometrium
  - Inguinal lymph nodes
    - Squamous cell carcinoma of penis (men)
    - Squamous cell carcinoma of vulva (women)
    - Malignant melanoma of lower extremity
  - Retroperitoneum
    - Real cell carcinoma
    - Testicular germ cell tumors
  - Perigastric
    - Adenocarcinoma of stomach

Endosalpingiosis (Müllerian Inclusions)

- In women, benign tubular epithelium can be found in lymph nodes
  - May be associated with psammoma body calcifications
  - Very rarely present in males
  - Usually in capsule or medullary sinuses
- Tubules are lined by single layer of low cuboidal cells
  - Nuclei are small with inconspicuous nuclei
  - Cilia may be present
- Squamous metaplasia can occur

Ectopic Decidua

- Stromal tissue, under influence of progesterone during pregnancy, can undergo decidual changes
  - Changes can occur in lymph nodes, omentum, and peritoneum
  - May be present in pregnant or postpartum women
- Stromal cells resemble epithelial cells
  - Large cells with abundant granular eosinophilic cytoplasm
  - Present in solid nests in subcapsular sinuses of node
  - Loosely cohesive, but clustering can create impression of sheets of epithelial cells
  - Oval to round nuclei with prominent nucleoli
  - May be associated with myxoid stroma
- Cytoplasm can also have marked vacuolization
  - Can closely resemble signet ring cells &/or mucinous carcinoma &/or squamous cell carcinoma
- May be present in multiple nodes in single patient

Mesothelial Inclusions

- May be associated with effusions or mesothelial hyperplasia of peritoneum
  - Very rare in abdomen
- Present as single cells and small clusters
  - Located in sinuses and limited to node

Lymphoma

- Multiple enlarged nodes with fleshy, uniform appearance are most suggestive of lymphoma
  - Hodgkin lymphoma can be associated with prominent granulomatous reaction
- Cytologic preparations are typically highly cellular with monomorphic population
  - Intraoperative diagnosis of "suspicious for lymphoproliferative disorder" can be sufficient
  - Tissue is triaged for special studies
  - Cytologic evaluation is best method to preserve tissue for ancillary studies
- If lymphoma is suspected, non-cryostat-frozen tissue should be reserved for ancillary studies if possible
  - Special fixatives (B-Plus and others)
  - RPMI or other preservative for flow cytometry

- Snap-frozen tissue for molecular studies (depending on institution)
- Stained/unstained touch imprints for Romanowsky-stained slides

Reactive Changes

- Enlarged nodes may be reaction to prior surgery, inflammation, trauma, or disease
- Large germinal centers cause outer contour of node to be lobulated
- Lymph node sinuses should be open
- Various patterns of reactive change include but are not limited to
  - Follicular hyperplasia
  - Sinus histiocytosis
  - Granulomatous lymphadenitis
  - Dermatopathic lymphadenopathy
  - Vascular transformation
- Clinically enlarged nodes may be due to fatty replacement

Epiploic Appendage

- Outpouchings of peritoneum can twist and infarct
  - Resulting area of fat necrosis often calcifies
  - Area feels like hard mass to surgeon, similar to metastatic carcinoma to lymph node
- Due to dense calcification, it may not be possible to section mass
  - In these cases, presumptive diagnosis of infarcted epiploic appendage can be made

Endometriosis

- More common in lymph nodes in patients with pelvic endometriosis
- Well-formed endometrial glands are associated with stroma
- Hemosiderin is often present

Sarcoidosis

- Results in enlarged, firm nodes due to confluent noncaseating granulomas
- Metastatic seminoma and Hodgkin disease can also be associated with granulomatous reaction
- When possible, tissue should be submitted for culture

Tuberculosis

- Peritoneal tuberculosis can mimic advanced ovarian carcinoma
  - Patients may present with adnexal mass, ascites, enlarged lymph nodes, and peritoneal involvement
- Tissue should be submitted for microbiological culture when possible

Nevus Cell Nests

- Benign epithelioid to spindle cells with bland nuclei present in capsule of lymph node
  - Rarely within lymph node septa

Endothelial Cells

- Prominent endothelial cells can mimic metastasis when close to peripheral sinus of lymph node
  - Can mimic tubules or solid nests of cells when lumen is not seen
- Cells can have moderate amount of cytoplasm, large nuclei, and small nucleoli
- On deeper levels, blood cells can sometimes be seen within lumen
- Should be similar in appearance to adjacent more obvious blood vessels

Lymphangiomyomatosis

- Rare disease occurring predominantly in young women
- Abnormal proliferation of smooth muscle around dilated lymphatic channels
- Most commonly involves lung but can also involve uterus and adjacent lymph nodes
- Involvement of nodes could be mistaken for metastatic leiomyosarcoma

REPORTING

Frozen Section

- Report "metastatic carcinoma" for cases with known primary carcinoma
  - For cases without diagnosed primary carcinoma, additional information concerning most likely primary site can be helpful to surgeon
- For nodes without metastatic carcinoma, preliminary diagnosis is usually sufficient
  - Report "suspicious for lymphoproliferative disorder; tissue taken for ancillary studies" if findings suggest lymphoma
  - Report "noncaseating granulomas; tissue taken for microbiologic culture" if findings suggest infection

Cytology

- If node is grossly abnormal, diagnosis can usually be provided

PITFALLS

Carcinoma vs. Benign Inclusions

- Possibility of benign inclusion instead of metastatic carcinoma should always be considered, especially in women
- Metastases almost always resemble primary carcinoma

Granulomas Obscuring Tumor

- Some malignant tumors are associated with marked granulomatous response
  - Most frequently seen with seminoma and Hodgkin lymphoma

SELECTED REFERENCES

1. Deng X et al: Abdominal radical trachelectomy guided by sentinel lymph node biopsy for stage IB1 cervical cancer with tumors >2 cm. Oncotarget. 8(2):3422-3429, 2017
2. Tempfer CB et al: Lymphatic spread of endometriosis to pelvic sentinel lymph nodes: a prospective clinical study. Fertil Steril. 96(3):692-6, 2011
3. Acikalin MF et al: Mesothelial pelvic lymph node inclusion in a patient with ovarian microinvasive borderline mucinous tumor: case report with review of the literature. Int J Gynecol Cancer. 17(4):917-21, 2007
4. Wu DC et al: Ectopic decidua of pelvic lymph nodes: a potential diagnostic pitfall. Arch Pathol Lab Med. 129(5):e117-20, 2005
5. Argani P et al: Hyperplastic mesothelial cells in lymph nodes: report of six cases of a benign process that can stimulate metastatic involvement by mesothelioma or carcinoma. Hum Pathol. 29(4):339-46, 1998

Metastatic Pancreatic Carcinoma

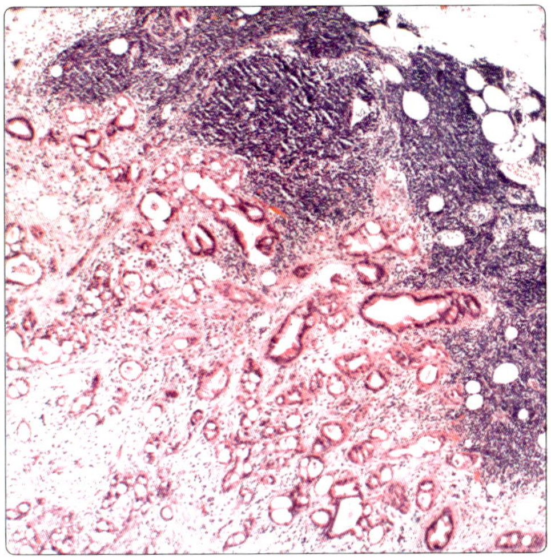

Metastatic Pancreatic Neuroendocrine Carcinoma

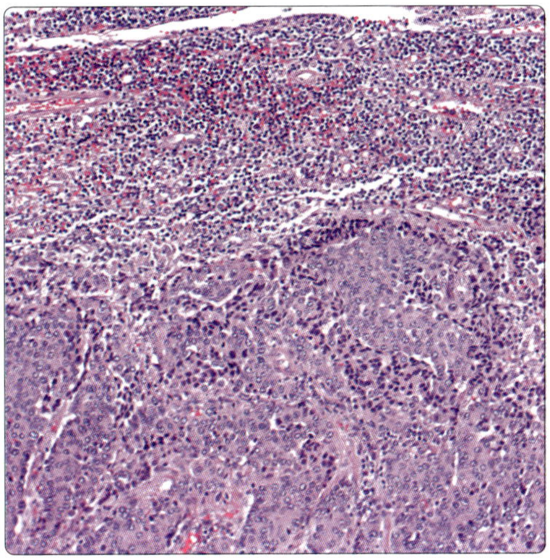

(Left) *Metastatic pancreatic carcinoma consists of small acini, usually with bland nuclei. Columnar cells with mucin may be present. The presence of metastatic pancreatic carcinoma usually precludes any benefit from resection of the pancreas.* **(Right)** *This high-grade metastatic neuroendocrine carcinoma of the pancreas shows a nested pattern and is comprised of large epithelioid cells with relatively uniform nuclei. Mitoses are readily observed.*

Metastatic Colon Carcinoma

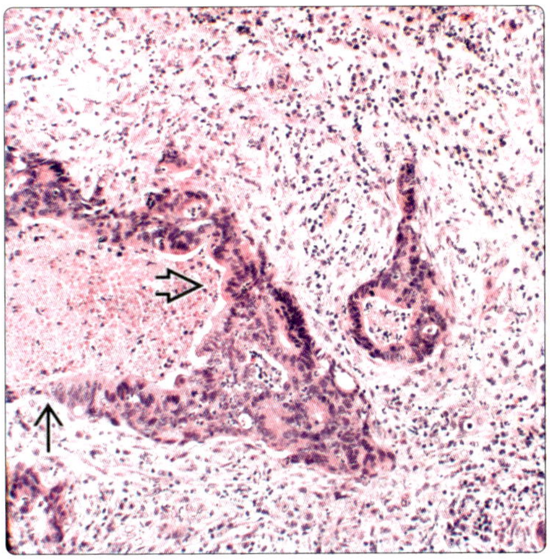

Metastatic Mucinous Adenocarcinoma

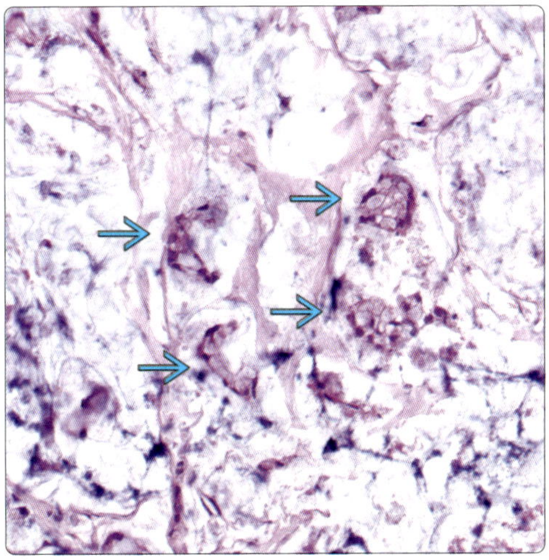

(Left) *The most likely primary site of a carcinoma in a patient without known malignancy can often be predicted based on the histologic appearance of a metastasis. Metastatic colon carcinoma is characterized by tall columnar cells ⇨ and gland walls destroyed by dirty necrosis →.* **(Right)** *This colon primary tumor maintained its histologic character as a metastatic lesion, with clusters of glands formed by atypical goblet cells in a mucinous background →.*

Metastatic Hepatocellular Carcinoma

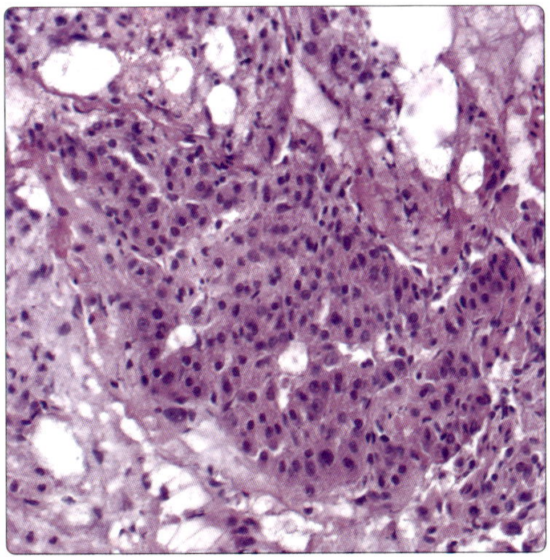

Metastatic Gastric Signet Ring Cell Adenocarcinoma

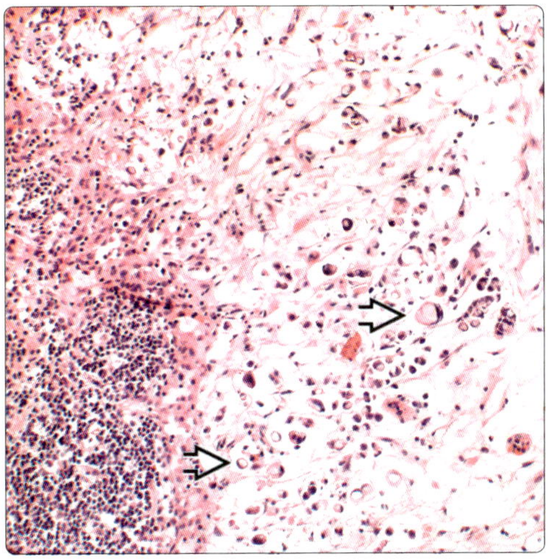

(Left) *It is unusual for hepatocellular carcinoma to metastasize. This tumor deposit shows packeted cuboidal epithelial cells with moderate granular eosinophilic cytoplasm and centrally placed nuclei with prominent nucleoli.* **(Right)** *Metastatic signet ring cell carcinoma of the stomach can be quite subtle when only rare signet ring cells ⇨ are present. Metastatic lobular carcinoma of the breast should also be considered, particularly if the primary site is unknown.*

Contents

(Left) *Metastatic clear cell renal cell carcinoma is usually easily identified in a lymph node . The presence of blood lakes due to the delicate vasculature are very characteristic of this tumor.* **(Right)** *Metastatic renal cell carcinoma is often associated with blood lakes , both grossly and microscopically. This is due to the delicate vasculature within the tumor. The tumor cells often appear quite bland.*

Metastatic Renal Cell Carcinoma

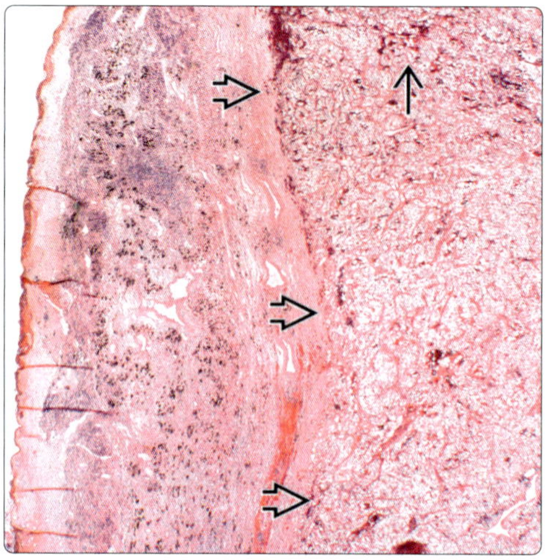

Metastatic Renal Cell Carcinoma

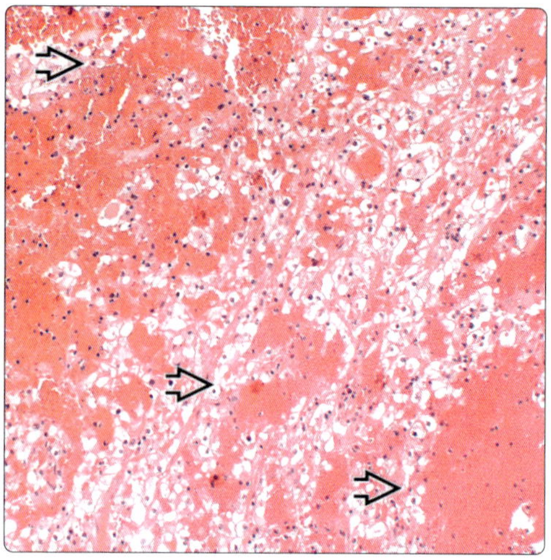

(Left) *Seminoma can be associated with a granulomatous response . The tumor cells are located between the granulomas and can be focal and easily missed . Hodgkin disease can also be associated with granulomas.* **(Right)** *Seminomas consist of dyscohesive cells with large nuclei and large boxcar-shaped nucleoli . When associated with a granulomatous response, the tumor cells may be difficult to see.*

Metastatic Seminoma: Granulomatous Response

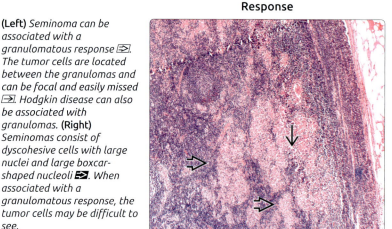

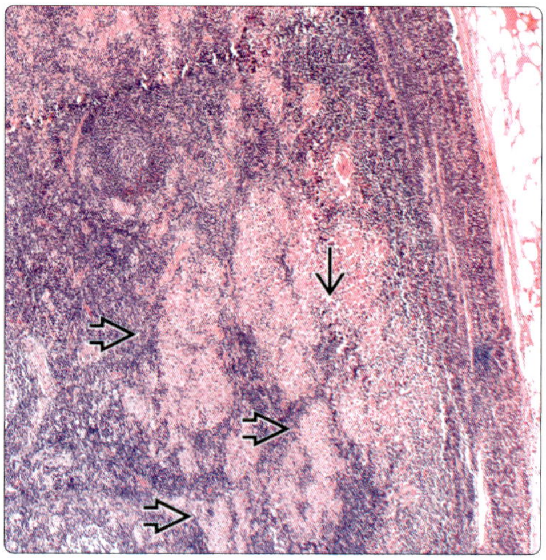

Metastatic Seminoma

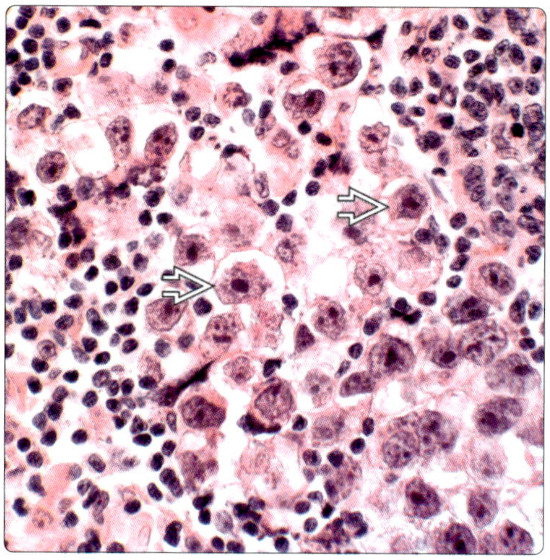

(Left) *Metastatic germ cell tumors can have multiple patterns. In this node, both embryonal carcinoma and a yolk sac tumor are present.* **(Right)** *There is extensive replacement of this node by metastatic prostate carcinoma with crisply formed glands comprised of columnar cells with abundant light pink cytoplasm and basally oriented nuclei with prominent nucleoli.*

Metastatic Embryonal Cell Carcinoma

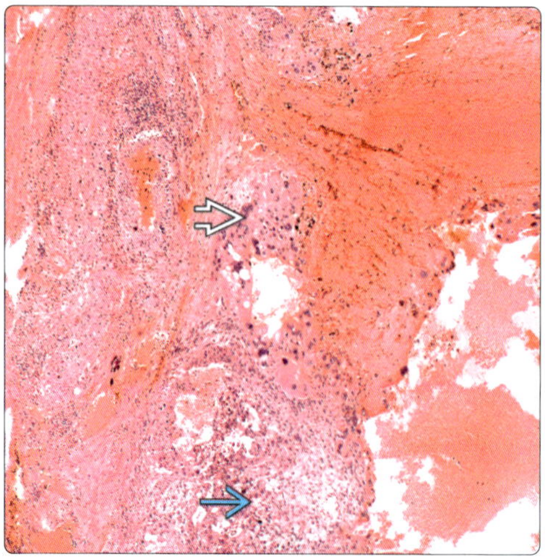

Metastatic Prostate Carcinoma

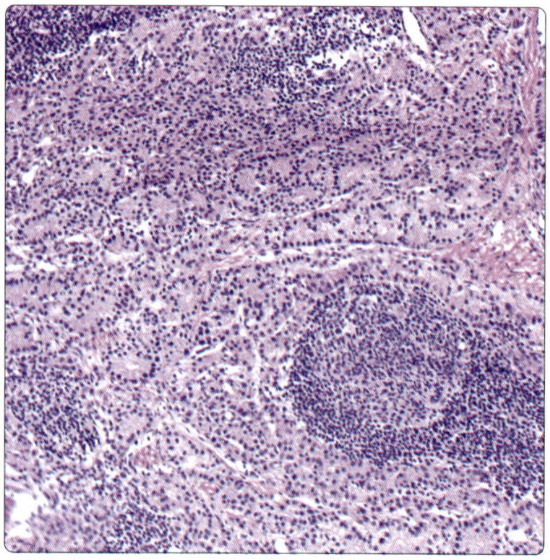

Metastatic Müllerian Serous Carcinoma

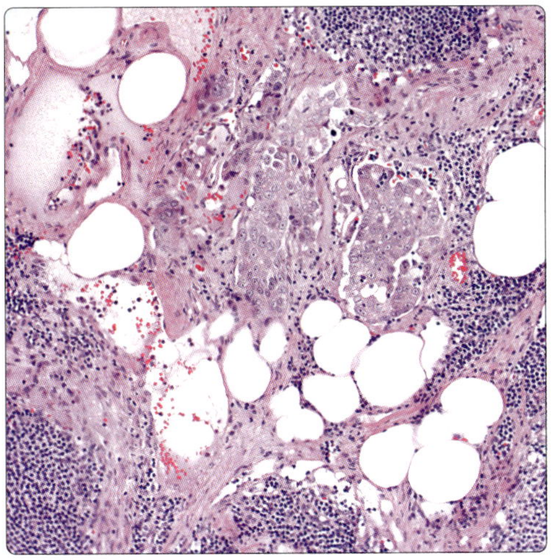

Metastatic Müllerian Serous Carcinoma

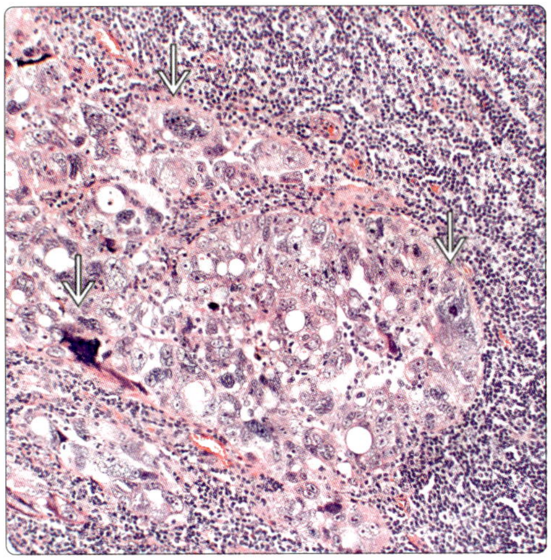

(Left) *This lymph node shows, in addition to fatty replacement, nests of markedly atypical large epithelioid cells with moderate eosinophilic cytoplasm, and large nuclei with vesicular chromatin and prominent nucleoli. There is abortive gland formation, and clefting between tumor nests and adjacent lymph node stroma.* **(Right)** *Metastatic papillary serous carcinoma typically has markedly enlarged and pleomorphic nuclei* ➡. *Psammoma body calcifications may be present.*

Metastatic Cervical Clear Cell Carcinoma

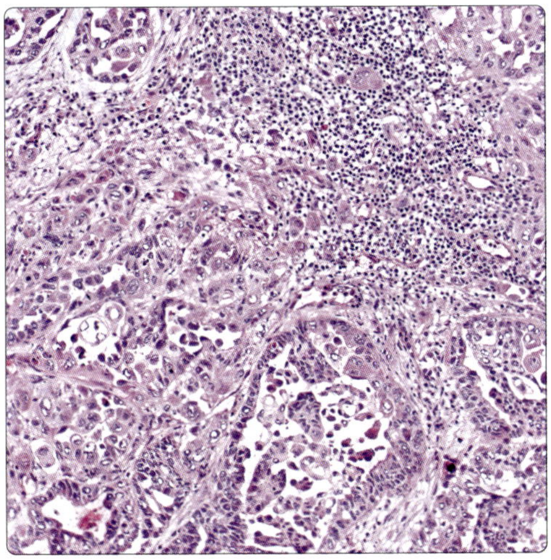

Metastatic Endometrioid Adenocarcinoma

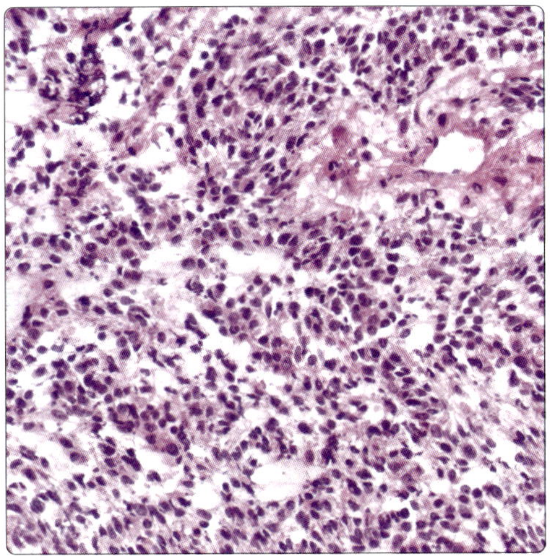

(Left) *This clear cell carcinoma, showing glandular and micropapillary growth of clear and hobnail cells with markedly atypical nuclei, originated in the uterine cervix.* **(Right)** *Lymph node sampling remains a standard procedure for staging of endometrial carcinoma, although frozen sections are rarely submitted. This endometrioid carcinoma shows a solid growth pattern, consistent with FIGO grade 3.*

Decidua

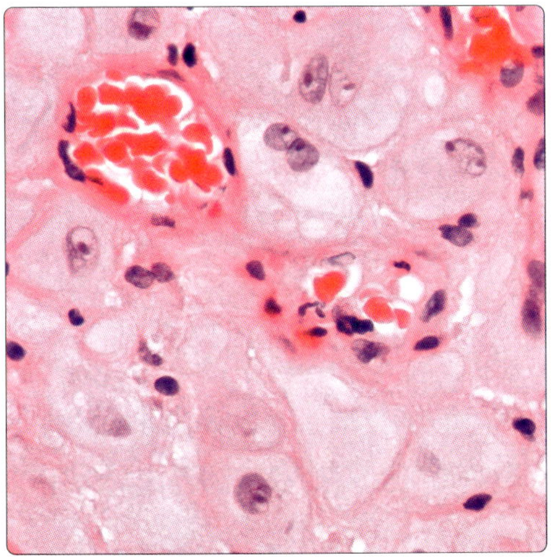

Decidual Reaction With Vacuolization

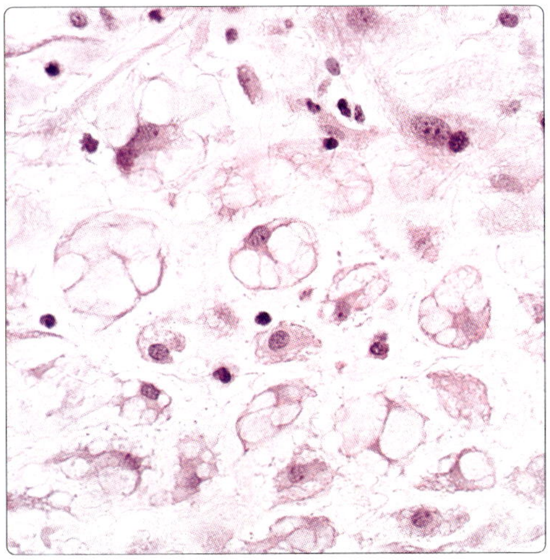

(Left) *In pregnant women, cells in lymph nodes, omentum, and peritoneum can undergo decidualization. The cells have an epithelioid appearance with enlarged nuclei, prominent nucleoli, and abundant cytoplasm. (Courtesy M. Nucci, MD.)* **(Right)** *Ectopic decidua can show prominent cytoplasmic vacuolization and can closely resemble metastatic mucinous adenocarcinoma. Note that the cells have a low nuclear:cytoplasmic ratio and the nuclei have bland cytomorphologic features. (Courtesy M. Nucci, MD.)*

Small Lymphocytic Lymphoma/Chronic Lymphocytic Leukemia

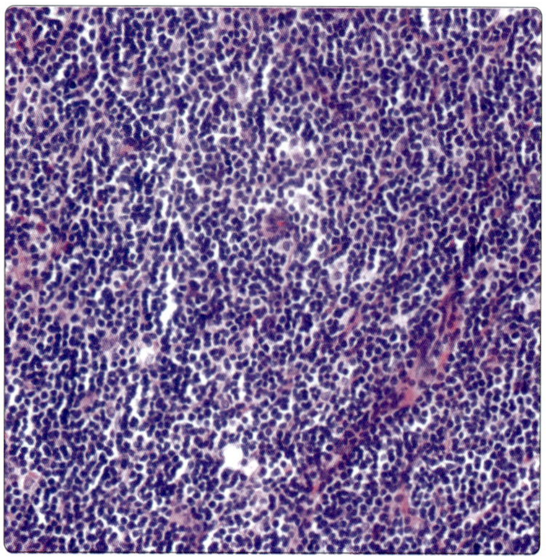

Mantle Cell Lymphoma

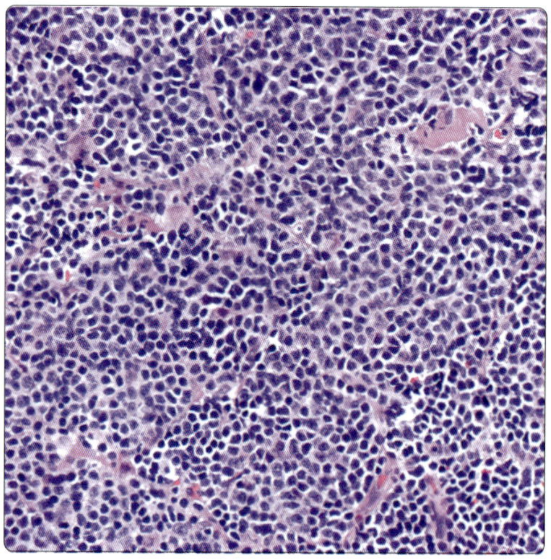

(Left) *In this case, there is effacement of nodal architecture by a monomorphic population of small mature lymphocytes. Touch preps may be helpful. A definite intraoperative diagnosis is not required, but tissue for flow cytometry may be highly useful.* **(Right)** *In this mantle cell lymphoma, there is diffuse effacement of the nodal architecture by a proliferation of slightly enlarged lymphocytes with "intermediate" features between those of lymphocytic lymphoma and the cleaved cells of follicular lymphoma.*

Diffuse Large B-Cell Lymphoma

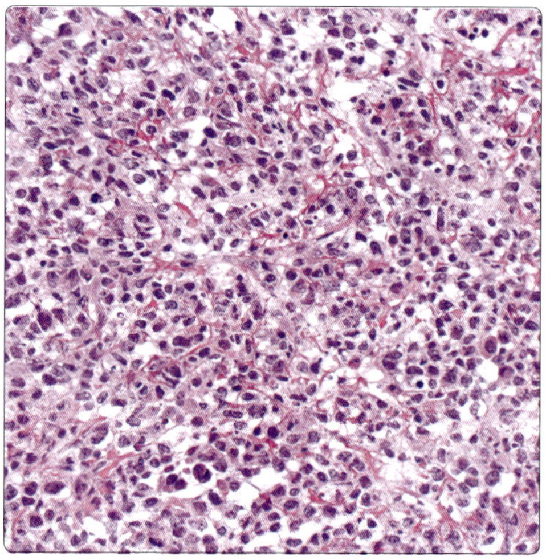

Follicular Lymphoma: High Grade

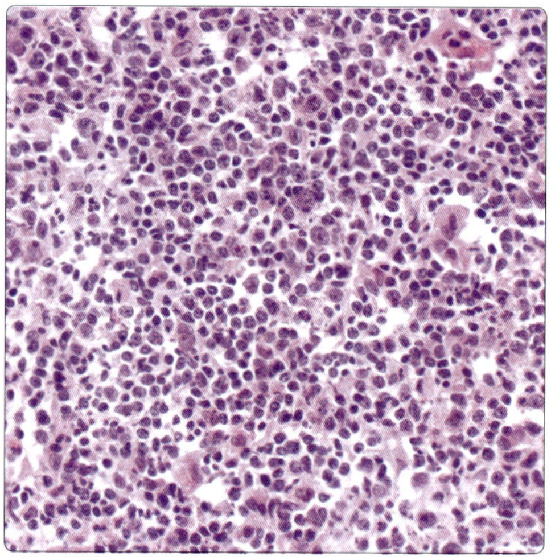

(Left) *This lymph node shows complete replacement by sheets of large, malignant epithelioid cells with prominent nucleoli. No secondary structures to suggest epithelial differentiation are seen in this diffuse large B-cell lymphoma.* **(Right)** *There is diffuse effacement of the nodal architecture by a mixed population of small, lymphocytes with "cleaved" dark nuclei, and larger, atypical epithelioid lymphocytes with more open chromatin and distinct nucleoli in this follicular lymphoma.*

Anaplastic Large Cell Lymphoma

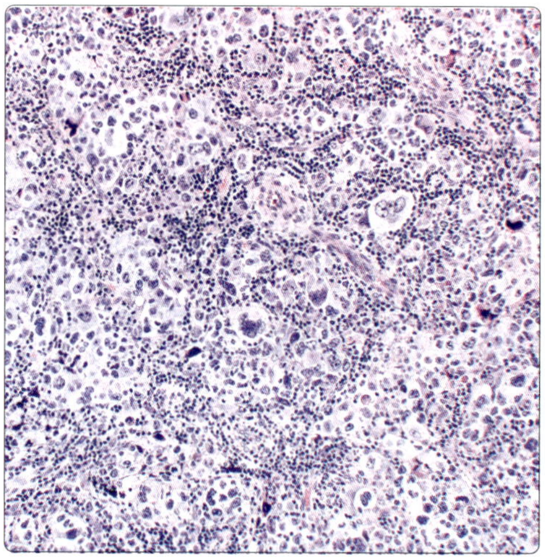

Metastatic Melanoma

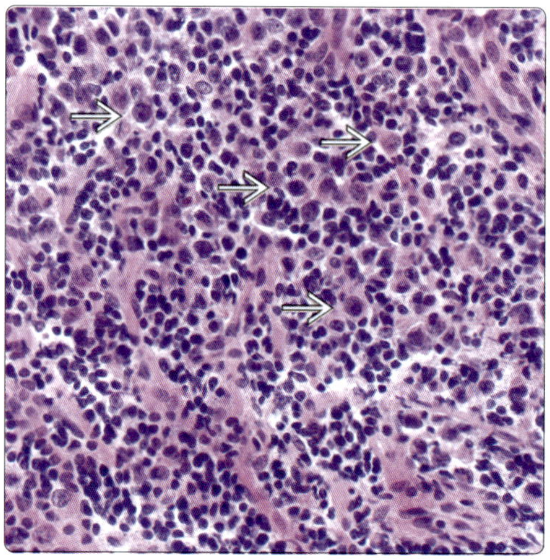

(Left) *Anaplastic large cell lymphoma consists of large cells with abundant cytoplasm and markedly pleomorphic nuclei and can closely resemble metastatic carcinoma. Cytologic preparations may suggest lymphoma due to the dyscohesion of the cells.* **(Right)** *This nodal metastasis of melanoma shows singly dispersed malignant epithelioid ➡ cells in a lymphoid background. The differential diagnosis includes carcinomas (particularly gastric or breast origin) and large cell lymphoma.*

Contents

Reactive Lymph Node

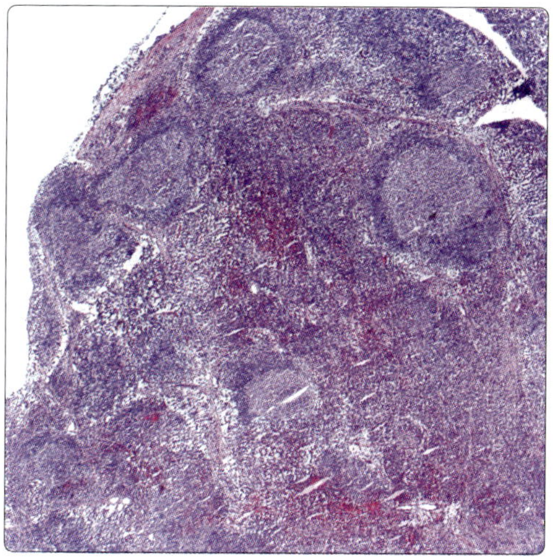

Reactive Lymph Node

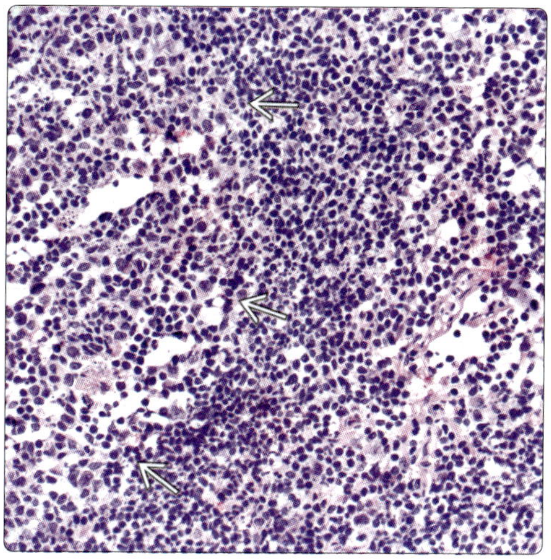

(Left) *In a perfect world (for the pathologist), all reactive lymph nodes will show this accentuation of nodal architecture with prominent germinal centers and marginal zones with bland interfollicular lymphocytes.* **(Right)** *Careful examination of lymph nodes at low magnification is important to assess architecture. Overreliance on high magnification can lead to overinterpretation of transformed, reactive lymphocytes, like those seen in this reactive germinal center* .

Endosalpingiosis

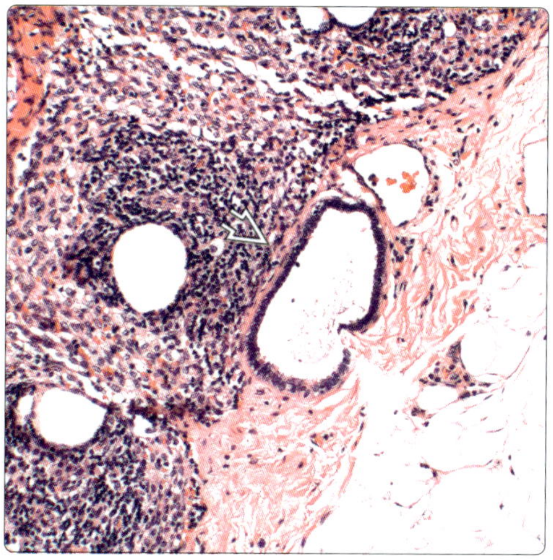

Sarcoidosis

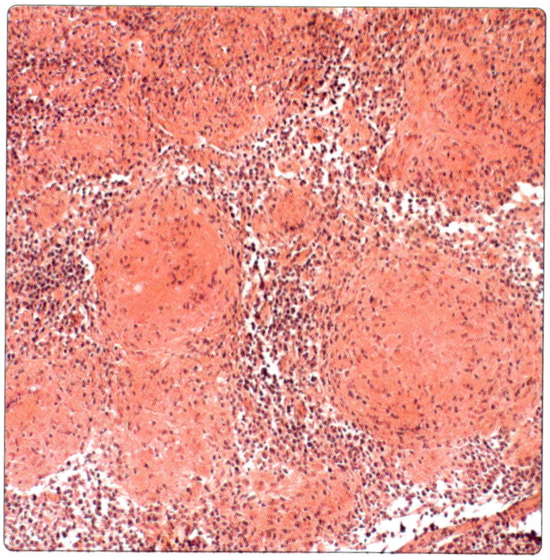

(Left) *Benign inclusions should be considered when epithelioid cells in nodes do not resemble a known primary carcinoma. Endosalpingiosis , decidual reaction, and mesothelial cells should be considered.* **(Right)** *Abdominal sarcoid can involve lymph nodes &/or the omentum. Necrosis is more common in infectious diseases but can also be seen in sarcoid. Tissue for culture should be taken, if possible.*

Calcification in Lymph Node

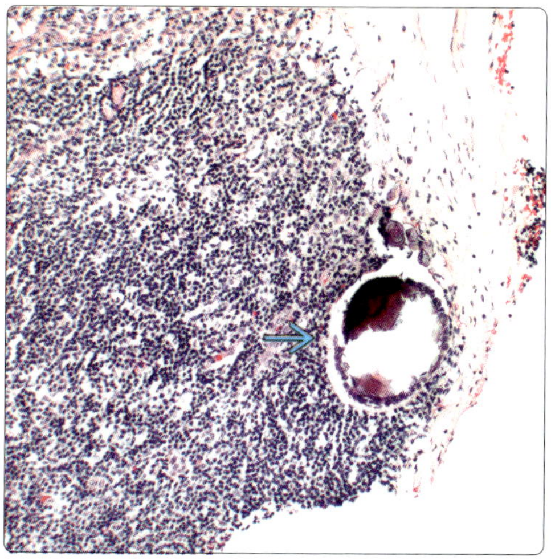

Infarcted Epiploic Appendage

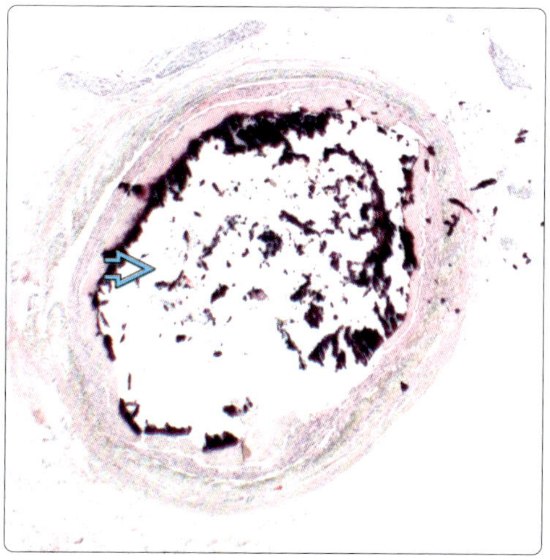

(Left) *Psammoma body calcifications in a peritoneal lymph node could be due to metastatic ovarian carcinoma or endosalpingiosis. Deeper levels into the tissue block may reveal diagnostic areas of the associated epithelial cells.* **(Right)** *When epiploic appendages infarct, the fat necrosis often calcifies and forms a hard nodule. To a surgeon, the lesion is grossly similar to a node with metastatic carcinoma. A gross diagnosis is sufficient when a nodule is too calcified to be cut by a scalpel.*

SURGICAL/CLINICAL CONSIDERATIONS

Goal of Consultation

- Preliminary diagnosis of pathogenesis underlying lymphadenopathy
- Confirmation that diagnostic/lesional tissue is present
  - Precise classification of lymphoproliferative disorders on frozen section (FS) can be challenging and is often not necessary at time of intraoperative consultation (IOC)
- Allocation of tissue for ancillary studies needed for eventual diagnosis

Change in Patient Management

- Additional nodes may be biopsied if initial specimen is nonlesional or inadequate

Clinical Setting

- Lymphadenopathy can be due to infection, autoimmune conditions, or malignancy
  - Optimal IOC for lymph nodes depends on whether IOC is for staging of known malignancy or primary diagnosis
    - Reason for consultation must be clear before examining specimen

SPECIMEN EVALUATION

Gross

- Lymph nodes are delicate and should be handled with care
  - Avoid crushing nodes during gross inspection
  - Moisten tissue with saline to prevent air-drying artifact
- Specimen should be kept sterile
  - Tissue may be taken for culture if infection is suspected
- Describe number of nodes and size of each node
  - Describe capsule (smooth or disrupted)
  - Number of involved and uninvolved nodes is very important for accurate cancer staging
- Thinly slice each node (2-3 mm)
  - Nodes may be inked different colors to identify each portion after sectioning
  - Use sharp blade to avoid crushing
  - Examine all slices for focal lesions
- Describe cut surface of node(s)
  - Lymphoma: Fleshy, white, homogeneous, sometimes nodular
  - Nodular sclerosis Hodgkin lymphoma: Fleshy nodules divided by fibrous bands
  - Metastatic carcinoma: Hard white mass, often partially involving node
  - Sarcoid: Firm white mass involving entire node
  - Infection: Mottled appearance with focal necrosis
- Tissue should be allocated for ancillary studies according to most likely diagnosis
  - Flow cytometry: Submit tissue if non-Hodgkin lymphoma is in differential diagnosis
  - Cytogenetic studies: Useful for chromosome analysis and ploidy studies
    - FISH studies can also be performed on formalin-fixed, paraffin-embedded tissue sections
  - Hematopathology fixatives that enhance cytologic detail: B-Plus, others
  - Snap freezing: Useful for molecular testing &/or tumor banking
    - Many molecular studies can also be performed on formalin-fixed, paraffin-embedded tissue
    - If amount of tissue is scant, block used for FS can be kept frozen
      - □ Surface of block with tissue should be covered with additional embedding medium and frozen
      - □ This protects tissue from thawing during specimen transfers
  - Microbiologic culture: Useful for suspected infectious etiologies or to rule out infection in cases of sarcoidosis
  - Permanent sections: Tissue not used for ancillary studies should be fixed promptly in formalin

Frozen Section

- If FS is for staging of carcinoma to guide surgery, entire node should be frozen
  - Reason for IOC should be clear before freezing tissue
- If FS is to guide tissue allocation, entire specimen should not be frozen

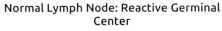

Normal Lymph Node: Reactive Germinal Center

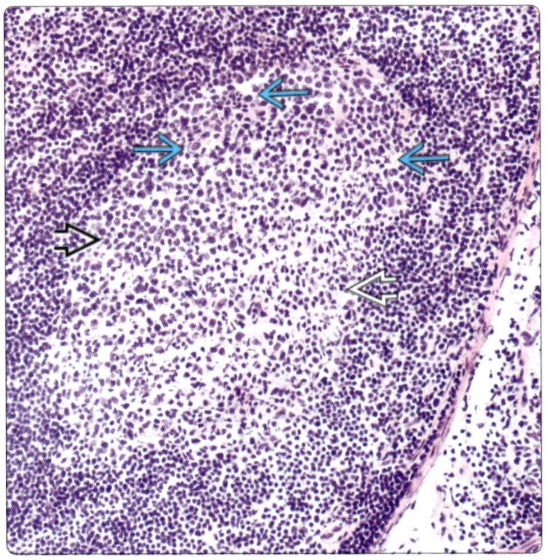

Normal Lymph Node: Cytologic Preparation

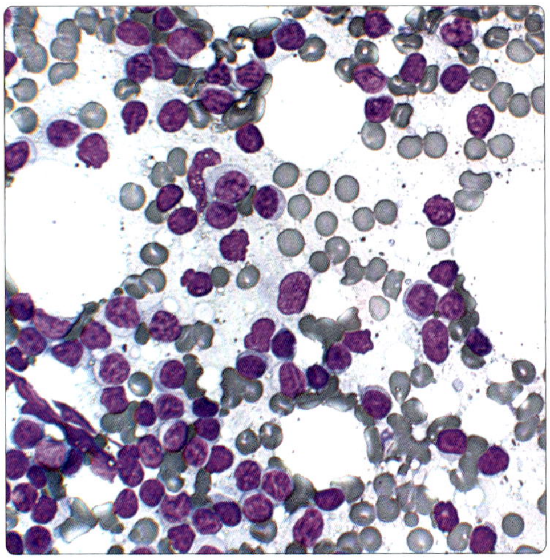

(Left) *Reactive germinal centers contain a mixture of cell types, including tingible body macrophages ➡, and show light ➡ and dark ➡ zones. They are helpful indications of a benign reactive enlarged lymph node.* **(Right)** *A normal lymph node smear should show multiple cell types. If the node is grossly abnormal in appearance, a frozen section should also be performed, as malignant cells associated with fibrosis or sclerosis might be difficult to dislodge from the node.*

- Nonfrozen tissue should be conserved for permanent sections and ancillary studies
- Cytologic preparations often provide superior cytologic detail and are adequate to provide provisional diagnosis
  - If cytologic preparation shows only normal cells, FS may be helpful to look for more specific diagnosis
  - Lesions with dense fibrosis may yield paucicellular cytologic preparations
    - Hodgkin lymphoma, mediastinal lymphomas, sarcoidosis
- Surrounding adipose tissue should be carefully removed from outside of node
  - Adipose tissue freezes poorly and creates difficult to cut sections

Cytology

- Cytologic preparations are preferable if lymphoma or infection are suspected
  - Cytologic detail superior to that seen in FS
  - Avoids contamination of cryostats with infectious agents and minimizes exposure of personnel
- Cut surface of node can be scraped or slides can be touched to surface
  - If evaluation is for possible metastatic carcinoma, all surfaces should be sampled
  - Scrape preparations are preferred if carcinoma is suspected or node has gross sclerotic appearance
  - Touch preparations are preferred if lymphoma is suspected and resulting preparations are highly cellular
- Both rapid-fixed hematoxylin and eosin and air-dried Romanowsky (Diff-Quik) preparations are often prepared to provide nuclear and cytoplasmic detail, respectively
  - Cells appear larger on air-dried preparations

COMMON DIAGNOSES

Reactive Follicular Hyperplasia

- Characterized by node with numerous follicles of varying sizes
- Germinal centers have reactive features
  - Germinal center polarization (dark and light zones)
  - Multiple cell types present within germinal centers (centrocytes, centroblasts, tingible body macrophages)
  - Germinal centers typically bulge out, creating lobulated outer surface to node
    - Lymphoproliferative disorders typically expand node, resulting in rounded shape
- Mixed population in interfollicular areas (small lymphocytes, plasma cells, histiocytes)
- Normal capsule without thickening and with open sinuses

Non-Hodgkin Lymphoma

- Patients are typically older (median age at diagnosis: 66 years)
- Lymph node is diffusely enlarged
- Effacement of normal lymph node architecture is helpful in identifying lesional tissue
- Cytology preparations are helpful for evaluation of malignant cell population
  - Preserves tissue that can be used for permanent sections and ancillary studies
- Ancillary studies are helpful for eventual diagnosis
  - Flow cytometry for surface markers
  - Fresh viable tissue for cytogenetic analysis
  - Frozen tissue for molecular analysis and tumor banking
- Lymphomas with small- to intermediate-sized cells may be difficult to recognize
  - Atypical nodal features should raise possibility of lymphoma
    - Lack of open sinuses; smooth outer contour
    - Small germinal centers with expanded marginal or mantle zones
    - Effacement of normal architecture with absence of normal germinal centers
      - Monotonous population of small lymphocytes (e.g., in chronic lymphocytic leukemia)
      - Nodular architecture with closely packed/back-to-back follicles (e.g., in follicular lymphoma)
  - Definitive diagnosis is not necessary intraoperatively
- Large cell lymphomas are often easily recognized as malignant
  - Often show dyscohesive growth pattern
    - Metastatic melanoma and signet ring cell carcinoma (including lobular breast cancer) also consist of dyscohesive cells
      - Patients will often have clinical history of malignancy
      - In other cases, primary carcinoma is clinically occult and 1st diagnosis is of metastatic disease
  - Sheets of large, atypical cells, often with frequent mitoses
  - Lymphomas of mediastinum and retroperitoneum can be associated with dense fibrosis
    - Can resemble carcinomas with desmoplasia or fibrosing diseases
    - Flow cytometry is often low yield for lesions with dense fibrosis
  - Consider lymphoblastic lymphoma in young patient with mediastinal mass
    - Cytologic preparations are often helpful in diagnosing lymphoblastic lymphoma
- Lymph nodes from patients with known low-grade lymphoma may be submitted to determine if there has been progression to large cell lymphoma
  - If original specimen shows only small cells, additional lymph nodes may be biopsied

Hodgkin Lymphoma

- Incidence shows bimodal age distribution with 1st peak in young patients (20s to 30s) and 2nd peak in older adults (after age 55)
  - Symptoms (night sweats, fever, pruritus, weight loss) present in some
- Lymph node is diffusely enlarged
  - Nodular sclerosis type characterized by fibrous bands surrounding fleshy nodules
  - Interfollicular expansion between normal germinal centers is suspicious
- Cytology preparations may only reveal background of normal lymphocytes
  - Diagnostic Reed-Sternberg cells may be rare and difficult to identify

Contents

- If Hodgkin lymphoma is strongly suspected and tissue is limited, tissue for flow cytometry, which will characterize the background inflammatory infiltrate, is of low priority

Acute Lymphoblastic Leukemia/Lymphoma

- Neoplasm of precursor cells (lymphoblasts) that most commonly occurs in children but can be seen at any age
  - T-cell acute lymphoblastic leukemia/lymphoma (ALL/LBL) is most common in adolescent males and often presents with large mediastinal mass; lymph nodes and extranodal sites may also be involved
  - B-cell ALL/LBL is most common in children under 6 and less frequently involves mediastinum; however, extramedullary involvement is common, particularly in CNS, lymph nodes, spleen, liver, testes, skin, soft tissue, and bone
- Specific diagnosis is helpful during IOC if possible, as mediastinal masses can show rapid growth resulting in respiratory emergency
- Lymphoblasts in B-cell ALL/LBL and T-cell ALL/LBL are morphologically indistinguishable
- Blast morphology can vary from small cells with condensed chromatin, indistinct nucleoli, and scant cytoplasm to medium-sized cells with finely dispersed chromatin, variably prominent nucleoli, and moderate amounts of occasionally vacuolated cytoplasm
  - Nuclear contours may be round to irregular to convoluted
  - Cytologic preparations are often helpful in examining blast morphology, especially chromatin texture and presence of nucleoli
- Tissue sections can provide helpful information in addition to cytologic appearance of cells
  - Blasts often show single-file infiltration of soft tissues
  - Frequent tingible body macrophages may give starry-sky appearance
  - Mitotic figures are often numerous
- Depending on blast morphology, it may be difficult to distinguish ALL/LBL from mature or high-grade lymphoma
  - Clinical scenario and site of involvement are often helpful in suggesting ALL/LBL, and immunophenotyping may be necessary to confirm diagnosis
- Allocate tissue for flow cytometry and cytogenetic studies
  - If tissue is limited, many cytogenetic lesions can be identified by FISH analysis on paraffin-embedded tissue

Metastatic Cancer

- Patients are usually older (> 60 years)
  - Important to know any history of prior cancer, including type of cancer
- Most common clinical settings of patients presenting with lymphadenopathy and occult primary include
  - Breast cancer metastatic to axillary node (predominantly lobular breast cancer)
  - Lung cancer metastatic to cervical node
  - Thyroid cancer metastatic to cervical node
  - Abdominal cavity carcinomas metastatic to left supraclavicular node (Virchow node), inguinal node (sometimes mistaken for inguinal hernia), or umbilicus (Sister Mary Joseph node)
  - Squamous cell carcinoma of oropharynx (HPV-related) metastatic to cervical node
- Lymph nodes may be completely or only partially involved
  - Partial gross involvement strongly favors metastasis over lymphoma
    - Some high-grade lymphomas grossly resemble metastatic carcinoma
  - Metastases are most commonly present in subcapsular sinus but can also involve central portion of node
- Cytologic preparations show clumps of malignant cells
  - Exceptions are melanoma and signet ring cell carcinomas of stomach and breast (lobular)

Sarcoidosis

- Most common in men and women in their 20s and women > 50
- Multiple nodes usually involved
- Node is completely replaced by confluent noncaseating granulomas
  - Small foci of necrosis do not exclude sarcoid
- Infectious disease is always in differential diagnosis
  - Sterile tissue should be saved for microbiological culture
- Hodgkin lymphoma and metastatic seminoma can be associated with granulomas
  - Nodal areas between granulomas should be carefully examined for malignant cells

Infection

- Patients are usually symptomatic
  - Symptoms can mimic those associated with some forms of lymphoma (fever, night sweats)
- Nodes with mottled appearance and punctate necrosis favor infectious process
  - Cytologic preparations are preferred to avoid contaminating cryostats and exposing personnel
  - Mixed inflammatory cells with necrosis suggest infection
- Infectious mononucleosis can be mistaken for lymphoma due to numerous large immunoblasts
- Sterile tissue should be saved for microbiological culture

Rosai-Dorfman Disease

- Also known as sinus histiocytosis with massive lymphadenopathy
  - Cause unknown
- Most common in children < 10 years of age but can occur in adults
- Cervical nodes are most commonly involved but also occurs in other nodal groups and extranodal sites (skin, sinuses)
- Lymph node is expanded by population of histiocytes with abundant eosinophilic granular cytoplasm

Kikuchi Disease

- Kikuchi disease (also known as Kikuchi-Fujimoto disease or histiocytic necrotizing lymphadenitis) usually involves cervical nodes in young adults (20s, 30s)
- Clinical course is benign; lymphadenopathy usually resolves spontaneously within weeks to months
- Foci of necrosis are surrounded by collections of numerous immunoblasts and histiocytes
  - Immunoblasts with prominent nucleoli can be mistaken for malignancy
  - Neutrophils and eosinophils are typically absent
- Very difficult to distinguish from lymphoma or infection on IOC

- Generally better to defer diagnoses to permanent sections
- Tissue should be preserved for possible lymphoma work-up and sent for microbiologic culture

REPORTING

Frozen Section and Cytology

- If IOC is for cancer staging, diagnoses of "metastatic carcinoma" or "no carcinoma seen" are sufficient
- If IOC is for evaluation of lymphadenopathy, definitive diagnosis is not necessary
  - Diagnoses of "suspicious for lymphoproliferative disorder" or "lesional tissue present" are sufficient
  - Allocation of tissue for ancillary studies is documented

PITFALLS

Missed Lymphoma

- Lymphomas can be missed if low grade or if lymphoma only partially involves node
- Typically occurs when node is biopsied for staging purposes for known carcinoma and lymphoma is not suspected clinically
- Lymph nodes involved by metastatic carcinoma can show concurrent involvement by lymphoma

Misdiagnosis

- Cells with Reed-Sternberg-like morphology can be seen in other types of lymphoma, poorly differentiated carcinomas, and infectious mononucleosis
- Anaplastic large cell lymphoma often grows within lymph node sinuses and may mimic metastatic carcinoma
- Kikuchi disease can be difficult or impossible to distinguish from lymphoma or infection on IOC

Normal Nodal Structures Mistaken for Malignancy

- Reactive follicular hyperplasia with increased numbers of follicles with large germinal centers may be mistaken for follicular lymphoma
  - Normal features are helpful to recognize (germinal center polarization, tingible body macrophages)
- Some germinal centers can appear to be near or within peripheral sinus
  - Large lymphocytes, mitotic figures, and apoptotic cells within germinal centers can be mistaken for malignant features
- Prominent vascular structures can resemble glands of metastatic adenocarcinoma
  - Endothelial nuclei can look enlarged on FS but lack pleomorphism of most carcinomas
  - Blood cells in lumen are important feature of blood vessels

Freezing Entire Node in Cases of Lymphoma or Infection

- Ancillary studies may be required for final &/or optimal diagnosis
- Cytologic preparations are preferable to narrow differential diagnosis and conserve tissue

Crush and Cauterization Artifact

- Lymph nodes are delicate and easily crushed during removal or during gross evaluation
- It can be difficult to impossible to determine if crushed blue cells are lymphoma, small cell carcinoma, carcinoid tumor, or normal lymphocytes
  - Definitive diagnosis should not be made if artifact precludes optimal evaluation
- Additional specimens should be requested from surgeon

SELECTED REFERENCES

1. Solomon AC et al: Frozen sections in hematopathology. Semin Diagn Pathol. 19(4):255-62, 2002
2. Guo LR et al: Incidental malignancy in internal thoracic artery lymph nodes. Ann Thorac Surg. 72(2):625-7, 2001
3. Wilkerson JA: Intraoperative cytology of lymph nodes and lymphoid lesions. Diagn Cytopathol. 1(1):46-52, 1985

Low-Grade Lymphoma: Nodal Effacement

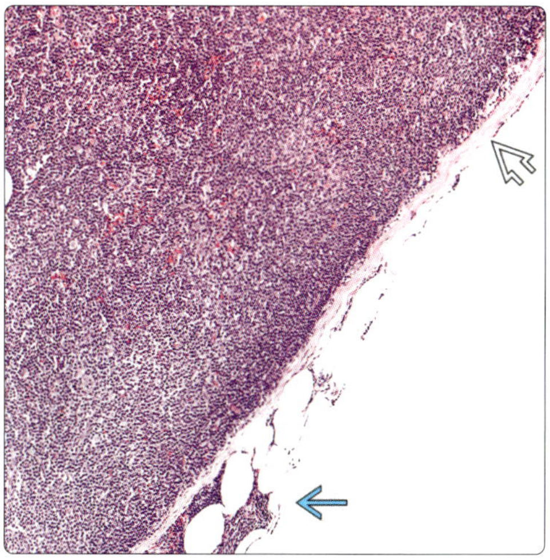

Low-Grade Lymphoma: Cytologic Preparation

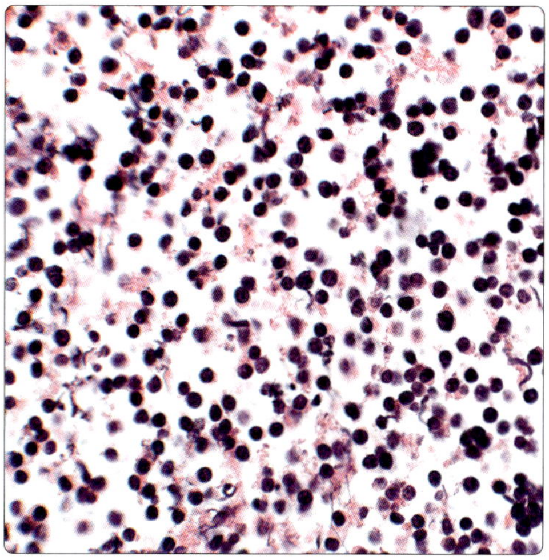

(Left) *Lymphomas often efface normal nodal architecture (including germinal centers), filling the node & causing a smooth outer contour ➡. Lesional cells may infiltrate perinodal adipose tissue ⇨.* **(Right)** *Low-grade lymphoproliferative diseases, like this chronic lymphocytic leukemia (CLL)/small lymphocytic lymphoma (SLL), are composed of small uniform cells. Definitive diagnosis of lymphoma may not be possible & is not required intraoperatively. Tissue should be allocated for special studies.*

(Left) *CLL/SLL often shows effacement of normal architecture by sheets of small cells. Note the lack of normal germinal centers. The abnormal cell population may be easier to appreciate on frozen section rather than on cytologic preparations.* **(Right)** *Intraoperative consultation may be requested for patients with CLL/SLL to determine if there has been a transformation to large cell lymphoma (Richter transformation). If not diagnosed in the initial biopsy, additional nodes may be biopsied.*

Chronic Lymphocytic Leukemia/Small Lymphocytic Lymphoma: Frozen Section

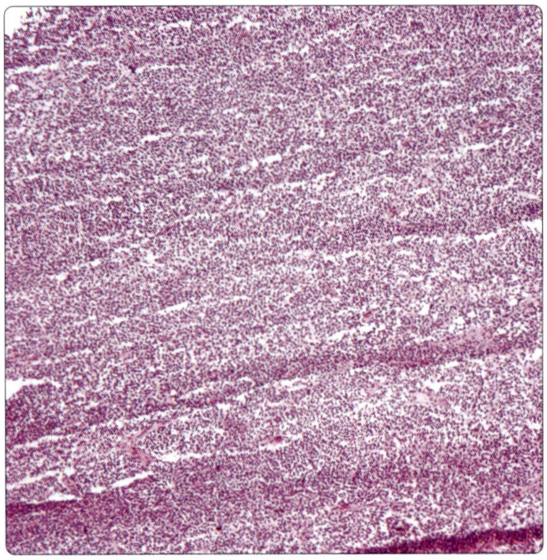

Chronic Lymphocytic Leukemia/Small Lymphocytic Lymphoma: Frozen Section

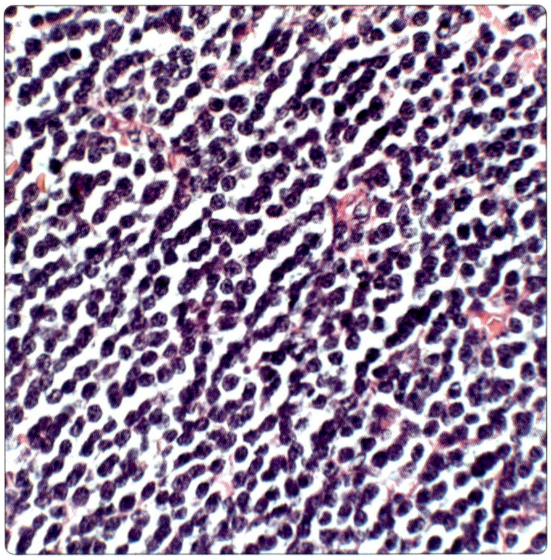

(Left) *Follicular lymphoma shows a nodular infiltrate composed of closely packed follicles with germinal centers that lack polarization or tingible body macrophages.* **(Right)** *Reactive follicular hyperplasia can be mistaken for follicular lymphoma. Note reactive-appearing follicles of varying sizes with polarized germinal centers ➔ containing tingible body macrophages and well-developed mantle zones ➔ as well as patent lymph node sinuses ➔.*

Follicular Lymphoma

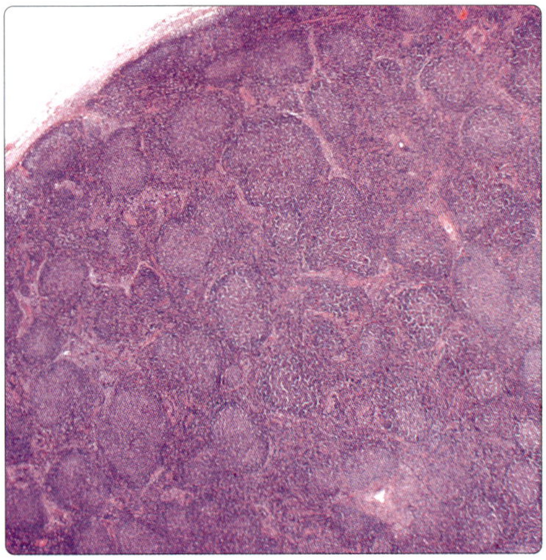

Reactive Follicular Hyperplasia

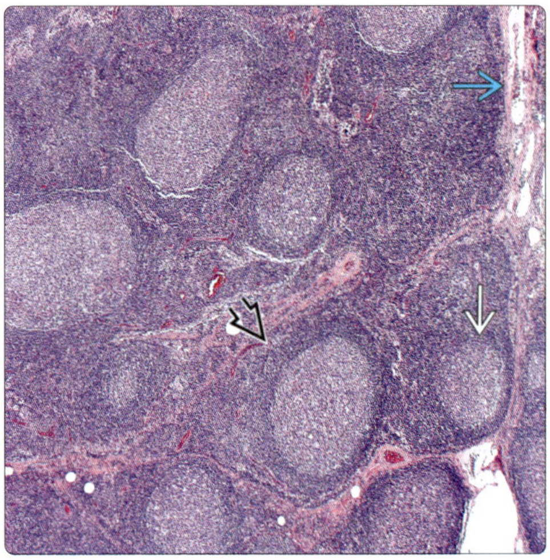

(Left) *Diffuse large B-cell lymphoma is composed of sheets of intermediate- to large-sized cells with oval to irregular nuclei and prominent nucleoli, with occasional cells showing increased pleomorphism ➔.* **(Right)** *Large cell lymphomas can usually be recognized as malignant on cytologic preparations, which often show dyscohesive intermediate- to large-sized cells ➔ with oval to irregular nuclei and prominent nucleoli admixed with background small lymphocytes ➔.*

Diffuse Large Cell Lymphoma

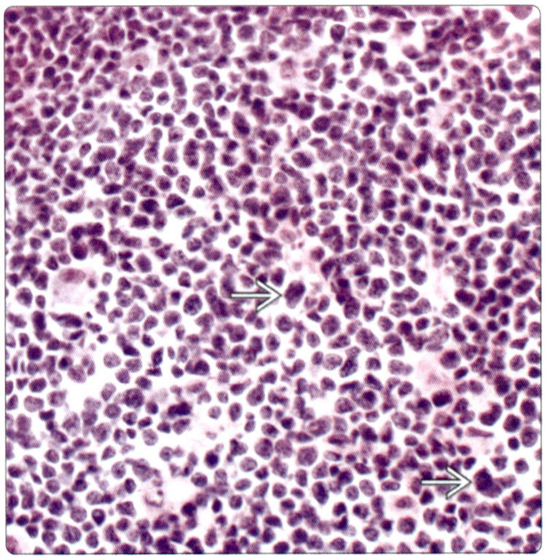

Diffuse Large Cell Lymphoma: Touch Imprint

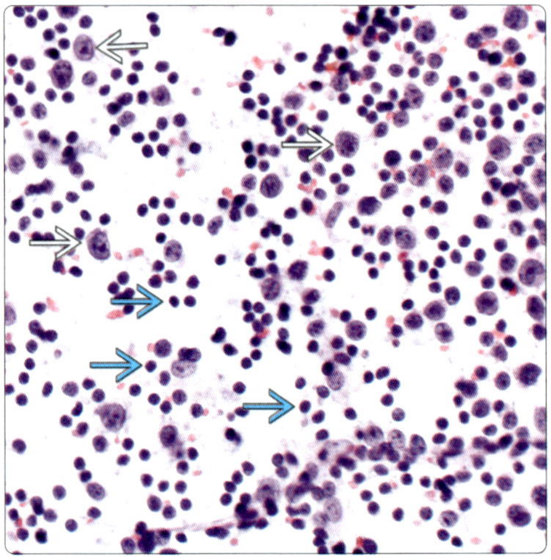

High-Grade B-Cell Lymphoma

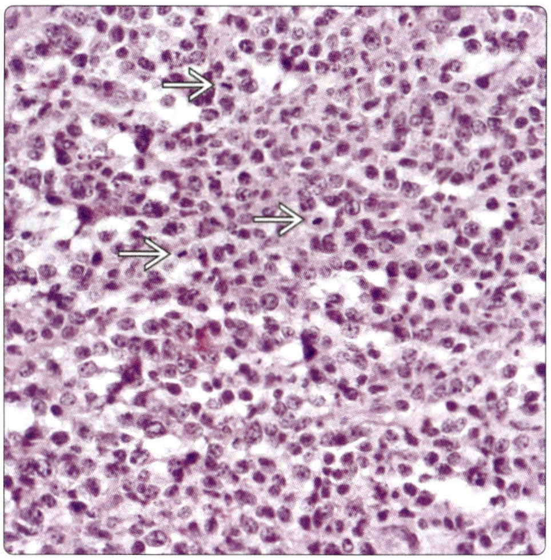

High-Grade B-Cell Lymphoma: Touch Imprint

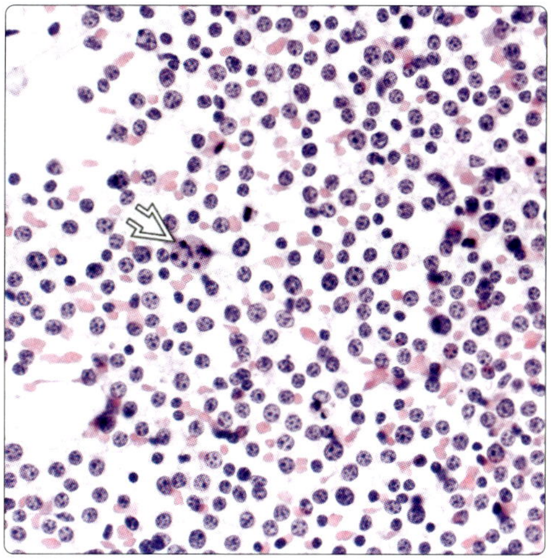

(Left) *High-grade B-cell lymphoma shows sheets of intermediate- to large-sized cells that are often relatively monomorphic with dispersed chromatin and prominent nucleoli as well as frequent mitotic figures* ➔. **(Right)** *High-grade B-cell lymphomas are often relatively monomorphous with intermediate-sized cells with prominent nucleoli. Tingible body macrophages* ➔ *may be present, creating a starry-sky appearance on tissue sections.*

Anaplastic Large Cell Lymphoma

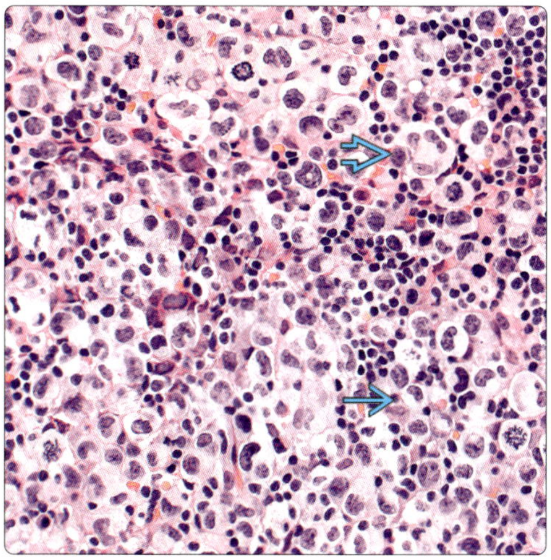

Anaplastic Large Cell Lymphoma: Touch Imprint

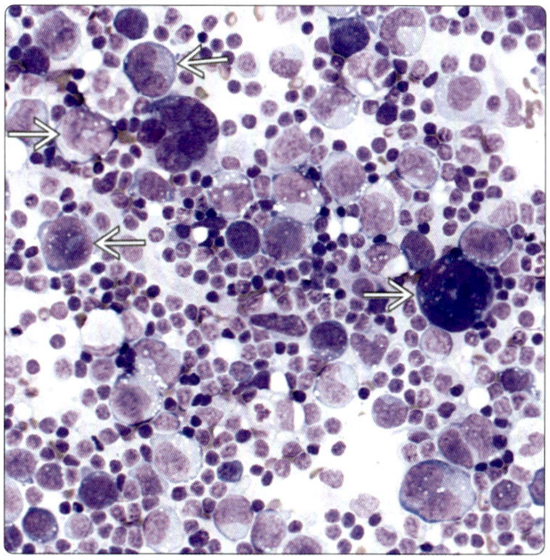

(Left) *Cells in anaplastic large cell lymphoma can show a range of morphologies, from intermediate-sized cells with kidney-shaped nuclei* ➔ *to very large cells with markedly irregular nuclei and abundant cytoplasm* ➔. **(Right)** *This case of anaplastic large cell lymphoma shows large-sized cells with a range of morphologies, including a variable number of large cells with kidney-, horseshoe-, or wreath-shaped nuclei, so-called "hallmark cells"* ➔.

Classic Hodgkin Lymphoma

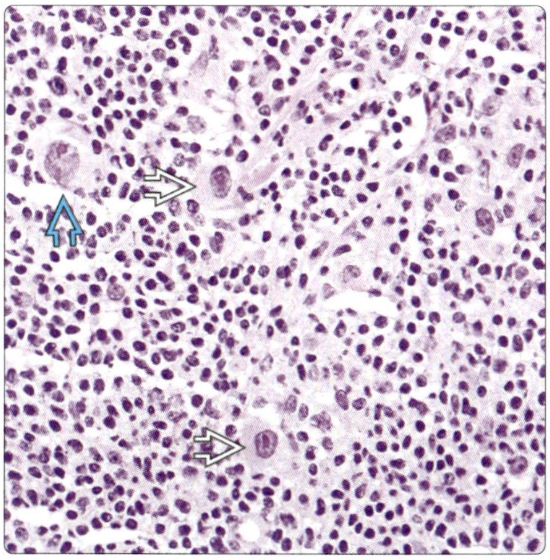

Classic Hodgkin Lymphoma: Touch Imprint

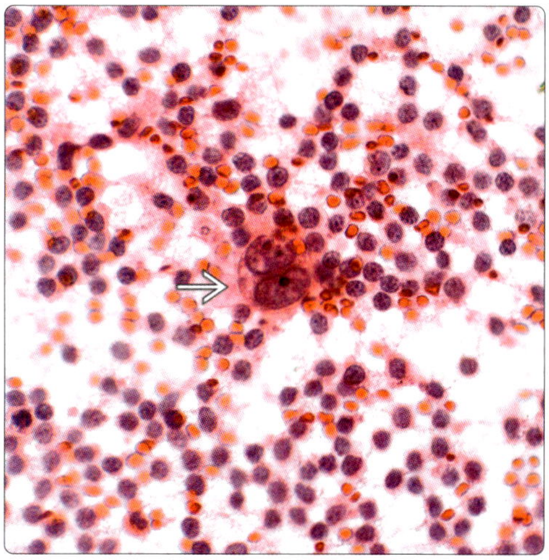

(Left) *Reed-Sternberg cells* ➔ *and mononuclear variants* ➔, *with large nuclei, prominent nucleoli, and abundant cytoplasm, are present in a background of small lymphocytes in this case of classic Hodgkin disease.* **(Right)** *Hodgkin lymphoma can be difficult to diagnose because only rare diagnostic cells may be present in a background of benign lymphocytes. A single Reed-Sternberg cell* ➔ *is seen in this touch imprint.*

Acute Lymphoblastic Leukemia/Lymphoma

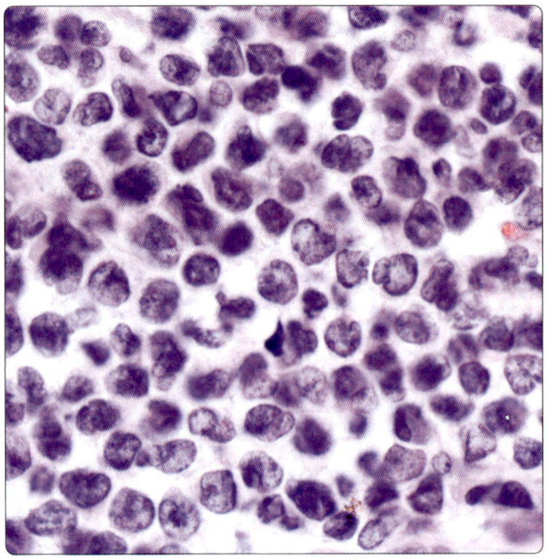

Acute Lymphoblastic Leukemia/Lymphoma

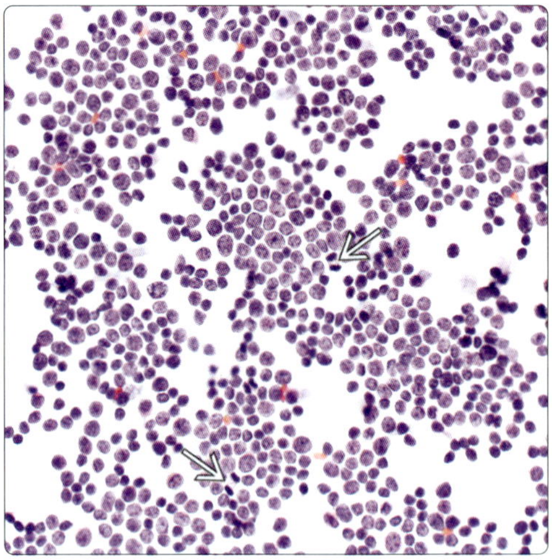

(Left) *Blasts of ALL/LBL have irregular nuclei, finely dispersed chromatin, variably distinct nucleoli, and scant cytoplasm. Although high-grade lymphomas may also show sheets of intermediate-sized cells with a high mitotic rate, blasts often show more finely dispersed chromatin and less prominent nucleoli.* **(Right)** *Touch preparations from ALL/LBL are often highly cellular and show a monotonous population of immature-appearing cells with fine chromatin. Mitotic figures* ➡ *may be frequent.*

Acute Lymphoblastic Leukemia/Lymphoma

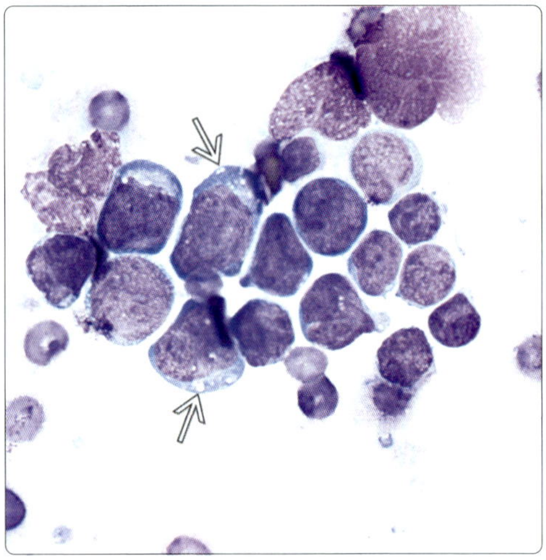

High-Grade B-Cell Lymphoma

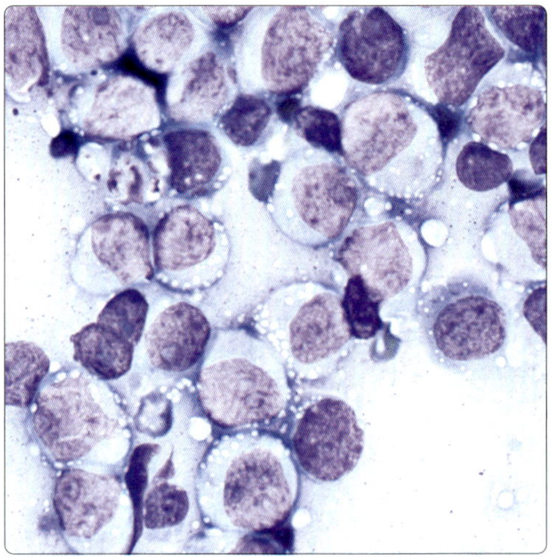

(Left) *These blasts show relatively small amounts of basophilic cytoplasm containing cytoplasmic vacuoles* ➡*. Cytoplasmic vacuoles are not specific to ALL/LBL and can be seen in other high-grade lymphoid processes, such as high-grade B-cell lymphoma and Burkitt lymphoma.* **(Right)** *This case of high-grade B-cell lymphoma shows frequent cytoplasmic vacuoles, which can also be seen in ALL/LBL. The cells in this case show more abundant cytoplasm than is typical for lymphoblasts.*

T-Lymphoblastic Lymphoma

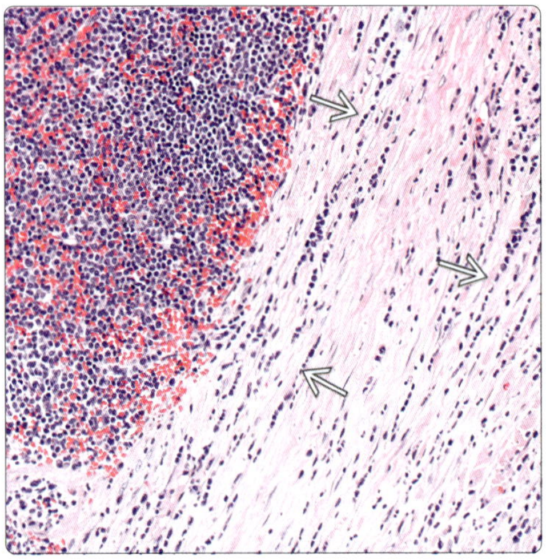

T-Lymphoblastic Lymphoma

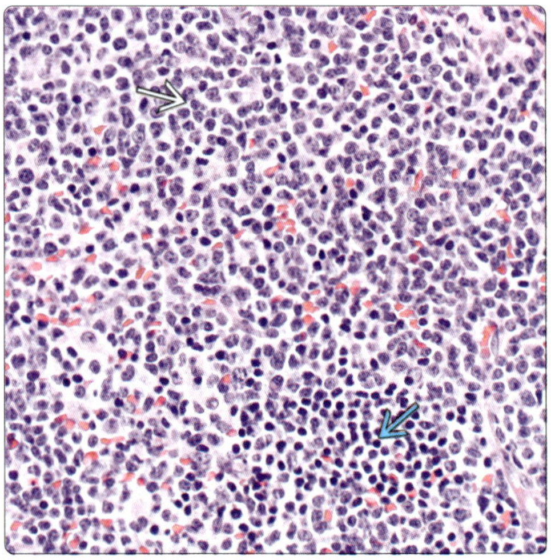

(Left) *In this case of T-lymphoblastic lymphoma in a lymph node, sheets of lymphoblasts efface the nodal architecture. Note the single-file arrangement* ➡ *of blasts infiltrating the lymph node capsule.* **(Right)** *The lymphoblasts* ➡ *of this T-lymphoblastic lymphoma involving a lymph node are larger than the background mature lymphocytes* ➡ *and show more finely dispersed chromatin.*

Metastatic Carcinoma and Lymphoma

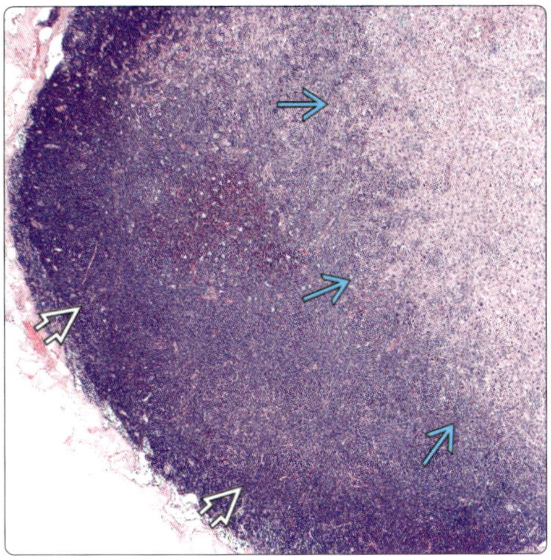

Metastatic Carcinoma: Cytologic Preparations

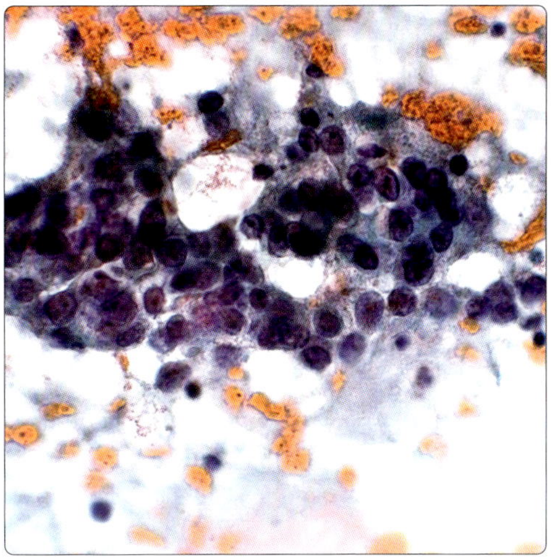

(Left) *Lymph nodes can show concurrent involvement by 2 neoplastic processes. This node is involved by squamous cell carcinoma and chronic lymphocytic leukemia/small lymphocytic lymphoma. Note the effacement of nodal architecture in the areas not involved by metastatic carcinoma.* **(Right)** *Metastatic carcinomas typically form cohesive clusters on cytologic preparations, allowing them to be distinguished from high-grade lymphomas. However, some carcinomas (e.g., signet ring cell carcinoma) are dyscohesive.*

Metastatic Carcinoma

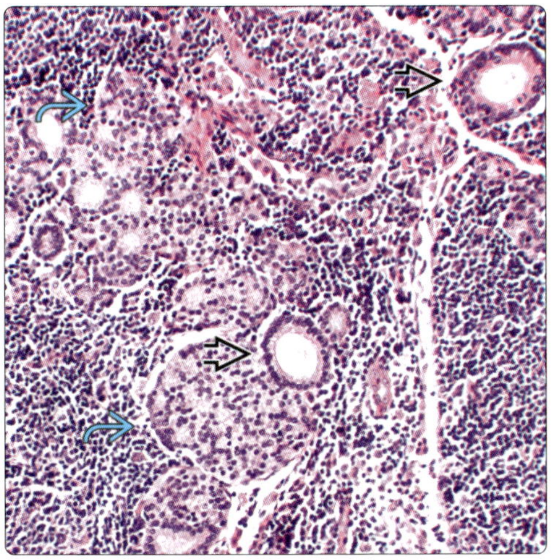

Anaplastic Large Cell Lymphoma Mimicking Metastatic Carcinoma

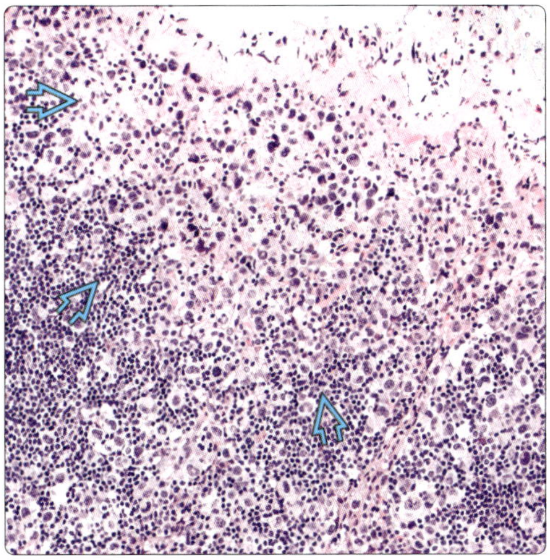

(Left) *Both metastatic colon carcinoma and metastatic prostate carcinoma are present in this lymph node. It is always important when performing a frozen section on a lymph node to know if the patient has a history of prior malignancies.* **(Right)** *Anaplastic large cell lymphoma consists of large pleomorphic cells that often show a sinusoidal pattern of lymph node involvement. This pattern can closely mimic metastatic carcinoma.*

Diffuse Large B-Cell Lymphoma Mimicking Metastatic Carcinoma

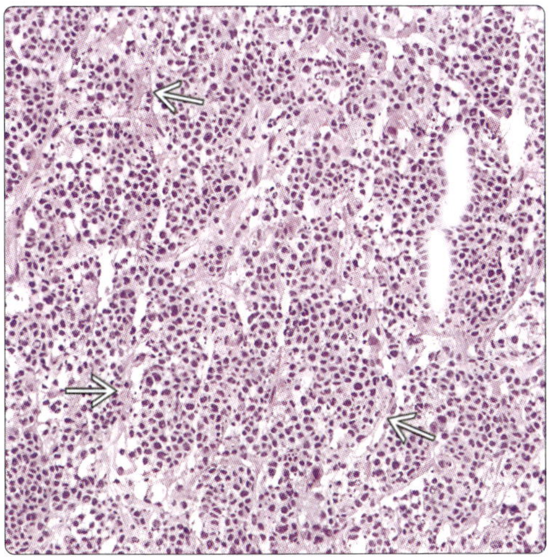

Metastatic Melanoma

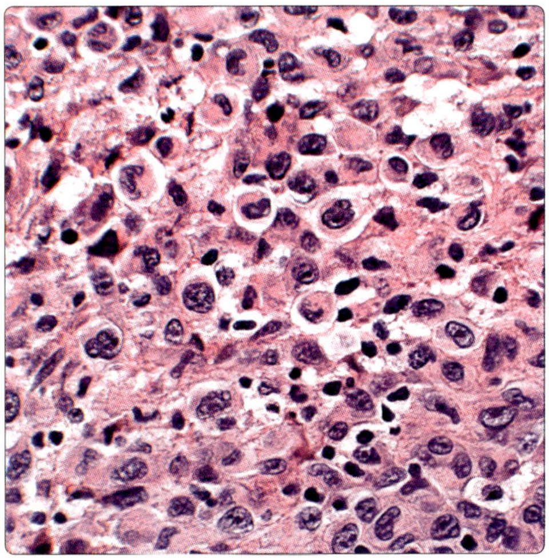

(Left) *Strands of fibrosis within this diffuse large B-cell lymphoma create a cohesive, nested appearance, mimicking high-grade carcinoma. A cytologic preparation could aid in the diagnosis of lymphoma.* **(Right)** *The cells of some malignancies are dyscohesive. Melanoma (seen here), signet ring cell carcinomas of stomach and breast (lobular), and lymphoma are the most common.*

(Left) *Granulomas with central necrosis are often evident grossly and are highly suggestive of tuberculosis. Tissue should be taken for culture, and appropriate notification of exposed personnel is critical.* **(Right)** *Infection should always be considered in evaluating lymphadenopathy. Cytologic preparations are preferred. Necrotic debris and Langhans giant cells are highly suggestive of tuberculosis.*

Necrotizing Granulomas

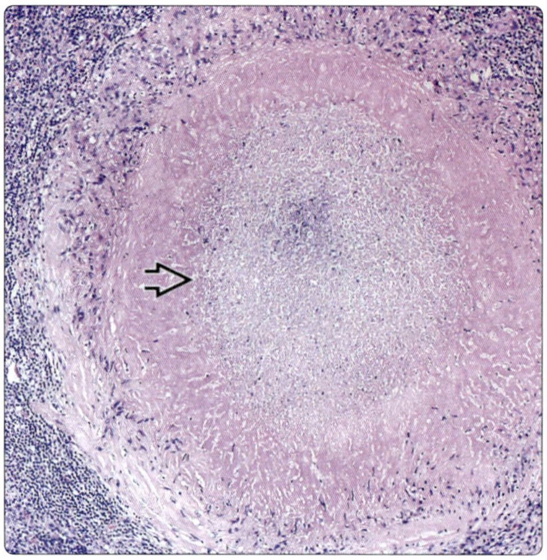

Tuberculosis: Cytologic Preparation

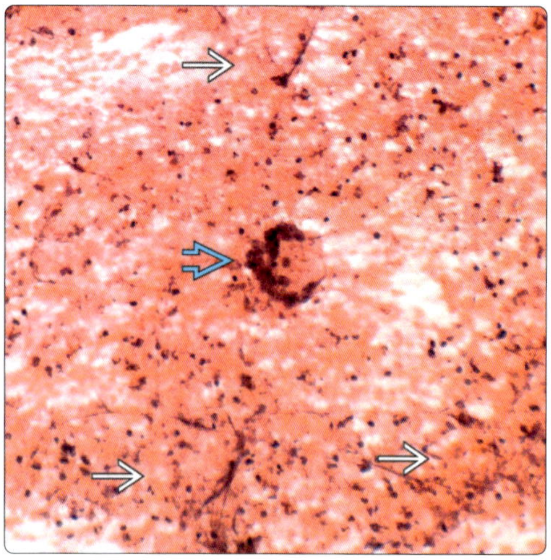

(Left) *Hodgkin lymphoma can be associated with granulomas in lymph nodes. In this case, multiple Reed-Sternberg cells and mononuclear variants are present in the areas between the granulomas.* **(Right)** *Metastatic seminoma to a lymph node can be associated with a granulomatous response. The area between the granulomas should be examined for tumor cells. The tumor cells have prominent nuclei and characteristic rectangular nucleoli (boxcar-shaped).*

Hodgkin Lymphoma With Noncaseating Granulomas

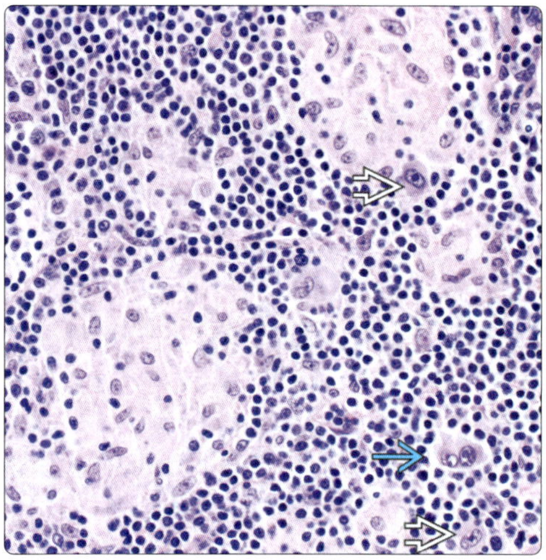

Metastatic Seminoma

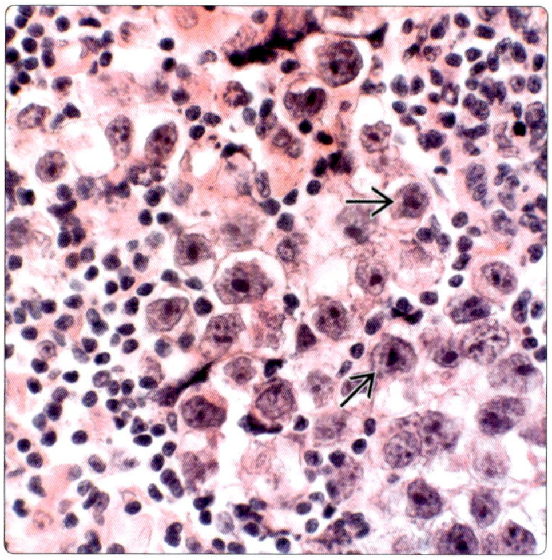

(Left) *Sarcoidosis is characterized by confluent noncaseating granulomas. Hodgkin lymphoma or seminoma with granulomas should be excluded by examining the tissue between the granulomas.* **(Right)** *Crush and cautery artifact have caused coagulative necrosis and distortion of normal lymphocytes at the periphery of this lymph node. This is the area most likely to harbor small metastases. In addition, the artifactual distortion of the cells could be mistaken for a metastasis.*

Sarcoidosis

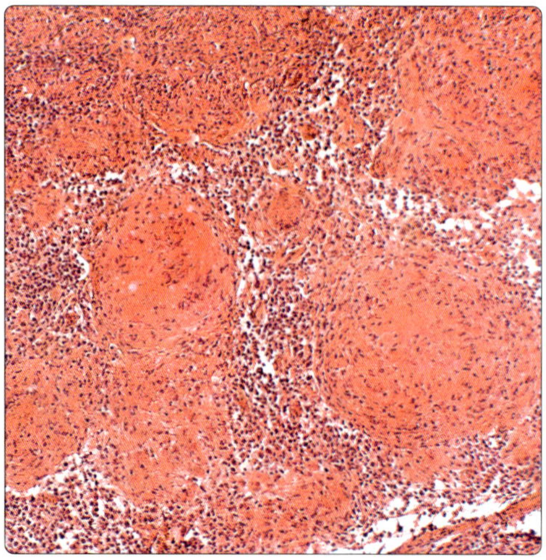

Crush and Cautery Artifact

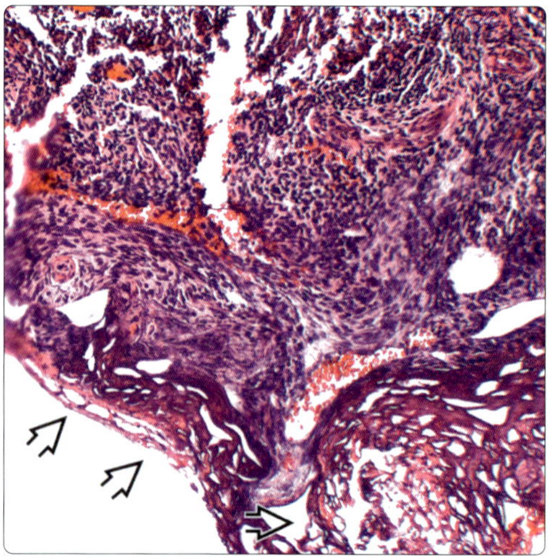

Epstein-Barr Virus Lymphadenitis: Reed Sternberg-Like Cells

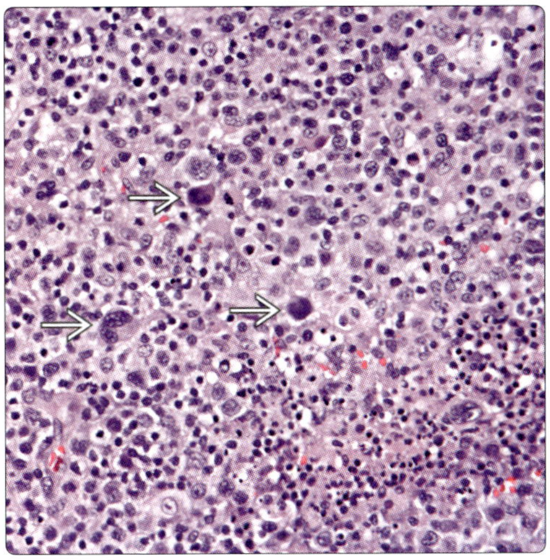

Kikuchi-Fujimoto Disease

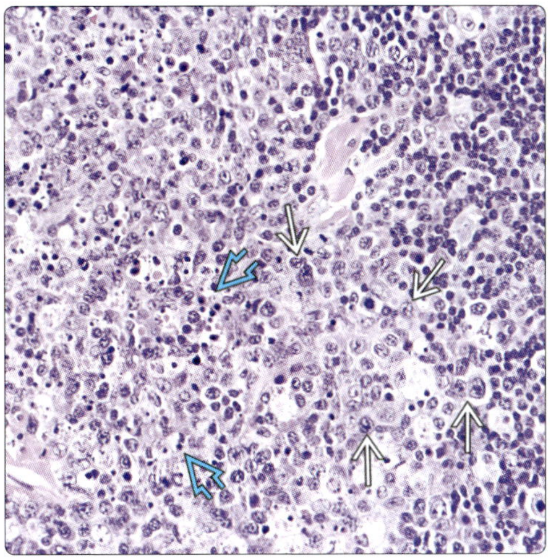

(Left) Reed-Sternberg-like cells ➡ are seen in a background of marked lymphoid proliferation and focal necrosis in this case of Epstein-Barr virus lymphadenitis. This could cause confusion with Hodgkin lymphoma. **(Right)** *This lymph node involved by Kikuchi-Fujimoto disease shows apoptotic cells ➡ with incipient necrosis as well as a proliferation of histiocytes and large immunoblasts ➡, which may be mistaken for lymphoma. Note the lack of neutrophils.*

Rosai-Dorfman Disease

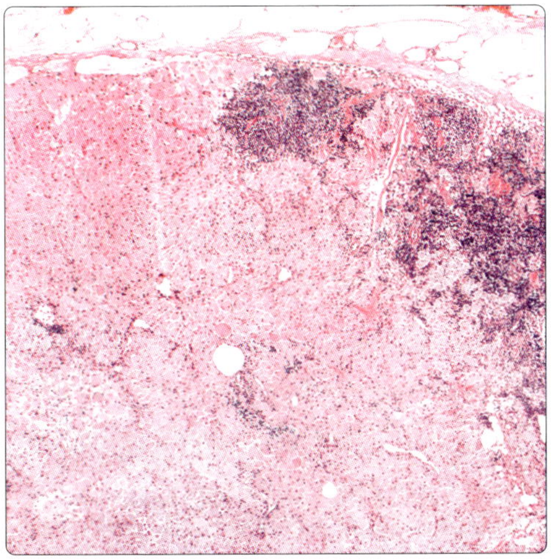

Rosai-Dorfman Disease

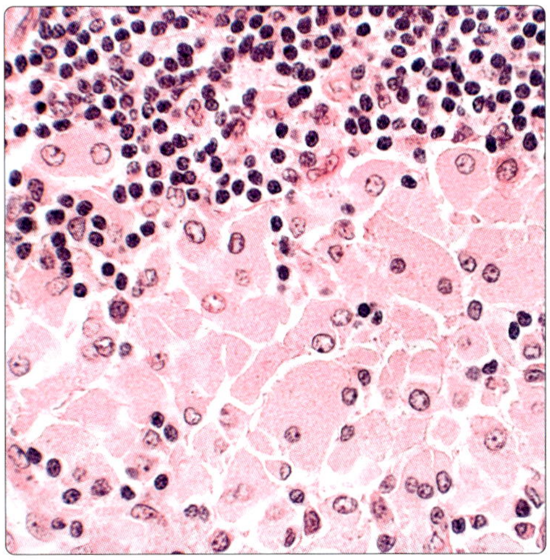

(Left) *Rosai-Dorfman disease or sinus histiocytosis with massive lymphadenopathy most commonly involves the cervical lymph nodes. The nodes are filled with abundant histiocytes.* **(Right)** *Sheets of histiocytes causing lymphadenopathy are characteristic of Rosai-Dorfman disease. Emperipolesis (the presence of intact cells within another cell) is also a feature and may be seen best in cytologic preparations. The abundant pink, granular cytoplasm and relatively small, round nuclei are typical.*

Silicone

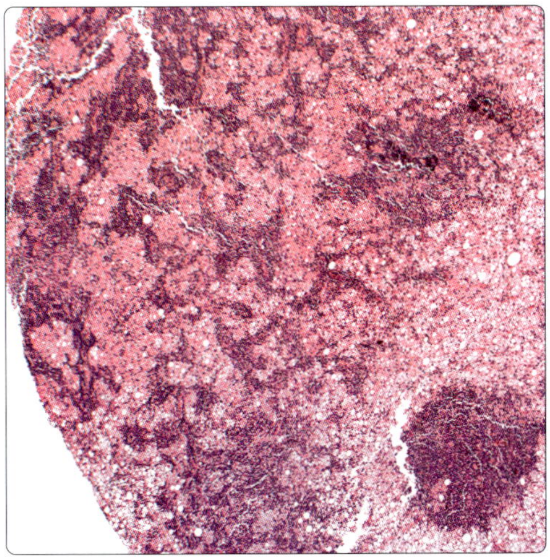

Silicone

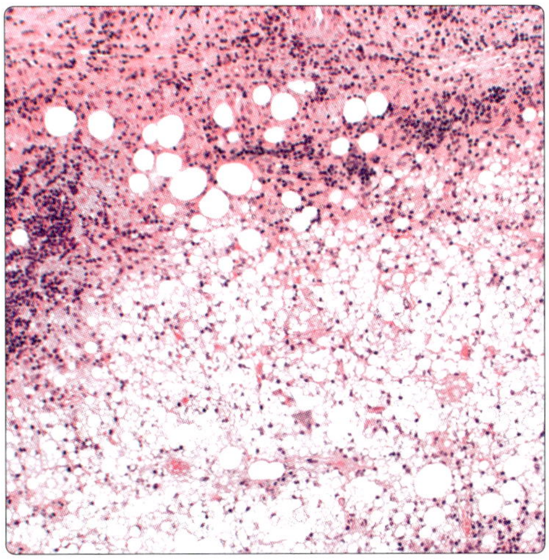

(Left) *Silicone in a lymph node is most commonly seen in the axillary nodes of women with silicone breast implants. It usually occurs after rupture, although silicone can "bleed" through an intact implant. The nodes can be very hard and gritty when sectioned, closely mimicking carcinoma.* **(Right)** *Histiocytes filled with silicone have clear or bubbly cytoplasm and the nuclei can be indented by the cytoplasmic inclusions. The appearance can mimic a liposarcoma if the clinical setting is not known.*

SURGICAL/CLINICAL CONSIDERATIONS

Goal of Consultation

- Determine if metastatic tumor is present in lymph nodes of patients with known malignancy
- Evaluate lymphadenopathy of unknown etiology and allocate tissue for ancillary studies

Change in Patient Management

- Additional nodes may not be biopsied
- Plan for surgery with curative intent may be altered

Clinical Setting

- Patients with known carcinoma may undergo biopsy with intraoperative evaluation prior to definitive surgical treatment
- Patients with lymphadenopathy of unknown etiology require biopsy for diagnosis
- Important to obtain clinical history

SPECIMEN EVALUATION

Gross

- Number of nodes is identified and recorded
  - Number of involved and uninvolved nodes is often important for staging and prognosis
  - Each node must be identifiable for accurate count
    - Nodes can be inked in separate colors
    - Each node can be kept in separate cassette
- Nodes are serially sectioned and examined
  - Metastatic carcinoma usually focally involves node as firm white-tan mass
    - Note if grossly apparent, extranodal spread is seen
  - Lymphoma generally shows diffuse nodal involvement and has uniform fleshy or nodular appearance
  - Infection may cause mottled appearance with necrosis

Frozen Section

- Representative section of most suspicious area for metastasis can be frozen if lymph node appears grossly positive
  - If negative, remainder of lymph node should be frozen
- If gross appearance is suggestive of lymphoma or infection, cytologic preparations (smears) are preferable

Cytology

- Scrape or touch preparations can detect carcinoma
- For potential lymphoproliferative disorders, cytology smears provide superior nuclear detail and preserve fresh tissue for ancillary studies
- Granulomatous disease can be detected with cytology without risk of cryostat contamination

Ancillary Studies

- Tissue is triaged depending on favored diagnosis
  - Most molecular and genetic tests can be performed on formalin-fixed paraffin-embedded tissue sections
- Microbiologic cultures: Suspected infection (vs. sarcoidosis)
- Hematopathology fixatives: Suspected lymphoma
- Flow cytometry: Suspected non-Hodgkin lymphoma
- Cytogenetics for karyotype: Suspected lymphoma or sarcoma (fresh viable tissue)

MOST COMMON DIAGNOSES

Metastatic Carcinoma

- Up to 90% of cervical lymph node metastases are head and neck squamous cell carcinoma
- At least 10% of patients who present with nodal metastasis have unknown primary
- **Metastatic squamous cell carcinoma**
  - Conventional squamous cell carcinomas are typically keratinizing
    - May arise from mucosal or cutaneous sites
  - If no previously known primary, most are HPV-associated oropharyngeal primaries
    - Characteristically cystic
    - Nonkeratinizing, basaloid morphology
    - Undifferentiated variant morphologically identical to nasopharyngeal carcinoma
      - Most commonly involve level II and III nodes
- **Metastatic nasopharyngeal carcinoma**

Metastatic HPV Squamous Cell Carcinoma

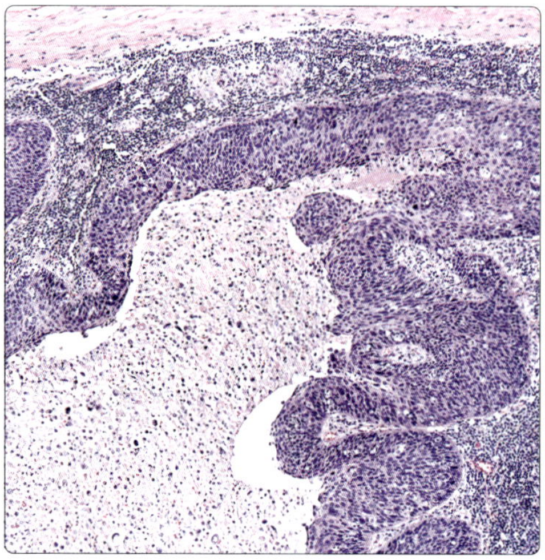

Metastatic Nasopharyngeal Carcinoma

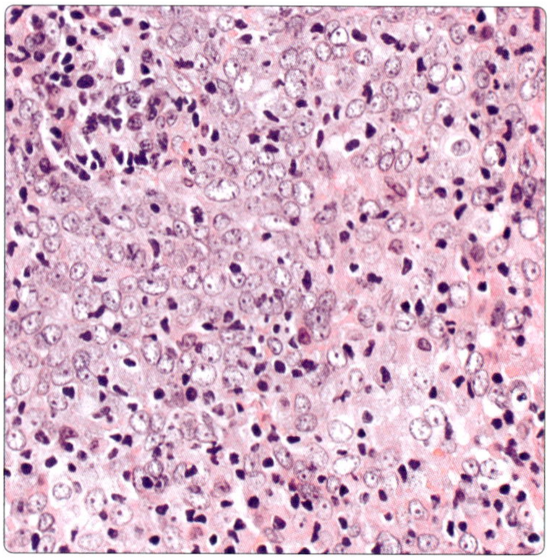

(Left) *Metastatic HPV-associated squamous cell carcinomas from the oropharynx are frequently cystic. This pattern is an important clue when presenting as carcinoma of unknown primary but may lead to diagnostic pitfalls.* **(Right)** *Metastatic undifferentiated carcinoma to neck nodes is a frequent presentation for EBV-associated nasopharyngeal carcinoma, but it may also be associated with high-risk HPV.*

- Nonkeratinizing with differentiated or undifferentiated morphology
  - Differentiated pattern has appearance of nonkeratinizing squamous cell carcinoma
  - Undifferentiated pattern has syncytial clusters or individual cells with large nuclei having vesicular chromatin and prominent nucleoli
- May involve posterior triangle (level V) nodes, unusual for other head and neck primaries

- **Metastatic papillary thyroid carcinoma**
  - Papillary architecture, occasionally follicular pattern
  - Enlarged nuclei have irregular nuclear membranes, grooves, clearing, pale chromatin, delicate nucleoli, pseudoinclusions
  - Psammoma bodies may be present
    - If only calcification is seen, levels should be performed to identify carcinoma
- **Adenocarcinoma**
  - Consider lung and gastrointestinal tract primaries
- **Metastatic neuroendocrine neoplasms**
  - Clinical correlation needed to identify primary site
    - Metastatic breast and prostate carcinoma can often have neuroendocrine appearance
  - Carcinoid (typical and atypical) tumors from lung may present in cervical nodes
  - Medullary thyroid carcinoma may present initially with nodal neck metastasis
  - Distinguish from similar-appearing tumors including paraganglioma and parathyroid gland

Metastatic Malignant Melanoma

- May show spindled or epithelioid morphology

Sarcoidosis

- Tightly formed, often confluent, nonnecrotizing granulomata

Lymphoma

- Non-Hodgkin lymphoma
  - Normal nodal architecture is often effaced with monotonous population of lymphoid cells
    - Small lymphocytes in chronic lymphocytic leukemia/small lymphocytic lymphoma (CLL/SLL)
    - Large cells in large cell lymphoma
  - Prominent nodular architecture lacking polymorphous population of benign reactive germinal center is seen in follicular lymphoma
  - Differential diagnosis for round cell neoplasms includes sarcomas (e.g., alveolar rhabdomyosarcoma) and metastases (e.g., olfactory neuroblastoma)
- Hodgkin lymphoma
  - Sclerosis and mixed inflammatory infiltrate including eosinophils are clues to search for characteristic Reed-Sternberg cells

Reactive Changes

- Polymorphous lymphoid population with reactive germinal centers
  - Tingible-body macrophages are also present
- If clinical suspicion for lymphoma is high, tissue should be allocated for ancillary studies

REPORTING

Frozen Section

- Presence or absence of metastatic malignancy
  - If possible, report tumor type
- Extranodal extension for metastasis is associated with worse outcome for many tumors and should be noted if present
- Report presence of granulomatous inflammation and whether or not it is necrotizing
- If lymphoma suspected, sufficient to report as atypical lymphoid infiltrate and defer classification to permanent sections

PITFALLS

Nodular Hashimoto Thyroiditis

- May have parasitic thyroid nodules that appear to be lymph nodes to surgeon
  - Follicular cells with oncocytic change, lymphoid infiltrate with reactive germinal centers, and variable fibrosis
  - Lacks papillary carcinoma nuclear features and nodal architecture
  - Helpful to know nodule proximity to thyroid

Benign Developmental Cysts

- Thyroglossal duct (midline) and branchial cleft (lateral) cysts may mimic enlarged nodes clinically
- Epithelial lining can be squamous or respiratory type
- Squamous epithelial lined cysts must be distinguished from cystic metastatic squamous cell carcinoma
  - Be cautious in diagnosing branchial cleft cysts on frozen section in adults
  - Look for overtly malignant cytologic features

Lymphoid Response to Salivary Tumor

- Salivary gland tumors with prominent lymphoid response may be difficult to distinguish from nodal metastasis
- Capsule and subcapsular sinus help identify lymph nodes

Thymic Tissue

- Thymic remnants may mimic lymph nodes, and Hassall corpuscles may be mistaken for metastatic squamous cell carcinoma
- Thymus lacks capsular structure with medullary sinus and reactive germinal centers of lymph node
- Hassall corpuscles have characteristic squamous whorls with keratohyaline granules but lack cytologic atypia

Benign Inclusions

- Benign salivary structures within intra- or periparotid lymph nodes as well as nevus cell rests
- Lack morphologic features of malignancy and are often not in subcapsular sinus location
- Significance of incidental thyroid epithelium in lymph node is controversial, but this finding should be assumed to represent metastasis
  - Thyroid should be evaluated for occult primary

SELECTED REFERENCES

1. Goldenberg D et al: Cystic lymph node metastasis in patients with head and neck cancer: an HPV-associated phenomenon. Head Neck. 30(7):898-903, 2008

(Left) *Atypia, mitotic figures* ➡*, and single cell necrosis are present in this metastatic squamous cell carcinoma. High-risk HPV was subsequently detected, and a tonsillar primary was later identified.* **(Right)** *Cytologic smears can be helpful in intraoperative consultation. This smear of a cystic metastatic squamous cell carcinoma shows abundant necrotic keratin debris in the background. Viable tumor cells* ➡ *may be sparse, but their large, hyperchromatic nuclei are diagnostic of malignancy.*

Metastatic HPV Squamous Cell Carcinoma

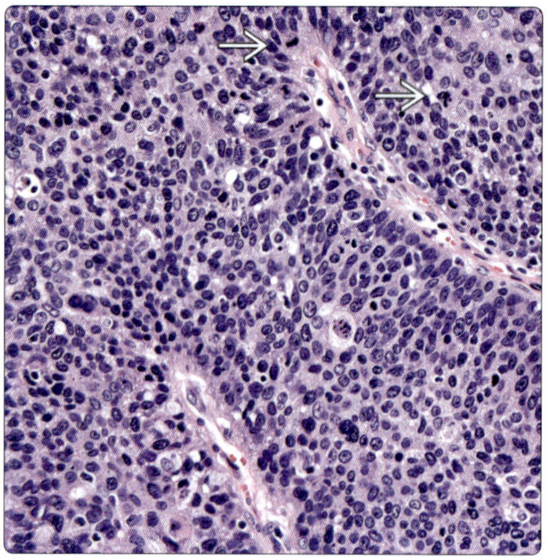

Metastatic Squamous Cell Carcinoma

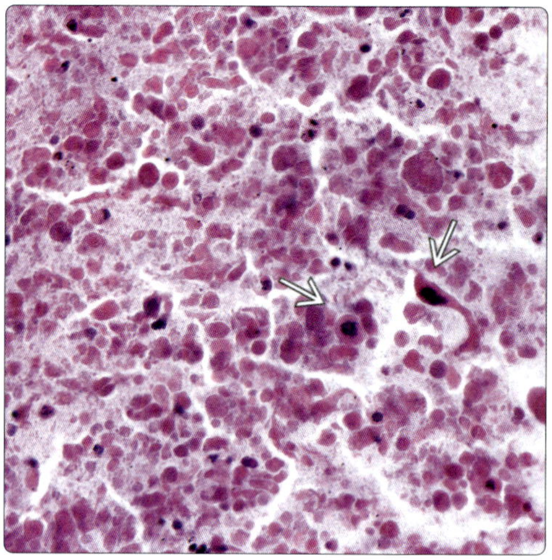

(Left) *Benign developmental cysts, such as this one, contain a reactive lymphoid stroma in the cyst wall that may mimic the appearance of a lymph node. The lining of squamous epithelium raises concern for a cystic metastatic squamous cell carcinoma.* **(Right)** *The branchial cleft cyst lining in this example is squamous but lacks any cytologic atypia that would raise concern for malignancy. The epithelium is strictly confined to the cyst lumen without evidence of invading into the cyst wall.*

Branchial Cleft Cyst

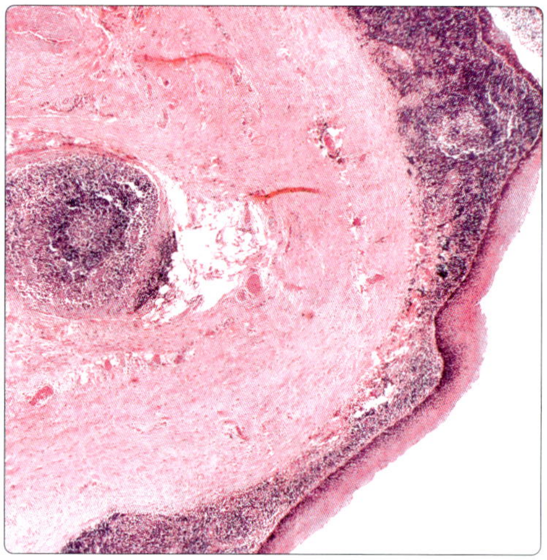

Branchial Cleft Cyst

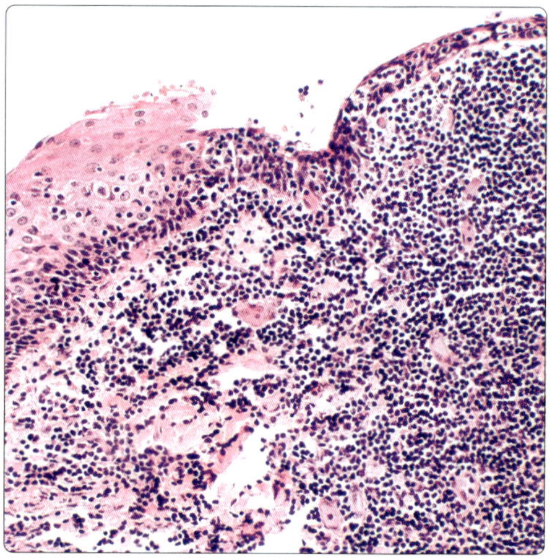

(Left) *Metastatic malignant melanoma shows a nested growth pattern of epithelioid (as shown here) or spindle cells with large nuclei and prominent nucleoli. Many metastases lack pigmentation, such as this example.* **(Right)** *Acinic cell carcinoma and mucoepidermoid carcinoma frequently have an associated prominent reactive lymphoid infiltrate that can mimic nodal metastasis.*

Metastatic Malignant Melanoma

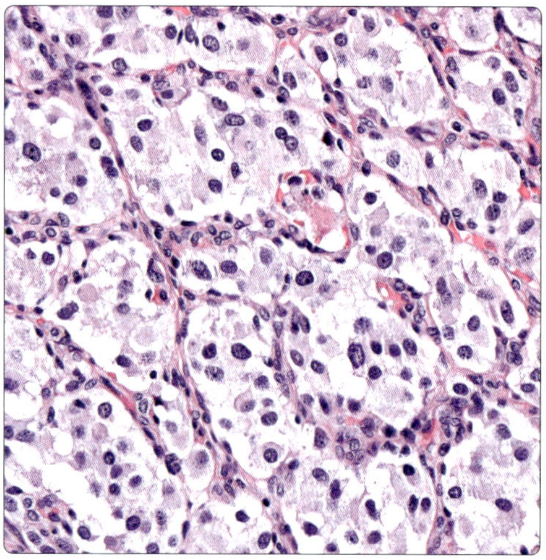

Acinic Cell Carcinoma

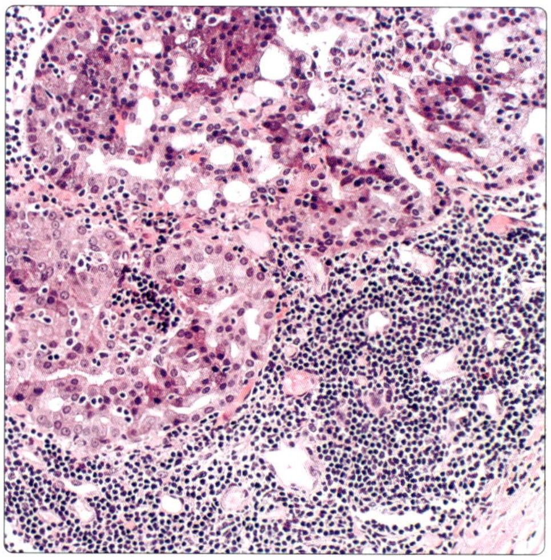

Normal Germinal Center

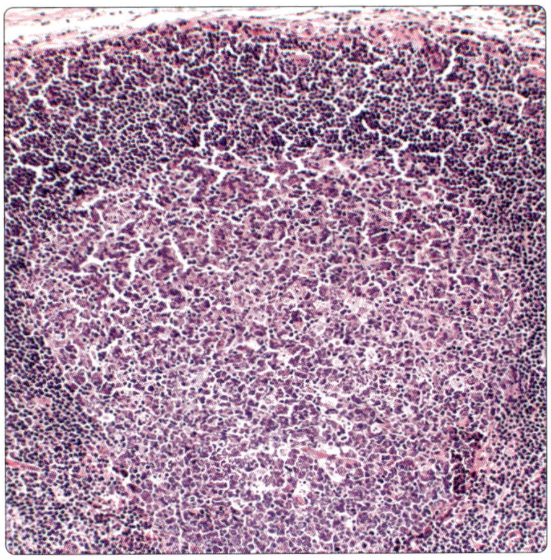

Small Lymphocytic Lymphoma

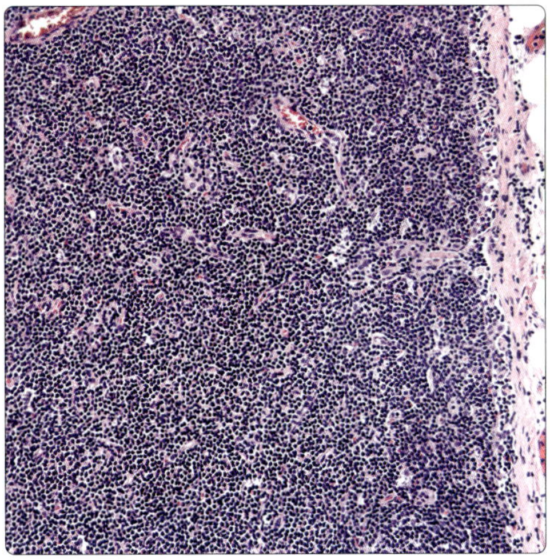

(Left) *Identification of normal germinal centers is helpful in assessing a lymph node for a lymphoma. Effacement of normal nodal architecture is an important clue to the diagnosis of lymphoma. The presence of altered germinal centers lacking the polymorphous population of cells seen in reactive adenopathy is a feature of follicular lymphoma.* **(Right)** *This small lymphocytic lymphoma diffusely involves the node with effacement of the normal architecture by monotonous small lymphocytes.*

Follicular Lymphoma

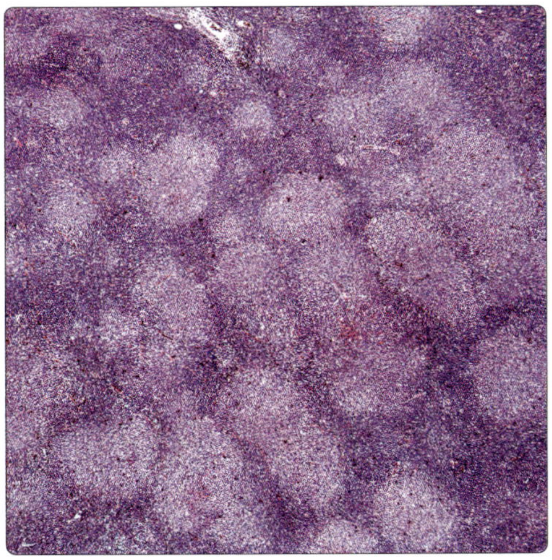

Follicular Lymphoma

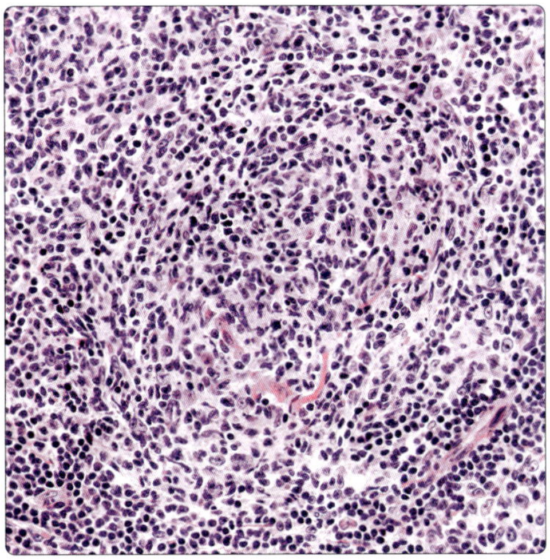

(Left) *A follicular lymphoma has a nodular configuration with numerous haphazardly arranged neoplastic follicles that could be mistaken for reactive germinal centers at low power.* **(Right)** *Follicular lymphomas form nodular lymphoid aggregates with a predominance of small- to medium-sized lymphoid cells with irregular and occasionally folded nuclei. The polymorphous lymphoid population with tingible body macrophages typical of a reactive germinal center is not seen. (Courtesy O. Pozdnyakova, MD.)*

Large Cell Lymphoma

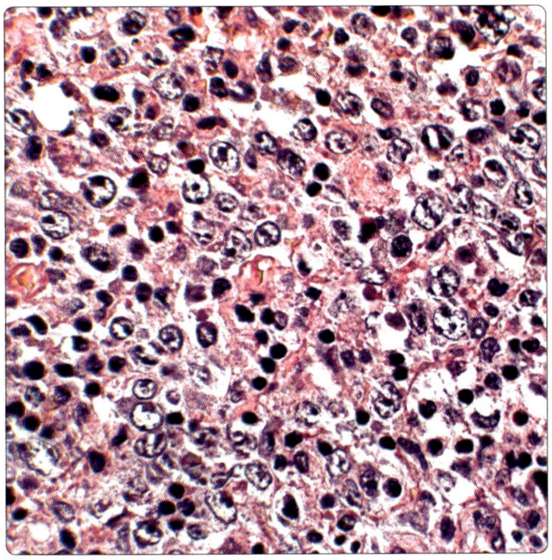

Classic Hodgkin Lymphoma

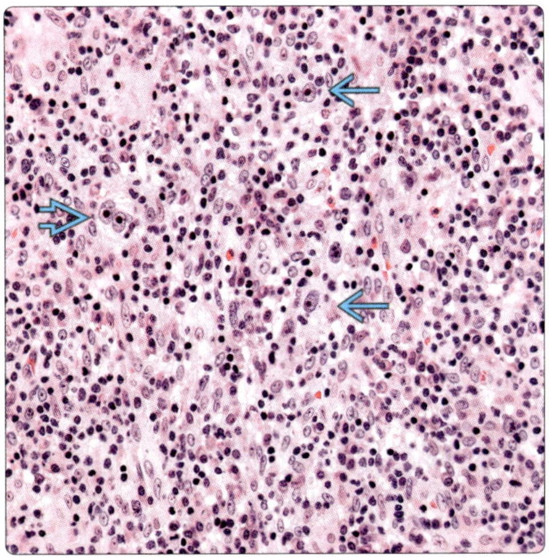

(Left) *The malignant cells in this large cell lymphoma have large nuclei with vesicular chromatin and prominent nucleoli. This specimen was initially interpreted as being metastatic carcinoma, but it proved to be a diffuse large B-cell lymphoma.* **(Right)** *Classic Hodgkin lymphoma exhibits mixed cellularity with eosinophils, plasma cells, and small lymphocytes admixed with rare Reed-Sternberg cells ⇨ and variants →. (Courtesy O. Pozdnyakova, MD.)*

Contents

(Left) *The diagnostic nuclear features of metastatic papillary carcinoma are nuclear enlargement, overlapping, and nuclear inclusions or grooves. If absent, the possibility of the biopsy being of nodular thyroid tissue involved by lymphocytic thyroiditis should be considered, as this finding can be mistaken for a metastasis to a lymph node.* **(Right)** *This metastatic classic papillary thyroid carcinoma shows numerous papillae with fibrovascular cores and abundant psammoma bodies.*

Metastatic Papillary Thyroid Carcinoma

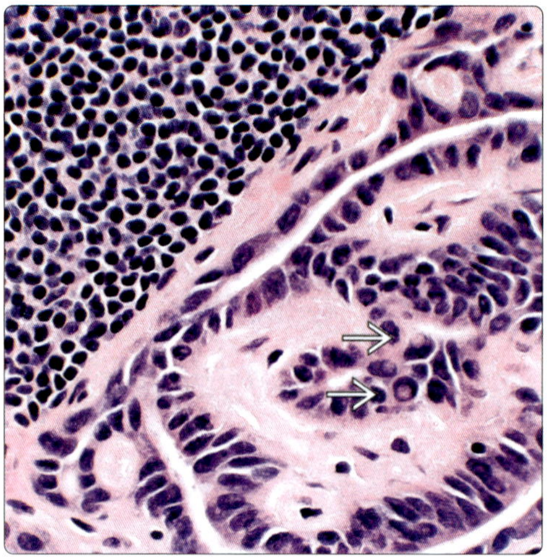

Metastatic Papillary Thyroid Carcinoma

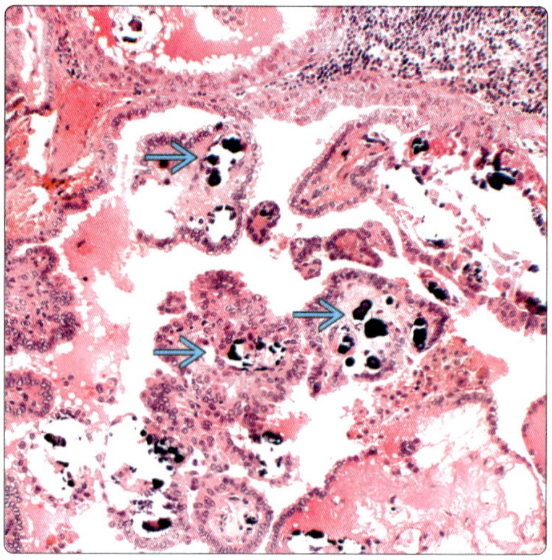

(Left) *A psammoma body in a lymph node in the head and neck region is usually due to metastatic papillary thyroid carcinoma. Deeper levels often reveal diagnostic foci of carcinoma. (Courtesy J. Barletta, MD.)* **(Right)** *Follicular variant of papillary carcinoma often shows a microfollicular growth pattern with more subtle cytologic features. Careful examination for diagnostic nuclear features is necessary.*

Psammoma Body in Lymph Node

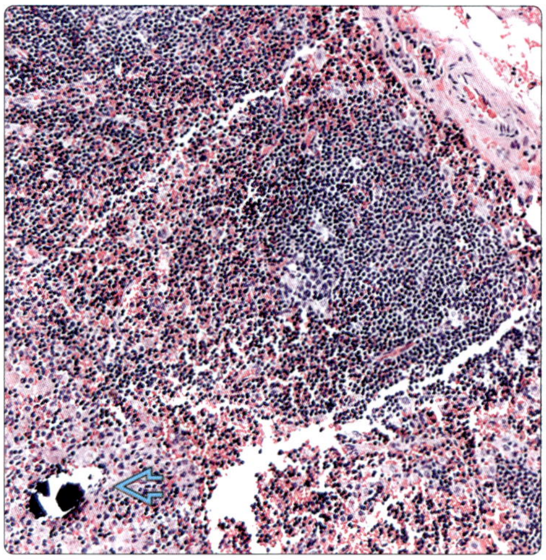

Metastatic Papillary Thyroid Carcinoma, Follicular Variant

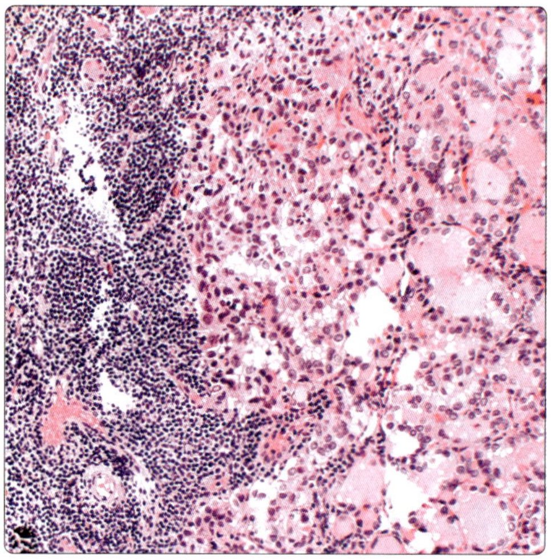

(Left) *Medullary carcinoma of the thyroid may initially present as a lymph node metastasis. Amorphous pink amyloid is often difficult to visualize by frozen section.* **(Right)** *Identification of the primary site for metastatic neuroendocrine tumors, such as this carcinoid tumor from the lung, requires clinical correlation and possibly ancillary studies. Metastatic breast cancer and prostate cancer can often closely resemble carcinoid tumor, and all 3 can be strongly positive for chromogranin.*

Metastatic Medullary Thyroid Carcinoma

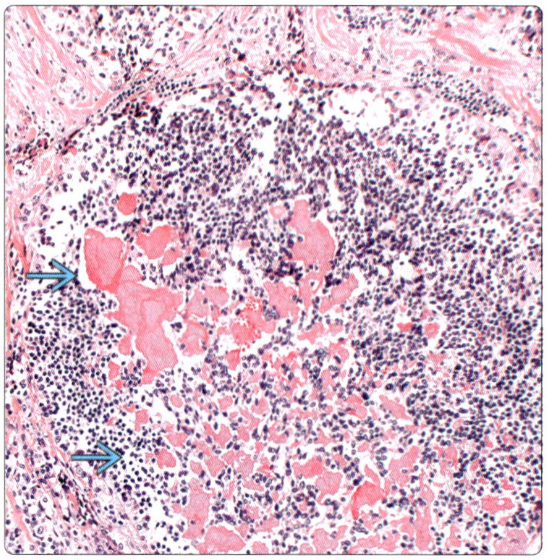

Metastatic Pulmonary Carcinoid Tumor

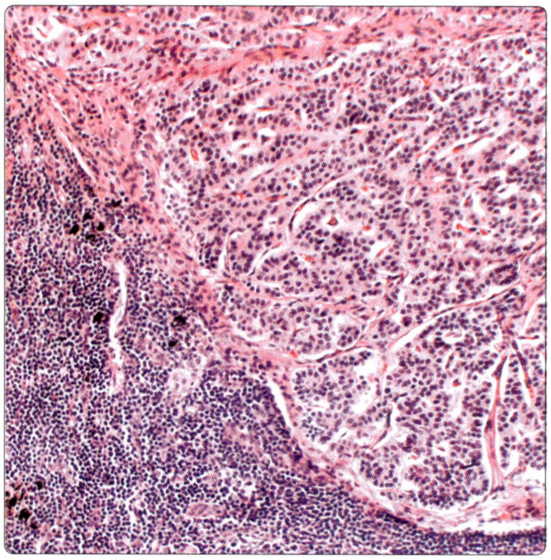

Intraparotid Lymph Node

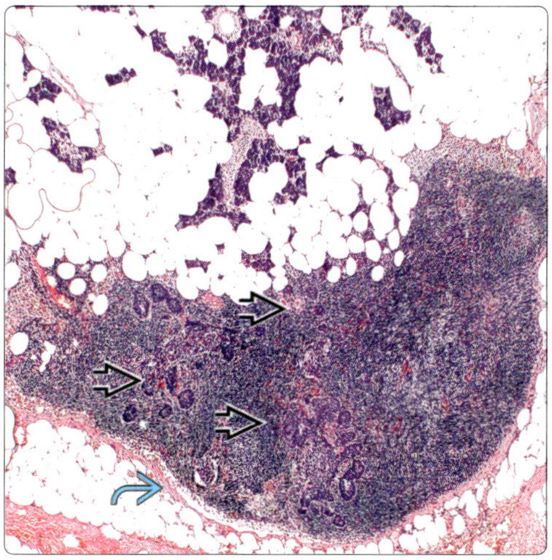

Intraparotid Lymph Node

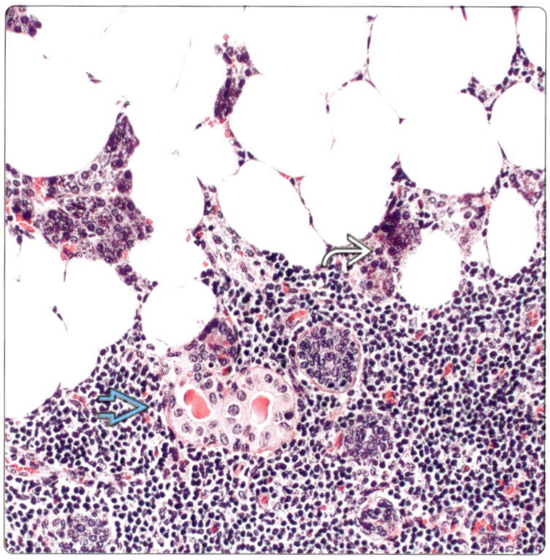

(Left) *Epithelial inclusions in intraparotid lymph nodes may be mistaken for metastatic carcinoma. This lymph node is only partially encapsulated and contains epithelial islands within the nodal parenchyma.* **(Right)** *The epithelial islands appear benign in this intraparotid lymph node. Ductal and acinar cells as well as eosinophilic striated ducts are seen and are indistinguishable from their extranodal counterparts, confirming the benign nature of these cells.*

Normal Thymus

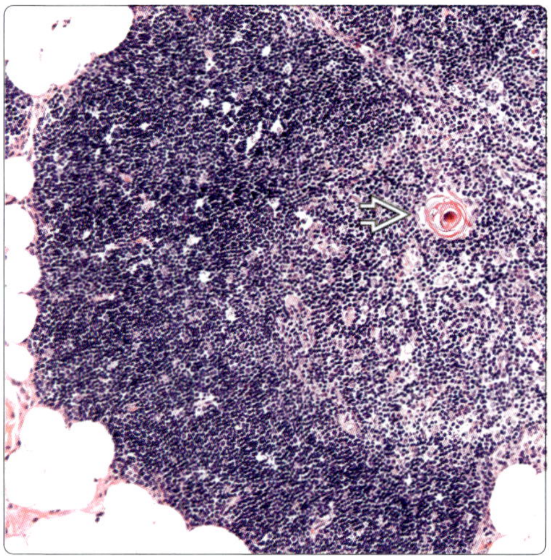

Sarcoidosis

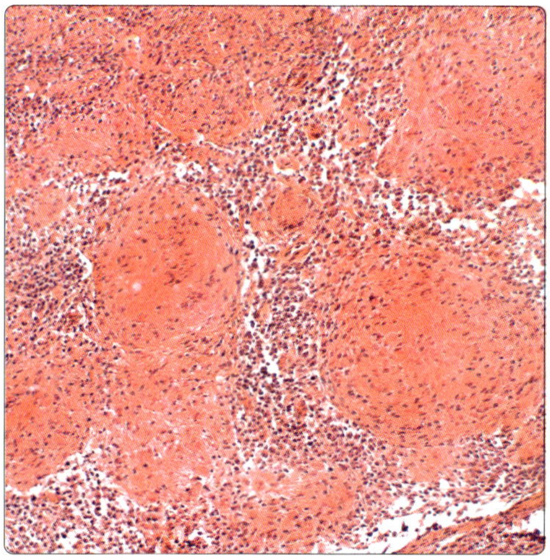

(Left) *Thymic remnants in the neck can mimic the appearance of a lymph node. Note the absence of a capsule and germinal centers. Hassall corpuscles, with their squamoid whorls, aid in recognition as thymus but must not be mistaken for deposits of metastatic squamous cell carcinoma. (Courtesy O. Pozdnyakova, MD.)* **(Right)** *Confluent nonnecrotizing granulomas are nonspecific but consistent with sarcoidosis. When identified, fresh tissue should be sent for cultures to exclude an infection.*

Paraganglioma

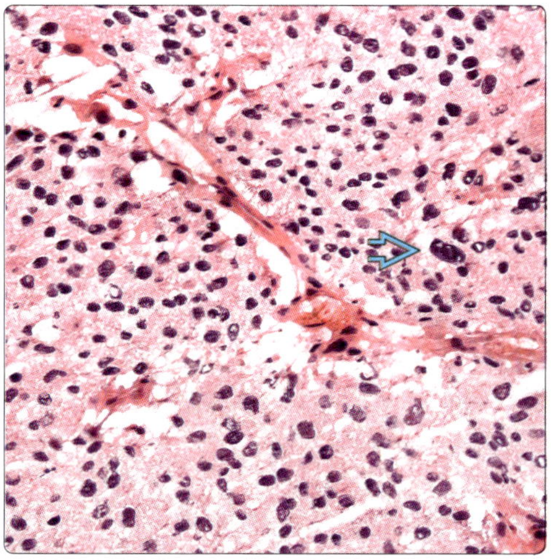

Nevus Cell Nest

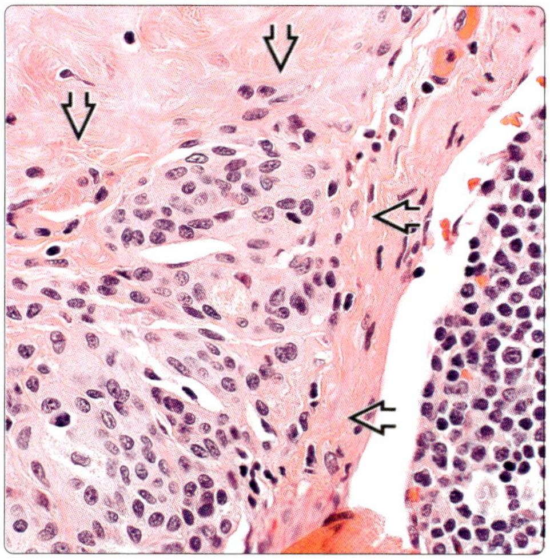

(Left) *Paragangliomas can mimic lymph nodes at surgery. The presence of endocrine atypia may be worrisome for malignancy. Distinction of paraganglioma from its mimics may require immunohistochemistry and a definitive diagnosis is deferred to permanent section.* **(Right)** *Nevus cell nests are benign rests that may be identified within lymph nodes. When seen in a capsular location, as in this example, they are readily recognized as not representing metastatic melanoma or carcinoma.*

SURGICAL/CLINICAL CONSIDERATIONS

Goal of Consultation

- For patients with lung mass, to determine if lung carcinoma resectable
  - Patients with non-small cell carcinoma and no nodal disease or only ipsilateral peribronchial metastases candidates for immediate resection
  - Patients with small cell carcinoma or metastatic non-small cell carcinoma to mediastinum may receive systemic treatment and may or may not later undergo resection
  - After positive lymph node identified, additional sampling generally not necessary
- For patients without lung mass, to determine etiology of mediastinal lymphadenopathy
  - Sufficient lesional tissue should be taken to arrive at specific diagnosis
  - Institutional protocols helpful to determine how tissue will be allocated

Change in Patient Management

- Patients with lung mass and no contralateral metastases may proceed to definitive resection
- Patients with lung mass and contralateral metastasis will not undergo immediate resection
- Patients with lymphadenopathy may undergo changes in immediate management based on preliminary frozen section diagnosis
  - If tuberculosis suspected
    - Operating room personnel notified
    - Patient placed under special infectious disease precautions
    - Treatment may be initiated depending on status of patient
  - If metastatic carcinoma or lymphoma diagnosed
    - Patient may undergo additional diagnostic procedures
    - Treatment may be initiated if patient severely ill

Clinical Setting

- For patients with lung mass, mediastinal lymphadenopathy usually due to metastatic carcinoma
  - Patients generally older and have history of tobacco use
- For patients without lung mass, mediastinal lymphadenopathy often not metastatic carcinoma
  - Patients generally younger and do not have history of tobacco use
    - Sarcoidosis: ~ 25%
    - Lymphoma: ~ 25%
    - Necrotizing granulomas: ~ 25%
    - Metastatic carcinoma: ~ 25% (majority have history of carcinoma)

SPECIMEN EVALUATION

Gross

- Lymph nodes dissected away from adipose tissue
  - If possible, nonfrozen tissue should be kept sterile in case infectious disease suspected
    - Cases of suspected infection should have tissue collected by operating team and sent for culture directly
  - Number, size, and appearance of nodes recorded
  - Larger nodes thinly sectioned (2-mm width)

Frozen Section

- Patients with lung mass
  - Grossly negative nodes
    - Portion or all nodal tissue may be used for frozen section
      - Entire face of embedded tissue should be represented on slides; deeper levels may be necessary in some cases
    - If only portion of node frozen and only nodal tissue present, remainder of specimen should be examined by frozen section
    - If only portion of node used for frozen section and lesional tissue present, nonfrozen tissue may be triaged for ancillary studies or tumor banking
  - Grossly positive nodes

Metastatic Pulmonary Mucinous Adenocarcinoma

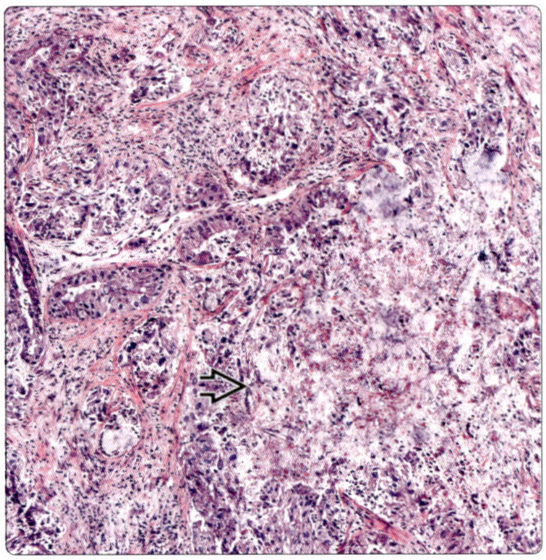

Metastatic Pulmonary Squamous Cell Carcinoma

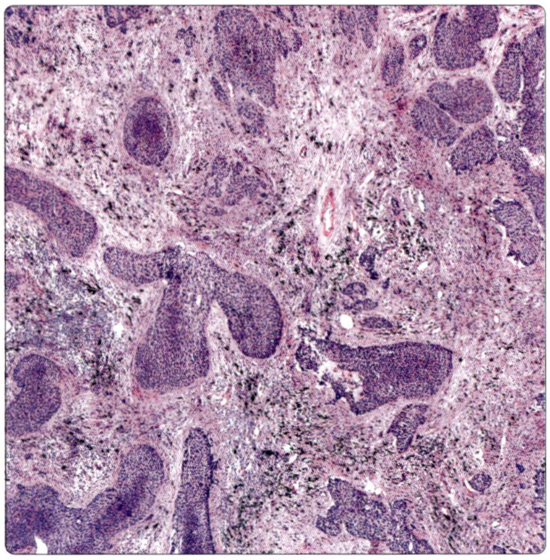

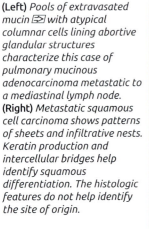

(Left) *Pools of extravasated mucin ⇨ with atypical columnar cells lining abortive glandular structures characterize this case of pulmonary mucinous adenocarcinoma metastatic to a mediastinal lymph node.* **(Right)** *Metastatic squamous cell carcinoma shows patterns of sheets and infiltrative nests. Keratin production and intercellular bridges help identify squamous differentiation. The histologic features do not help identify the site of origin.*

        - Only representative portion need be used for frozen section
        - Cytologic touch preparations can also be used to document positive node
- Patients without lung mass
    - Nonfrozen tissue should be reserved in case granulomatous or other infectious disease or lymphoma is suspected
    - Representative portions of most abnormal appearing node or nodes may be frozen
    - If frozen portion shows only normal nodal tissue, remainder of specimen should be frozen

Cytology

- Mottled gross appearance with punctate necrosis suggestive of infectious etiology
- Cytologic preparations particularly useful for granulomatous disease
    - Avoids contamination of cryostat
    - Less likely to expose personnel by puncture wounds or aerosolization
    - Tissue can be kept sterile for microbiologic culture

MOST COMMON DIAGNOSES

Metastatic Non-Small Cell Carcinoma

- Most common etiology for mediastinal lymphadenopathy
- Morphology dependent on differentiation (squamous vs. glandular) and grade
    - Usually identical or similar to primary carcinoma
- Range of variants possible; consider nonpulmonary sites in differential diagnosis
    - Appearance of pulmonary non-small cell carcinoma often nonspecific
        - Squamous carcinoma from various sites cannot be distinguished
    - Consider other sites when adenocarcinoma well differentiated
        - Review of clinical records, pathology reports, or previous slides often helpful
        - Knowledge of previous histologic type useful (e.g., papillary, signet ring cell, mucinous, or other types)

Metastatic Small Cell Carcinoma

- Often metastatic at time of diagnosis
    - Generally treated with systemic chemotherapy rather than surgery
- Small blue cell tumor
    - Cells 3-4x size of lymphocyte
    - Scant cytoplasm
    - Nuclear molding
    - Nuclei with dispersed (salt-and-pepper) chromatin and inconspicuous nucleoli
    - Necrosis usually present as discrete foci or apoptotic cells
    - Mitotic figures usually present
    - Lacks desmoplastic response
        - Crush artifact common and characteristic
- In frozen sections, may be difficult to distinguish from lymphoma and carcinoid
    - Cytoplasmic preparations may provide better cytologic detail

Carcinoid Tumor

- Patients somewhat younger than those typically seen with lung carcinoma
    - May present with centrally located intrabronchial lesion, causing obstruction
- Typical carcinoid tumor
    - Insular, trabecular, cribriform patterns possible
        - Can resemble well-differentiated adenocarcinoma from other sites
        - Prostate and breast cancer can closely resemble carcinoid
    - Less commonly has spindle cell pattern
    - Uniform nuclei with salt-and-pepper chromatin
- Atypical carcinoid tumor
    - Defined by mitotic rate > 2 per 10 HPF
    - May show atypia &/or focal necrosis
    - May be impossible to distinguish from carcinoid on frozen section
- Important to distinguish from small cell carcinoma

Lymphoma

- Hodgkin and non-Hodgkin lymphoma can present as mediastinal adenopathy
- Based on gross examination, nodes should be selectively sampled
    - Nodes involved by lymphoma usually have homogeneous fleshy appearance
- Tissue triage of primary importance for optimum management
    - Nonfrozen tissue for optimal histologic evaluation
        - Formalin as well as special hematologic fixatives (B-Plus and others)
    - Ancillary studies
        - Flow cytometry
        - Frozen tissue for molecular studies
            - Many studies can be performed on fixed tissue
    - If tissue limited, communication with surgeon important to assess risks/benefits of obtaining more for ancillary studies

Granulomatous Inflammation

- Both caseating and noncaseating granulomata may be seen
- In cases of suspected granulomatous disease, touch preps may be confirmatory and avoid cryostat contamination
- Sarcoid: Typically noncaseating rounded epithelioid granulomata
    - Sarcoid occasionally has focal necrosis
    - Tuberculosis may not show central necrosis
- Sterile tissue for culture should be saved when possible

REPORTING

Frozen Section

- For patients with lung mass
    - If non-small cell carcinoma present, diagnosis of "metastatic carcinoma" sufficient
        - Subclassification of type of carcinoma not necessary or expected intraoperatively but important for final diagnosis
        - If nonpulmonary primary origin suspected, this should be discussed with surgeon

- Metastatic small cell carcinoma should be specifically reported
  - Patients often will not undergo additional surgery
- For patients without lung mass
  - Most common diagnoses lymphoma, necrotizing granulomas, and granulomas consistent with sarcoid
    - If lymphoma suspected, tissue should be allocated for hematopathologic studies (special fixatives, flow cytometry, possibly saved frozen)
    - If granulomas present, tissue should be sent for mycobacterial and fungal cultures

Cytology

- Positive or negative for carcinoma
- Features suggestive of infectious process
  - Giant cells &/or necrosis

Reliability for Metastatic Carcinoma

- False-positive results very rare (< 5%)
  - Pleural adhesions and mesothelial cells may be mistaken for carcinoma
  - Benign mesothelial cells rarely present in lymph nodes
  - Prominent histiocytes in marginal sinus can mimic carcinoma
- False-negative results occur in ~ 2% of cases
  - Usually due to failure to freeze entire node or to obtain deep enough sections to represent all tissue in block

PITFALLS

Failure to Freeze All Nodal Tissue in Patients With Lung Masses

- Metastasis can be missed if only portion of node is frozen
- All macrometastases (> 2 mm) should be detected by freezing all tissue; smaller metastases may or may not be seen

Small Cell Carcinoma vs. Lymphocytes

- Tumor cells may be mistaken for lymphocytes
  - May be difficult if cells crushed or cauterized
  - Cytologic preparations may provide preparation for evaluation of tumor cells
- Necrosis and numerous mitoses should not be present in benign lymphocytes
- Cells of small cell carcinoma 3-4x size of lymphocytes
  - Can be difficult to determine if node completely replaced by carcinoma

Metastatic Carcinoid vs. Carcinoma

- Can be mistaken for small cell carcinoma in small crushed biopsies
  - Small cell carcinoma should not be diagnosed unless mitoses and necrosis present
- Patients with carcinoid generally younger with central peri- or intrabronchial masses

Pulmonary vs. Nonpulmonary Metastasis

- Site of origin of poorly differentiated tumors may be difficult to determine
- Review of preoperative history and (if available) slides can be of great assistance
- Recognition of invasion patterns or cytologic features unusual for lung cancer can raise index of suspicion
  - Signet ring cells and linear invasive pattern typical of lobular breast cancer
  - Pigmented cells and single cell pattern suggestive of melanoma

Prominent Histiocytes

- Can be mistaken for metastatic carcinoma, lymphoma, or melanoma
- Histologic features distinguish these cells from most carcinomas
  - Abundant foamy and usually clear cytoplasm
  - Bland round nuclei with small nucleoli
  - May contain intracytoplasmic anthracotic pigment or hemosiderin
- Typically scattered throughout node rather than forming discrete masses

Mesothelial Cells

- Can be mistaken for carcinoma when present in adhesions or within lymph nodes
  - Almost always found in patients with pericarditis or pleuritis
- Mesothelial cells in pleural adhesions adjacent to adipose tissue can be mistaken for metastatic adenocarcinoma
- Single cells or small clusters of mesothelial cells can be present in peripheral sinuses of draining lymph nodes
  - Glandular or papillary architecture generally not seen
  - Cells have bland nuclei and can resemble histiocytes
- Potential source of false-positive results if immunohistochemical studies for keratin used on permanent sections

Thymic Tissue

- Normal thymus may be biopsied
- Lacks outer capsule and germinal centers
- Hassall corpuscles can be mistaken for metastatic squamous carcinoma if not recognized
  - Squamous whorls
  - Keratohyaline granules
  - Lack nuclear atypia seen in squamous carcinomas

SELECTED REFERENCES

1. Yang XN et al: A lobe-specific lymphadenectomy protocol for solitary pulmonary nodules in non-small cell lung cancer. Chin J Cancer Res. 27(6):538-44, 2015
2. Jakubiak M et al: Fast cytological evaluation of lymphatic nodes obtained during transcervical extended mediastinal lymphadenectomy. Eur J Cardiothorac Surg. 43(2):297-301, 2013
3. Colebatch A et al: Benign mesothelial cells as confounders when cytokeratin immunohistochemistry is used in sentinel lymph nodes. Hum Pathol. 42(8):1209-10; author reply 1210-1, 2011
4. Lewis AL et al: Benign salivary gland tissue inclusion in a pulmonary hilar lymph node from a patient with invasive well-differentiated adenocarcinoma of the lung: a potential misinterpretation for the staging of carcinoma. Int J Surg Pathol. 19(3):382-5, 2011

Metastatic Pulmonary Adenocarcinoma

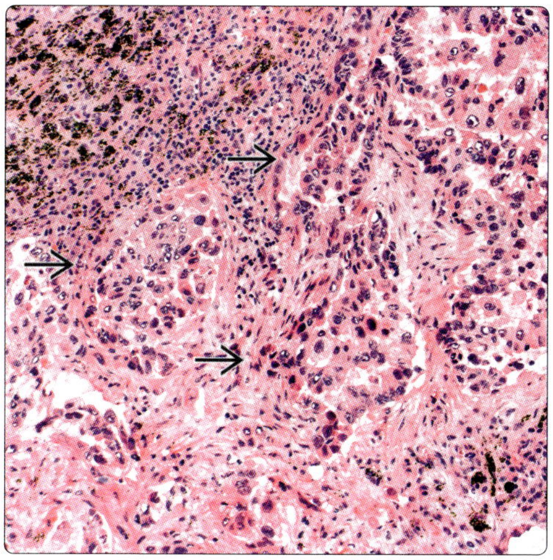

Metastatic Pulmonary Adenocarcinoma: Cytologic Preparation

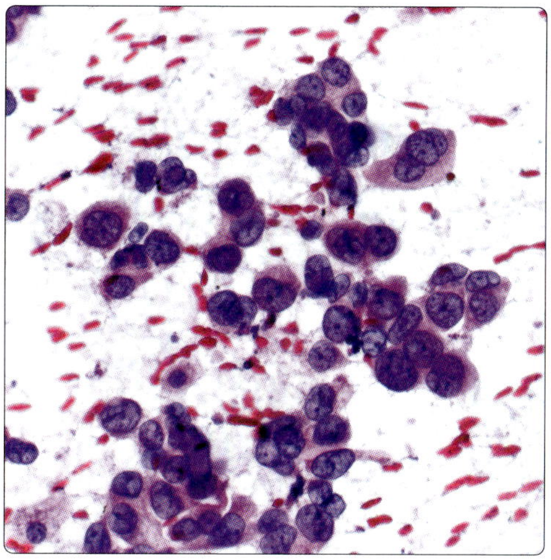

(Left) *This pattern of lung adenocarcinoma metastatic to a lymph node is commonly encountered. Nests and poorly formed glands → composed of pleomorphic epithelial cells invade desmoplastic stroma.* **(Right)** *Touch prep cytology may be used as an adjunct or (particularly with grossly visible lesions) a tissue-preserving replacement for standard frozen section of a lymph node. Clusters of malignant cells are diagnostic of metastatic carcinoma, in this case pulmonary adenocarcinoma.*

Metastatic Pulmonary Squamous Cell Carcinoma

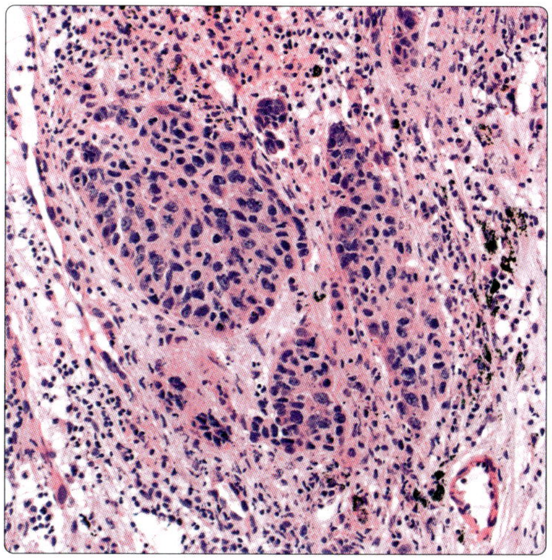

Metastatic Pulmonary Squamous Cell Carcinoma: Cytologic Preparation

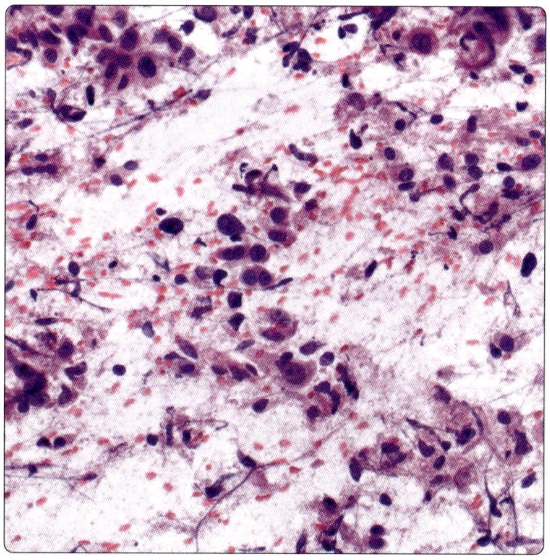

(Left) *Metastatic squamous cell carcinomas typically form well-defined nests. Although keratin formation is not seen, the dense eosinophilic cytoplasm represents cytoplasmic keratinization. In addition, intercellular bridges on higher magnification are additional evidence of squamous differentiation.* **(Right)** *Scrape preparations of a lymph node show malignant epithelioid cells with dense eosinophilic cytoplasm and a "dirty" background in this case of metastatic pulmonary squamous cell carcinoma.*

Metastatic Pulmonary Non-Small Cell Carcinoma

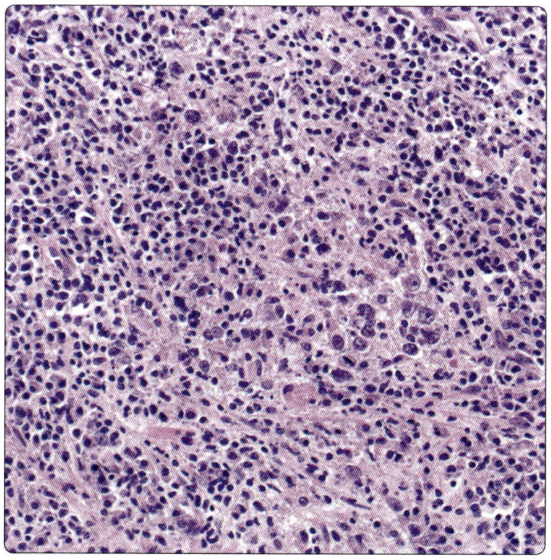

Metastatic Pulmonary Sarcomatoid Carcinoma

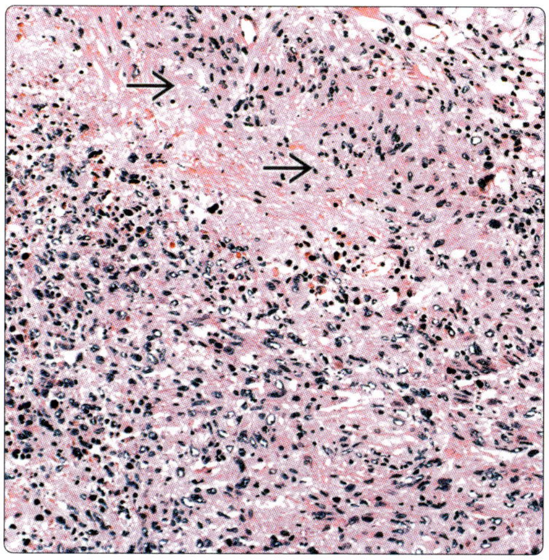

(Left) *Not infrequently, lung metastases may be sufficiently poorly differentiated to defy further subclassification. Intraoperatively, it should be sufficient for surgical management to confirm metastatic non-small cell carcinoma.* **(Right)** *Sarcomatoid lung carcinoma metastatic to a lymph node may elicit an exuberant granulomatous response → that can mimic sarcoid or infection. Knowledge of the histologic type of the primary carcinoma, when known, is very helpful.*

(Left) *This lymph node is effaced by small cell carcinoma consisting of a subtly nested proliferation of highly malignant small blue cells, with apoptosis, mitoses, crush artifact (Azzopardi effect)* ➡, *and focal nuclear molding.* **(Right)** *Cytologic features of small cell carcinoma include nuclear crowding, overlap, molding, extremely scant cytoplasm, and dark but relatively even chromatin. The clusters of cells help exclude a diagnosis of lymphoma.*

Metastatic Pulmonary Small Cell Carcinoma

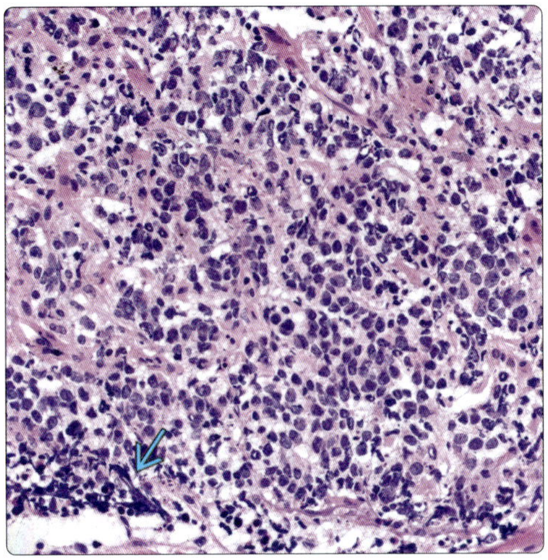

Metastatic Pulmonary Small Cell Carcinoma: Cytologic Features

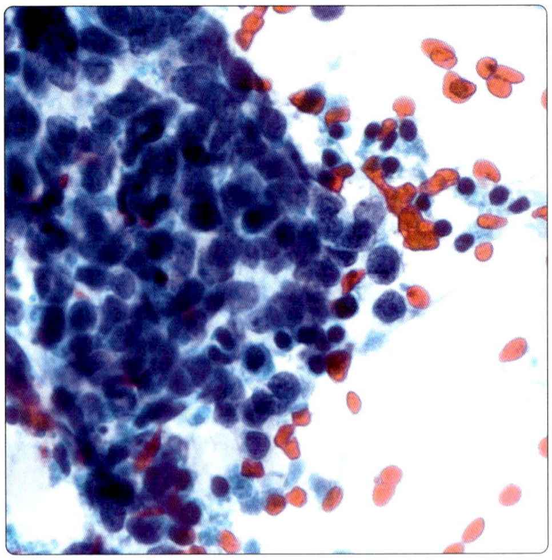

(Left) *Metastatic carcinoid tumor may show a cribriform growth pattern similar to prostate carcinoma or well-differentiated breast carcinoma. Preoperative review of clinical history, prior pathology reports, and slides may help to avoid pitfalls.* **(Right)** *Cytologic preparations may show finer nuclear detail than frozen section. This case of carcinoid tumor metastatic to a mediastinal lymph node shows round to ovoid, monotonous nuclei with salt and pepper chromatin. When cytoplasm is intact, cells may appear plasmacytoid.*

Metastatic Carcinoid Tumor

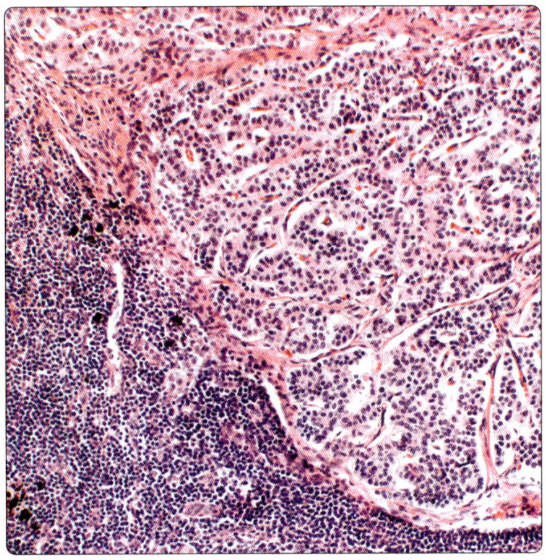

Metastatic Carcinoid Tumor: Cytologic Features

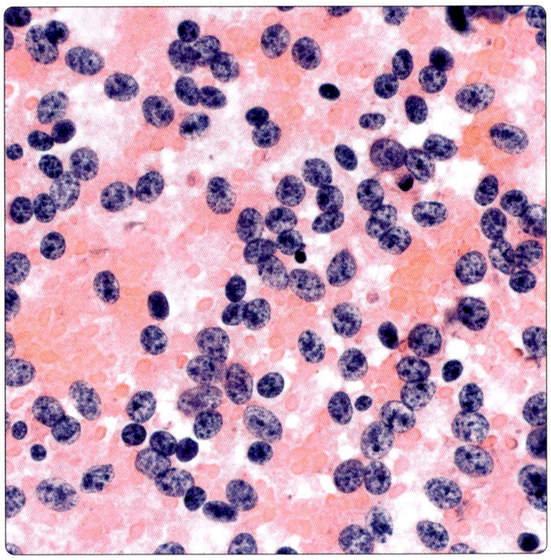

(Left) *On frozen section, carcinoid tumor may appear very glandular, and neuroendocrine (salt and pepper) chromatin may not be evident. Nuclear uniformity is a clue to diagnosis, and touch preparations may also be useful.* **(Right)** *This case of atypical carcinoid of lung metastatic to a mediastinal lymph node shows nested growth, moderate nuclear pleomorphism, and salt and pepper chromatin. Nuclear pleomorphism is moderate. Mitotic figures and focal necrosis can be present.*

Metastatic Carcinoid Tumor

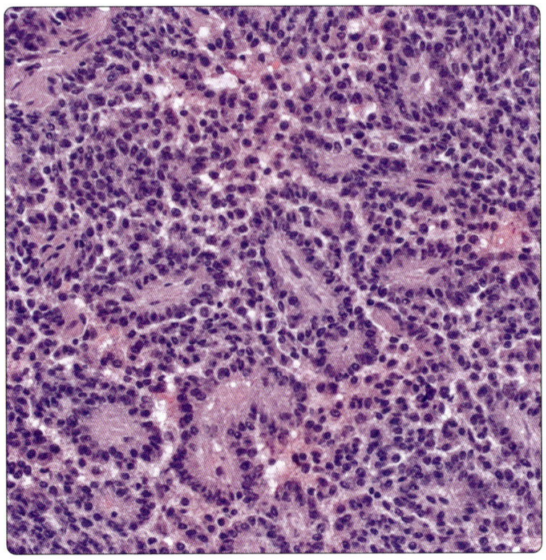

Metastatic Atypical Carcinoid Tumor

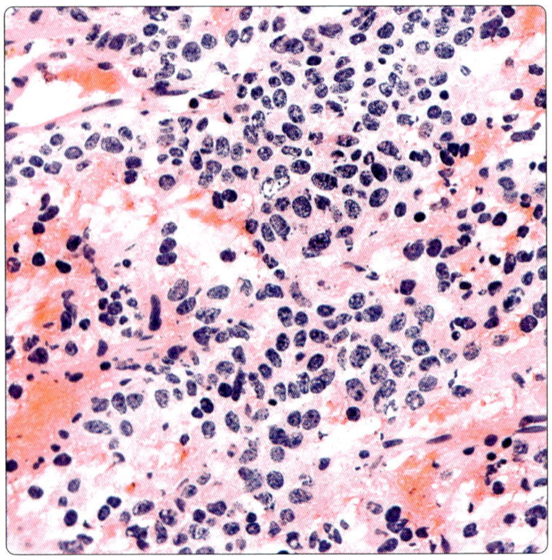

Metastatic Pulmonary Non-Small Cell Carcinoma Simulating Granuloma

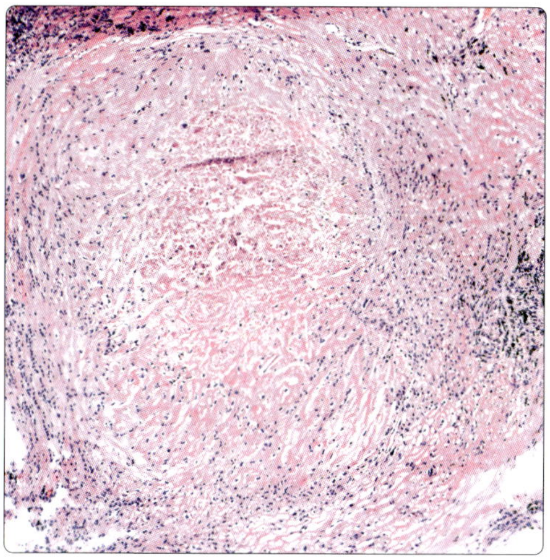

Metastatic Breast Carcinoma

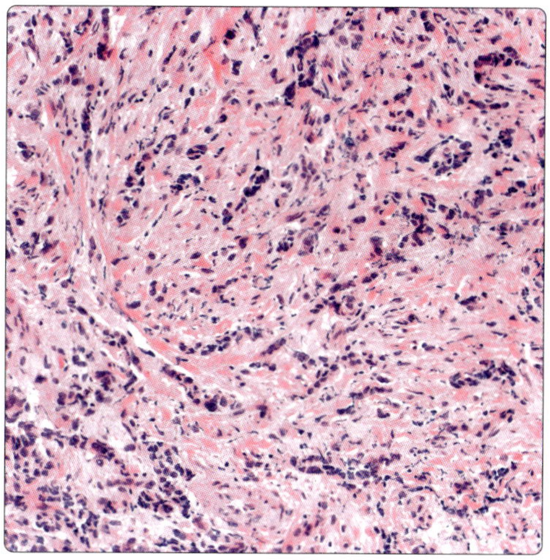

(Left) *This pulmonary non-small cell carcinoma metastatic to anthracotic lymph node shows extensive cellular necrosis simulating granulomatous disease. Viable tumor cells are quite sparse. Prior treatment may also cause necrosis of tumor cells in lymph nodes.* **(Right)** *This metastatic breast carcinoma shows nests and cords of atypical cells invading in fibrous stroma. Breast carcinomas can have a wide range of histologic appearances. Knowledge of the prior histologic type is very helpful.*

Metastatic Mesothelioma

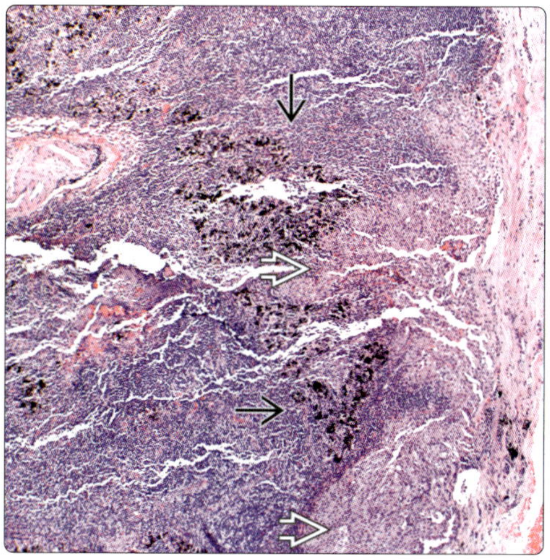

Metastatic Melanoma

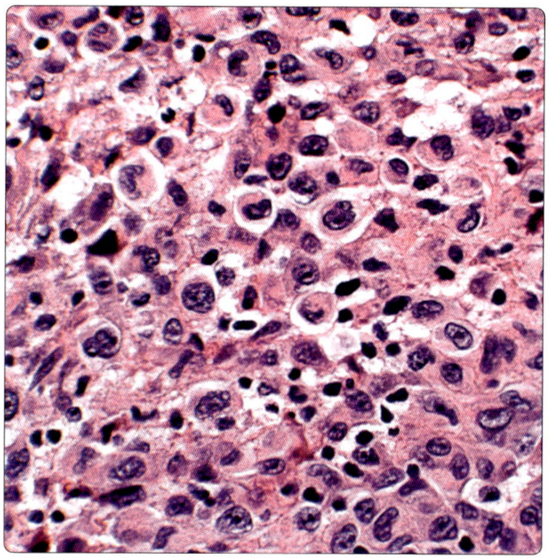

(Left) *Metastatic mesothelioma ➔ is rarely seen in lymph nodes. The cells can fill the peripheral sinuses and resemble histiocytes. Note that the malignant cell population excludes the anthracotic pigment ⇨ that is present in the true histiocytes.* **(Right)** *Metastatic melanoma in lymph nodes may have a nested pattern that simulates carcinoma or can be dyscohesive, resembling lymphoma. Pigment and intranuclear inclusions may serve as diagnostic clues. Patients usually have a history of melanoma.*

Diffuse Large B-Cell Lymphoma

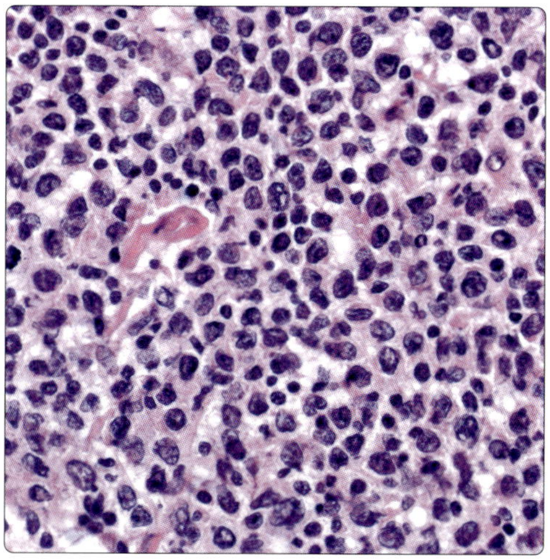

Follicular Lymphoma

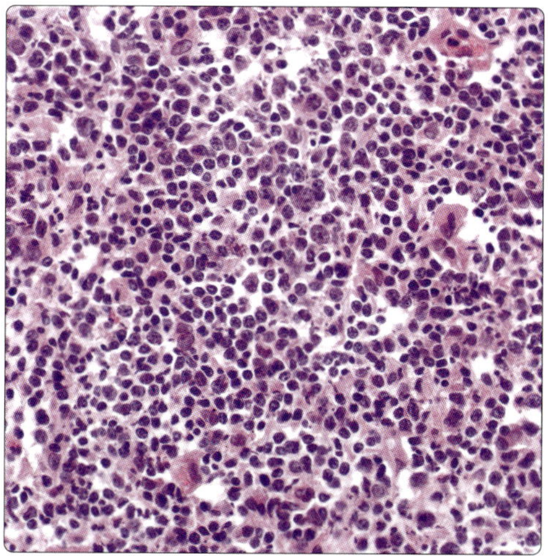

(Left) *Diffuse large B-cell lymphoma shows effacement of the nodal architecture by large atypical lymphocytes. Recognition as malignancy is usually not a problem, but small specimens with crush artifact may be difficult to distinguish from small cell carcinoma.* **(Right)** *This follicular lymphoma shows an admixture of large, atypical transformed lymphocytes and a subpopulation of smaller cells with cleaved, irregular nuclear membranes.*

(Left) *In small lymphocytic lymphoma, there is a uniform population of small cells lacking true germinal centers but showing pale "proliferation zones." The outer sinuses are filled, and the node has a rounded (rather than normal lobulated) contour.* **(Right)** *This node has been filled with a very uniform and monomorphic population of lymphocytes characteristic of small lymphocytic lymphoma. No germinal centers were present.*

Small Lymphocytic Lymphoma

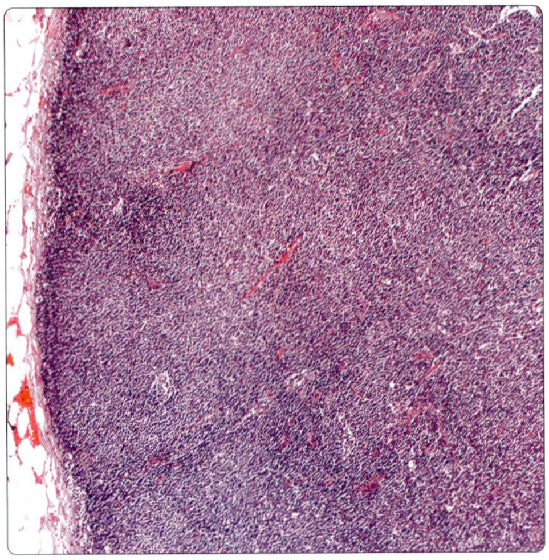

Small Lymphocytic Lymphoma

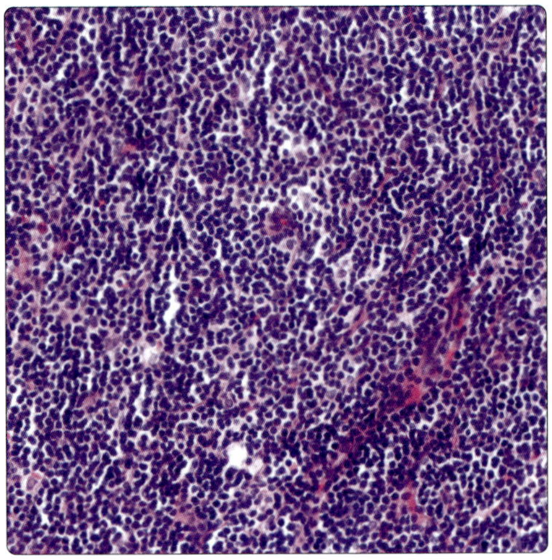

(Left) *The normal nodal architecture is effaced by a proliferation of slightly enlarged lymphocytes with nuclear features "intermediate" between those of the small mature cells of small lymphocytic lymphoma and the cleaved nuclei of follicular lymphomas. This is characteristic of mantle cell lymphoma.* **(Right)** *This case of Hodgkin lymphoma shows readily identifiable Reed-Sternberg cells and variants in a background of small, mature lymphocytes and occasional eosinophils.*

Mantle Cell Lymphoma

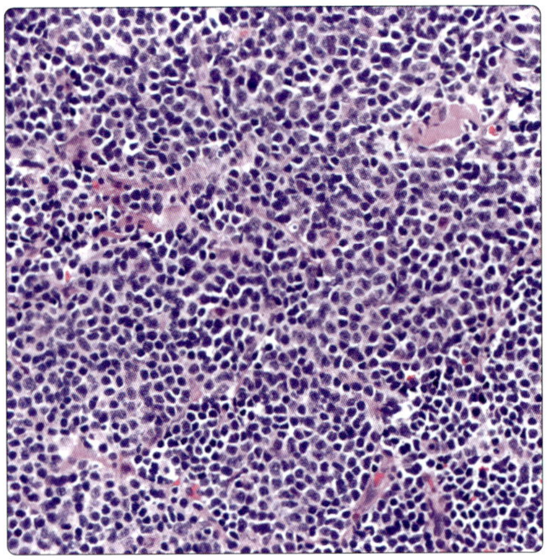

Hodgkin Lymphoma, Classic Type

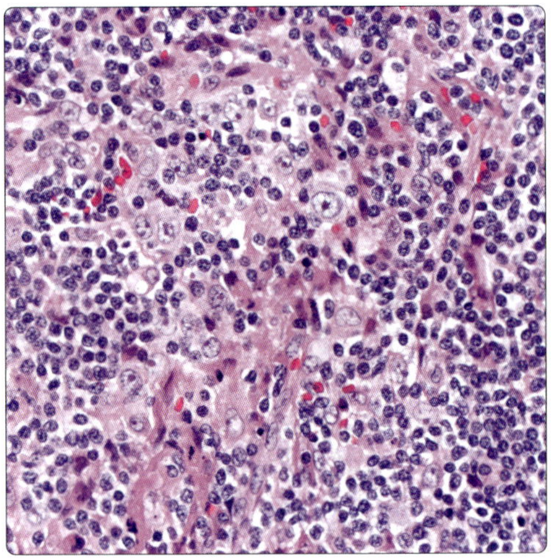

(Left) *This mediastinal nodal architecture is effaced by a proliferation of small mature lymphocytes and larger pale cells. Scattered larger cells with dark nuclei are the diagnostic Reed-Sternberg cells of Hodgkin lymphoma.* **(Right)** *Large, mononuclear Hodgkin cells with polylobate or multiple nuclei with prominent nucleoli and abundant cytoplasm* → *are seen in a background of mature lymphocytes. In some cases, tumor cells are very sparse, raising the possibility of benign reactive change in the differential diagnosis.*

Nodular Lymphocyte-Predominant Hodgkin Lymphoma

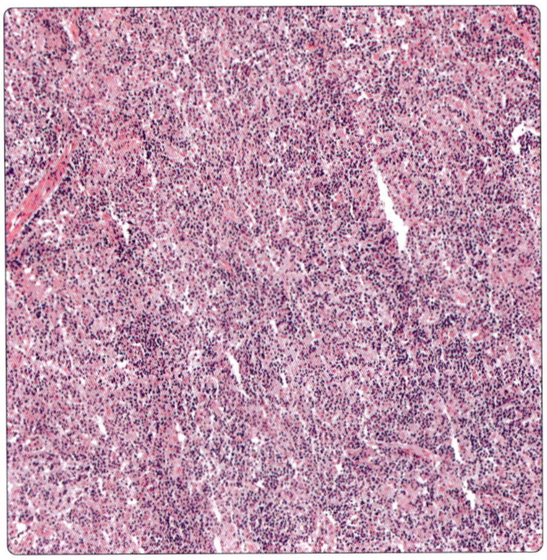

Nodular Lymphocyte-Predominant Hodgkin Lymphoma

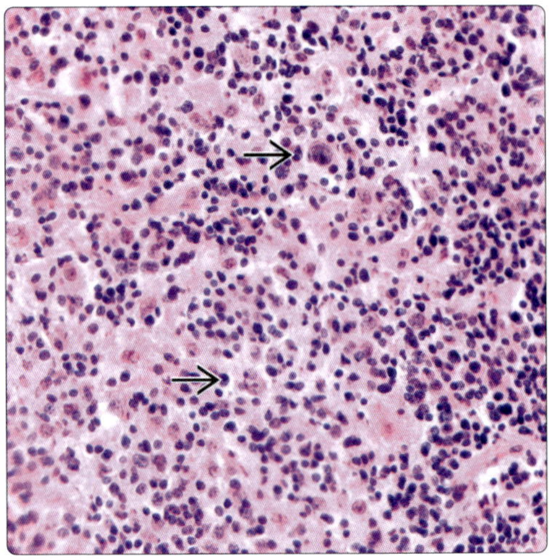

Metastatic Epithelioid Angiosarcoma

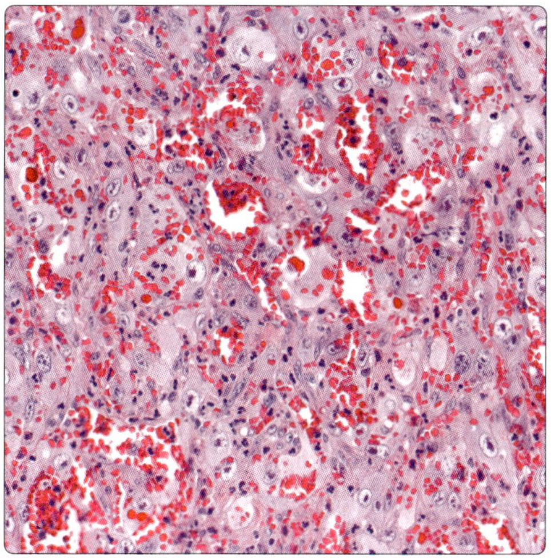

Vascular Transformation of Lymph Node

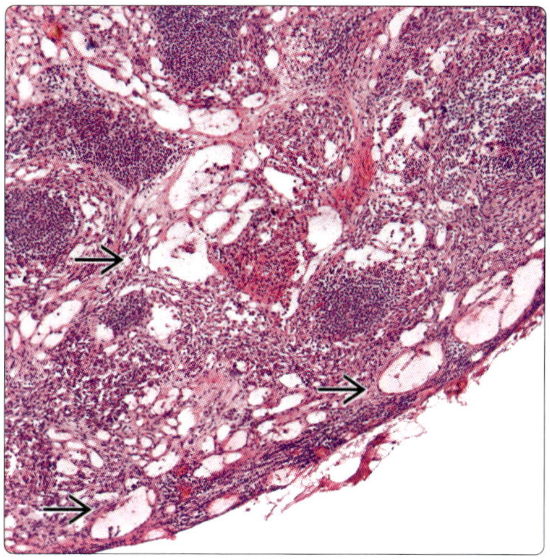

(Left) *Clinical history can be essential for patients with unusual primary malignancies. This rare metastatic epithelioid angiosarcoma would be very difficult to classify on frozen section alone.* **(Right)** *Vascular transformation ⇒ of sinuses is a rare finding in lymph nodes, usually in the abdomen. This is a very rare case in a mediastinal lymph node. This finding needs to be distinguished from rare metastasizing malignant vascular sarcomas.*

Noncaseating Granulomatous Lymphadenitis

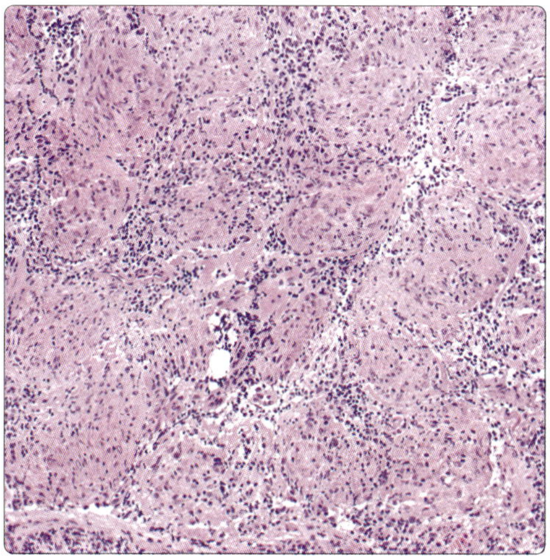

Necrotizing Granulomas

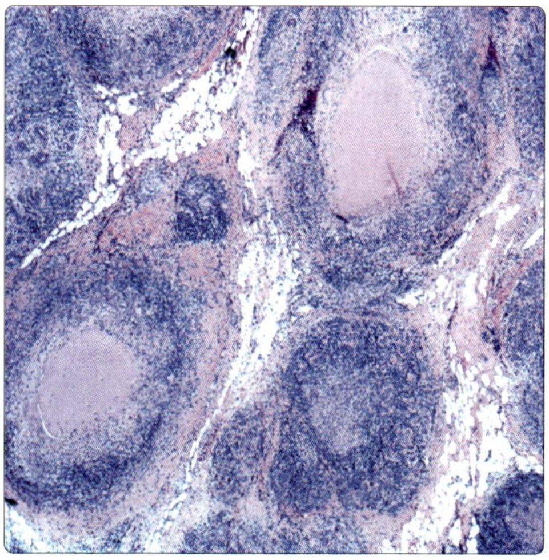

(Left) *Granulomatous inflammation is most commonly due to sarcoid in the US but may also be associated with infections and rarely with some tumors. Special handling precautions should be used in case infection is identified.* **(Right)** *Necrotizing granulomas are most commonly seen associated with mycobacterial infections. Tissue should be sent for culture, and special procedures to protect hospital staff and other patients are necessary (e.g., respirator masks and cryostat decontamination).*

Crush Artifact

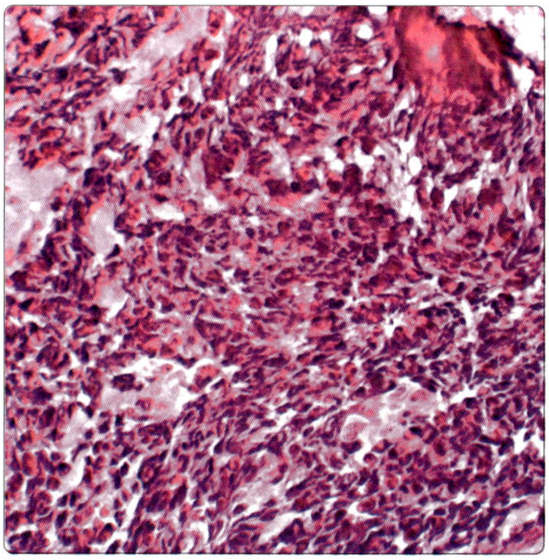

Prominent Histiocytes in Lymph Node

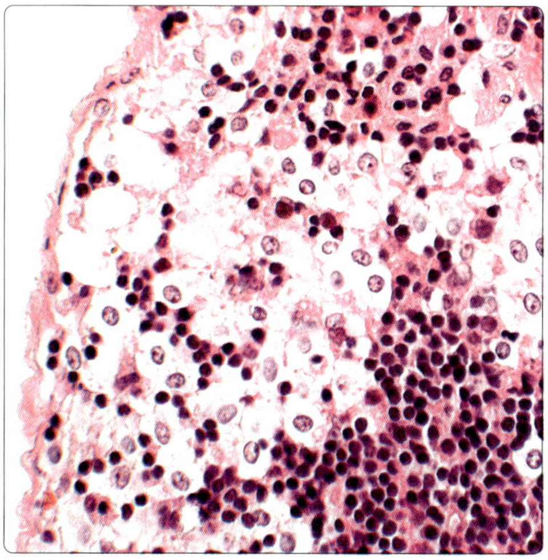

(Left) *Lymphocytes, lymphoma, carcinoid tumor, and small cell carcinoma are all susceptible to crush artifact due to the lack of supporting stroma. Diagnosis was deferred on frozen section in this case. The final diagnosis was metastatic small cell carcinoma.* **(Right)** *Prominent histiocytes can sometimes mimic metastatic carcinoma, lymphoma, or melanoma. The cells have abundant foamy cytoplasm and rounded bland nuclei with small nucleoli. Some cells may contain hemosiderin or anthracotic pigment.*

SURGICAL/CLINICAL CONSIDERATIONS

Goal of Consultation

- Diagnosis of meningeal mass or other process
- Provisional diagnosis aids in allocation of tissue for ancillary studies (molecular)

Change in Patient Management

- Diagnosis of meningioma could result in complete resection for definitive treatment
  - Dependent on location of tumor and involvement of other structures (dural sinuses, bone)
  - Occasionally, dural margins may be sent for adequacy of excision
- Other types of lesions will generally not undergo resection
  - Metastasis, lymphoma, infectious or inflammatory process

Clinical Setting

- Usual presentation headache, seizure, or focal neurologic deficit
- Patients with germline mutations can present with meningeal masses
  - Meningiomas: Neurofibromatosis type 2, multiple meningioma syndrome
  - Hemangioblastoma: von Hippel-Lindau syndrome
  - Meningioangiomatosis: Neurofibromatosis type 2
- Prior radiation for other conditions of central nervous system (acute lymphocytic leukemia, pituitary adenoma) can increase risk for developing meningioma
  - Secondary meningiomas typically radiation induced and often atypical or malignant

SPECIMEN EVALUATION

Gross

- Nodular, plaque-like, or fragmented appearance, ± dural attachments
- May be calcified or gritty in texture

Frozen Section

- Initial specimen often small biopsy, which can be used for cytologic preparations, and remainder frozen
- If larger resection specimen received, representative area can be frozen
- Cytologic preparations sometimes better for evaluation of meningiomas
  - If specimen very fibrous and paucicellular on cytologic preparations, frozen section can be helpful

Cytology

- May be difficult to smear
- Touch preparations best for calcified lesions
- Scrape preparations useful for fibrous lesions
- Important adjunct to diagnosis of
  - Lymphoproliferative lesions
  - Bony or fibrous lesions difficult to cut (touch preparations helpful)
  - Cysts, as lining cells may be better preserved
- May spare contamination of cryostat in cases suspected to be infectious

MOST COMMON DIAGNOSES

Meningioma and Variants

- Main goal: Identification as meningioma
  - Meningiomas will generally be resected
  - Other processes will generally not be resected (metastasis or inflammatory lesions)
- Architecture varies with subtype
- Detection of anaplasia useful if all features present
  - May be indication for more extensive resection
- **Meningioma, WHO grade I**
  - Subtypes
    - Fibrous, meningothelial, transitional, psammomatous, secretory, angiomatous, microcystic
    - Not necessary to distinguish among subtypes during intraoperative consultation
  - Meningothelial whorls with psammoma bodies may be seen on touch prep

Meningioma: Location

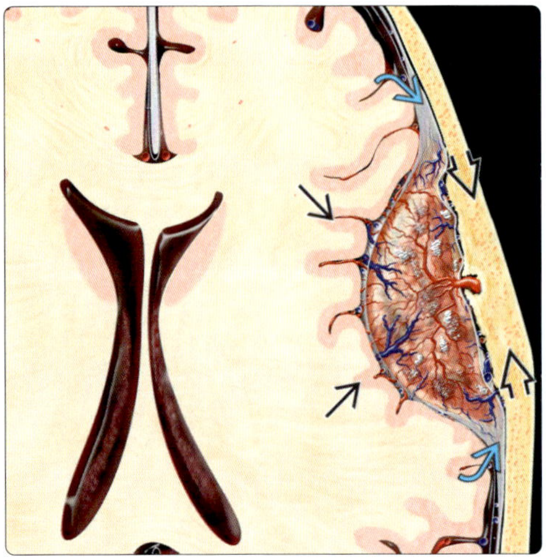

Meningioma: MR Appearance

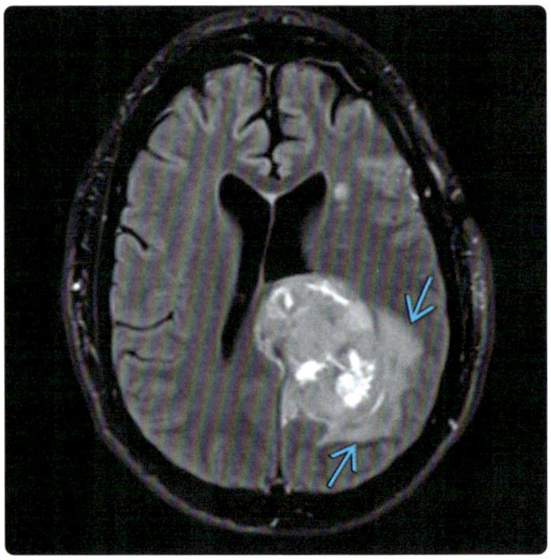

(Left) *Meningiomas arise from the cranial dura ➙ and derive their blood supply from it. The underlying brain is compressed ➙. Hyperostosis ➙ of adjacent cranial bone is a common feature.* **(Right)** *Axial FLAIR MR shows a left posterior falcine extraaxial mass ➙ most compatible with meningioma. The lesion shows increased associated edema, mass effect, and midline shift.*

  - Syncytial groupings of cells with broad, flat, eosinophilic cytoplasm, nuclei with fine dusty chromatin, and smooth nuclear borders
- **Atypical meningioma, WHO grade II**
  - Frozen section or smear
    - Requires 4 mitoses/10 HPF **or** 3 of following
      - Sheet-like growth (disordered architecture)
      - Small cell change
      - Prominent nucleoli
      - Hypercellularity
      - Necrosis (if lesion has not been embolized)
    - **Or** chordoid or clear cell morphology
  - Not necessary to determine grade at intraoperative consultation
  - Report as "meningioma with atypical features, grading deferred"
- **Anaplastic meningioma, WHO grade III**
  - Frozen section or smear
    - ≥ 20 mitoses/10 HPF
    - **Or** atypia in excess of that seen in grade II (resembling carcinoma, melanoma, or sarcoma)
    - **Or** rhabdoid or papillary features in majority of tumor
  - Not necessary to determine grade at intraoperative consultation
  - Report as "meningioma with atypical features, grading deferred" or "malignant neoplasm, type to be determined"
- **Meningioangiomatosis**
  - 1/2 of cases arise in setting of neurofibromatosis type 2
  - Frozen and smear: Perivascular meningothelial whorls and spindle cells in superficial cortex
  - Sometimes calcified or fibrotic

Solitary Fibrous Tumor/Hemangiopericytoma

- Currently, solitary fibrous tumor and hemangiopericytoma considered to be same entity (WHO 2016)
- Identical to those tumors arising in pleural or other soft tissue sites
- Frozen and smear
  - Epithelioid or spindle cells with intervening wire-like collagen
  - Staghorn vessels
  - Mitotic activity variable (> 4 mitoses/HPF indicates atypical solitary fibrous tumor)
- Usually treated with resection
  - Distinction from meningioma on frozen section not critical for intraoperative management
  - Tumor often extremely hemorrhagic during surgery

Dural Fibrosarcoma

- Identical to those arising in other soft tissue sites
- Frozen and smear: Spindle cells in herringbone or fascicular growth pattern, variable pleomorphism and mitotic activity

Metastatic Carcinoma or Lymphoma

- Single deposit may mimic meningioma
  - Dural-based, circumscribed mass with dural tail
- Leptomeningeal carcinomatosis or diffuse involvement by lymphoma has widespread enhancement on MR
- Frozen and smear
  - Features indicating primary origin
    - Cytoplasmic clearing or vacuoles
      - Glands identify adenocarcinoma
    - Small cell vs. non-small cell for metastatic lung carcinoma
    - Single-file cells for lobular breast carcinoma
    - Dyscohesive atypical lymphoid cells for lymphoma
  - History of prior malignancy critically important for correct interpretation

Hemangioblastoma

- Dural-based nodule in posterior fossa or spinal cord
- Frozen section and smear
  - Multivacuolated cells (oil red O positive) amid fine capillary stroma
  - Often striking nuclear atypia without mitoses
  - Microcystic changes
- Pitfall
  - Strong resemblance to metastatic renal clear cell carcinoma

Infection/Inflammatory Lesions

- Pachymeningitis (inflammation of dura mater) may have infectious or autoimmune cause
  - Tuberculosis (in developing world)
    - Smear and frozen: Typical necrotizing granulomas with giant cells
  - Idiopathic hypertrophic pachymeningitis is usually autoimmune
    - IgG4 disease
    - Rheumatoid conditions
    - Smear and frozen: Abundant lymphoplasmacytic infiltrates, collagen deposition
  - Sarcoidosis
    - Hard granulomas with giant cells
  - Biopsied when localized, mimicking meningioma
- In leptomeninges, almost always infectious cause, although paraneoplastic process is in differential diagnosis
  - Bacterial
    - Neutrophilic exudates in acute bacterial meningitis
    - Lymphocytes and giant cells in tuberculous meningitis
  - Fungal
    - Mononuclear or mixed inflammatory infiltrates
    - Organisms (*Cryptococcus*, *Coccidioides*, or (rarely) *Aspergillus* or *Candida*) detectable on smear and frozen
  - Viral
    - Mononuclear infiltrates
    - In herpes encephalitis, biopsy may include involved brain, showing macrophages and necrosis
    - Viral cytopathic effect rarely visible
  - Biopsied rarely, as cerebrospinal fluid testing often diagnostic
  - Material should be sent for specific cultures

Cysts

- Infrequently sent for intraoperative consultation, as imaging and gross appearance to surgeon sufficient for diagnosis
- Lining cells may be scarce relative to contents
  - Arachnoid cyst: Flattened meningothelial cells and variably thick collagen wall

- Dermoid/epidermoid cyst: Squamous cells, abundant keratin debris
- Enterogenous cyst: Ciliated columnar cells, mucoid material

Vascular Malformation

- Arteriovenous malformation
  - Usually extends into underlying parenchyma (cortex and white matter)
  - Angiography diagnostic
  - Frozen section usually not requested unless appearance atypical intraoperatively
- Dural cavernous hemangioma
  - May mimic meningioma, prompting intraoperative consultation
  - Sponge-like appearance of dilated vessels
- Dural venous anomaly
  - Rarely biopsied, unless change detected on serial imaging
  - Adjacent brain may show ischemic changes ("steal phenomenon")

REPORTING

Frozen Section

- Diagnosis of meningioma or solitary fibrous tumor/hemangiopericytoma should be made when possible to allow complete resection in same procedure
- Provisional diagnosis of another type of lesion allows appropriate tissue allocation for ancillary studies and eventual diagnosis

Cytology

- Diagnosis provided to extent possible, as for frozen sections

PITFALLS

Preoperative Embolization in Meningioma

- Embolization of this highly vascular tumor facilitates excision and reduces blood loss
  - Embolic agents (such as isopropyl alcohol/methacrylate) introduced via catheter
- Causes necrosis and mitotic activity
- Grading of tumor should be deferred to permanent sections
  - Grading can be difficult, even with optimal formalin-fixed permanent sections

Tumors in von Hippel-Lindau Patients

- Difficult distinction between hemangioblastoma and metastatic renal cell carcinoma
- May require immunohistochemical studies on permanent sections

Lymphoproliferative Disorders

- May be difficult to distinguish from infectious/inflammatory lesions
- Provisional diagnosis critical for appropriate allocation for flow cytometric and molecular studies

SELECTED REFERENCES

1. Karthigeyan M et al: Frozen section can 'sharpen' or 'sand off' the surgeon's knife: two case Illustrations with skull base meningioma mimics. World Neurosurg. ePub, 2017
2. Louis DN et al: The 2016 World Health Organization Classification of Tumors of the Central Nervous System: a summary. Acta Neuropathol. 131(6):803-20, 2016
3. Han SH et al: Cytologic features of pigmented atypical meningioma mimicking melanoma on intraoperative crush preparations. Diagn Cytopathol. 43(2):149-52, 2015
4. Savage NM et al: Dural-based metastatic carcinomas mimicking primary CNS neoplasia: report of 7 cases emphasizing the role of timely surgery and accurate pathologic evaluation. Int J Clin Exp Pathol. 4(5):530-40, 2011
5. Siddiqui MT et al: Cytologic features of meningiomas on crush preparations: a review. Diagn Cytopathol. 36(4):202-6, 2008
6. Johnson MD et al: Dural lesions mimicking meningiomas. Hum Pathol. 33(12):1211-26, 2002
7. Folkerth RD: Smears and frozen sections in the intraoperative diagnosis of central nervous system lesions. Neurosurg Clin N Am. 5(1):1-18, 1994

Meningioma: Gross Appearance

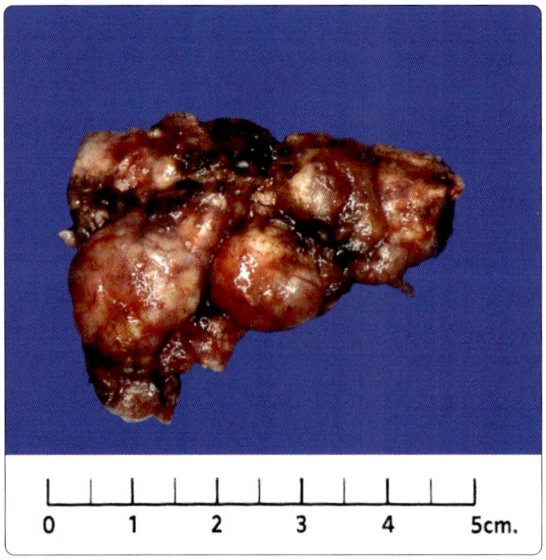

Meningioma: Gross Appearance

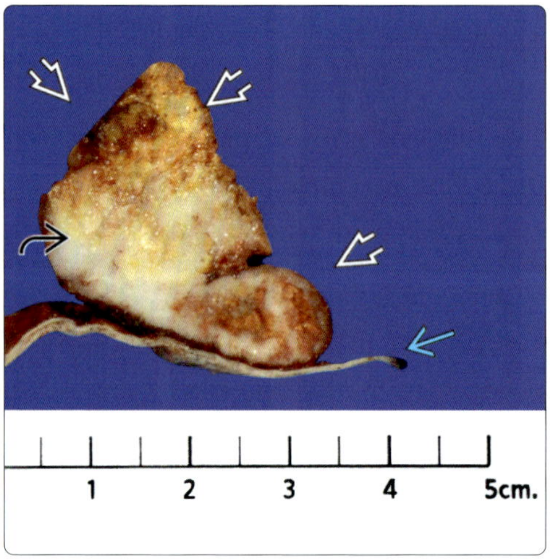

(Left) *Meningiomas grossly form multilobulated masses with a pink, reddish glistening surface.* **(Right)** *This meningioma* ➡ *shows a variable surface with firm, white, fibrous areas, more tan and reddish hemorrhagic areas, and yellow foci of necrosis* ↷. *Dural* ➡ *attachment is typical.*

Contents

Meningioma: Cytologic Appearance

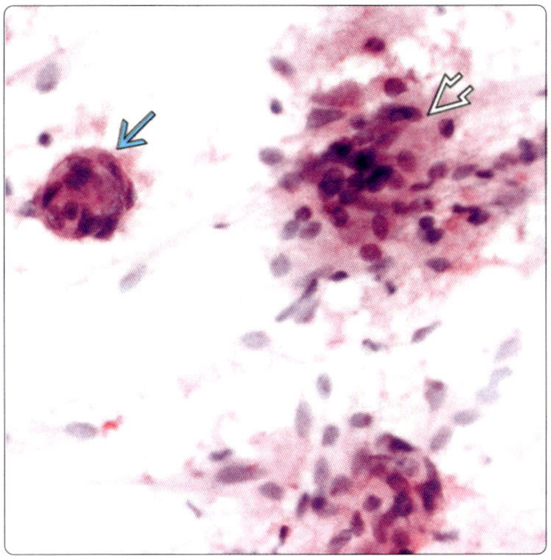

Meningioma: Psammoma Bodies

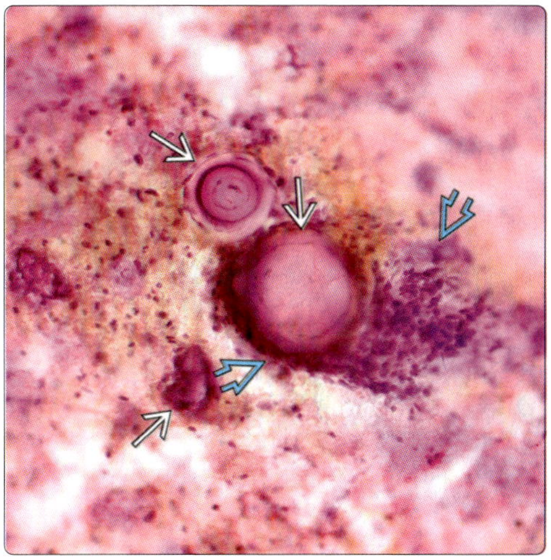

(Left) *Meningiomas can be difficult to smear as cells tend to stick together* *and, sometimes, only rare meningothelial whorls can be identified* . **(Right)** *Psammoma bodies (concentric calcification)* *surrounded by meningothelial cells* *feel like sand during the preparation of smears and impart a gritty sensation.*

Meningioma: Atypical Features

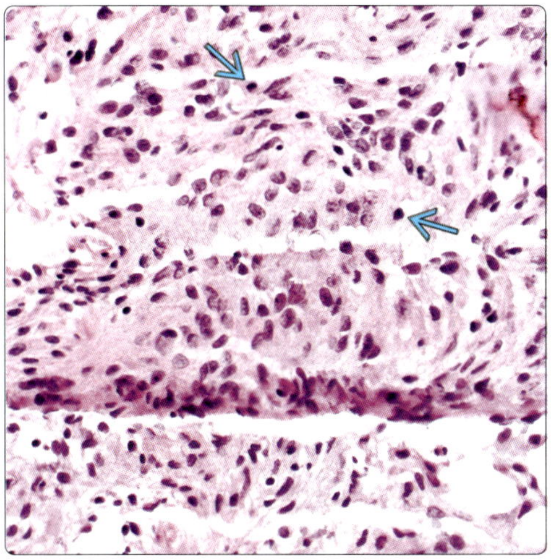

Meningioma/Brain Interface

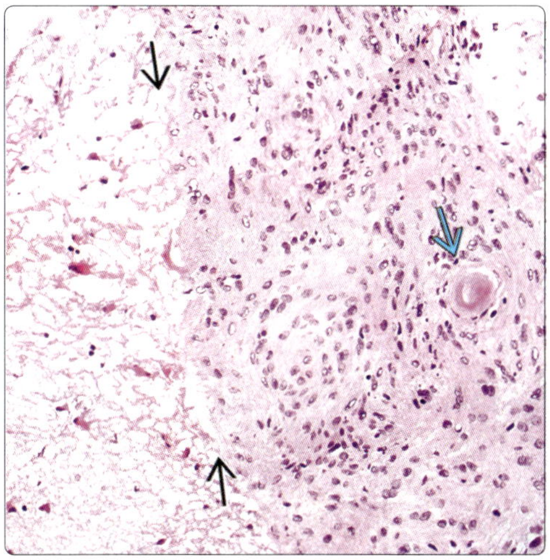

(Left) *Patternless growth and sheets of cells with mitotic figures* *are suggestive of atypical meningioma.* **(Right)** *If the interface with normal brain* *is present in the frozen section of meningioma, it should be carefully inspected for brain invasion. Invasion is not observed here. A psammoma body is present* .

Meningioma: Embolizing Material

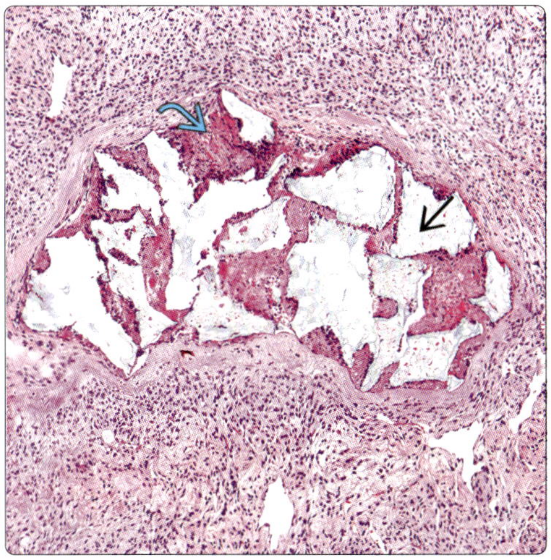

Anaplastic Meningioma

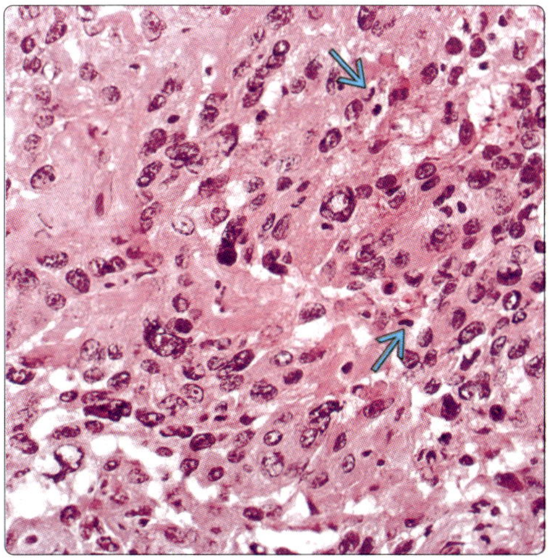

(Left) *This meningioma underwent preoperative embolization to facilitate removal. An intratumoral blood vessel is distended by embolizing material* *intermixed with fibrin* . *Embolized tumors may have increased atypia, mitotic activity, and necrosis and are difficult to grade.* **(Right)** *Anaplastic meningioma is characterized by pleomorphic cells, a high mitotic rate* , *and necrosis. Differential diagnosis includes metastatic carcinoma and sarcoma.*

(Left) *A large, extraaxial, dural-based mass ➡ arising from the anterior aspect of the right frontal convexity with mass effect and vasogenic edema ➡ is shown. There is 1 cm of leftward midline shift. The findings are consistent with a solitary fibrous tumor/hemangiopericytoma.* **(Right)** *This solitary fibrous tumor/hemangiopericytoma shows moderate cellularity and an abundant fibroblastic background.*

Solitary Fibrous Tumor/Hemangiopericytoma

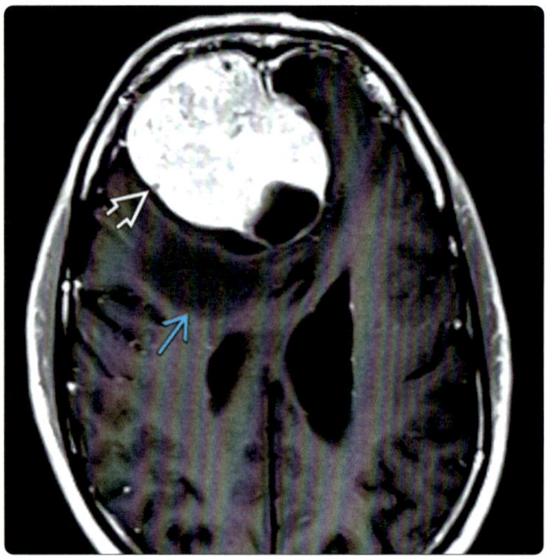

Solitary Fibrous Tumor/Hemangiopericytoma

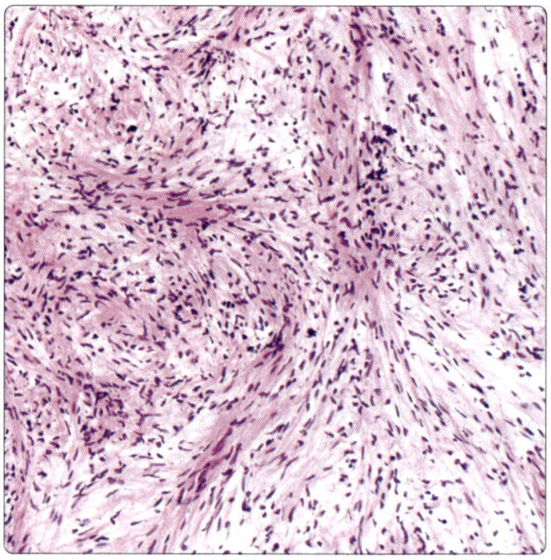

(Left) *Solitary fibrous tumor/hemangiocytoma has irregular staghorn vessels ➡ and spindled cells with intervening collagen bundles ➡. If atypical, mitoses and necrosis may be seen.* **(Right)** *On this cytologic smear, solitary fibrous tumor/hemangiopericytoma shows epithelioid to spindled cells with intervening ➡ collagen fibers. The distinction from meningioma may be quite difficult intraoperatively.*

Solitary Fibrous Tumor/Hemangiopericytoma

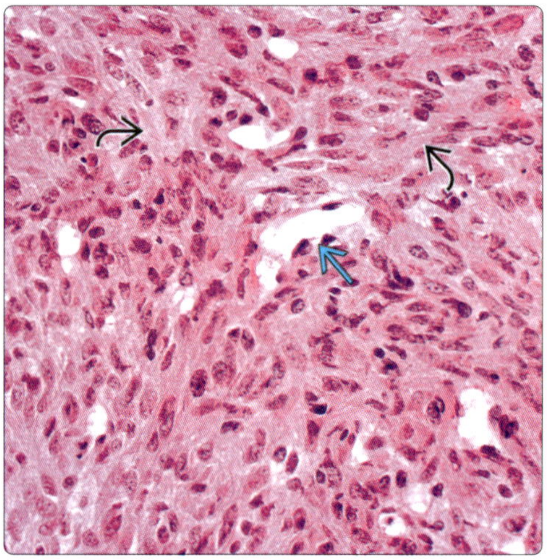

Solitary Fibrous Tumor/Hemangiopericytoma

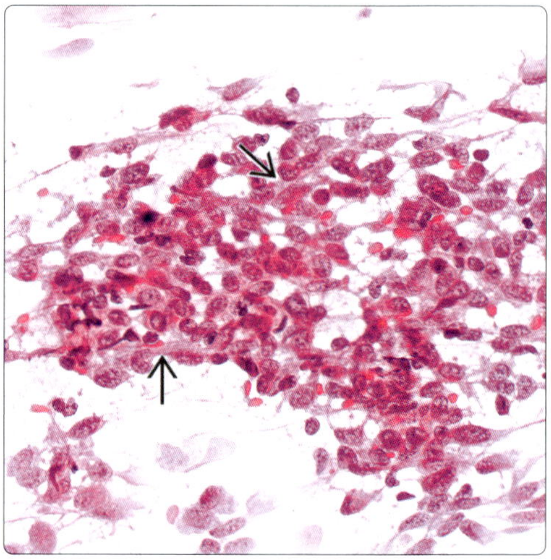

(Left) *Solitary fibrous tumor/hemangiopericytoma consists of sheets of cells and characteristic staghorn blood vessels ➡. This tumor showed a very high mitotic rate, diagnostic of anaplastic solitary fibrous tumor/hemangiopericytoma.* **(Right)** *Anaplastic solitary fibrous tumor/hemangiopericytoma is characterized by high cellularity and relatively monomorphic cells.*

Solitary Fibrous Tumor/Hemangiopericytoma

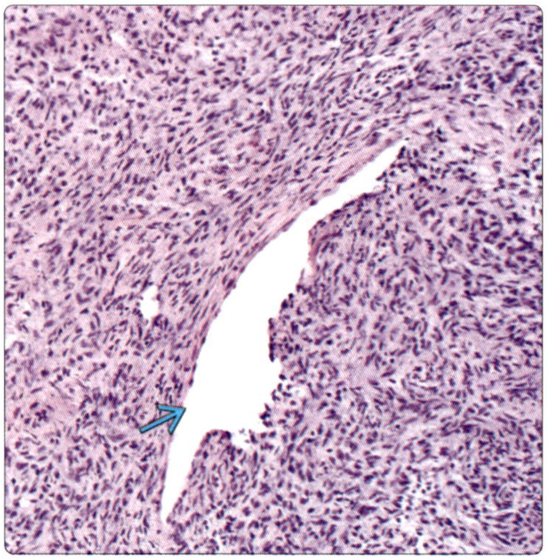

Anaplastic Solitary Fibrous Tumor/Hemangiopericytoma

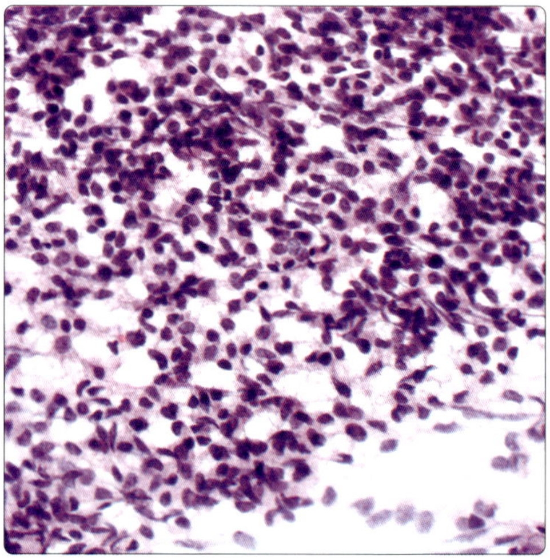

Hemangioblastoma

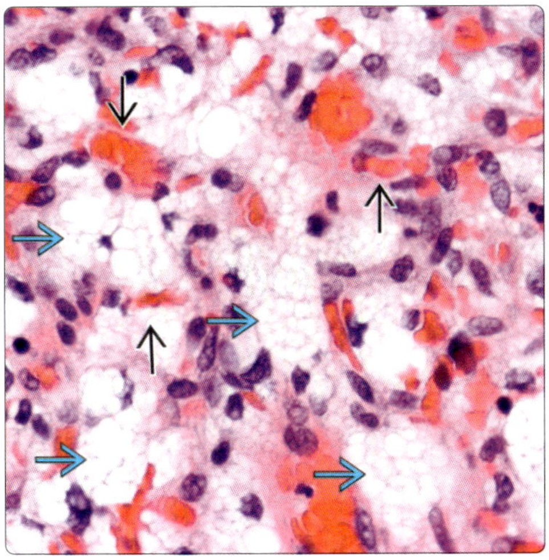

Meningeal Carcinomatosis: MR Appearance

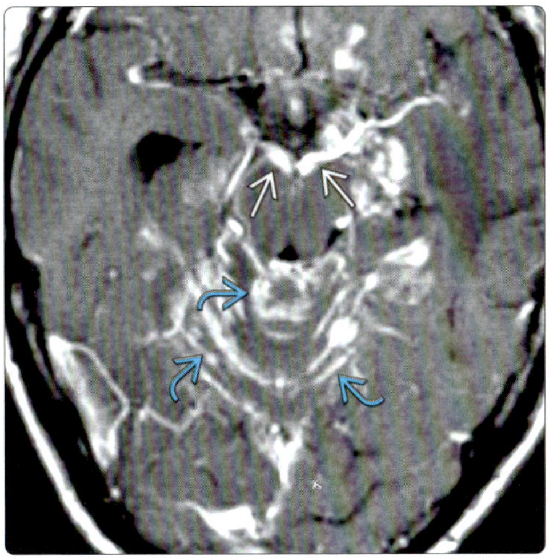

(Left) *Foamy stromal cells → and fine capillary network → are typical of hemangioblastoma. It can be very difficult to distinguish this tumor from metastatic renal cell carcinoma on frozen section.* **(Right)** *Axial T1 C+ MR shows linear and nodular metastases extending throughout the cerebellar folia and basal cisterns ↗. Note the nodular thickening at the exit of both oculomotor nerves from the midbrain ➡.*

Meningeal Carcinomatosis

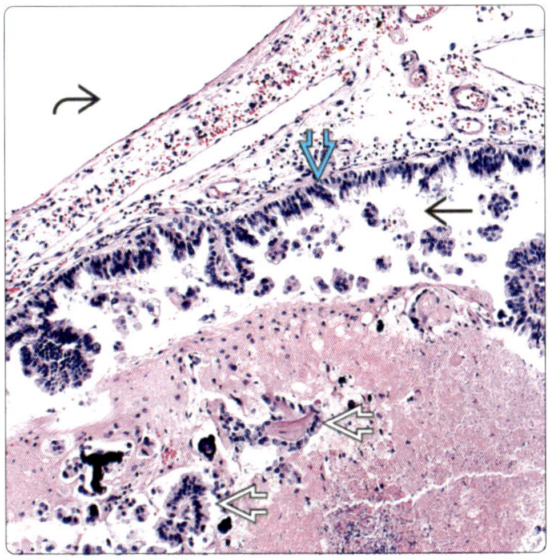

Metastatic Carcinoma in Dura

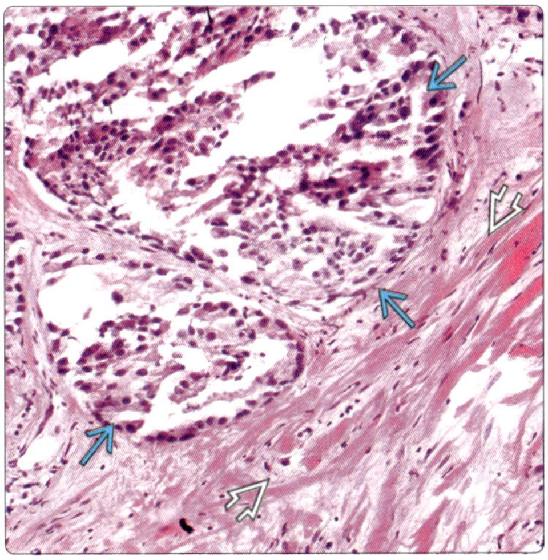

(Left) *This metastatic adenocarcinoma of the lung occupies the subarachnoid space → along the inner surface of the meninges ⇒. The tumor grows in the perivascular spaces of superficial cortical blood vessels ➡ beneath the subdural space ↗.* **(Right)** *This metastatic prostatic adenocarcinoma → is embedded in dense dural collagen ➡. It is very important for the pathologist to know relevant clinical history, including prior diagnoses of malignancy.*

Neurosarcoidosis

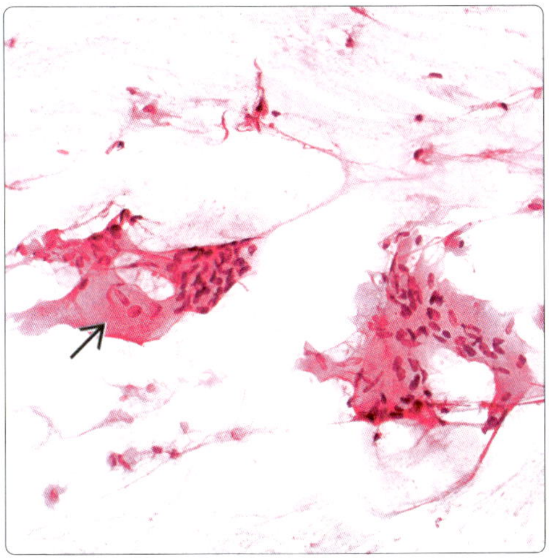

Neurosarcoidosis

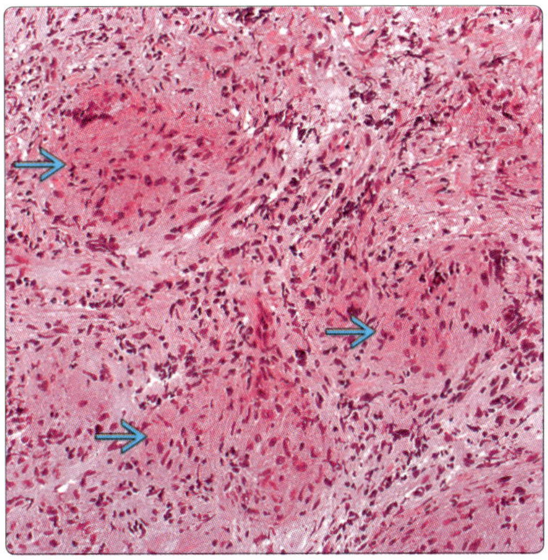

(Left) *A smear from neurosarcoidosis shows clusters of epithelioid histiocytes and giant cells →. Variable lymphocytic infiltrates may be seen (not shown).* **(Right)** *Sarcoidal granulomas → are detected on frozen section as aggregates of epithelioid histiocytes and giant cells without central necrosis in neurosarcoidosis. Fibrosis and lymphocytic infiltrates are common. As in any intraoperative diagnosis of a granulomatous process, tissue should be sent for microbiology.*

(Left) *Axial T1 C+ MR shows a focus of pachymeningitis (inflammation of the meninges) causing meningeal thickening and mimicking meningioma. Note the dural tail and indistinct margin with the underlying brain.* **(Right)** *A mixed chronic inflammation in the dura is seen here as small lymphocytes and macrophages on touch imprint. This may be due to an autoimmune or infectious process. Material should be sent for microbiologic studies.*

Pachymeningitis: MR Appearance

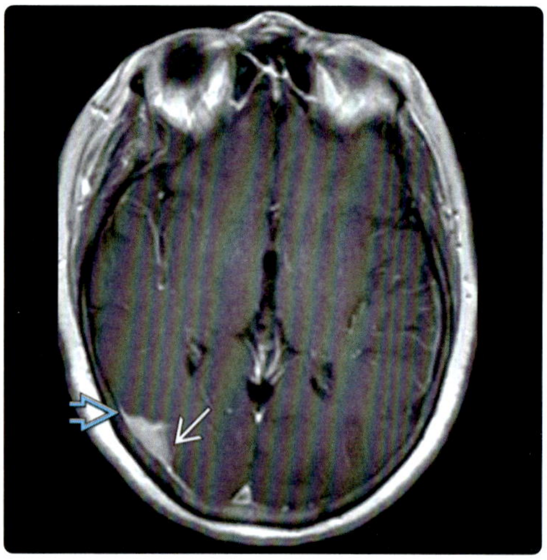

Pachymeningitis: Cytologic Features

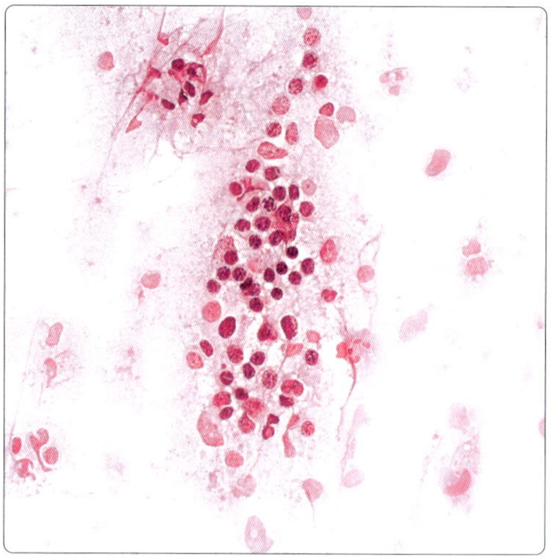

(Left) *On frozen section of pachymeningitis, small lymphocytes and macrophages are noted, occasionally forming vague germinal centers amid the dural collagen fibers. In specific infections, such as mycobacterium, giant cells may be a clue to the nature of the process.* **(Right)** *A germinal center is present in this case of dural inflammation. Intraoperative evaluation of lesions thickening the meninges is required to distinguish meningiomas that will be resected from inflammatory diseases.*

Pachymeningitis

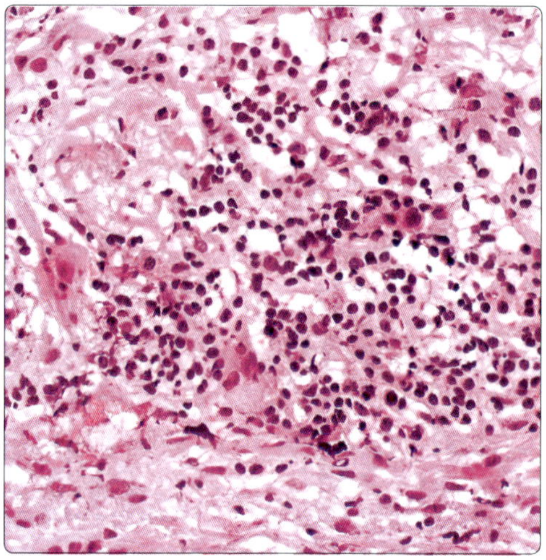

Pachymeningitis

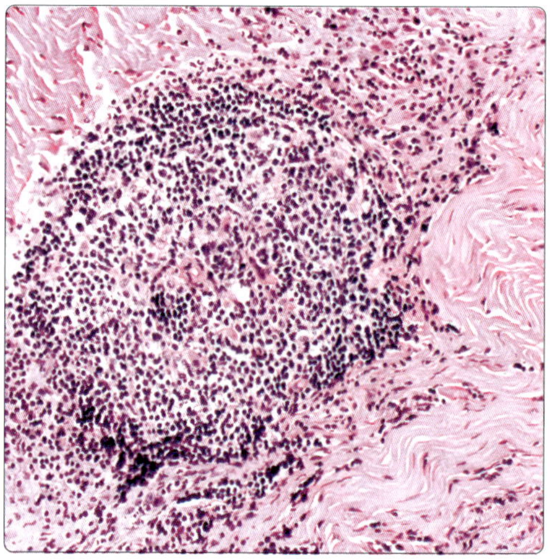

(Left) *Frozen sections of lesions thickening the dura, such as this case of pachymeningitis, are performed to distinguish them from neoplasms (e.g., meningioma). If an inflammatory lesion is identified, tissue should be sent for culture.* **(Right)** *Multiple small capillaries are noted with abundant spindle cell fibroblasts in collagenous stroma in this organizing subdural hematoma. Mitotic figures can be present and should not be mistaken for malignancy.*

Pachymeningitis

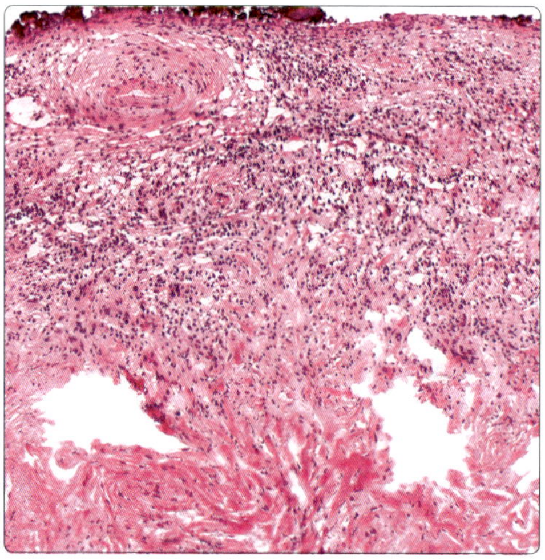

Organizing Subdural Hematoma

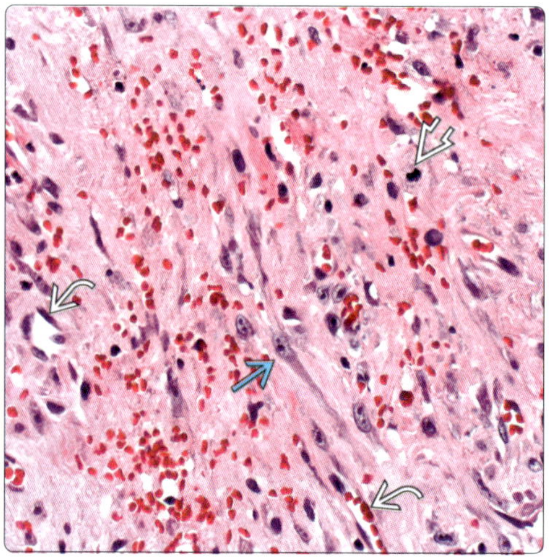

Arachnoid Cyst: MR Appearance

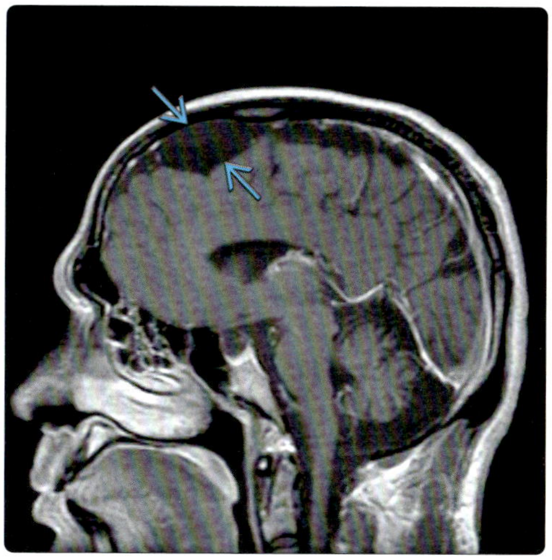

Arachnoid Cyst

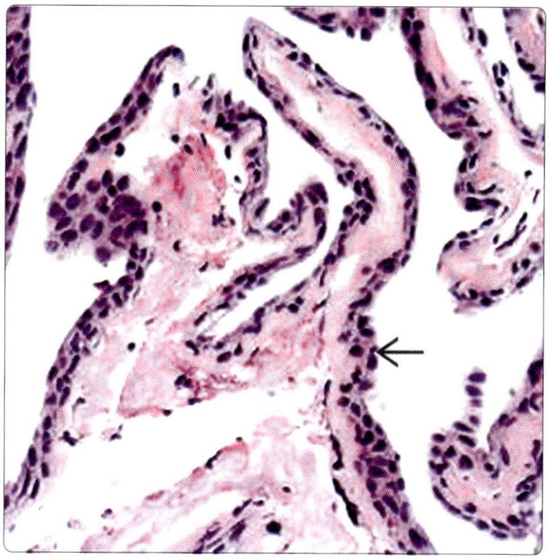

(Left) *Sagittal T1 C+ MR shows a frontal, oval, well-circumscribed cyst. The cyst's content resembles cerebrospinal fluid when compared to the ventricles.* **(Right)** *Arachnoid cysts are lined by flattened meningothelial cells with a fibrous wall of variable thickness. (Courtesy R. Hewlett, PhD.)*

Basilar Meningitis: Location

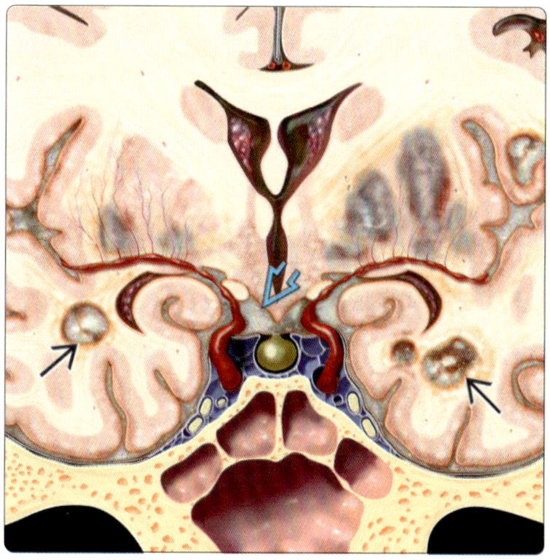

Basilar Meningitis: Gross Appearance

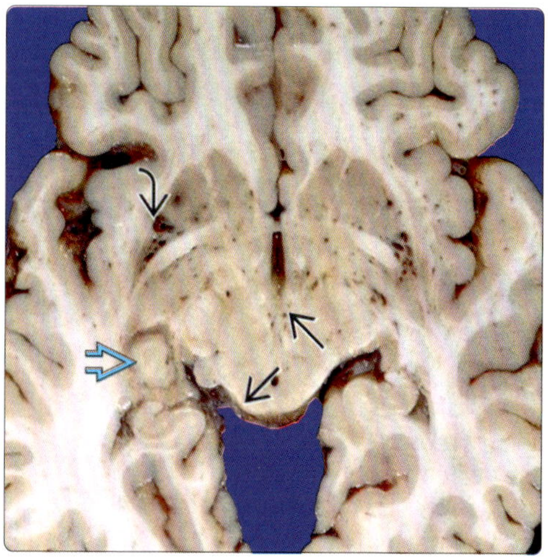

(Left) *Basilar TB meningitis and tuberculomas often coexist. Note the vessel irregularity and early basal ganglia ischemia related to arteritis.* **(Right)** *Brain section at autopsy shows numerous features of central nervous system tuberculosis. Exudates with meningitis in the basilar cisterns, tuberculoma, and vasculitic changes are all present. (Courtesy R. Hewlett, PhD.)*

Purulent Meningitis

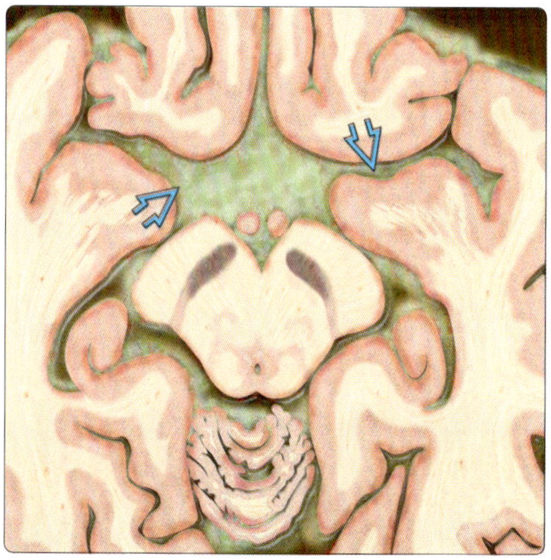

Tumors of Cerebellopontine Angle

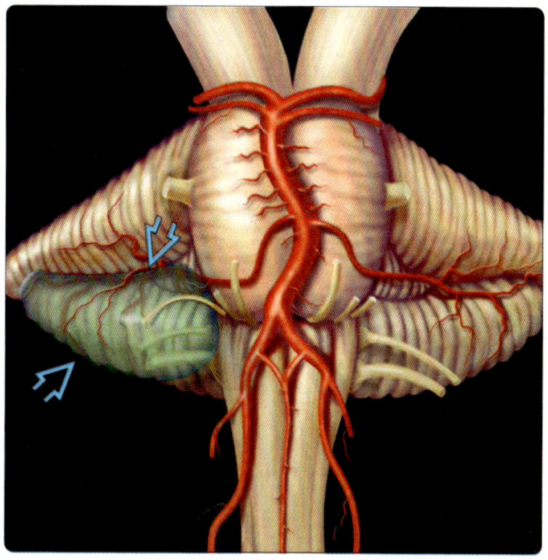

(Left) *A collection of neutrophils and microorganisms is filling the subarachnoid space in this case of purulent meningitis.* **(Right)** *In adults, tumors of the cerebellopontine angle are common. Differential diagnosis includes schwannoma, meningioma, and epidermoid cyst.*

Contents

SPECIMEN/CLINICAL CONSIDERATIONS

Goal of Consultation

- Determine if diagnostic features of acute invasive fungal rhinosinusitis are present

Change in Patient Management

- Extensive debridement of involved tissues
  - Frozen section may help guide extent of debridement
  - Vascular obstruction by fungi may restrict bleeding from involved tissue
    - This is important observation that can be made by surgeon
    - Active bleeding is sign of viable tissue but is not entirely specific for absence of organisms
  - Orbital exenteration may be necessary in some cases
- Systemic antifungal treatment can be initiated based on frozen section diagnosis

Clinical Setting

- Difficult to diagnose preoperatively
  - Other noninfectious processes can have similar radiographic features
- Acute invasive fungal rhinosinusitis
  - Almost all patients are immunocompromised
    - Hematologic malignancies, immunosuppressive therapy, diabetes, etc.
    - However, also rarely reported in patients with HIV/AIDS
  - Most commonly caused by *Aspergillus* or *Mucor*
  - Initial symptoms are nonspecific (fever of unknown origin, nasal obstruction, facial pain, headache)
  - Rapid onset and aggressive clinical course
    - Destruction of involved sinuses within days
  - Later symptoms may include proptosis, ophthalmoplegia, visual loss, decreasing mental status, seizures
    - Poor survival with intracranial involvement and cranial neuropathy
  - Clinical exam may show mucosal discoloration, ulceration, black crust
  - Life-threatening condition
    - Survival rate in USA is ~ 50%
    - Early diagnosis and treatment improves outcome
  - Treatment
    - Immediately perform extensive tissue debridement with attempt for wide surgical excision
    - Systemic antifungal therapy initiated urgently
- Chronic invasive fungal rhinosinusitis
  - Rare in USA (< 10% of invasive fungal rhinosinusitis)
    - Usually due to *Aspergillus*
  - Patients may have subtle immune system abnormalities
    - Also occurs in immunocompetent patients in endemic areas (e.g., Middle East, Africa)
  - Defined by symptoms persisting longer than 12 weeks
  - Fungal tissue invasion but no granulomatous inflammation
  - Managed conservatively

SPECIMEN EVALUATION

Gross

- Usually small biopsy
- May have dry and black appearance
- Microbial cultures for exact species determination should be submitted directly from operating room by surgeon
  - Fungi are identified in only ~ 70% of cases by culture

Frozen Section

- Entire specimen may be frozen

MOST COMMON DIAGNOSES

Invasive Fungal Sinusitis

- Acute fulminant form shows fungal organisms within viable or necrotic submucosal tissue
  - Necrosis is often present
  - Fungi within vessels or vessel walls (angioinvasion)
  - Perineural invasion
- Chronic granulomatous fungal sinusitis shows fungal invasion with fibrosis, chronic inflammation, and possibly ulceration

Invasive *Aspergillus*

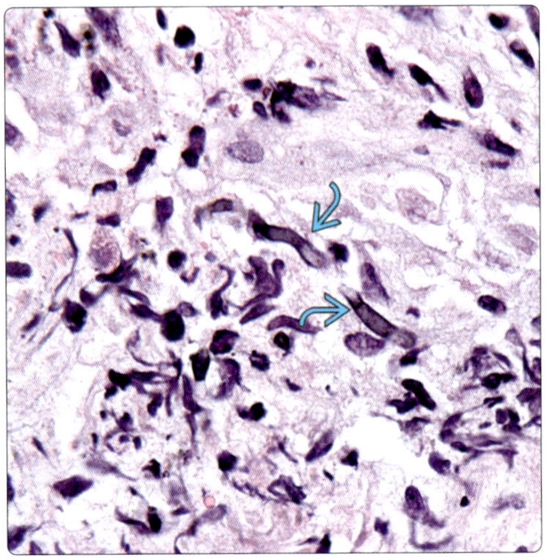

Invasive *Mucor*

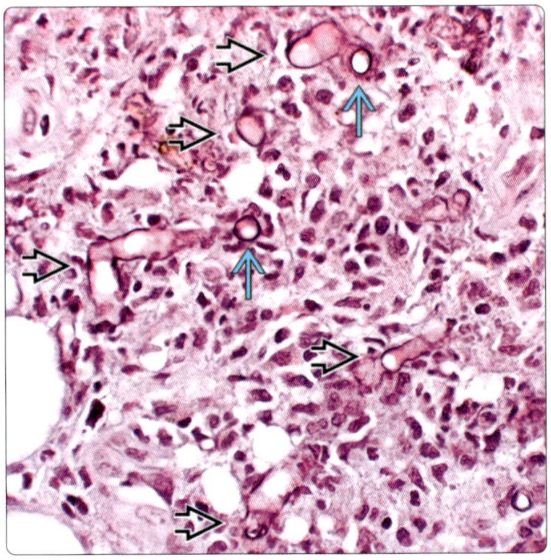

(Left) *Invasive Aspergillus is identified by the presence of narrow hyphae with septation ➚ in viable or necrotic tissue. Immediate aggressive medical treatment is required. (Courtesy W. Faquin, MD.)* **(Right)** *Numerous fungal forms are visible on H&E, invading in tissue. The fungi can be identified as Mucor due to the broad nonseptate hyphae ⇨. In cross section, the hyphae appear as hollow tubes with distinct borders →.*

- Granulomata distinguish chronic from acute sinusitis
- No prominent angioinvasion is seen

- *Aspergillus*
  - Most common type
  - Smaller and narrower hyphae
  - Hyphae have septations and acute angle (45°) branching
- *Mucor*
  - 2nd most common type
  - Larger/broader hyphae (up to 20 μm)
    - Often has twisted appearance
  - Hyphae do not have septations and have variable angle branching

Mycetoma (a.k.a. Fungus Ball)

- Presents with nasal stuffiness, discharge, and facial pain
- Most commonly *Aspergillus* (aspergilloma)
  - Dematiaceous (melanin-forming) fungi also reported
- Numerous tightly packed fungal forms
  - Grows within sinuses
  - Tissue invasion is **not** present
  - Fruiting heads (conidial heads) may be seen
- No prominent allergic mucin
  - In some cases, both allergic sinusitis and mycetoma are present

Allergic Fungal Sinusitis

- Chronic allergic result to presence of fungal colonization within sinus(es)
  - Reaction to fungal antigens and not true infection
- Presents with chronic sinusitis, discharge, headache, and facial pain
  - Usually have nasal polyps
- Edematous and often polypoid sinonasal mucosa, usually with prominent eosinophils within chronic inflammation
- Allergic (eosinophilic) mucin shows layering/lamination with inflammatory cells (often degranulated eosinophils) and Charcot-Leyden crystals
- Occasional fungal forms can be seen within allergic mucin, not within tissue
  - However, forms are typically not prominent and identification usually requires special stains
- Most commonly dematiaceous fungi (e.g. *Alternaria, Curvularia, Cladosporium*), but *Aspergillus* is more common in some geographic areas

Granulomatosis With Polyangiitis (Formerly Wegener Granulomatosis)

- Vasculitis, necrosis, and occasionally giant cells
- No fungal forms present
- Diagnosis not typically made on frozen section
  - May require serologic correlation (antineutrophil cytoplasmic antibodies)

Hematolymphoid Malignancy

- Patients with acute leukemia and lymphoma are at risk for invasive fungal sinusitis
- Nasal symptoms may be due to tumor involvement rather than infection
  - If suspected, appropriate tissue allocation should be performed
    - Flow cytometry (fresh), cytogenetics (fresh and sterile), special fixatives, frozen tissue (molecular studies)

REPORTING

Frozen Section

- Reporting absence or presence of invasive fungal forms is usually sufficient
  - If present, further classification may be deferred to permanent sections and culture

Reliability

- Reported sensitivity ranges from 75-86% with reported specificity of 100% in 1 study (although case numbers were low)
- Identification of fungal forms on frozen section is highly predictive of invasive disease and should lead to prompt surgical debridement

PITFALLS

False-Positive Diagnosis

- Folds in mucin and bone dust can create appearance of fungal forms
- Fungal forms are present but not within tissue
  - Mycetoma
  - Allergic fungal sinusitis

False-Negative Diagnosis

- Fungal forms can be scant in some cases
  - GMS or PAS stain on permanent sections better visualizes fungal forms, especially *Aspergillus*
  - May require immunohistochemistry or sequencing
- *Mucor* is usually more easily detectable on H&E and may be difficult to see on GMS

Fungal Identification

- *Mucor* and *Aspergillus* usually have different appearances on H&E
  - It is important to identify species to select most appropriate antifungal therapy
- In some cases, identification of fungal type may not be possible
  - Degenerative fungal forms due to treatment or necrosis
    - Can cause *Aspergillus* to have swollen hyphae that resemble *Mucor*
  - Some cases due to other fungal types such as dematiaceous fungi
- Culture is better method for identification but shows lower sensitivity than frozen section
  - ~ 30% of cases of known fungal infection have negative cultures
- Speciation may require ancillary studies
  - Immunohistochemical identification of antigens
  - Molecular studies may be required

SELECTED REFERENCES

1. Pagella F et al: Invasive fungal rhinosinusitis in adult patients: our experience in diagnosis and management. J Craniomaxillofac Surg. 44(4):512-20, 2016
2. Ghadiali MT et al: Frozen-section biopsy analysis for acute invasive fungal rhinosinusitis. Otolaryngol Head Neck Surg. 136(5):714-9, 2007
3. Taxy JB et al: Acute fungal sinusitis: natural history and the role of frozen section. Am J Clin Pathol. 132(1):86-93, 2009

(Left) *Numerous fungal forms are present, filling and obstructing a blood vessel. The hyphae are narrow and septate and, therefore, most consistent with Aspergillus. Infarction has caused the surrounding tissue to become necrotic.* **(Right)** *Invasion of blood vessels by fungi causes obstruction and infarction to create a favorable environment for their growth. In this case, Mucor is seen invading into a blood vessel. The hyphae branch at a 90° angle, and there are no septations. (Courtesy W. Faquin, MD.)*

Angioinvasive *Aspergillus*

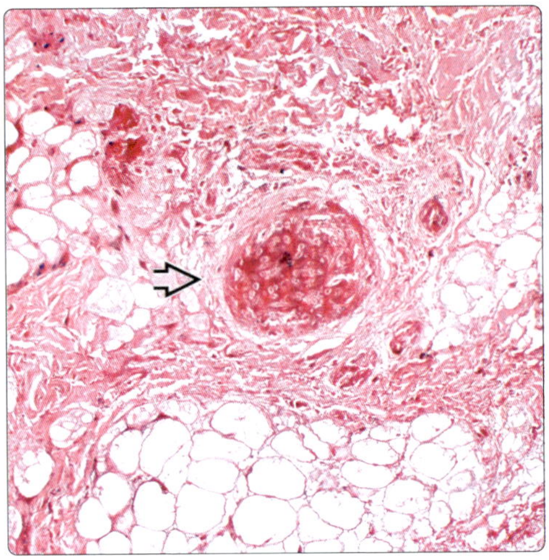

Angioinvasive *Mucor*

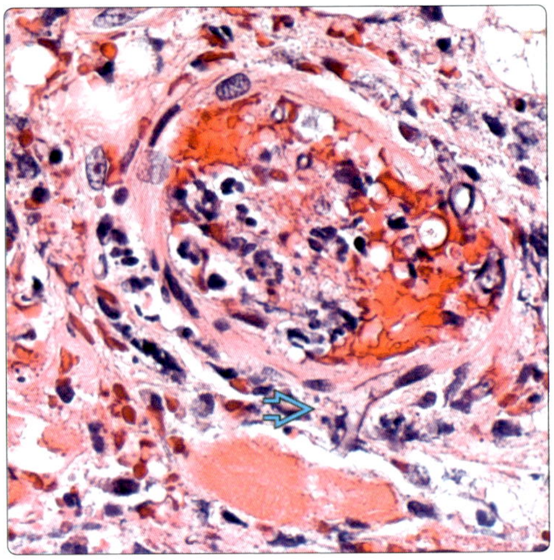

(Left) *Invasive Mucor has broad nonseptated hyphae with thin walls and 90° branching. The hyphae may appear twisted. The fungal forms are large and can generally be identified on H&E stain without the need for special stains.* **(Right)** *Mucor can be identified in frozen sections by the large size of the hyphae. Fungal forms should be uniform in caliber as opposed to other structures that will vary in size. Fungi may be found in and around blood vessels and nerves.*

Invasive *Mucor*

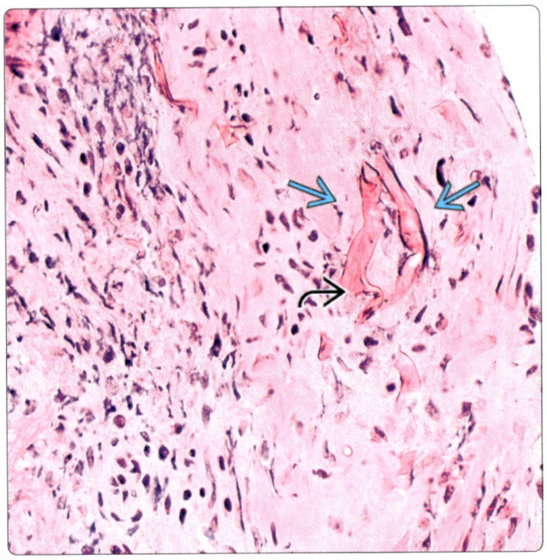

Invasive *Mucor*

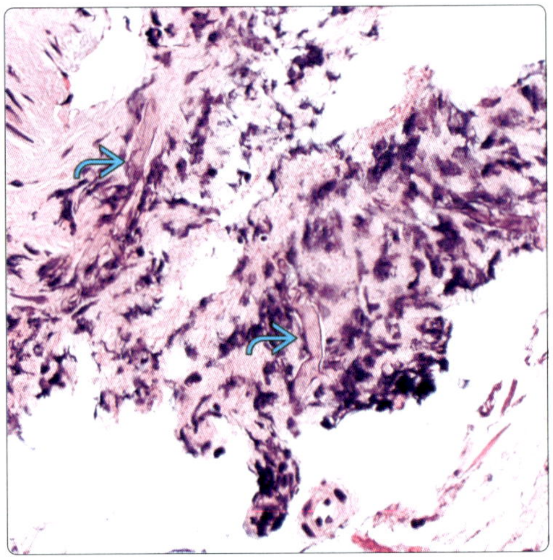

(Left) *Broad, thin-walled, and nonseptated hyphae, some twisted, identify this fungus as Mucor. An adjacent obstructed blood vessel is an important feature associated with invasive fungal infection.* **(Right)** *Patients with acute leukemia and lymphoma are at risk for invasive fungal infections. The nasal symptoms may be due to local involvement by the patient's tumor, such as this NK-/T-cell lymphoma. If a hematologic malignancy is suspected on frozen section, tissue should be allocated for appropriate ancillary studies.*

Invasive *Mucor*

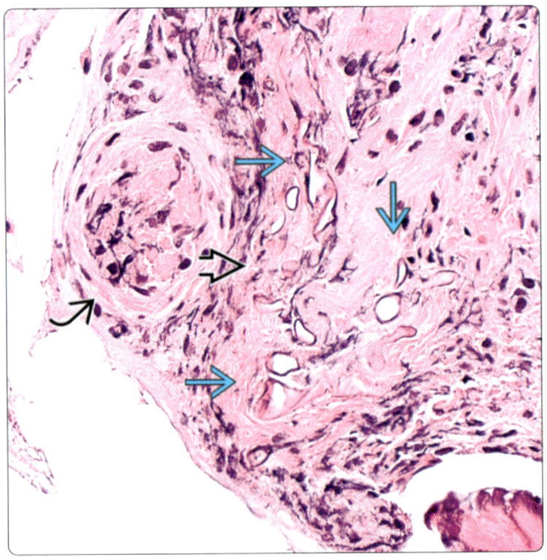

NK-/T-Cell Lymphoma

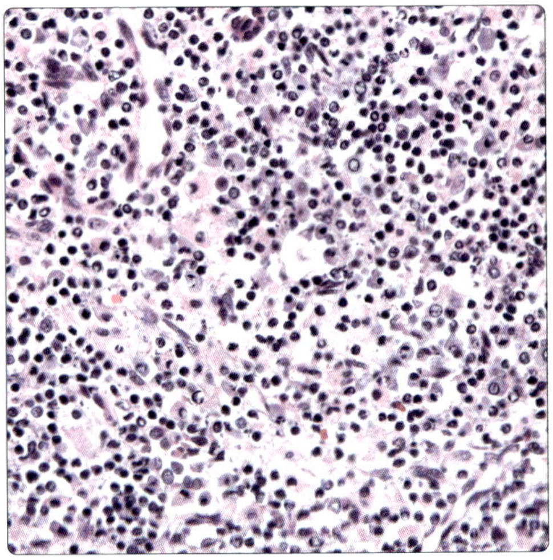

Mycetoma

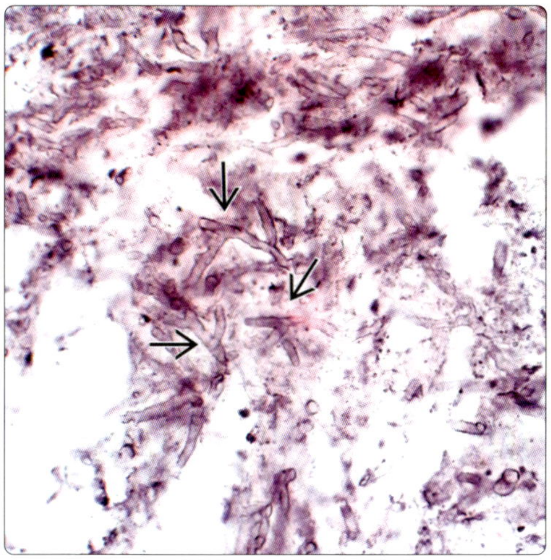

Mycetoma

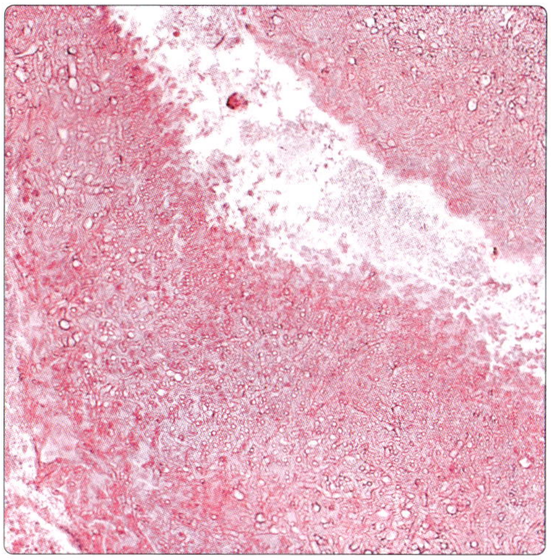

(Left) *Aspergillus and other species can be found as a noninvasive fungal ball in the sinuses that causes obstruction. The narrow hyphae and 45° angle branching ⇒ are typical for Aspergillus.* **(Right)** *Aspergillus can grow within a sinus as a fungus ball without tissue invasion. Sheets of fungal hyphae are easily recognized on H&E stain. This finding is a cause of chronic sinusitis and does not require surgical debridement or systemic therapy.*

Allergic Fungal Sinusitis: Eosinophils

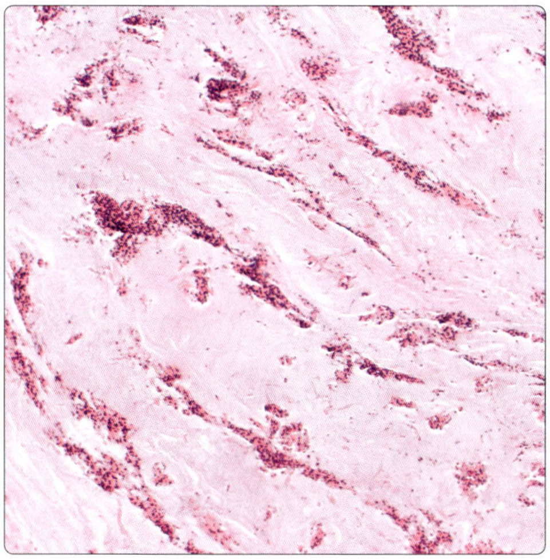

Allergic Fungal Sinusitis: Charcot-Leyden Crystals

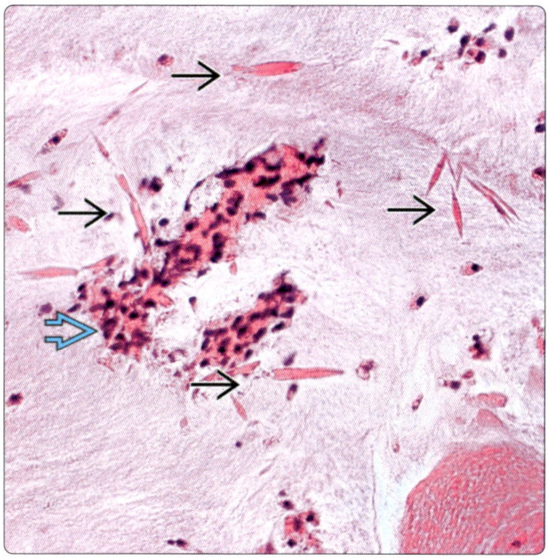

(Left) *Allergic mucin is densely eosinophilic and has a layered appearance. Sloughed epithelial cells and inflammatory cells, including eosinophils, are intermingled. Fungal forms may be sparse and require histologic stains for identification. This finding does not require surgical debridement.* **(Right)** *Charcot-Leyden crystals ⇒ are eosinophilic angular structures consisting of lysophospholipase released from eosinophils ⇨. They are characteristic of allergic mucin (but not entirely specific).*

Nasal Biopsy With Necrosis

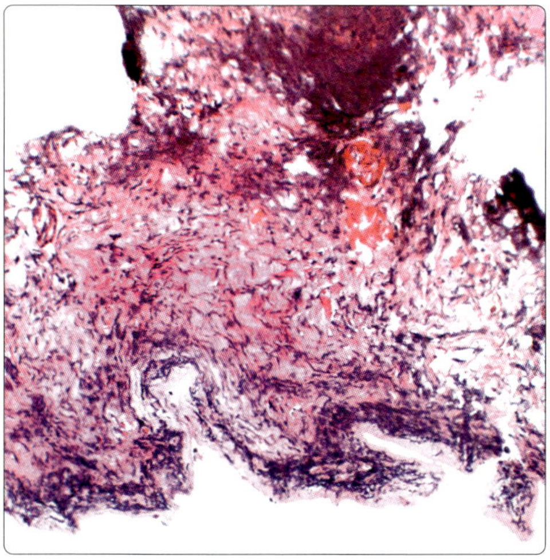

Calcifications

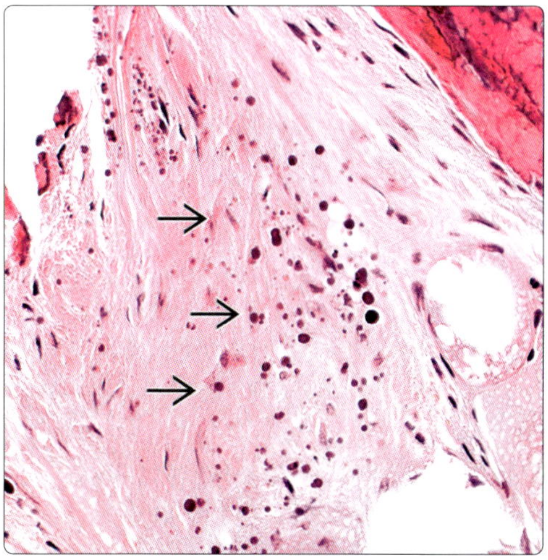

(Left) *This nasal biopsy from a patient with bacterial sepsis shows extensive tissue necrosis. No fungal forms were identified on the frozen sections. The intraoperative observation of brisk bleeding from the biopsy site supported that the necrosis was not due to fungal infection.* **(Right)** *Calcifications (likely from a previous procedure) can form ovoid or angulated structures ⇒ that could be mistaken for fungal forms. Variable size and the absence of hyphae are clues for the correct diagnosis.*

SURGICAL/CLINICAL CONSIDERATIONS

Goals of Consultation

- Determine if malignancy or neoplasia is present
- Assess margins for carcinoma or extent of involvement by sinonasal papilloma

Change in Patient Management

- Presence of malignancy may lead to further surgery, depending on type of malignancy (e.g., carcinoma)
  - Ancillary studies are often required for definitive classification
- Absence of malignancy may halt further surgery
- Involvement of different anatomic structures by sinonasal papilloma may determine further surgery

Clinical Setting

- Sinonasal mass with unknown diagnosis
- Known history of sinonasal papilloma with question of recurrence or malignant transformation
- Incidental finding during surgery for chronic rhinosinusitis with question of sinonasal papilloma

SPECIMEN EVALUATION

Gross

- Typically, small biopsies or fragmented excision specimens
- If complete resection specimen for margins, orientation by surgeon may be helpful
- If sinonasal papilloma is found, entire specimen should be submitted for permanent sections

Frozen Section

- Representative section should be frozen if biopsy is larger and diagnosis is unknown (to allow for possible tissue allocation for ancillary studies)
  - If biopsy is small, entire specimen is frozen
- If biopsy is performed to determine margins or anatomic involvement, entire specimen should be frozen
  - Submit margins as perpendicular sections

Cytology

- Touch preps may be useful, especially with small round cell neoplasms or lymphoma

MOST COMMON DIAGNOSES

Sinonasal (Schneiderian) Papilloma

- Benign neoplasm arising from specialized sinonasal (schneiderian) mucosa
- Complete surgical excision, usually by endoscopic sinus surgery, is necessary to prevent recurrence or malignant transformation
  - Recurrence rates of 20-30% after incomplete removal
- 3 types: Inverted, oncocytic, and exophytic
  - All lack significant cytologic atypia
- **Inverted sinonasal papilloma**
  - Most common type
  - M:F = 3:1
  - Often arises from lateral nasal wall or maxillary sinus
  - Have activating *EGFR* mutations
  - Histologic findings
    - Thickened epithelium with endophytic growth
    - Transitional, ciliated columnar, and squamous epithelium
    - Mixed inflammatory infiltrate with intraepithelial neutrophils
    - Admixed mucocytes and microcysts within epithelium
    - Intact basement membrane around epithelium
    - Mitoses limited to basal and parabasal layers; no atypical forms
  - 5-32% malignant transformation
- **Oncocytic sinonasal papilloma**
  - Most commonly arises from lateral nasal wall
  - Men and women equally affected
  - Harbor activating *KRAS* mutations
  - Histologic findings
    - Exophytic and endophytic growth patterns
    - Columnar cells with granular eosinophilic cytoplasm, occasionally ciliated
    - Intraepithelial mucocytes and microcysts

Keratinizing Squamous Cell Carcinoma

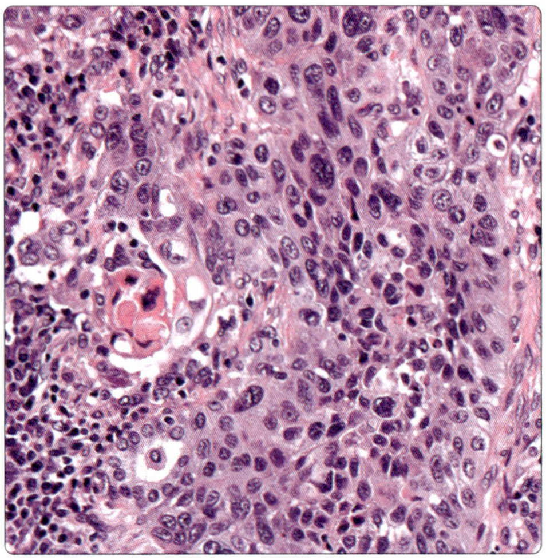

Nonkeratinizing Squamous Cell Carcinoma

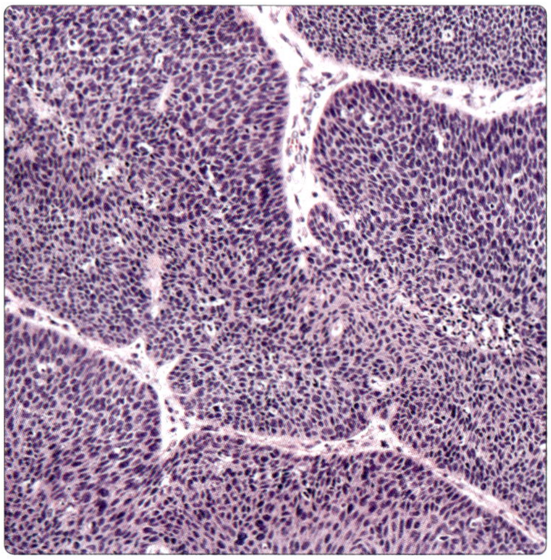

(Left) *Squamous cell carcinoma is the most common sinonasal malignancy. Most squamous cell carcinomas such as this keratinizing example are associated with conventional risk factors such as tobacco use and industrial exposure (e.g., wood or leather dust) and may rarely arise secondary to a sinonasal papilloma.* **(Right)** *In the sinonasal tract, up to 50% of nonkeratinizing squamous cell carcinomas are associated with high-risk HPV.*

- 10-17% malignant transformation
- **Exophytic sinonasal papilloma**
  - Almost always arises from septum
  - Malignant transformation very rare
  - Histologic findings
    - Papillary growth of thickened epithelium with fibrovascular cores
    - Squamous and ciliated columnar epithelium admixed with mucocytes and microcysts
      - Surface keratinization is rare, unless traumatized
- Malignant transformation
  - Most commonly to squamous cell carcinoma
    - In situ or invasive carcinoma in association with preexisting papilloma (occasionally no residual papilloma is seen)
  - No reliable histologic predictors of transformation, although dysplasia may be present in papilloma

Squamous Cell Carcinoma

- Most common malignancy (70%) in sinonasal tract
- Complete surgical resection is necessary, possibly with adjuvant radiotherapy
- Most are keratinizing or nonkeratinizing
  - Also papillary, sarcomatoid/spindle cell, undifferentiated
- Keratinizing squamous cell carcinoma is related to conventional risk factors (tobacco abuse)
  - < 5% associated with high-risk HPV or EBV

HPV-Associated Squamous Cell Carcinoma

- In head and neck, sinonasal tract is 2nd in frequency for high-risk HPV carcinomas, after oropharynx
- Morphologic appearances
  - Nonkeratinizing: Nests and trabeculae of immature epithelium, often with pushing border
  - Papillary: Exophytic growth of transitional-appearing epithelium, fibrovascular cores, often with invasive endophytic component
  - Undifferentiated: Sheets of epithelioid cells with vesicular chromatin and prominent nucleoli, resembling lymphoepithelial carcinoma
- Detection of high-risk HPV via p16 immunohistochemistry and confirmatory direct HPV testing (e.g. in situ hybridization, PCR)
- **HPV-related carcinoma with adenoid cystic-like features**
  - Morphologic features of both surface-derived squamous cell carcinoma and high-grade adenoid cystic carcinoma
  - Solid nests of basaloid cells, often with cribriform architecture
  - Adenoid cystic carcinoma-like morphology with true ductal and myoepithelial differentiation
  - Surface squamous dysplasia present in subset
  - Perineural invasion is rare, in contrast to adenoid cystic carcinoma

Lymphoepithelial Carcinoma

- Term for EBV-positive nonkeratinizing, undifferentiated squamous cell carcinoma arising in sinonasal tract
  - Analogous to nonkeratinizing, undifferentiated nasopharyngeal carcinoma
  - Exclude extension from primary nasopharyngeal carcinoma
- Large tumor cells with large vesicular nuclei and large nucleolus, often showing syncytial growth
- EBV can be detected by in situ hybridization for EBV-encoded mRNA

NUT Carcinoma

- Aggressive, poorly differentiated carcinoma frequently showing squamous differentiation
  - Median survival of ~ 9.8 months
- Common presentation as rapidly growing mass in early adulthood
- Histologic appearance of poorly differentiated or undifferentiated squamous cell carcinoma
- Sheets of undifferentiated cells with abrupt foci of squamous differentiation
  - Round vesicular nuclei with prominent nucleolus and scant or clear cytoplasm
- Mitotic activity and necrosis frequent
- Defined by *NUTMI* rearrangements (encoded on chromosome 15q14)
  - Most common fusion partner is *BRD4*
  - Immunohistochemistry for NUT protein is useful diagnostic tool
  - FISH or RT-PCR to detect translocation or fusion gene

Sinonasal Adenocarcinoma, Intestinal Type

- Predominantly locally aggressive tumors
  - Some due to environmental exposure (hardwood sawdust and leather dust)
- Resembles intestinal adenocarcinoma
  - Colonic (most common), papillary, solid, mucinous, and mixed types
- Immunohistochemistry: Majority positive for CK20 and CDX-2; many also express CK7

Sinonasal Adenocarcinoma, Nonintestinal Type

- Does not show intestinal or minor salivary gland phenotype
- Separated into low- and high-grade tumors
  - **Low grade** (relatively favorable prognosis)
    - Tubular &/or papillary growth patterns
    - Uniform back-to-back glandular structures lined by columnar to cuboidal cells with relatively mild cytologic atypia
    - Rare subset resemble clear cell renal cell carcinoma
    - No necrosis
  - **High grade** (aggressive)
    - Sheets of invasive tumor cells with marked atypia, occasional glandular structures, or mucous cells
    - Mitotic activity and necrosis common
- Mucicarmine stain or immunohistochemistry may be necessary for final diagnosis
  - Negative for CK20, CDX-2, pax-8, and neuroendocrine markers

Neuroendocrine Carcinoma

- Overall uncommon, < 3% of all sinonasal tumors
- Encompasses both **small cell carcinoma** and **large cell neuroendocrine carcinoma**
- May be associated with squamous cell carcinoma or adenocarcinoma
- Rare examples associated with high-risk HPV or prior irradiation

- Immunohistochemistry: Positive for keratin (perinuclear dot-like pattern), synaptophysin, chromogranin

Olfactory Neuroblastoma

- Arise in areas of olfactory epithelium: Cribriform plate, superior turbinate, superior 1/2 of nasal septum
- Histologic appearance
  - Uniform small- to intermediate-sized round and ovoid tumor cells with scant cytoplasm
  - Nests, lobules, or sheets with fibrovascular stroma
  - Delicate fibrillary neural matrix
  - Subset show rosettes (Homer Wright or Flexner-Wintersteiner)
- High-grade tumors show necrosis, pleomorphism, increased mitoses, decreased neuropil, less lobular growth
- Definitive diagnosis is often not possible on frozen section
  - Differential diagnosis includes all small round cell neoplasms (carcinoma, sarcoma, lymphoma)
  - Final diagnosis often requires ancillary studies
    - Immunohistochemistry: Positive for synaptophysin and chromogranin; negative for keratin
      - S100 and GFAP will highlight sustentacular cells (not visible on H&E)

Sinonasal Undifferentiated Carcinoma

- Rare, very aggressive undifferentiated malignancy
  - < 20% 5-year survival
  - Poorly responsive to chemotherapy and radiation
- No obvious line of differentiation, other than expression of epithelial markers (keratin, EMA)
- This is diagnosis of exclusion and requires ancillary studies
  - Must exclude HPV, EBV, NUT carcinoma, neuroendocrine carcinoma, olfactory neuroblastoma, etc.
- Histologic findings
  - Various growth patterns (trabecular, solid, organoid)
  - Medium- to large-sized cells with large round nuclei, often vesicular with prominent nucleoli, and little to moderate amount of cytoplasm
  - Frequently show high mitotic activity and necrosis
- Genetic subsets have been recognized and are currently provisional entities
  - **SMARCB1 (INI1)-deficient carcinoma**
  - Activating *IDH1/2* mutations

Extranodal NK-/T-Cell Lymphoma

- Aggressive extranodal lymphoma with cytotoxic phenotype
- Strong association with EBV
- Most common in endemic Asia and South America
- Histologic findings
  - Polymorphous infiltrate with variable cytomorphology
  - Angioinvasive with necrosis
- Ancillary studies required for final diagnosis

Ewing Sarcoma

- May arise as osseous primary (skull or jaw) or as extraosseous primary in sinonasal tract
  - More common in children and young adults
  - Extraosseous tumors account for most older patients
- Harbor *EWSR1* gene rearrangements with members of ETS family of transcription factors
  - *EWSR1-FLI1* fusion most common
- Histologic findings
  - Sheets of small or intermediate-sized round cells with high nuclear:cytoplasmic ratio
  - Round to ovoid nuclei with powdery chromatin, smooth nuclear membrane, and inconspicuous to small nucleoli
  - **Adamantinoma-like variant**
    - Nested growth, fibrous or sclerotic stroma
    - May see pseudorosettes or foci of keratinization
    - Diffuse keratin and p63/p40 expression
- Final diagnosis requires ancillary studies
  - Immunohistochemistry: Diffuse membranous CD99 reactivity, nuclear FLI-1 and NKX2.2 positivity
  - Molecular studies: FISH to confirm *EWS* rearrangement or PCR to detect fusion protein

Rhabdomyosarcoma

- Often arise in head and neck sites
- Predominantly affects children and young adults
- Major subtypes
  - **Embryonal**: Myxoid stroma, variation in cellularity with atypical tumor cells in varying stages of myogenesis (spindle cells, spider cells, round cells)
  - **Alveolar**: Large round cells with hyperchromatic nuclei, often arranged in dyscohesive nests
    - Multinucleated giant tumor cells may be seen
    - *FOXO1* gene rearrangements with either *PAX3* or *PAX7* fusion partners
  - **Pleomorphic**: Older patients, pleomorphic malignant neoplasm
  - **Spindle cell/sclerosing**: Spindle cells in long fascicles &/or in dense sclerotic stroma
- Final diagnosis usually requires ancillary studies
  - Immunohistochemistry: Positive for desmin, myogenin/myf4, MYOD1

Sinonasal Glomangiopericytoma

- Relatively indolent tumor, 40% recur with incomplete excision
- Uniform bland tumor cells with spindled or ovoid nuclei arranged in short fascicles, whorls, or palisades, with frequent pervicascular growth
- Cytologic atypia absent or at most mild; necrosis is rare
- Harbor *CTNNB1* mutations
- Immunohistochemistry: Positive for SMA, HHF-35, and β-catenin

Biphenotypic Sinonasal Sarcoma

- Low-grade spindle cell sarcoma showing dual myoid and neural differentiation
- Arise in adulthood, often infiltrative and locally aggressive mass
  - Recurrence (30-40%), metastases rare/exceptional
- Short fascicles of mildly atypical spindle cells and hemangiopericytoma-like vessels
  - Bone invasion is frequent
- Frequent entrapment and proliferation of benign respiratory epithelium
- Focal rhabdomyoblastic differentiation may be seen
- Final diagnosis requires ancillary studies
  - Need to distinguish from malignant peripheral nerve sheath tumor and synovial sarcoma
  - Immunohistochemistry: Coexpression of S100 and SMA/MSA, desmin

- Myogenin positive in foci or rhabdomyoblastic differentiation
- *PAX3* gene rearrangement in most cases

Mucosal Melanoma

- Rare, very aggressive, commonly arising in nasal cavity or septum
  - More commonly primary tumor rather than metastasis
- Histologic findings
  - Typically epithelioid or spindle cell morphology
  - Surface ulceration and necrosis common
  - May lack in situ component or pigmentation
- Immunohistochemistry for melanocytic markers necessary for diagnosis

Sinonasal Inflammatory Polyp

- Nonneoplastic inflammatory lesions
- May be solitary or multiple with involvement of both nasal cavity and sinuses
- **Antrochoanal polyp** is variant that originates in maxillary sinus and extends into nasal cavity via stalk
- Histologic findings
  - Polypoid lesion with respiratory ciliated epithelium (may show squamous metaplasia), thickened basement membrane, and stromal edema
  - Absent or scant mucous glands
  - Eosinophil-rich mixed inflammatory infiltrate
  - Reactive atypical stromal cells may be seen, especially in antrochoanal polyps

REPORTING

Frozen Section

- Report absence or presence of neoplasia/malignancy and type if possible (e.g., squamous cell carcinoma)
- Most sinonasal neoplasms require ancillary studies for definitive diagnosis
- If definitive diagnosis is not possible, report as following
  - Poorly differentiated carcinoma, classification deferred to permanent sections
  - Malignant epithelioid neoplasm, classification deferred to permanent sections
  - Round cell neoplasm, classification deferred to permanent sections
  - Spindle cell neoplasm, classification deferred to permanent sections
- Document allocation of tissue for ancillary studies
- Reliability: False-negative rates for frozen section margins in sinonasal malignancies is 6.5%

PITFALLS

Ectopic Pituitary Adenoma

- Epithelial cell proliferation with salt and pepper nuclei that may mimic malignant round cell neoplasms
  - Lacks significant atypia; rarely have mitoses and necrosis

Benign Salivary Gland Neoplasms

- May be confused with nonintestinal sinonasal adenocarcinoma
  - Myoepithelial cells present as basal layer in benign neoplasms
  - Immunohistochemical studies may be necessary to confirm myoepithelial cells (e.g., p63)

Respiratory Epithelial Adenomatoid Hamartoma

- Benign proliferation of medium to large sinonasal glands connected to surface epithelium
- Glands lined by ciliated respiratory epithelium with multiple cell layers and admixed mucous cells
- Stromal hyalinization with thickened basement membrane
- Must be differentiated from inverted sinonasal papilloma, which does not show prominent glands
- Must be differentiated from low-grade nonintestinal adenocarcinoma, which shows more complex growth pattern with back-to-back glands and does not originate from surface epithelium

Seromucinous Hamartoma

- May mimic nonintestinal sinonasal adenocarcinoma
- Proliferation of small seromucinous glands with occasional larger, cystic glands
- Lacks complex architecture
- Positive for S100, but lacks basal or myoepithelial cells (confirmed by absent p63 staining)

Mucosal Melanoma

- Absence of in situ component or pigmentation should not exclude melanoma
- In situ melanoma can be very extensive but difficult to detect, especially in respiratory mucosa, and may extend into seromucous glands
  - False-negative rate for frozen section margin evaluation: 25%
  - Assessment of margins is best performed on permanent sections

Inflammatory Polyp

- Must be distinguished from sinonasal papilloma
  - Polyps lack marked epithelial thickening, inverted growth pattern, and prominent microcysts
- Reactive atypia due to trauma should not lead to misdiagnosis as squamous cell carcinoma

Inverted Sinonasal Papilloma

- Endophytic growth may be pitfall for invasive squamous cell carcinoma
- Lacks significant cytologic atypia
- Intact basement membrane, no single cell invasion

Exophytic Sinonasal Papilloma

- Surface keratinization and reactive atypia from trauma may mimic papillary squamous cell carcinoma
- Lacks full-thickness severe cytologic atypia, mitotic figures in superficial epithelium, and atypical mitotic forms

SELECTED REFERENCES

1. Bishop JA et al: Human papillomavirus-related carcinomas of the sinonasal tract. Am J Surg Pathol. 37(2):185-92, 2013
2. Johncilla M et al: Soft tissue tumors of the sinonasal tract. Semin Diagn Pathol. 33(2):81-90, 2016
3. Lewis JS Jr: Sinonasal squamous cell carcinoma: a review with emphasis on emerging histologic subtypes and the role of human papillomavirus. Head Neck Pathol. 10(1):60-7, 2016
4. Mochel MC et al: Primary mucosal melanoma of the sinonasal tract: a clinicopathologic and immunohistochemical study of thirty-two cases. Head Neck Pathol. 9(2):236-43, 2015

(Left) *The most common type of sinonasal papilloma is inverted papilloma, which is characterized by an inverted growth pattern and loss of underlying seromucinous glands. The thickened epithelium is squamous, transitional, or ciliated columnar.* **(Right)** *Inverted sinonasal papilloma has a thickened transitional epithelium, transmigrating neutrophils, and microcysts →. Inverted papillomas may recur if incompletely excised and rarely show malignant transformation.*

Inverted Sinonasal Papilloma

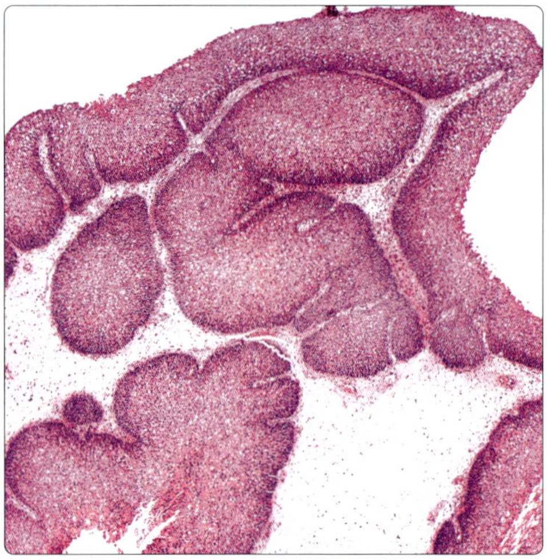

Inverted Sinonasal Papilloma

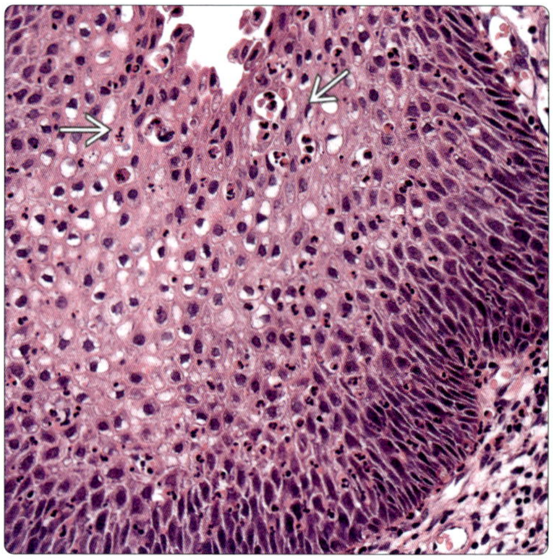

(Left) *This oncocytic papilloma on frozen section has an inverted growth pattern and is composed of a thickened oncocytic epithelium with interspersed mucous cells. Microcysts and mucocytes may also be present.* **(Right)** *Exophytic sinonasal papilloma has fibrovascular cores and thickened squamous epithelium with microcysts ↷ and mucous cells →. Note the lack of cytologic atypia, which distinguishes exophytic papilloma from papillary squamous cell carcinoma.*

Oncocytic Sinonasal Papilloma

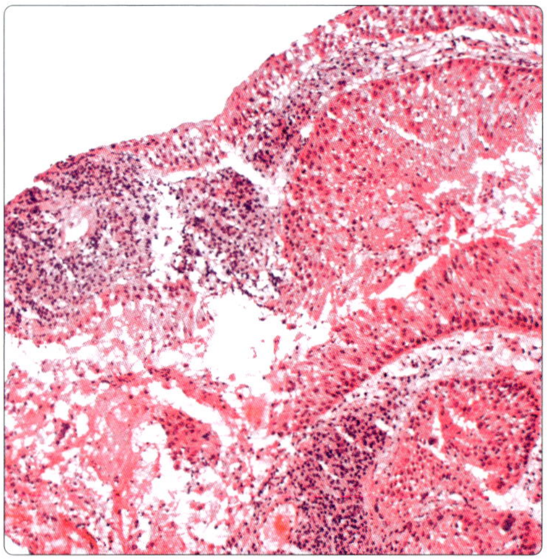

Exophytic Sinonasal Papilloma

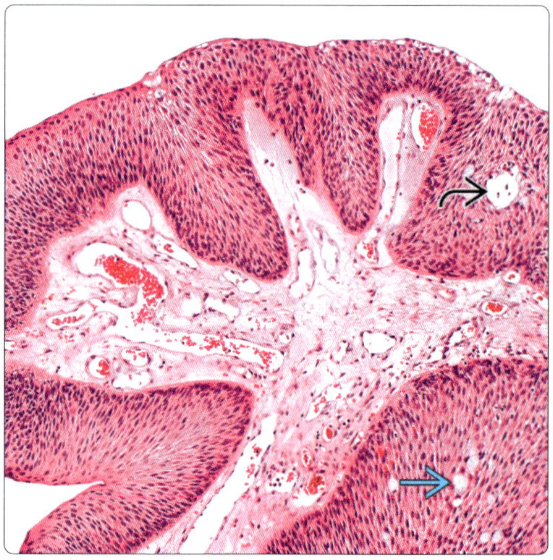

(Left) *Inverted sinonasal papillomas ⇨ should be completely excised with negative margins to prevent recurrence because some lesions give rise to squamous cell carcinoma →. There are no reliable predictive factors for recurrence or progression.* **(Right)** *This inflammatory polyp on frozen section is lined by respiratory epithelium of normal thickness →, in contrast to the thickened epithelium in a sinonasal papilloma. The underlying edematous stroma has scattered inflammatory cells. Glands are rare or absent.*

Invasive Squamous Cell Carcinoma Arising in Inverted Sinonasal Papilloma

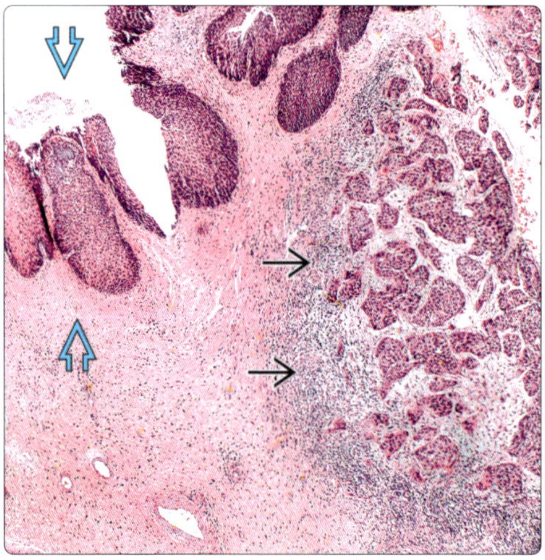

Sinonasal Inflammatory Polyp

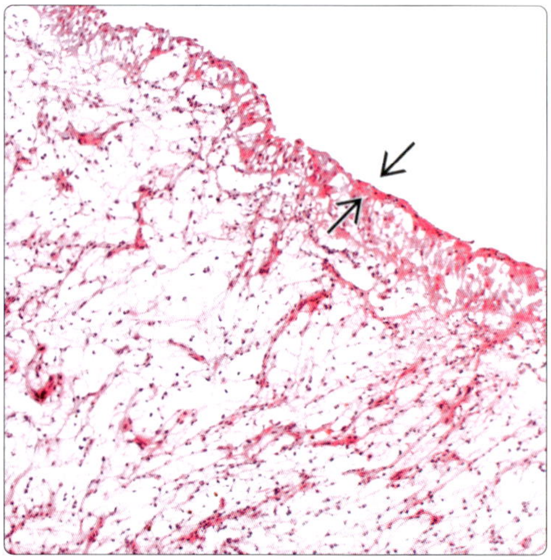

Papillary Squamous Cell Carcinoma

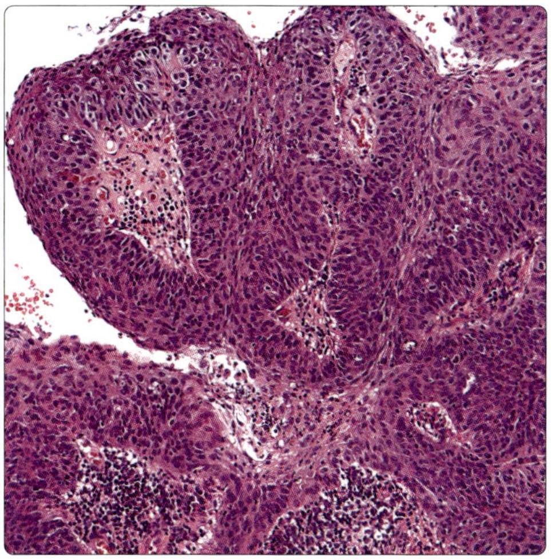

Papillary Squamous Cell Carcinoma

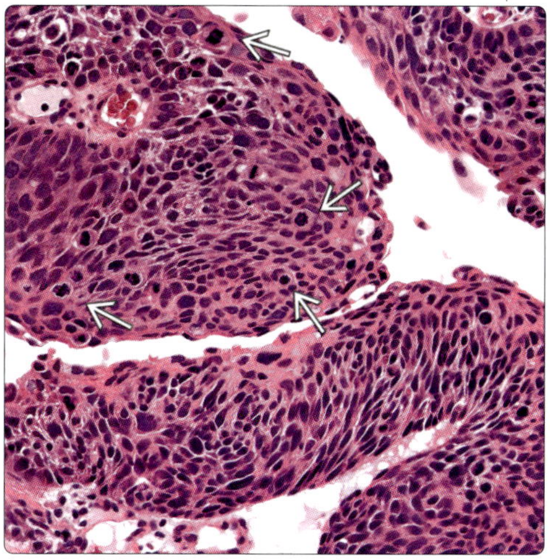

(Left) *Papillary squamous cell carcinoma shows an exophytic growth of immature-appearing atypical squamous epithelium growing around fibrovascular cores. Approximately 80% of papillary squamous cell carcinomas in the sinonasal tract are associated with high-risk HPV.* **(Right)** *Note the severe cytologic atypia and frequent mitotic figures ➔ towards the epithelial surface. These tumors may also show an invasive endophytic component resembling nonkeratinizing squamous cell carcinoma.*

HPV-Related Carcinoma With Adenoid Cystic-Like Features

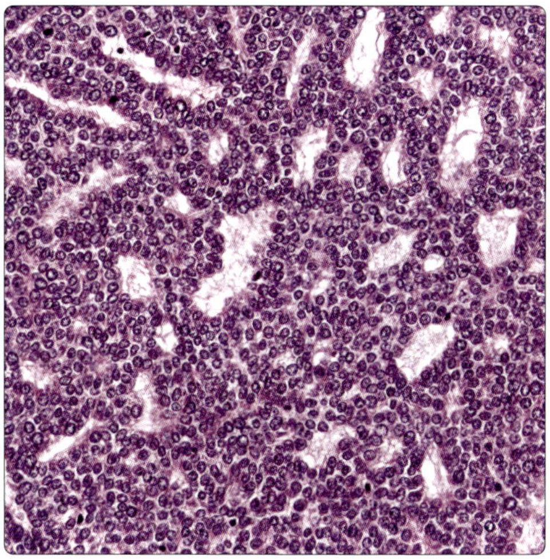

HPV-Related Carcinoma With Adenoid Cystic-Like Features

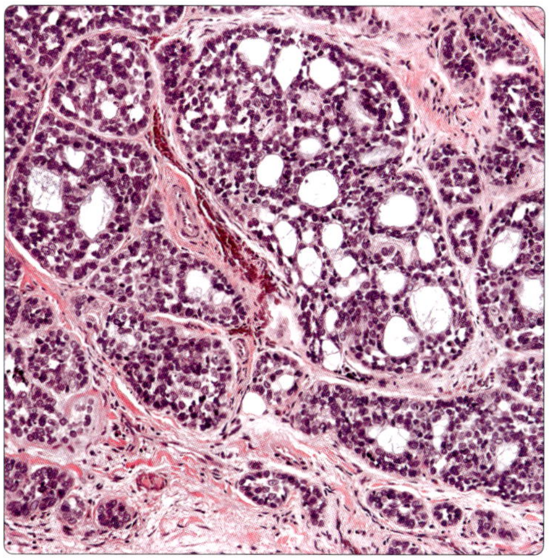

(Left) *HPV-related carcinoma with adenoid cystic-like features has features of both surface-derived squamous carcinoma and salivary gland carcinoma, with multilobular growth of sheets of basaloid cells with frequent cribriform structures.* **(Right)** *Some areas with cribriform and microcystic structures strongly resemble salivary adenoid cystic carcinoma and show true ductal and myoepithelial differentiation. However, these tumors lack MYB gene rearrangement that characterizes adenoid cystic carcinoma.*

NUT Carcinoma

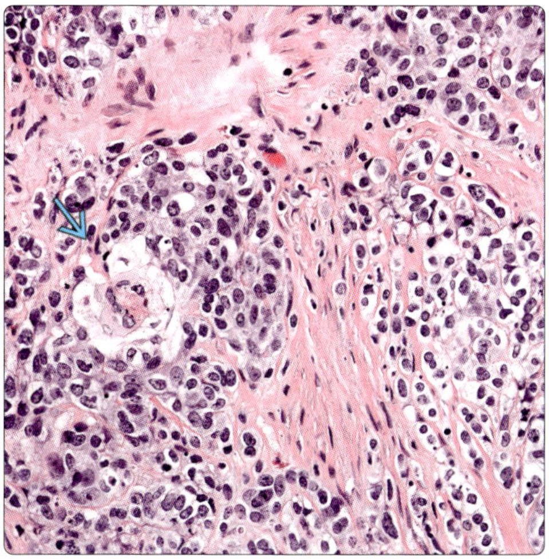

Sinonasal Neuroendocrine Carcinoma

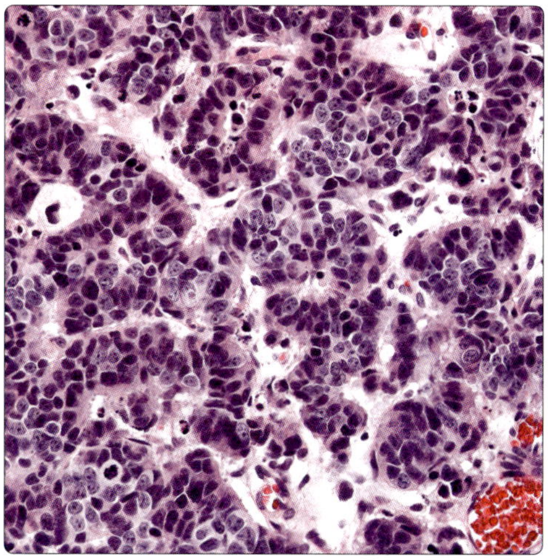

(Left) *NUT carcinoma is characterized by NUTM1 rearrangement. Tumors show sheets of undifferentiated or poorly differentiated tumor cells with large vesicular nuclei and scant to moderate cytoplasm that is occasionally clear. Foci of abrupt keratinization ➔ are typical.* **(Right)** *Neuroendocrine carcinomas encompass large cell (pictured) or small cell morphologies. Tumors show strong diffuse staining for neuroendocrine markers and keratin, though many mimics should be excluded. Some are associated with high-risk HPV.*

Contents

Sinonasal Intestinal-Type Adenocarcinoma

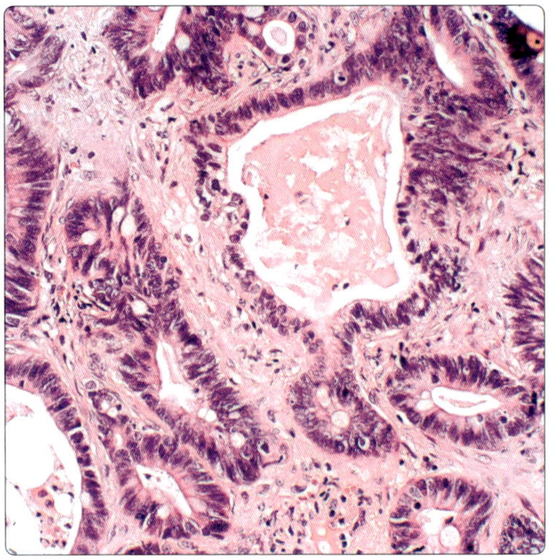

Sinonasal High-Grade Nonintestinal-Type Adenocarcinoma

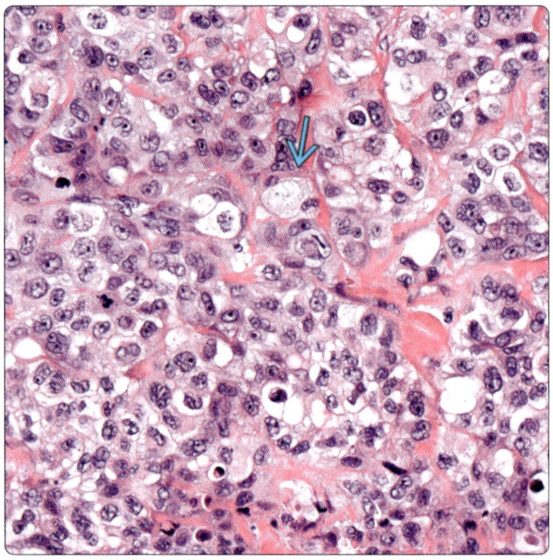

(Left) *This sinonasal adenocarcinoma is composed of glands and tubules resembling colonic adenocarcinoma. The tumor cells are columnar and have atypical hyperchromatic nuclei.* **(Right)** *This high-grade sinonasal adenocarcinoma appears as a poorly differentiated malignancy with solid growth of malignant cells. While there is no overt gland formation, the presence of individual mucocytes → confirms glandular differentiation. These tumors lack intestinal or salivary differentiation.*

Sinonasal Low-Grade Nonintestinal-Type Adenocarcinoma

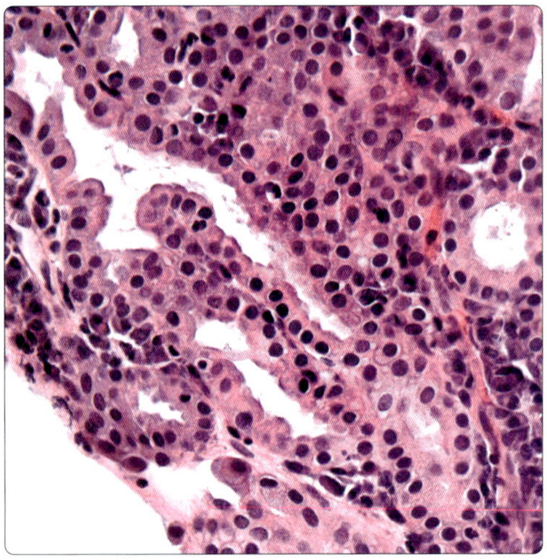

Respiratory Epithelial Adenomatoid Hamartoma

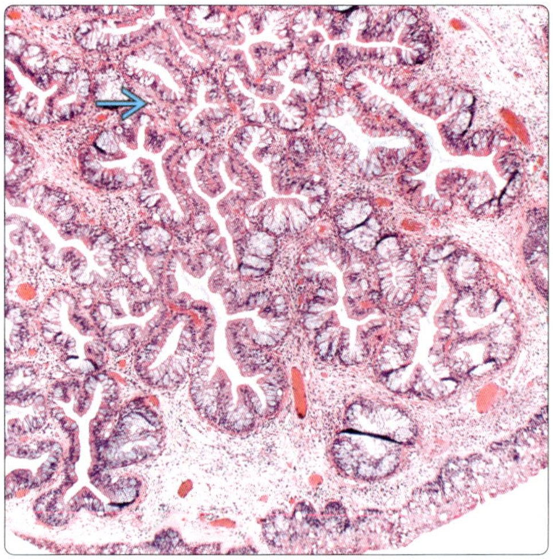

(Left) *This low-grade adenocarcinoma consists of a proliferation of back-to-back glands. The single layer of uniform columnar to cuboidal cells have basally oriented nuclei and mild atypia. No cilia are seen. (Courtesy W. Faquin, MD.)* **(Right)** *Respiratory epithelial adenomatoid hamartoma consists of a glandular proliferation. The presence of 2 cell types (epithelial and mucous cells) is an important feature. Glands are evenly spaced apart with areas of stromal hyalinization with thickened basement membranes →.*

Olfactory Neuroblastoma

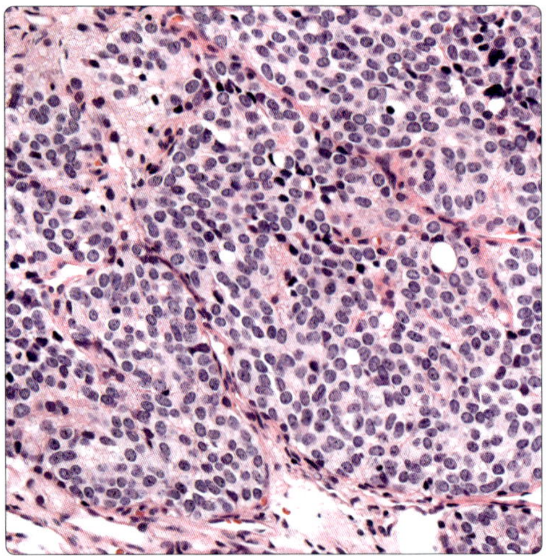

Olfactory Neuroblastoma

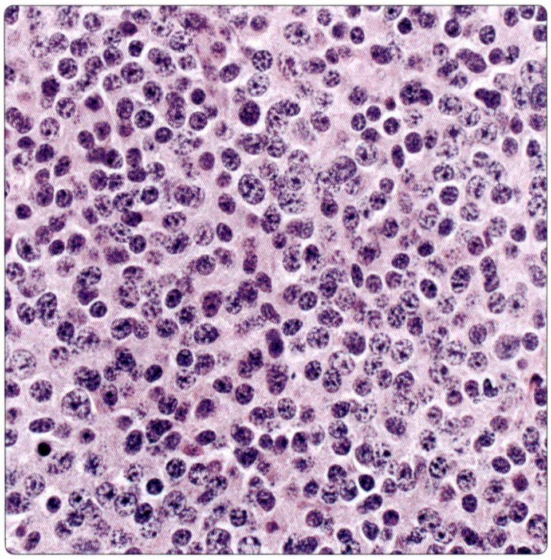

(Left) *Olfactory neuroblastoma has a multilobular growth pattern of small- to medium-sized cells with round or ovoid nuclei. Ancillary studies may be necessary to distinguish these tumors from other small round cell tumors.* **(Right)** *The tumor cell nuclei of olfactory neuroblastoma often show a salt and pepper chromatin and occasional nucleoli. Scant pale eosinophilic fibrillary material is present in the background. Rosette formation is seen in ~ 25% of cases.*

Sinonasal Undifferentiated Carcinoma

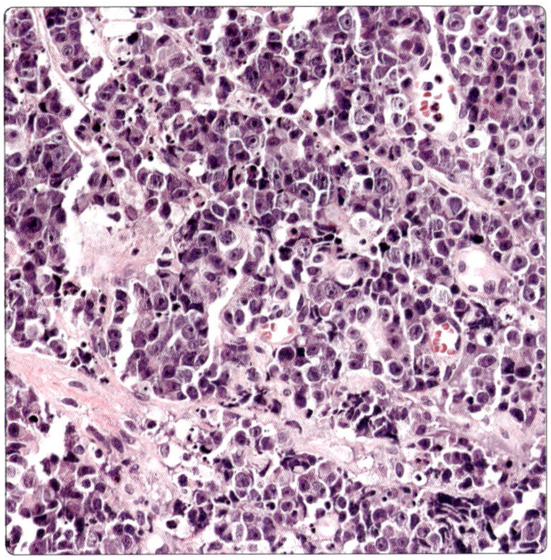

SMARCB1 (INI1)-Deficient Sinonasal Carcinoma

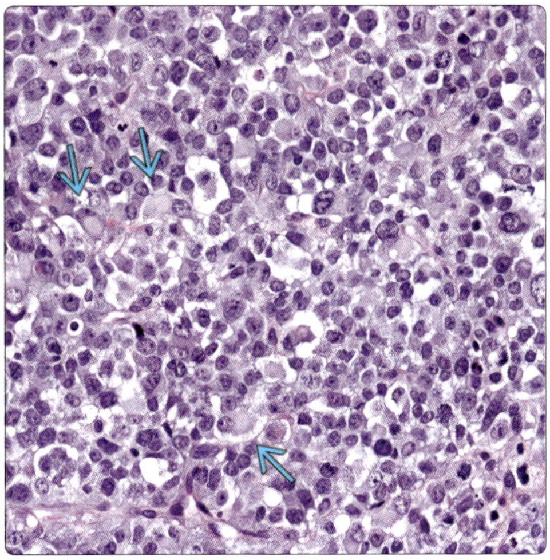

(Left) *Sinonasal undifferentiated carcinoma is a diagnosis of exclusion. Tumors are comprised of sheets, nests, and trabeculae of relatively uniform tumor cells that have large round hyperchromatic nuclei with prominent nucleoli and varying cytoplasm.* **(Right)** *A subset of undifferentiated carcinomas show SMARCB1/INI1 loss (which can be detected by immunohistochemistry). These tumors often show rhabdoid features with dense eosinophilic cytoplasmic inclusions* →.

Sinonasal Mucosal Melanoma

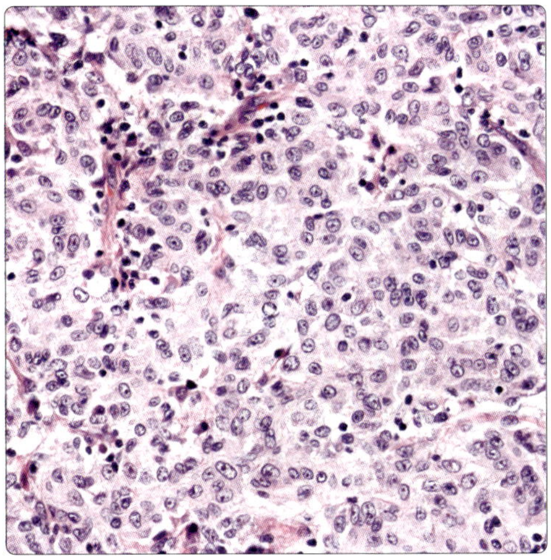

Ewing Sarcoma, Adamantinoma-Like

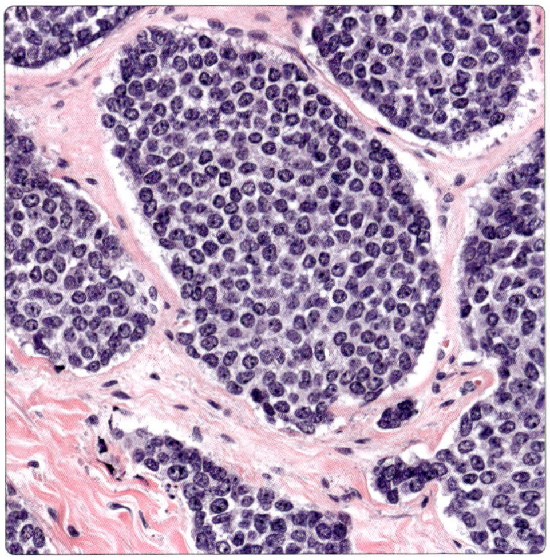

(Left) *An epithelioid sinonasal melanoma may be difficult to recognize due to a lack of an in situ component or pigmentation. Helpful features for diagnosis are the nested growth pattern, large nucleoli, and amphophilic cytoplasm.* **(Right)** *The adamantinoma-like variant of Ewing sarcoma may be difficult to recognize in the head and neck, appearing as a small round cell neoplasm with prominent nested architecture and expression of keratin and p40. Confirmation of EWSR1 gene rearrangement is diagnostic.*

Alveolar Rhabdomyosarcoma

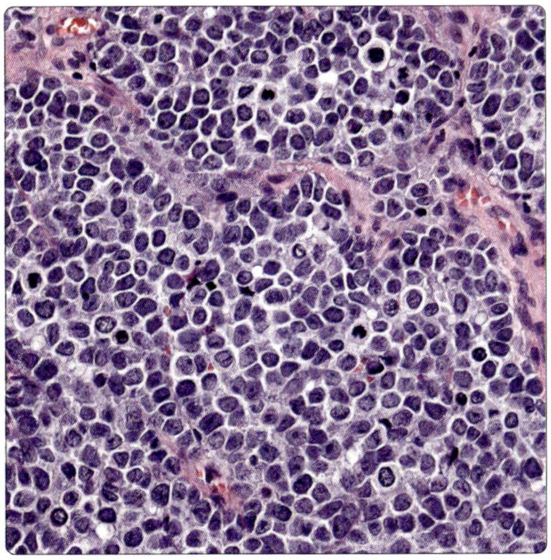

Biphenotypic Sinonasal Sarcoma

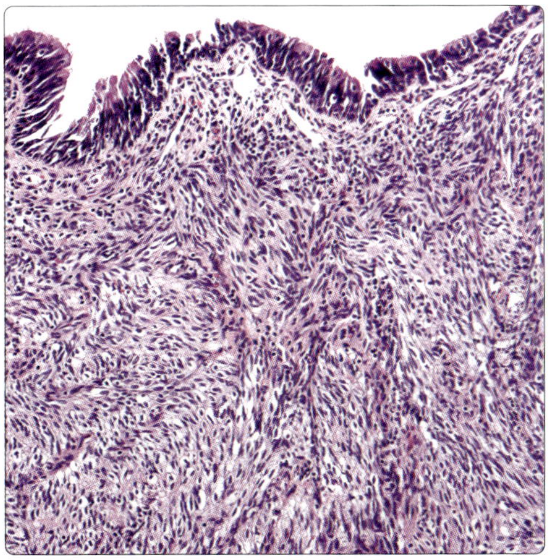

(Left) *A specific diagnosis for most small round cell neoplasms cannot be rendered on frozen section, and tissue should be allocated for ancillary studies. Diffuse desmin and myogenin expression and presence of FOXO1 gene rearrangement confirm the diagnosis of alveolar rhabdomyosarcoma.* **(Right)** *Biphenotypic sinonasal sarcoma is composed of fascicles of mildly atypical spindle cells with pale eosinophilic cytoplasm. Tumors coexpress neural and myoid markers and harbor PAX3 gene rearrangements.*

SURGICAL/CLINICAL CONSIDERATIONS

Goal of Consultation

- Determine if carcinoma is present, most commonly squamous cell carcinoma (SCC)
- Identify potential cases of lymphoma and allocate tissue as needed for definitive evaluation (e.g., fresh tissue for flow cytometry)

Change in Patient Management

- Additional biopsies to find primary carcinoma may be unnecessary
- If surgical excision of primary is planned, additional biopsies to map extent of disease may be performed once diagnosis is established
- For potential lymphoma cases, additional biopsies may be needed if lesional tissue is not identified or if more tissue is needed for ancillary studies

Clinical Setting

- Oropharyngeal SCC and nasopharyngeal carcinoma often initially present with cervical lymph node metastasis with occult primary
- Extensive upper aerodigestive tract evaluation with multiple biopsies may be undertaken to identify primary carcinoma
- Patients presenting with nasopharyngeal or oropharyngeal mass may undergo biopsies to evaluate for carcinoma or lymphoma
- Biopsies may be obtained specifically to assess human papilloma virus (HPV) status, since HPV-associated SCCs are associated with more favorable prognosis

SPECIMEN EVALUATION

Gross

- Biopsies usually consist of ≥ 1 small fragments of pink/tan soft tissue
- Sometimes larger excision specimens are submitted for carcinoma of unknown primary
  - Serially section and submit entirely for frozen section

Frozen Section

- If goal is to identify primary carcinoma in setting of lymph node metastasis, it is usually appropriate to freeze entire specimen
- If goal is to evaluate mass for lymphoma vs. reactive process, only portion of specimen should be frozen
  - Tissue should be reserved for ancillary studies, if possible
- If in doubt, consult with surgeon about availability of additional tissue for diagnosis and ancillary studies

Cytology

- Touch preps and smears may be helpful in evaluating potential lymphoproliferative disorders
- For carcinomas, malignant cells may be less obscured by lymphoid cells on cytologic preparation
- Cytologic evaluation preserves valuable tissue for permanent sections and ancillary studies

MOST COMMON DIAGNOSES

Oropharyngeal Squamous Cell Carcinoma

- Most are HPV associated and arise in palatine tonsils or tongue base (lingual tonsil)
- Small primary tumors may give rise to bulky lymph node metastases that are frequently cystic
- Arise in specialized reticulated epithelium lining of tonsillar crypts
  - Not typically associated with surface dysplasia
  - Considered invasive when arising in crypts
- Typically has nonkeratinizing, basaloid morphology
  - Immature appearance resembles specialized crypt-lining epithelium
  - All regarded as highly differentiated carcinomas
- May also have papillary architecture
  - Moderate to severe cytologic atypia with maturation loss, mitoses in upper portions of epithelium, and atypical mitoses
- Majority are positive for high-risk HPV, most frequently HPV type 16
  - Comprise majority (80%) of HPV-associated carcinomas across all head and neck sites

Oropharyngeal Squamous Cell Carcinoma: HPV Positive

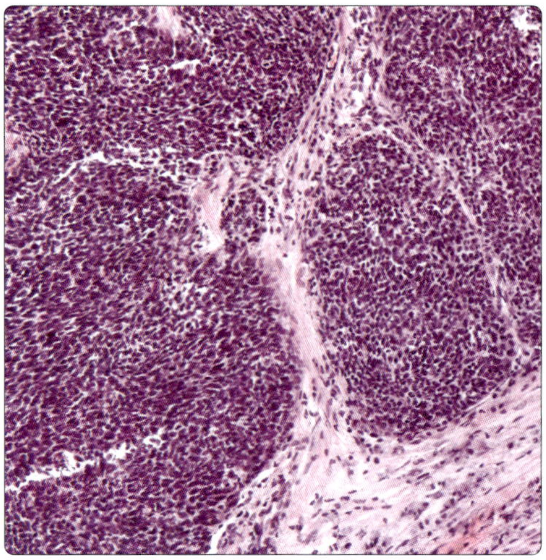

Oropharyngeal Squamous Cell Carcinoma: HPV Positive

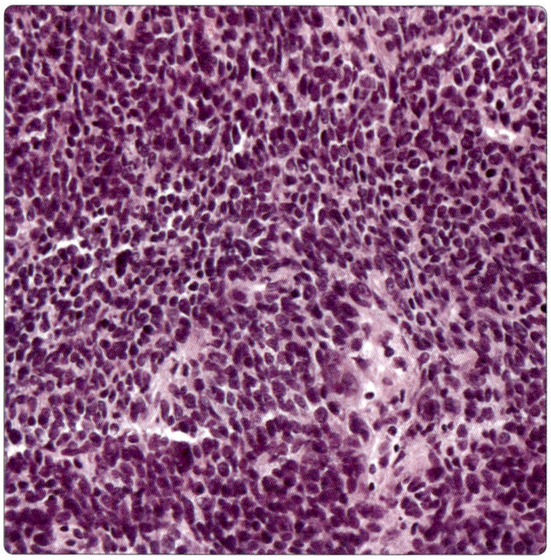

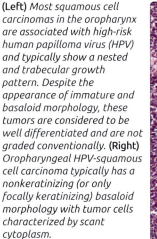

(Left) *Most squamous cell carcinomas in the oropharynx are associated with high-risk human papilloma virus (HPV) and typically show a nested and trabecular growth pattern. Despite the appearance of immature and basaloid morphology, these tumors are considered to be well differentiated and are not graded conventionally.* **(Right)** *Oropharyngeal HPV-squamous cell carcinoma typically has a nonkeratinizing (or only focally keratinizing) basaloid morphology with tumor cells characterized by scant cytoplasm.*

Contents

- All oropharyngeal SCC should be tested for high-risk HPV on permanent section
  - p16 immunohistochemistry is sensitive surrogate marker
  - Many laboratories also perform direct HPV testing (in situ hybridization or sequencing)
- Other rare types of HPV-positive carcinoma may occur
  - Includes adenosquamous, neuroendocrine/small cell, undifferentiated, and sarcomatoid carcinoma

Nasopharyngeal Carcinoma

- Term retained for all SCC in nasopharynx
- **Nonkeratinizing nasopharyngeal carcinoma**
  - Undifferentiated type: Atypical epithelioid or spindle cells with vesicular nuclei and prominent nucleolus
    - Syncytial growth within lymphoid stroma most common
    - Single-cell pattern difficult to distinguish from large B-cell lymphoma or Hodgkin lymphoma
  - Differentiated type: Nests or cords of cohesive cells
  - Both patterns can be seen in single lesion and need not be distinguished for clinical purposes
  - Associated with Epstein-Barr virus (EBV)
- **Keratinizing nasopharyngeal carcinoma**
  - Classic keratinizing SCC morphology
  - Minority are EBV associated
  - Worse prognosis than nonkeratinizing type due to lower radiosensitivity

Reactive Lymphoid Follicular Hyperplasia

- Common in Waldeyer tonsillar ring, such as palatine tonsils and nasopharyngeal tonsils ("tonsil/adenoid hypertrophy"), especially in younger patients
- Distinction from low-grade lymphoma may require appropriate tissue allocation for ancillary tests

Lymphoma

- Non-Hodgkin lymphoma is predominant category
  - Diffuse large B-cell lymphoma is most common type
    - Sheets of intermediate to large cells with vesicular nuclei, prominent nucleoli, and marked mitotic activity
  - Other high-grade non-Hodgkin lymphomas include Burkitt lymphoma, extranodal NK-/T-cell lymphoma, and anaplastic large cell lymphoma
  - Mantle cell lymphoma may be seen in extranodal sites of the Waldeyer ring
  - Low-grade lymphomas
    - Extranodal marginal zone lymphoma (or mucosa-associated lymphoid tissue lymphoma) most often involves tonsils
    - Extranodal follicular lymphoma is very uncommon
- Hodgkin lymphoma is rare in extranodal head and neck sites

Squamous Papilloma

- Benign, often associated with low-risk HPV (types 6 or 11)
- Papillary squamous growth with fibrovascular cores
  - Bland or mildly atypical squamous cells, sometimes with koilocytic change
  - Mitoses absent or only in basal layer; no atypical forms
- Must be differentiated from papillary SCC

REPORTING

Frozen Section

- Presence or absence of carcinoma should be reported and type given, if possible
- Lymphoid lesions
  - Definitive diagnosis on frozen section is usually difficult
  - Appropriate tissue allocation for ancillary studies is most important goal
  - If reactive process is favored, it is sufficient to remain descriptive with comment that reactive process is favored, but further work-up will be undertaken
  - Report "atypical lymphoid infiltrate, final diagnosis deferred to permanent sections" if low-grade non-Hodgkin lymphoma is suspected
  - Report "poorly differentiated malignant epithelioid neoplasm, final diagnosis deferred to permanent sections" if high-grade non-Hodgkin lymphoma is suspected
    - It can be difficult to differentiate lymphoma from carcinoma or sarcoma on frozen section

PITFALLS

Oropharyngeal Squamous Cell Carcinoma

- Primary lesions may be quite small with subtle distortion of crypt architecture
  - Normal tonsillar crypts can be pitfall
- HPV-associated SCC often shows large nests or cystic spaces
  - Complexity of architecture (bulky nests, etc.) is clue
- Immunohistochemical studies on permanent sections may be helpful in distinguishing neoplasia from reactive epithelium
  - p16 positivity (> 70% tumor cells) and Ki-67 reactivity throughout all epithelial layers
- Benign lymphoid aggregates may mimic mass lesion

Sialometaplasia

- Evaluation for residual/recurrent SCC after chemoradiation may be complicated by presence of extensive sialometaplasia with atypia
- Sialometaplasia exhibits extensive squamous metaplasia within preexisting salivary gland parenchyma and adjacent tissue necrosis
- Definitive diagnosis is often not required at time of frozen section
  - Additional tissue sampling and p16 immunohistochemistry may be helpful

Nasopharyngeal Carcinoma

- Nonkeratinizing carcinoma can be difficult to detect due to presence of single tumor cells or small clusters merging with lymphoid stroma and absent desmoplastic response
- Appropriate tissue allocation should be considered to exclude lymphoma
- Keratin or p40 immunohistochemical stains may be necessary for definitive diagnosis

SELECTED REFERENCES

1. Carpenter DH et al: Undifferentiated carcinoma of the oropharynx: a human papillomavirus-associated tumor with a favorable prognosis. Mod Pathol. 24(10):1306-12, 2011

Contents

(Left) *Tonsillar squamous cell carcinoma arises from the surface epithelium ➩ and shows keratinization, in keeping with conventional squamous cell carcinoma. These morphologic features are unlikely to be associated with HPV.* (Right) *Complex architecture and bulky nests of this squamous cell carcinoma ➩ aid in identifying it as invasive rather than in situ carcinoma within tonsillar crypts. The overlying mucosa is not involved ➩. This basaloid morphology is highly associated with HPV.*

Invasive Keratinizing Squamous Cell Carcinoma of Tonsil

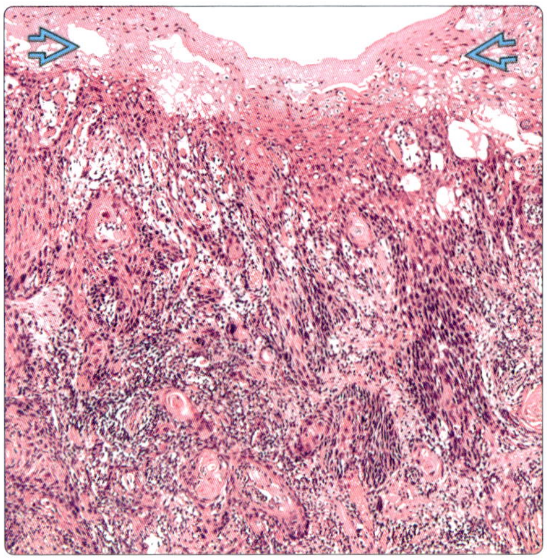

Invasive Nonkeratinizing Squamous Cell Carcinoma of Tonsil

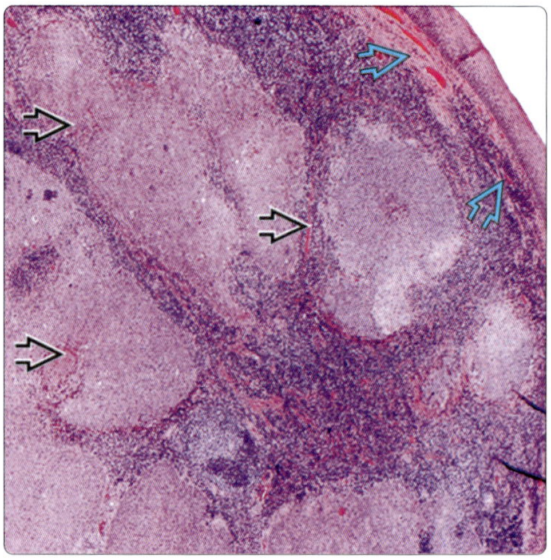

(Left) *Complex architecture and bulky nested growth of immature epithelium is characteristic of oropharyngeal HPV-squamous carcinoma. In this example, there is focal keratinization present →.* (Right) *Papillary squamous cell carcinoma shows atypical squamous epithelium growing around fibrovascular cores with loss of stratification and nuclear atypia. In the oropharynx, the majority are associated with high-risk HPV.*

Oropharyngeal HPV-Squamous Cell Carcinoma

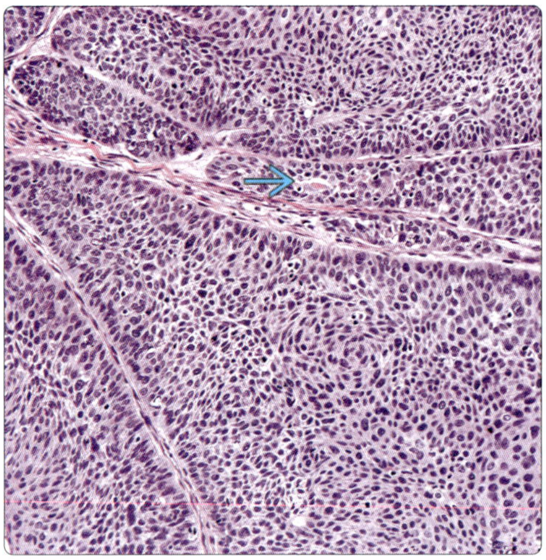

Papillary Squamous Cell Carcinoma

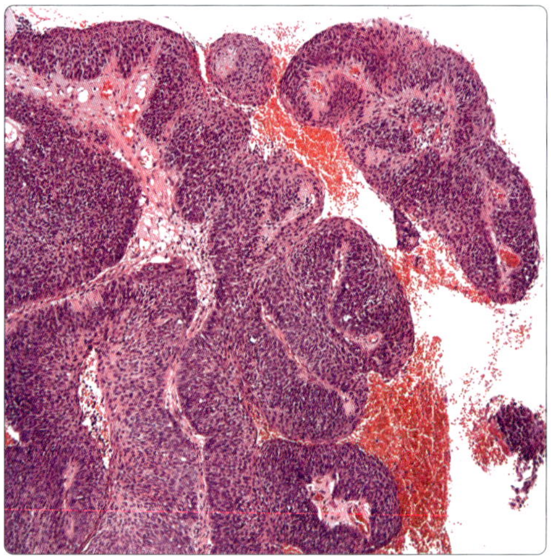

(Left) *Papillary squamous cell carcinoma exhibits full-thickness atypia, loss of polarity, and lack of maturation. Mitoses can be seen in the upper 1/2 of the epithelium ➩. These features distinguish this lesion from a benign squamous papilloma.* (Right) *Squamous papilloma is a papillary lesion lined by bland squamous epithelium. These lesions are common in the oral cavity but may also be seen in the oropharynx (especially uvula and tonsils) and nasopharynx. These are associated with low-risk HPV (types 6 or 11).*

Papillary Squamous Cell Carcinoma

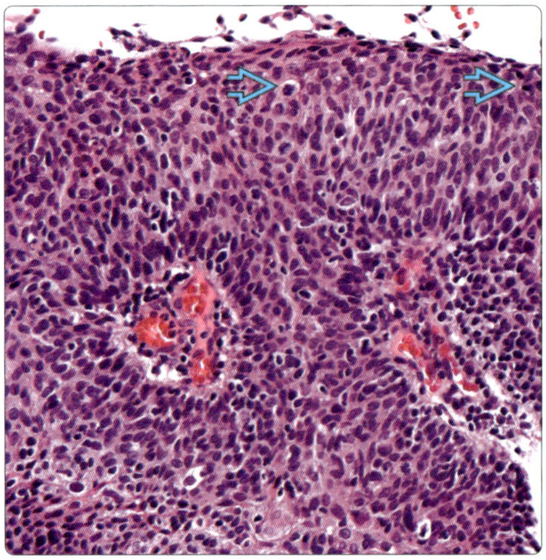

Squamous Papilloma

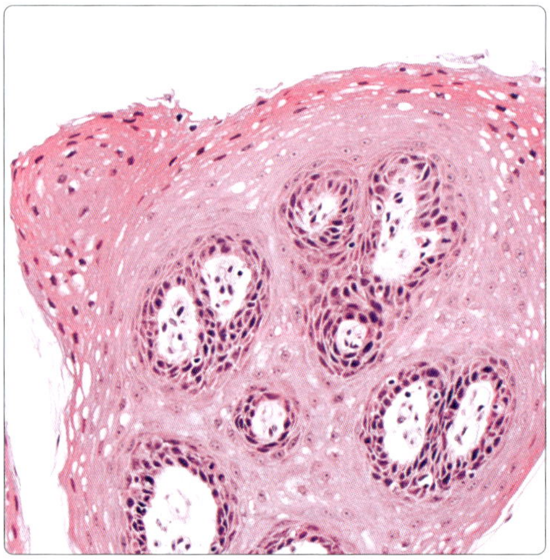

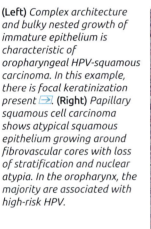

Nasopharyngeal Carcinoma, Nonkeratinizing Type

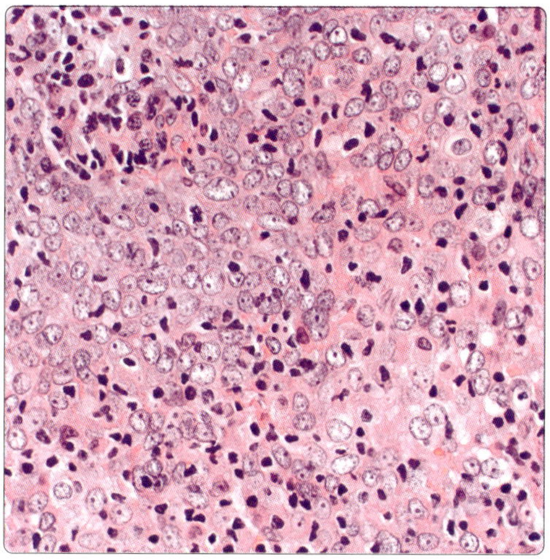

Nasopharyngeal Carcinoma, Nonkeratinizing Type

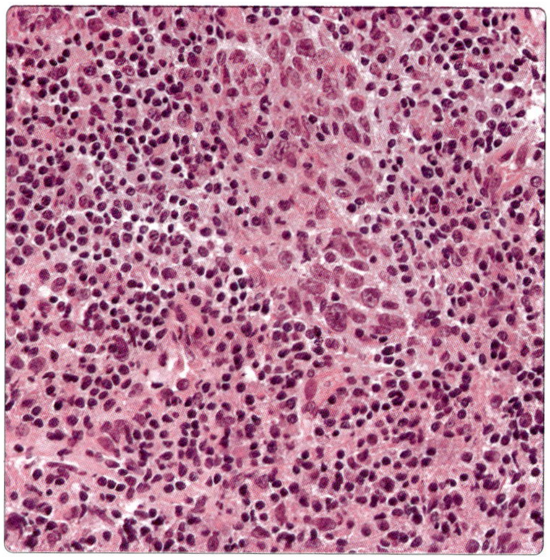

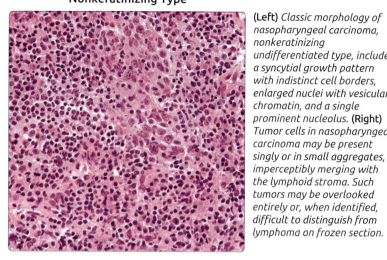

(Left) *Classic morphology of nasopharyngeal carcinoma, nonkeratinizing undifferentiated type, includes a syncytial growth pattern with indistinct cell borders, enlarged nuclei with vesicular chromatin, and a single prominent nucleolus.* (Right) *Tumor cells in nasopharyngeal carcinoma may be present singly or in small aggregates, imperceptibly merging with the lymphoid stroma. Such tumors may be overlooked entirely or, when identified, difficult to distinguish from lymphoma on frozen section.*

Nasopharyngeal Carcinoma, Nonkeratinizing Type

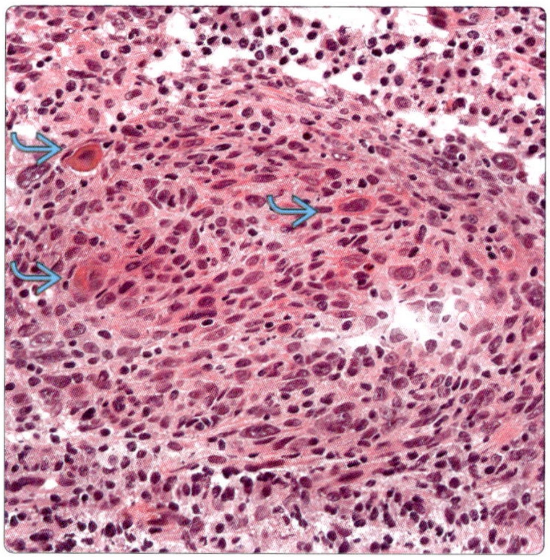

Nasopharyngeal Carcinoma, Nonkeratinizing Type

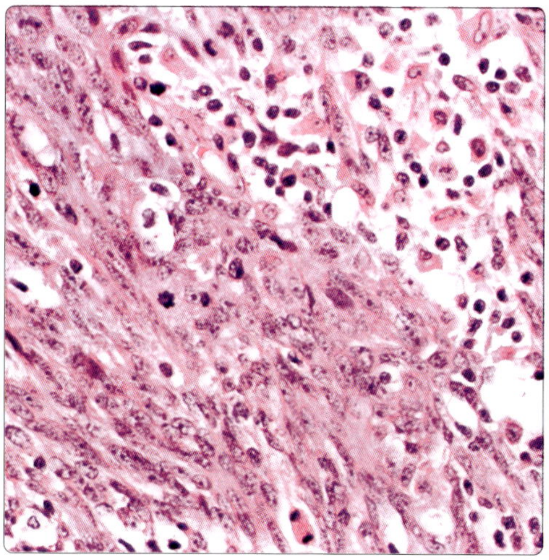

(Left) *Some nasopharyngeal carcinomas show cohesive groups of cells, although both differentiated and undifferentiated patterns may be present within a single tumor. Note the focal keratinization* ➙ *in this example.* (Right) *Nasopharyngeal carcinoma, nonkeratinizing undifferentiated type, is Epstein-Barr virus (EBV) associated and has syncytial growth. Both spindle cells (such as in this case) and epithelioid cells can be seen.*

Normal Tonsillar Crypt

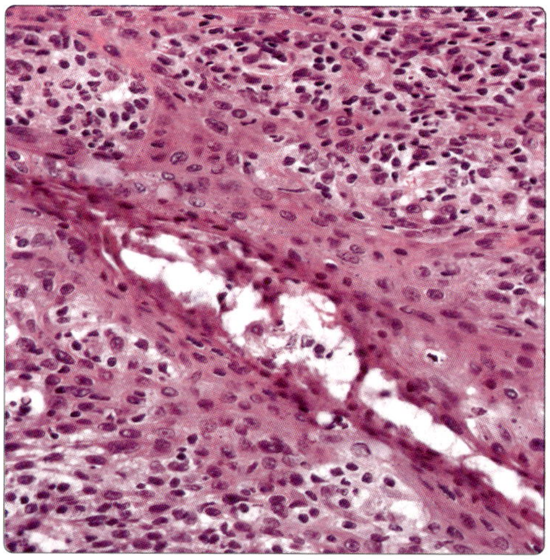

Reactive Lymphoid Tissue

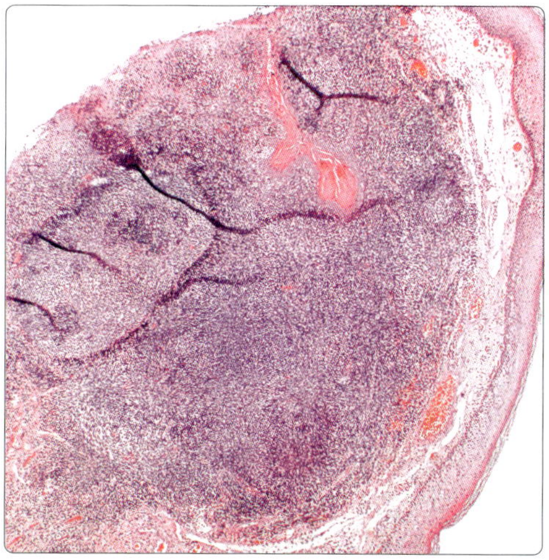

(Left) *Normal tonsillar crypts are lined by specialized reticular epithelium and may be difficult to distinguish from subtle squamous cell carcinomas. Normal crypts are lined by thin layers of benign-appearing squamous epithelium with squamous cells having more cytoplasm and lacking atypia.* (Right) *Prominent lymphoid aggregate creates the clinical impression of a small nodule in the tongue base. Some examples may need to be distinguished from low-grade non-Hodgkin lymphoma by ancillary studies.*

SURGICAL/CLINICAL CONSIDERATIONS

Goal of Consultation

- Determine if ovarian lesion is benign or malignant
  - Malignant mucinous carcinomas are evaluated for likelihood of metastasis vs. primary carcinoma
- Accurately stage patients with carcinoma
  - For patients with uterine carcinoma, involvement of ovaries increases stage
  - For patients with ovarian carcinoma, surface involvement of ovary may alter stage

Change in Patient Management

- If malignancy is identified, appropriate staging biopsies and definitive surgery may be performed
  - Total abdominal hysterectomy and bilateral salpingo-oophorectomy
  - Debulking of large tumors
  - Peritoneal washings
  - Lymph node biopsies
- If no malignancy is identified, no additional surgery is required
  - Fertility can be preserved in premenopausal women
- If metastasis to ovary is suspected and there is no prior history of carcinoma, peritoneal cavity is inspected for possible primary sites
  - Appendix is possible site and may be resected

Clinical Setting

- It is difficult to determine if ovarian mass is benign or malignant preoperatively
  - Imaging findings are often nonspecific
  - Needle biopsy is contraindicated due to risk of spillage of malignant cells into peritoneal cavity
- Malignancy is more common in women > age 40
  - Ovarian lesions in women < age 40 are generally benign
    - Preservation of fertility is frequent goal in young women

SPECIMEN EVALUATION

Gross

- Great care should be used in examining outer surface of ovary as involvement may alter stage
  - Surface must not be rubbed or abraded
  - Any irregularities to surface are noted
    - May be due to carcinoma penetrating capsule or to serosal metastasis
- Selectively ink surface, including any possible excrescences or metastasis
- Ovary is serially sectioned
  - Cysts with fluid under pressure can appear to be solid masses by palpation
    - These cysts should be opened with caution and with proper eye protection to avoid uncontrolled release of contents
    - Small incision directed away from prosector is made into cyst
      - Adequate surgical drapes, pan, or sink should be available to dispose of cyst fluid
    - If multilocular, all cysts should be opened
- Evaluate appearance of solid masses and cysts
  - Inner surface of cysts must not be touched as this may dislodge diagnostic cells
  - Bilateral involvement or multiple nodules within single ovary may be seen in metastatic disease
  - It is noted whether contents are serous (freely flowing) or mucinous (viscous and sticky)
- **Unilocular cyst with smooth inner lining**
  - Almost always benign
    - Typical diagnoses are cystadenoma, follicle cyst, or luteal cyst
  - Gross examination is sufficient
- **Cystic lesion filled with sebaceous material and hair**
  - Mature cystic teratoma (dermoid cyst)
  - Almost always benign
  - Gross examination is sufficient unless there is substantial solid area or cyst has ruptured
    - Rare tumors have malignant component

Endometrioma: Gross Appearance

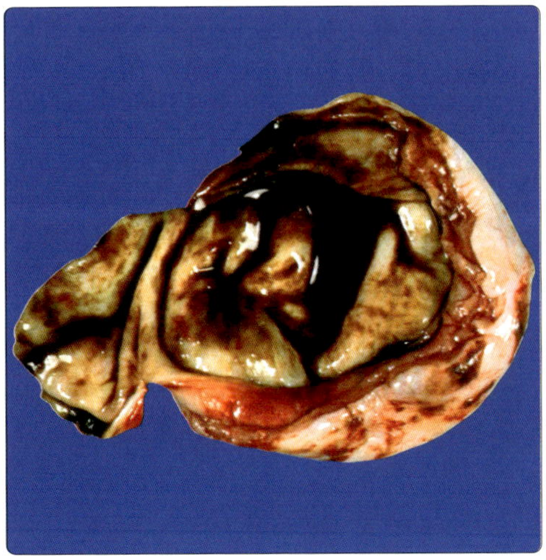

Endometrioma

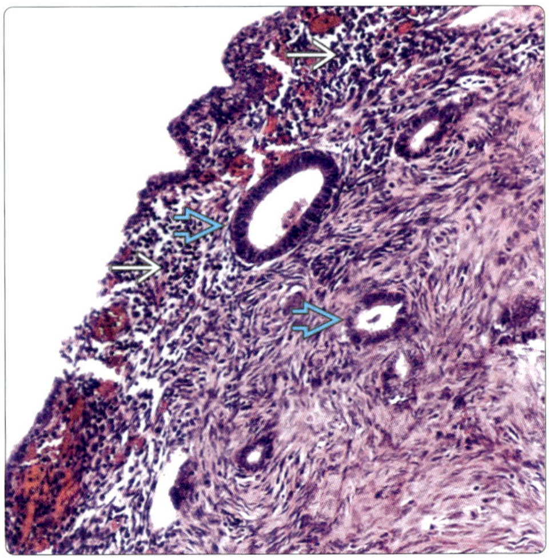

(Left) *A typical endometrioma, or "chocolate cyst," of the ovary has a flat, velvety lining and is filled with a thick, brown fluid. Carcinomas arising in these lesions may form solid masses or papillary areas.* **(Right)** *Endometrial glands ➡ &/or endometrial stroma ➡ are the characteristic components of an endometrioma. Hemorrhage and hemosiderin-laden macrophages are usually present.*

- **Unilocular or multilocular cysts with irregular or solid areas**
  - Lining is inspected
    - Inner lining should never be touched as this may dislodge diagnostic lining epithelial cells
    - Minute papillary excrescences or solid/nodular areas are suspicious for borderline tumors or malignancy
  - Most suspicious area may be selected for frozen section
- **Hemorrhagic mass**
  - Most common diagnoses are ovarian torsion, endometrioma, and nongestational choriocarcinoma
    - Tumors are sometimes cause of torsion
    - Carcinomas may arise in endometriomas in older women
  - Solid areas suspicious for carcinoma may be selected for frozen section
- **Solid mass**
  - Majority are benign, but many malignancies have this appearance
  - Carcinomas typically have homogeneous appearance with variable amounts of necrosis, hemorrhage, and cystic degeneration
    - Extensive necrosis is suggestive of metastatic colon carcinoma

Frozen Section

- 1-2 representative sections of area most likely to show malignancy may be frozen
- 2 frozen sections may be performed in cases of suspected borderline tumor (both mucinous and serous) or mucinous carcinoma
  - If definite diagnostic features are not seen, lesion is best evaluated by extensive sampling on permanent sections

MOST COMMON DIAGNOSES

Mature Cystic Teratoma (Dermoid)

- Most common tumor of ovary
  - 10-15% are bilateral
  - Most common in premenopausal women
- Unilocular cystic mass filled with sebaceous material, keratin, and hair
  - Nodule projecting into cyst (Rokitansky protuberance) may contain bone or teeth
  - Struma ovarii consists of thyroid tissue and is red-brown with small colloid-filled cysts
- Rare tumors have immature elements (immature teratoma)
  - Appear as homogeneous, fleshy or solid areas
    - Foci of necrosis may be present
    - May be intermingled with mature areas
  - Spontaneous rupture is suspicious for underlying malignancy
  - Cellular immature areas need to be distinguished from differentiated neural tissue (e.g., retina or cerebellum)
  - Difficult to make malignant diagnosis on frozen section
- Gross examination may be sufficient if no suspicious areas are identified and pathologic and clinical impressions agree

Serous Tumors

- ~ 5-10% borderline, 20-25% malignant, and remainder benign
- May be unilocular or multilocular
  - Cysts are filled with clear, watery serous fluid
  - Psammoma bodies may be present
- Benign tumors have thin cyst walls with smooth inner linings
- Borderline lesions have numerous small papillary projections in inner cyst lining
- Carcinomas have areas of solid &/or papillary growth
  - Most common type of ovarian malignancy
  - Malignant features are generally present throughout tumor
  - Necrosis often present
  - Surface involvement common
  - May be extensive
    - May invade adjacent structures
    - 25-30% bilateral
    - 30% associated with extraovarian implants

Mucinous Tumors

- ~ 10-15% borderline, 10% malignant, and remainder benign
  - Benign and borderline tumors tend to be large (≥ 20 cm)
  - Carcinomas are generally smaller
  - 5% of benign lesions are bilateral and 20% of carcinomas are bilateral
    - May be difficult to distinguish from metastatic carcinomas
- Cysts filled with viscous gelatinous fluid
- Benign tumors usually simple cysts with thin, delicate cyst walls and smooth inner lining
- Borderline tumors are usually multilocular
  - May only have focal areas of papillary projections within cyst wall
- Carcinomas are often multilocular with solid areas and necrosis
  - Diagnostic features of malignancy can be very focal
    - May be difficult to document malignancy on limited sampling by frozen section
    - At least 2 frozen sections should be examined
  - Surface involvement is less common compared to serous carcinomas

Fibroma

- Well-circumscribed, firm mass with homogeneous chalky white, whorled surface
  - May have calcifications
- Almost all bilateral
- Fibrosarcomas are rare
  - Softer with areas of necrosis and hemorrhage

Thecoma

- Large (often > 10 cm), lobulated, solid, yellow tumor
  - Calcifications, cysts, hemorrhage, and necrosis may be present
- Majority are unilateral
- Endometrial hyperplasia may be present due to secretion of estrogen by tumor

Endometrioid Neoplasms

- Usually mixture of solid and cystic areas
  - 40% are bilateral
  - Cysts filled with hemorrhagic or mucinous fluid
- Majority are malignant

  - Metaplasia is common (squamous, secretory, oxyphilic)
  - Wide variety of histologic patterns occur (including spindle, adenoid cystic, microglandular)
  - Can resemble metastatic colon carcinoma
- 15-20% are associated with endometriosis

Brenner Tumor

- Typically small (< 2 cm), well-circumscribed, white to yellow masses
  - Occasionally, unilocular mucinous cyst with solid fibrous component
- ~ 1/4 of cases are associated with 2nd tumor (usually mucinous cystadenoma)
  - Combination can mimic malignancy

Germ Cell Tumors

- More common in children and young adults
- Dysgerminoma: Large, solid masses with creamy white "cerebriform" cut surface
- Embryonal carcinoma: Solid, soft, heterogeneous mass with abundant hemorrhage and necrosis and occasional cysts
- Yolk sac tumor: Large tumors with solid and cystic cut surface, usually associated with hemorrhage and necrosis
  - Serum α-fetoprotein may be elevated
- Nongestational choriocarcinoma: Rare in its pure form, typically presents as solid, unilateral hemorrhagic mass
  - Usually component of mixed germ cell tumor
  - Serum human chorionic gonadotropin (hCG) may be elevated

Clear Cell Carcinoma

- May be solid or cystic
  - Swiss cheese appearance
- Usually unilateral or only minimally involves surface of contralateral ovary
- Can arise as fleshy nodule in endometriotic cyst
- Can mimic low-grade mucinous and serous tumors
  - Clear cells may not be as apparent on frozen section as they are on permanent sections
  - Due to tumor heterogeneity, marked nuclear atypia and mitotic figures may not be seen

Granulosa Cell Tumor

- Large (often > 12 cm), soft solid, and cystic yellow-brown masses
  - Hemorrhagic cysts or necrosis may be present
- Majority are unilateral; 5% are bilateral
- Have tendency to rupture preoperatively, leading to surgical emergency
- Endometrial hyperplasia may be present due to estrogen production by tumor
- Monotonous cell population: Nuclear grooves and scant cytoplasm
  - Cytologic preparations can be helpful to identify nuclear features
  - Call-Exner bodies: Small spaces filled with eosinophilic material

Endometrioma

- Usually found in premenopausal women
- Cystic mass with shaggy or velvety lining and hemorrhagic contents
  - Thick, brown, chocolate-like blood within cyst
  - Surface usually covered by fibrous adhesions
- Carcinoma should be suspected in older women
  - Polypoid masses or solid areas may indicate malignancy (but are most often benign)
  - Usually endometrioid carcinoma or clear cell carcinoma

Metastatic Carcinoma

- May diffusely involve ovary, giving homogeneous appearance, or be present as multiple nodules
  - Very large tumors (> 10 cm) are more likely to be primary ovarian carcinomas
- ~ 2/3 involve both ovaries
  - Some primary ovarian tumors may be bilateral
- Most commonly from gastrointestinal tract
  - History of prior malignancy should be provided
  - If patient has not been diagnosed with cancer and metastasis is suspected, surgeon should closely inspect peritoneal cavity, including appendix
- Unusual histologic patterns suggest metastasis
  - Infiltrative invasive pattern by small glands or single cells is highly suggestive of metastasis
  - Tall columnar cells with dirty necrosis are typical of metastatic colon carcinoma
  - Signet ring cell carcinoma may be metastatic from stomach or breast (Krukenberg tumor)
    - May be associated with stromal hyperplasia and simulate fibrous lesion
  - Pseudomyxoma peritonei may involve 1 or both ovaries and mimic primary ovarian mucinous tumor
    - Most cases are due to appendiceal primary

Ovarian Masses During Pregnancy

- Masses may enlarge secondary to hormonal stimulation, leading to torsion or rupture of ovary
- Some lesions are present due to pregnancy
  - Luteoma of pregnancy, luteal cyst, corpus luteum of pregnancy, stromal hyperthecosis, stromal hyperplasia
- Tumors may be altered by pregnant state
  - Luteinized granulosa cell tumor
  - Stromal luteinization of metastatic carcinoma
  - Peritoneal implants may be associated with stromal decidual change and mesothelial hyperplasia

Ovarian Torsion

- Enlarged, rubbery ovary with hemorrhage and red to brown discoloration
  - Gelatinous, "weeping" cut surface
  - Massive edema may be seen in early stages of ovarian torsion, typically in younger patients
- Careful gross examination is important to determine if mass has caused torsion
  - ~ 1/2 associated with benign neoplasms
  - ~ 1/3 associated with other types of lesions (endometrioma, corpus luteum, cysts)
  - Rarely (< 5%) associated with carcinoma
    - ~ 1/4 of postmenopausal women with torsion will have malignancy

Follicular Cyst

- Small (< 2 cm), thin-walled, unilocular cyst with smooth inner lining

- May contain clear or blood-tinged serous fluid
- Cysts have inner layer of granulosa cells with basally located luteinized theca cells

Luteal Cyst

- Small, thin-walled cyst with slightly convoluted yellow inner lining
- Usually contains blood, although clear fluid may be present
- May become large during pregnancy, and multiple cysts may be present

Cystadenoma

- Typically unilocular with flat lining
- Small firm excrescences are indicative of cystadenofibroma

Corpus Luteum

- Yellow/orange 1.5- to 2-cm ovoid mass with convoluted borders and central hemorrhage
- Enlarges during pregnancy to fill up to 1/2 ovary
  - Brighter yellow and with cystic center

Corpora Albicantia

- Normal regressed form of corpus luteum
- Small, fibrotic, white lobulated masses
- Usually multiple in both ovaries

Lutein Cyst (Theca Lutein Cyst)

- Bilateral functional cysts that form due to elevated hCG
  - Multifetal gestation
  - Molar pregnancy
- Filled with clear yellow fluid
- Yellow areas in cyst wall correspond to luteinized cells
  - Layer of fibrin and blood is present

Benign Stromal Changes

- Stromal hyperthecosis: Bilateral ovarian enlargement with homogeneous, yellow cut surface
- Stromal hyperplasia: Normal to slightly enlarged ovaries with uniform, occasionally nodular, expansion of ovarian medulla

Pelvic Actinomycosis

- Uncommon infection usually associated with intrauterine device
- Clinical systems and multiple pelvic masses on imaging closely mimic malignancy
  - Majority of cases are diagnosed intraoperatively
  - Very important to recognize to avoid unnecessary surgery
  - May present as ovarian mass
- Most common pathogen is *Actinomyces israelii*
  - Anaerobic gram-positive bacillus
- Inflammatory response is suppurative and granulomatous
  - Presence of sulfur granules typical

REPORTING

Frozen Section

- Carcinoma
  - In cases of carcinoma where subtype (serous, mucinous, or endometrioid) is obvious, specific diagnosis is appropriate
    - Example: "Serous carcinoma, high grade, involving ovarian surface in 1 examined section"
  - Cases with ambiguous histologic features or mixed phenotypes may be reported as "carcinoma" with note describing tumor grade (low vs. high) and possible subtype
    - Example: "Adenocarcinoma, low grade, favor endometrioid in 1 examined section"
  - If lesion is possible metastasis, this should be reported
    - Example: "Adenocarcinoma with extensive necrosis, colorectal metastasis cannot be ruled out"
  - If definitive diagnosis of carcinoma is uncertain, it is best to defer to permanent sections
    - Patient can undergo definitive surgery in 2nd procedure if carcinoma is confirmed
- Borderline tumors
  - Use of phrase "at least" is appropriate to convey heterogeneous nature of these tumors
    - Up to 1/4 of cases will show areas of carcinoma after more extensive sampling on permanent sections
    - Example: "At least serous borderline tumor; ovarian surface negative in 2 examined sections"
  - Number of sections examined should be communicated to surgeon
- Solid spindle cell tumors
  - Fibromas and leiomyomas may appear similar on frozen section
    - Therefore, diagnosis of "benign spindle cell neoplasm" is appropriate
  - Presence of marked cellularity, atypia, and necrosis may indicate malignant sarcoma

PITFALLS

Adequate Sampling of Large Tumors (> 10 cm)

- It may be difficult to exclude malignancy in very large ovarian masses

Mucinous Neoplasms

- Mucinous carcinomas can be very heterogeneous in appearance and can require extensive sampling for diagnosis
- Metastasis from gastrointestinal primary may mimic ovarian mucinous tumor

Borderline Tumors

- Up to 1/4 of tumors classified as borderline on frozen section will be reclassified as malignant after extensive sampling

SELECTED REFERENCES

1. García-García A et al: Pelvic actinomycosis. Can J Infect Dis Med Microbiol. 2017:9428650, 2017
2. Abudukadeer A et al: Accuracy of intra-operative frozen section and its role in the diagnostic evaluation of ovarian tumors. Eur J Gynaecol Oncol. 37(2):216-20, 2016
3. Bozdag H et al: The diagnostic value of frozen section for borderline ovarian tumours. J Obstet Gynaecol. 36(5):626-30, 2016
4. Hashmi AA et al: Accuracy of intraoperative frozen section for the evaluation of ovarian neoplasms: an institutional experience. World J Surg Oncol. 14:91, 2016
5. Lee KR et al: The distinction between primary and metastatic mucinous carcinomas of the ovary: gross and histologic findings in 50 cases. Am J Surg Pathol. 27(3):281-92, 2003

Ovarian Tumors: Frequency

Benign (80% of total)	Frequency	Malignant (20% of Total)	Frequency
Mature cystic teratoma (dermoid)	55%	Serous/mixed epithelial carcinoma	47%
Serous cystadenoma/cystadenofibroma	24%	Undifferentiated carcinoma	14%
Mucinous cystadenoma	11%	Endometrioid carcinoma	11%
Fibroma/thecoma	4%	Mucinous carcinoma	10%
Borderline serous tumor	3%	Sex cord-stromal tumors (all types)	7%
Borderline mucinous tumor	< 2%	Germ cell tumors (all types)	7%
Brenner tumor	1%	Clear cell carcinoma	4%

Ovarian Tumors: Frequency by Age

Tumor Type	< 30 Years of Age	30-64 Years of Age	≥ 65 Years of Age
Borderline tumors	28%	12%	4%
Malignant epithelial tumors	33%	84%	92%
Sex cord-stromal tumors	2%	1%	1%
Germ cell tumors	34%	2%	<1%
Other mesenchymal/soft tissue	1%	< < 1%	< 1%
Lymphoma	1%	< < 1%	< 1%
Unclassified	< 1%	1%	2%
All percentages rounded to the nearest whole number.			

Partridge EE et al: The National Cancer Database Report on Ovarian Cancer Treatment in United States Hospitals. *Cancer.* 78:2236-2246, 1996

Ovarian Tumors: Common Gross Appearances

Tumor	Typical Gross Appearance
Endometrioma	Typically cystic with velvety lining, which may be stained brown or red; thick brown fluid may be expressed; may occasionally be hemorrhagic
Mature cystic teratoma	Leathery cystic tumor with small solid areas and occasional calcification or bone formation; thick keratin debris and hair are common
Serous cystadenoma/ cystadenofibroma	Unilocular, thin-walled cyst; adenofibroma may demonstrate smooth, firm, fungiform excrescences; cyst fluid is typically thin and clear
High-grade serous carcinoma	Predominately solid with areas of friable papillary growth and tan, white, firm and gritty cut surface; necrosis may be present as well as peritoneal and contralateral adnexal involvement
Mucinous cystadenoma	Thin-walled cystic structure, which may be unilocular or multilocular; may reach massive sizes; cyst fluid may range from thin to mucoid and is typically clear
Serous borderline tumor	Cystic structures, usually unilocular, with delicate, fleshy papillary excrescences that may be on inner or outer surfaces; solid growth should be absent
Fibroma/thecoma/Brenner tumor/leiomyoma	Solid, unilateral, well-circumscribed, firm masses with tan/yellow (thecoma), smooth cut surface; leiomyomas have whorled, bulging cut surface
Endometrioid carcinoma	Cystic and solid masses with hemorrhage; cyst fluid, if present, is typically thin to mucoid and brown; up to 40% may be bilateral
Mucinous borderline tumor/carcinoma	Multilocular cystic masses with variable amounts of solid growth; solid growth and necrosis are associated with carcinomatous transformation
Granulosa cell tumor	Soft, cystic to solid, unilateral mass; hemorrhage, necrosis, and tumor rupture are common
Metastasis	Classically bilateral; mild to moderate enlargement of ovaries with relative preservation of gross architecture; metastatic mucinous carcinoma from colon or appendix may be multicystic with increased amounts of necrotic debris

Serous Cystadenoma: Gross Features

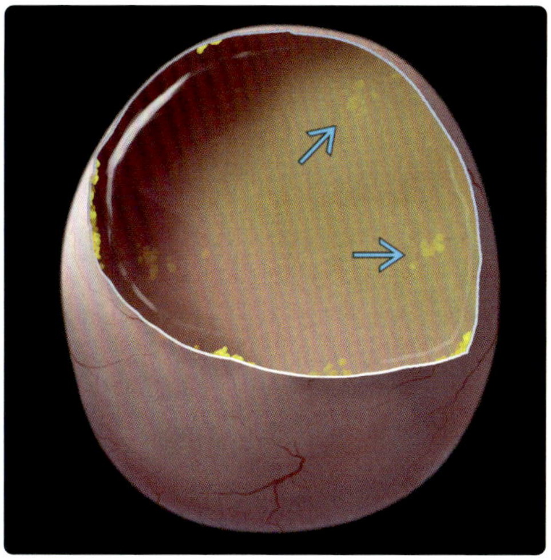

Serous Cystadenoma: Gross Appearance

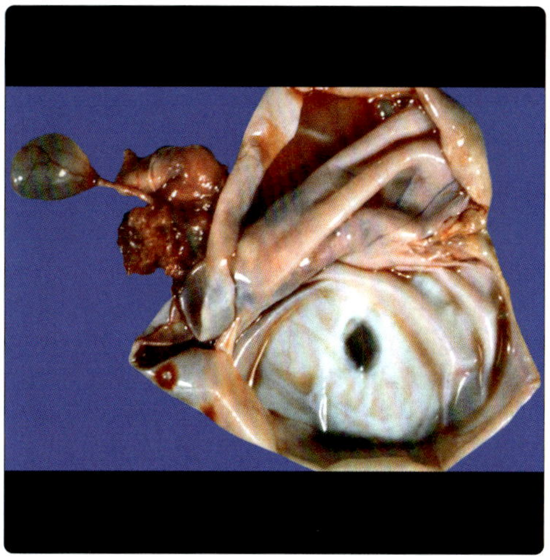

(Left) *Serous cystadenomas are a common cause of ovarian enlargement and typically consist of a unilocular, thin-walled cyst filled with a thin clear fluid. Solid areas and excrescences should be absent. If present ➡, a borderline tumor or cystadenofibroma should be suspected.* **(Right)** *Cystadenomas may be unilocular or multilocular. The cyst wall is typically thin with no masses or excrescences. This serous cystadenoma is unilocular with a thin, simple lining and was filled with clear watery fluid.*

Serous Cystadenoma

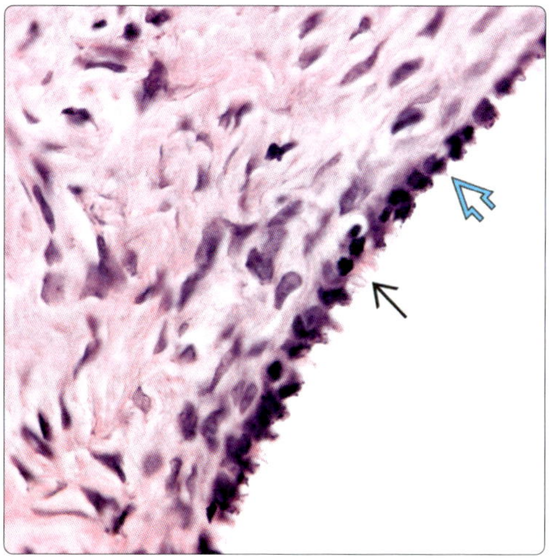

Mucinous Cystadenoma: Gross Features

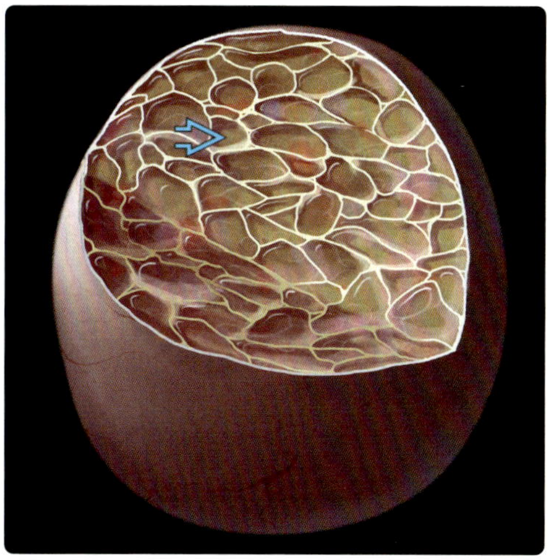

(Left) *Cystadenomas are lined by a single layer of epithelium ➡ with minimal (< 10%) epithelial stratification or tufting. Serous cystadenomas may be recognized by the lack of mucinous epithelium and the presence of occasional ciliated cells ➡.* **(Right)** *Mucinous lesions, as opposed to serous ones, typically have multiple cysts. Mucinous cystadenomas may be unilocular. However, many are composed of multiple thin-walled cysts ➡. Solid areas may represent borderline or carcinomatous transformation.*

Mucinous Cystadenoma: Gross Appearance

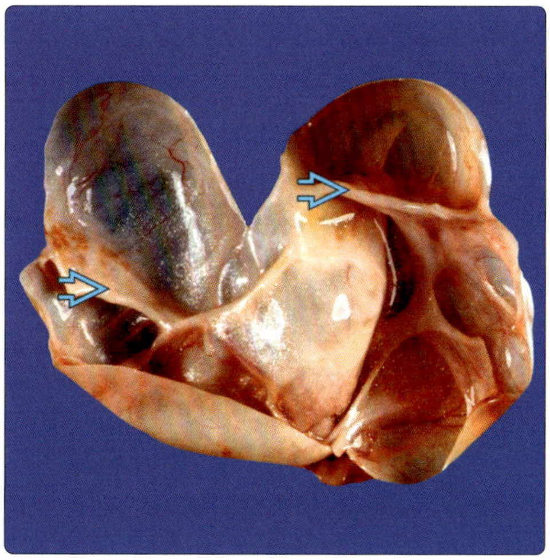

Mucinous Cystadenoma

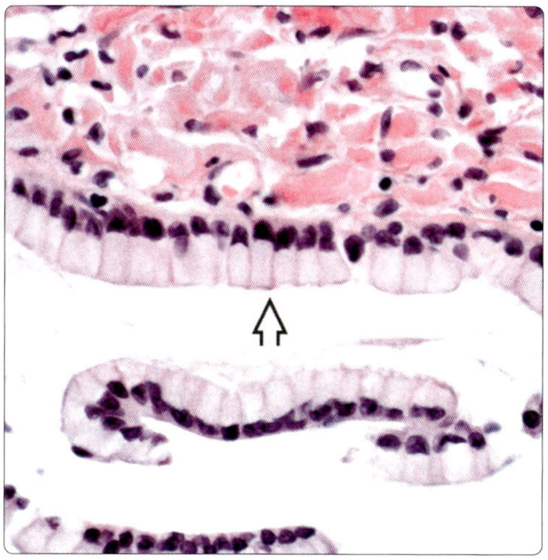

(Left) *Mucinous cystadenomas are usually large and multilocular. Occasional septations ➡ may be present. Gross features that favor a benign tumor are the thin-walled cystic spaces without the presence of masses or excrescences.* **(Right)** *The lining of a mucinous cystadenoma is composed of a single layer of mucinous epithelium ➡. Nuclear atypia should be absent to mild, and mitotic figures should be rare to absent. However, due to heterogeneity, at least 2 frozen sections should be performed.*

Cystadenofibroma: Gross Appearance

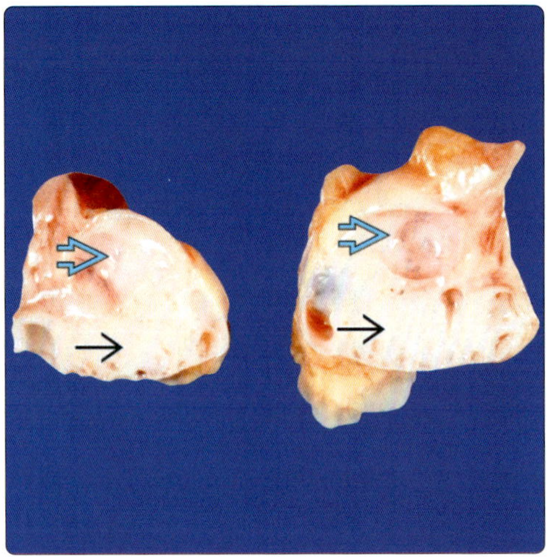

Cystadenofibroma

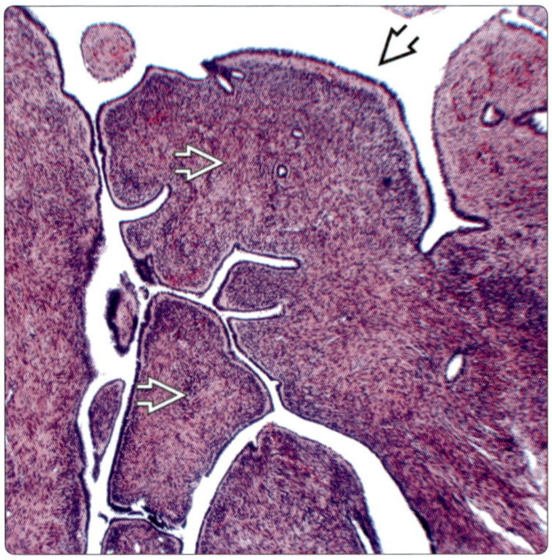

(Left) *Cystadenofibromas are identified by the presence of solid areas comprising varying amounts of the ovarian mass. In this example, a small cystic portion with a smooth lining is present ⇨ adjacent to a solid fibromatous region ⇨. A malignant component would most likely be within the fibromatous area.* **(Right)** *Cystadenofibromas are typically composed of broad, bulbous papillae ⇨ lined by a simple serous or mucinous epithelium ⇨. Occasional excrescences may mimic borderline tumors.*

Follicle Cyst: Gross Appearance

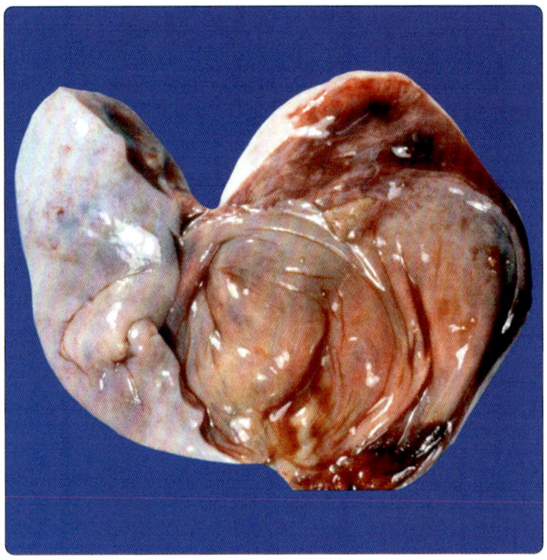

Follicle Cyst

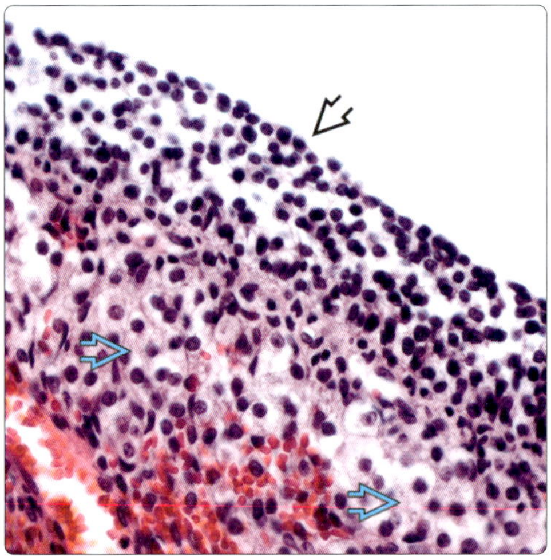

(Left) *A follicle cyst has a smooth inner lining and thin cyst walls. The cyst is typically filled with clear or blood-tinged fluid. Usually, these cysts are small. The presence of a large cyst (> 10 cm) may be seen in pregnancy, or rarely, with unilocular granulosa cell tumors.* **(Right)** *The lining of a follicle cyst is composed of several layers of granulosa cells ⇨ and underlying luteinized theca cells ⇨. Both cell types may be seen in a granulosa cell tumor but are usually more disorganized.*

Lutein Cyst: Gross Appearance

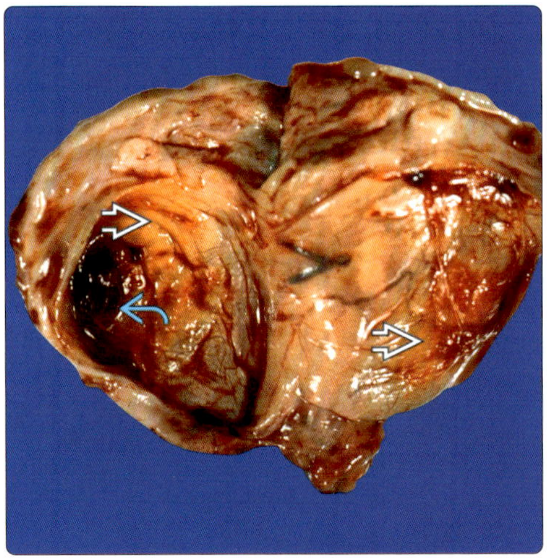

Lutein Cyst

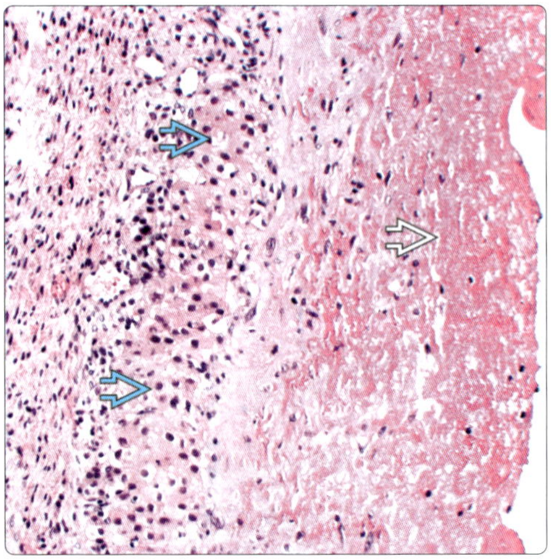

(Left) *Lutein cysts form in response to elevated human chorionic gonadotropin (hCG). The yellow areas ⇨ correspond to the luteinized cells seen microscopically. Hemorrhage ⇨ may be present. These cysts are typically small. However, they may become large and simulate a neoplasm clinically.* **(Right)** *The lining of a lutein cyst is composed of luteinized cells ⇨ that have abundant, eosinophilic cytoplasm (corresponding to the yellow areas seen grossly) and a layer of acellular blood and fibrin ⇨.*

Lutein Cyst of Pregnancy: Gross Appearance

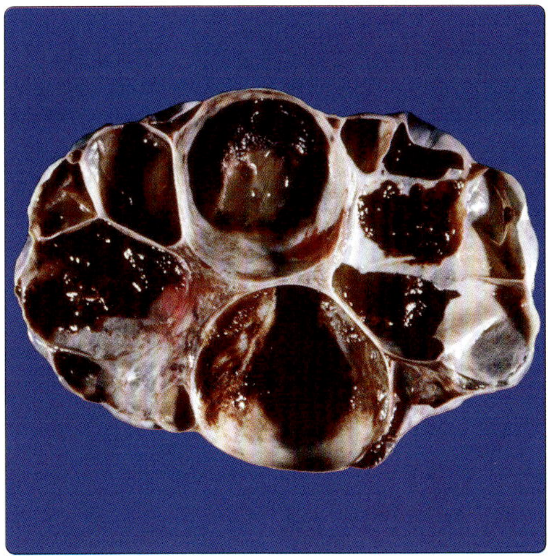

Dermoid Cyst: Gross Appearance

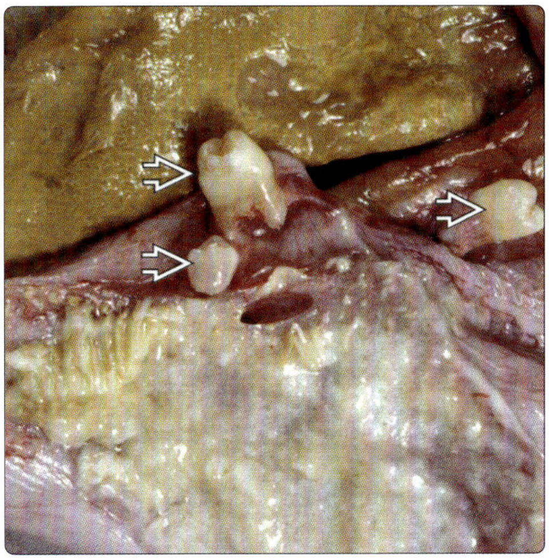

(Left) *In pregnancy, lutein cysts may become enlarged and occasionally multiloculated, which may be clinically concerning for a borderline tumor or malignancy. Histologic examination will reveal an unremarkable convoluted lutein cyst lining.* **(Right)** *Bone and rudimentary teeth may be identified in a mature cystic teratoma. Areas of solid growth with a homogeneous, fleshy cut surface should be selected for sectioning as they may represent immature mesenchymal (neural) elements.*

Dermoid Cyst: Gross Appearance

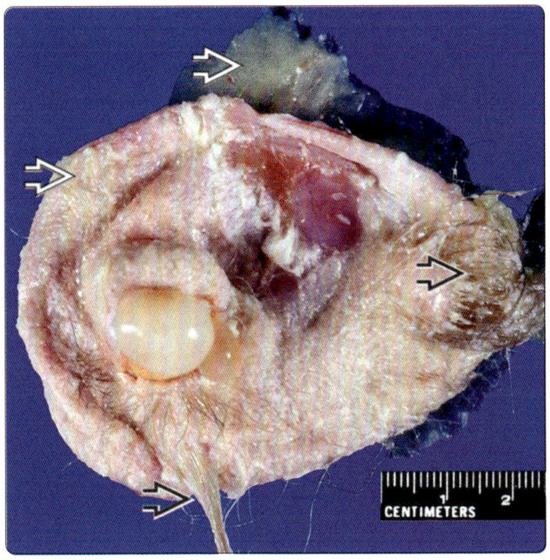

Immature Neural Tissue

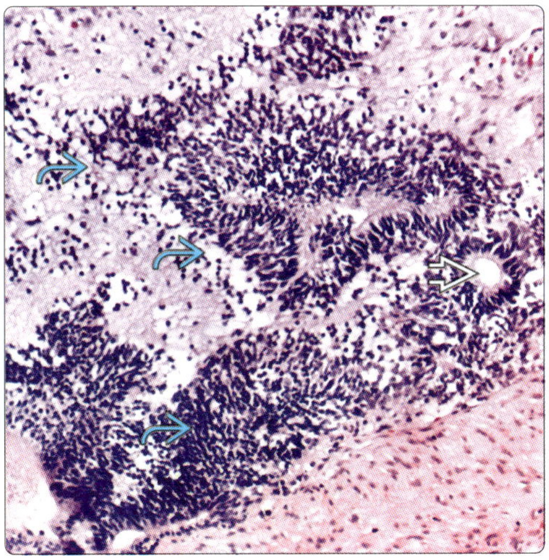

(Left) *Mature cystic teratomas (dermoid cysts) usually have a simple lining and are filled with hair and caseous material. If no solid, fleshy areas are present, gross evaluation may suffice.* **(Right)** *Immature neural tissue is composed of hyperchromatic, crowded cells and occasional rosettes. Numerous mitotic figures are present. The immature tissue may be intermingled with mature elements. Mature cerebellar tissue and retinal tissue can have a similar cellular appearance.*

Serous Borderline Tumor: Gross Features

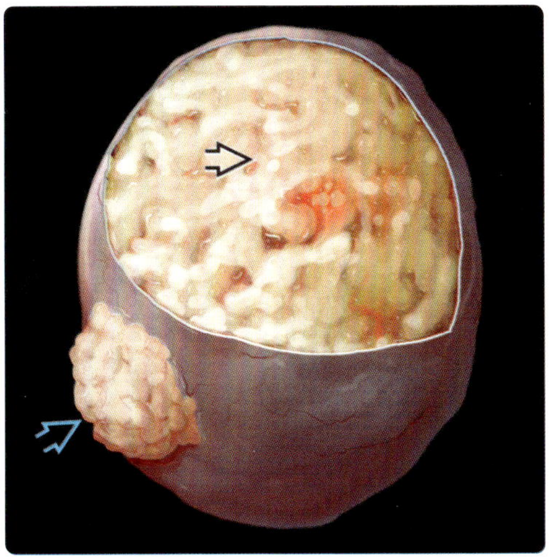

Serous Borderline Tumor: Gross Appearance

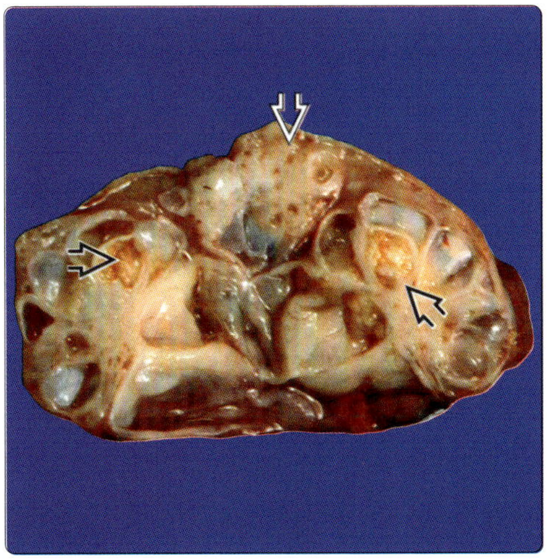

(Left) *Serous borderline tumors are often filled with soft, fleshy excrescences. Areas of surface involvement should be carefully sought for and differentially inked and sectioned for staging purposes.* **(Right)** *Serous borderline tumors may be unilocular or multiloculated (as in this case). The cysts may display delicate excrescences that can have a soft velvety texture. Solid areas are correlated with a fibromatous component.*

(Left) *Fine papillary excrescences cover the surface of the ovary in this borderline tumor. Note the fallopian tube in the upper right. Surface involvement is more common in serous tumors.* **(Right)** *The typical histologic features of borderline tumors include a hierarchical branching pattern consisting of progressively smaller papillae. Small tufts of cells may be seen at the terminal end of the papillae or "free floating" within the cyst.*

Serous Borderline Tumor: Gross Appearance

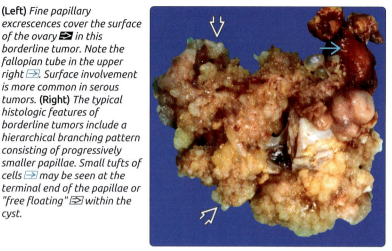

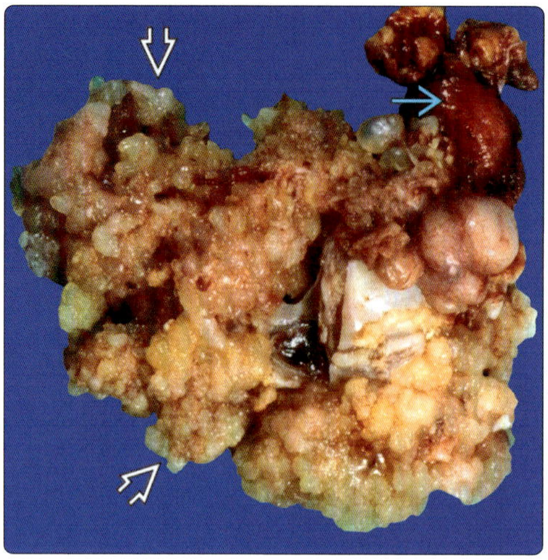

Serous Borderline Tumor

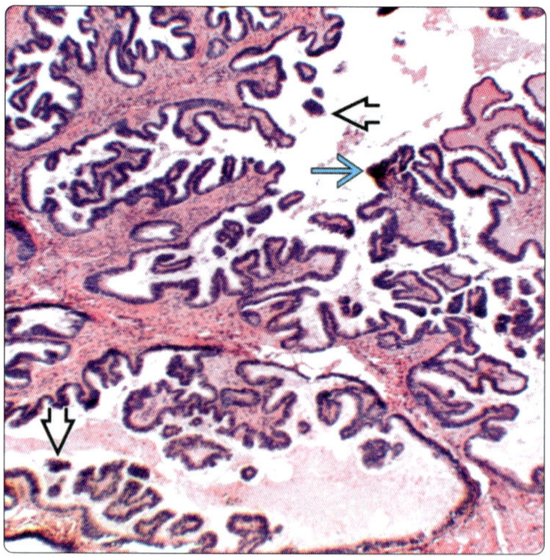

(Left) *Typical histologic features of serous borderline tumors include cellular stratification and tufting, mild to moderate nuclear atypia, and the occasional presence of a columnar-type epithelium with scattered ciliated cells, similar to the epithelium present within the fallopian tube.* **(Right)** *Benign, borderline (pictured here), and malignant mucinous cystic tumors have similar features and cannot always be distinguished by gross examination alone. Borderline tumors, as well as carcinomas, tend to be multiloculated.*

Serous Borderline Tumor

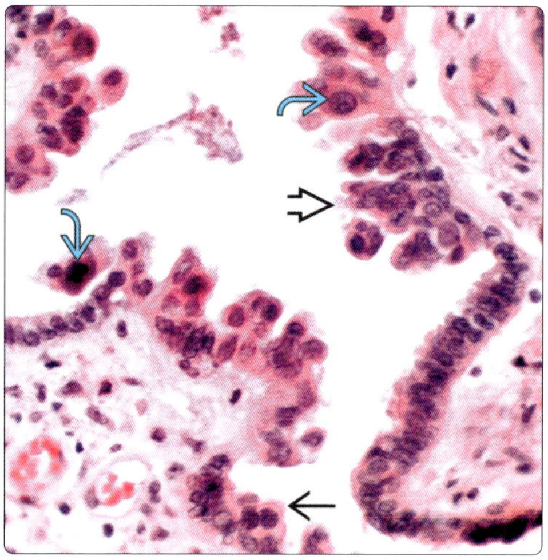

Mucinous Borderline Tumor: Gross Appearance

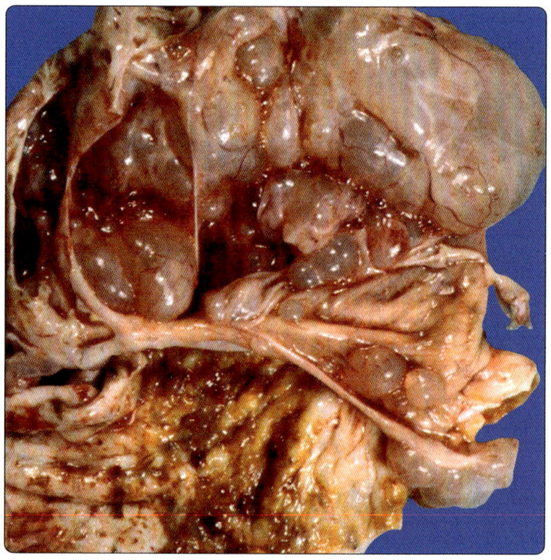

(Left) *The cytologic features of a mucinous tumor can vary from benign areas to areas of subtle nuclear stratification and early tufting, identifying this lesion as a borderline tumor. Extensive sampling may be necessary to exclude malignancy.* **(Right)** *Adult granulosa cell tumors often form large (> 12 cm), soft masses. The color may be yellow, correlating with the production of estrogens. Cystic change is common. The cysts are usually filled with a clear or blood-tinged fluid.*

Mucinous Borderline Tumor

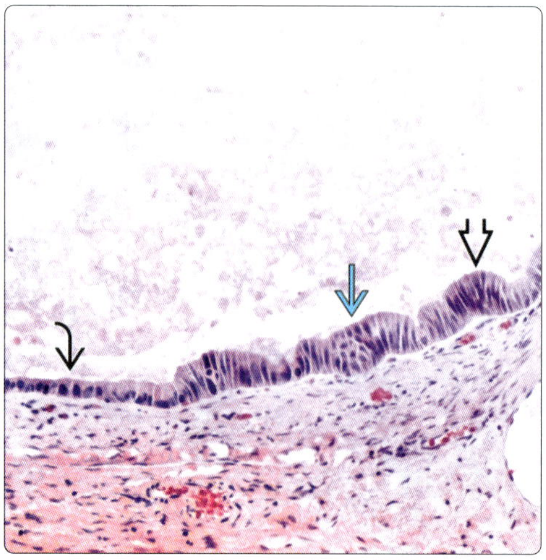

Adult Granulosa Cell Tumor: Gross Appearance

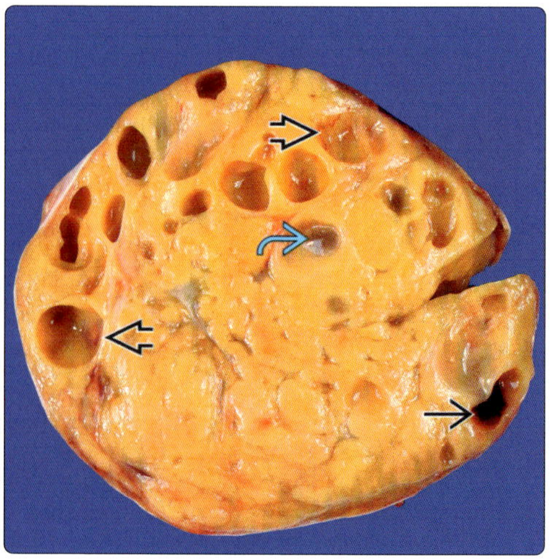

Adult Granulosa Cell Tumor: Gross Appearance

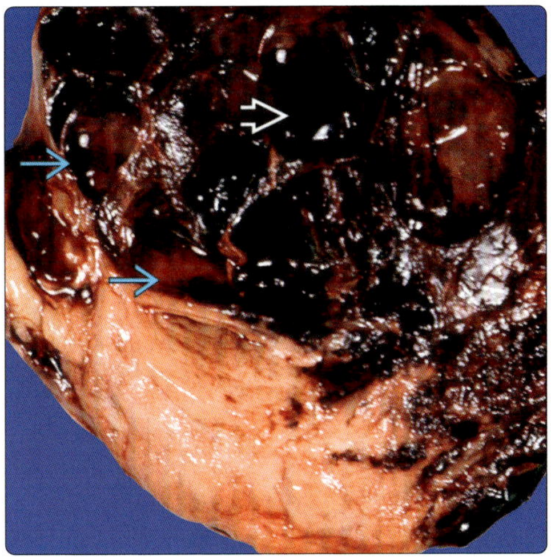

Adult Granulosa Cell Tumor

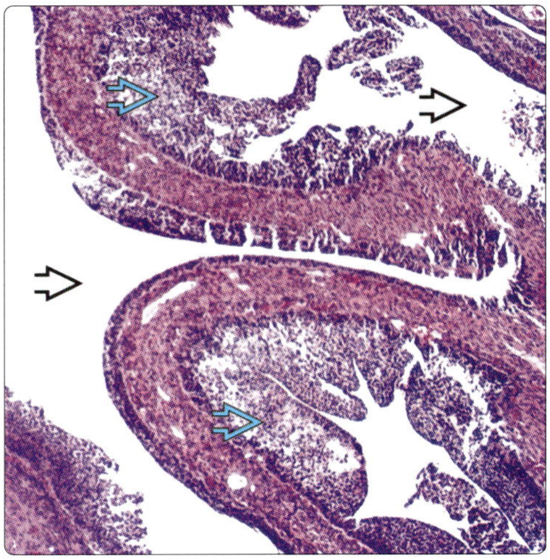

(Left) *Occasional granulosa cell tumors may be extensively cystic and hemorrhagic. Granulosa cell tumors have a tendency to spontaneously rupture, leading to an acute abdomen.* **(Right)** *The histologic appearance of adult granulosa cell tumors is highly variable. At low power, the neoplastic cells in the majority of tumors appear as "small blue cells". Here, the neoplastic cells can be seen lining large cystic cavities.*

Adult Granulosa Cell Tumor

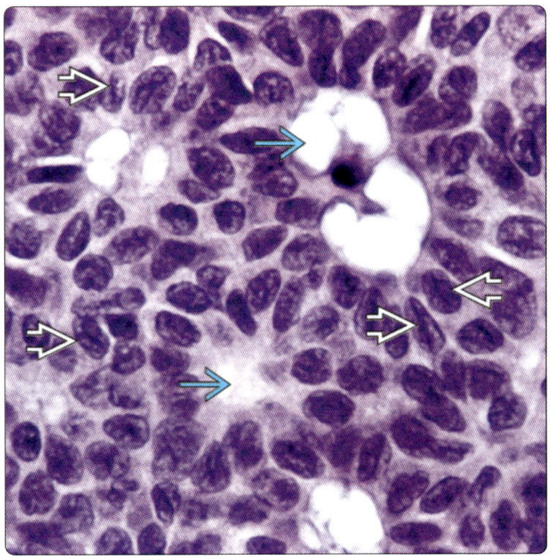

Yolk Sac Tumor: Gross Appearance

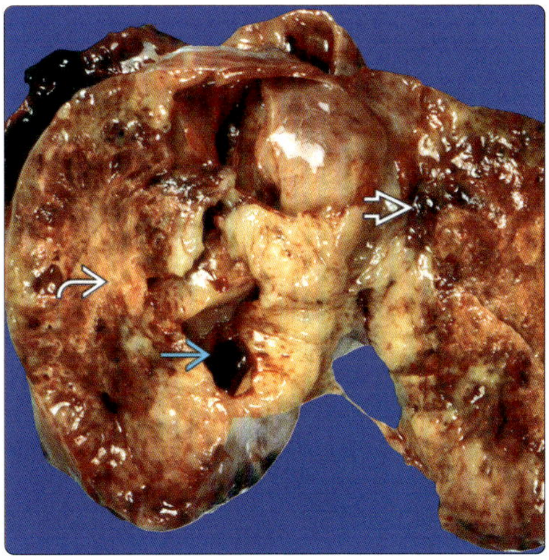

(Left) *Call-Exner bodies consist of small pseudoglandular spaces or microfollicles that are present in areas of granulosa cells. The nuclei of these tumor cells are commonly described as coffee-bean-shaped and may display grooved nuclei. These features are more easily appreciated on cytologic preparations.* **(Right)** *Yolk sac tumors are typically soft, yellow to gray masses that often display areas of hemorrhage, cystic degeneration, and necrosis.*

Yolk Sac Tumor

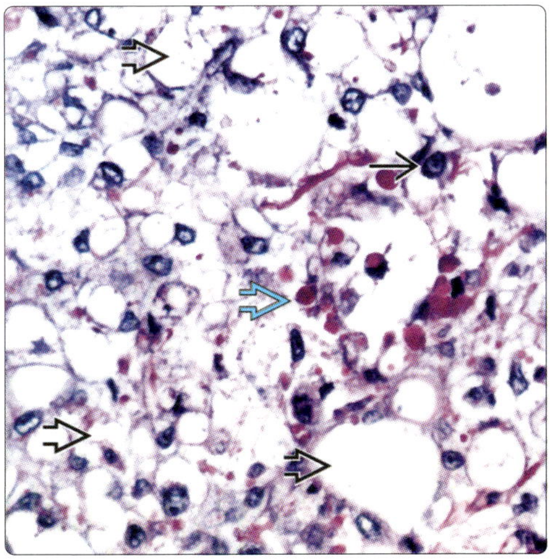

High-Grade Serous Carcinoma: Gross Appearance

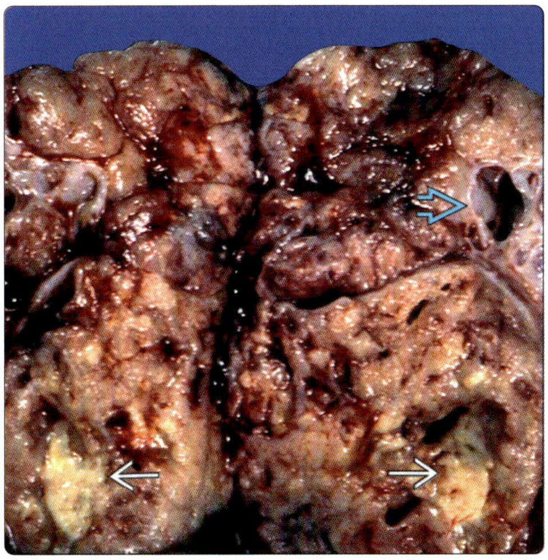

(Left) *The most common pattern in yolk sac tumors is the microcystic pattern. It is composed of variably sized cystic spaces bordered by primitive cells with nuclear pleomorphism and prominent nucleoli. Hyaline bodies may be seen but are not specific for this tumor.* **(Right)** *Serous carcinoma is often indistinguishable from other high-grade carcinomas grossly. They are often bulky, predominately solid with cystic degeneration and necrosis. Rarely, they may be predominately cystic with excrescences.*

(Left) *High-grade serous carcinomas often display cleft-like glandular spaces ➡ formed by cells with marked nuclear pleomorphism and violaceous nucleoli. These carcinomas have a high mitotic rate.* (Right) *Mucinous carcinoma typically presents as solid growth ➡ within a background of a multicystic neoplasm. Surface involvement ➡ should be identified, differentially inked, and sampled.*

High-Grade Serous Carcinoma

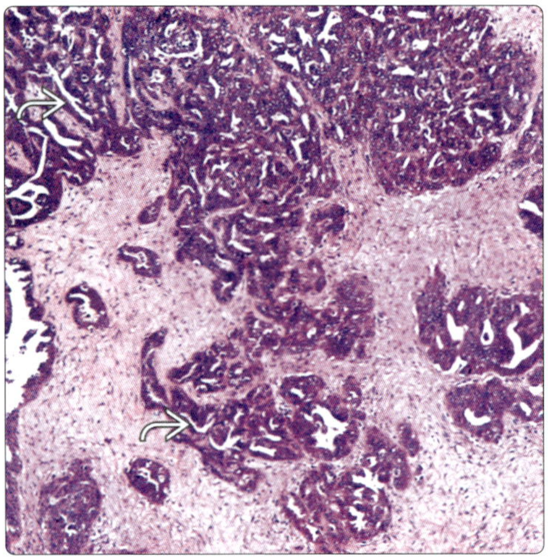

Mucinous Carcinoma: Gross Features

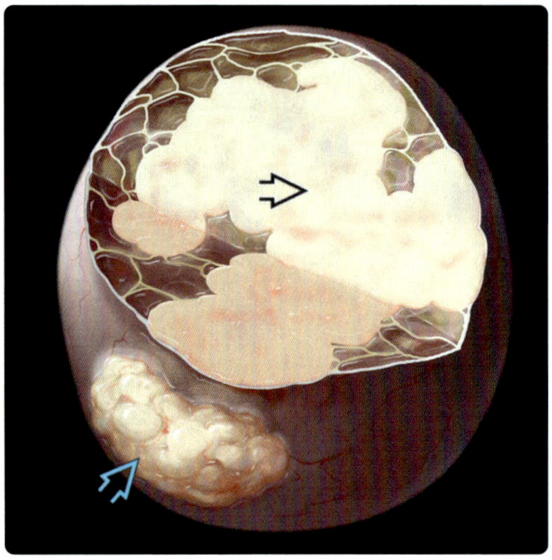

(Left) *Mucinous carcinomas tend to be smaller and more solid than their benign and borderline counterparts. The masses will often display fleshy solid areas ➡ and necrosis ➡ set within a multiloculated cystic background ➡. Metastasis to the ovary should always be considered.* (Right) *Mucinous carcinoma can most easily be identified when there is an infiltrative growth pattern. Small nests of glands as well as single glands ➡ are scattered throughout the stroma in a haphazard manner.*

Mucinous Carcinoma: Gross Appearance

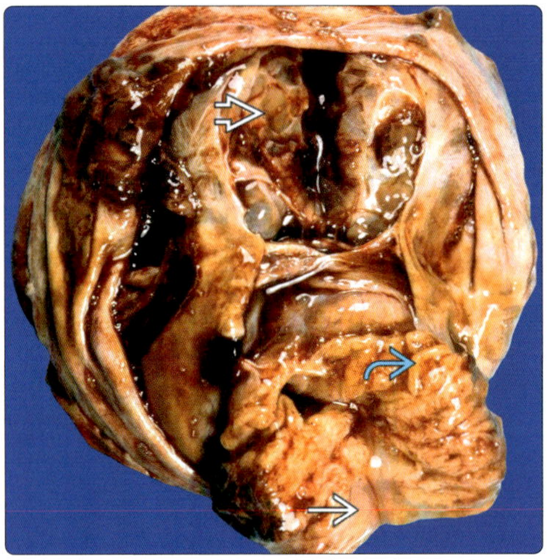

Mucinous Carcinoma

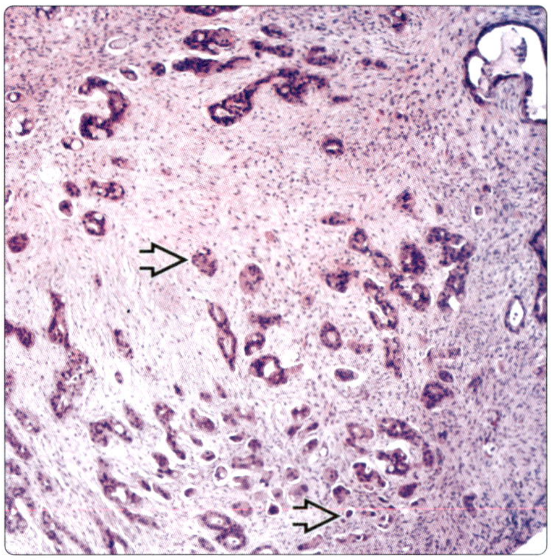

(Left) *Bilateral moderate enlargement of both ovaries (as compared to large unilateral masses) and surface involvement suggests the possibility of metastatic disease. The cut surface of the ovary on the right shows areas of necrosis ➡.* (Right) *Dilated glandular spaces with abundant necrosis ➡ are suggestive of metastasis from gastrointestinal primaries, most commonly colonic adenocarcinoma. The surgeon should be notified of the possibility of a metastasis when abundant necrosis is encountered.*

Bilateral Ovarian Disease: Gross Appearance

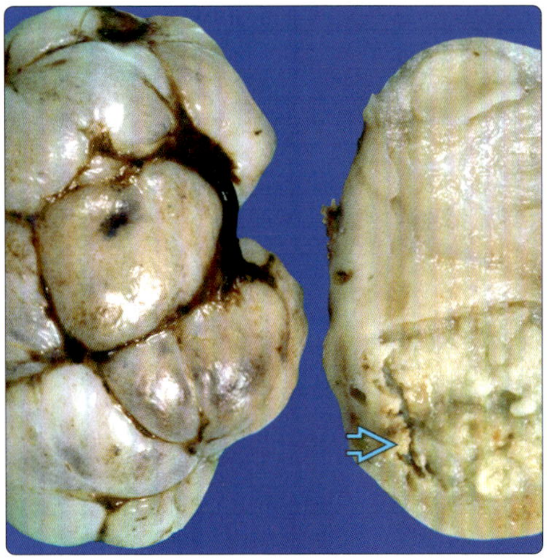

Metastatic Mucinous Carcinoma

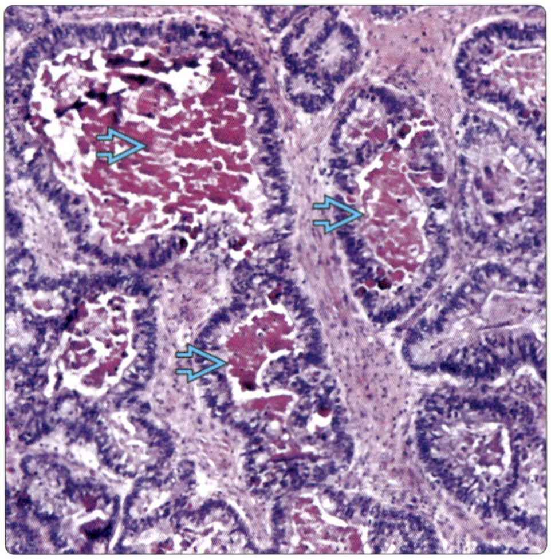

Endometrioid Adenocarcinoma in Endometriotic Cyst: Gross Appearance

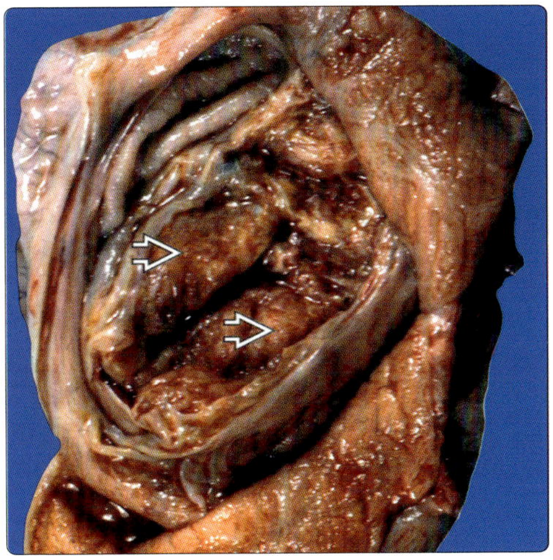

Endometrioid Adenocarcinoma

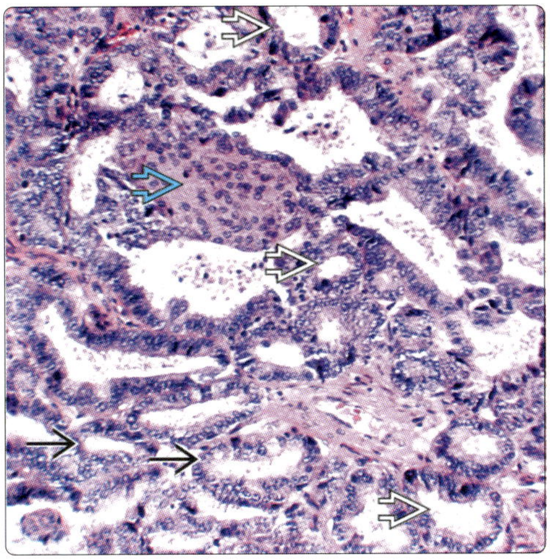

(Left) *Endometrioid adenocarcinoma can arise within an endometriotic cyst. Solid or papillary areas within endometriotic cysts should be sampled at the time of intraoperative consultation to evaluate the possibility of adenocarcinoma.* **(Right)** *Endometrioid adenocarcinoma is typically composed of back-to-back glands that have more rounded lumina when compared to the cleft or slit-like spaces in high-grade serous carcinoma. Squamous morules are a helpful feature and would not be seen in metastatic colon carcinoma.*

Clear Cell Carcinoma in Endometriotic Cyst: Gross Appearance

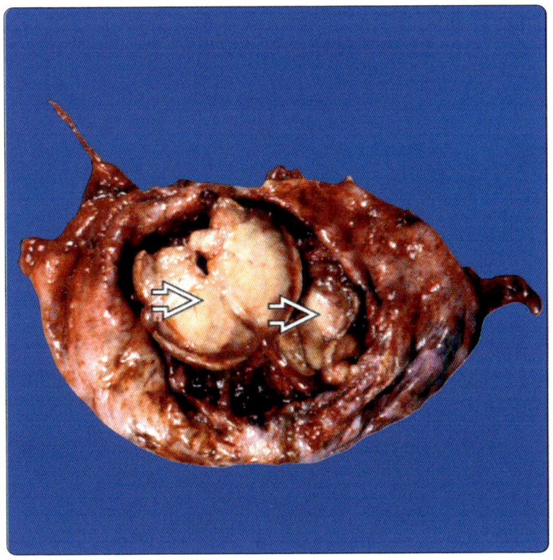

Clear Cell Carcinoma

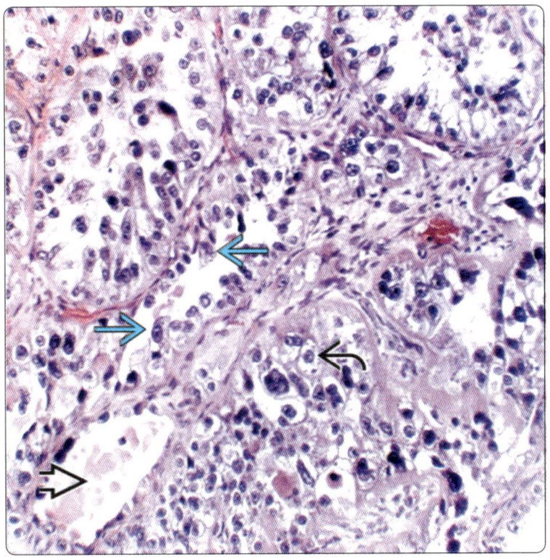

(Left) *Clear cell carcinoma arise as masses within an endometriotic cyst. As a result, all hemorrhagic cysts must be thoroughly searched for solid components at the time of gross evaluation.* **(Right)** *Clear cell carcinoma commonly displays a tubulocystic pattern composed of small glands (tubules) and variably sized cystic spaces. The pleomorphic cells project in a hobnail fashion into the spaces. Cytoplasmic clearing may be present, but this is not always seen.*

Massive Ovarian Edema: Gross Appearance

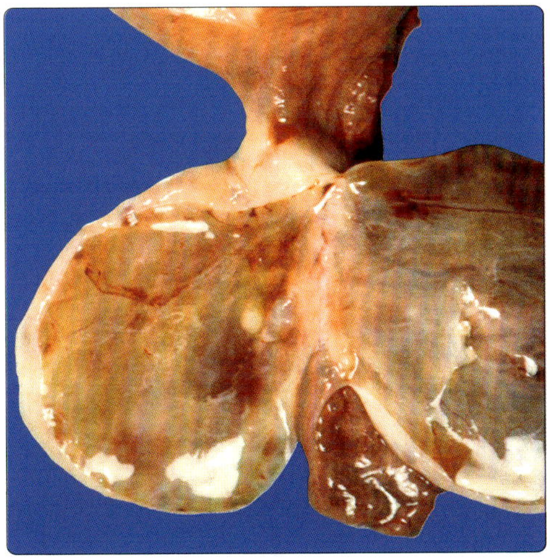

Stromal Hyperthecosis: Gross Appearance

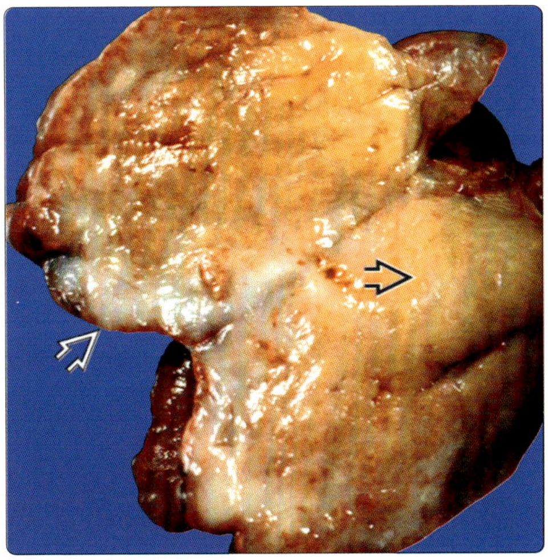

(Left) *Moderate (10 cm) to massive (> 30 cm) enlargement of the ovary may be seen. This may be a cause of ovarian torsion. The cut surface of the ovary typically shows a gelatinous, wet surface.* **(Right)** *Bilateral ovarian involvement in stromal hyperthecosis is common. The ovaries may be slightly enlarged and show replacement with firm white to yellow fibrous tissue. Elevated serum estrone levels may lead to concurrent endometrial hyperplasia. Elevated androgen levels can lead to virilization.*

(Left) *Typically seen in perimenopausal or postmenopausal patients, stromal hyperplasia may lead to slight ovarian enlargement. The cut surface of the ovary demonstrates an ill-defined area of white to yellow discoloration* → *. Multiple nodules may be present, and they may involve the cortex or medulla of the ovary.* **(Right)** *Areas involved by stromal hyperplasia are replaced by a cellular proliferation of bland spindle cells with scant cytoplasm. The histologic features are similar to that seen in cellular fibroma.*

Stromal Hyperplasia: Gross Appearance

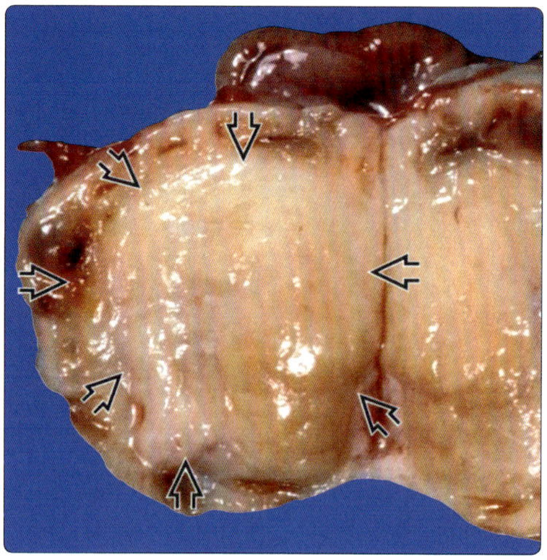

Stromal Hyperplasia

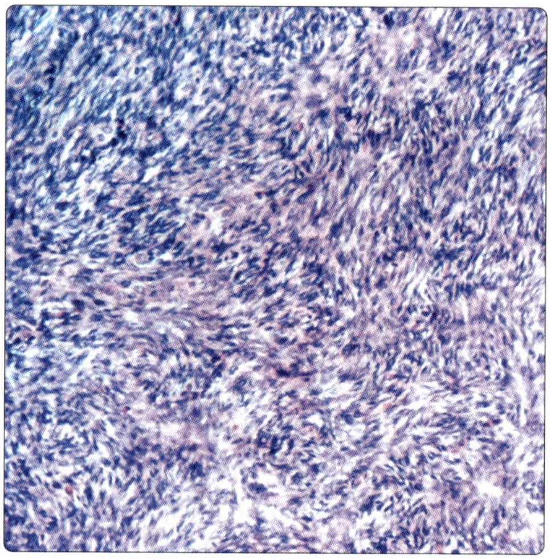

(Left) *Brenner tumors* → *are often small incidental findings and > 95% are benign. They have a firm, white to yellow cut surface. They may be seen in association with other tumors, most commonly mucinous tumors, as seen in this example.* **(Right)** *Brenner tumors are composed of a biphasic population of transitional epithelium* → *and cellular stroma* → *. Small, centrally located cysts may contain an eosinophilic substance. The epithelial nests may include mucinous, ciliated, or squamous cells.*

Brenner Tumor: Gross Appearance

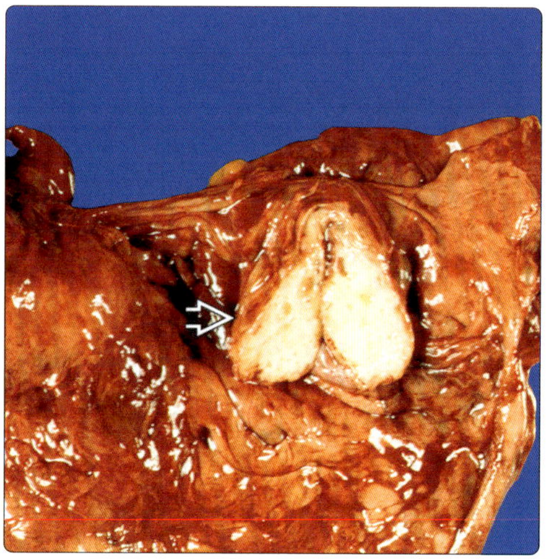

Brenner Tumor

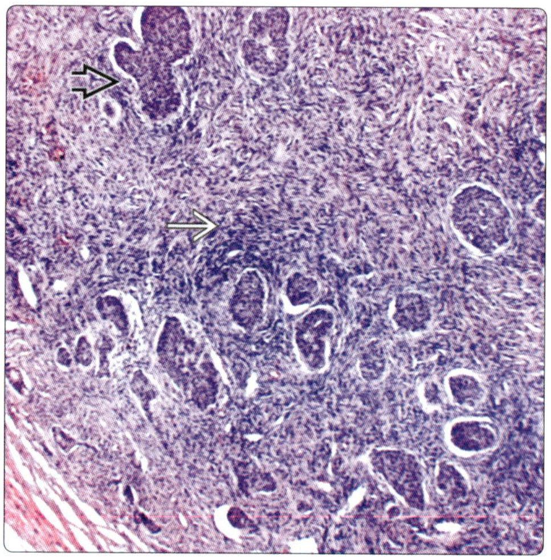

(Left) *Fibromas are typically small (≤ 5 cm) and firm. They have a white cut surface with occasional calcification, cyst formation, or edema. More cellular lesions tend to be softer during sectioning. Fibrosarcomas are very rare.* **(Right)** *Fibromas may display sparse to highly cellular morphologies. The tumors are composed of bland, spindled cells* → *arranged in fascicles. Mitotic figures are uncommon; however, cellular variants may have upwards of 4 mitoses per 10 HPF.*

Fibroma: Gross Appearance

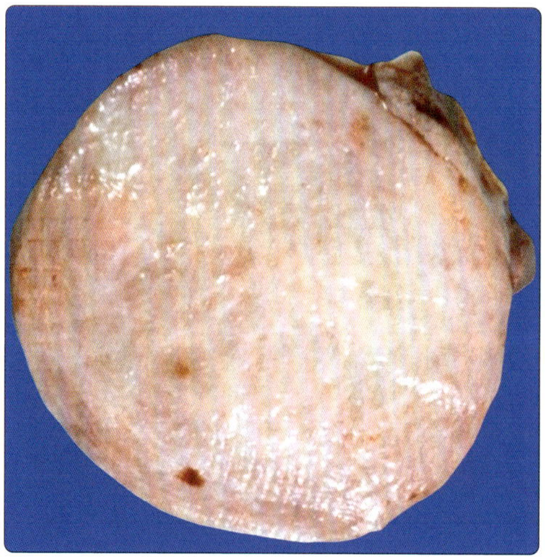

Fibroma

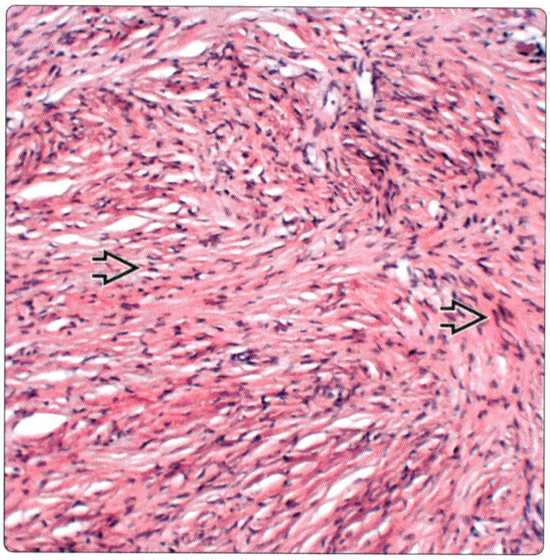

Steroid Cell Tumor: Gross Appearance

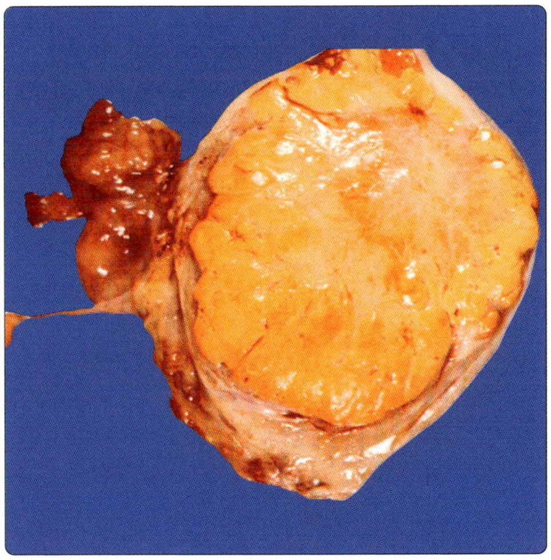

Steroid Cell Tumor

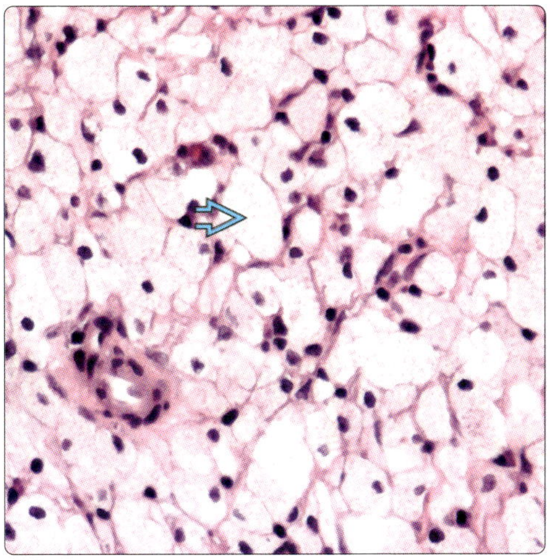

(Left) *Steroid cell tumors are uncommon but easily recognized due to their bright yellow color. They may be classified as luteomas or Leydig cell tumors, but the most common type does not have specific features ("not otherwise specified").* **(Right)** *The cells that compose steroid cell tumors are often pale to eosinophilic and have abundant, lipid-rich cytoplasm, imparting their yellow color. The cells usually form sheets, but nests and cords of cells may be present as well. Necrosis may be seen in malignant tumors.*

Dysgerminoma: Gross Appearance

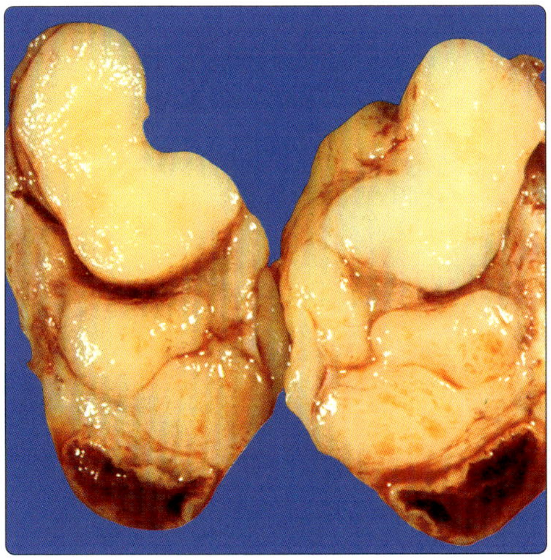

Dysgerminoma

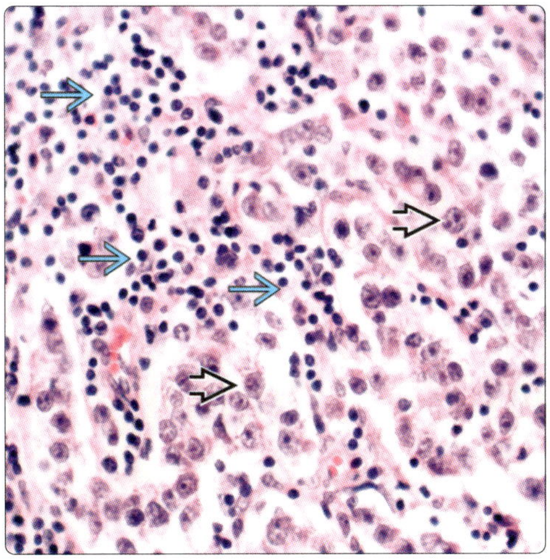

(Left) *Dysgerminomas tend to be large, averaging > 15 cm. They have a cerebriform cut surface with a white to creamy yellow fleshy texture. Areas of cystic degeneration or hemorrhage may be present.* **(Right)** *Cells comprising a dysgerminoma are large, primitive cells with prominent nucleoli. These cells may be arranged in sheets, cords, nests, or tubules. Scattered lymphocytes are typically present. Occasionally, giant cells, granulomas, or syncytiotrophoblasts may be identified.*

Embryonal Carcinoma: Gross Appearance

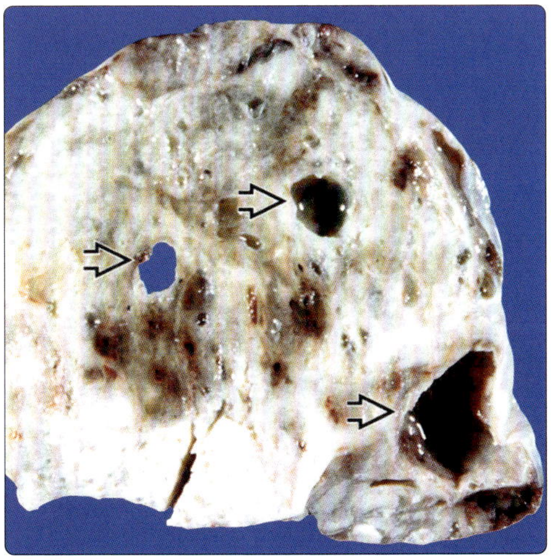

Embryonal Carcinoma

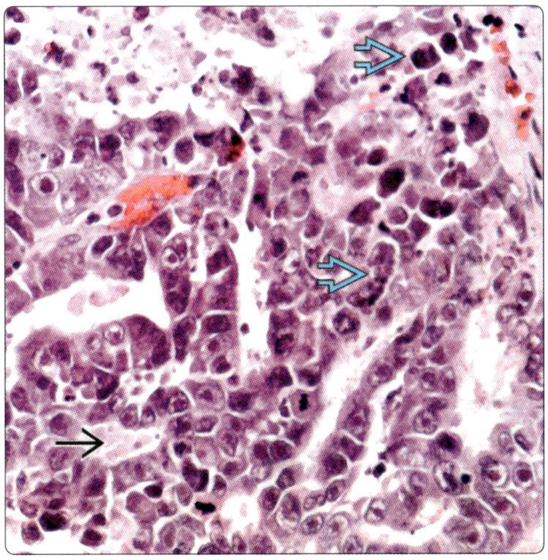

(Left) *Embryonal carcinoma presents as large (usually > 15 cm) masses with white to gray to yellow cut surfaces with scattered cysts. Hemorrhage and necrosis are common. The cysts are often filled with thick, mucoid fluid.* **(Right)** *Embryonal carcinomas consist of large primitive cells with pleomorphic nuclei. The cells are arranged in sheets or poorly formed "glands." Necrosis is usually present. Syncytiotrophoblasts are typically present and hyaline bodies may be identified.*

SURGICAL/CLINICAL CONSIDERATIONS

Goal of Consultation

- Determine if pancreatic mass is due to pancreatic duct adenocarcinoma or benign inflammatory process

Change in Patient Management

- Resection with curative intent performed for neoplastic lesions

Clinical Setting

- Scarring from chronic pancreatitis can be difficult to distinguish from pancreatic carcinoma on imaging studies
- Sclerosis in autoimmune pancreatitis often extends beyond pancreas and mimics pancreatic cancer
- Tissue cores obtained are usually small in length or very thin in order to minimize morbidity
- Biopsies are difficult to obtain percutaneously

SPECIMEN EVALUATION

Frozen Section

- Entire specimen is frozen

MOST COMMON DIAGNOSES

Pancreatic Adenocarcinoma

- Definitive diagnosis of pancreatic adenocarcinoma will usually depend on
  - Architectural &/or cytologic features of proliferating ducts that are compatible with carcinoma
  - Glandular structures next to thick-walled blood vessels or surrounded by desmoplastic stroma
  - Evidence of perineural or lymph-vascular invasion
    - Of these, perineural invasion is most easily assessed in pancreatic biopsies
- Approach to pancreatic cancer diagnosis in biopsies is best considered under 2 distinct scenarios
  - **Poorly differentiated (high-grade) cytomorphology**
    - Glands show marked nuclear enlargement and hyperchromasia
      - Nuclei vary in size and may have irregular contours
      - Enlarged nucleoli may be present
    - Typical and atypical mitoses are often present
    - Only differential diagnosis in this setting is pancreatic intraepithelial neoplasm (high grade) (PanIN-3)
      - Ducts with PanIN-3 retain more compact stroma around them compared to loose desmoplastic stroma around invasive adenocarcinoma
      - Prominent clear cell change is more common in carcinomas and makes PanIN-3 less likely
  - **Well-differentiated (low-grade) cytomorphology**
    - Differential diagnosis is with reactive/inflammatory process
    - Architectural criteria for malignancy and desmoplastic stromal response are helpful findings
    - Loss of lobular configuration of proliferating ducts, small angular duct profiles, and fused glands favor cancer
    - Proximity of ducts to medium-sized arterioles or large vessels also favors cancer

Chronic Pancreatitis

- Diagnosis is now used more as morphologic descriptor rather than specific disease entity
  - Broad umbrella term "chronic pancreatitis" includes cases with alcoholic, hereditary, autoimmune, and obstructive pancreatitis
- Specific features of these disease categories lends more certainty of benign diagnosis when ruling out diagnosis of pancreatic carcinoma
  - Alcoholic pancreatitis
    - Ectatic ducts with secretions
    - Pseudocysts often present on imaging or macroscopic examination
  - Autoimmune pancreatitis
    - Periductal lymphoplasmacytic infiltrate
    - Storiform fibrosis
    - Obliterative phlebitis
- Lobular architecture is usually preserved
  - In some cases, fibrotic stroma can distort lobules and mimic desmoplastic stroma

Chronic Pancreatitis

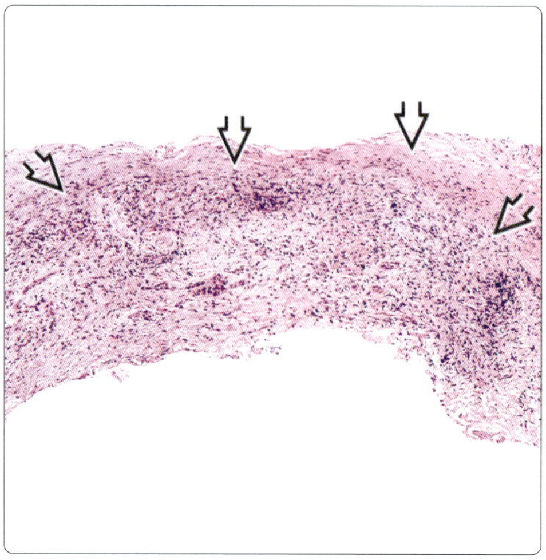

Pancreatic Carcinoma

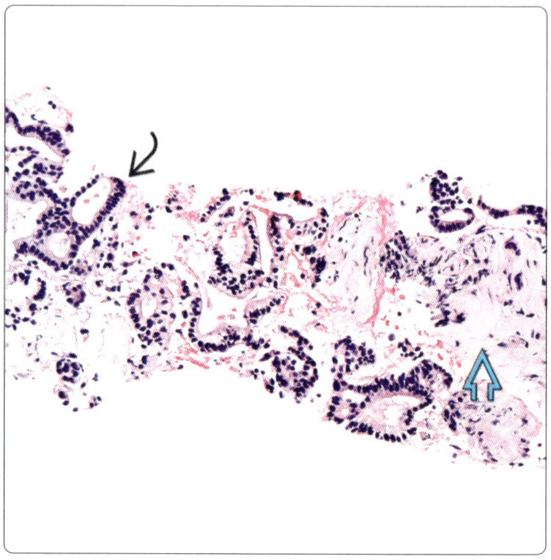

(Left) *In severe acinar atrophy in chronic pancreatitis, only residual small ductules may be present. However, the normal lobular configuration can still be discerned ⇨ and supports that this is a benign process.* **(Right)** *In contrast to chronic pancreatitis, pancreatic duct carcinoma shows a haphazard proliferation of small, angulated duct profiles that may be fused together ⇨ and are surrounded by abundant desmoplastic stroma ⇨.*

Features Distinguishing Pancreatic Carcinoma From Chronic Pancreatitis

Feature	Pancreatic Carcinoma	Chronic Pancreatitis
Architecture		
Lobular configuration	Lost	Preserved
Ducts in proximity to arterioles/large vessels	Present	Absent (except in postneoadjuvant treatment)
Duct contours	Irregular, angulated, confluent	Smooth, undulating, dilated, with secretions
Single cell infiltration	Present	Absent
Stroma	Abundant desmoplastic stroma	Hyalinized stroma, calcification
Cytologic Changes		
Nuclear atypia	Variable (may be subtle)	Typically mild
Cytoplasm	Variable, but clear cell cytoplasmic change is common	Typically mucinous
Evidence of Invasion		
Perineural	May be present	May abut, but not encircle, nerves
Vascular	May be present	Absent
Duodenal wall	May be present	Absent

  - Residual islets in fibrotic stroma can mimic solid nests of tumor cells

REPORTING

Frozen Section

- Definitive diagnosis of malignancy should be made when possible
- When definitive features of malignancy are not seen, it may be appropriate to defer diagnosis to permanent sections
  - Additional biopsies for frozen section may be helpful when there is high clinical suspicion of malignancy

Reliability

- False-positive diagnoses are rare
  - Most pathologists prefer undercalling lesion to prevent unnecessary surgery
- False-negative diagnoses are more common (2-30%)
  - Due to both sampling errors and errors in interpretation

PITFALLS

Failure to Diagnose Carcinoma

- Foci of perineural or lymph-vascular invasion overlooked
- Well-differentiated adenocarcinoma misinterpreted as benign glandular epithelium
- Relying on any single feature instead of constellation of features to make definitive diagnosis of cancer

Paraduodenal or Groove Pancreatitis vs. Carcinoma

- Inflammation is typically around accessory pancreatic duct with inflammation in wall of duodenum
- Ectatic ducts with inspissated secretions and prominent smooth muscular proliferation mimicking mesenchymal neoplasm may be present

Perineural Invasion vs. Benign Glands Next to Nerves

- Typically occurs in setting of marked acinar atrophy in severe chronic pancreatitis when benign ducts may be juxtaposed adjacent to nerves
  - This phenomenon is extremely rare, and diagnosis of pseudoperineural invasion must be made with extreme caution
- Atypical glands encircling nerves are only seen in cases of carcinoma

Islet Cells vs. Carcinoma

- Islet cell proliferation in chronic pancreatitis may appear as solid foci in small biopsy and misinterpreted as carcinoma
- Pancreatic adenocarcinoma often does not destroy islets as it invades through parenchyma
  - Presence of entrapped islets cannot be used to differentiate benign lesions from carcinoma

Autoimmune Pancreatitis vs. Carcinoma

- Prominent periductal lymphoplasmacytic infiltration with storiform fibrosis and obliterative phlebitis seen in autoimmune pancreatitis
- Process is often more diffuse in autoimmune pancreatitis than in pancreatic carcinoma

Alcoholic Pancreatitis vs. Carcinoma

- Alcoholic pancreatitis commonly shows ectatic ducts with inspissated secretions
- Pseudocysts are often present on imaging or macroscopic examination

SELECTED REFERENCES

1. Nelson DW et al: Examining the accuracy and clinical usefulness of intraoperative frozen section analysis in the management of pancreatic lesions. Am J Surg. 205(5):613-7; discussion 617, 2013
2. Bandyopadhyay S et al: Isolated solitary ducts (naked ducts) in adipose tissue: a specific but underappreciated finding of pancreatic adenocarcinoma and one of the potential reasons of understaging and high recurrence rate. Am J Surg Pathol. 33(3):425-9, 2009
3. Doucas H et al: Frozen section diagnosis of pancreatic malignancy: a sensitive diagnostic technique. Pancreatology. 6(3):210-3; discussion 214, 2006
4. Lechago J: Frozen section examination of liver, gallbladder, and pancreas. Arch Pathol Lab Med. 129(12):1610-8, 2005
5. Adsay NV et al: Chronic pancreatitis or pancreatic ductal adenocarcinoma? Semin Diagn Pathol. 21(4):268-76, 2004
6. Cioc AM et al: Frozen section diagnosis of pancreatic lesions. Arch Pathol Lab Med. 126(10):1169-73, 2002

(Left) *Pancreatic adenocarcinoma* ➮ *infiltrates in interlobular stroma outside the confines of the pancreatic acinar lobules* ➮. *Loss of lobular configuration is a useful feature in distinguishing well-differentiated carcinoma from a benign reactive proliferation.* **(Right)** *Malignant glands and single cells* ➮ *invade in abundant desmoplastic stroma* ➮ *in this carcinoma. The duct with pancreatic intraepithelial neoplasm (PanIN-3)* ➮ *also shows marked atypia but is rimmed by a more compact collagenous stroma* ➮.

Pancreatic Carcinoma: Loss of Normal Architecture

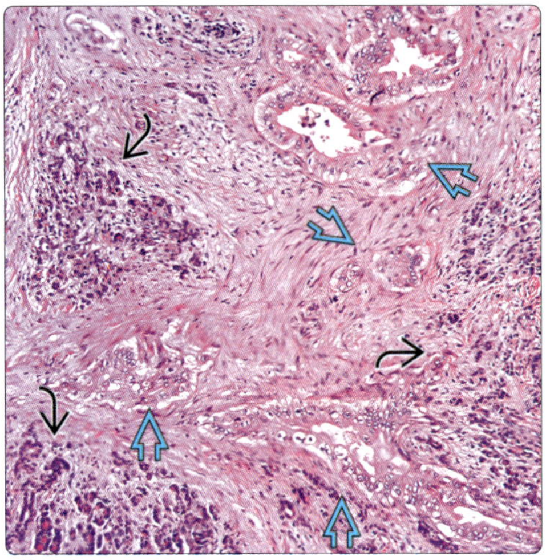

Pancreatic Carcinoma: Desmoplastic Stroma

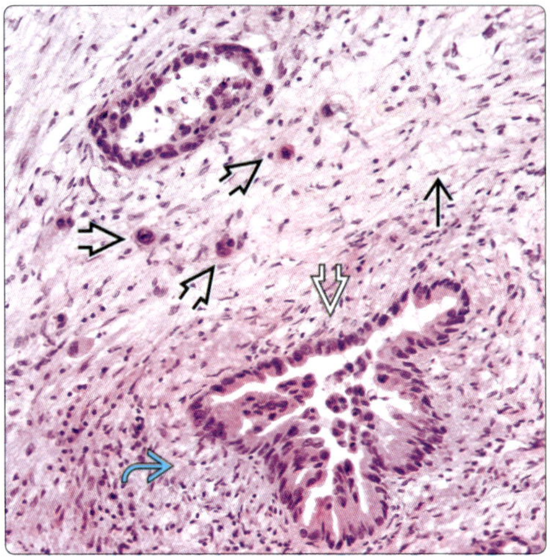

(Left) *Invasive carcinomas are characterized by irregular angulated glands formed by atypical epithelial cells. The sharp angulated edges* ➮ *of the malignant glands often give off little buds and single cells that infiltrate into the surrounding stroma* ➮. **(Right)** *Cytoplasm with prominent clear cell change is rarely seen in PanIN lesions but is common in invasive duct carcinoma.*

Pancreatic Carcinoma: Angulated Glands

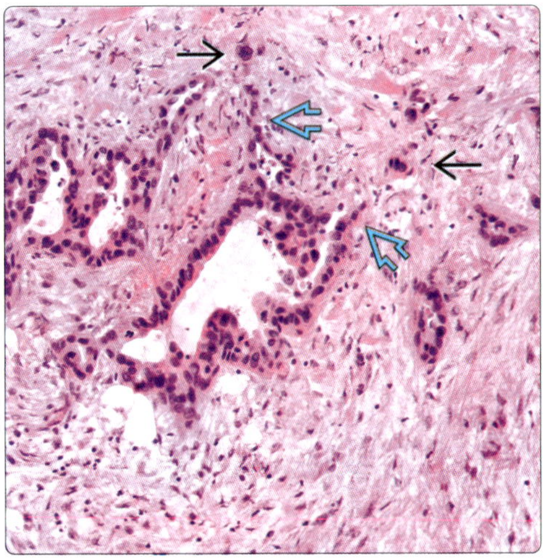

Pancreatic Carcinoma: Clear Cell Change

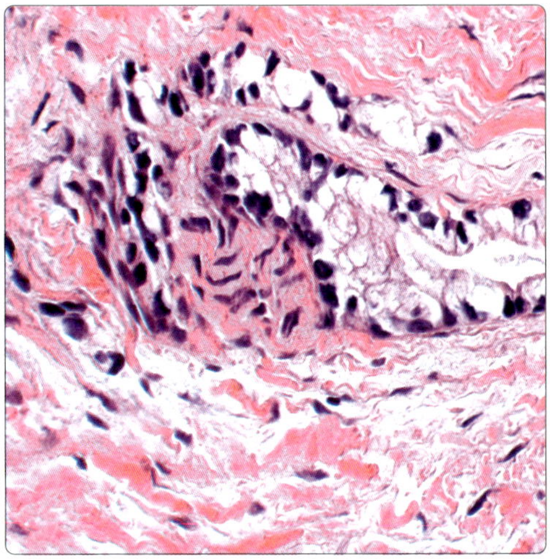

(Left) *The large duct pattern of infiltration of pancreatic carcinoma can be mistaken for an intraductal papillary mucinous neoplasm. The malignant glands* ➮ *are cystically dilated but still show markedly irregular contours and are filled with necrotic debris.* **(Right)** *Infiltration into the muscularis propria of the duodenum* ➮ *is diagnostic of adenocarcinoma, but such areas are seldom included in pancreatic mass biopsies, limiting the utility of this feature.*

Pancreatic Carcinoma: Large Duct Pattern

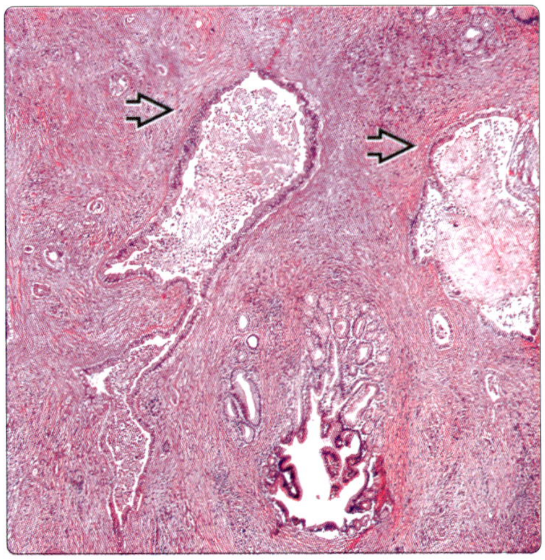

Pancreatic Carcinoma: Muscle Invasion

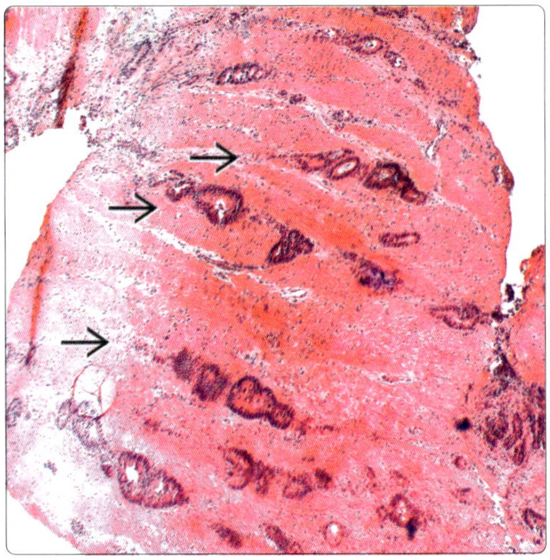

Pancreatic Carcinoma: Blood Vessels

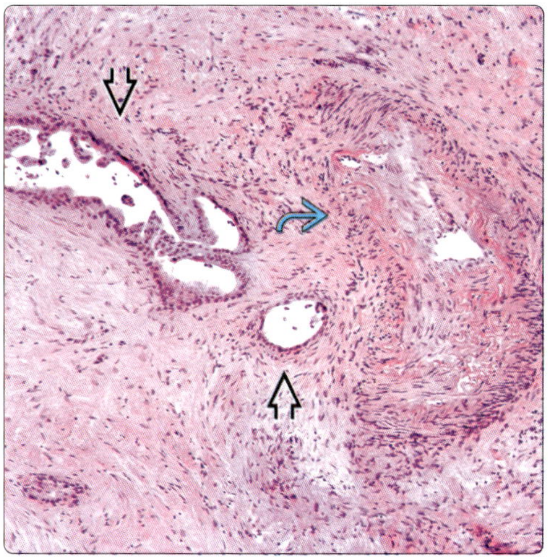

Pancreatic Carcinoma: Perineural Invasion

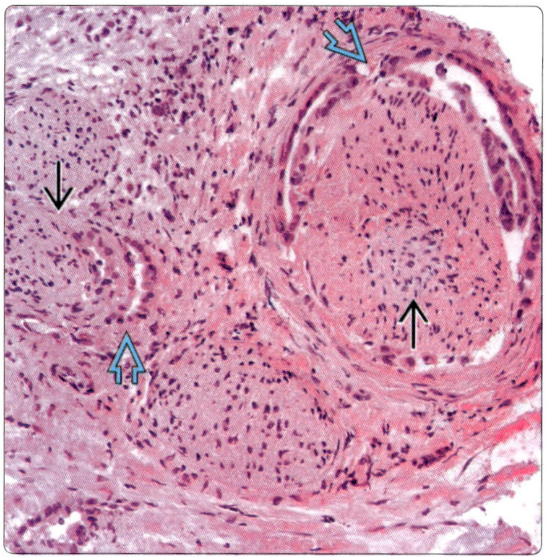

(Left) *Proliferating glands adjacent to large muscular blood vessels are a useful sign of malignancy in well-differentiated tumors. Rarely, benign ducts may also show this phenomenon but only in severe chronic pancreatitis or after neoadjuvant chemotherapy.* **(Right)** *Perineural invasion is common in pancreatic adenocarcinoma. The wrapping of malignant glands around nerves is diagnostic of malignancy. Benign glands may push against nerves but do not encircle them in this manner.*

Chronic Pancreatitis: Reactive Atypia

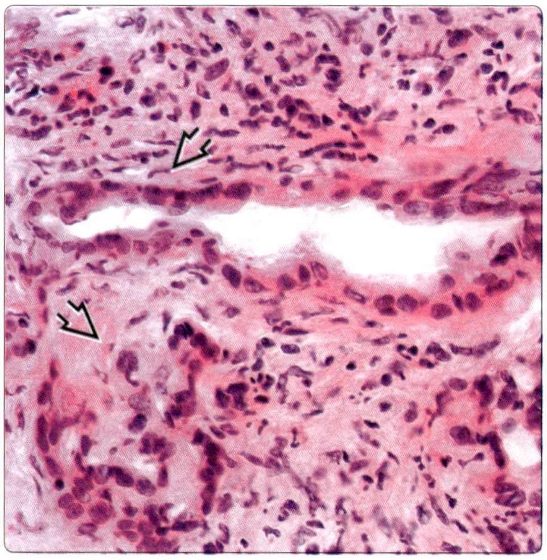

Chronic Pancreatitis: Acinar Atrophy

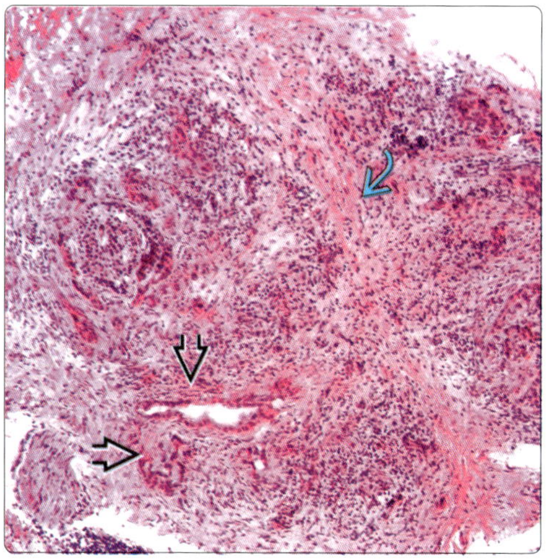

(Left) *Reactive atypia in inflamed ducts in chronic pancreatitis may be difficult to distinguish from carcinoma. The angulated duct profiles and nuclear enlargement are worrisome for malignancy. In such cases, it is useful to consider the overall architecture of the glands.* **(Right)** *The atypical ducts in the same case are confined within the lobule and are surrounded by marked acinar atrophy. The interlobular stroma is also devoid of proliferating glands, further supporting a benign diagnosis.*

Autoimmune Pancreatitis: Lymphoplasmacytic Infiltration

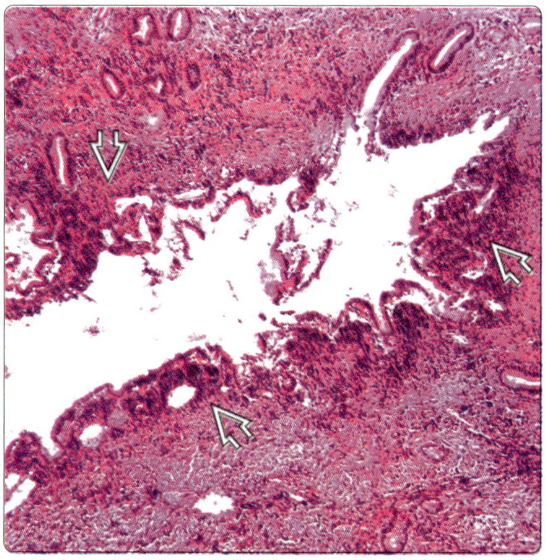

Autoimmune Pancreatitis: Obilterative Phlebitis

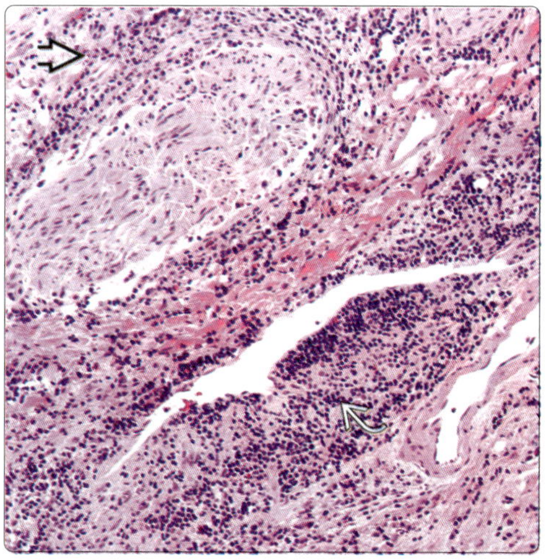

(Left) *Autoimmune pancreatitis (AIP) is a perfect mimic of pancreatic cancer on imaging and gross examination. Marked lymphoplasmacytic infiltration centered around large ducts, ± granulocytic lesions, and prominent sclerosis extending into peripancreatic soft tissue are typically seen in AIP.* **(Right)** *Obliterative phlebitis and perineural lymphoid infiltration are useful features for supporting a diagnosis of autoimmune pancreatitis.*

SURGICAL/CLINICAL CONSIDERATIONS

Goal of Consultation

- Evaluate pancreatic parenchymal and bile duct margins for tumor
- Provide/confirm diagnosis

Change in Patient Management

- Additional tissue may be taken to ensure tumor-free margins

Clinical Setting

- Pancreatic tumors can be difficult to diagnose preoperatively
  - Needle biopsies may be difficult to perform, especially for small lesions
    - A small number are associated with complications such as pancreatitis, hemorrhage, and infection
  - Endoscopic biopsies may provide diagnosis in some cases
- May not be possible to establish diagnosis for some patients prior to surgery
- Clinical information can provide most likely diagnosis prior to surgery
  - Age & gender
    - Majority (90%) of patients > 45 years of age
    - Adenocarcinomas most common from age 60-80 with slight male predominance
    - Endocrine tumors equally common in men and women from age 30-60
    - Mucinous cystic neoplasms most commonly occur in women in their 40s-50s
    - Solid pseudopapillary tumors most commonly occur in women in their 20s-30s
  - Imaging findings
    - Head of pancreas: Bile duct obstruction and jaundice may lead to early detection
    - Tail of pancreas: Fewer symptoms and thus may present at more advanced stage
    - Mucinous cystic neoplasms occur most commonly in tail
    - Connection to duct system typical for intraductal papillary mucinous neoplasms (IPMN)
- Complete (Whipple procedure) or distal pancreatectomy may be performed for potential cure or palliation
  - Biopsies will be taken of lymph nodes, liver, or other possible sites of metastases
    - If metastatic carcinoma found, surgery for cure no longer possible
    - Patients with other types of metastatic pancreatic tumors may benefit from resection

SPECIMEN EVALUATION

Gross

- Identify all structures present (not all will be present in all resections)
  - Distal stomach (missing in pylorus preserving pancreatico-duodenectomies)
    - Usually far from carcinoma and not evaluated by frozen section
  - Proximal duodenum
    - Distal margin of duodenum usually far from carcinoma and not evaluated by frozen section
  - Pancreas (head, tail, or complete pancreatectomy)
  - Spleen
    - Involvement by carcinoma would be exceedingly unusual; not generally evaluated by frozen section
  - Great vessels: Superior mesenteric artery (SMA)
    - Not resected; soft tissue around SMA may be sent to document cancer
- Examine outer aspects to identify any areas of likely tumor involvement
- Open stomach along greater curvature and duodenal wall opposite pancreatic head
- If partial pancreatectomy has been performed, identify pancreatic parenchymal margin and pancreatic duct
  - Ink margin a specific designated color to distinguish it from other margins
  - Take en face section for margin evaluation
- Identify common bile duct margin as it exits pancreas and passes behind proximal duodenum

Whipple Procedure

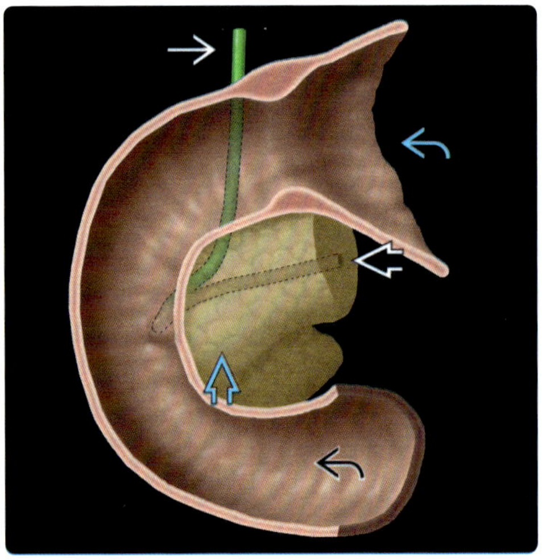

Distal Pancreatectomy

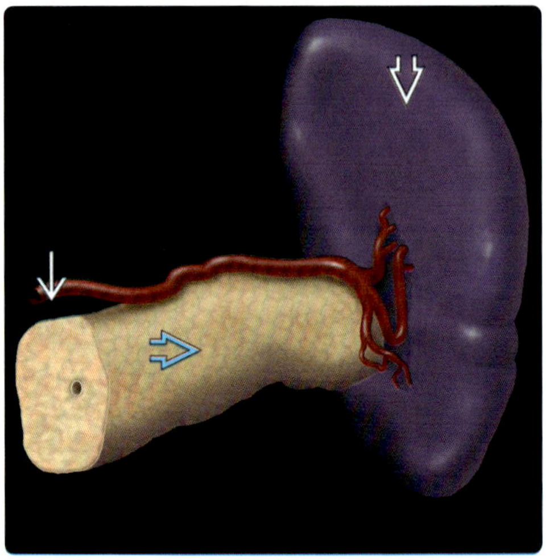

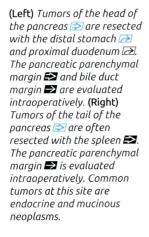

(Left) *Tumors of the head of the pancreas* ➡ *are resected with the distal stomach* ➡ *and proximal duodenum* ➡*. The pancreatic parenchymal margin* ➡ *and bile duct margin* ➡ *are evaluated intraoperatively.* **(Right)** *Tumors of the tail of the pancreas* ➡ *are often resected with the spleen* ➡*. The pancreatic parenchymal margin* ➡ *is evaluated intraoperatively. Common tumors at this site are endocrine and mucinous neoplasms.*

  - Ink proximal common bile duct margin
  - Take en face section for margin evaluation
- Identify uncinate process (posterior) margin
  - This is a nonperitonealized portion of pancreas lying directly on superior mesenteric vessels for 3-4 cm
  - Surgeon must separate pancreas from blood vessels and surrounding autonomic nerve plexus
  - This is an important margin and should be inked a specific color for evaluation on permanent sections
  - The margin is not typically evaluated by frozen section because it is fatty and 1 section is not likely to give an accurate evaluation of margin status
- **Partial pancreatectomy (head of pancreas)**
  - Probes are placed within major ducts
  - Probe in common bile duct should exit through ampulla of Vater in duodenum
  - Probe in main pancreatic duct advanced as far as possible
    - Duct may be obstructed by carcinoma
- Pancreatic head sectioned along plane of both probes
  - Area of duct obstruction may be identified
    - Carcinomas firm and white and efface normal parenchyma
    - Intraductal papillary mucinous neoplasm (IPMN) is mucinous and papillary in appearance and fills main duct and side branch ducts
- **Distal pancreatectomy**
  - Parenchymal margin taken as en face section
  - Pancreas serially sectioned perpendicular to long axis
  - Size, color, borders, and relationship to margins of lesions recorded
- **Separate en face parenchymal margin submitted by surgeon**
  - Recommended that margin be taken from specimen by pathologist
  - If submitted separately, pathologist cannot evaluate distance of gross lesion involving main duct from margin

Frozen Section

- **Pancreatic parenchymal margin**
  - True margin embedded face up
    - 1st section is true margin
  - If too large for single frozen section, divide tissue into 2 frozen sections
    - Entire duct profile should be within one tissue block
- **Bile duct margin**
  - True margin embedded face up
    - 1st section is true margin
- **Uncinate margin**
  - Not usually examined by frozen section
  - If examination requested, take as perpendicular section with ink indicating margin

MOST COMMON DIAGNOSES

Adenocarcinoma

- Most common pancreatic tumor (> 90% of total)
- Carcinomas eligible for resection usually in head of pancreas
- Often associated with secondary acinar atrophy and fibrosis
  - Gland may be fibrotic due to scarring
  - Carcinomas may not be apparent as discrete mass in all cases
- Carcinomas best identified by sectioning along main ducts
  - Area of duct obstruction may be seen as narrowing of lumen
    - Duct distal to obstruction may be dilated
- Carcinomas efface normal architecture
  - Often small and diffusely infiltrative
  - Consist of small tubules or nests of cells
  - Cytologic atypia may be minimal

Endocrine Tumors

- 2nd most common pancreatic tumor (3-5% of total)
  - ~ 10% occur in patients with germline mutation
  - Patients with multiple endocrine neoplasia type 1 (MEN1) develop multiple nonfunctioning endocrine microadenomas (< 0.5 cm)
    - 20-70% develop functional tumor
- Usually arise in tail of pancreas
- Well-circumscribed, encapsulated, fleshy yellow to red masses
  - Necrosis, cysts, and hemorrhage may be present
- Uniform cells in nests, sheets, or trabeculae
  - Monomorphic nuclei with dispersed (salt and pepper) chromatin
  - Rare or absent mitoses
  - Small nucleoli
  - Scant granular cytoplasm

Solid Pseudopapillary Neoplasm

- Most common in young women (20s-30s)
- May involve any part of pancreas
- Well-circumscribed unilocular or multilocular cystic tumor
  - Central necrosis common
- Pseudopapillae form around blood vessels
  - Nuclei uniform and grooved
  - Cells dyscohesive
  - Cytoplasmic eosinophilic hyaline globules may be present

Mucinous Cystic Neoplasm

- Most common in women (40s-50s)
  - ~ 1/3 malignant, usually in older individuals
- Mucinous cystadenoma and cystadenocarcinoma most common in tail of pancreas
- Grow as thin-walled cystic tumors containing mucin
  - Tumors with solid areas or papillary excrescences in cyst wall more likely to be carcinomas
  - Do not communicate with duct system
- Cysts lined by tall columnar mucin-producing epithelium
- Ovarian-type stroma lining cyst wall diagnostic feature distinguishing from IPMN

Serous Cystic Neoplasm

- More common in women
  - Usually benign
- Occurs at any site in pancreas
- Grows as circumscribed area of small, thin-walled cysts
  - Central stellate scar may be present
  - Calcifications may be present
- Cysts lined by low cuboidal cells with uniform nuclei

Intraductal Papillary Mucinous Neoplasm

- Macroscopic lesions that grow within duct system of pancreas
  - Defined as ≥ 1 cm in size
    - Often extend microscopically beyond grossly evident mass
  - Multifocal in 40% of cases
  - Subset associated with invasive carcinoma
- Usually involve main pancreatic duct
  - Majority are in head of pancreas
  - Can involve entire length of duct as well as common bile duct and ampulla of Vater
  - Associated pancreas with chronic obstructive pancreatitis
- IPMN in branch duct usually forms cystic mass in uncinate process
  - Mucinous cysts ranges 1-10 cm
  - Cyst walls thin and have flat or papillary lining
  - Adjacent pancreas normal
  - Lower risk of high-grade dysplasia and invasive carcinoma compared to tumors involving main duct
- Histologic types
  - **Gastric type**
    - Usually involves branch ducts
    - Tall columnar cells with basal nuclei and abundant pale mucinous cytoplasm
      - Resembles gastric foveolar epithelium
    - Low- or intermediate-grade dysplasia most common
  - **Intestinal type**
    - Usually involves main duct
    - Papillae lined by tall columnar cells with basophilic cytoplasm and apical mucin
      - Resembles colonic villous adenoma
    - May be associated with invasive colloid (mucinous) carcinoma (large extracellular mucin pools containing tumor cells)
    - Intermediate- to high-grade dysplasia most common
  - **Pancreaticobiliary type**
    - Usually involve main duct
    - Thin, branching papillae lined by cells resembling native pancreaticobiliary epithelium
  - **Oncocytic type**
    - Form large (5-6 cm), tan, nodular papillary tumors in large pancreatic ducts
    - Complex branching papillae and solid nests with lumen
    - Enlarged round nuclei with prominent nucleoli and abundant eosinophilic granular cytoplasm
    - High-grade dysplasia most common
- Not associated with ovarian-type stroma
  - This type of stroma characteristic of mucinous cystic neoplasms

Pancreatic Intraepithelial Neoplasia

- Not detected clinically and not seen on gross examination
  - Majority < 0.5 cm
- Short papillae
  - Architecture becomes complex in PanIN-3 (severe dysplasia)
- Cuboidal to columnar cells with varying amounts of mucin
- Divided into grades according to cytologic and architectural atypia
  - PanIN-1: Mild dysplasia
  - PanIN-2: Moderate dysplasia
  - PanIN-3: Severe dysplasia
    - Papillary or micropapillary architecture
    - Cribriform growth with appearance of small clusters of epithelial cells budding off into lumen
    - Marked nuclear abnormalities including loss of polarity, nuclear crowding, enlarged and irregular nucleoli, hyperchromasia, enlarged nuclei, and dystrophic goblet cells

Acinar Cell Carcinoma

- Occurs at any site in pancreas
- Multiple soft, well-circumscribed, red to brown nodules separated by fibrous septa
  - May be cystic
- Solid or cribriform patterns
- Granular cytoplasm
- Basally located nuclei
  - Uniform with minimal pleomorphism and single prominent nucleolus
- ~ 15% associated with metastatic fat necrosis due to increased serum lipase

Pancreatoblastoma

- Most common pancreatic tumor of childhood (mean age: 10 years)
- Occurs at any site in pancreas
- Large, soft, encapsulated mass
- Consists of acinar cells and squamous nests
  - Mesenchymal, ductal, and endocrine areas can also be present

Chronic Pancreatitis and Pseudocysts

- Normal pancreas is replaced by very hard fibrotic scar tissue
  - Fat necrosis often present
- Calculi may be present in pancreatic duct
- Pseudocysts may form in peripancreatic soft tissue
  - Form when tissues digested by pancreatic enzymes
  - May be filled with blood and necrotic material
- Small, irregular ducts in fibrotic stroma maintain their lumina
  - Nuclei may be enlarged but are uniform in size
  - Mitoses rare or absent
  - Vascular and perineural invasion not present
- Lymphocytic sclerosing pancreatitis can result in mass or diffuse enlargement of head of pancreas
  - Fibrosis and inflammation can involve adjacent tissue
  - Dense lymphoplasmacytic infiltrate present
  - Can be very difficult to distinguish from carcinoma clinically, grossly, and on frozen section

REPORTING

Gross

- Grossly evident tumors, chiefly IPMN, present at margin should be reported
  - Resection would be considered, regardless of grade of dysplasia

Intraductal Papillary Mucinous Neoplasm: Grade

Dysplasia	Architecture	Nuclei	Cytoplasm
Low grade (mild dysplasia)	Mild intraluminal papillary proliferation	Small, basal, ovoid	Gastric phenotype
Intermediate grade (moderate dysplasia)	Florid intraluminal papillary proliferation	Pencillate, hyperchromatic, stratified	Intestinal (goblet cell) phenotype
High grade (severe dysplasia)	Florid intraluminal papillary proliferation, with solid/cribriform areas	Marked pleomorphism, prominent nucleoli	HIgh nuclear:cytoplasmic ratio, no specific line of differentiation

Frozen Section

- **Diagnosis**
  - Definitive diagnosis of carcinoma should be made, when possible
    - If definite features not seen, diagnosis of "atypical glands" may be more appropriate
  - In absence of definite carcinoma, other tumors can be given provisional diagnosis
    - Type of tumor generally does not alter surgical approach
- **Pancreatic parenchymal margin**
  - Invasive carcinoma should be reported if present at margin
  - If margin shows normal pancreatic tissue
    - "Normal parenchyma; negative for PanIN and carcinoma"
  - If low- or moderate-grade lesion present in duct at margin
    - "Negative for carcinoma; focal PanIN1-2 present, involving main/side branch pancreatic ducts"
  - If high-grade lesion present in duct at margin
    - "Negative for carcinoma; PanIN-3 present, involving main/side branch pancreatic ducts"
  - If no epithelium present in main duct at margin
    - "Denuded main duct epithelium, unable to evaluate PanIN"
- **Bile duct margin**
  - Positive or negative for invasive carcinoma

Reliability

- False-positive diagnoses of primary lesions rare, as pathologists tend to be very conservative in making diagnosis of carcinoma with very poor prognosis
- However, false-negative diagnoses more common with negative predictive value of ~ 50%
- Accuracy for evaluation of margins much higher (> 95%)

PITFALLS

Chronic Pancreatitis vs. Carcinoma

- Pancreatic carcinoma is a difficult diagnosis to make on frozen section
- Both pancreatitis and carcinoma can consist of small tubules in fibrotic stroma
- Features favoring malignancy
  - Disorganized distribution of ducts
  - Ducts present in interlobular stroma or adjacent to thick-walled arteries/veins
  - Ducts in peripancreatic soft tissue
  - Perineural invasion

Bile Duct Accessory Glands vs. Carcinoma

- Bile duct has numerous peribiliary glands
  - May be difficult to distinguish from well-differentiated adenocarcinomas
  - Clustered in lobular pattern in wall of duct
  - Nuclear pleomorphism and mitoses should not be present
  - Should not be located near large blood vessels

Reactive Changes in Bile Duct

- Stent may be placed in bile duct in patients with obstruction
  - Inflammation can cause reactive changes
- Resulting changes may be difficult to distinguish from neoplasia
  - Papillary architecture
  - Cytologic atypia (enlarged nuclei with nucleoli)
  - Pyloric gland metaplasia
  - Ulceration

Invasive Carcinoma in Bile Duct

- Usually present in deeper tissue, located away from duct lumen
- Entire wall must be examined for carcinoma
- Nerves should be carefully examined for perineural invasion

Crushing and Cautery Artifact

- Distortion of tissue at margin may preclude definitive diagnosis
  - Deeper sections may show better preservation of tissue
- Gross distance of tumor from margin can be helpful to determine likelihood of probable involvement
- Additional tissue can be requested from surgeon

SELECTED REFERENCES

1. Barreto SG et al: Does revision of resection margins based on frozen section improve overall survival following pancreatoduodenectomy for pancreatic ductal adenocarcinoma? A meta-analysis. HPB (Oxford). 19(7):573-579, 2017
2. Maksymov V et al: An anatomical-based mapping analysis of the pancreaticoduodenectomy retroperitoneal margin highlights the urgent need for standardized assessment. HPB (Oxford). 15(3):218-23, 2013
3. Nelson DW et al: Examining the accuracy and clinical usefulness of intraoperative frozen section analysis in the management of pancreatic lesions. Am J Surg. 205(5):613-7; discussion 617, 2013
4. Verbeke CS: Resection margins in pancreatic cancer. Surg Clin North Am. 93(3):647-62, 2013
5. Tanaka M et al: International consensus guidelines 2012 for the management of IPMN and MCN of the pancreas. Pancreatology. 12(3):183-97, 2012
6. Verbeke CS et al: Resection margin involvement and tumour origin in pancreatic head cancer. Br J Surg. 99(8):1036-49, 2012
7. Sauvanet A et al: Role of frozen section assessment for intraductal papillary and mucinous tumor of the pancreas. World J Gastrointest Surg. 2(10):352-8, 2010

(Left) *The pancreatic neck margin contains the opening of the main pancreatic duct. The smooth, indented surface behind it is the vascular groove, and the ragged soft tissue with sutures is the posterior soft tissue (uncinate) margin.* **(Right)** *The pancreatic neck margin sections must include the main pancreatic duct in order to evaluate involvement by PanIN or IPMN. Much of the lining epithelium in this duct is flat and monolayered, but a discrete focus of PanIN-3 involving the duct is present.*

Whipple Procedure: Margins

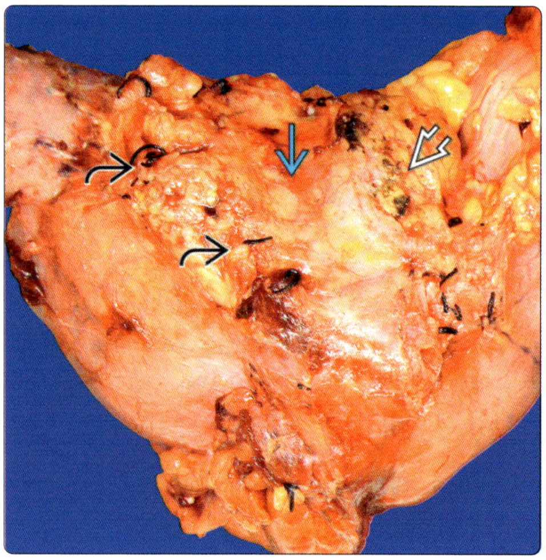

Pancreatic Neck Margin

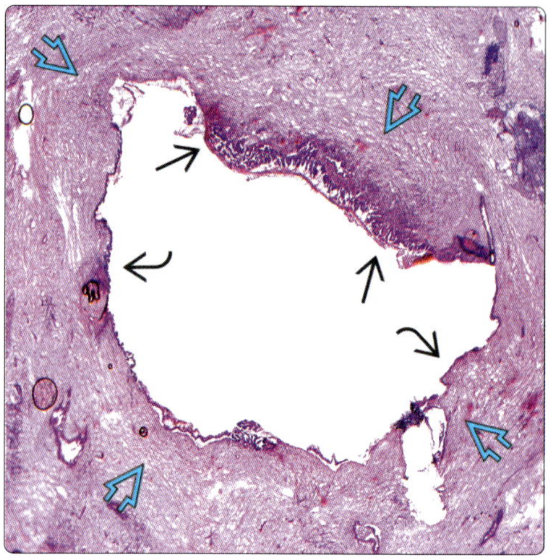

(Left) *The luminal lining epithelium of the pancreatic duct shows a papillary proliferation lined by cells with a high nuclear:cytoplasmic ratio and hyperchromatic nuclei. Despite the presence of inflammation, the degree of atypia is beyond what one would expect in reactive change.* **(Right)** *This pancreatic duct margin shows papillae lined by cells with a high nuclear:cytoplasmic ratio and markedly hyperchromatic nuclei diagnostic of PanIN-3. This finding at the margin may not lead to additional surgery.*

Pancreatic Duct Margin: PanIN-3

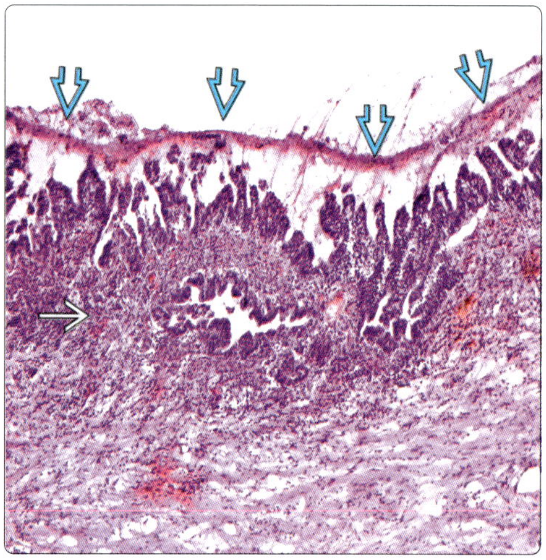

Pancreatic Duct Margin: PanIN-3

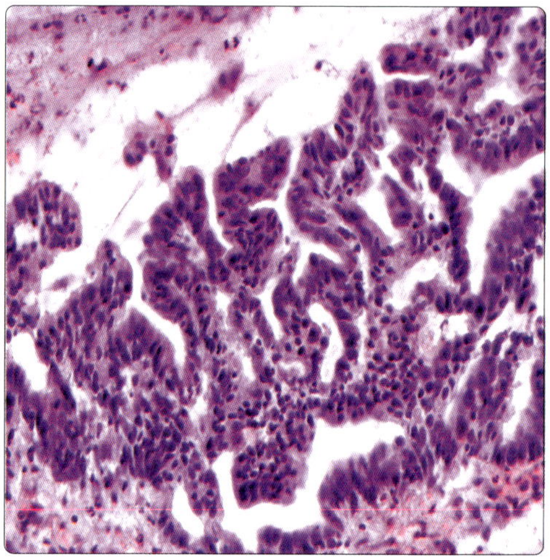

(Left) *Reactive epithelial change can be difficult to separate from neoplastic ducts in frozen sections of the pancreatic duct. The presence of acute inflammation and nuclei with open chromatin favor reactive change. The low-power appearance is helpful in making this distinction.* **(Right)** *The main pancreatic duct is present in atrophic and inflamed parenchyma. In this setting, a small atypical duct in close proximity to the parent duct is unlikely to be neoplastic.*

Pancreatic Duct Margin: Reactive Atypia

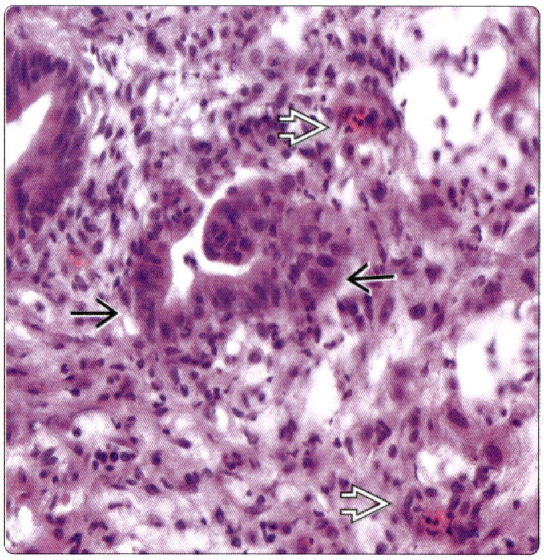

Pancreatic Duct Margin: Reactive Atypia

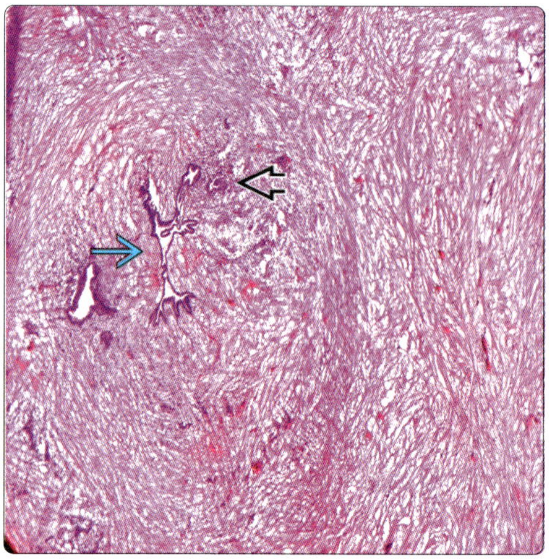

Chronic Pancreatitis

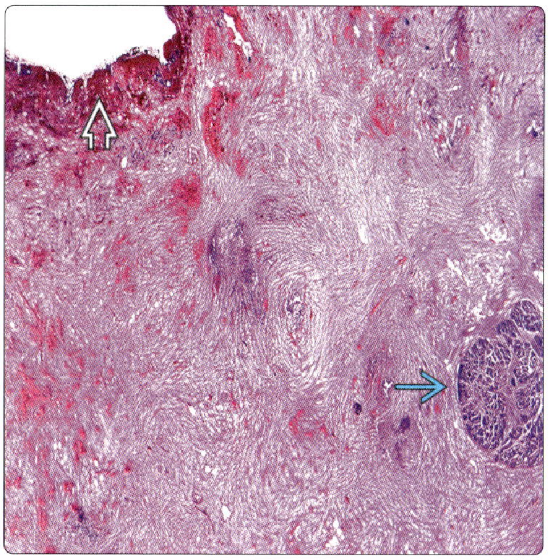

Chronic Pancreatitis

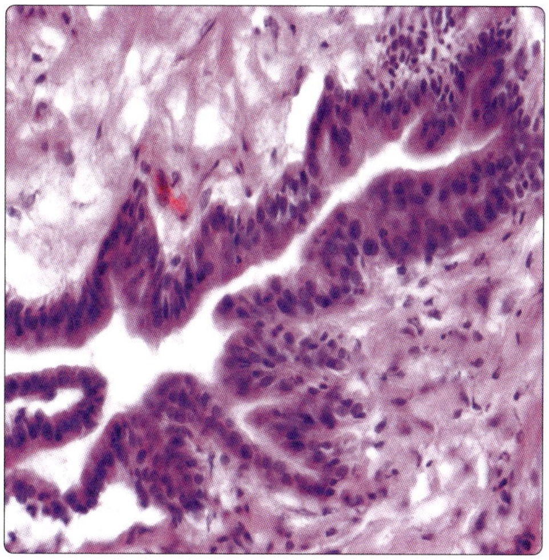

(Left) *Chronic pancreatitis can present as a mass-forming lesion mimicking pancreatic cancer. Marked atrophy and fibrosis is usually present in these cases. The main duct* ➡ *and residual pancreatic acinar parenchyma* → *will be present in the areas of fibrosis.* **(Right)** *Reactive changes in chronic pancreatitis can mimic neoplasia. Although the nuclei show some stratification, there is lack of papillary formations, and the nuclei show open chromatin with small nucleoli consistent with reactive atypia.*

Pancreatic Carcinoma After Neoadjuvant Chemotherapy: Gross Appearance

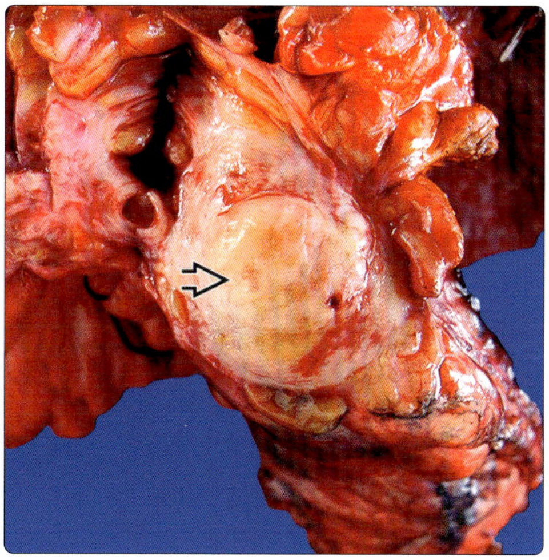

Post Neoadjuvant Pancreatic Carcinoma

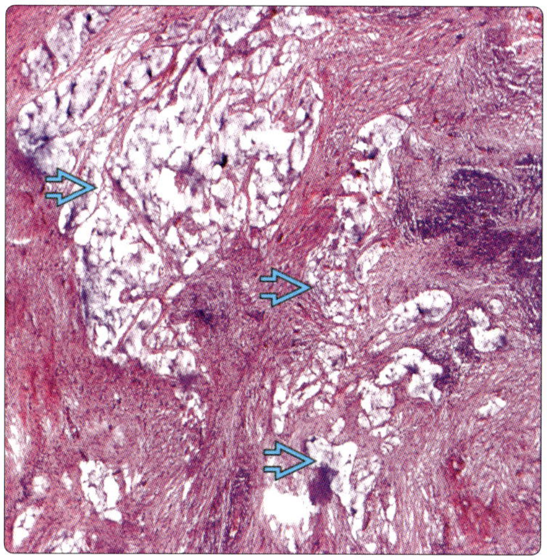

(Left) *Pancreatic carcinomas* ⇨ *may be difficult to recognize grossly after neoadjuvant therapy due to the surrounding pancreatitis with fibrosis and effacement of the normal glandular architecture.* **(Right)** *Carcinomas can be paucicellular and difficult to detect after treatment. In this case, mucin pools* ⇨ *without residual viable tumor cells are present in this pancreatic cancer resection after neoadjuvant chemotherapy.*

Intraductal Papillary Mucinous Neoplasm: Gross Appearance

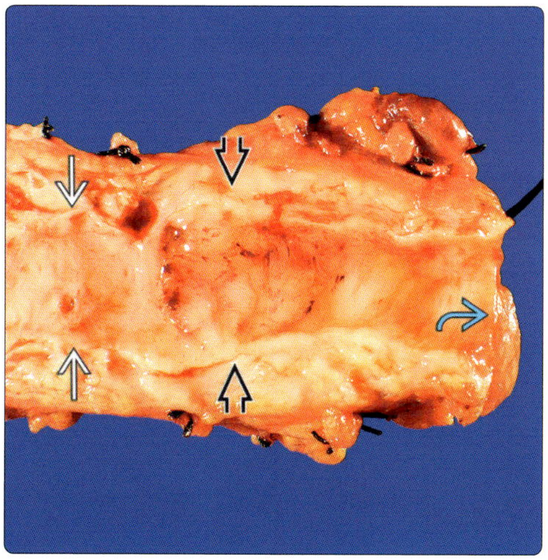

Intraductal Papillary Mucinous Neoplasm

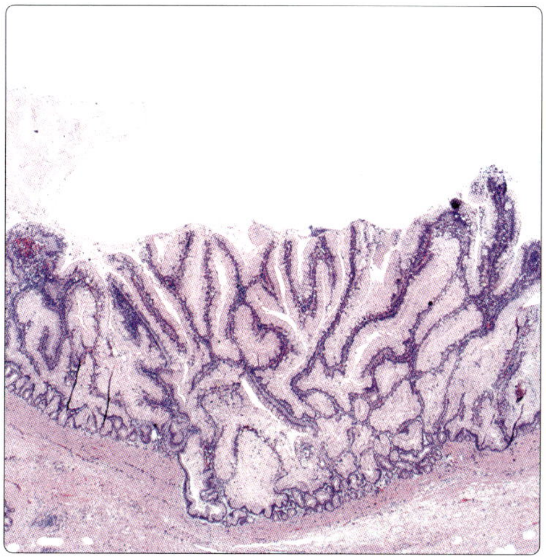

(Left) *This IPMN with a glistening mucinous appearance is present in the main branch of the pancreatic duct and has caused marked ductal dilatation* ⇨ *compared to the adjacent duct* ➡*. The lesion extends to the proximal margin of resection* ↪ *on gross examination.* **(Right)** *This intraductal papillary proliferation involves the main pancreatic duct, which is markedly dilated. The finding of a grossly evident lesion in the main duct is diagnostic of IPMN.*

(Left) *IPMNs and pancreatic intraepithelial neoplasias are both characterized by an intraductal papillary proliferation of mucinous epithelium and lack of ovarian-type stroma. Marked duct dilatation and extension of the papillary proliferation into contiguous ducts, as seen here, are key features for diagnosing IPMN.* **(Right)** *The degree of cytologic and architectural atypia in IPMNs is variable and classified as mild, moderate, or severe dysplasia. High-grade IPMNs are usually resected if at the margin.*

Intraductal Papillary Mucinous Neoplasm

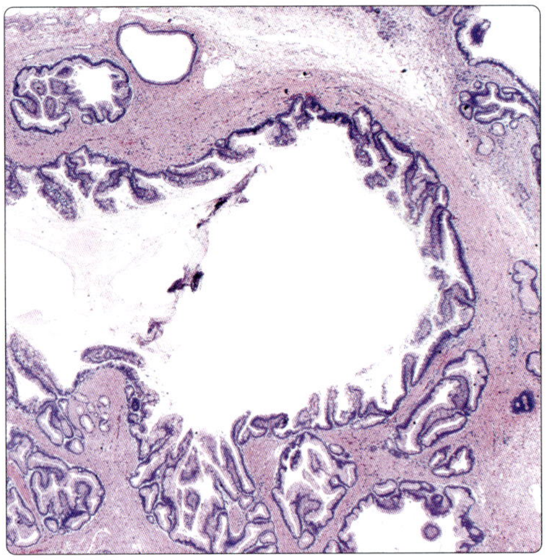

Intraductal Papillary Mucinous Neoplasm

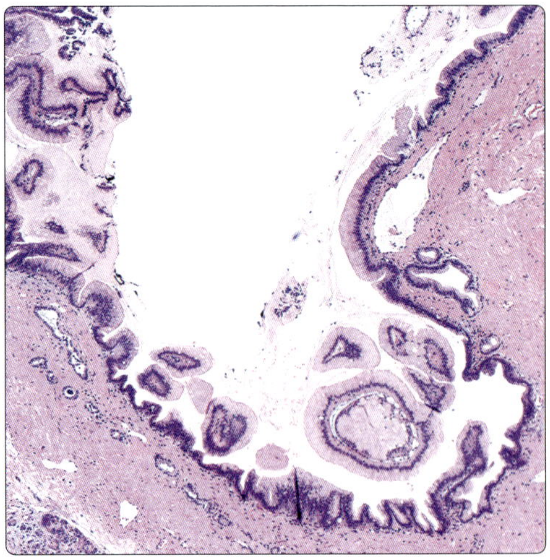

(Left) *This endocrine neoplasm ➡ has a well-circumscribed border and a fleshy tan appearance. The majority are found in the tail of the pancreas. Approximately 10% of patients have germline mutations.* **(Right)** *Some endocrine tumors have a cystic appearance. The cytologic appearance of tumor cells in these cases, however, is the same as typical noncystic endocrine tumors. Solid pseudopapillary tumors of the pancreas also show cystic change but have a different cytologic appearance.*

Pancreatic Endocrine Tumor: Gross Appearance

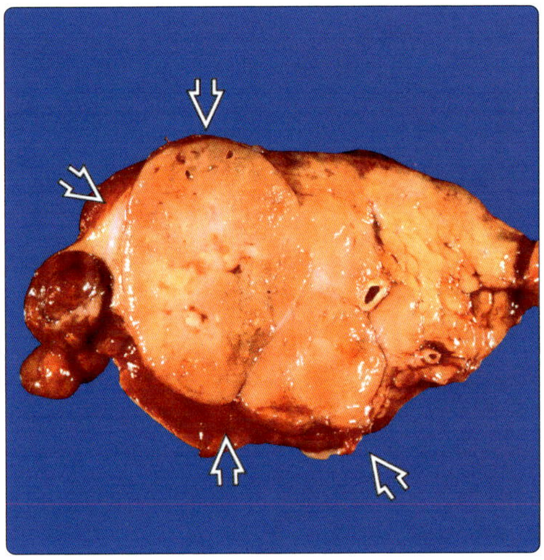

Pancreatic Endocrine Tumor: Cystic Pattern

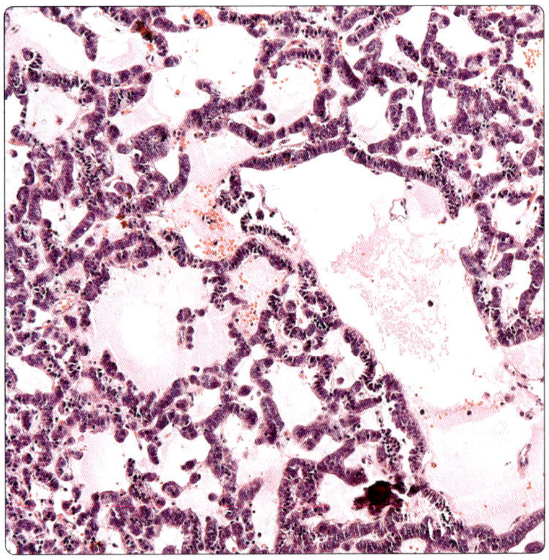

(Left) *Solid pseudopapillary tumors of the pancreas occur in adolescent and young women and are typically large (~ 9 cm), encapsulated tumors with zones of necrosis and cystic degeneration.* **(Right)** *As the name implies, solid pseudopapillary tumors are characterized by solid ➡ and pseudopapillary ➡ growth patterns. The neoplastic cells have bland, grooved, or indented nuclei and pale-clear cytoplasm. Foamy macrophages are abundant in areas of cystic degeneration.*

Solid Pseudopapillary Tumor: Gross Appearance

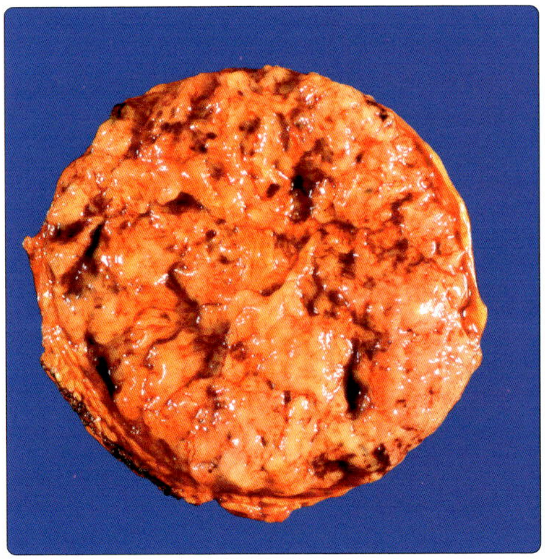

Solid Pseudopapillary Tumor

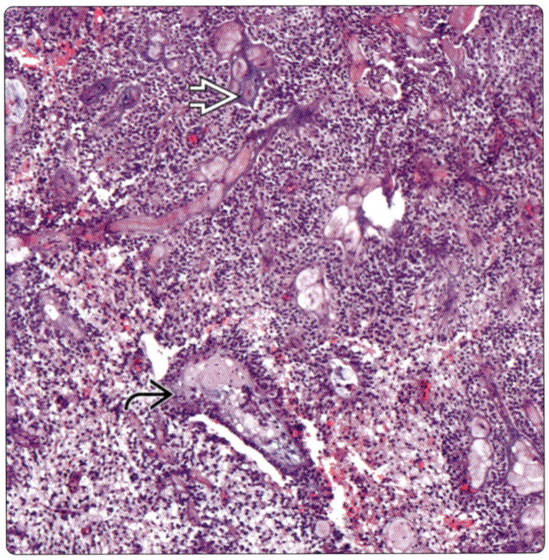

Serous Cystadenoma: Gross Appearance

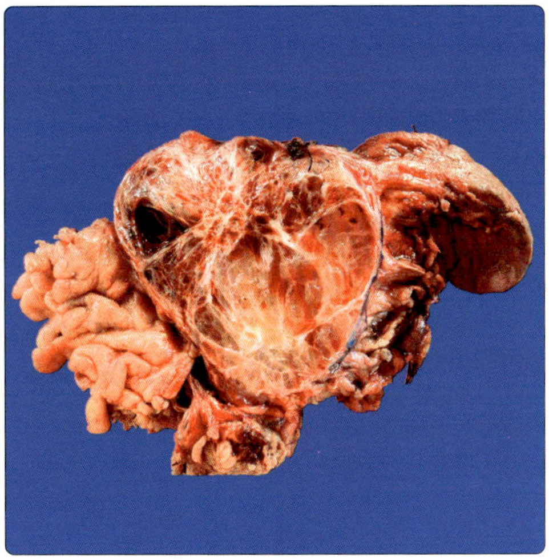

Serous Cystadenoma

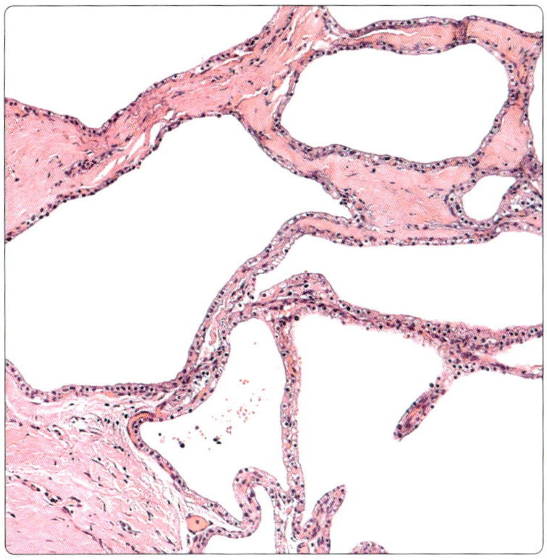

(Left) *Serous cystadenomas are benign lesions that usually occur in women. The tumors are typically large (~ 11 cm) and consist of a well-circumscribed mass of multiple thin-walled cysts, giving the tumor a sponge-like appearance. Excision is usually curative.* **(Right)** *The cysts in serous cystadenoma are lined by low cuboidal cells with bland nuclei and pale-clear cytoplasm that is rich in glycogen. Other names for this tumor are microcystic adenoma and glycogen-rich cystadenoma.*

Mucinous Cystic Neoplasm: Gross Appearance

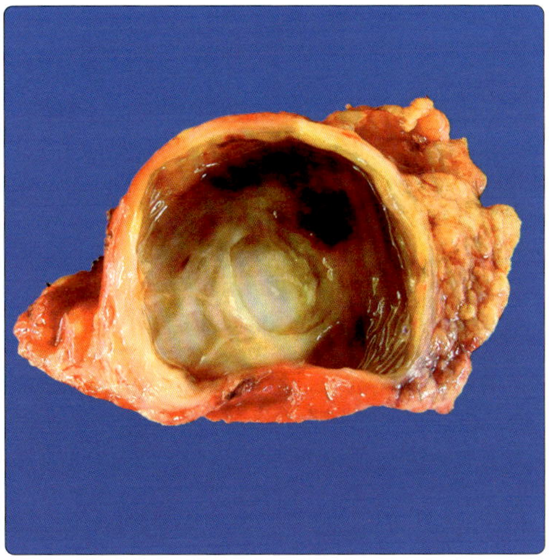

Mucinous Cystic Neoplasm

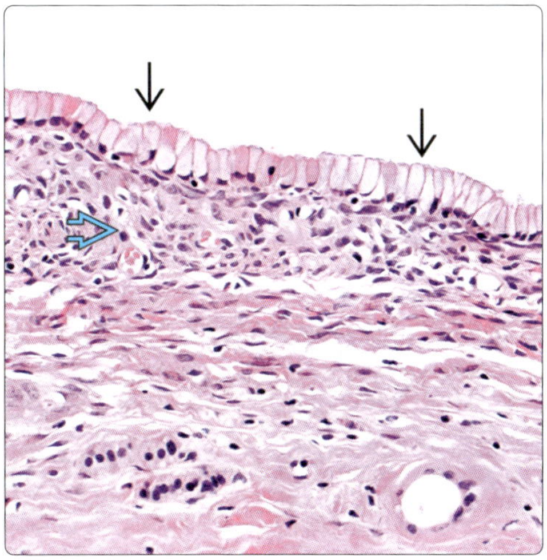

(Left) *Mucinous cystic neoplasms are benign or low-grade malignant tumors that usually occur in women in their 40s. The tumors are generally large (~ 10 cm) and may be unilocular or multilocular. The tumors do not communicate with the main pancreatic duct.* **(Right)** *The cysts in mucinous cystic neoplasms are lined by tall, columnar, mucin-producing cells →. The main diagnostic feature distinguishing them from IPMNs is the presence of ovarian-type stroma → underneath the mucinous-lining epithelium.*

Colloid (Mucinous Noncystic) Carcinoma: Gross Appearance

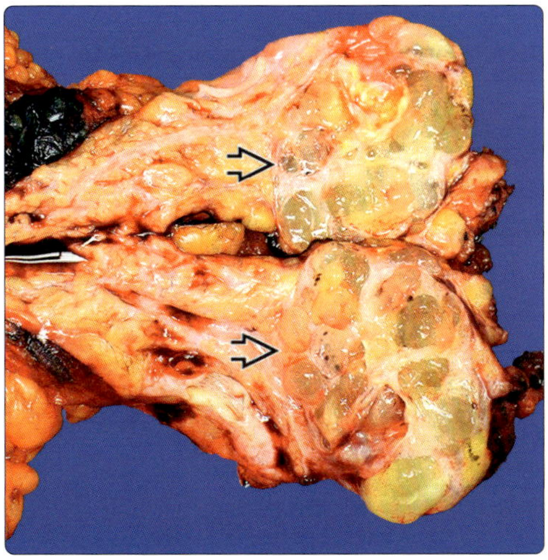

Pancreatoblastoma

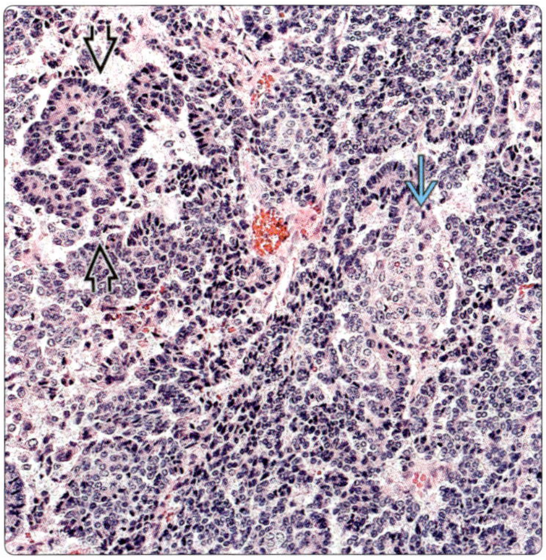

(Left) *Colloid carcinomas occur in both men and women at older ages. They arise in IPMNs and are characterized by abundant extracellular pools of mucin → that dissect through normal parenchyma. Unlike mucinous cystic carcinomas, these tumors do involve the main pancreatic duct.* **(Right)** *Pancreatoblastoma is the most common pancreatic tumor in children. The tumor consists of acinar cells → and squamoid morules →. These tumors may be difficult to distinguish from acinar cell carcinomas.*

SURGICAL/CLINICAL CONSIDERATIONS

Goal of Consultation

- Confirm parathyroid tissue has been removed as entire gland or as biopsy
- Confirm abnormal parathyroid gland has been removed

Change in Patient Management

- After removal of parathyroid gland(s) or biopsy confirmed, additional surgery is not necessary
  - Differentiation of adenoma, primary hyperplasia, and normal parathyroid may be used to guide surgery
- In rare cases, confirmation of parathyroid carcinoma can guide completion of surgery

Clinical Setting

- **Primary hyperparathyroidism**
  - Defined as disease as result of abnormal gland function
  - Patients usually diagnosed with hypercalcemia on serum tests and found to have elevated parathyroid hormone (PTH)
    - Less commonly, patients present with symptoms of osteoporosis or renal calculi
  - ~ 80% have solitary adenoma
    - 2 adenomas occur in ~ 10%
    - Involvement of 3 or 4 glands is considered primary hyperplasia and occurs in ~ 10%
- **Secondary hyperparathyroidism**
  - Defined as increase in normal gland function in response to another disease state
  - Parathyroid glands become enlarged and hyperfunctioning in response to low calcium levels
    - Most commonly due to renal failure
    - Causes debilitating loss of calcium from bones
- **Tertiary hyperparathyroidism**
  - After secondary hyperplasia, glands can start to function autonomously
  - Serum calcium becomes elevated

Surgical Approaches

- **Preoperative Imaging**
  - Parathyroid glands can be difficult for surgeon to identify
    - Normal glands are very small
    - Number and location of glands can vary
      - Most people have 4 parathyroid glands, 10% have ≥ 5, and 3% have < 4
      - 15% are found in unusual locations: Mediastinum, within thyroid, other sites
    - Lymph nodes, thymic tissue, thyroid nodules, and other areas of nodular tissue may resemble glands grossly
  - Number and location of abnormally enlarged glands can usually be identified by preoperative imaging
    - Ultrasound: Most common
      - Also used to evaluate thyroid for abnormalities prior to surgery
    - Sestamibi scan
      - Technetium Tc-99m is taken up by hyperfunctioning glands
      - Useful to identify adenomas in unusual locations
      - Less useful to detect multiple hyperplastic glands
    - 4-dimensional computed tomography
  - Minimally invasive surgery may be used when location of abnormal gland or glands is known
- **Surgery for adenoma with intraoperative PTH (IOPTH) assay**
  - Serum PTH is evaluated during surgery
    - PTH has half-life of < 5 minutes
    - Decreased PTH occurs within 10- to 15-minutes after removal of hyperfunctioning parathyroid tissue
  - If PTH decreases by > 50% after removal of adenoma, further surgery is not necessary
    - Frozen section is not necessary for confirmation of parathyroid tissue
    - If PTH is not decreased, surgeon will search for 2nd adenoma
  - IOPTH assays have largely replaced frozen section when available
    - IOPTH on fine-needle biopsy of excised tissue can be used to document it is parathyroid tissue

Parathyroid Adenoma: Gross Appearance

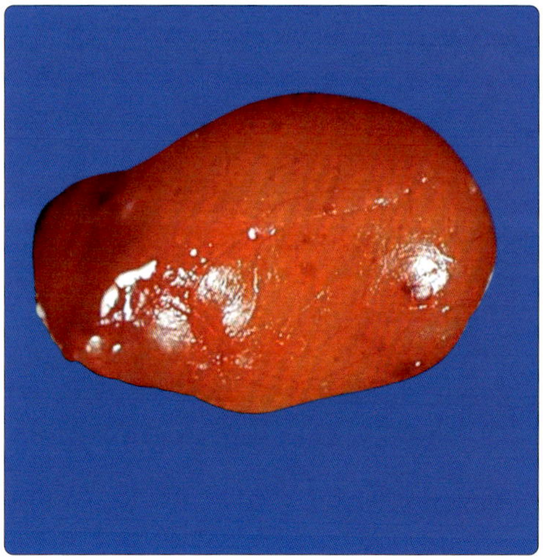

Parathyroid Hyperplasia: Gross Appearance

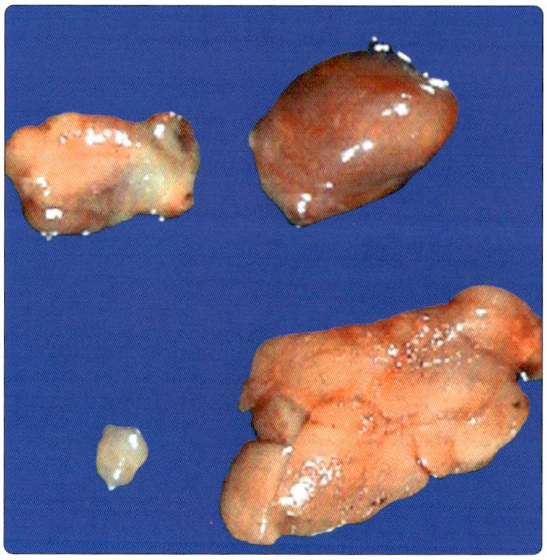

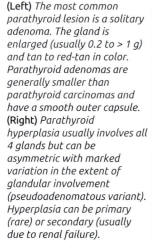

(Left) *The most common parathyroid lesion is a solitary adenoma. The gland is enlarged (usually 0.2 to > 1 g) and tan to red-tan in color. Parathyroid adenomas are generally smaller than parathyroid carcinomas and have a smooth outer capsule.* **(Right)** *Parathyroid hyperplasia usually involves all 4 glands but can be asymmetric with marked variation in the extent of glandular involvement (pseudoadenomatous variant). Hyperplasia can be primary (rare) or secondary (usually due to renal failure).*

- **Surgery for adenoma without IOPTH assay**
  - Surgeon visualizes all 4 parathyroid glands
  - Abnormally enlarged glands are removed
  - Removed glands are examined by frozen section
- **Surgery for secondary or tertiary hyperplasia**
  - 3 glands are removed
  - 4th gland is biopsied to ensure parathyroid tissue has been identified and left in situ
- **Current uses of frozen section**
  - IOPTH not available
  - Initial IOPTH level is normal
    - More common when there is multigland disease
  - Confirmation of parathyroid tissue prior to autotransplantation

SPECIMEN EVALUATION

Gross

- Specimen is identified as biopsy or resection of entire gland
  - Complete gland is ovoid and has smooth glistening capsule (size and shape of kidney bean)
    - Size and weight are measured
      - Important parameters to identify and document abnormal glands
      - Remove normal adipose tissue before measurements, if present
  - Adenoma: Single enlarged gland
    - Rim of normal tissue may be identifiable on cut section
  - Hyperplasia: Multiple enlarged glands
  - Biopsies are small irregular fragments of tissue
- Inking is unnecessary unless carcinoma is suspected clinically or grossly
  - Carcinomas are generally large (> 2 cm)
  - Surgeon may remove additional adherent tissue
- Complete glands are serially sectioned

Frozen Section

- Representative section of complete gland is frozen
- Biopsies are completely frozen

Cytology

- Most helpful when used in combination with frozen section
  - Highest sensitivity and specificity for correctly identifying parathyroid tissue
  - As single test, frozen section alone is superior to cytological preparations
- Useful to differentiate parathyroid cells from thyroid follicular cells or lymphocytes

Special Stains

- Oil red O
  - Parenchymal cells in normal glands contain large amount of intracytoplasmic lipid droplets
  - Intracellular and extracellular parenchymal lipid content is decreased to absent in hyperfunctioning parathyroid cells
  - Rim of normocellular parathyroid can be highlighted by this stain, confirming diagnosis of parathyroid adenoma

MOST COMMON DIAGNOSES

Normal Parathyroid Glands

- Normal size
  - 4-6 mm x 2-4 mm x 0.5-2 mm
- Normal weight
  - Men: 30 ± 3.5 mg
  - Women: 35 ± 5.2 mg
  - Any gland > 60 mg is enlarged
- Normal glands can show significant variation in cellularity, even in single individual
  - Age, gender, constitutional factors (body fat, etc.) affect cellularity
    - Cellularity is high in infants and children
    - Cellularity decreases with age
  - Adipose tissue
    - Stromal fat constitutes 10-30% of parathyroid
    - Increases with age
    - Not reliable feature to distinguish normal glands from adenomas or hyperplasia
    - More stromal fat in polar regions of parathyroid than central

Parathyroid Adenoma

- ~ 85% of surgical cases are to resect adenoma
- Majority (~ 96%) of adenomas are solitary
  - Rare cases of ≥ 2 adenomas can occur
- Size: 1-3 cm
- Weight: 300 mg to several grams
- Light tan color
- Usually < 5% adipose tissue
  - However, some adenomas have intracellular fat and adipose tissue
- Spontaneous infarction may result in adjacent inflammatory changes and adherence to surrounding tissue
- Normal-appearing parenchyma may be seen compressed to 1 side in ~ 50%
  - Can also be seen in some cases of hyperplasia
- Solid growth pattern most common
  - Macropseudofollicular growth pattern with colloid-like material may be seen
    - This pattern may mimic thyroid follicles
- Multiple cell types typically present
  - Chief cells (usually predominant), oxyphil cells, water-clear cells
  - Variant types of adenomas consist predominantly of oxyphil or water-clear cells
  - Scattered cells with marked nuclear atypia may be present
    - Not diagnostic feature of malignancy
- Ectopic parathyroid adenoma: Located at abnormal sites
  - Intrathyroidal, mediastinum, thymus, soft tissue behind esophagus and pharynx
- Rarely associated with genetic syndromes such as hyperparathyroidism-jaw tumor syndrome (HPT-JT) and familial hypercalcemic hypercalciuria
- **Cytologic features**
  - Cohesive cell clusters
    - Microfollicles can be present
  - Multiple cell types

 - Chief cells: Small cells with moderate to scant cytoplasm
 - Oxyphil cells: Larger nuclei with abundant eosinophilic granular cytoplasm
 - Adipocytes
- Stripped nuclei are common due to delicate cytoplasm

Parathyroid Adenoma Variants

- Parathyroid microadenoma: Weight < 0.1 g
- Oxyphil parathyroid adenoma: Composed of > 90% mitochondria-rich oncocytes
- Water-clear cell parathyroid adenoma: Composed of cells with extensively vacuolated clear cytoplasm
- Parathyroid lipoadenoma: Composed of abundant adipose tissue with scattered nests of parenchymal chief cells
- Cystic parathyroid adenoma
  - Varying degrees of cystic change can be seen in parathyroid adenomas
  - Particularly common in larger parathyroid adenomas
  - Associated with HPT-JT
    - Autosomal dominant disorder caused by inactivating mutations in *HRPT2* tumor suppressor gene that encodes parafibromin

Primary Hyperplasia

- Very rare
- Usually all 4 glands are enlarged
  - In some cases not all glands are abnormal
- 20% of patients will have germline syndrome
  - Generally multiple endocrine neoplasia type1 (MEN1), MEN2A, or isolated familial hyperparathyroidism
- Recurrence of hypercalcemia is more common than for single adenomas

Secondary Hyperplasia

- All 4 glands are usually enlarged, but enlargement may not connote level of involvement
  - Each, some, or all 4 glands may be multinodular
  - Asymmetric enlargement can resemble adenoma or adenomas (pseudoadenomatous variant)
- Nodular growth pattern is common
  - Cell populations typically consist of multiple types with nodules of chief cells, oxyphil cells, and clear cells
  - Scattered fat cells are usually present
    - Usually diminished compared to normal glands
  - Adipose tissue may be decreased and rarely absent
- It may not be possible to distinguish adenoma from hyperplasia if only 1 gland is examined and clinical history is not provided

Atypical Parathyroid Adenoma

- Parathyroid neoplasm composed of chief cells with variable oxyphil cells, transitional cells, and water-clear cells with some features of parathyroid carcinoma
  - Adherence to adjacent structures
  - Mitotic activity
  - Fibrosis
  - Trabecular growth
  - Tumor cells in capsule
- No definitive invasion into capsule, adjacent structures, nerves, or vessels is seen

Parathyroid Carcinoma

- Majority are functional and cause hyperparathyroidism
- Very rare (~ 1-2% of cases)
- Usually in older adults (4th-6th decades)
- Generally large: 2-6 cm, over 40 grams
- Parathyroid carcinoma usually necessitates en bloc resection
  - En bloc resection is necessary because carcinomas adhere to/infiltrate adjacent tissues
  - Removed with attached skeletal muscle and adjacent thyroid
  - Specimen should be inked and margins evaluated
- Histologic features
  - Monotonous or trabecular growth patterns
  - Invasion into adjacent structures, vessels, perineural space
  - ~ 2/3 have marked nuclear pleomorphism present throughout carcinoma
    - High nuclear:cytoplasmic ratio
    - Prominent nucleoli
    - Numerous mitoses
  - Thick capsule may be invaded
  - Necrosis
  - Lymph-vascular or perineural invasion
  - Dense fibrous bands
    - Fibrosis and fibrous bands but can be seen in both parathyroid adenoma and carcinoma

Thyroid Lesion

- Ectopic nodule of multinodular thyroid hyperplasia may grossly mimic parathyroid gland
- Thyroid tissue usually has follicular growth pattern with colloid
- Normal and abnormal thyroid tissue typically
  - Have colloid and calcium oxylate crystals (highlighted by polarization)
  - Lack adipose tissue
  - Lack intracytoplasmic lipid
  - Lack well-defined cytoplasmic membranes characteristic of parathyroid cells
- Lymphocytic infiltrate may be seen within thyroid

Metastatic Carcinoma

- Rarely identified during life
- Autopsy studies show up to 12% of patients with known cancer have parathyroid involvement
- Metastases are usually from breast, prostate, liver, lung, and hematolymphoid malignancies
- Also may be involved from direct extension from thyroid tumor or head and neck neoplasm

REPORTING

Frozen Section

- Document that parathyroid tissue is present
  - If entire gland has been removed, size and weight are reported
- Report if ≥ 1 gland(s) are hypercellular
  - % of adipose tissue should be reported
    - Specific diagnosis of adenoma or hyperplasia is not necessary and is often not possible

Types of Hyperparathyroidism

Type	Usual Cause	Number of Glands Involved	Serum Calcium
Primary	Solitary adenoma (common)	Usually 1, rarely ≥ 2	Elevated
Primary	Primary hyperplasia (rare)	2-4	Elevated
Secondary	Chronic renal failure	4: All glands involved	Decreased
Tertiary	Chronic renal failure	4: All glands involved	Elevated

Comparison of Normal and Abnormal Parathyroid Glands

Feature	Normal Glands	Abnormal Glands
Number	Usually 4 glands	Up to 12 glands, ectopic location, intrathyroidal or intrathymic
Weight	~ 30 mg each	Any gland > 60 mg
Size	Up to 6 mm	> 6 mm
% adipose tissue	Usually > 25%, increases with age	< 5%
Intracytoplasmic lipid	Abundant	Lack of intracellular and intercellular lipid deposition (negative oil red O stain)

- If single gland is enlarged and if rim of normocellular parathyroid, diagnosis of adenoma may be rendered
- Presence or absence of intracellular and extracellular lipid on oil red O stain (when used)

Cytology

- Reported in conjunction with gross and frozen section findings

ACCURACY OF INTRAOPERATIVE DIAGNOSIS

Distinguishing Parathyroid From Other Tissues

- Highly reliable means of identifying parathyroid origin during parathyroid exploration
  - Accuracy rate in diagnosing normal or abnormal parathyroid and distinguishing from other tissues: > 99%
- Deferral rate and incorrect diagnosis are very low (usually < 0.5%) and are usually due to
  - Distinguishing parathyroid from thyroid
  - Sampling error
  - Frozen section artifact
  - Interpretation errors

PITFALLS

Parathyroid Mistaken for Thyroid

- Parathyroid parenchyma can resemble thyroid parenchyma
  - Pseudofollicular and trabecular structures can be present
  - Pseudofollicles can contain eosinophilic material that simulates colloid
  - Oxyphilic cells can resemble Hürthle cell nodule of thyroid
- Features helpful to identify true parathyroid parenchyma
  - Well-defined cytoplasmic membranes
  - Cytoplasmic lipid (fat droplets) common
  - Cells smaller and more vacuolated than thyroid cells
  - Nuclei have rounder and denser chromatin than thyroid nuclei
  - Pseudofollicles lack true colloid
    - Lack birefringent and polarizable calcium oxalate crystals seen in thyroid
    - Pseudofollicles can contain material that closely mimics colloid
  - Clusters of oxyphil cells

Thyroid Mistaken for Parathyroid

- Thyroid parenchyma can resemble parathyroid parenchyma
  - Stromal edema or ice crystal artifact can simulate adipose tissue
    - Rarely, true adipose metaplasia can be present within thyroid tissue
  - Hürthle cells of thyroid can be mistaken for oxyphil cells

Lymph Node vs. Parathyroid Gland

- Ice crystal artifact can mimic adipose tissue within lymph node and mimic parathyroid gland
- Parathyroid tissue has more cytoplasm than lymphocytes

Assessment of Cellularity

- Assessing cellularity in small biopsies can be difficult
  - Variable within parathyroid glands and among glands in single individual
  - Polar regions of parathyroid more cellular than central
  - Cellularity increases with age and varies with gender, ethnicity, and body habitus

SELECTED REFERENCES

1. Coan KE et al: Intraoperative ex vivo parathyroid aspiration: A point-of-care test to confirm parathyroid tissue. Surgery. 160(4):850-7, 2016
2. Wei S et al: Images in endocrine pathology: parathyroid adenoma with frozen section artifact mimics thyroid papillary carcinoma. Endocr Pathol. 26(2):185-6, 2015
3. Wong KS et al: Utility of birefringent crystal identification by polarized light microscopy in distinguishing thyroid from parathyroid tissue on intraoperative frozen sections. Am J Surg Pathol. 38(9):1212-9, 2014
4. Anton RC et al: Frozen section of thyroid and parathyroid specimens. Arch Pathol Lab Med. 129(12):1575-84, 2005
5. Shidham VB et al: Intraoperative cytology increases the diagnostic accuracy of frozen sections for the confirmation of various tissues in the parathyroid region. Am J Clin Pathol. 118(6):895-902, 2002

(Left) *This coronal view demonstrates the normal posterior anatomic position of the parathyroid glands ➡ and the relationship with the thyroid ➡ and larynx ➡, along with the nerves and vessels. These glands are small and can be difficult for the surgeon to identify.* (Right) *This axial view shows the thyroid lobes and the isthmus ➡ in the anterior visceral space. A normal parathyroid gland ➡ and a markedly enlarged parathyroid adenoma ➡ are present in the area of the tracheoesophageal groove.*

Normal Parathyroid Gland Topography

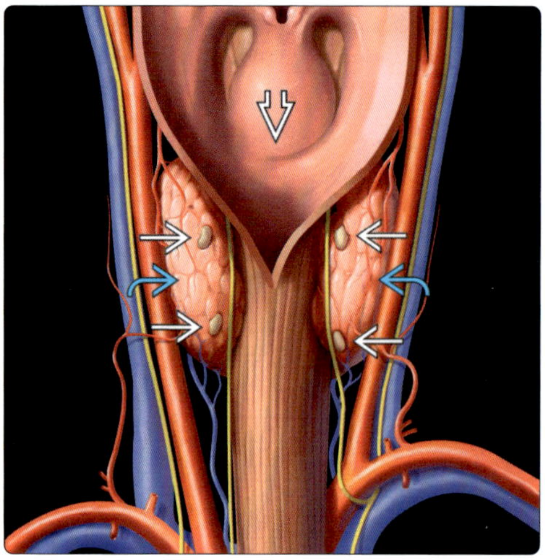

Parathyroid Adenoma: Anatomic Location

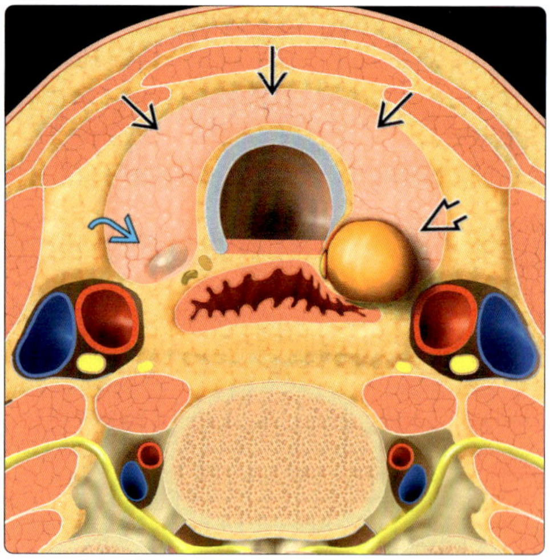

(Left) *Parathyroid lesions are often identified by imaging prior to surgery. If a single abnormal gland is present, minimally invasive surgery can be attempted. In this case, the patient has enlarged left ➡ and right ➡ parathyroid glands.* (Right) *Hyperfunctioning right ➡ and left ➡ parathyroid glands have taken up technetium Tc-99m on this sestamibi scan. These scans can be helpful to identify the number and location of abnormal glands. In general, these scans are less helpful for multigland disease.*

Parathyroid Masses: CT Scan

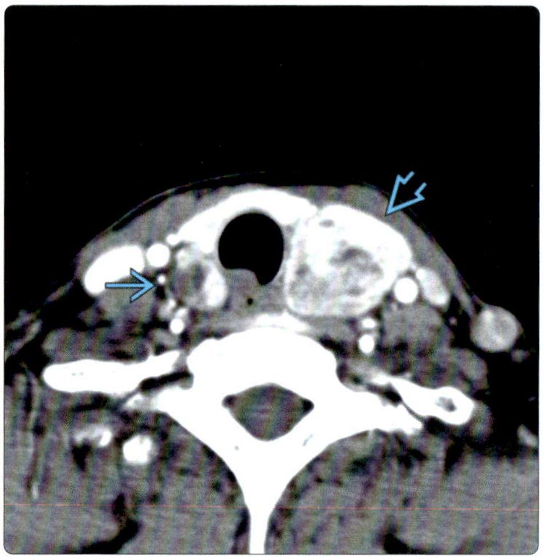

Parathyroid Masses: Sestamibi Scan

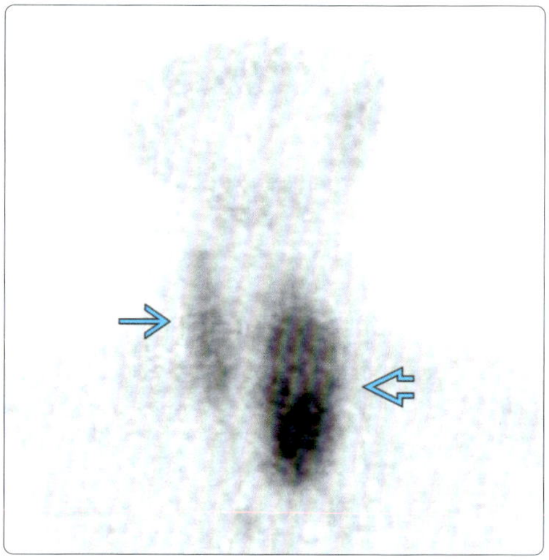

(Left) *This parathyroid carcinoma has a firm yellow nodular surface and is larger than a typical adenoma. The surgeon often removes additional tissue due to infiltration into and adherence to surrounding structures.* (Right) *Parathyroid carcinomas usually present clinically as large, functional, locally invasive tumors. Vascular invasion ➡ is 1 of the most definitive histologic features of malignancy, but it occurs in a minority of cases. Nuclear pleomorphism is often present, but is not indicative of carcinoma in isolation.*

Parathyroid Carcinoma: Gross Appearance

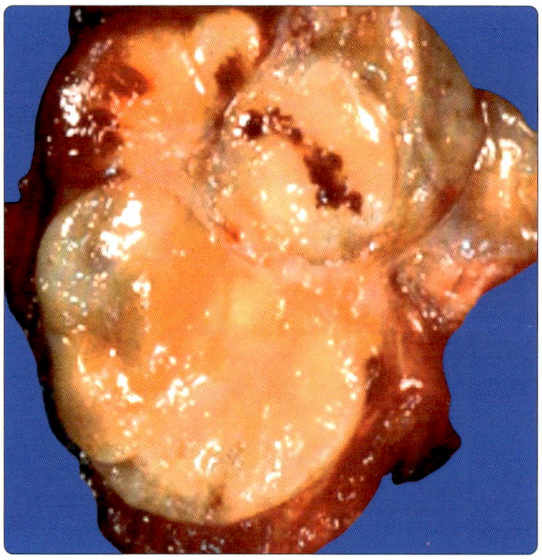

Parathyroid Carcinoma: Lymph-Vascular Invasion

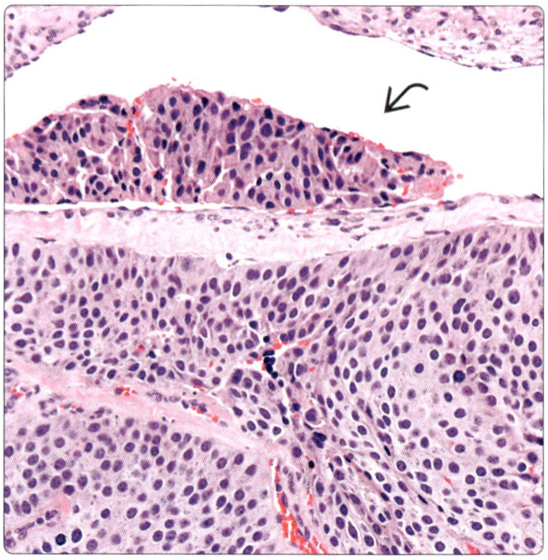

Normal Parathyroid Gland and Hyperplasia

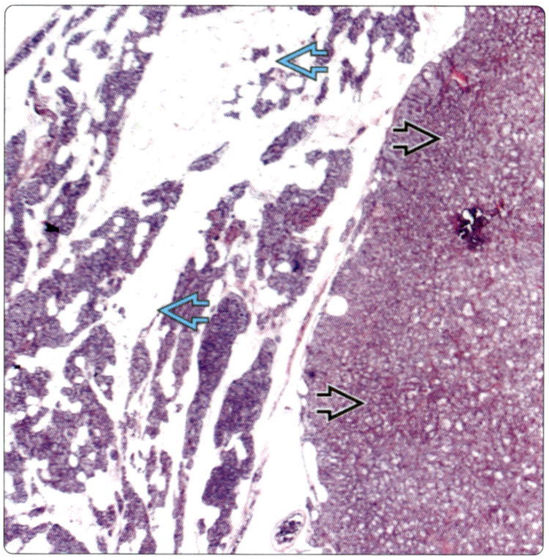

Normal Parathyroid: Presence of Fat

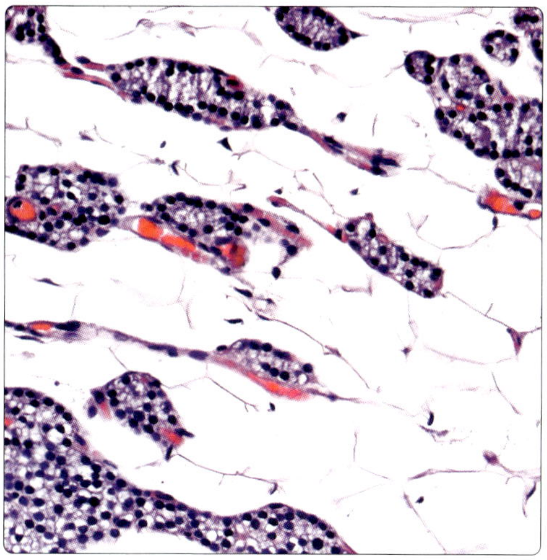

(Left) *Normal parathyroid tissue has a prominent component of adipose tissue ⇨. In contrast, adenomas generally lack adipose tissue and areas of hyperplasia ⇨ have diminished adipose tissue.* **(Right)** *The presence of abundant adipose tissue in a parathyroid gland favors a normal gland. On occasion, a normal gland can be mistaken for adipose tissue. Rare lipoadenomas have adipose tissue and must be recognized by the abnormal large size.*

Parathyroid Adenoma: Absence of Fat

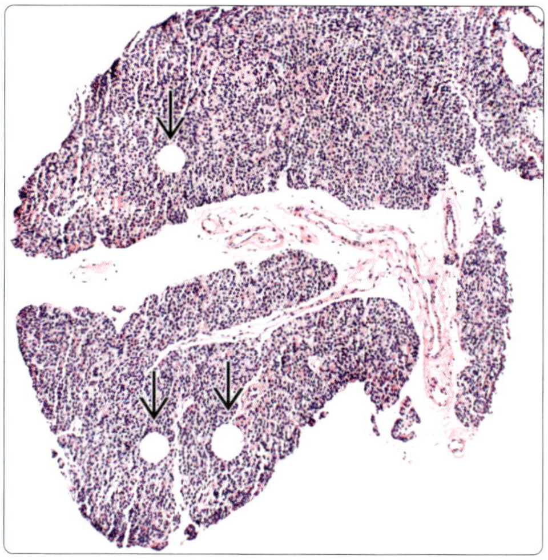

Parathyroid Adenoma: Absence of Fat

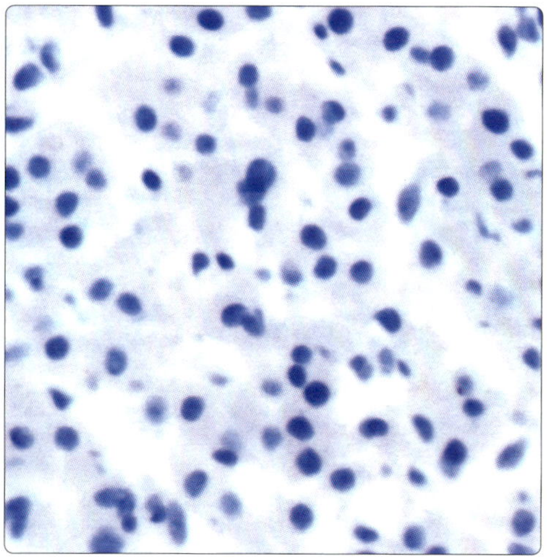

(Left) *Parathyroid adenomas usually lack adipose tissue, whereas normal parathyroid glands contain adipose tissue. Artifactual spaces → and ice crystal artifact can sometimes mimic adipose tissue and can make estimates of cellularity difficult.* **(Right)** *These chief cells in a parathyroid adenoma stained by oil red O during frozen section show a complete absence of intracytoplasmic fat. Parenchymal fat was also absent. This is characteristic of a hyperfunctioning chief cell proliferation.*

Parathyroid Hyperplasia: Decreased Fat

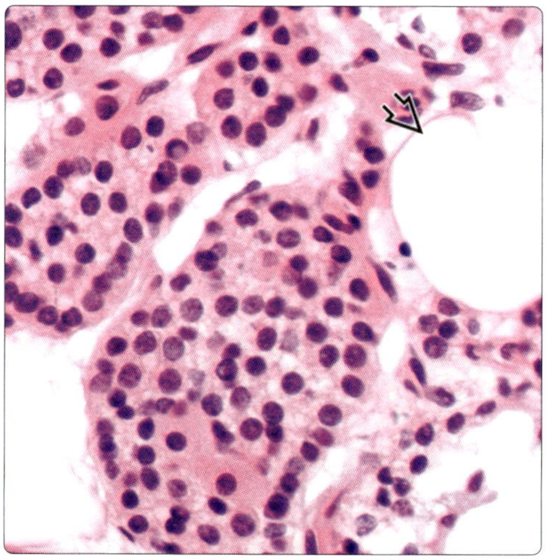

Parathyroid Hyperplasia: Decreased Fat

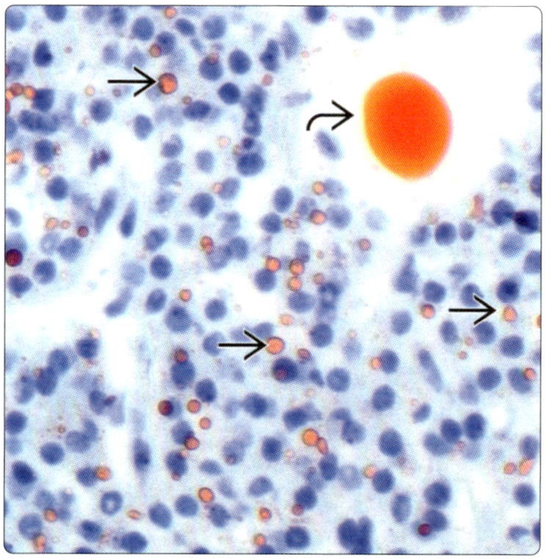

(Left) *Hyperplastic glands in response to renal failure are hypercellular and usually show a reduced amount of intraparenchymal adipose tissue ⇨. Intracytoplasmic fat is also generally reduced.* **(Right)** *This oil red O stain of a hyperplastic gland shows the parenchymal cells with small amounts of intracellular fat → and a droplet of extracellular fat ↷. Although fat is generally reduced in cases of hyperplasia, this is not a reliable feature to distinguish hyperplasia from normal glands.*

(Left) *Parathyroid adenoma is a benign neoplasm and is most commonly solitary. The tumor is covered by a thin capsule. The tissue is homogeneous tan to orange-tan in color. An intact gland is ovoid in shape with a smooth outer surface.* **(Right)** *The parenchyma of a parathyroid adenoma has a homogeneous tan-orange surface with focal areas of hemorrhage. A small rim of normal parathyroid tissue is compressed to the side of the adenoma. The size and weight of glands are important features to record.*

Parathyroid Adenoma: Gross Appearance

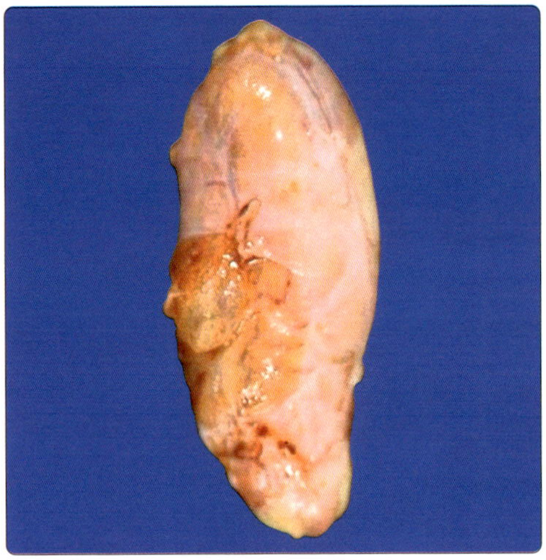

Parathyroid Adenoma: Gross Appearance

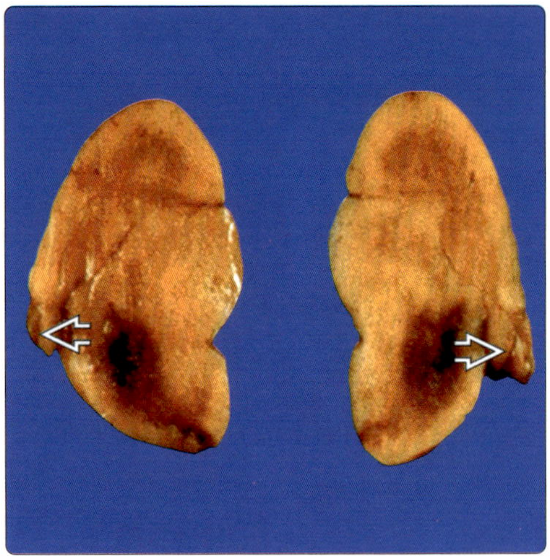

(Left) *A chief cell adenoma shows an adjacent area of normal parenchyma also comprised of chief cells but with adipose tissue. The presence of a rim of normocellular parathyroid adjacent to a singe hypercellular enlarged parathyroid gland supports the diagnosis of an adenoma.* **(Right)** *The normal parathyroid chief cell nuclei are uniformly small and round with dense chromatin. The cells can resemble small lymphocytes on frozen section. However, parathyroid cells have a rim of cytoplasm.*

Parathyroid Adenoma: Chief Cells

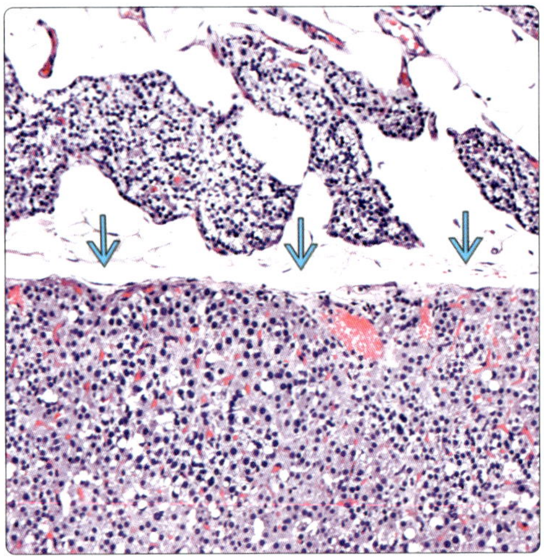

Parathyroid Adenoma: Chief Cells

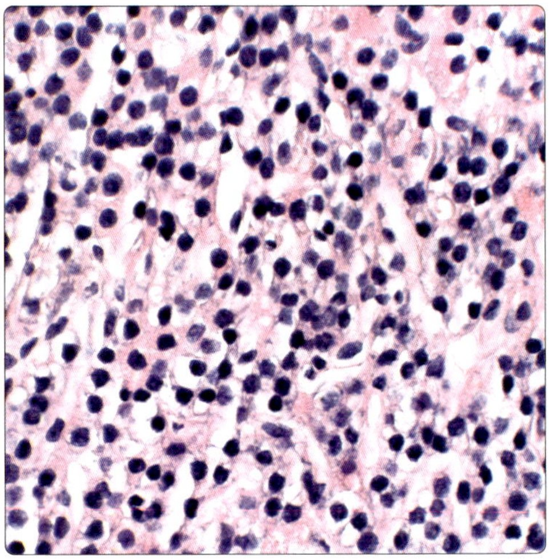

(Left) *This oxyphil adenoma is comprised of cells with round hyperchromatic nuclei and abundant eosinophilic granular cytoplasm. An adjacent area of normal parenchyma shows chief cells and adipose tissue.* **(Right)** *Oxyphil adenomas are composed almost exclusively of mitochondria-rich oxyphil cells. These tumors may show slight nuclear pleomorphism, so-called endocrine atypia. These cells augment the sensitivity of technetium sestamibi scans.*

Parathyroid Adenoma: Oxyphil Variant

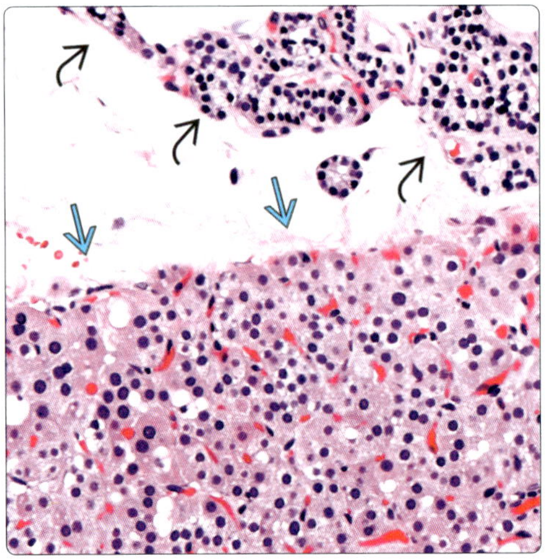

Parathyroid Adenoma: Oxyphil Variant

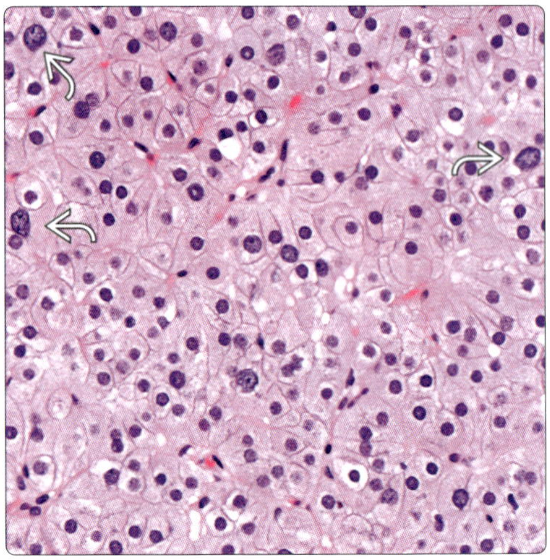

Parathyroid Adenoma: Follicular Pattern

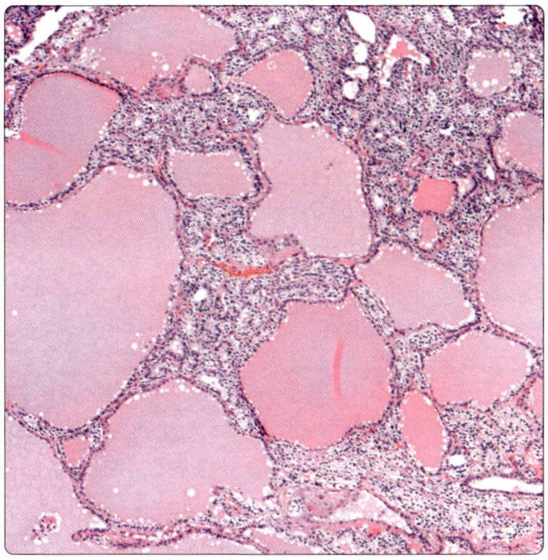

Parathyroid Adenoma: Follicular Adenoma

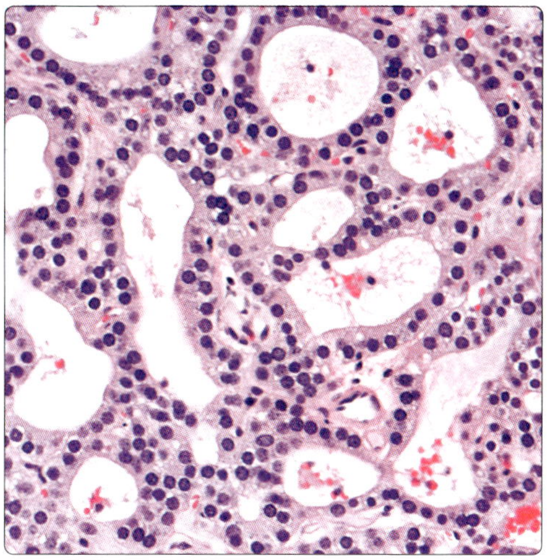

(Left) *Predominantly macrofollicular growth patterns with colloid-like material are relatively common in parathyroid adenomas. This pattern can be mistaken for thyroid tissue at frozen section. Real thyroid tissue often has polarizable calcium oxalate in follicles.* **(Right)** *This chief cell parathyroid adenoma has a follicular growth pattern. In this case, the spaces appear empty.*

Parathyroid Adenoma: Follicular Pattern With Chief Cells

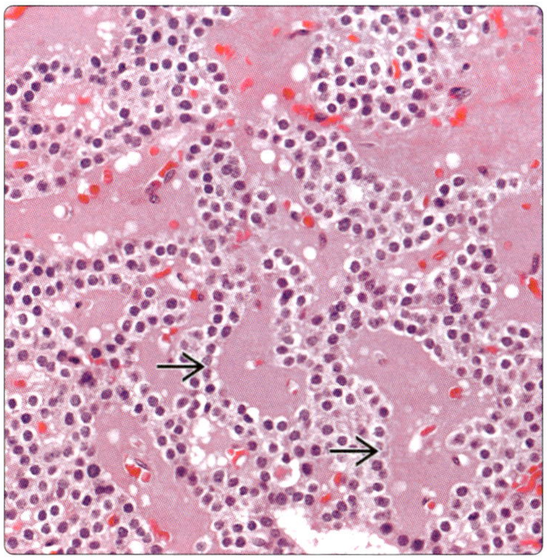

Parathyroid Adenoma: Follicular and Microfollicular Patterns

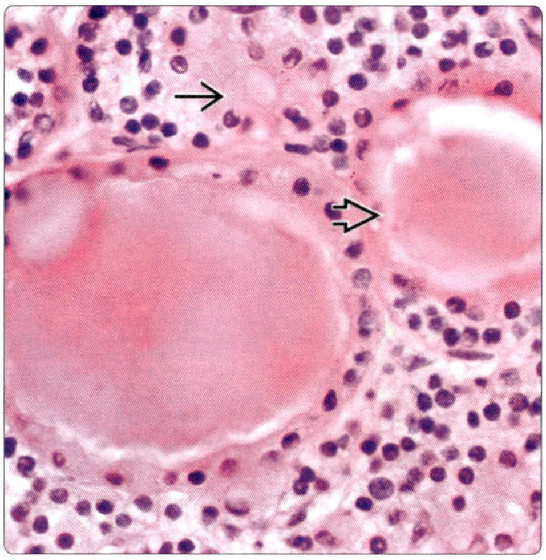

(Left) *This chief cell adenoma has a follicular growth pattern and the follicles are filled with colloid-like material ➙.* **(Right)** *A parathyroid adenoma with a predominantly follicular ➙ and microfollicular ➙ pattern may contain colloid-like material and strongly resemble thyroid. The presence of more typical parathyroid elsewhere within the lesion may help with the diagnosis.*

Parathyroid Adenoma: Water-Clear Cell Variant

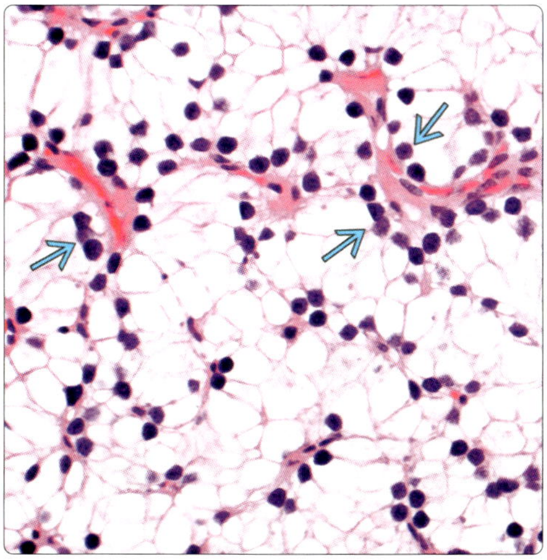

Parathyroid Adenoma: Touch Imprint

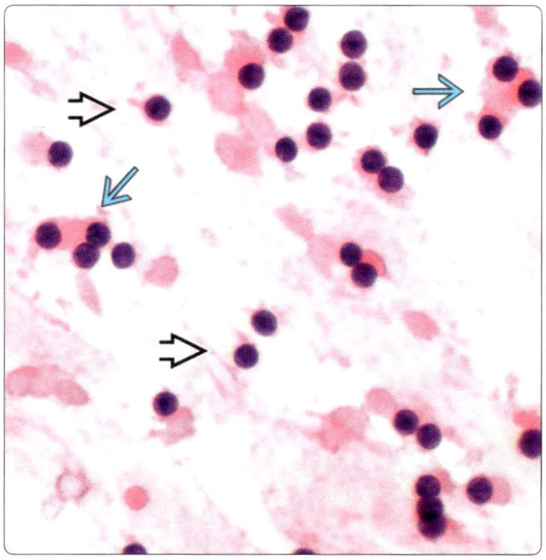

(Left) *Water-clear cell parathyroid adenoma involves only 1 parathyroid gland, unlike the very rare water-clear cell hyperplasia, which involves multiple glands. Nuclei can be basally located next to stroma and vessels, as demonstrated here ➙.* **(Right)** *Cytological preparations may be used to identify parathyroid tissue. However, they lack architectural features and yield many bare nuclei ➙ that are not identifiable as to cell type. Clusters of cells and the presence of cytoplasm help distinguish parathyroid cells from lymphocytes ➙.*

(Left) *This parathyroid gland has been replaced by a tan-yellow soft mass involving almost the entire gland, leaving only a small rim of normal parathyroid tissue. This appearance is characteristic of a lipoadenoma.* (Right) *This enlarged parathyroid gland shows a marked increase in stromal fat cells surrounding nests of chief stromal cells. These findings can be seen in parathyroid lipoadenoma and lipohyperplasia and must be distinguished from normal parathyroid.*

Parathyroid Lipoadenoma: Gross Appearance

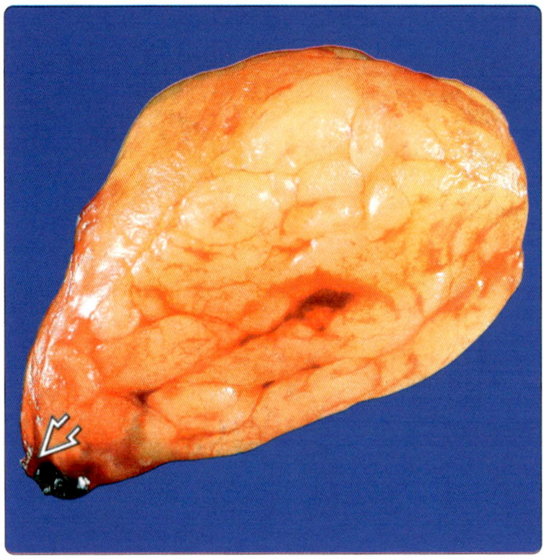

Parathyroid Lipoadenoma

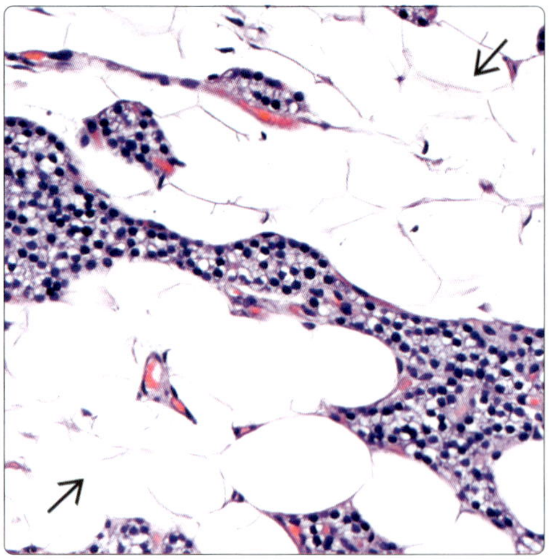

(Left) *This parathyroid lipoadenoma shows small nests of parathyroid chief cells and abundant fat cells. The fat cells lack the cytoplasmic vacuolization seen in water-clear cells of water-clear cell parathyroid adenomas.* (Right) *Varying degrees of cystic change can be seen in parathyroid adenomas. Cystic changes are particularly common in larger parathyroid adenomas and in those associated with hyperparathyroidism-jaw tumor syndrome.*

Parathyroid Lipoadenoma: Nests of Chief Cells

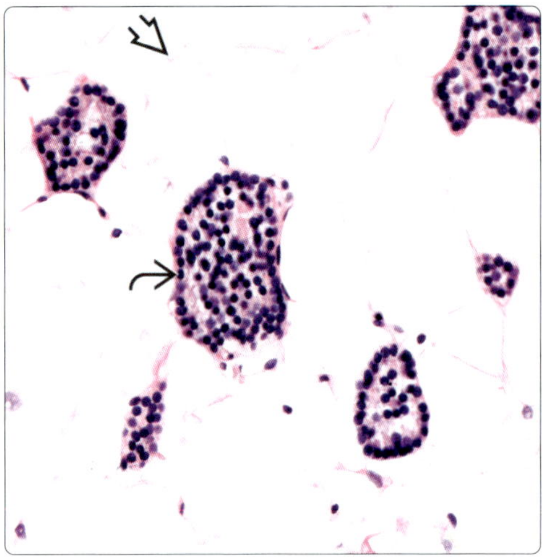

Parathyroid Adenoma: Cystic Change

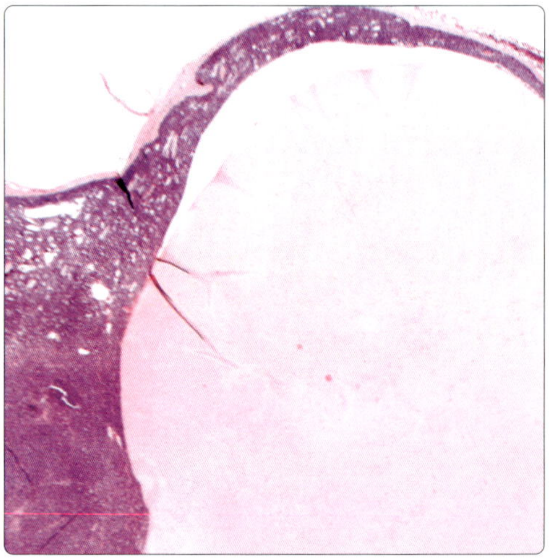

(Left) *Approximately 15% of parathyroid glands are located at unusual sites. This parathyroid adenoma was identified by frozen section within the thyroid gland after the thyroid was removed during surgery for hyperparathyroidism.* (Right) *A parathyroid adenoma can be located within the thyroid, as both develop from the 4th branchial pouch. The small dark nuclei of the chief cells can be compared to the more dispersed chromatin of the thyroid nuclei.*

Parathyroid Adenoma: Intrathyroidal Location

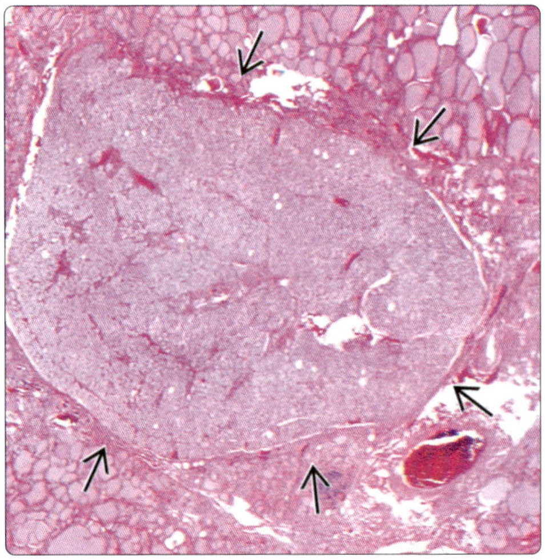

Parathyroid Adenoma: Intrathyroidal Location

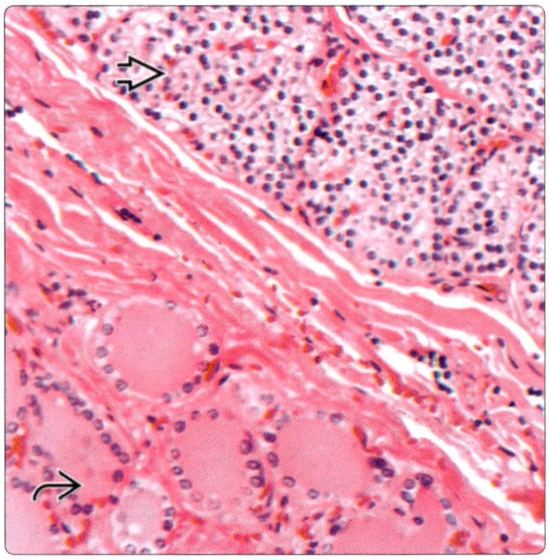

Parathyroid Hyperplasia: Gross Appearance

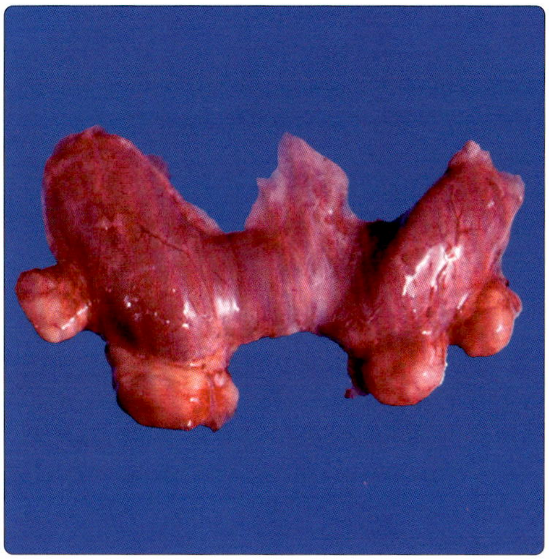

Parathyroid Hyperplasia: Fibrosis and Calcifications

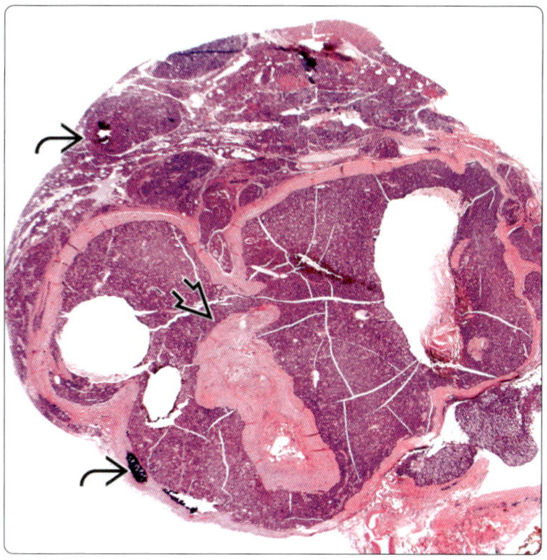

(Left) *Parathyroid hyperplasia can be characterized by asymmetric hyperplasia with marked variation in the extent of glandular involvement (pseudoadenomatous variant). The asymmetric hyperplasia is easily confused with a single adenoma or multiple adenomas.* **(Right)** *This hyperplastic parathyroid gland shows degenerative changes, including fibrosis ⇨ and calcifications ↷, features seen in longstanding hyperplastic parathyroid glands. The presence of dense fibrous bands would raise concern for carcinoma.*

Parathyroid Hyperplasia: Nodular Pattern

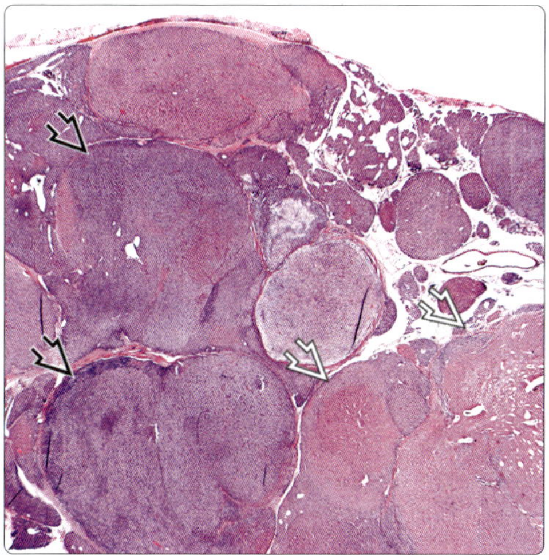

Parathyroid Hyperplasia: Decreased Fat

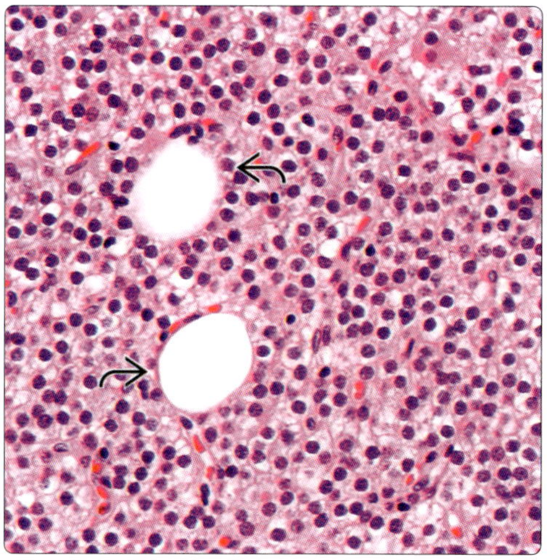

(Left) *Parathyroid hyperplasia usually shows a nodular growth pattern, whereas adenomas generally have a more uniform growth pattern. The nodules are composed of populations of chief cells ⇨, which predominate, as well as nodules of oxyphil cells ➡.* **(Right)** *Parathyroid glands involved by primary hyperplasia can be composed primarily of chief cells, as seen in this gland. Scattered fat cells ↷ are present but are less numerous than those seen in normal glands.*

Parathyroid Hyperplasia: Multiple Cell Types

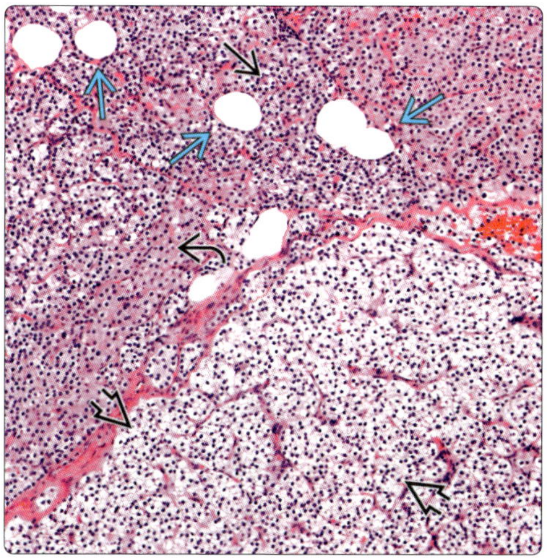

Parathyroid Hyperplasia: Follicular Pattern

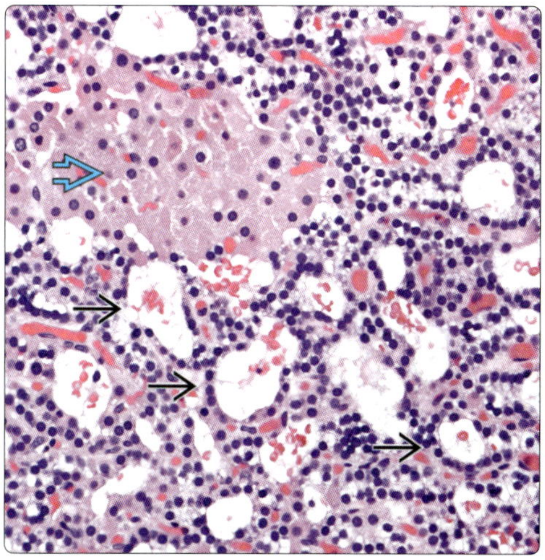

(Left) *A nodular growth pattern is usually seen in parathyroid hyperplasia. The cell populations can consist of multiple types with nodules of chief cells →, oxyphil cells ↷, and water-clear cells ⇨. Scattered fat cells are present →.* **(Right)** *Parathyroid glands involved by hyperplasia are composed by chief and oxyphil cells ⇨. The chief cells are usually in a diffuse pattern. When in a follicular pattern →, the tissue may be mistaken as thyroid during frozen section.*

Peripheral Nerve and Skeletal Muscle: Allocation of Tissue for Special Studies

SURGICAL/CLINICAL CONSIDERATIONS

Goal of Consultation

- Confirm presence of nerve or muscle
- Confirm sufficient size of the specimen
- Allocate fresh tissue for special studies

Change in Patient Management

- Additional nerve or muscle may be resected if specimen is inadequate
- Crushed or torn specimen requires additional sampling
- It should be possible to orient and identify longitudinal axis of specimen for accurate sectioning

Clinical Setting

- Nerve: For peripheral neuropathy
  - Inherited primary nerve disorders
  - Inflammatory demyelinating disorders
  - Secondary involvement (e.g., diabetes, vasculitis, amyloidosis)
- Muscle: For primary and secondary myopathies
  - Inherited myopathies/dystrophies
  - Inflammatory myopathies
  - Neurogenic atrophy
  - Toxic myopathies (e.g., statin, chloroquine)
  - Systemic processes (e.g., vasculitis, amyloidosis)

SPECIMEN EVALUATION

Gross

- Nerve (allocations in order of importance)
  - Electron microscopy
    - Longitudinal and cross sections fixed in glutaraldehyde
    - Processed for 1-µm sections and ultrastructural analysis as indicated
  - Frozen tissue
    - Small cross section snap frozen in embedding medium
    - Processed for immunofluorescence for immunoglobulins, as indicated (e.g., collagen-vascular disease, vasculitis)
  - Teased fiber preparation
    - Longitudinal section fixed in glutaraldehyde
    - Processed by technician by separating individual nerve fibers under dissecting microscope
    - Fibers placed on coverslip and stained with osmium
    - Evaluates segmental de- and remyelination
  - Light microscopy
    - Remaining tissue fixed in formalin
    - 2-3 H&E levels and trichrome stain
- Muscle (allocations in order of importance)
  - Frozen tissue
    - Cross and longitudinal sections
    - Snap frozen in liquid nitrogen-cooled isopentane
    - Processed for histochemistry (ATPase, NADH, SDH, COX, trichrome, PAS, oil red O)
    - Portion stored frozen for biochemical or mutational analyses
  - Electron microscopy
    - Longitudinal and cross sections, fixed in glutaraldehyde
    - Processed for 1-µm sections and ultrastructural analysis, if indicated
  - Light microscopy
    - Remaining tissue fixed in formalin
    - 3 H&E levels

REPORTING

Gross Examination

- Describe size of submitted specimen
- Determine tissue adequacy for special studies

Frozen Section

- Performed if surgeon is uncertain if nerve or muscle is present
- Only presence of nerve or muscle need be reported

SELECTED REFERENCES

1. Pestronk A: Neuromuscular Disease Center. http://neuromuscular.wustl.edu. Updated July 2017. Accessed August 4, 2017

Sural Nerve Biopsy Site

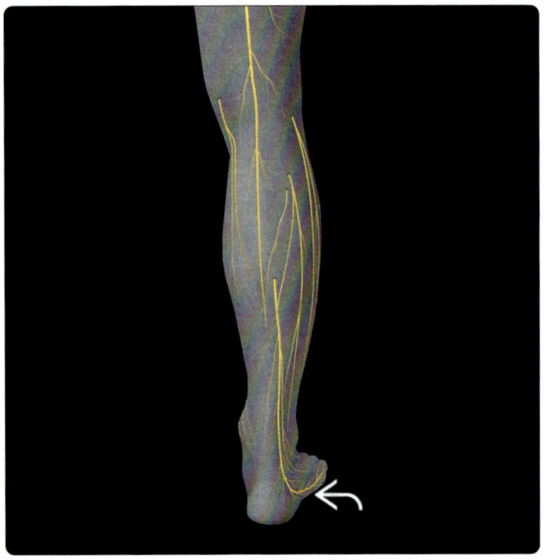

Muscle Biopsy Site

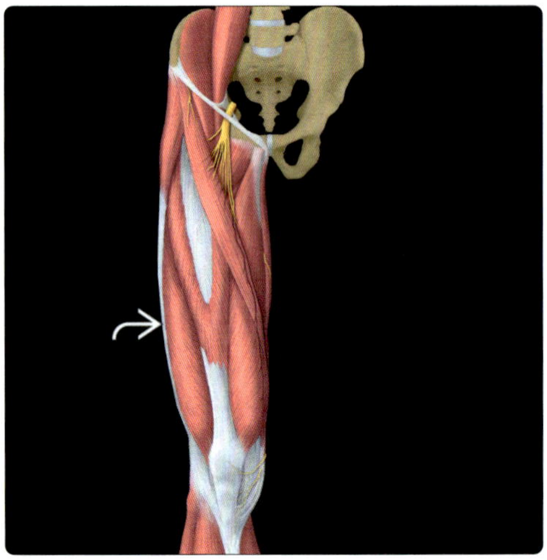

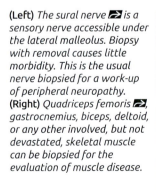

(Left) *The sural nerve* ➡ *is a sensory nerve accessible under the lateral malleolus. Biopsy with removal causes little morbidity. This is the usual nerve biopsied for a work-up of peripheral neuropathy.* **(Right)** *Quadriceps femoris* ➡, *gastrocnemius, biceps, deltoid, or any other involved, but not devastated, skeletal muscle can be biopsied for the evaluation of muscle disease.*

Nerve Biopsy Allocation

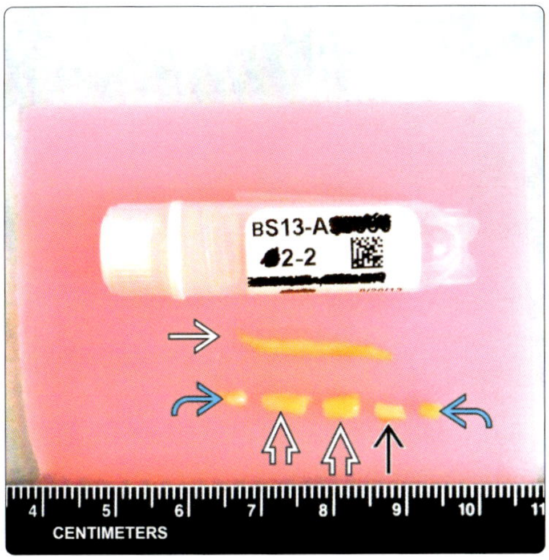

Skeletal Muscle Biopsy Allocation

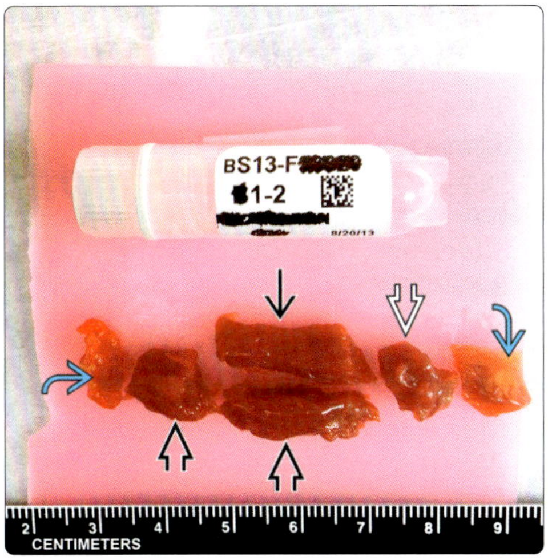

(Left) *One longitudinal fascicle of a peripheral nerve segment is saved for teased fiber preparation. The remainder of the specimen is divided for electron microscopy cross and longitudinal sections, paraffin cross and longitudinal sections, and snap freezing.* **(Right)** *This segment of muscle has been divided for freezing for biochemistry/molecular studies, cross and longitudinal sections for snap freezing for histochemistry, electron microscopy, and paraffin embedding.*

Nerve Biopsy: Snap Freezing

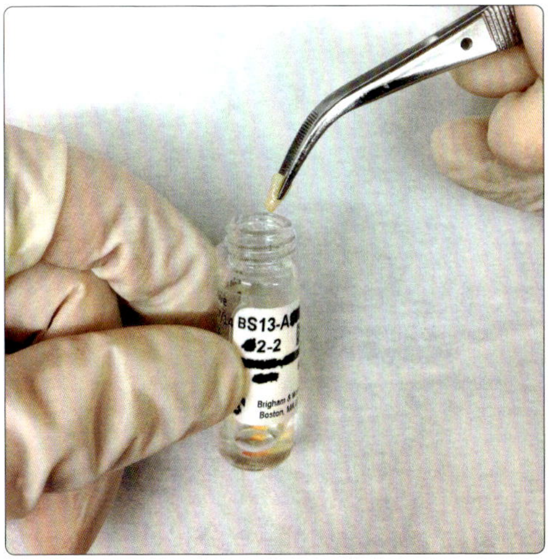

Skeletal Muscle Biopsy: Snap Freezing

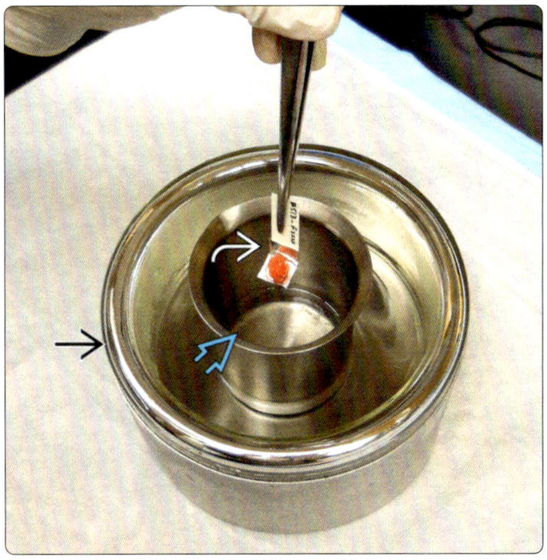

(Left) *Cross sections and longitudinal sections of a peripheral nerve biopsy are placed in glutaraldehyde for processing for electron microscopy. The tissue should be handled very gently with forceps to avoid crushing.* **(Right)** *A muscle biopsy is gently placed on a labeled cardboard tab and then submerged in isopentane that has been precooled in a liquid nitrogen bath in order to snap freeze the tissue. The tissue is then stored at -80°C until sectioning for muscle enzyme histochemistry.*

Peripheral Nerve Biopsy

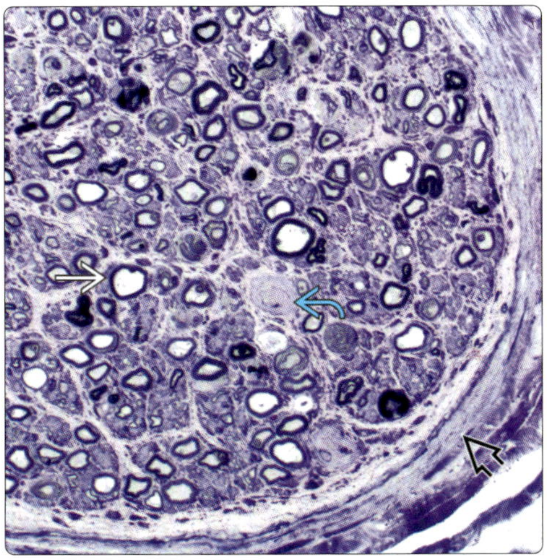

Skeletal Muscle Biopsy: Inclusion Body Myositis

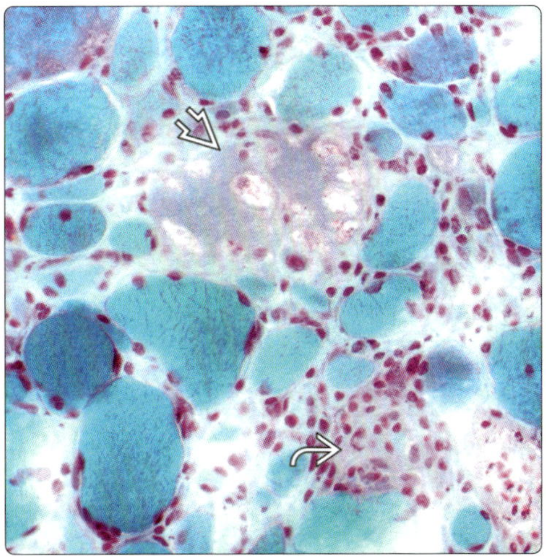

(Left) *A 1-µm plastic-embedded section of glutaraldehyde-fixed sural nerve shows myelinated axons, endoneurial blood vessels, and perineurium. From this block, ultrathin sections are cut for electron microscopy and diagnosis.* **(Right)** *Trichrome stain on a frozen section shows the features of inclusion body myositis, including variability in fiber diameter, fibers with rimmed vacuoles (granular debris in vacuoles), myophagocytosis, and endomysial chronic inflammation.*

SURGICAL/CLINICAL CONSIDERATIONS

Goal of Consultation

- Identify mass within peritoneum as benign or malignant

Change in Patient Management

- Planned surgery may be altered if malignancy is identified
  - If presence of malignancy is unexpected, search for primary site may be undertaken
  - In cases of known malignancy, presence of metastatic disease may change type of planned surgery
- For women with ovarian lesions, peritoneum or omentum may be sampled to determine if invasive implant is present
  - If found, surgeon may choose to place port for chemotherapy

Clinical Setting

- During abdominal surgery for benign or malignant conditions, surgeon routinely explores abdominal cavity
- It is important to determine if any masses found are benign or malignant to guide subsequent surgery

SPECIMEN EVALUATION

Gross

- Masses are generally completely removed as small excisional biopsies
  - In patient with ovarian mass, omentum may be removed and sent for intraoperative consultation to assess presence and types of implants
- In general, mass does not need to be inked as primary isolated malignancies of peritoneum are exceedingly rare
- Tissue is serially sectioned
  - Focal lesions are identified
    - Size, number, color, and borders of lesions are recorded

Frozen Section

- Small biopsies are completely frozen
- In large samples, areas of fleshy tumor growth should be preferentially sampled
  - Areas of extensive necrosis or mucin should be avoided as they are often nondiagnostic
  - Diffusely infiltrative carcinomas in omentum may be slightly paler and firmer than normal adipose tissue
  - Frozen section evaluation of grossly normal specimen is low yield and generally contraindicated

MOST COMMON DIAGNOSES

Metastatic Carcinoma (Nonovarian)

- If patient has history of malignancy, or known current malignancy, it is important to know histologic type and whether or not patient has been treated
- Tumors of gastrointestinal tract often metastasize to peritoneum and have variety of histologic presentations
  - Colon cancer is typically composed of glands with varying degrees of cystic dilation
    - Tall columnar tumor cells line glands
    - Extensive central "dirty" necrosis is common
  - Pancreatic carcinomas are often metastatic at time of surgery
    - Presence of mucinous glands, desmoplasia, and perineural invasion are often helpful features in identifying this tumor
    - Surgery for curative intent is often aborted if metastatic disease is identified
  - Signet ring cell gastric carcinoma may metastasize widely
    - Small tumor cells with little cytoplasmic mucin may resemble histiocytes or lymphocytes and be difficult to identify
    - Enlarged cells with abundant mucin vacuoles that displace nuclei are easier to identify
    - Lobular carcinoma of breast may have strikingly similar appearance and should be included in differential diagnosis if primary is unknown
    - These carcinomas are typically not associated with desmoplastic response
      - Infiltrated adipose tissue may be slightly paler and firmer than normal tissue
      - Tumor cells can mimic reactive mesothelial cells

Peritoneal Inclusion Cysts

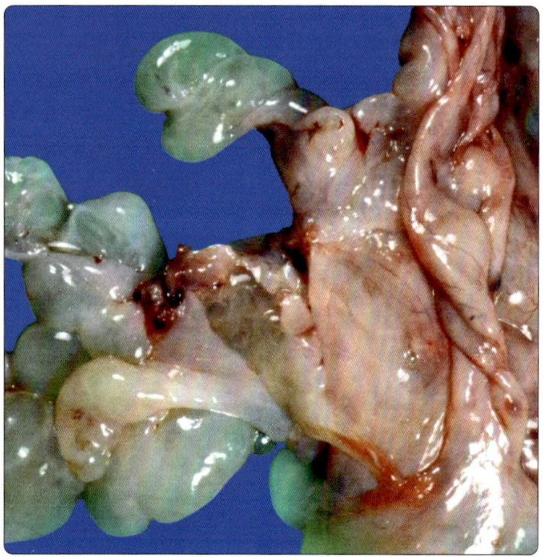

Peritoneal Inclusion Cyst

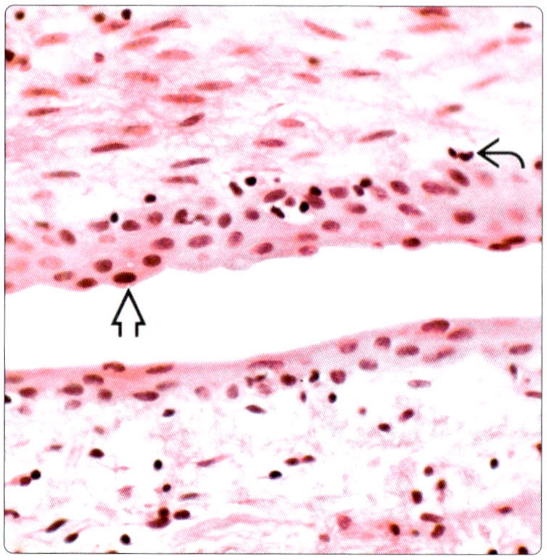

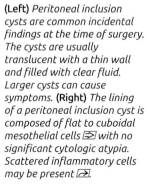

(Left) *Peritoneal inclusion cysts are common incidental findings at the time of surgery. The cysts are usually translucent with a thin wall and filled with clear fluid. Larger cysts can cause symptoms.* **(Right)** *The lining of a peritoneal inclusion cyst is composed of flat to cuboidal mesothelial cells ⇨ with no significant cytologic atypia. Scattered inflammatory cells may be present ⇨.*

- Pseudomyxoma peritonei is often secondary to appendiceal primary
  - Specimen is primarily composed of mucin
  - Only scant foci of mucinous epithelium may be present and may not be seen on frozen section
- Neuroendocrine tumors are typically composed of nests, cords, or trabeculae of tumor cells, which display vesicular (i.e., "salt and pepper") chromatin
- Cancers from nonabdominal sites also metastasize to abdomen but are less common

Ovarian Carcinoma

- In women with ovarian masses, serous tumors (borderline, low grade, and high grade) are most likely to be associated with metastases
  - High-grade carcinomas frequently display striking nuclear atypia, increased mitotic activity, and widespread dissemination
  - Low-grade carcinomas often show destructive invasion of underlying structures but are cytologically bland compared to their high-grade counterparts
- Women with tumors of low malignant potential (borderline tumors) may have extraovarian implants at time of surgery
  - Type of implant is important prognostic factor
- **Noninvasive implant (borderline tumor)**
  - Desmoplastic: Associated with marked stromal reaction
    - Form smoothly contoured foci of glands surrounded by fibrous stroma
    - Papillae and glandular structures often present
  - Epithelial: Not associated with marked stromal reaction
    - Circumscribed clusters of glands
    - May have branching papillae and detached cell clusters
- **Invasive implant (low-grade serous carcinoma)**
  - Shows definite, irregular, destructive invasion with desmoplasia into normal underlying tissue structures
- If invasive implant is definitively identified on frozen section, surgeon may opt to place catheter for chemotherapy at time of surgery

Mesothelial Lesions

- **Mesothelial hyperplasia**
  - Reactive mesothelial hyperplasia is relatively common finding
    - Inciting source of irritation, such as peritonitis or endometriosis, is often present
    - By definition, invasion into underlying tissue is not present
    - Numerous patterns can be seen
      - Tufts
      - Papillae
      - Spindle cells
      - Tubules
      - Solid nests
      - Single cells
    - Mesothelial cells generally show minimal nuclear atypia
      - Mitoses are absent or rare
      - Usually have abundant cytoplasm
    - Necrosis can be present
- **Low-grade (well-differentiated) mesothelioma**
  - May present as cystic or papillary masses
    - More common in women
    - Generally detected as incidental finding during surgery
    - Usually < 2 cm in size (although rare lesions are diffuse)
    - Papillae have simple architecture
      - Single cell layer
      - Monomorphic nuclei with minimal to no atypia
      - Mitotic figures are rare or absent
    - Invasion is not present
    - Reactive and low-grade mesothelial lesions may be impossible to differentiate on frozen section, and extensive sampling for permanent sections should be performed
- **Malignant mesothelioma**
  - May present with myriad histologic patterns, including papillary, tubulopapillary, solid, sarcomatoid, and epithelioid
    - Tumors are often bulky and widespread and display invasion, necrosis, increased mitotic activity, and nuclear atypia
    - However, areas may be low grade in appearance and mimic a well-differentiated or reactive tumor
    - These tumors are typically readily evident at surgery

Adenomatoid Tumor

- Benign proliferation of mesothelial cells
- Can occur in subserosa of uterus and in fallopian tube as well as testis and epididymis
  - Also rarely occurs at extragenital sites, such as mesentery or omentum
- Form firm, gray-tan nodules that are usually small but can be as large as 3 cm
  - Lymphocytic infiltrate or germinal centers are common findings
- Cells line tubular spaces or form cords
  - Borders can be infiltrative
  - May be present in smooth muscle or dense stroma
- Cells have low cuboidal epithelium with prominent cell borders
  - Vacuoles can mimic mucin vacuoles
  - Nuclear atypia should be minimal and mitoses rare

Peritoneal Inclusion Cysts

- Usually occur in young to middle-aged women
- Can be single or multiple
- Cysts are typically unilocular with thin walls
  - Lined by single layer of bland mesothelial cells
  - Filled with clear fluid
- Small cysts are common incidental findings
- Large cysts can be symptomatic
  - Some are multilocular
  - Squamous metaplasia may be present

Endometriosis

- Occurs in women of reproductive age
- Grossly forms red to black masses (has appearance of powder burns)
  - Hemorrhage and inflammation can lead to adhesions
- Definitive diagnosis requires 3 components

- Endometrial glands
  - Tall columnar cells in single layer
- Endometrial-type stroma
  - Short spindle cells
  - Can be decidualized
- Hemosiderin-laden macrophages due to hemorrhage

- Glands may be difficult to identify in some cases
  - Presence of endometrial-type stroma and stigmata of hemorrhage are consistent with endometriosis
- Polypoid endometriosis forms large cystic masses in bowel wall
- Pseudoxanthomatous endometriosis has central necrosis and surrounding chronic inflammation
  - Pseudoxanthoma cells contain hemofuscin

Endosalpingiosis

- Occurs in women
  - Usually incidental finding
  - Less commonly forms small, white or yellow solid nodules or cysts on peritoneum
  - May also be found in lymph nodes
- Consists of small, scattered, simple glands lined by tubal-type epithelium
  - Occasionally, larger cysts, simple intraluminal papillae, or cellular stratification may be present
  - Lined by secretory-type cells, peg cells, and ciliated cells
  - Unlike endometriosis, glands are not accompanied by specific stroma

Endocervicosis

- Benign endocervical-type glands found in cul-de-sac and posterior uterine serosa
  - Mucinous glands display basally oriented nuclei and abundant, eosinophilic mucinous cytoplasm

Decidual Reaction

- Commonly encountered in pregnant women undergoing cesarean section
  - Also occurs with persistent corpus luteum or exogenous hormone use
- Forms white masses, plaques, or polypoid masses in peritoneum or in lymph nodes
- Consists of small collections of large, polygonal, eosinophilic cells with central round nuclei
  - Should not be mistaken for squamous cell carcinoma

Gliomatosis

- Presence of mature glial tissue on peritoneal surfaces
  - Ectopic tissue is identical to mature glial tissue in central nervous system
    - Small round nuclei
    - Abundant eosinophilic fibrillary cytoplasm
- May be associated with ovarian teratoma
  - Does not alter prognosis

Splenosis

- Often associated with prior abdominal trauma
- Splenosis presents as single accessory spleen or scattered, red to brown nodules
- Histologically identical to splenic parenchyma

Peritoneal Leiomyomatosis

- May be primary or secondary to morcellation of uterine leiomyomas
- Only occurs in women
- Histologically similar to uterine leiomyomas
  - Composed of bland, spindled cells with cigar-shaped nuclei arranged in intersecting fascicles

Developmental Remnants

- Mesonephric remnants are found near fallopian tube
  - Scattered glandular structures surrounded by small bundles of smooth muscle and lined by low cuboidal epithelium
    - Eosinophilic secretions may be present in glandular lumina
- Displaced pancreatic tissue can be present in wall of small intestine
- Urachal remnants occur in dome of urinary bladder

Fat Necrosis

- May present as circumscribed or irregular firm mass that may be calcified
  - Varying sized fat droplets, macrophages, and calcifications (depending on chronicity)

Infarcted Epiploic Appendage

- Generally round and firm with gritty cut surface due to calcification
  - Fat necrosis and calcification are diagnostic findings
- Nodule may be too calcified to cut on cryostat
  - In such cases, presumptive diagnosis can be made based on gross appearance

Granulomatous Peritonitis

- Granulomas can be found in peritoneum for many reasons
- Keratin
  - May be due to inflammatory changes with squamous metaplasia
  - Also associated with ruptured mature teratomas or endometrioid adenocarcinomas with squamous differentiation
- Infections
  - *Mycobacterium tuberculosis*
    - Rare in USA
    - May not have pulmonary disease and may have negative skin test
  - Fungi
- Foreign material
  - Barium or plant material can be dispersed into peritoneum after bowel perforation
    - Barium has appearance of gold granular material in histiocytes
    - Plant material has thick cell walls
      - Can be recognized as refractile material by lowering condenser
  - After healing, can form firm peritoneal nodules
  - Polarization is helpful to identify foreign material
- Sarcoidosis

Actinomycetes

- Formation of multiple peritoneal necrotic masses closely mimics carcinoma clinically

- Diagnosis is usually made only after surgery
- Associated with long-term use of intrauterine devices
- Abscess formation with acute inflammation is typical
  - Sulfur granules consist of filamentous bodies
  - Reactive fibrosis and necrosis can be marked
- Bacteria are anaerobic and require special culture

Sclerosing Mesenteritis

- Reactive condition that mimics malignancy
  - Often patients present with abdominal pain, weight loss, and bowel obstruction
  - Large masses or scattered nodular masses may be present in mesentery
- Lesion has lobular architecture divided by fibrous bands
  - Lobules are composed of varying amounts of fat cells (many of which are undergoing fat necrosis), chronic inflammatory cells, and scattered calcifications

Liver Capsule Lesions

- **Bile duct hamartoma**
  - Also termed von Meyenburg complex
  - Forms white capsular nodules that are often multiple and usually small (< 0.5 cm)
  - Lesion consists of circumscribed proliferation of well-formed ducts
    - Often has intraluminal bile
    - Stroma can be loose or sclerotic
    - Cells are cuboidal without atypia, mitoses, or architectural atypia
- **Bile duct adenoma**
  - Forms capsular mass that is usually solitary and small (< 1 cm) but can be large (up to 4 cm)
  - Consists of circumscribed proliferation of small tubules
    - May have intraluminal mucin
    - Stroma is fibrous
    - Cells are cuboidal without atypia or mitoses
    - Tubules may be in closely packed, back-to-back pattern
- Prior treatment can cause cytologic atypia that can make distinction from malignancy difficult
  - Surgeon should provide pathologist with information about treatment

REPORTING

Frozen Section

- **Known primary malignancy**
  - If histologic features of the primary tumor and the peritoneal tumor are similar, specimen may be confidently diagnosed as metastasis
- **Unknown primary**
  - In cases in which a primary neoplasm is undefined, reporting "adenocarcinoma, not otherwise specified" is appropriate
  - If characteristic histologic features are present, an attempt to identify primary site may be appropriate
    - e.g., report "adenocarcinoma with 'dirty' necrosis, suggestive of colonic origin"
- **Lesions of indeterminate malignancy**
  - In cases of unknown malignant potential, the phrase "at least" should be utilized to convey minimum potential of lesion
    - Report "at least reactive mesothelial hyperplasia, low-grade mesothelioma cannot be completely excluded, final diagnosis deferred to permanent sections" if lesion is not definitely benign
- **Benign, identifiable lesions**
  - Common, benign lesions should be simply stated to avoid confusion (e.g., endometriosis)
- **Ovarian implants**
  - If implant shows clear obvious invasion, this can be reported
  - If features of invasion are not definitive, it is preferable to defer classification to permanent sections

PITFALLS

Metastatic Carcinoma vs. Benign Lesions

- There are many lesions that form benign glands or pseudoglands in peritoneum
- If patient has known malignancy, it is very helpful to compare histologic appearances
  - Metastases usually closely resemble primary carcinoma
- If definitive diagnosis of malignancy cannot be made, it may be preferable to defer diagnosis to permanent sections

SELECTED REFERENCES

1. Baker PM et al: Selected topics in peritoneal pathology. Int J Gynecol Pathol. 33(4):393-401, 2014
2. Churg A et al: The separation of benign and malignant mesothelial proliferations. Arch Pathol Lab Med. 136(10):1217-26, 2012
3. Malpica A et al: Well-differentiated papillary mesothelioma of the female peritoneum: a clinicopathologic study of 26 cases. Am J Surg Pathol. 36(1):117-27, 2012
4. Vlachos K et al: Sclerosing mesenteritis: diverse clinical presentations and dissimilar treatment options. a case series and review of the literature. Int Arch Med. 4:17, 2011
5. Miedema JR et al: Practical issues for frozen section diagnosis in gastrointestinal and liver diseases. J Gastrointestin Liver Dis. 19(2):181-5, 2010
6. Clement PB: The pathology of endometriosis: a survey of the many faces of a common disease emphasizing diagnostic pitfalls and unusual and newly appreciated aspects. Adv Anat Pathol. 14(4):241-60, 2007
7. Rakha E et al: Accuracy of frozen section in the diagnosis of liver mass lesions. J Clin Pathol. 59(4):352-4, 2006
8. Hoekstra AV et al: Well-differentiated papillary mesothelioma of the peritoneum: a pathological analysis and review of the literature. Gynecol Oncol. 98(1):161-7, 2005
9. Longacre TA et al: Ovarian serous tumors of low malignant potential (borderline tumors): outcome-based study of 276 patients with long-term (> or =5-year) follow-up. Am J Surg Pathol. 29(6):707-23, 2005
10. Lunca S et al: Abdominal wall actinomycosis associated with prolonged use of an intrauterine device: a case report and review of the literature. Int Surg. 90(4):236-40, 2005
11. Younes M: Frozen section of the gastrointestinal tract, appendix, and peritoneum. Arch Pathol Lab Med. 129(12):1558-64, 2005
12. Coban A et al: Abdominal actinomycosis: a case report. Acta Chir Belg. 103(5):521-3, 2003
13. Wagenlehner FM et al: Abdominal actinomycosis. Clin Microbiol Infect. 9(8):881-5, 2003
14. Daya D et al: Pathology of the peritoneum: a review of selected topics. Semin Diagn Pathol. 8(4):277-89, 1991
15. Bell DA et al: Peritoneal implants of ovarian serous borderline tumors. histologic features and prognosis. Cancer. 62(10):2212-22, 1988

(Left) *The glands of endosalpingiosis are lined by fallopian tube-type cells. The glands can be found in the fibroadipose tissue of the peritoneum and omentum or within lymph nodes. The majority of lesions are incidental findings, but some are large and multicystic and can mimic malignancy.* **(Right)** *The benign glands of endosalpingiosis are lined by tubal secretory-type cells. The presence of ciliated cells ➔ is an important feature to identify the benign nature of the glands.*

Endosalpingiosis

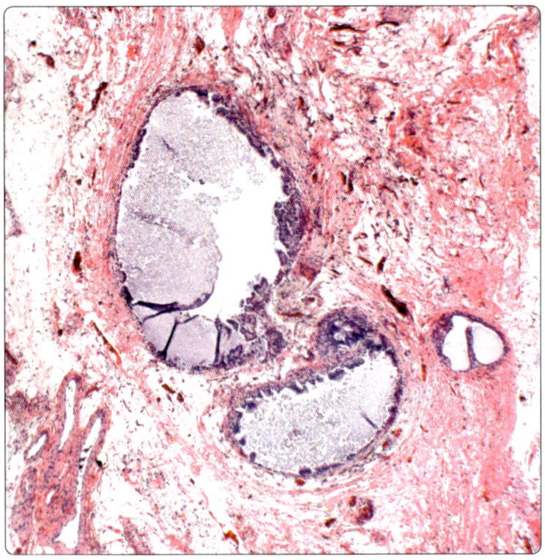

Endosalpingiosis

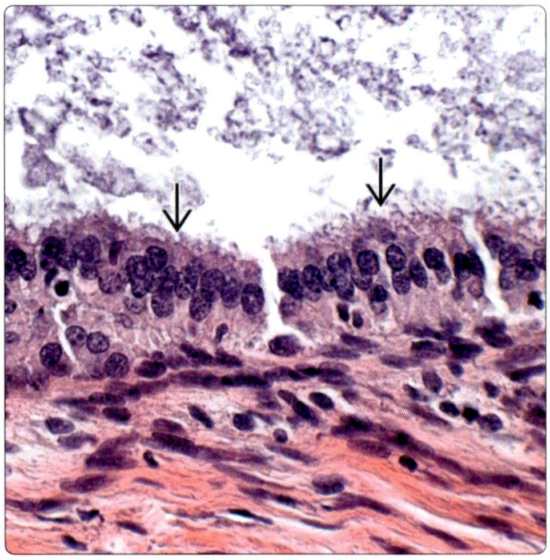

(Left) *Endocervicosis is the presence of benign glands in ectopic locations lined by mucin-producing cells that resemble the cells of the endocervix. If the cysts rupture, the extravasated mucin can cause inflammation, fibrosis, and adhesions.* **(Right)** *Mesonephric remnants are often found in the region of the adnexa and are composed of smooth muscle stroma ➔ with scattered glands with a flat to cuboidal lining ➚. Eosinophilic secretions ➔ may be present and are a helpful diagnostic feature.*

Endocervicosis

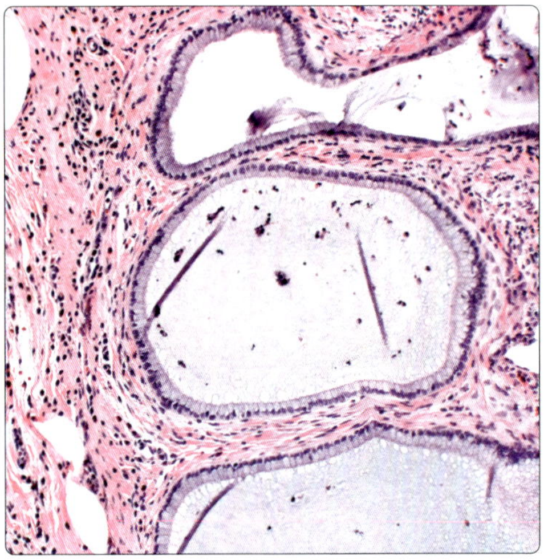

Mesonephric Remnant

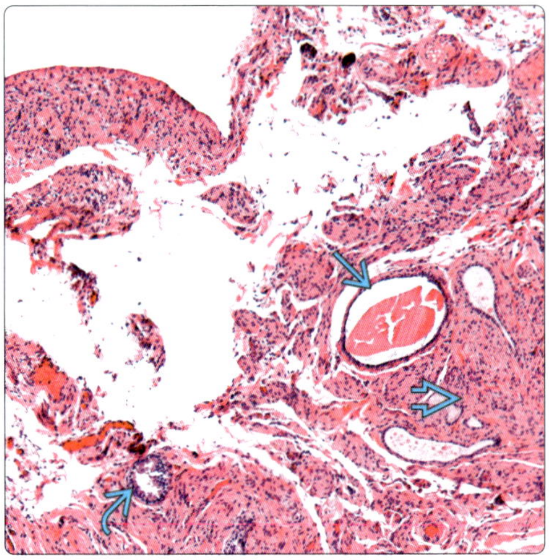

(Left) *Endometriosis appears as blue to brown to black lesions on the peritoneal surface and is composed of endometrial glands ➔ and stroma ➔. Decidual change (deciduosis) may result from high levels of progesterone. Extensively decidualized endometriosis may consist of small glands that are hard to see.* **(Right)** *Hemosiderin ➔ may be seen in the stroma of endometriotic lesions due to cyclic breakdown and hemorrhage. This is a helpful feature to identify this lesion in difficult cases.*

Endometriosis

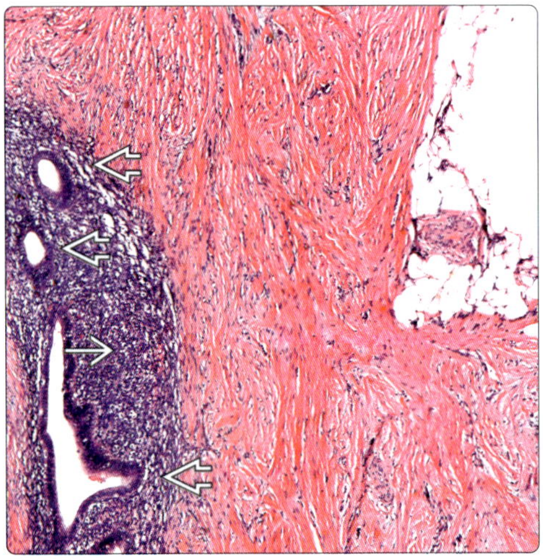

Endometriosis With Hemosiderin

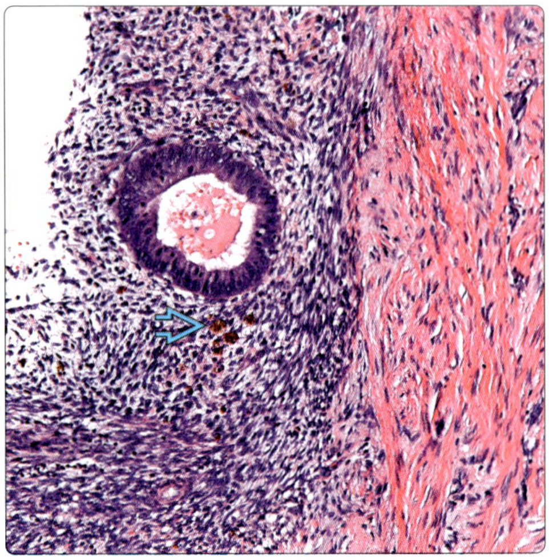

Gliomatosis

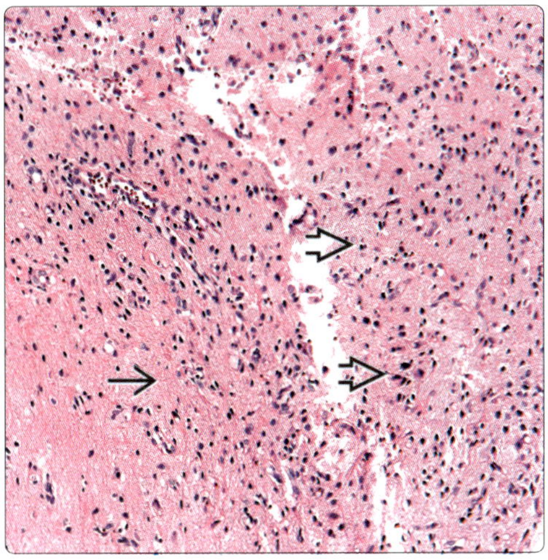

Keratin Granuloma

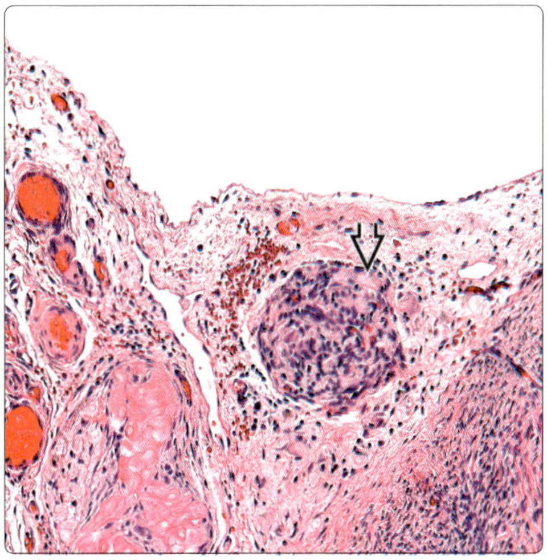

(Left) *Gliomatosis is a rare condition consisting of mature glial tissue in the peritoneum. The cells have small dark nuclei ➲ and abundant fibrillary, eosinophilic cytoplasm →. Gliomatosis is often associated with the presence of a mature cystic teratoma.* **(Right)** *Keratin granulomas are composed of sloughed keratinocytes and macrophages ➲. They are benign but may be associated with mature cystic teratomas or endometrioid adenocarcinomas of the ovary with squamous differentiation.*

Splenosis

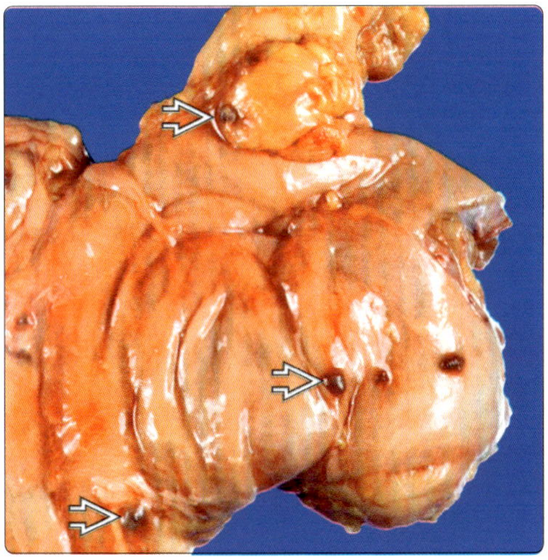

Sclerosing Mesenteritis

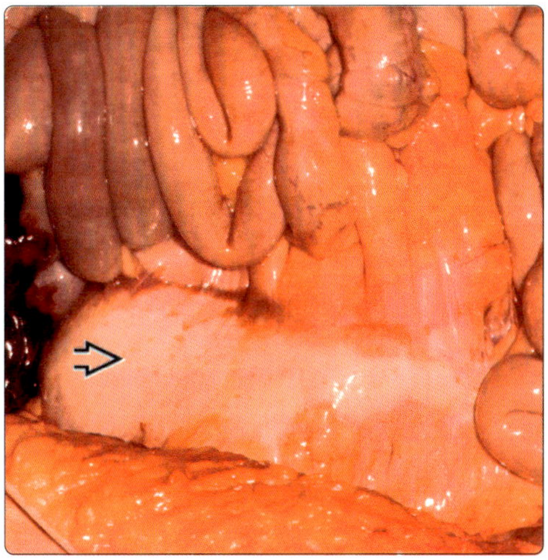

(Left) *Accessory spleens or scattered foci of splenic tissue ➲ (splenosis) may mimic metastatic malignancy and be sent for intraoperative consultation. Histologically, the nodules are composed of unremarkable splenic tissue. They often arise secondary to trauma.* **(Right)** *Sclerosing mesenteritis is a reactive condition that often mimics malignancy. Large masses ➲ or scattered nodules may be present in the mesentery. Often, patients present with abdominal pain, weight loss, and bowel obstruction.*

Sclerosing Mesenteritis

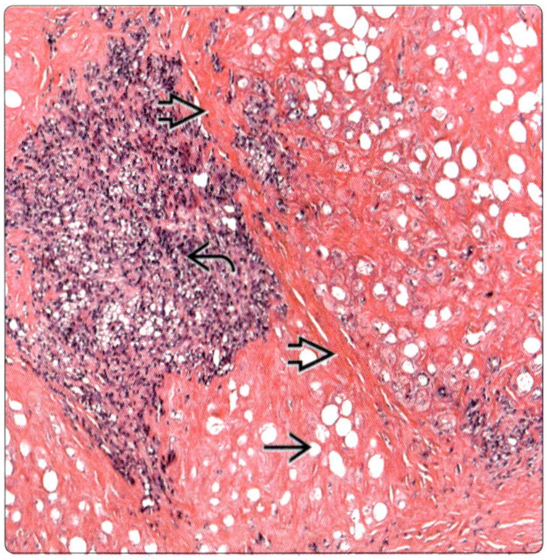

Sclerosing Mesenteritis

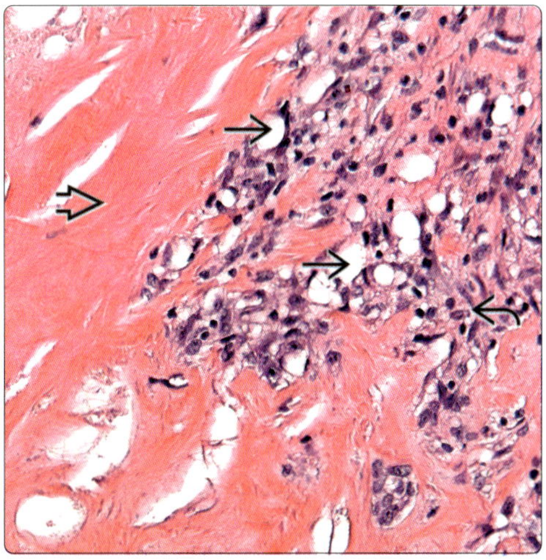

(Left) *Sclerosing mesenteritis has a lobular architecture divided by fibrous bands ➲. The lobules are often composed of varying amounts of fat cells → (many of which are undergoing fat necrosis), chronic inflammatory cells ↩, and scattered calcifications.* **(Right)** *Dense collagen ➲ with admixed adipocytes → and macrophages ↩ are common findings in sclerosing mesenteritis. Scattered lymphocytes and plasma cells are typically present as well.*

(Left) *Inflammatory conditions (e.g., endometriosis ➡) may cause mesothelial hyperplasia. Hyperplasia may be solid, papillary ➡, tubulopapillary, or have a spindled appearance. The lining cells are bland with small nucleoli.* **(Right)** *Well-differentiated papillary mesothelioma is composed of complex papillary structures ➡ that do not invade into the underlying peritoneal structures. These lesions are more common in women and in patients with asbestos exposure.*

Mesothelial Hyperplasia

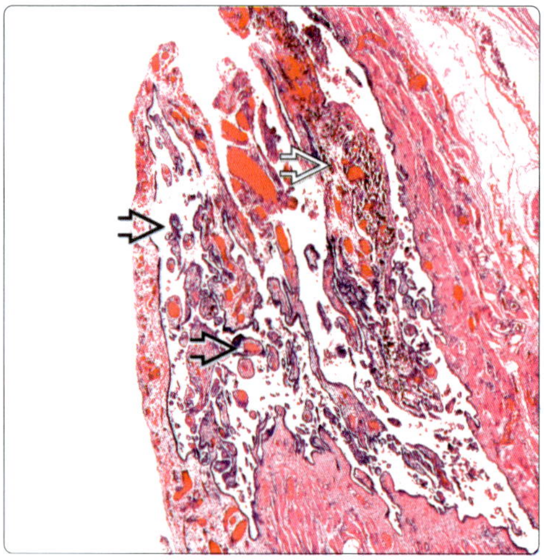

Well-Differentiated Papillary Mesothelioma

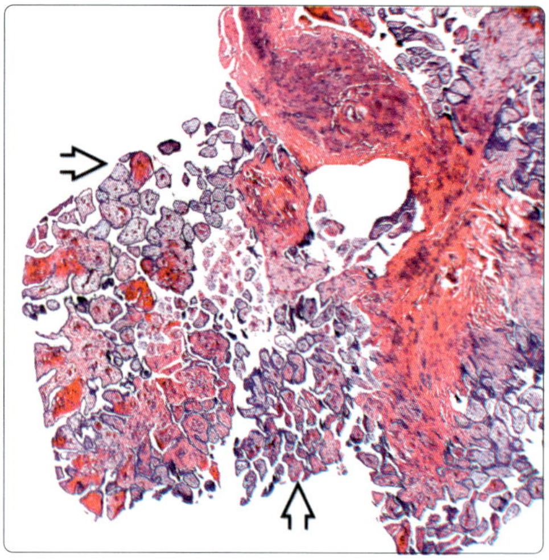

(Left) *The cells that line the papillae of a well-differentiated papillary mesothelioma are low cuboidal ➡ with little to no cytologic atypia or mitotic activity. These cells are essentially indistinguishable from those seen in benign mesothelial hyperplasia.* **(Right)** *This malignant mesothelioma is composed of a prominent papillary component ➡. Invasion of the underlying tissue is one of the most helpful features used in differentiating benign from malignant mesothelioma.*

Well-Differentiated Papillary Mesothelioma

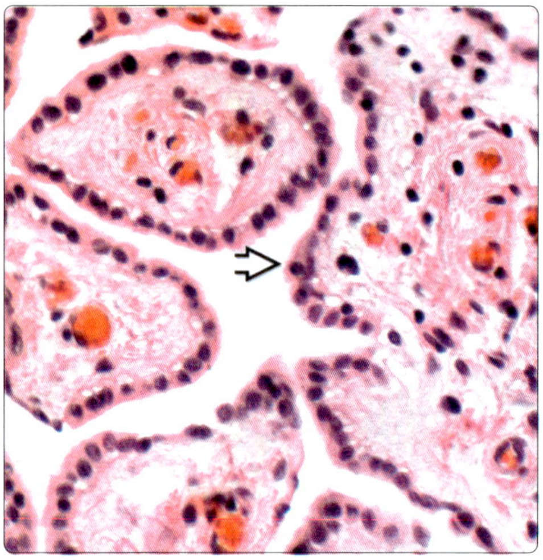

Malignant Mesothelioma

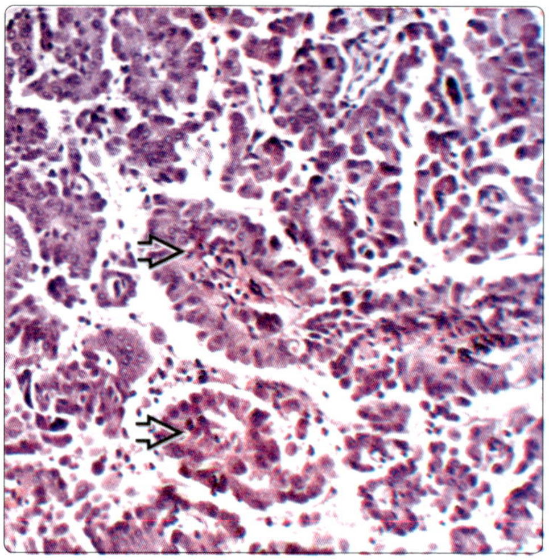

(Left) *Malignant mesothelioma has numerous growth patterns, including solid ➡, papillary ➡, tubular, and tubulopapillary. Psammoma bodies ➡ may be present but occur in benign lesions as well.* **(Right)** *A common histologic appearance of malignant mesothelioma is the sarcomatoid growth pattern. Here, the tumor cells display a spindle cell tumor morphology with elongated cells with oval nuclei ➡. Atypia ➡ and mitotic figures ➡ are often easy to identify.*

Malignant Mesothelioma

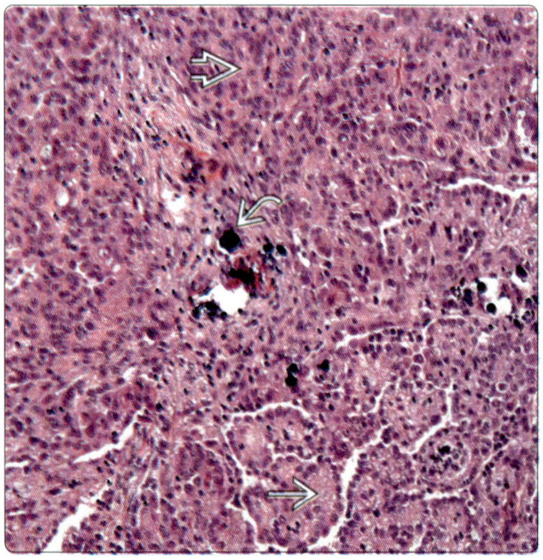

Malignant Mesothelioma: Sarcomatoid Pattern

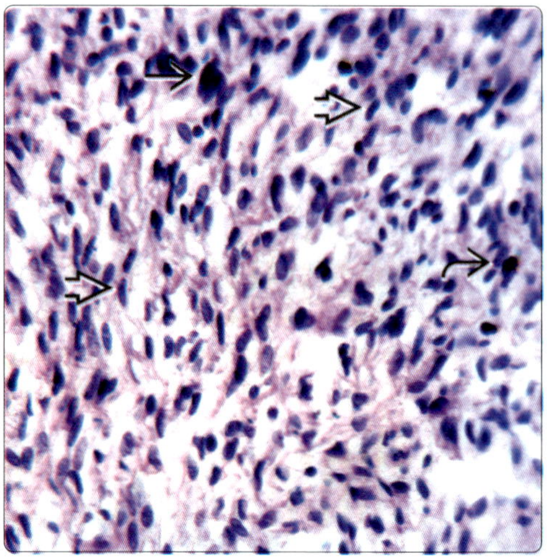

Serous Ovarian Carcinoma

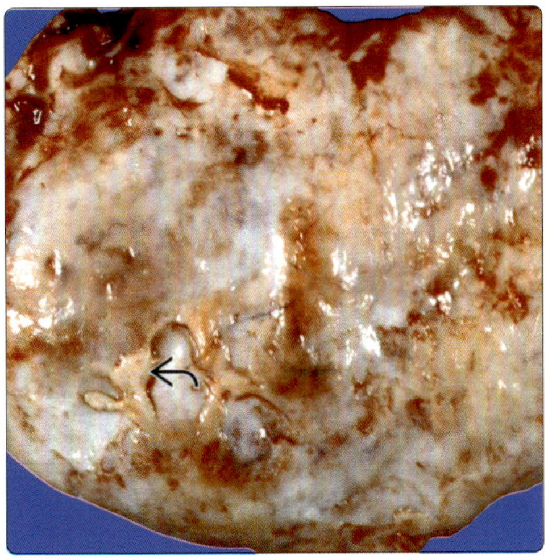

Serous Carcinoma of Ovary

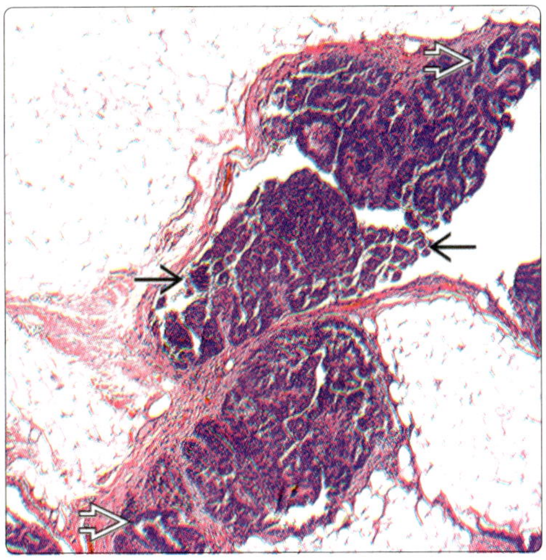

(Left) *High-grade carcinoma, in this case of serous ovarian carcinoma can lead to diffuse thickening of the omentum (so-called omental cake). The omental fat is replaced by a tan-white mass with a firm, gritty texture. Yellow areas correspond to necrosis.* **(Right)** *One of the most commonly encountered tumors involving the omentum is metastatic high-grade serous carcinoma. At low power, the tumor is composed of slit-like glandular spaces and papillary structures.*

Serous Carcinoma of Ovary

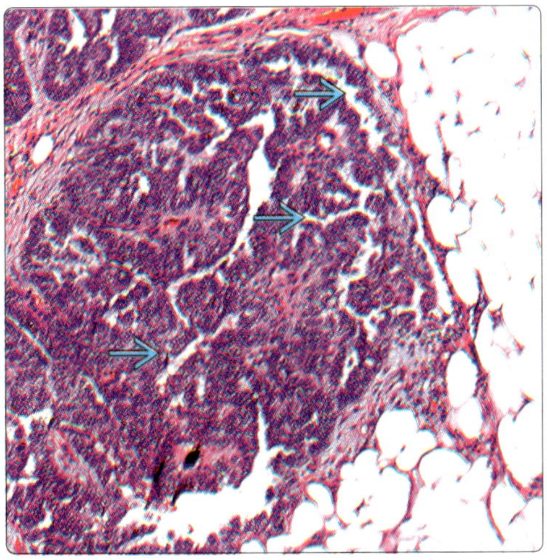

Serous Carcinoma of Ovary

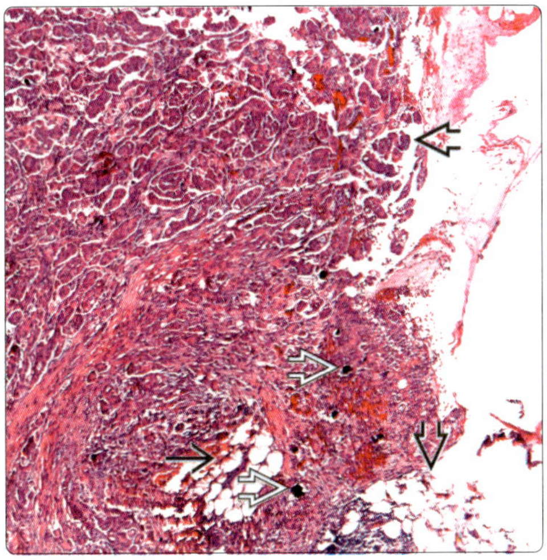

(Left) *The papillary structures in high-grade serous carcinoma often grow together to form nodules with clefted or jagged lumina. This is in contrast to the rounded glandular lumina seen in colonic or endometrioid adenocarcinomas.* **(Right)** *Low-grade serous ovarian carcinoma is typically composed of small papillae and variable numbers of psammoma bodies. The differential diagnosis includes malignant mesothelioma. This carcinoma invades into the adipose tissue.*

Serous Ovarian Carcinoma: Invasive Implant

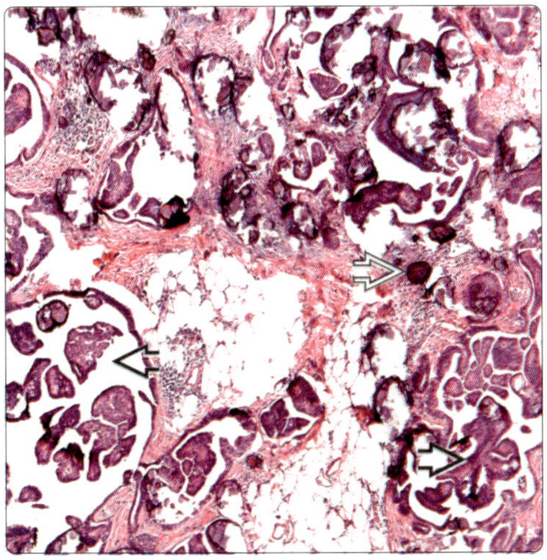

Borderline Ovarian Tumor: Noninvasive Implant

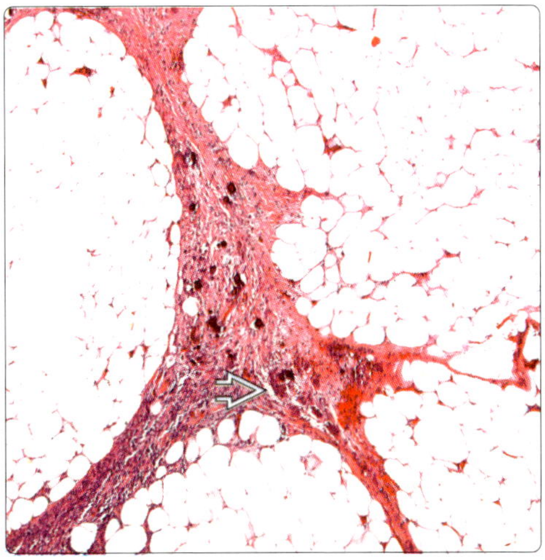

(Left) *This invasive implant from a low-grade serous ovarian carcinoma destroys the normal omental architecture. Numerous papillae and psammoma bodies are usually present. These tumors may be impossible to differentiate from mesothelioma on omental sampling alone.* **(Right)** *A common finding in women with borderline malignancies of the ovary is a noninvasive implant in the omentum. The tumor cells do not invade into the lobules of fat and are limited to the fibrous septa.*

(Left) *Pancreatic carcinoma commonly metastasizes early in its course. Rounded to angulated mucinous glands ⇨ and perineural invasion are common features. Extensive surgery is generally not performed when metastasis is identified.* **(Right)** *Rarely, prostatic adenocarcinoma metastasizes to the peritoneum. Numerous small round glands ⇨ lined by cells with bland nuclei are typical. Luminal basophilic mucin may be present. The appearance can closely mimic metastatic carcinoid tumor.*

Metastatic Pancreatic Carcinoma

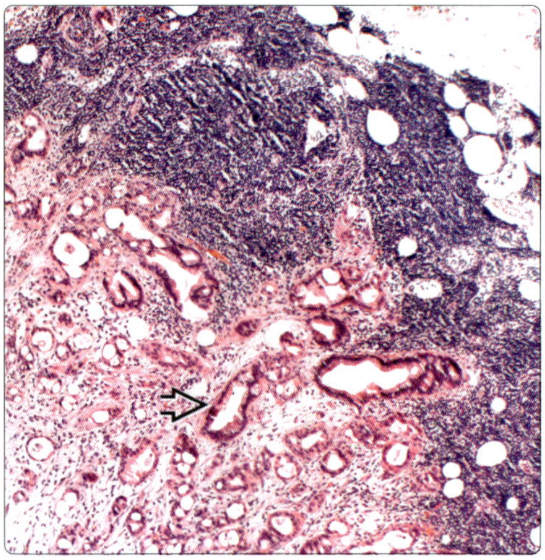

Metastatic Prostate Carcinoma

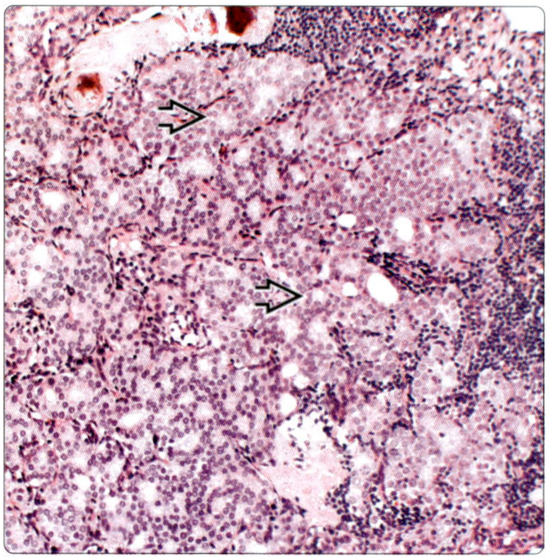

(Left) *Neuroendocrine tumors from the gastrointestinal tract may metastasize to the peritoneum. The presence of cords, nests, or trabeculae ⇨ is a helpful architectural clue. Higher power examination often reveals the traditional salt and pepper stippled nuclear chromatin pattern of a neuroendocrine tumor.* **(Right)** *Spindle cell lesions of the peritoneum can be benign (mesothelial hyperplasia, leiomyomatosis) or malignant (mesothelioma, sarcoma, or carcinoma). This is a case of leiomyosarcoma.*

Metastatic Neuroendocrine Tumor

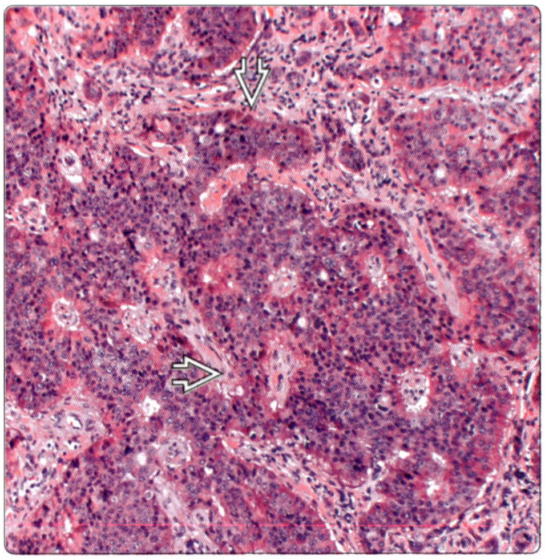

Metastatic Leiomyosarcoma

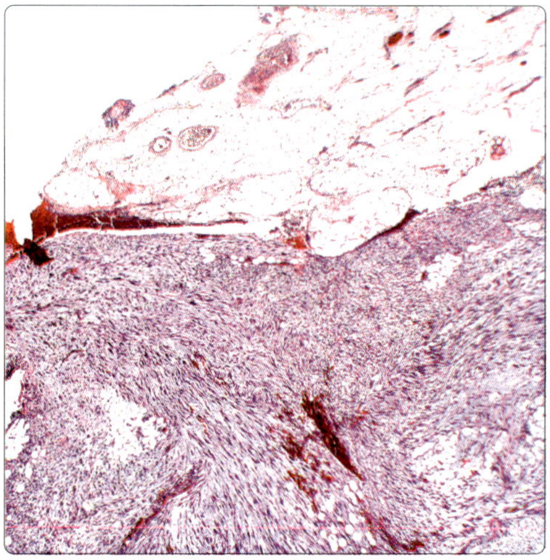

(Left) *Metastatic lobular carcinoma of the breast is easily recognized when numerous cells are present ⇨. However, if only scattered tumor cells are seen →, it may be difficult or impossible to distinguish them from lymphocytes or histiocytes without special studies.* **(Right)** *This metastatic lobular carcinoma → was not initially seen as the cells were obscured by associated inflammation and mesothelial hyperplasia ⇨. Lobular carcinomas can line serosal surfaces and be difficult to detect.*

Metastatic Lobular Carcinoma

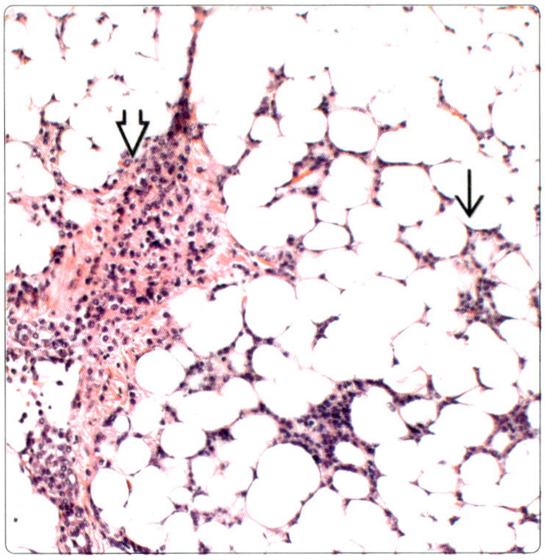

Metastatic Lobular Carcinoma to Peritoneum

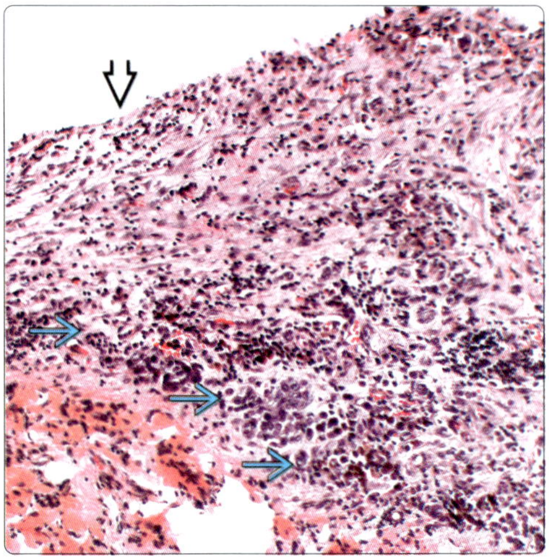

Metastatic Adenocarcinoma

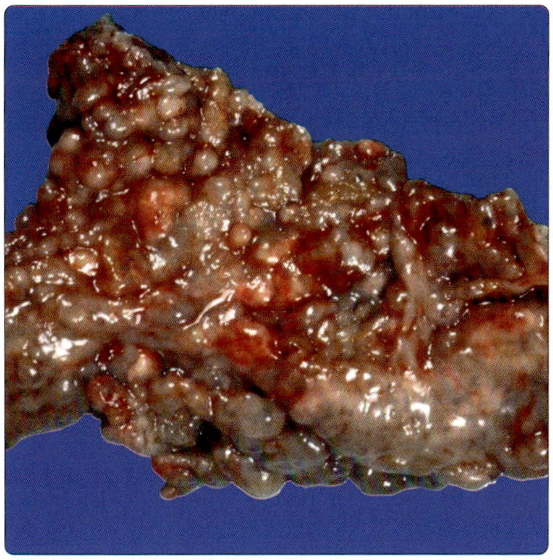

Metastatic Colon Carcinoma

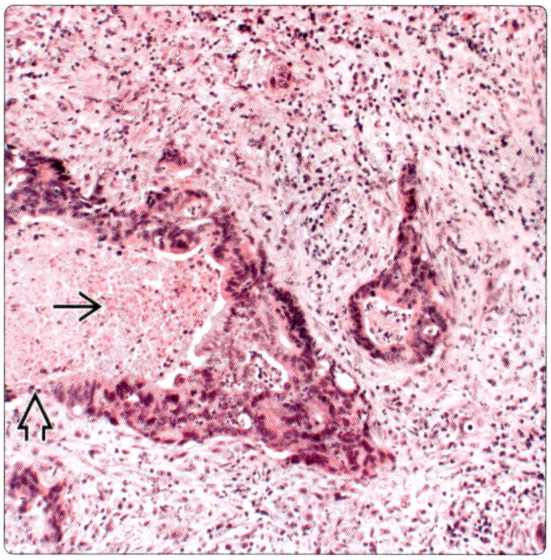

(Left) *Metastatic adenocarcinomas to the omentum tend to have a tan to red and granular surface. Gross mucin and abundant necrosis may be present.* **(Right)** *Metastatic colonic carcinoma typically consists of glands with cystic dilation and central "dirty" necrosis ⇨ composed of necrotic tumor cells and inflammation. The glandular epithelium that lines the cystic spaces may become thinned ⇨ and ribbon-like and is said to resemble a garland. The tumor cells are typically tall and columnar.*

Pseudomyxoma Peritonei

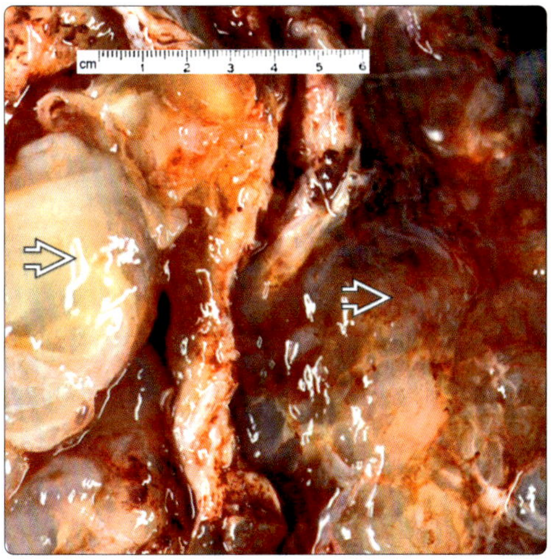

Gastric Signet Ring Cell Carcinoma

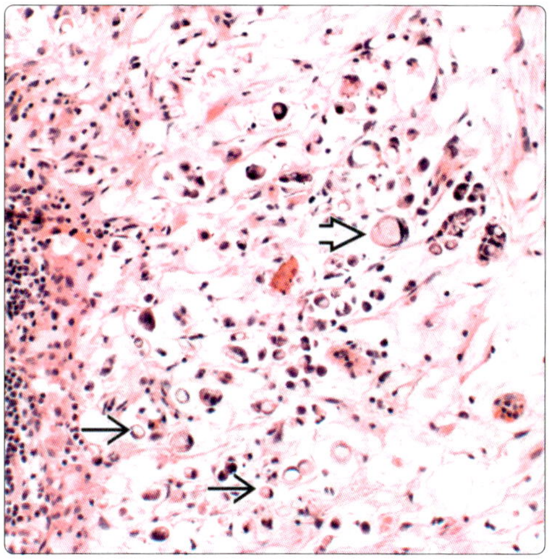

(Left) *Specimens from patients with pseudomyxoma peritonei typically consist of thick mucus ➡ with little to no identifiable gross tumor. (Courtesy G. F. Gray, Jr., MD.)* **(Right)** *Signet ring cell carcinoma may be easily missed. Smaller signet ring cells ⇨ can be mistaken for histiocytes or inflammatory cells. The presence of larger tumor cells ⇨ with intracellular mucin and eccentrically displaced and compressed nuclei are more obvious. Metastatic lobular carcinoma should also be considered.*

Pseudomyxoma Peritonei

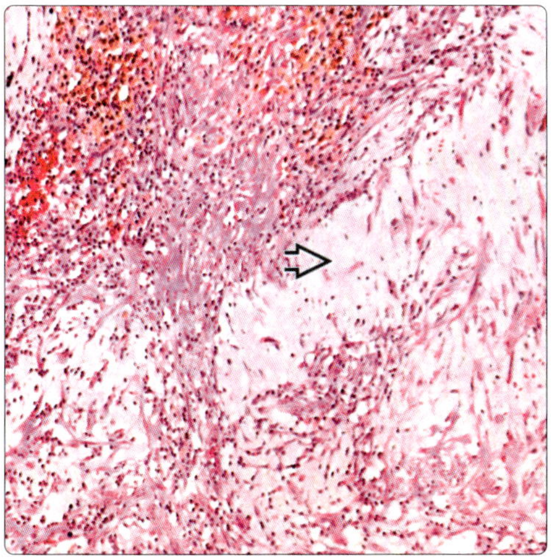

Pseudomyxoma Peritonei

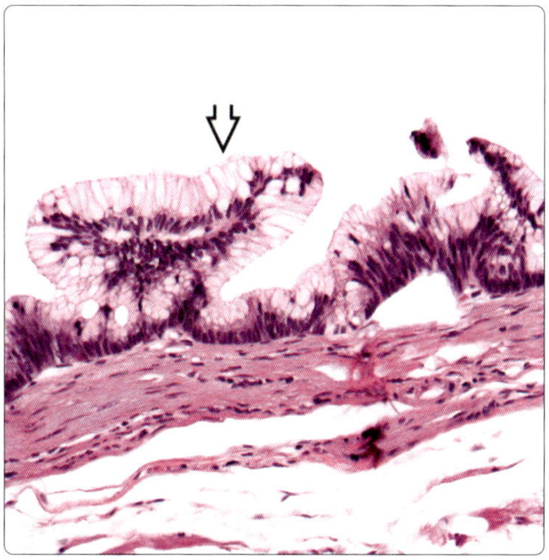

(Left) *Examination of the mucin in cases of pseudomyxoma by intraoperative consultation is generally a low-yield undertaking. In the majority of cases, acellular mucin ⇨ with inflammatory cells is the only finding. It is preferable to extensively sample the specimen for permanent sections. (Courtesy G. F. Gray, Jr., MD.)* **(Right)** *Bland mucinous epithelium ⇨ within mucin pools of pseudomyxoma peritonei confer a worse prognosis than cases without tumor cells. (Courtesy G. F. Gray, Jr., MD.)*

(Left) *Colonic epiploica may infarct, leading to fat necrosis, fibrosis, and central calcification →. The hard spherical mass mimics a metastasis to a lymph node or a tumor implant. These lesions are often too hard to cut without prior decalcification.* **(Right)** *Fat necrosis has a firm, pale cut surface and is composed of an admixture of fat cells of varying sizes → and macrophages → (± calcifications). Masses can form at the site of injury and may mimic a malignant tumor implant.*

Infarcted Epiploic Appendage

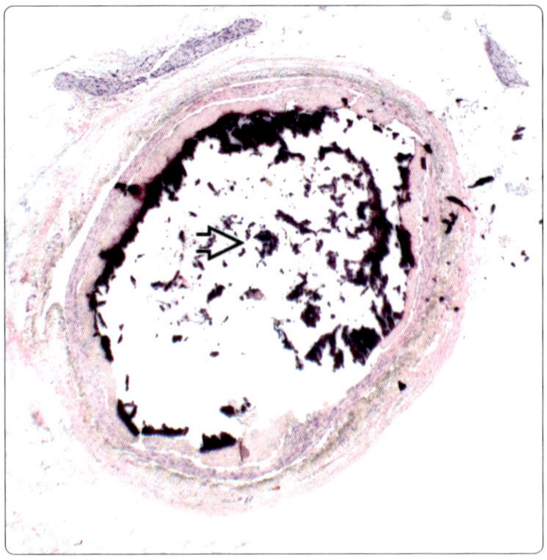

Fat Necrosis

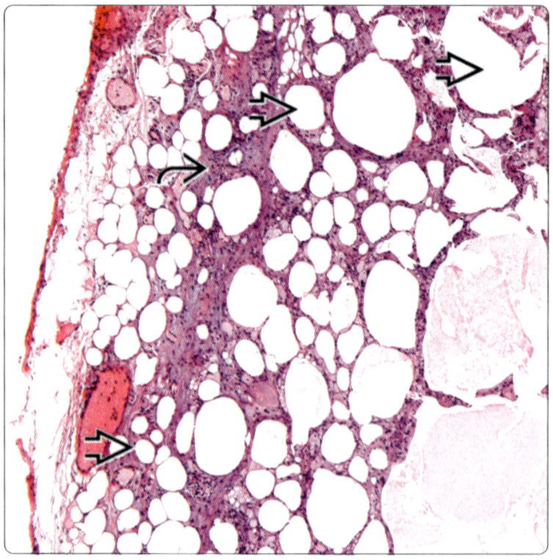

(Left) *Patients often undergo presurgical imaging with barium enemas. If there is a bowel perforation, barium → (refractile and gold in color) may cause inflammation and masses in the abdomen.* **(Right)** *Plant material can be recognized by thick cell walls that are refractive. When present in the peritoneum, it is indicative of a prior bowel perforation. Foreign material can result in the formation of fibrotic nodules and adhesions.*

Barium

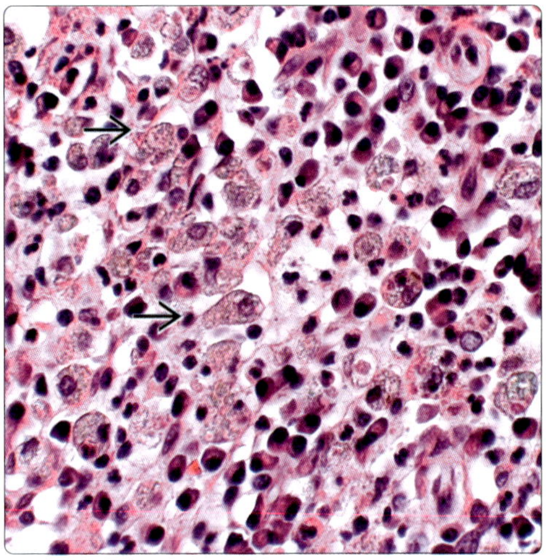

Foreign Material

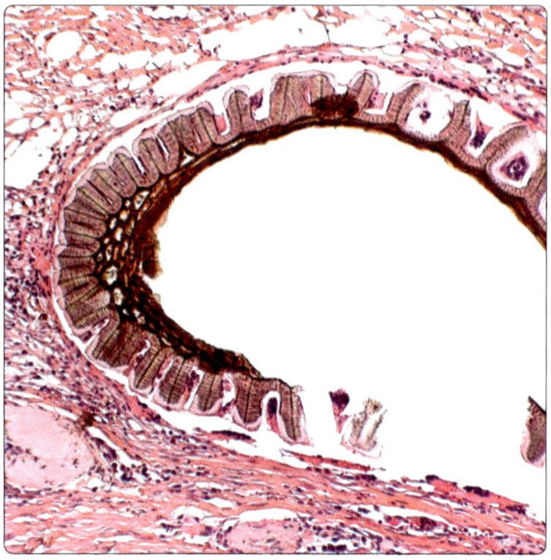

(Left) *Deciduosis presents as yellow, red, or white plaques on the peritoneal surface. They are typically found incidentally at the time of cesarean section. The cells are large, polygonal, and eosinophilic → with no nuclear atypia.* **(Right)** *Decidual change in stromal cells is recognized by the abundant eosinophilic cytoplasm and the round uniform nuclei. This change can mimic squamous cell carcinoma. (Courtesy M. Nucci, MD.)*

Deciduosis

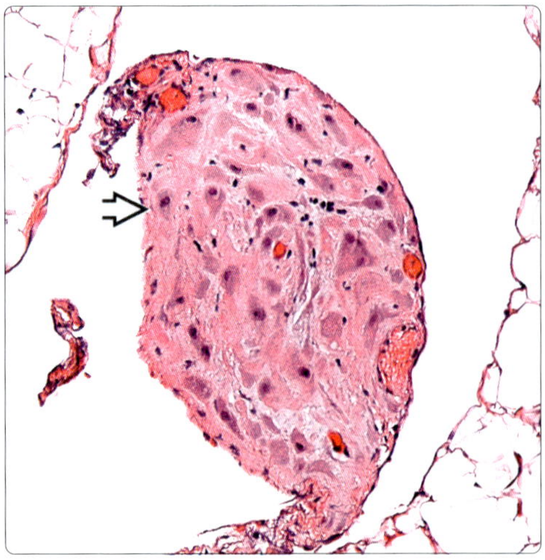

Deciduosis

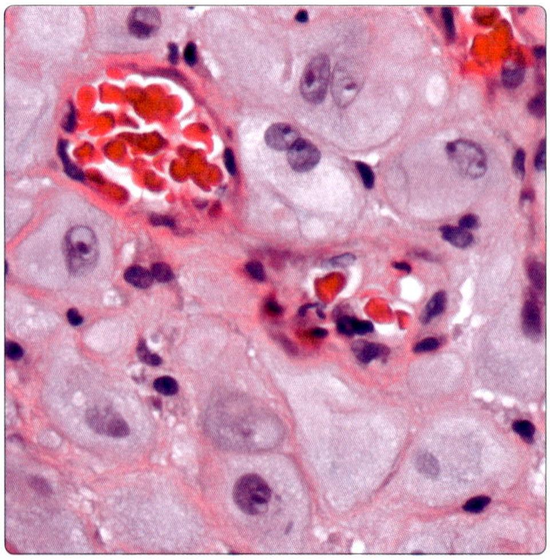

Deciduosis With Vacuolization

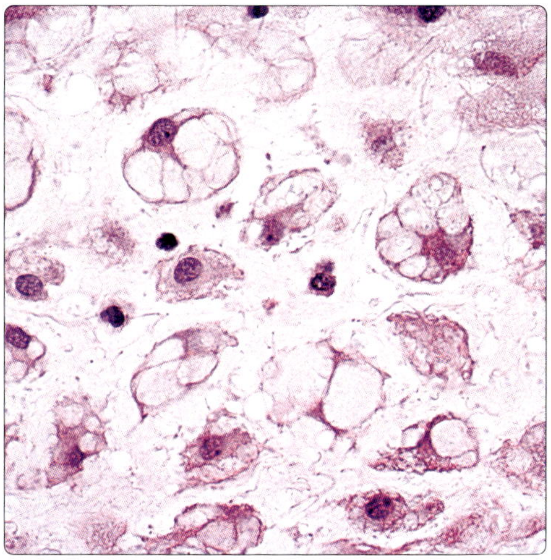

Actinomycetes

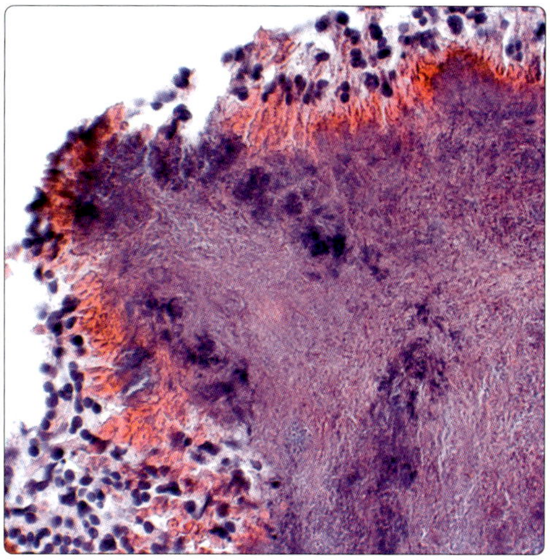

(Left) *Decidua can show marked vacuolization and closely mimic a mucinous signet ring cell carcinoma. The abundant cytoplasm and the bland nuclear appearance are important features. (Courtesy M. Nucci, MD.)* **(Right)** *Infection with actinomycetes can cause fever, abdominal pain, weight loss, and multiple hard abdominal masses that are often thought to be due to advanced malignancy until biopsied. Tissue specimens show acute inflammation and conglomerations of filamentous organisms known as sulfur granules.*

Adenomatoid Tumor: Permanent Section

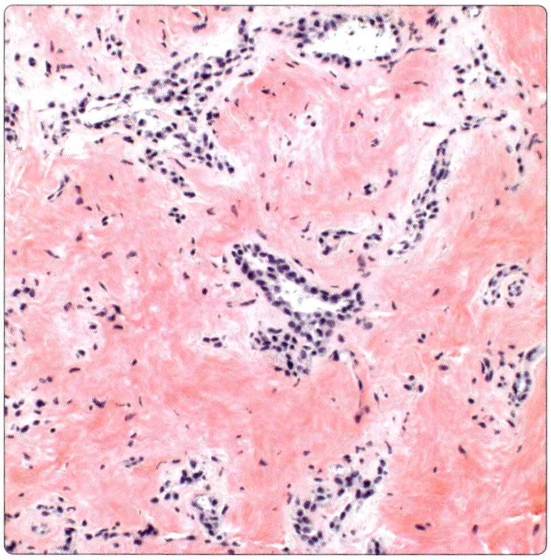

Adenomatoid Tumor: Frozen Section

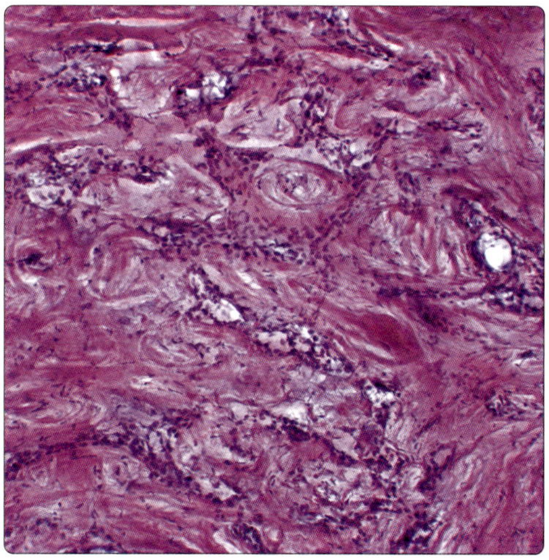

(Left) *Adenomatoid tumors consist of bland cells lining spaces in dense stroma. The appearance can mimic the tubules of adenocarcinoma in desmoplastic stroma.* **(Right)** *On frozen section, the benign features of an adenomatoid tumor are more difficult to appreciate. The thickness of the section obscures the nuclear features. If the patient has a known malignancy, comparison of the histologic appearances is helpful to determine if a nodule sent for frozen section resembles a metastasis.*

Adenomatoid Tumor

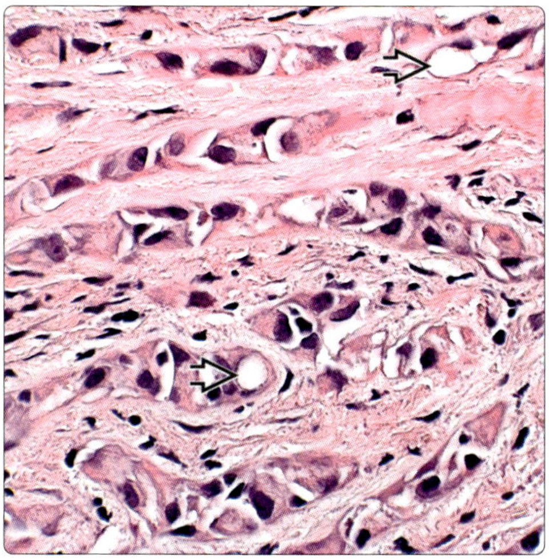

Mesonephric Remnants

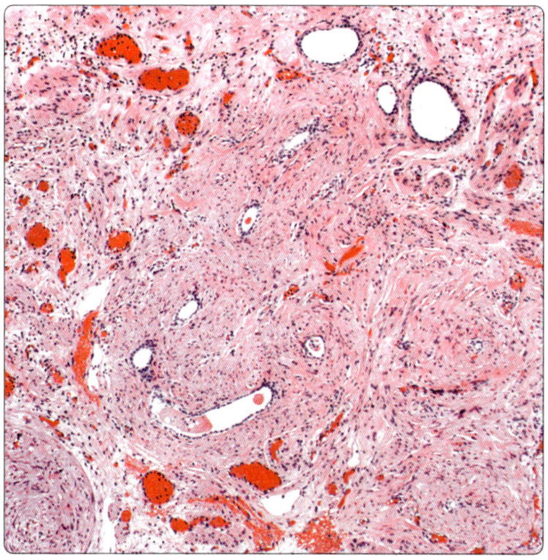

(Left) *Adenomatoid tumors are benign proliferations of mesothelial cells that can form gland-like spaces and infiltrate in fibrous tissue with irregular borders mimicking adenocarcinoma. The presence of vacuoles in some cells ⇨ can resemble mucin.* **(Right)** *Mesonephric remnants are usually found around the reproductive organs or the bladder. The small, well-formed tubules lined by bland cells are associated with smooth muscle.*

Contents

SURGICAL/CLINICAL CONSIDERATIONS

Goal of Consultation

- Ensure diagnostic tissue has been obtained
- Render diagnosis when possible
  - Identify microadenomas
- Ensure completeness of resection

Change in Patient Management

- Additional tissue will be biopsied until diagnostic tissue is obtained
- Lesions causing symptoms due to mass effect will be completely excised, if possible
- Specific diagnosis can help guide surgery
  - **Functional tumors**
    - Pituitary adenomas (including microadenomas), pituitary hyperplasia
    - Diagnosed prior to surgery due to symptoms and elevated serum levels of hormones
    - Adenoma cannot be distinguished from hyperplasia preoperatively
    - Diagnosis can be confirmed intraoperatively
    - If tumor is not completely resected, radiation therapy may be required for treatment
  - **Tumors with high risk of recurrence**
    - Rathke cleft cyst, spindle cell oncocytoma, meningioma, craniopharyngioma, invasive pituitary adenoma
    - May require resection of adjacent structures to prevent recurrence
    - Absence of cavernous sinus invasion may stop surgery for invasive pituitary adenomas
  - **Tumors with low risk of recurrence**
    - Epidermoid and dermoid cysts, paraganglioma, gangliocytoma
    - Removal of main tumor mass is often sufficient for cure
  - **Lesions not requiring surgical resection**
    - Plasmacytoma, lymphoma
    - Treated systemically
- Specimens are small, and frozen section artifact can preclude optimal evaluation
  - Tissue should only be frozen if diagnosis will alter surgical procedure or if surgeon encounters unexpected finding

Clinical Setting

- Patients with pituitary tumors usually present with symptoms due to abnormal function, compression of adjacent structures, or both
- Overproduction of hormones
  - Adrenocorticotrophic hormone (ACTH): Causes adrenal glands to make cortisol (Cushing syndrome)
    - Fat accumulation and upper back hump
    - Hypertension
    - Thin skin and striae
    - Hyperglycemia
    - Anxiety, irritability, or depression
  - Growth hormone (GH)
    - Gigantism: Accelerated and excessive growth in children and adolescents
    - Acromegaly: Coarsened facial features and enlarged hands and feet in adults
    - Hyperglycemia
  - Prolactin (PRL)
    - Can be caused by adenoma or any lesion obstructing pituitary stalk (blood flow normally resulting in inhibition is diminished)
    - Decrease in sex hormones
    - Women: Galactorrhea, irregular or absent menstrual periods
    - Men: Loss of sex drive, infertility
  - Thyroid-stimulating hormone (TSH)
    - Hyperthyroidism: Tachycardia, weight loss, hyperthermia
- Compression of adjacent structures &/or pituitary
  - Headache, nausea, and vomiting
  - Vision loss, especially peripheral vision
  - Pituitary hormone deficiency

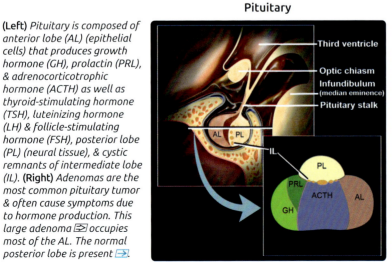

Pituitary

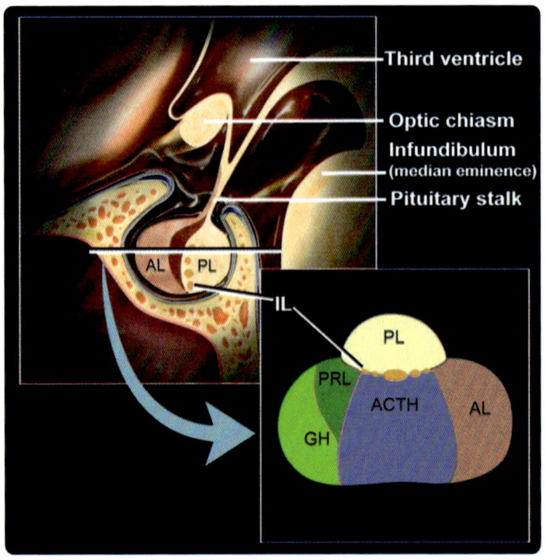

Pituitary Adenoma

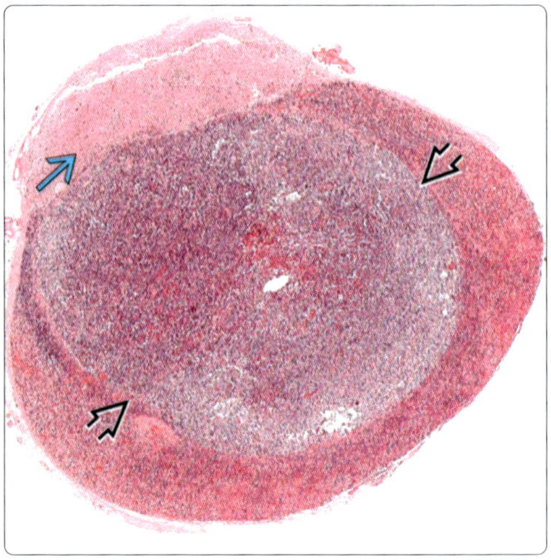

(Left) *Pituitary is composed of anterior lobe (AL) (epithelial cells) that produces growth hormone (GH), prolactin (PRL), & adrenocorticotrophic hormone (ACTH) as well as thyroid-stimulating hormone (TSH), luteinizing hormone (LH) & follicle-stimulating hormone (FSH), posterior lobe (PL) (neural tissue), & cystic remnants of intermediate lobe (IL).* **(Right)** *Adenomas are the most common pituitary tumor & often cause symptoms due to hormone production. This large adenoma ⇨ occupies most of the AL. The normal posterior lobe is present ➔.*

SPECIMEN EVALUATION

Gross

- Pituitary lesions are typically resected as multiple small fragments
  - Adenomas often have soft white, creamy appearance
- Specimen does not need to be inked
- Document size, number of fragments, and color

Frozen Section

- Tissue can be completely frozen after making cytologic preparations
  - Frozen section is best technique to demonstrate architectural pattern
    - Lobular pattern of normal gland
    - Diffuse lobular expansion of adenoma
  - Nuclei of adenomas can appear to be pleomorphic due to frozen section artifact
- If sufficient tissue is present, nonfrozen tissue should be saved for permanent sections and possible ancillary studies

Cytology

- Cytologic preparations (smear or touch preparations) are very helpful to evaluate pituitary adenomas
  - Delicate, loosely cohesive cells
  - Typical neuroendocrine (salt and pepper) chromatin pattern readily appreciated
  - Monomorphic population
- Squash preparations can lead to disintegration of cytoplasm and naked nuclei due to delicate nature of adenomas

MOST COMMON DIAGNOSES

Pituitary Adenoma

- 90% of lesions of sellar region are pituitary adenomas
  - Symptoms often due to overproduction of pituitary hormones
  - Diagnosis is usually known prior to surgery
- Classification as to type of adenoma is not important for intraoperative consultation
- Architectural features
  - Diffuse lobular expansion
    - Normal glands are organized in lobules
  - Epithelial cords and sheets with dyscohesive ends, acini, and papillary formations are seen on cytology
  - Solid, diffuse, trabecular, sinusoidal, and papillary growth patterns are common
    - Perivascular pseudorosette formation and solid papillary growth patterns are usually seen in gonadotroph adenomas
  - Cystic changes can occur
    - Lack of calcifications distinguish cystic adenomas from craniopharyngioma
- Nuclear features
  - Typical neuroendocrine appearance (finely dispersed chromatin with distinct nucleoli)
  - Mild cellular pleomorphism and binucleate forms are common
  - Monomorphic appearance
- Cytoplasmic features
  - Cytoplasmic granularity and staining identifies 3 morphologically distinct cell types
    - Eosinophilic: Characteristic of acidophilic adenomas that produce GH (somatotroph adenomas) or PRL (lactotroph adenomas) but can be nonfunctional
    - Basophilic: These adenomas produce ACTH (corticotrophic adenomas), luteinizing hormone, and follicle-stimulating hormone (gonadotrophic adenomas) or TSH (thyrotropic adenomas) but can be nonfunctional
    - Chromophobic: These adenomas are usually nonfunctional but may produce TSH
  - Normal pituitary glands are composed of all 3 cell types: Eosinophilic, basophilic, and chromophobic
    - Adenomas are composed of single cell population
  - Cytoplasmic contents, depending on functional status, are variably clear with vacuolation or eosinophilic bodies and occasional paranuclear bodies
- Necrosis and mitoses are uncommon
- Psammoma bodies may be present
  - Most common in adenomas producing TSH or PRL
- Invasive adenomas
  - Local extension can involve bone, posterior lobe, dura mater, or respiratory mucosa
  - Not indication of malignancy or capacity for metastasis
    - May recur locally
  - Cytologic features do not predict invasiveness
- Microadenoma
  - < 1 cm in size
  - May be functional or nonfunctional ("incidentaloma")
- Crooke cell adenoma
  - Corticotroph (producing ACTH) adenoma
  - Cytokeratin accumulates in cytoplasm in response to increased glucocorticoids (Crooke hyaline change)
  - 3/4 are invasive and > 1/2 recur locally

Pituitary Hyperplasia

- Occurs secondary to hypersecretion of stimulating hormone by either physiologic or pathologic mechanisms
  - Most common cause is hypothyroidism
- Gland is enlarged and lacks well-defined mass distinguishable from surrounding normal gland
  - May be diffuse within gland or focal with formation of nodules
- Anterior gland is composed of enlarged acini, composed mostly of single cell type
  - Focal or diffuse expansion of acini with preservation of reticulin pattern (reticulin stain)

Posterior Pituitary Lesions

- Anatomically consists of pars nervosa and infundibular stalk
- Composed of axons of magnocellular neurosecretory cells
  - Axons store and release oxytocin and vasopressin
  - Pituicytes are specialized glial cells resembling astrocytes that function in storage and release of hormones
- Symptoms can be due to loss of pituitary function, compression of adjacent structures (e.g., visual disturbance), or (less commonly) increase in pituitary hormones
- Lesions of this region include
  - Granular cell tumor

- Hypothalamic hamartoma
- Sarcoidosis
  - Presents with hypopituitarism
  - Almost all patients have systemic sarcoidosis
  - Only 1% have lesions limited to central nervous system
- Langerhans cell histiocytosis
- Pituicytoma
  - Low-grade glioma
  - Mitoses rare
- Hypothalamic or optic pathway astrocytomas

Craniopharyngioma

- Benign, slow-growing, suprasellar solid and cystic tumor arising from embryologic remnants of Rathke pouch
  - Growth due to increase in tumor cells
  - Symptoms of headache, pituitary dysfunction, and visual disturbances are due to impingement on adjacent structures
    - Leakage of contents can cause aseptic meningitis
  - May recur if entire tumor is not removed
  - Can be adherent to adjacent structures
- Cytologic features are "wet" keratin and clusters of squamous cells with palisaded border
- **2 histologic variants**
  - **Adamantinomatous craniopharyngioma**
    - Usually in children but also adults
    - Composed of cords or islands of epithelial cells in loose fibrous stroma with intervening cysts
    - Resemble adamantinoma (most common type of tooth tumor)
    - Outer layer of epithelium is palisaded
    - "Wet" keratin associated with nuclear dropout to form ghost keratinocytes
    - Cholesterol clefts, desquamated keratin, calcification
    - Calcifications can be seen on imaging and are helpful for diagnosis
    - Occasional inflammatory component and gliosis
  - **Papillary craniopharyngioma**
    - Almost all in adults
    - Stratified squamous epithelium with papillary projections
    - Solid growth pattern
    - Usually has smooth outer surface and is not adherent to adjacent structures
    - Lacks palisading, fibrosis, "wet" keratinization, and calcifications

Rathke Cleft Cyst

- Benign fluid-filled cyst formed if Rathke pouch does not develop normally
  - Symptoms occur due to compression of adjacent structures
    - Growth occurs due to fluid accumulation
  - Visual disturbances are most common, followed by pituitary dysfunction
- Lined by columnar cells with cilia and goblet cells
  - Cytology shows scattered clusters of cuboidal cells with prominent cilia
- Presence of extensive squamous change can mimic craniopharyngioma
- Hypocellular cystic craniopharyngiomas can be mistaken for epidermoid or Rathke cleft cysts

Epidermoid Cysts

- Arise from embryological remnants
  - Growth due to accumulation of keratin debris
  - Usually present in young adults (20-40 years of age)
  - Symptoms due to compression of adjacent structures
- Unilocular cysts lined by orderly stratified squamous epithelium
- Calcification is rare in epidermoid cysts

Neuronal Cell Tumors

- Relatively rare lesions
- Neuronal tumors of sellar region include paraganglioma, gangliocytoma, glioma, spindle cell oncocytoma, granular cell tumor, pituicytoma, schwannoma, meningioma, and neuroblastoma

Inflammatory Hypophysitis

- **Primary inflammatory hypophysitis**
  - Rare disorder characterized by focal or diffuse inflammatory infiltration and ultimate destruction of pituitary gland
  - Thought to be autoimmune disease localized to pituitary
  - Can affect anterior lobe, posterior lobe, or both
    - Symptoms depend on areas of pituitary with loss of function
  - Diagnosis requires biopsy
- **3 histologic categories**
  - **Lymphocytic hypophysitis**
    - Infiltration of anterior pituitary by lymphocytes and plasma cells with occasional germinal centers
    - Parenchymal atrophy, variable degree of fibrosis, and residual lymphocytic infiltration at later stages of disease
  - **Granulomatous hypophysitis**
    - Well-formed, noncaseating granulomas associated with variable lymphocytic infiltrates
  - **Xanthomatous hypophysitis**
    - Variable lymphoplasmacytic inflammatory infiltrates
    - Foamy macrophages with giant cell formation, necrosis, and hemosiderin deposition
- **Secondary inflammatory hypophysitis**
  - Inflammation of pituitary secondary to inflammation of nearby structure or systemic disease
  - Local causes include
    - Rupture of sellar cystic lesion (craniopharyngioma, Rathke cleft cyst, epidermoid cyst)
    - Meningitis
    - Osteomyelitis of sphenoid bone

Gangliocytoma

- May present with acromegaly or mass effect symptoms
- Composed of large mature ganglion cells with abundant cytoplasm
- Proliferative glial stroma with Rosenthal fibers

Pituitary Carcinoma

- No combination of histologic features diagnostic of carcinoma

- Presence of invasion, cellular pleomorphism, mitosis, or necrosis are not sufficient for diagnosis of malignancy
- Diagnosis of pituitary carcinoma is dependent upon demonstration of metastases
- Mitotic activity is increased in carcinomas (up to 67%), but there is considerable overlap with adenomas

Metastatic Carcinoma

- Secondary tumors of pituitary gland result from either hematogenous spread or direct invasion
  - Tumor cells are large, with nuclear pleomorphism, and some with glandular arrangements
- Involvement of posterior lobe is more common
  - Portal nature of vascularization of adenohypophysis has been thought to form protective barrier
- ~ 3-27% of patients with disseminated malignancy develop pituitary metastasis
- Most common primary sites are breast, lung, and gastrointestinal tract

REPORTING

Frozen Section

- Definitive diagnosis of pituitary adenoma or other diagnosis is reported when diagnostic features are present
- Defer to permanent sections if not diagnostic

Cytology

- Reported in conjunction with frozen section

PITFALLS

Pituitary Adenoma Mimics

- Pituitary hyperplasia
- Paraganglioma
- Metastatic neuroendocrine carcinoma (NEC)
- Meningioma
- Spindle cell oncocytoma
- Granular cell tumor
- Plasmacytoma
- Lymphoma
- Metastatic carcinoma
- Gangliocytoma

Metastatic NEC vs. Pituitary Adenoma

- Metastatic NEC can mimic pituitary adenoma
- Distinction may require immunohistochemical studies
  - Pituitary adenomas do not usually express peptides of thyroid, gut, and pancreas

Crooke Cell Adenoma vs. Metastatic Carcinoma

- Large atypical keratin (+) cells of Crooke cell adenoma may mimic metastatic carcinoma
- Demonstration of ACTH along with Tpit is valuable; however, metastatic NEC may produce ectopic ACTH

Meningioma vs. Pituitary Adenoma

- Meningothelial variants feature whorls and indistinct cell borders
  - Uncommon in pituitary adenomas
- Transitional and psammomatous variants have prominent psammoma bodies similar to PRL- and TSH-producing adenomas

Spindle Cell Oncocytoma/Pituicytoma vs. Pituitary Adenoma

- Immunoperoxidase studies may be necessary for diagnosis

Granular Cell Tumor vs. Pituitary Adenoma

- May require immunoperoxidase studies
  - Granular cell tumors are positive for TTF-1 and negative for PIT-1

Plasmacytoma vs. Pituitary Adenoma

- Difficult differential diagnosis due to some pituitary adenomas being composed of plasmacytoid cells
- Chromatin pattern is helpful
  - Plasma cells have central prominent nucleolus surrounded by clumps of chromatin (clock face chromatin)
  - Pituitary adenoma cells have finely dispersed chromatin with small distinct nucleoli (salt and pepper chromatin)
- Immunoperoxidase studies may be necessary
  - Plasmacytomas are negative for PIT-1 and positive for plasma cell markers

Lymphoma vs. Pituitary Adenoma

- Pituitary adenomas treated with bromocriptine can mimic lymphoma due to small amount of cytoplasm and irregular hyperchromatic nuclei
- Immunoperoxidase studies may be necessary
  - Pituitary adenomas are positive for PIT-1 and ER

SELECTED REFERENCES

1. Noh S et al: Rapid reticulin fiber staining method is helpful for the diagnosis of pituitary adenoma in frozen section. Endocr Pathol. 26(2):178-84, 2015
2. Mete O et al: Therapeutic implications of accurate classification of pituitary adenomas. Semin Diagn Pathol. 30(3):158-64, 2013
3. Afroz N et al: Role of imprint cytology in the intraoperative diagnosis of pituitary adenomas. Diagn Cytopathol. 39(2):138-40, 2011
4. Nosé V et al: Protocol for the examination of specimens from patients with primary pituitary tumors. Arch Pathol Lab Med. 135(5):640-6, 2011
5. Zhang Y et al: Endocrine tumors as part of inherited tumor syndromes. Adv Anat Pathol. 18(3):206-18, 2011
6. Zada G et al: Craniopharyngioma and other cystic epithelial lesions of the sellar region: a review of clinical, imaging, and histopathological relationships. Neurosurg Focus. 28(4):E4, 2010
7. Asa SL: Practical pituitary pathology: what does the pathologist need to know? Arch Pathol Lab Med. 132(8):1231-40, 2008
8. Jagannathan J et al: Benign brain tumors: sellar/parasellar tumors. Neurol Clin. 25(4):1231-49, xi, 2007
9. Daneshbod Y et al: Intraoperative cytologic crush preparation findings in craniopharyngioma: a study of 72 cases. Acta Cytol. 49(1):7-10, 2005
10. Shin JL et al: Cystic lesions of the pituitary: clinicopathological features distinguishing craniopharyngioma, Rathke's cleft cyst, and arachnoid cyst. J Clin Endocrinol Metab. 84(11):3972-82, 1999
11. Smith AR et al: Intraoperative cytologic diagnosis of suprasellar and sellar cystic lesions. Diagn Cytopathol. 20(3):137-47, 1999

(Left) *Coronal graphic shows physiologic pituitary hyperplasia. The gland is uniformly enlarged ➔ and has a mildly convex superior margin. An increase in the number of lactotrophs during pregnancy increases the size of the anterior lobe by ~ 30%. The gland regresses after delivery, and sequelae of this normal change are rare.* **(Right)** *A reticulin stain of a normal adenohypophysis (anterior lobe) shows a relatively uniform distribution of acini surrounded by a reticulin network.*

Pituitary Hyperplasia

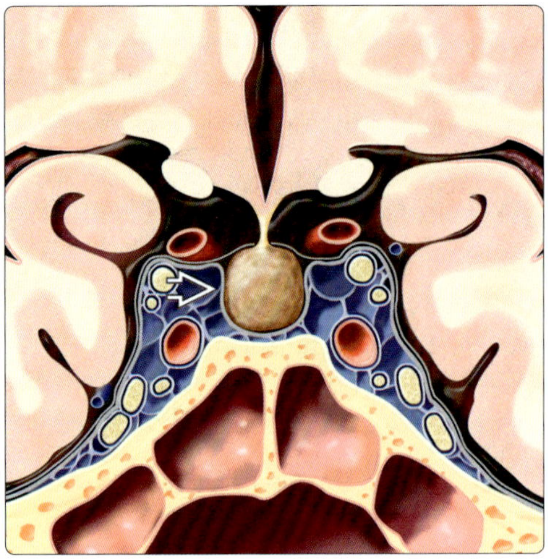

Normal Pituitary: Reticulin

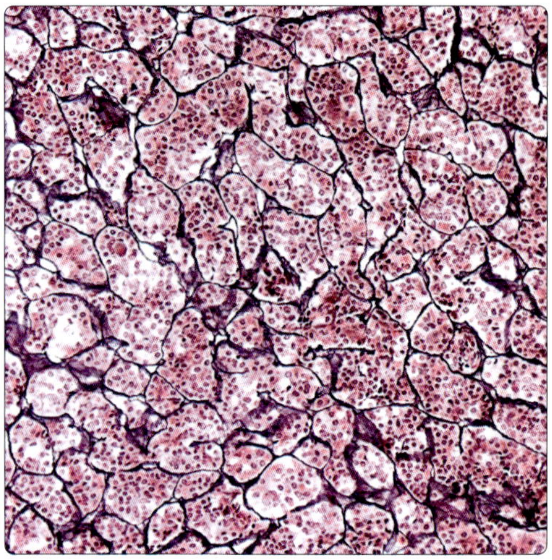

(Left) *This is a pituitary gland from a woman who died on the 2nd day of puerperium. The gland was enlarged and showed expansion of the acini that were entirely composed of acidophilic (lactotroph) cells. These cells produce prolactin and are stimulated to increase in number during pregnancy.* **(Right)** *A reticulin stain of a pituitary gland from a postpartum woman with prolactin cell hyperplasia confirms marked expansion of the acini with preservation of the reticulin pattern.*

Pituitary Hyperplasia

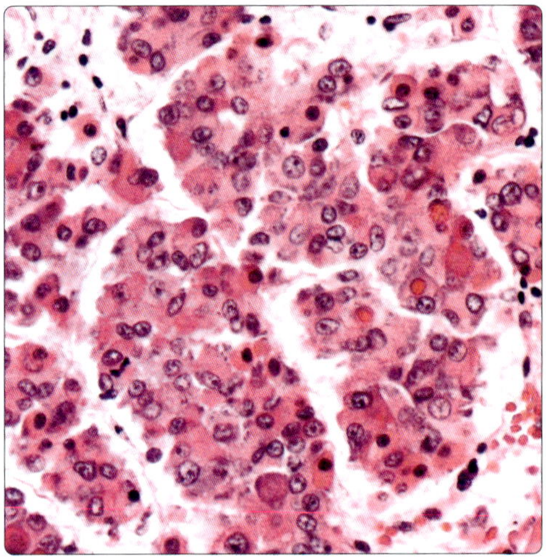

Pituitary Hyperplasia: Reticulin

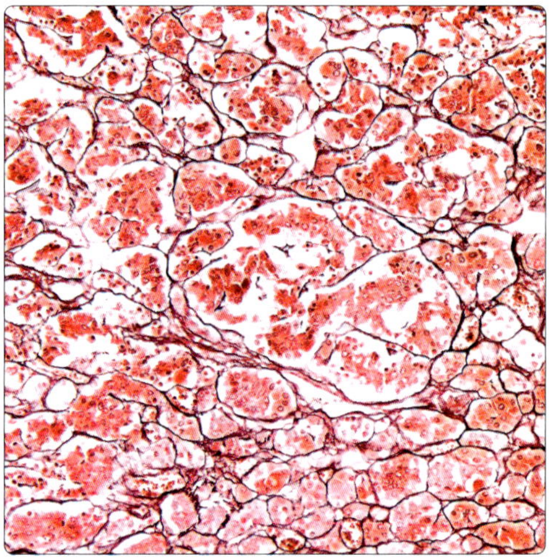

(Left) *This macroadenoma ➔ extends superiorly to compress the body of the chiasm ➔. Compression can cause loss of peripheral vision. Acute hemorrhage into the gland is termed pituitary apoplexy and frequently causes loss of pituitary function.* **(Right)** *This pituitary macroadenoma extends upward through the diaphragma sellae into the suprasellar cistern and laterally into the cavernous sinus, which is partially unroofed.*

Pituitary Macroadenoma

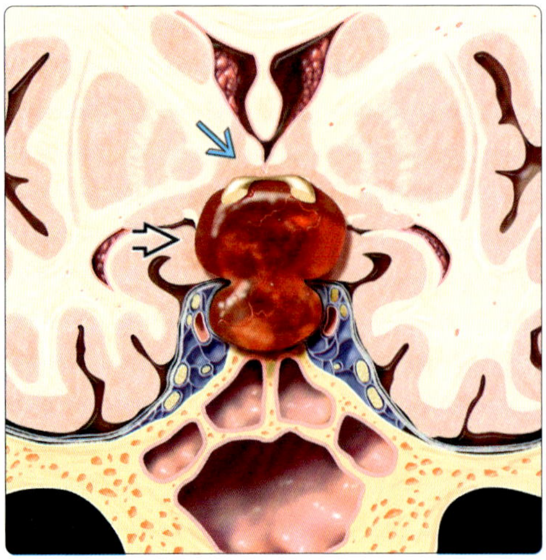

Pituitary Macroadenoma

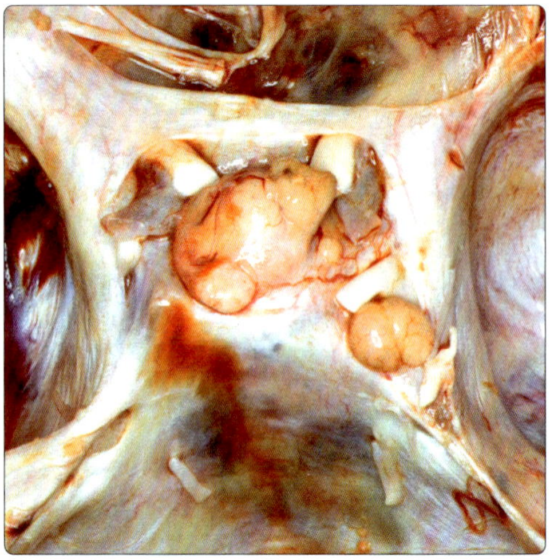

Pituitary Macroadenoma

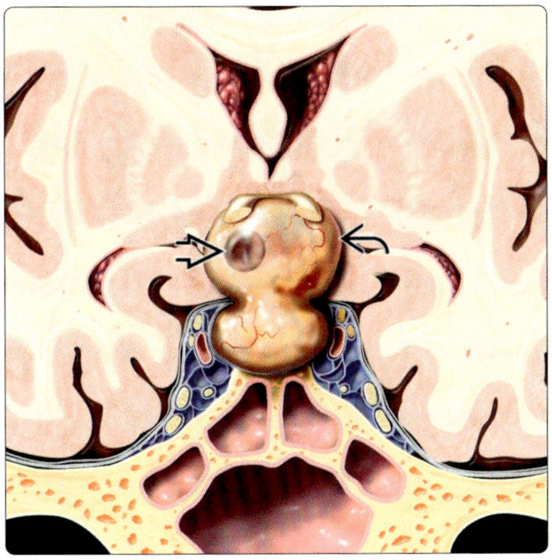

Pituitary Adenoma: Reticulin

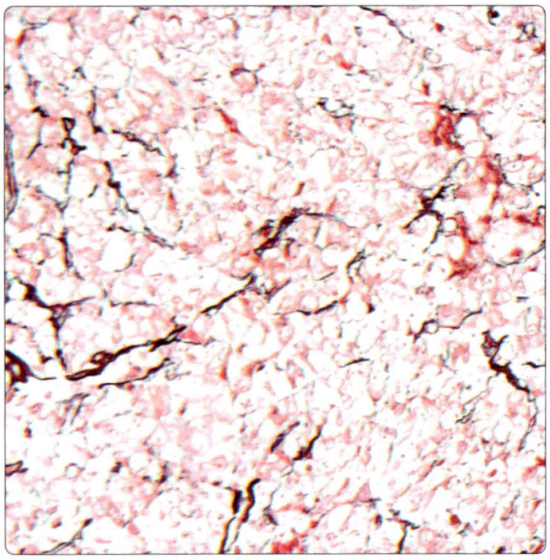

(Left) *This snowman-shaped or "figure of 8" sellar/suprasellar macroadenoma* ➜ *shows small foci of hemorrhage and cystic change* ➜*. The normal pituitary gland has been completely replaced by tumor. Adenomas can be locally invasive yet not be associated with metastases.* **(Right)** *Reticulin stain of a pituitary adenoma shows loss of the normal trabecular reticulin network. There are only rare residual reticulin fibers.*

Pituitary Microadenoma

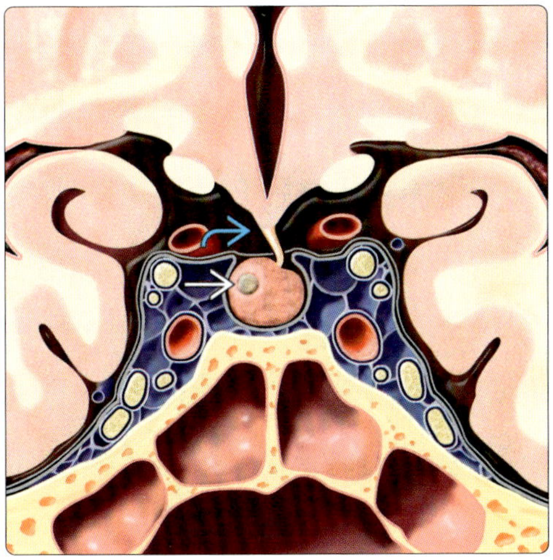

Pituitary Microadenoma: Reticulin

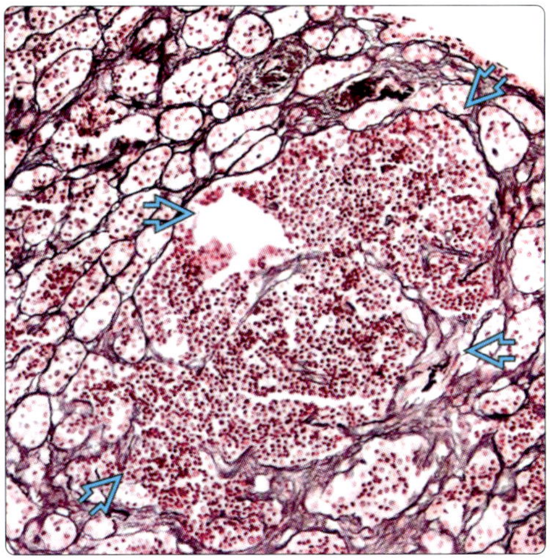

(Left) *This microadenoma* ➜ *slightly enlarges the right side of the pituitary gland and deviates the infundibulum* ➜ *toward the left. These small tumors (< 1 cm) may be functional or discovered incidentally.* **(Right)** *Reticulin stains are crucial for diagnosis of hyperplasia (expansion of the acini and preservation of the reticulin pattern) and its distinction from adenoma. An incidental prolactin-producing microadenoma is identified by disruption of acini and the reticulin network* ➜*. The normal pattern is seen in the adjacent gland.*

Pituitary Adenoma: Chromophobe Type

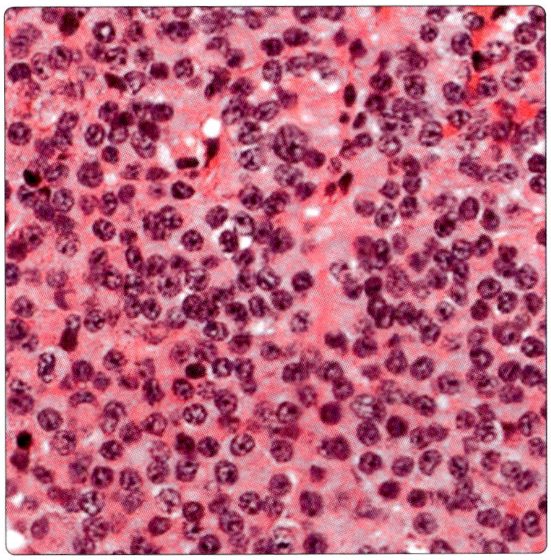

Pituitary Adenoma: Basophilic Type

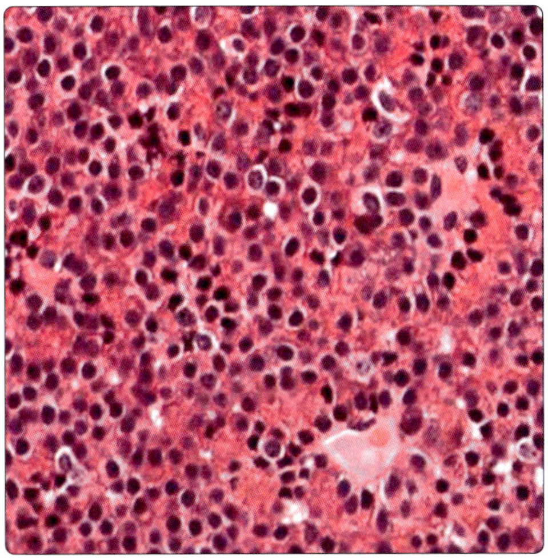

(Left) *This chromophobic adenoma is composed of cells that lack both acidophilic and basophilic granules. These tumors are most often nonfunctional but may produce thyroid-stimulating hormone.* **(Right)** *This basophilic pituitary adenoma is composed of cells that exhibit basophilic cytoplasm. These tumors may produce ACTH, gonadotropic hormones (LH or FSH), or TSH.*

(Left) *This sparsely granulated somatotroph adenoma is composed of eosinophilic cells. The nuclei tend to be eccentric, pushed to the cell periphery, and indented by the fibrous bodies ⇨. These tumors usually produce GH or PRL.* **(Right)** *Densely granulated somatotroph adenomas harbor numerous GH-containing secretory granules that correlate with their cytoplasmic eosinophilic appearance on H&E. Low-molecular-weight keratin (CAM5.2) reveals perinuclear staining ⇨.*

Somatotroph Pituitary Adenoma

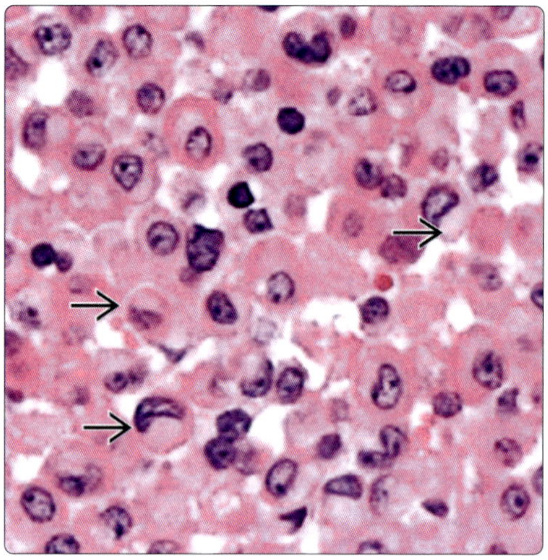

Somatotroph Pituitary Adenoma

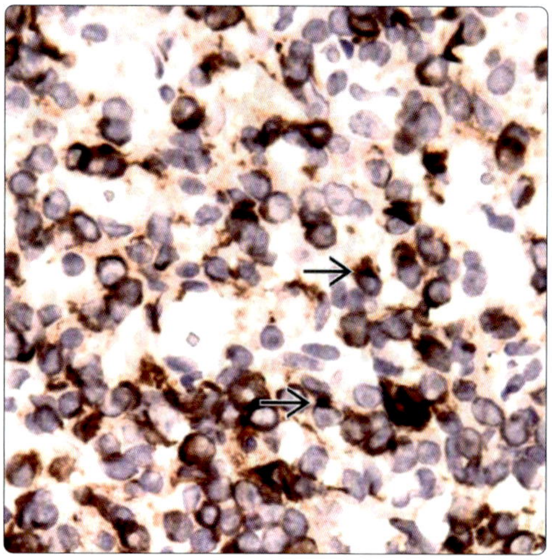

(Left) *Adenomas have neuroendocrine features with finely dispersed chromatin and distinct nucleoli. It may not be possible to distinguish an adenoma from metastatic neuroendocrine tumors on frozen section. The final diagnosis may require immunohistochemical studies.* **(Right)** *Immunohistochemistry plays a critical role in classification of adenomas on permanent sections. Sparsely granulated lactotroph adenomas are composed of chromophobic cells that reveal typical Golgi-type staining for PRL.*

Lactotroph Pituitary Adenoma

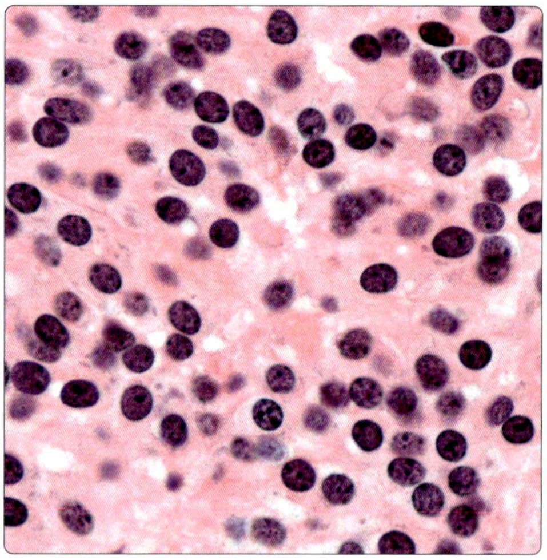

Lactotroph Pituitary Adenoma

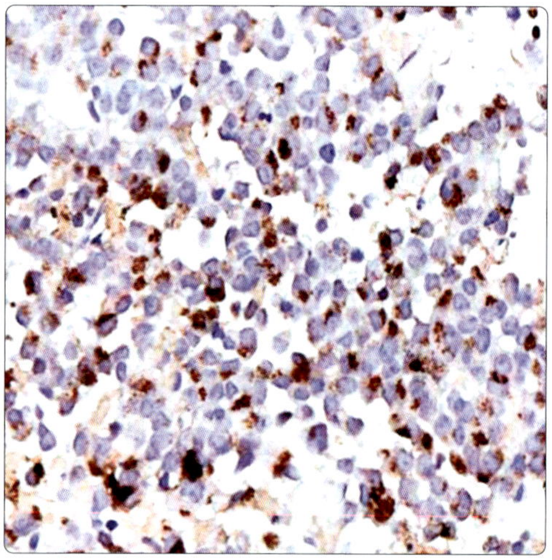

(Left) *Corticotroph adenomas usually have basophilic cytoplasm on H&E. A PAS stain highlights ACTH-containing secretory granules in corticotroph cells. Densely granulated corticotroph adenomas reveal strong PAS(+) granules ⇨.* **(Right)** *Regardless of the histological subtype, keratin CAM5.2 reveals strong cytoplasmic positivity in all corticotroph adenomas. This densely granulated corticotroph adenoma shows low-molecular-weight keratin positivity.*

Corticotroph Pituitary Adenoma

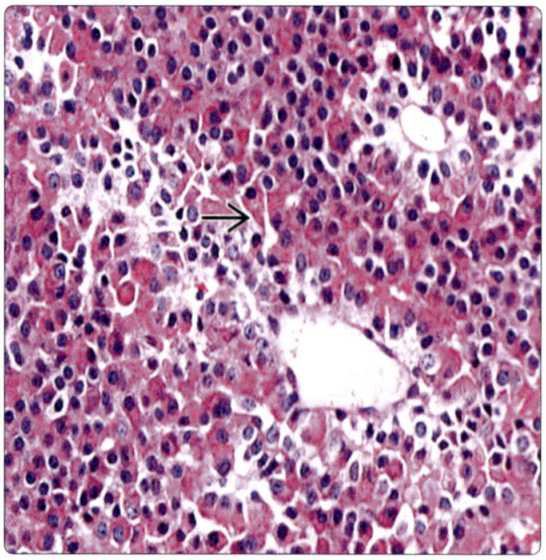

Corticotroph Pituitary Adenoma

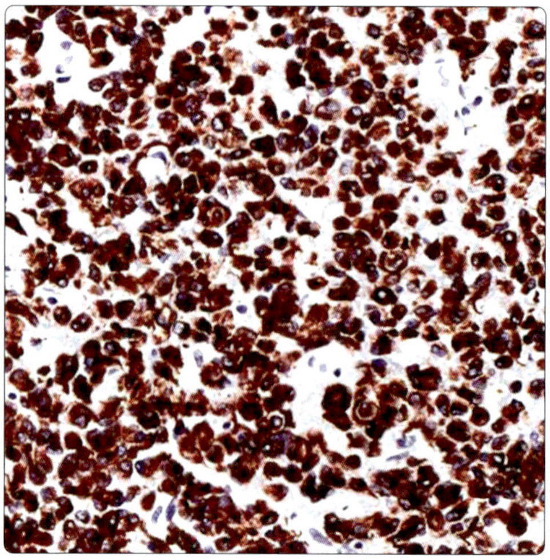

Pituitary Adenoma: Acidophilic Type

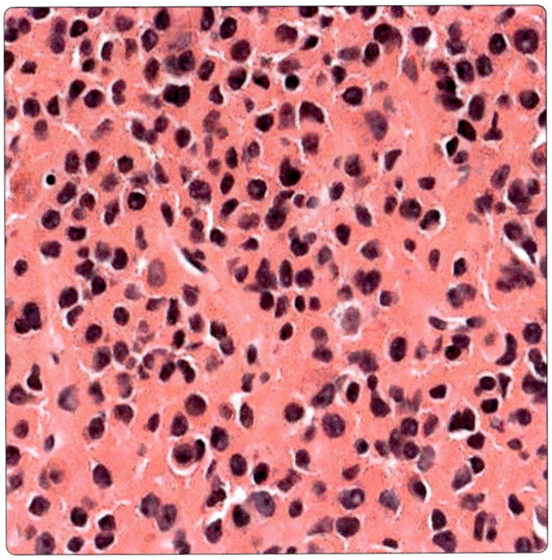

Pituitary Adenoma: Acidophil Stem Cell Type

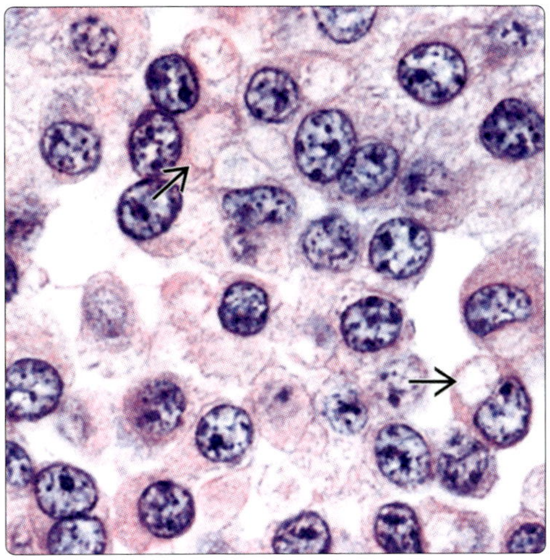

(Left) *Cytoplasmic granularity identifies 3 distinct cell types: Chromophobic, eosinophilic, & basophilic. This acidophilic adenoma is composed of cells with bright cytoplasmic eosinophilia that usually produce human growth hormone or PRL.* **(Right)** *Some adenomas, like acidophil stem cell adenomas, have unusual features. Large eosinophilic tumor cells exhibit cytoplasmic vacuolization ⇒ due to mitochondrial dilatation; thought to be precursor cells for cells producing GH or PRL, & tumors may or may not produce these hormones.*

Invasive Pituitary Adenoma

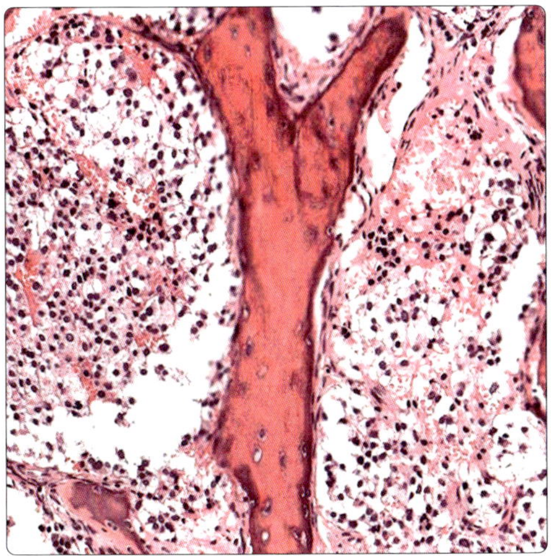

Atypia in Pituitary Carcinoma

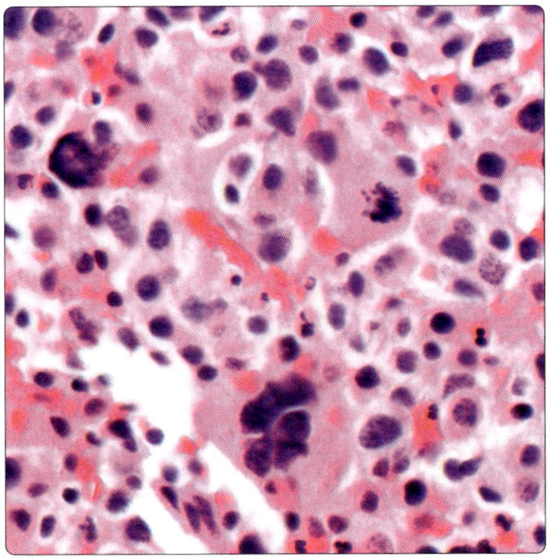

(Left) *Some pituitary adenomas are associated with invasive or aggressive behavior and are called "invasive pituitary adenomas." This invasive pituitary adenoma has invaded into the bone adjacent to the pituitary gland and is present within bone marrow.* **(Right)** *This touch imprint of a pituitary carcinoma shows cells with marked cytological atypia with pleomorphism, multinucleation, mitosis, and marked variability in nuclear size. However, metastatic behavior cannot be predicted by histologic features.*

Pleomorphic Cells in Pituitary Carcinoma

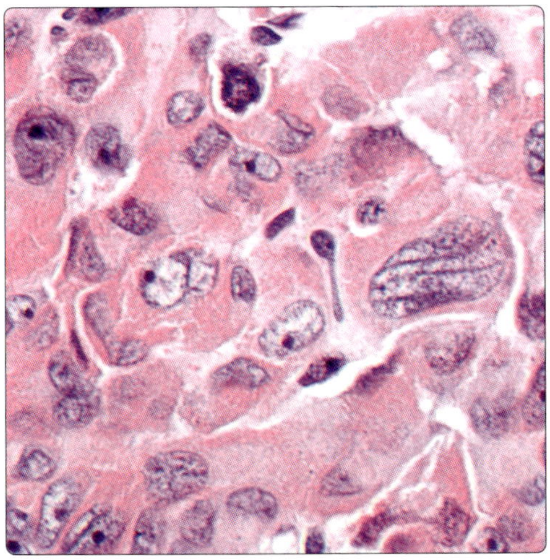

Crooke Hyaline

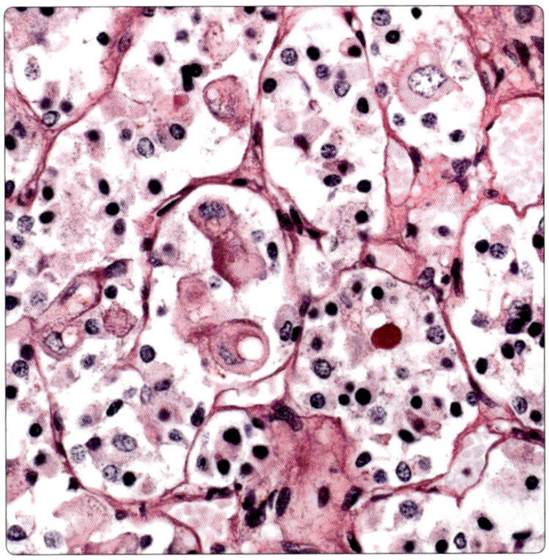

(Left) *This pituitary carcinoma shows a solid arrangement of pleomorphic cells with ample cytoplasm and exhibits cytologic atypia with cellular pleomorphism, distinct nucleoli, and irregular nuclear membranes. However, the diagnosis of carcinoma requires distant metastasis.* **(Right)** *Normal corticotrophs exposed to elevated glucocorticoids undergo Crooke hyaline change. This change results in relocation of the periodic acid-Schiff positive hormone to the cell periphery and to a juxtanuclear location.*

(Left) *Sagittal graphic depicts multiple intramedullary sarcoid granulomas in the brainstem →, upper cervical cord →, and pituitary stalk →. Almost all patients with neurosarcoidosis also have involvement of other organs. Disease isolated to the central nervous system only occurs in 1% of patients.* **(Right)** *Pituitary sarcoidosis is characterized by noncaseating granulomas with histiocytes and multinucleated giant cells diffusely infiltrating the gland. Hypopituitarism may result.*

Pituitary Stalk Sarcoidosis

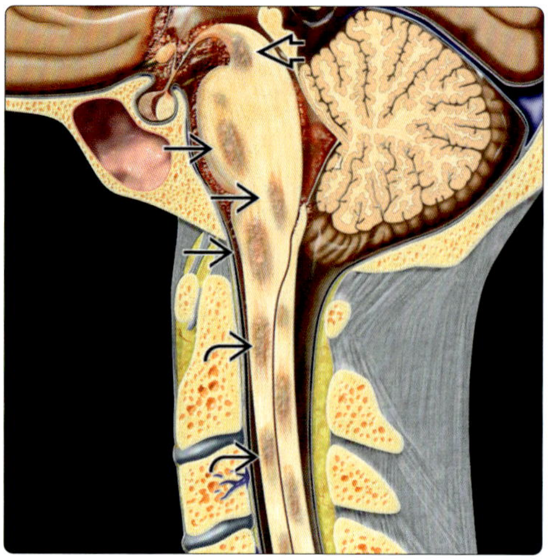

Giant Cells in Pituitary Sarcoidosis

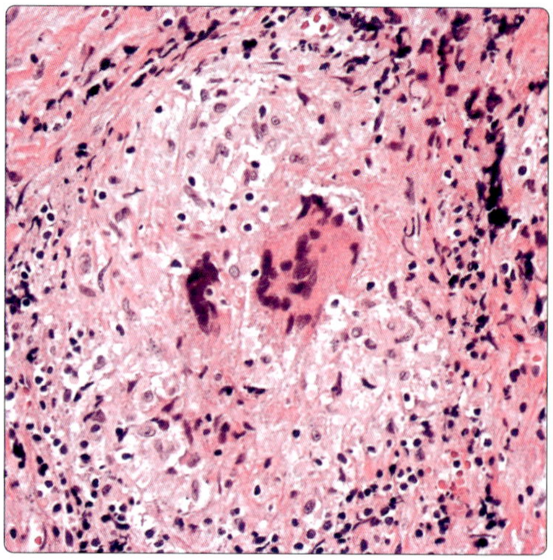

(Left) *Reticulin stain highlights the extensive fibrosis in a pituitary gland involved by sarcoidosis. Note the reticulin-free areas surrounding granulomas → and giant cells →. The normal reticulin pattern identifying acini has been lost.* **(Right)** *An immunohistochemical study for GH highlights normal GH-producing cells of the pituitary. The noncaseating granuloma → and giant cell → due to sarcoidosis are not immunoreactive.*

Pituitary Sarcoidosis: Reticulin

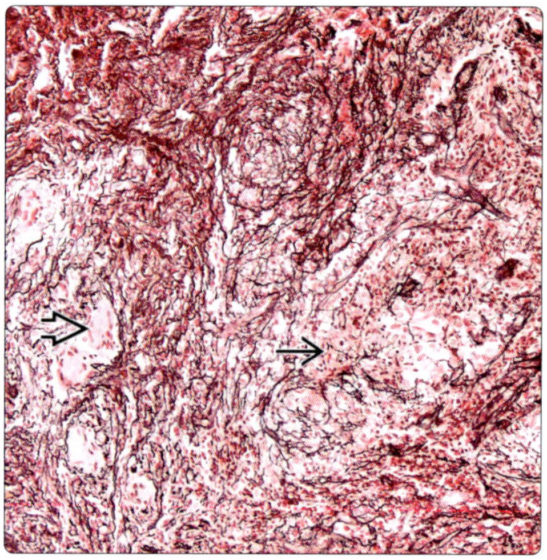

Growth Hormone in Pituitary Sarcoidosis

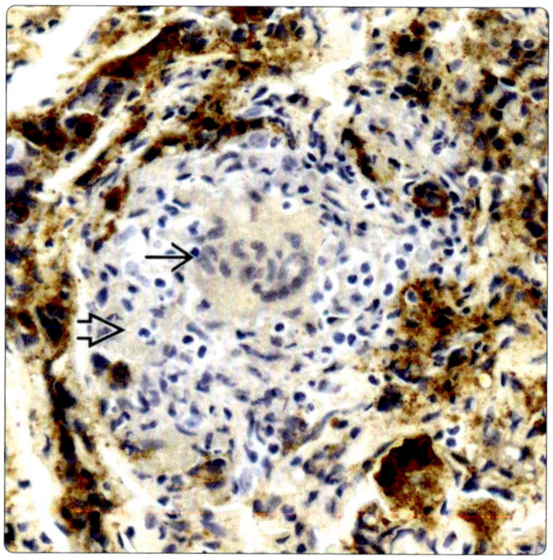

(Left) *Sagittal graphic shows lymphocytic hypophysitis. Note the thickening of the infundibulum → as well as infiltration into the AL of the pituitary gland →. The PL can also be affected. Symptoms of loss of pituitary function depend on the areas involved.* **(Right)** *Lymphocytic (autoimmune) hypophysitis is characterized by a dense infiltrate of lymphoplasmacytic inflammatory cells that diffusely infiltrate and damage the pituitary gland parenchyma →.*

Lymphocytic Hypophysitis

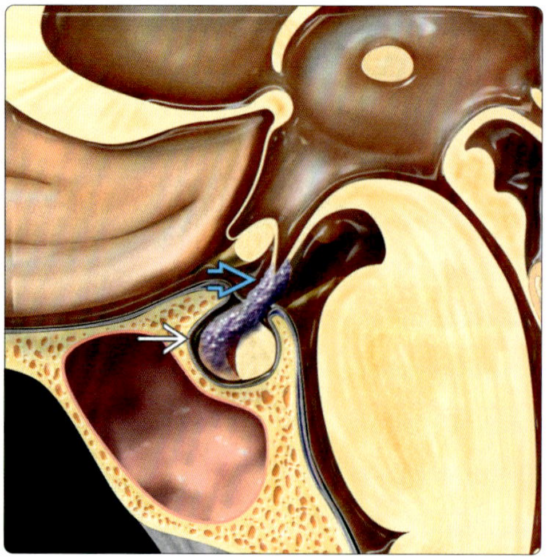

Lymphocytic Hypophysitis

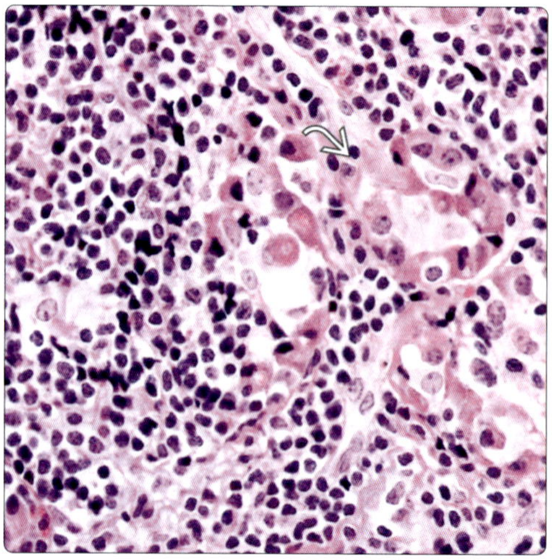

Rathke Cleft Cyst: MR Appearance

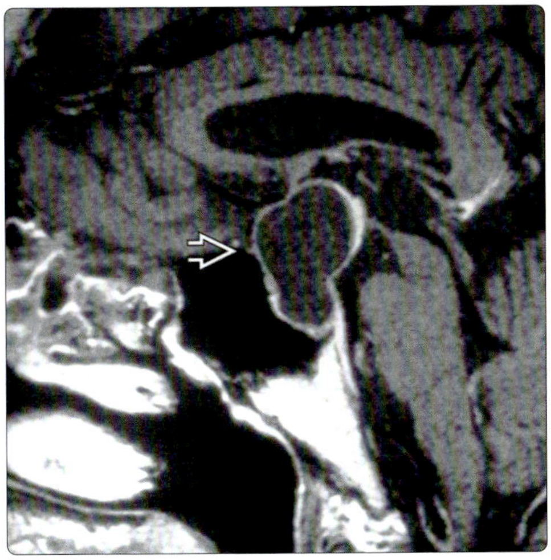

Rathke Cleft Cyst

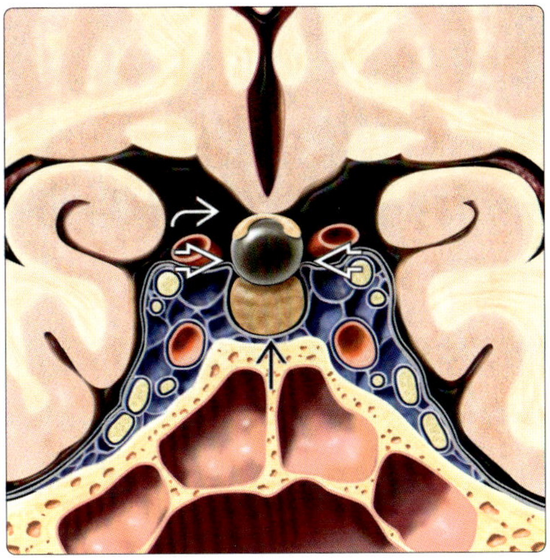

(Left) *Sagittal T1-weighted MR of a patient with vision loss shows a Rathke cleft cyst ➡ extending from the sella to the suprasellar area.* **(Right)** *Graphic of a coronal section shows a typical suprasellar fluid-filled Rathke cleft cyst ➡ interposed between the pituitary gland ➡ and the optic chiasm ➡. Symptoms of visual disturbances or pituitary dysfunction occur when these large benign cysts impinge on the adjacent structures. However, the majority of these cysts are small and do not cause symptoms.*

Rathke Cleft Cyst: Gross Appearance

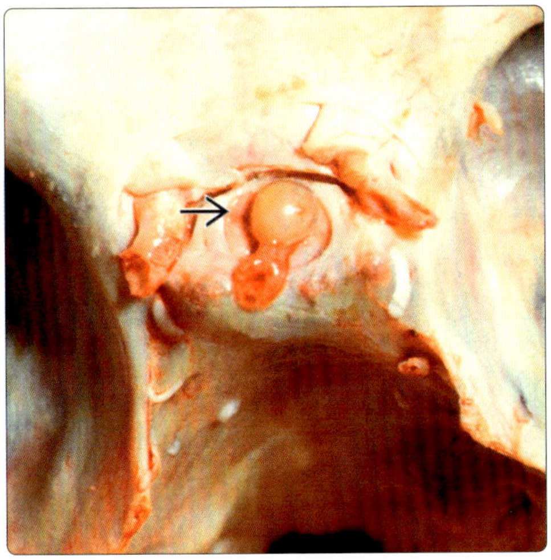

Rathke Cleft Cyst Lining

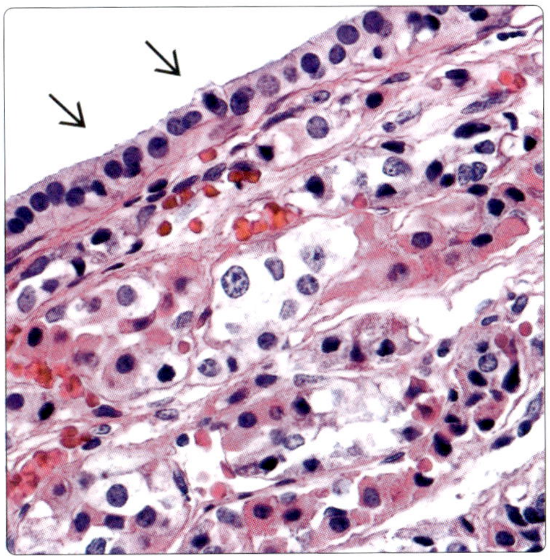

(Left) *Axial gross pathology shows a mucin-containing Rathke cleft cyst ➡ found at autopsy. The majority of these cysts are asymptomatic and are found incidentally at autopsy, as was this cyst. (Courtesy E. Hedley-Whyte, MD.)* **(Right)** *Rathke cleft cysts are lined by a thin wall composed of 3 types of epithelial cells. In this cyst, ciliated cuboidal to columnar cells ➡ line the wall. These cells within the pituitary are diagnostic of a Rathke cleft cyst.*

Rathke Cleft Cyst: Goblet Cells

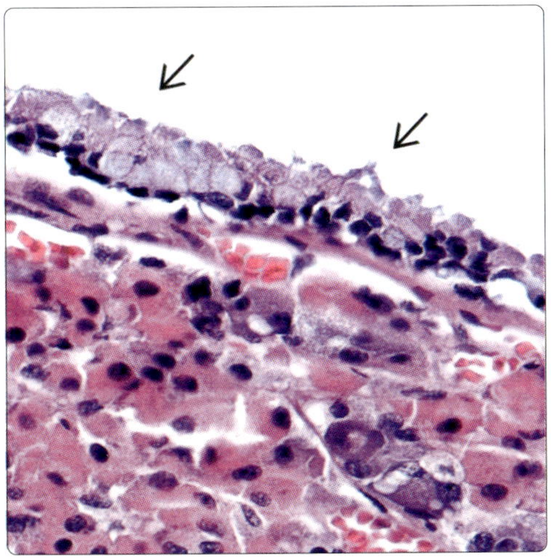

Rathke Cleft Cyst Wall

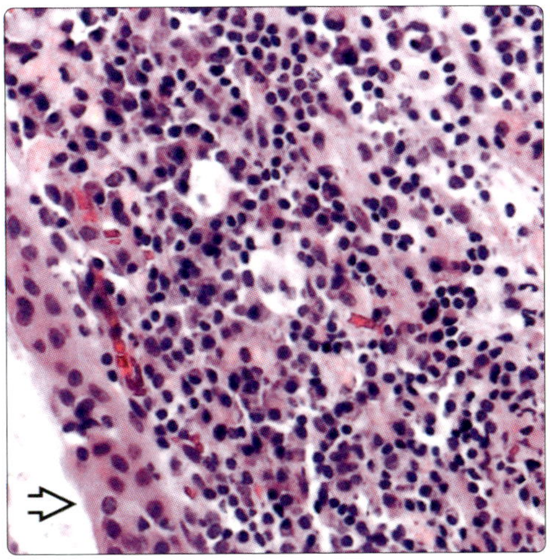

(Left) *Goblet cells (mucus-secreting cells) ➡ may be present in the epithelium of the Rathke cleft. These cells may be present alone or be intermixed with cuboidal to columnar cells, ± cilia. The contents of the cyst may be thick and gelatinous but can also be watery and thin.* **(Right)** *This Rathke cleft cyst shows focal squamous metaplasia ➡. The presence of squamous cells can mimic a craniopharyngioma. Lymphoplasmacytic inflammation involves the adjacent anterior pituitary gland.*

(Left) *T1-weighted MR of an epidermoid cyst is characterized by a large heterogeneous sellar and suprasellar mass with displacement of the optic chiasm.* **(Right)** *Epidermoid cysts arise from embryologic remnants in the central nervous system. This epidermoid cyst of the pituitary shows a stratified squamous epithelium lining resting upon a soft fibrous tissue stroma. The cysts slowly grow due to accumulation of keratin debris and do not cause symptoms until patients are 20-40 years old.*

Epidermoid Cyst: MR Appearance

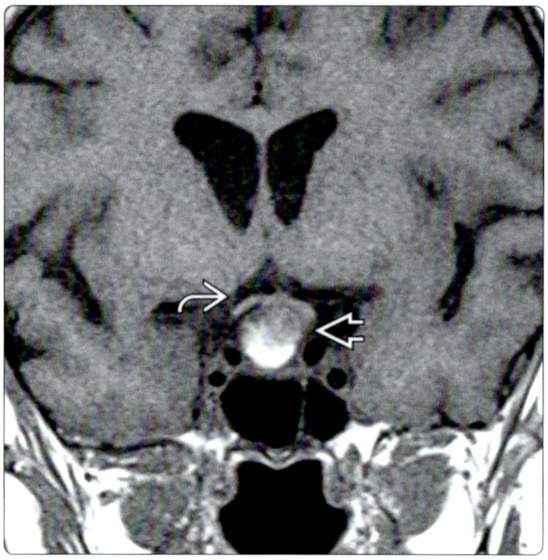

Epidermoid Cyst Wall

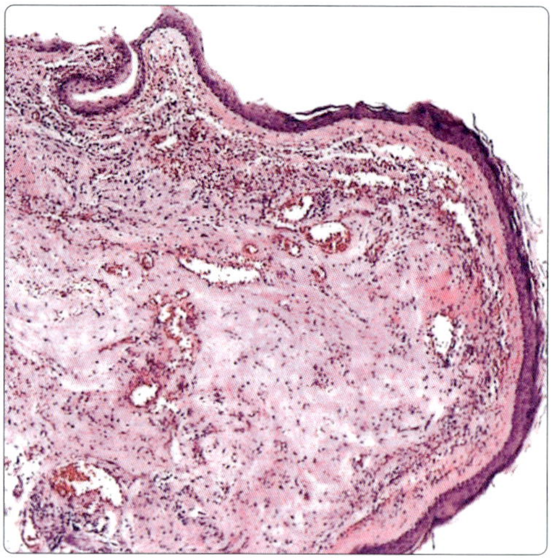

(Left) *Epithelial lining of an epidermoid cyst displays stratified squamous epithelium with a keratohyaline granular layer and dry (flaky) keratin formation. The keratin fills the cyst, causing it to slowly increase in size and eventually cause symptoms by impinging on adjacent structures.* **(Right)** *The contents of an epidermoid cyst are composed solely of dry (flaky) acellular keratin. Note the presence of eosinophilic and focally basophilic flakes.*

Epidermoid Cyst Lining Cells

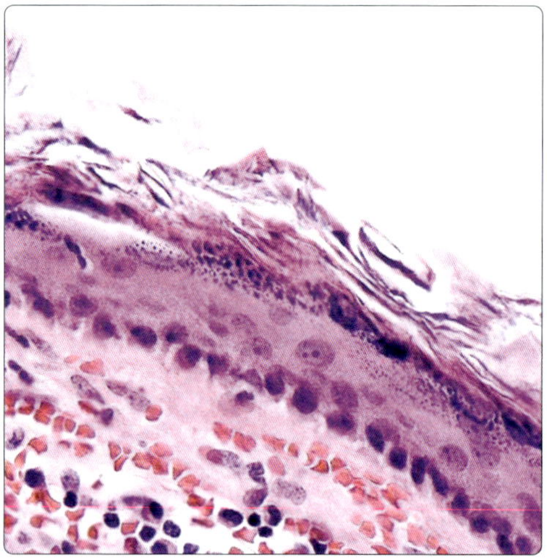

Acellular Keratin in Epidermoid Cyst

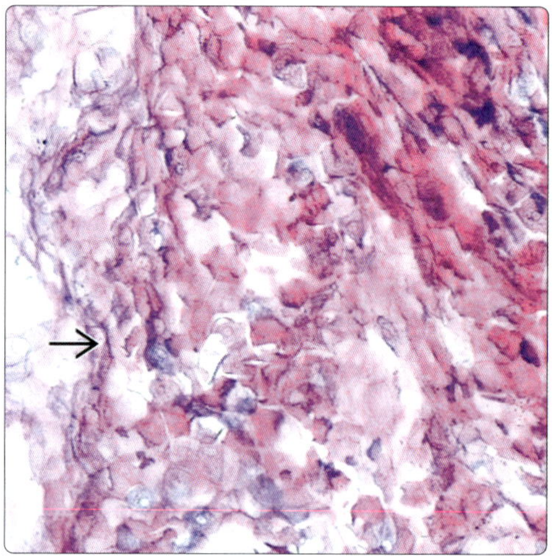

(Left) *Sheehan syndrome is hypopituitarism caused by blood loss and hypovolemic shock associated with childbirth. This whole mount from an autopsy of an affected patient shows an extensive area of infarction of the anterior lobe and hemorrhage of the posterior lobe.* **(Right)** *Anterior lobe of the pituitary of a patient with Sheehan syndrome shows extensive necrosis of the pituitary parenchyma with a small rim of viable cells.*

Pituitary in Sheehan Syndrome

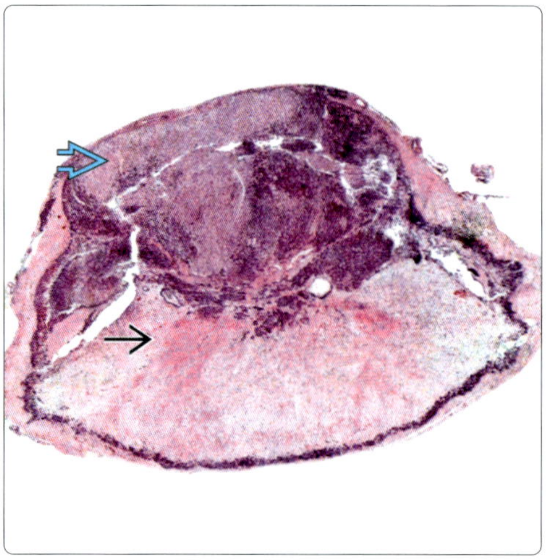

Sheehan Syndrome

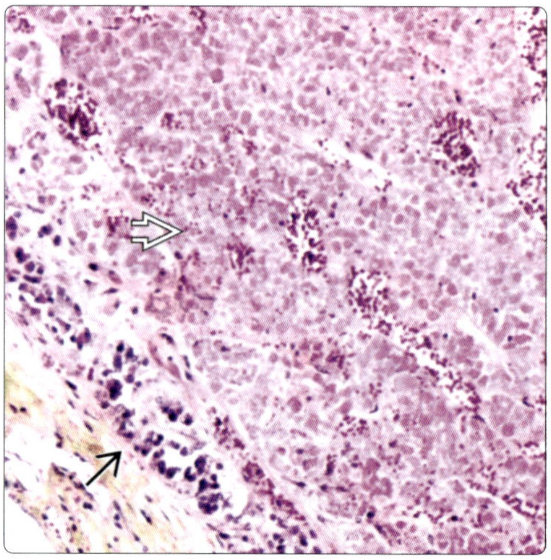

Palisading in Craniopharyngioma

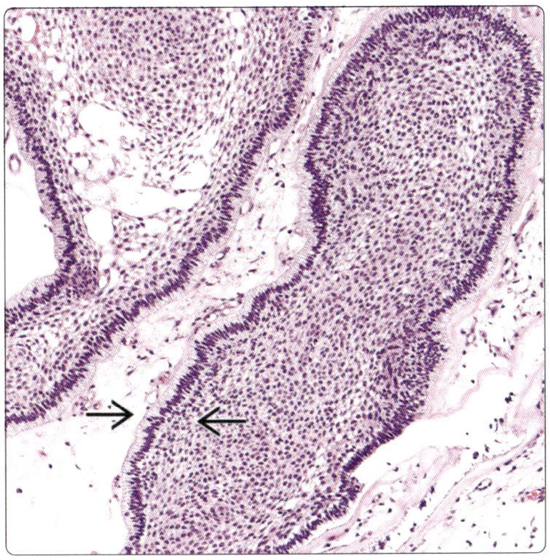

Papillary Craniopharyngioma

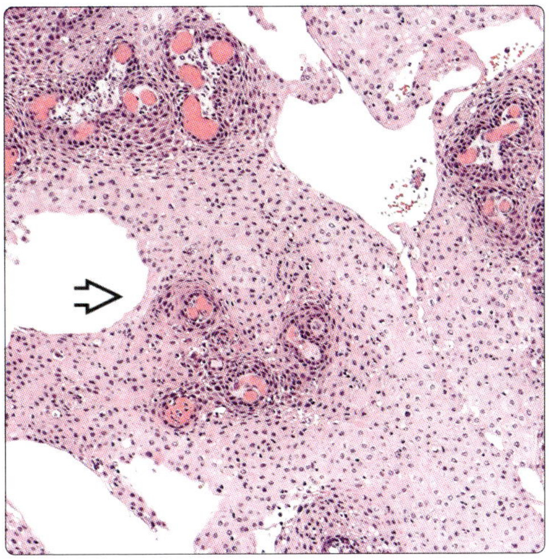

(Left) *Adamantinomatous craniopharyngioma is composed of cords or islands of epithelial cells in a loose fibrous stroma with intervening cysts resembling adamantinoma. The outer layer of epithelium shows palisading* →*.* **(Right)** *Papillary craniopharyngioma is composed of mature squamous epithelium* ⇨ *and lacks palisading, fibrosis, "wet" keratinization, and calcifications. These features distinguish this variant from adamantinomatous craniopharyngioma.*

Adamantinomatous Craniopharyngioma

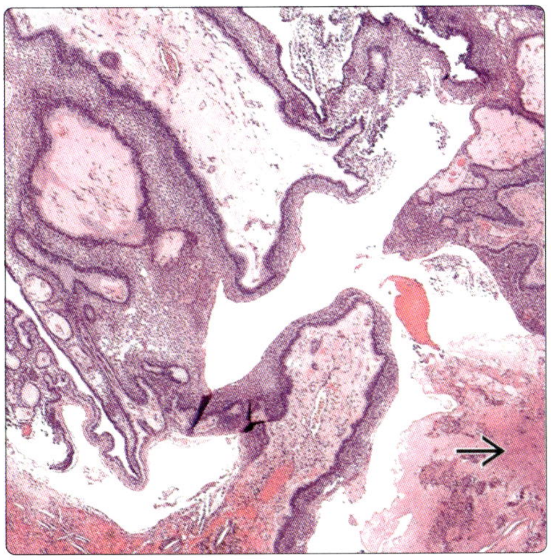

Craniopharyngioma

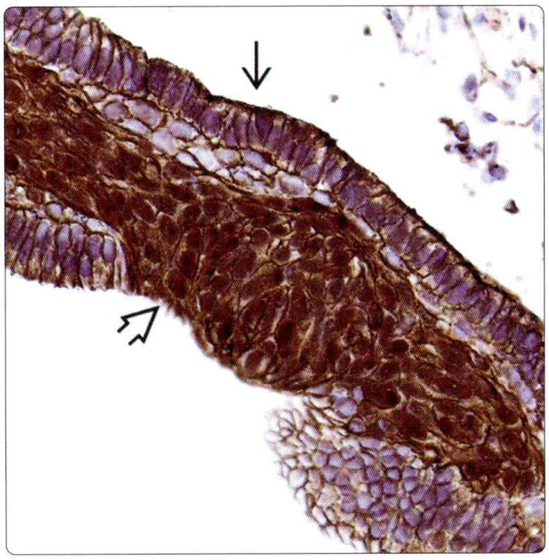

(Left) *One of the characteristic features of adamantinomatous craniopharyngioma is "wet" keratin* → *associated with nuclear dropout, forming ghost keratinocytes. Rupture with spillage of contents can cause aseptic meningitis.* **(Right)** *Adamantinomatous craniopharyngioma is characterized by aberrant nuclear β-catenin expression* ⇨*. Uninvolved cells show the normal membranous pattern* →*. Mutations in this gene are associated with protein overexpression in these tumors.*

Metastatic Carcinoma to Pituitary

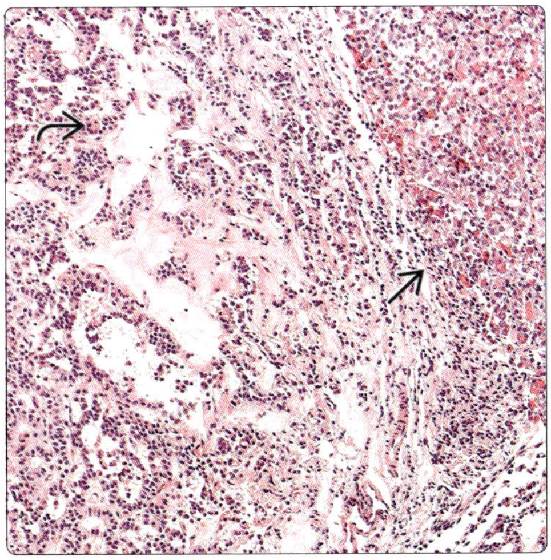

Metastatic Carcinoma to Pituitary

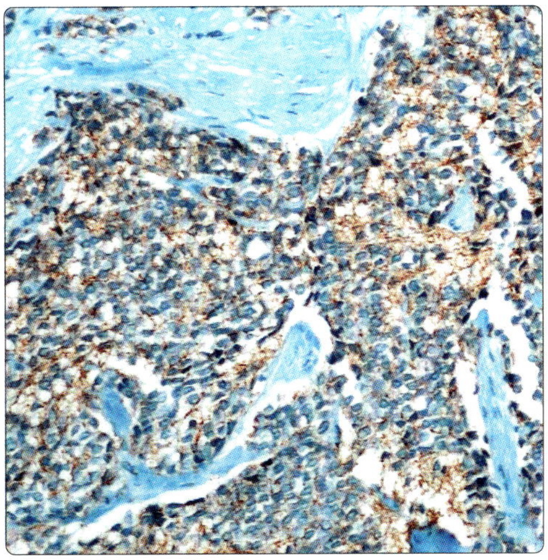

(Left) *Solid and acinar architecture in metastases* ↪ *may mimic pituitary adenomas. Metastatic neuroendocrine carcinoma to the anterior lobe of the pituitary* → *is illustrated. Metastases to the posterior lobe are more common.* **(Right)** *Small cell neuroendocrine carcinoma of lung may metastasize to the pituitary. This metastasis shows immunoreactivity for chromogranin-A, which can also be seen in some pituitary adenomas.*

SURGICAL/CLINICAL CONSIDERATIONS

Goal of Consultation

- Provide diagnosis for pleural lesion
- Determine if adequate tissue is present for further study

Change in Patient Management

- Additional biopsies may be taken until diagnostic tissue is provided
- If metastatic disease is present, surgery for curative intent may not be possible

Clinical Setting

- Patients with pleural effusions may have benign or malignant diseases
  - If there is a known diagnosis of lung cancer, pleural biopsy may be performed for staging
    - Pleural involvement usually precludes additional surgery
  - If there is no known malignancy, pleural biopsy is performed for diagnosis
    - It may be difficult or impossible to obtain definitive diagnosis using cytologic specimens
    - Multiple biopsies may be required to obtain sufficient tissue for diagnosis
- Biopsies may be performed during procedure to treat effusion (e.g., talc pleurodesis)

SPECIMEN EVALUATION

Gross

- Specimen usually consists of small fragments of tissue

Frozen Section

- Entire tissue sample is submitted for frozen section

MOST COMMON DIAGNOSES

Inflammatory Changes (Pleuritis)

- Often contains combination of fibrin, mixed inflammatory cells, granulation tissue, &/or fibrosis
- Zonation of cells is typical
  - Cellularity is greatest near pleural surface and becomes less cellular deeper
  - Cells are aligned parallel to pleural surface
- Can be associated with mesothelial hyperplasia
  - Reactive mesothelial cells can have enlarged nuclei and prominent nucleoli
  - Cells within fibrin can mimic invasion
- Overdiagnosis of malignancy should be avoided
  - Additional biopsies should be requested if diagnostic features of malignancy are not seen
  - In some cases, definitive diagnosis will need to be deferred
- If infection is suspected clinically or histologically, tissue for microbiologic cultures should be considered

Metastatic Carcinoma

- Patients usually have history of malignancy
  - Information about type of malignancy and review of slides can be helpful
- Definitive cytologic features of malignancy are usually present
- May show mucinous or signet ring cell features
- Can be very difficult to distinguish from mesothelioma histologically

Mesothelioma

- Mesothelioma is often difficult to diagnose on frozen section
  - Epithelioid mesotheliomas can be difficult to distinguish from reactive mesothelial cells and metastatic carcinoma
  - Desmoplastic mesothelioma can be difficult to distinguish from reactive pleuritis
- Features that favor malignancy rather than reactive mesothelial atypia
  - Invasion into stroma
    - Invasion into deeper structures, such as lung parenchyma or adipose tissue, is definitive for malignancy
      - Artifactual elongated spaces in collagen can mimic adipose tissue

Pleuritis

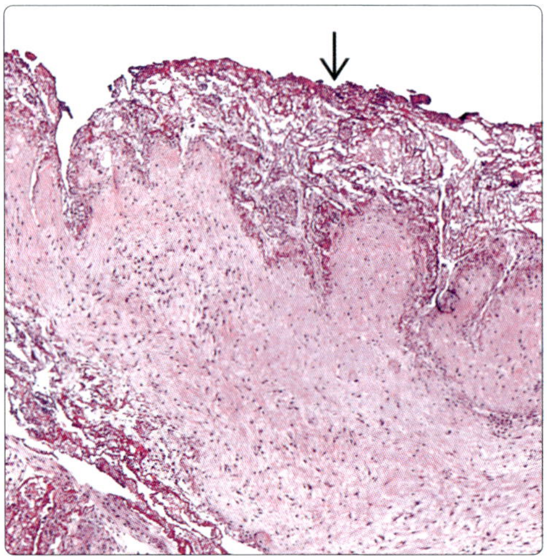

Metastatic Carcinoma

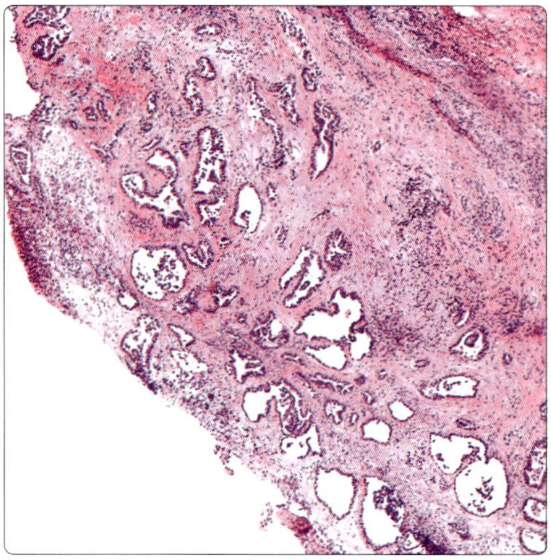

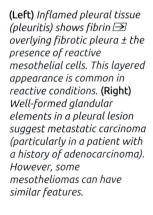

(Left) *Inflamed pleural tissue (pleuritis) shows fibrin ➙ overlying fibrotic pleura ± the presence of reactive mesothelial cells. This layered appearance is common in reactive conditions.* **(Right)** *Well-formed glandular elements in a pleural lesion suggest metastatic carcinoma (particularly in a patient with a history of adenocarcinoma). However, some mesotheliomas can have similar features.*

- Cells are present deep within tissue and are associated with stromal reaction
  - Papillary structures are lined by multiple cell layers in complex pattern
  - Cells have erratic pattern rather than appearing zonal in arrangement
    - Proliferation can be more cellular away from pleural surface
  - Desmoplastic mesotheliomas are present as haphazard arrangement
    - Reactive mesothelial cells often show layering parallel to pleural surface
- Marked nuclear atypia and enlargement may be present
  - However, many tumor cells can have small, bland nuclei and be monomorphic in appearance
  - Mitoses may be rare
- Necrosis favors diagnosis of malignancy
- Capillaries are in disorganized pattern, rather than being perpendicular to surface

Solitary Fibrous Tumor

- Grow as discrete solitary masses arising from pleura
  - May be sessile or pedunculated
- Bland spindle cell neoplasm with abundant collagen and ectatic staghorn vasculature
- Can mimic desmoplastic mesothelioma
  - However, desmoplastic mesotheliomas have diffuse infiltrative pattern in pleura
- Rare subset is histologically malignant and can show overlap with sarcomatoid mesothelioma and synovial sarcoma

Synovial Sarcoma

- Can show overlap with solitary fibrous tumor and sarcomatoid mesothelioma
- Intratumoral calcification in many cases can be helpful clue
- Diagnosis often requires immunohistochemical &/or molecular analysis

Lymphoma

- Systemic lymphomas can secondarily involve pleura
- Lymphoma would be very difficult to distinguish from pleuritis due to inflammatory diseases or infection
- If lymphomas is suspected, allocation for special studies should be considered (flow cytometric analysis, special fixatives)

REPORTING

Frozen Section

- Report "positive for malignancy, final diagnosis deferred to permanent sections" for cases of mesothelioma vs. carcinoma
- Report "diagnostic tissue obtained, final diagnosis deferred to permanent sections" for challenging diagnostic cases
  - Always request additional tissue if initial sample is sparse
- If it is unclear if definitive diagnosis can be determined on permanent sections with additional studies, request additional biopsies

PITFALLS

Mesothelioma vs. Metastatic Carcinoma/Sarcoma

- Can be extremely difficult to distinguish from one another without use of immunohistochemistry
- Clinical history and presentation are very valuable
  - History of prior malignancy and focal or multifocal pleural involvement favors metastatic carcinoma
    - Review of slides from prior malignancy is helpful
  - Known diffuse involvement and asbestos exposure favors mesothelioma
- Reporting as positive for malignancy and then deferring to permanent sections may be best approach in challenging cases

Reactive Mesothelial Cells vs. Mesothelioma

- Atypical mesothelial cells are very common in reactive conditions and can be mistaken for malignancy
- Intermixed inflammation often conspicuous and can make interpretation difficult
- Features that favor mesothelial hyperplasia with atypia rather than malignancy
  - Cells are confined to pleural surface
    - Papillary structures are lined by single layer
  - Cellular proliferation becomes less cellular away from pleural surface
  - Capillaries are arranged perpendicular to pleural surface
  - No stromal invasion is present
  - Cellular atypia is only present in areas of fibrin and organization
    - Mitoses can be frequent
  - Necrosis is absent or very rare (only within exudate)

SELECTED REFERENCES

1. Galateau-Salle F et al: The 2015 World Health Organization Classification of Tumors of the Pleura: advances since the 2004 classification. J Thorac Oncol. 11(2):142-54, 2016
2. Karpathiou G et al: Pleural neoplastic pathology. Respir Med. 109(8):931-43, 2015
3. Sirmali M et al: Utility of intraoperative frozen section examination in thoracic surgery. a review of 721 cases. J Cardiovasc Surg (Torino). 47(1):83-7, 2006
4. Cagle PT et al: Differential diagnosis of benign and malignant mesothelial proliferations on pleural biopsies. Arch Pathol Lab Med. 129(11):1421-7, 2005

Reactive Mesothelial Cells

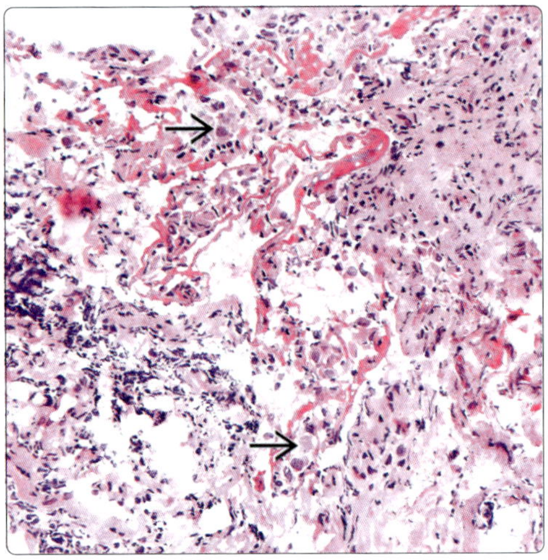

Reactive Mesothelial Cells: Cytologic Appearance

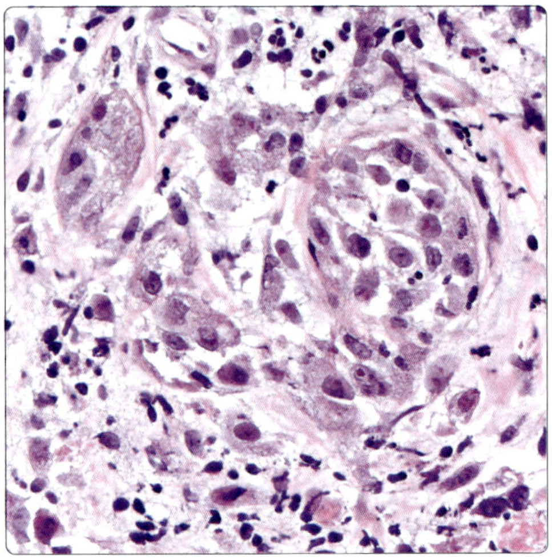

(Left) *This biopsy from a patient with pulmonary squamous cell carcinoma showed pink epithelioid cells* ⇒ *with stringy pink cytoplasm suspicious for carcinoma. However, these cells were identified as reactive mesothelial cells on permanent sections.* **(Right)** *Reactive mesothelial cells may form small nests or clusters that resemble carcinoma. Notably, these reactive cells often have granular cytoplasm on frozen section. A diagnosis of malignancy cannot be made based on cytologic features alone.*

Reactive Mesothelial Hyperplasia

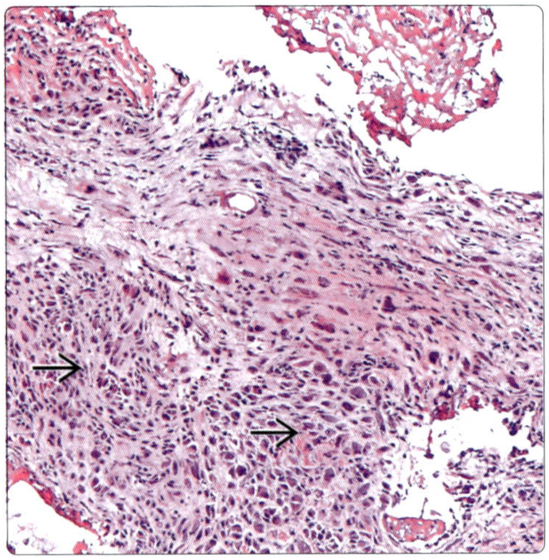

Reactive Mesothelial Cells

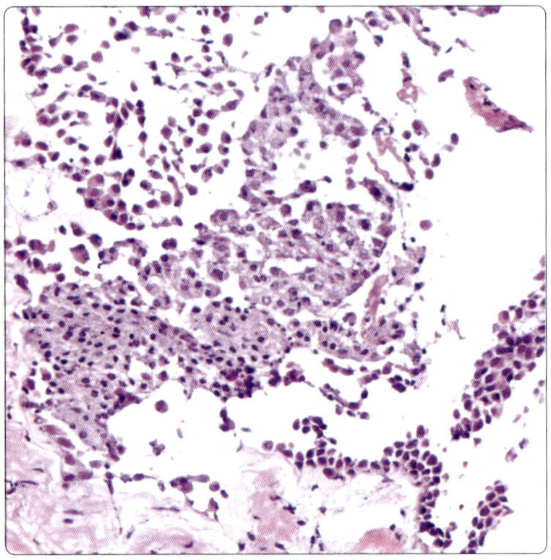

(Left) *Atypical mesothelial cells* ⇒ *are common in reactive pleura and may closely resemble malignancy. It is important to note the features that favor a reactive process: layered appearance with fibrin overlying the mesothelial cells as well as a lack of necrosis, no fat/muscle infiltration, and no complex architecture.* **(Right)** *Reactive mesothelial cells can form cellular sheets, particularly on the surface of the pleura, leading to confusion with malignant mesothelioma.*

Reactive Mesothelial Hyperplasia

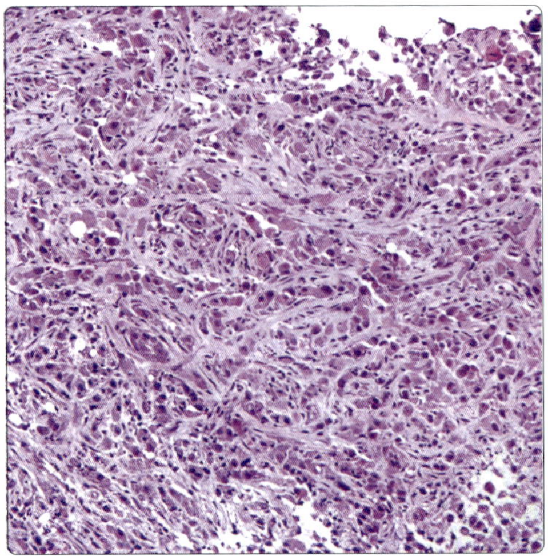

Malignant Mesothelioma

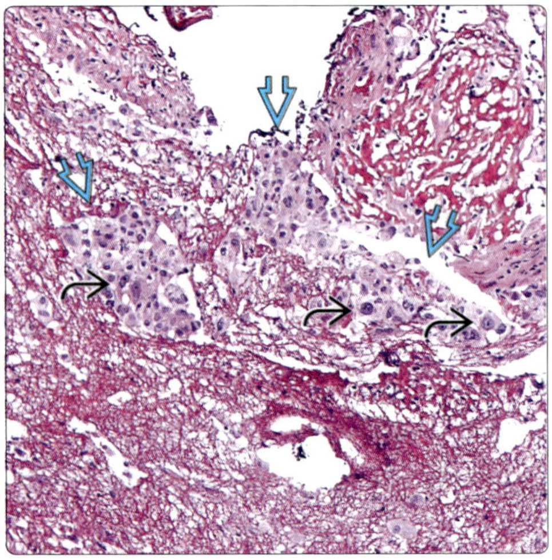

(Left) *Reactive mesothelial cells can have enlarged nuclei with prominent nucleoli. The cells can be intermingled in fibrin, fibrosis, &/or fibrin, making distinction from invasion difficult.* **(Right)** *These cell clusters* ⇒ *in fibrin show more variation in size and greater cytologic atypia* ⇒ *than usually seen in reactive mesothelial cells. Malignancy was suspected clinically. The final diagnosis was mesothelioma.*

Malignant Mesothelioma

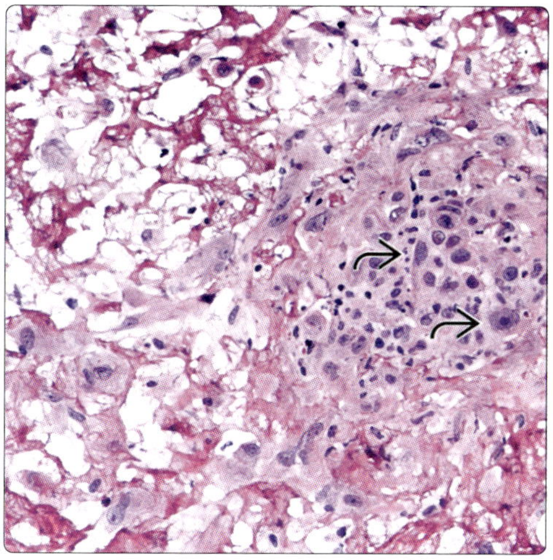

Malignant Mesothelioma

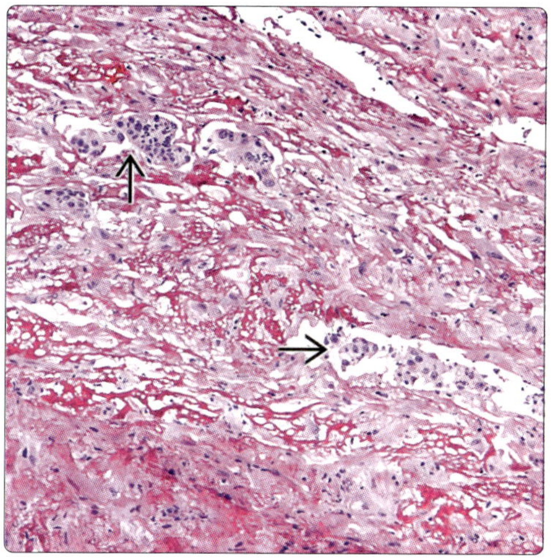

(Left) *The prominent enlarged nuclei with macronucleoli ➚ favor malignancy over reactive mesothelial atypia. There is also marked variation in the size of the cells. Immunohistochemical studies were required to identify this tumor as malignant mesothelioma rather than metastatic carcinoma.* **(Right)** *This malignant mesothelioma present in a biopsy as small nests of highly atypical cells resembles carcinoma with lymphatic space invasion ➙.*

Metastatic Sarcoma

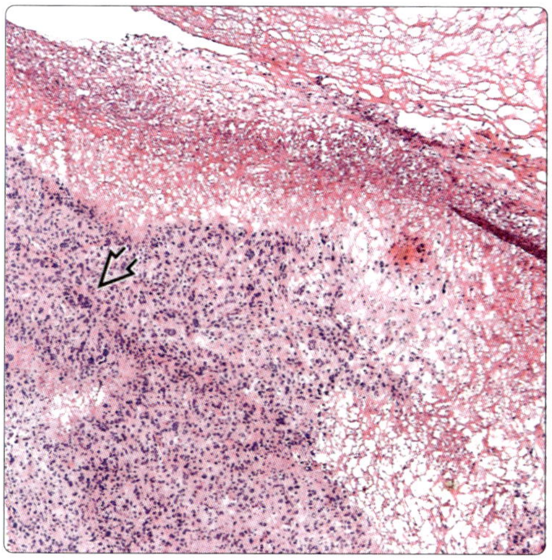

Solitary Fibrous Tumor

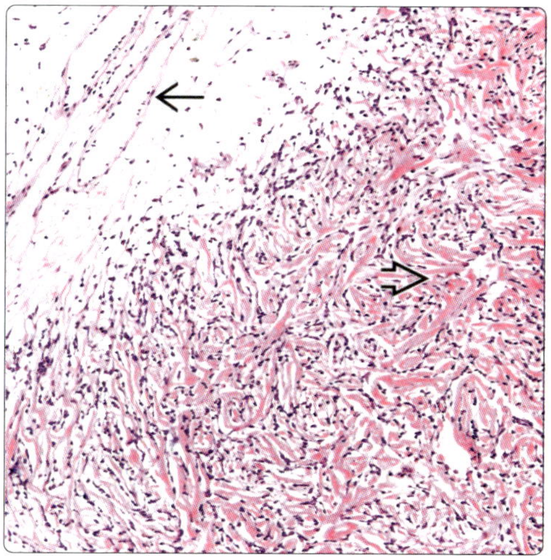

(Left) *Malignant cells ⇨ are identified in this case, but only a report of "positive for malignancy, defer" could be rendered. Final classification as metastatic sarcoma required ancillary stains and a history of a prior thigh mass.* **(Right)** *Solitary fibrous tumor is composed of bland spindle cells with stromal collagen ⇨ and ectatic blood vessels ➙. There is morphologic overlap with desmoplastic mesothelioma; however, the latter does not usually present as a localized or pedunculated lesion.*

Solitary Fibrous Tumor

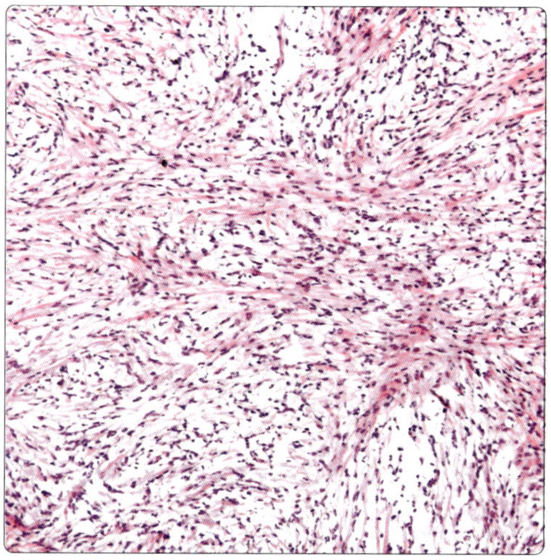

Solitary Fibrous Tumor

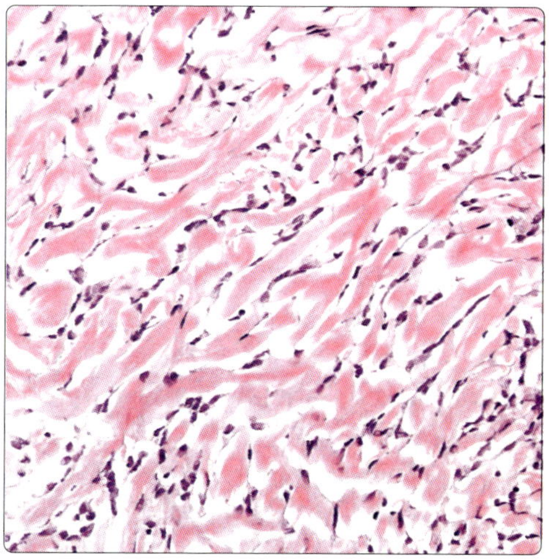

(Left) *Solitary fibrous tumors are bland spindle cell neoplasms with abundant collagen. They often form very localized (often pedunculated) tumors on the pleura.* **(Right)** *The stromal collagen in some examples of solitary fibrous tumor is very prominent and can raise the possibility of a sclerosing carcinoma or desmoplastic mesothelioma. However, the latter neoplasms will usually demonstrate more overt nuclear atypia and usually a more aggressive growth pattern.*

SURGICAL/CLINICAL CONSIDERATIONS

Goal of Consultation

- Determine if joint is infected

Change in Patient Management

- If infection is present, artificial joint may be removed and area drained
- New joint will not be placed until infection is cleared

Clinical Setting

- Can be difficult to distinguish mechanical from septic loosening of artificial joint
- Positive culture results may be due to contamination with skin bacteria

SPECIMEN EVALUATION

Gross

- Examine tissue to identify areas most suspicious for infection
    - Tan/pink to red/brown tissue (necrotic or hemorrhagic areas) should be selected
    - White fibrous tissue or fibrin are unlikely to show areas of diagnostic inflammation

Frozen Section

- At least 2 representative blocks of tissue should be frozen from most suspicious areas

MOST COMMON DIAGNOSES

Infected Artificial Joint

- Acute inflammatory cells (neutrophils) in periarticular connective tissue

Detritic Synovitis

- Inflammatory changes due to erosion/breakdown of joint
- Reaction to foreign material (e.g., silicone/metal shavings) is often present
- Chronic inflammation, but not acute inflammation, may be present

Diffuse-Type Tenosynovial Giant Cell Tumor

- Previously known as pigmented villonodular synovitis
- Papillary fronds containing sheets and nodules of epithelioid histiocytoid cells with eccentric reniform nuclei and variable numbers of multinucleated giant cells, pigment, and xanthomatous inflammation

REPORTING

Frozen Section

- Report only number of neutrophils per HPF; x 400
- Count at least 5 HPF in most inflamed areas of tissue
    - Average of ≥ 5 neutrophils over 5 HPF is suggestive of infection
- Recent metaanalysis has shown threshold of 10 neutrophils per HPF may have higher specificity
- Do not count neutrophils within fibrin, surface inflammatory infiltrates, or those marginated in vessels

Reliability

- Specificity is generally high if criteria are used and ≥ 2 blocks of tissue are frozen

PITFALLS

Rheumatoid Arthritis

- Neutrophils often present that are not related to infection; accurate evaluation may be impossible

Sampling Error

- Failure to freeze sufficient tissue may miss diagnostic areas

SELECTED REFERENCES

1. Zhao X et al: Ten versus five polymorphonuclear leukocytes as threshold in frozen section tests for periprosthetic infection: a meta-analysis. J Arthroplasty. 28(6):913-7, 2013
2. Tsaras G et al: Utility of intraoperative frozen section histopathology in the diagnosis of periprosthetic joint infection: a systematic review and meta-analysis. J Bone Joint Surg Am. 94(18):1700-11, 2012
3. Kanner WA et al: Reassessment of the usefulness of frozen section analysis for hip and knee joint revisions. Am J Clin Pathol. 130(3):363-8, 2008

Neutrophils

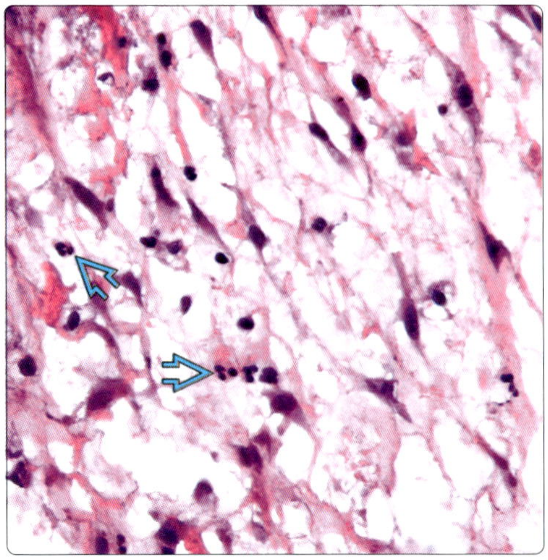

Nuclear Morphology

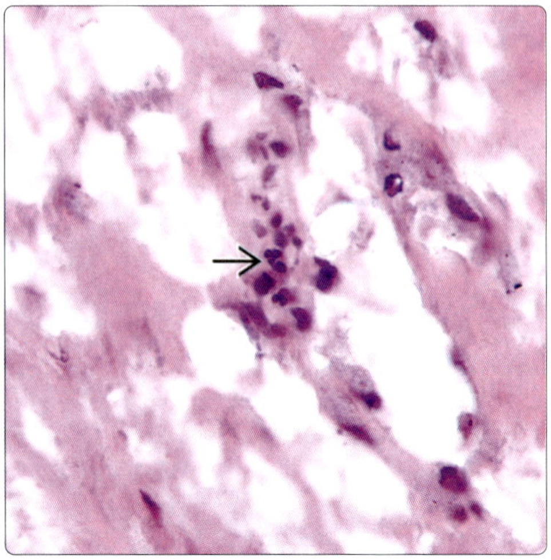

(Left) *To evaluate for infection in a revision arthroplasty case, count the number of neutrophils ⇨ per HPF, x 400 in at least 5 separate HPF, and report the average count.* **(Right)** *Neutrophils may be difficult to distinguish from crushed lymphocytes or apoptotic nuclei. The characteristic multilobated nuclear morphology → of this type of cell is the most reliable feature.*

Surface Inflammatory Infiltrates

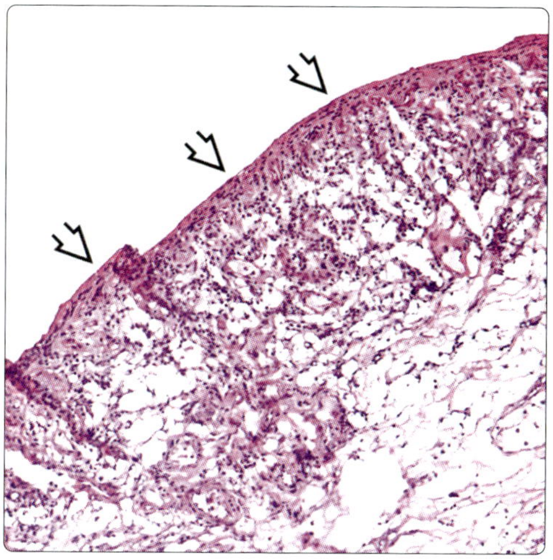

Neutrophils in Fibrin

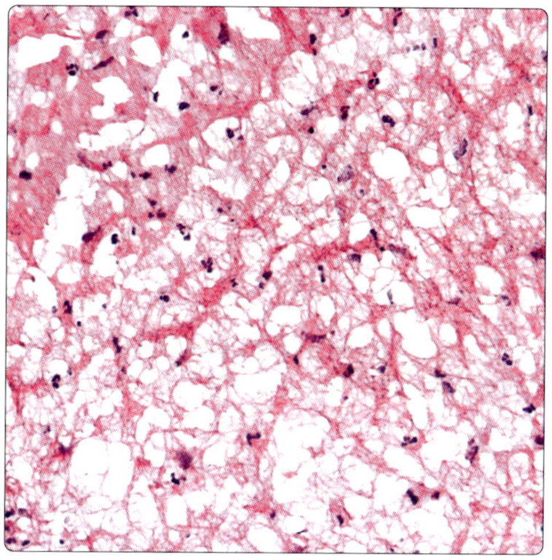

(Left) *Neutrophilic inflammatory infiltrates located at the tissue surface* → *should be ignored when counting neutrophils as their presence does not correlate well with true periprosthetic infection.* **(Right)** *Neutrophils located within surface fibrin do not correlate well with true periprosthetic infection and should be ignored when doing a formal count. This fibrin is often associated with blood related to the operative procedure. Only true connective tissue should be chosen for freezing.*

Margination of Neutrophils

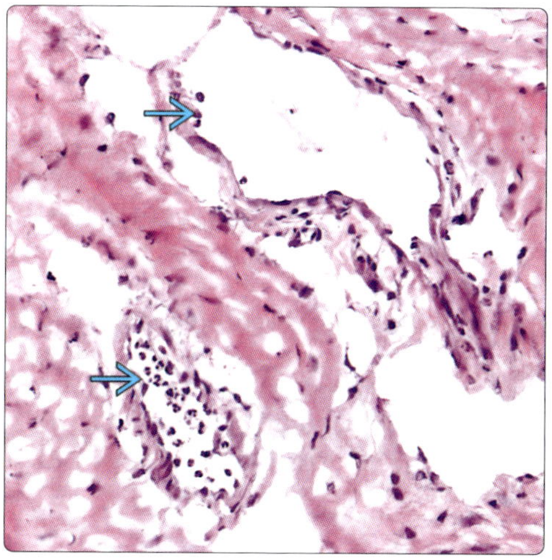

Detritic Synovitis

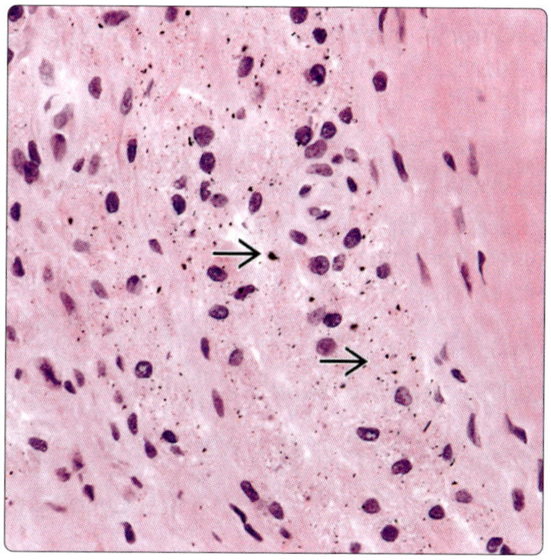

(Left) *Neutrophils may be present at the periphery of small blood vessels (known as margination* →*) in a variety of inflammatory states or due to the operation. This finding is nonspecific, and the cells should not be included in the count.* **(Right)** *In some patients, material* → *from a prosthesis will erode or flake off into the periarticular soft tissues, leading to a histiocytic inflammatory reaction (detritic synovitis). Although not common, this debris may somewhat resemble neutrophils.*

Diffuse-Type Tenosynovial Giant Cell Tumor

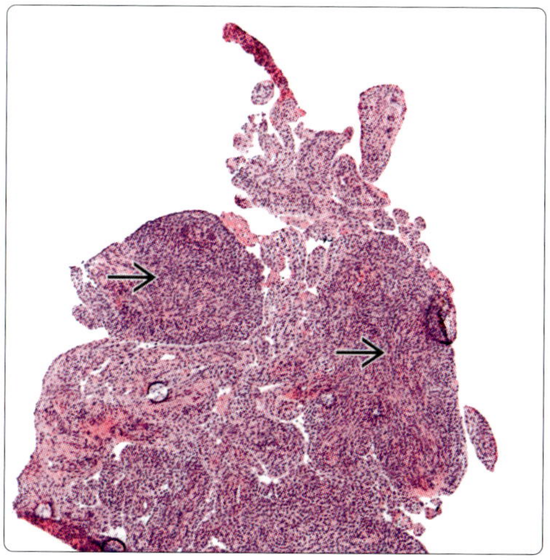

Diffuse-Type Tenosynovial Giant Cell Tumor

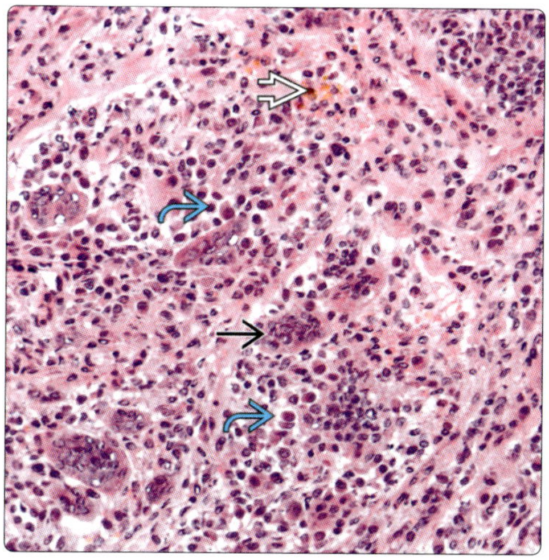

(Left) *Diffuse-type tenosynovial giant cell tumor (pigmented villonodular synovitis) usually has a much different clinical presentation than periarticular infection, but rare, clinically overlapping cases may occur. At low magnification, the papillary synovial structures are greatly expanded* → *by a mononuclear cell proliferation.* **(Right)** *Diffuse-type tenosynovial giant cell tumor is composed of a mixture of histiocytoid mononuclear cells* →*, multinucleated giant cells* →*, and pigment* →.

SURGICAL/CLINICAL CONSIDERATIONS

Goal of Consultation

- Determine if salivary gland mass is a high-grade malignancy
  - For parotid lesions, distinction of benign tumors from low-grade malignancies is not essential on frozen section as either will be treated with conservative excision
- Ensure margins free of tumor

Change in Patient Management

- If high-grade malignancy present, surgical procedure may be altered
  - In parotid, high-grade carcinoma often treated with total parotidectomy, requiring facial nerve dissection with associated morbidity
  - Neck lymph node dissection may be performed
  - Patients typically receive adjuvant radiation therapy, possibly combined with chemotherapy
- Positive margins may prompt additional surgery
- With increasing recognition of characteristic genetic alterations in salivary tumors, triage of fresh tissue for cytogenetics may be helpful in select cases
  - Characteristic translocations associated with pleomorphic adenoma, carcinoma ex pleomorphic adenoma, adenoid cystic carcinoma, mucoepidermoid carcinoma, secretory carcinoma, and clear cell carcinoma

Clinical Setting

- Salivary gland mass may not represent intrinsic lesion, particularly in parotid gland where peri- and intraparotid lymph nodes may be recipients of metastatic disease or involved by lymphoma
- Frozen section may be needed to resolve diagnostic uncertainty following fine-needle aspiration (FNA) of salivary gland mass
  - Distinction of basaloid neoplasms, including basal cell adenoma, basal cell adenocarcinoma, and adenoid cystic carcinoma, may not be possible on FNA
  - Cystic lesions may not yield diagnostic material
  - Atypia in pleomorphic adenoma raises concern about carcinoma ex pleomorphic adenoma
- High-grade malignancies (especially adenoid cystic carcinoma) may involve nerves with perineural spread well beyond grossly evident tumor

SPECIMEN EVALUATION

Gross

- Benign tumors typically circumscribed
- Benign and recurrent tumors may have multinodular growth
- High-grade carcinomas often grossly infiltrative
- If entire resection sent for margin evaluation, precise orientation essential
  - Direct consultation with surgeon can be very helpful to identify location of closest margins
  - Differential inking of margins with multiple colors can be helpful to maintain orientation
  - Entire specimen serially sectioned
- Margins may be sent as small biopsies from edges of surgical bed ("defect sampling") or may be taken from branches of facial nerve to determine extent of perineural involvement

Frozen Section

- Small biopsies may be completely frozen
- Sections should be taken perpendicular to margin
  - En face margins not capable of evaluating narrow (1-2 mm) but tumor-free margins
    - Narrow distance to margin may be clinically important and can only be assessed with perpendicular section
  - Infiltrative growth, perineural invasion, &/or lymph-vascular invasion indicative of malignancy even in tumors lacking significant atypia
    - Additional presence of pronounced cytologic atypia, necrosis, abundant mitotic activity, &/or atypical mitoses associated with high-grade carcinoma

Cytology

- Touch or scrape preps may be performed to evaluate tumors
- Cytology not routinely used for margin evaluation

Pleomorphic Adenoma

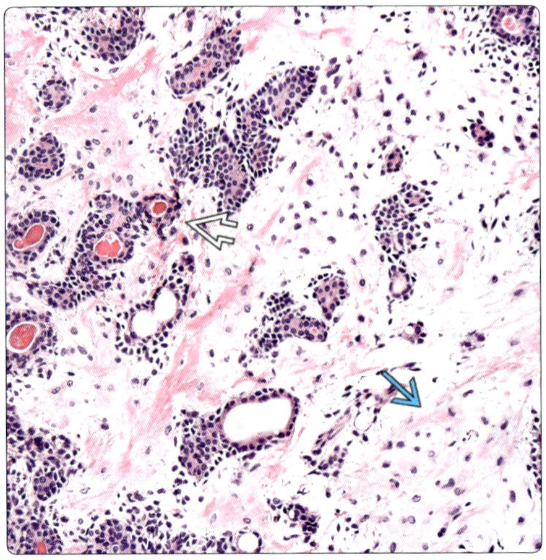

Adenoid Cystic Carcinoma

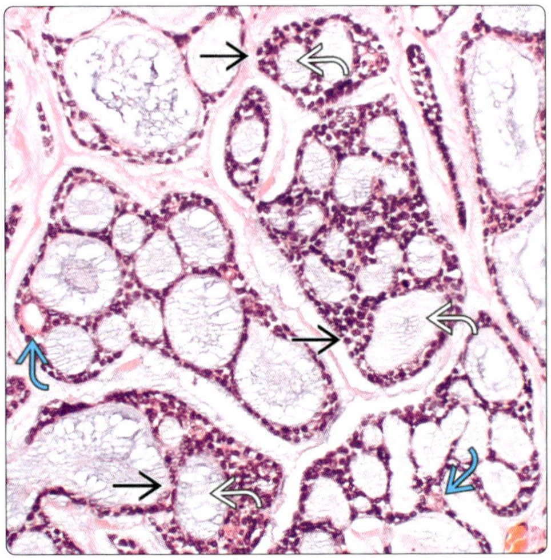

(Left) *Pleomorphic adenoma consists of ductal elements ➡ as well as spindled and ovoid myoepithelial cells ➡ embedded within the abundant chondromyxoid matrix that is characteristic of this tumor.* **(Right)** *Cribriform type of adenoid cystic carcinoma has basaloid myoepithelial cells ➡ surrounding acellular mucopolysaccharide matrix ➡. Rare ductal ➡ elements formed by luminal cells are present.*

MOST COMMON DIAGNOSES

Benign Tumors and Low-Grade Malignancies

- **Pleomorphic adenoma**
  - Most common benign tumor
  - Readily diagnosed by FNA in most cases
    - Frozen section analysis limited to tumors with unusual features
  - Cytologic atypia on FNA should prompt examination for malignant transformation and infiltrative growth
    - Noninvasive or minimally invasive (up to 4-6 mm) carcinoma ex pleomorphic adenoma has favorable clinical outcome compared to widely invasive tumor
  - Sparse chondromyxoid matrix results in appearance similar to basal cell adenoma or myoepithelioma
    - Distinction not critical among various possible benign tumor diagnoses on frozen section
  - Extensive metaplastic changes make distinction from other diagnoses challenging
    - May have squamous, mucinous, sebaceous, and oncocytic epithelial cells in addition to usual ductal and myoepithelial components
    - May have myxoid, chondroid, adipocytic, and osseous mesenchymal elements
    - Additional sampling of grossly distinct tumor areas may reveal more typical features of pleomorphic adenoma
- **Oncocytic and clear cell tumors**
  - Both oncocytic and clear cell features may be seen as nonspecific morphology in variety of tumors (including mucoepidermoid carcinoma and acinic cell carcinoma)
  - Prominent oncocytic features characteristic of certain tumors (Warthin tumor and oncocytoma), while clear cell features typical of other tumors (epithelial-myoepithelial carcinoma, clear cell carcinoma)
  - Wide sampling may be needed for final classification
    - Areas with features characteristic of specific tumor may be focal
  - Specific diagnosis usually not essential on frozen section as differential diagnosis is among benign tumors and low-grade malignancies that will be managed similarly vs. high-grade malignancies
  - **Warthin tumor**
    - Oncocytic epithelium lining lymphoid stroma
    - Almost exclusively in parotid gland
    - May be multifocal &/or bilateral
    - Extensive squamous metaplasia may raise concern for squamous cell carcinoma
  - **Oncocytoma**
    - Tumor composed predominantly of oncocytic cells with abundant eosinophilic cytoplasm
    - Clear cell change may be focal or prominent
    - Most common in parotid gland
    - Multifocal lesions in 1 or both parotid glands favor diagnosis of nodular oncocytic hyperplasia
  - **Low-grade mucoepidermoid carcinoma**
    - Mucoepidermoid carcinoma most common salivary gland malignancy in all age groups
    - Characteristic components are mucous cells, epidermoid cells, and intermediate cells
    - Low-grade tumors more cystic with more prominent mucous cell and intermediate cell components
    - Lack high-grade features, including solid growth, nuclear anaplasia, high mitotic rate, necrosis, perineural or lymph-vascular invasion, irregular invasive tumor front, and bone invasion
    - May have prominent lymphoid stroma
    - Prominent clear cell or oncocytic features may require additional sampling (or special stains) to identify characteristic cellular constituents
  - **Acinic cell carcinoma**
    - Tumor cells exhibit serous acinar cell differentiation with abundant granular basophilic cytoplasm
    - Solid, cystic, &/or papillary growth patterns
    - May have prominent lymphoid stroma
    - Most common in parotid gland
  - **Secretory carcinoma**
    - Previously termed mammary analogue secretory carcinoma
    - Microcystic, solid, tubular, follicular, &/or papillary growth patterns
    - Cells have eosinophilic cytoplasm that may be vacuolated or granular
    - Dense luminal colloid-like secretory material
    - Lack granular basophilic zymogen granules of acinic cell carcinoma
    - Most common in parotid gland but occurs elsewhere

Basaloid Neoplasms

- **Basal cell adenoma and basal cell adenocarcinoma**
  - Comprised of basaloid myoepithelial cells and ducts
  - Cellular areas exhibit peripheral palisading at interface with less cellular stromal component
  - Lacks characteristic chondromyxoid stroma of pleomorphic adenoma
  - Tubular, trabecular, solid, and membranous patterns
  - Benign and malignant counterparts are distinguished by presence of lymph-vascular invasion &/or infiltrative growth
  - Basal cell adenocarcinoma is low-grade malignancy
    - Distinction on frozen section not essential as surgical management similar for both tumors
  - Most common in parotid gland
- **Adenoid cystic carcinoma**
  - Solid variant most aggressive variant and challenging to recognize
    - Need to identify more typical areas with tubular or cribriform growth and typical acellular matrix spheres (may have mucoid or hyaline appearance)
    - Distinction of solid adenoid cystic carcinoma from other high-grade basaloid carcinomas (including primary or metastatic high-grade neuroendocrine carcinoma or basaloid squamous cell carcinoma) not essential on frozen section

High-Grade Carcinomas

- **Salivary duct carcinoma**
  - Nests and sheets of markedly atypical epithelioid cells with prominent mitotic activity and often central necrosis reminiscent of comedo-type ductal breast carcinoma

Contents

Immunohistochemical and Genetic Features of Common Salivary Neoplasms

Tumor Type	Immunohistochemistry	Genetic Alterations
Pleomorphic adenoma Carcinoma ex pleomorphic adenoma	PLAG1 HMGA2	Translocation of 8q12 (*PLAG1*) or 12q14-15 (*HMGA2*)
Basal cell adenoma	β-catenin (nuclear)	*CTNNB1* point mutation *CYLD* mutation (membranous type)
Salivary duct carcinoma	HER2 Androgen receptor	17q21.1 amplification (*ERBB2*) 3q26.32 mutation (*PIK3CA*)
Adenoid cystic carcinoma	MYB	t(6;9)(p21;q13); *MYB-NFIB* fusion gene
Mucoepidermoid carcinoma	p63 (multifocal staining)	t(11;19)(q21;p13) or t(11;15)(q21;q26); *CRCT1-MAML2* or *CRCT3-MAML2* fusion gene
Secretory carcinoma	Mammaglobin and S100	t(12;15)(p13;q25); *ETV6-NTRK3* fusion gene

  - Distinction from rare case of metastatic breast carcinoma requires clinicopathologic correlation
  - Arises de novo or as component of carcinoma ex pleomorphic adenoma
- **Carcinoma ex pleomorphic adenoma**
  - Must recognize preexisting pleomorphic adenoma for diagnosis
  - Malignant component most frequently salivary duct carcinoma
- **High-grade mucoepidermoid carcinoma**
  - Characterized by number of features, including solid growth, nuclear anaplasia, high mitotic rate, necrosis, perineural or lymph-vascular invasion, irregular invasive tumor front, and bone invasion
  - High-grade tumors tend to be squamoid with focal mucinous differentiation
  - Extensive keratinization indicates squamous cell carcinoma, likely of cutaneous origin, that has spread to and replaced parotid region lymph nodes
- **Poorly differentiated transformation ("dedifferentiation")**
  - High-grade component arising in association with differentiated carcinoma that no longer resembles precursor malignancy
  - Described in association with many tumors but most common with acinic cell carcinoma

Metastases

- Cutaneous squamous cell carcinoma of head and neck often metastasizes to intra- or periparotid lymph nodes
- Melanoma can also metastasize to salivary gland lymph nodes
- In setting of large mass with extranodal extension and replacement of lymphoid tissue, may be difficult to differentiate metastasis from primary carcinoma

REPORTING

Frozen Section

- Presence or absence of neoplasm (at margin, if applicable)
- Specific diagnosis when possible, but adequate to classify as low-grade salivary gland neoplasm or high-grade carcinoma
- Many differential diagnoses can be resolved by ancillary studies

PITFALLS

Squamous Metaplasia

- May be especially florid in pleomorphic adenoma and Warthin tumor, potentially causing confusion with squamous cell carcinoma or mucoepidermoid carcinoma
  - Look for characteristic chondromyxoid matrix of pleomorphic adenoma and oncocytic epithelium with reactive lymphoid stroma of Warthin tumor
- Sialometaplasia creates impression of invasive carcinoma
  - Changes seen in conjunction with ischemic changes in adjacent tissue, often after prior biopsy
  - Lobulated squamous metaplasia of salivary ducts without marked atypia aids in recognition

Cystic Lesions

- Distinction of nonneoplastic cysts from benign or low-grade malignant cystic lesions may be challenging
  - Epithelium may be poorly represented on frozen section
  - Differentiation (such as in cystic acinic cell carcinoma) may not be evident on frozen section or may require special stains (PAS with diastase for acinar differentiation, mucicarmine for mucoepidermoid carcinoma)
- Specific diagnosis intraoperatively not critical

Distinction of Normal Structures From Tumor

- Especially challenging when assessing margins where isolated glandular structures from well-differentiated carcinomas may mimic normal salivary gland elements
- Comparison with main tumor may help resolve uncertainty

SELECTED REFERENCES

1. Seethala RR et al: Update from the 4th edition of the World Health Organization Classification of Head and Neck Tumours: Tumors of the Salivary Gland. Head Neck Pathol. 11(1):55-67, 2017
2. Seethala RR et al: Molecular pathology: predictive, prognostic, and diagnostic markers in salivary gland tumors. Surg Pathol Clin. 9(3):339-52, 2016
3. Schmidt RL et al: A systematic review and meta-analysis of the diagnostic accuracy of frozen section for parotid gland lesions. Am J Clin Pathol. 136(5):729-38, 2011

Pleomorphic Adenoma

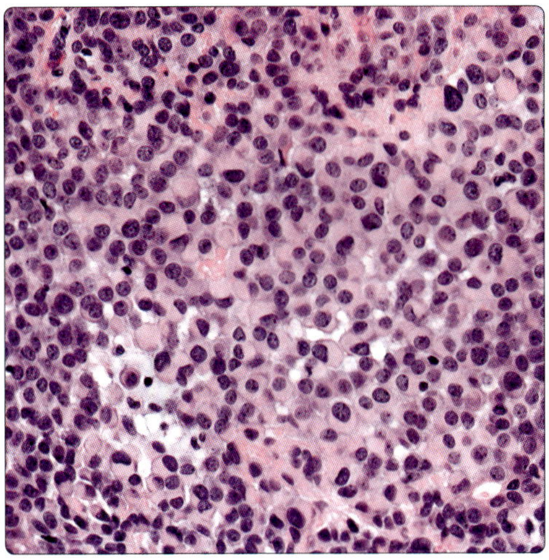

Pleomorphic Adenoma

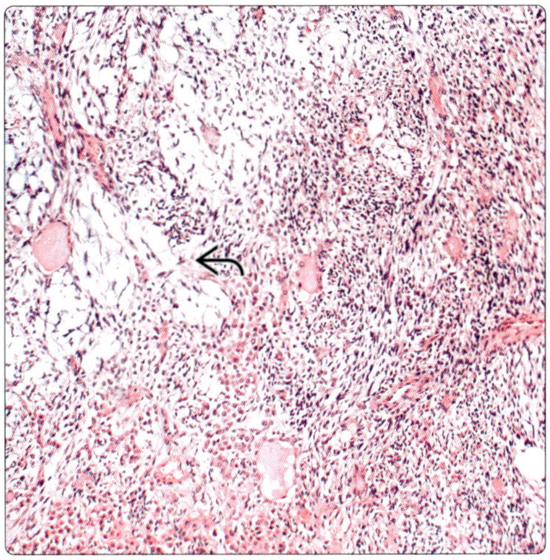

(Left) *Recognition of pleomorphic adenoma is difficult when the characteristic matrix material is sparse. Distinction of plasmacytoid myoepithelial cells from plasmacytoma may require immunohistochemical studies.* **(Right)** *In this pleomorphic adenoma, the predominant population of myoepithelial cells has a prominent spindle cell morphology, raising a differential diagnosis with spindled mesenchymal proliferations. Note the focal presence of chondromyxoid matrix material ⇨.*

Recurrent Pleomorphic Adenoma

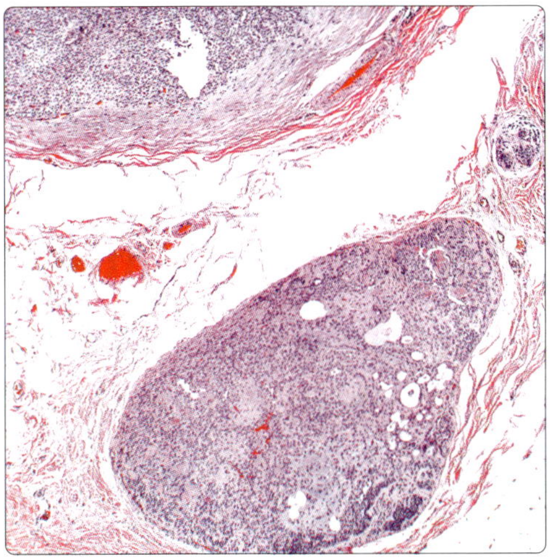

Pleomorphic Adenoma

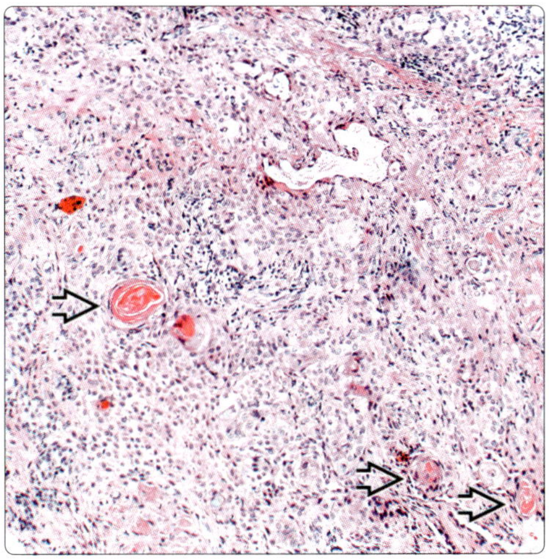

(Left) *Recurrent pleomorphic adenoma often presents as multiple discrete tumor nodules within soft tissue in the surgical bed. These nodules are circumscribed and should not be confused with the infiltrative growth seen with carcinoma ex pleomorphic adenoma.* **(Right)** *This incisional biopsy of a palatal pleomorphic adenoma shows foci of squamous metaplasia ⇨ within a largely solid sheet of myoepithelial cells. These findings were initially misinterpreted as representing an invasive squamous cell carcinoma.*

Carcinoma Ex Pleomorphic Adenoma

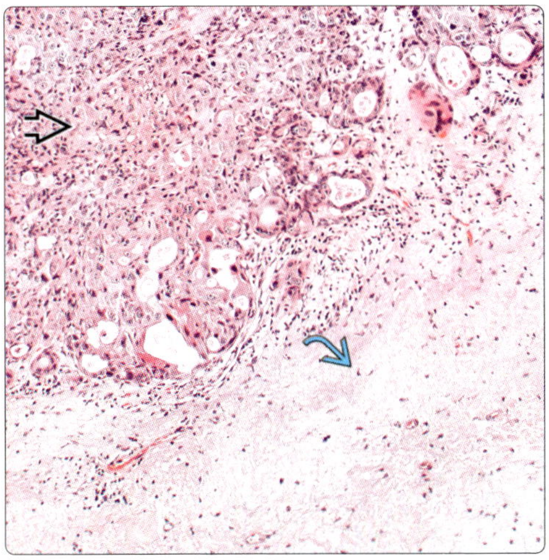

Carcinoma Ex Pleomorphic Adenoma

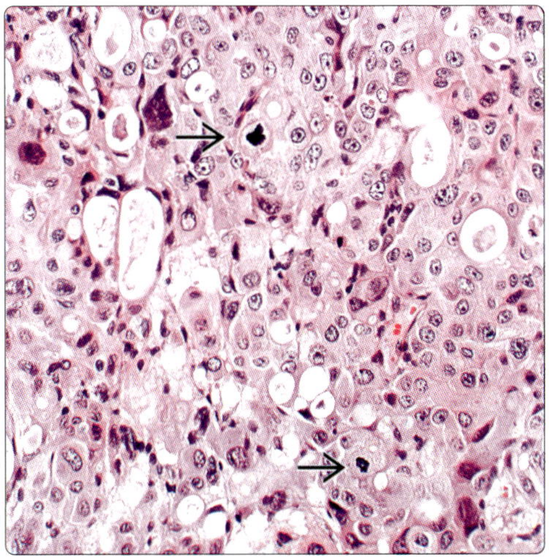

(Left) *A cellular solid and acinar proliferation of markedly atypical ductal cells ⇨ is present adjacent to the remnants of the preexisting paucicellular hyalinized pleomorphic adenoma ⇨ that has undergone malignant transformation.* **(Right)** *Carcinoma ex pleomorphic adenoma is a high-grade tumor with pleomorphic cells having hyperchromatic nuclei, prominent nucleoli, and atypical mitotic figures ⇨. The patient may present with sudden growth of a longstanding mass, pain, or facial paralysis.*

(Left) *In contrast to pleomorphic adenoma, basal cell adenoma lacks chondromyxoid extracellular matrix. Solid, trabecular, and tubular aggregates of basaloid cells with admixed ductal structures* → *are sharply delineated from the loose intervening stroma. Nuclei often palisade* → *at the periphery of these cell groups. Nuclear atypia is absent.* **(Right)** *Low-grade malignant counterpart of basal cell adenoma infiltrates into adjacent tissue. Perineural invasion may be present* →*.*

Basal Cell Adenoma

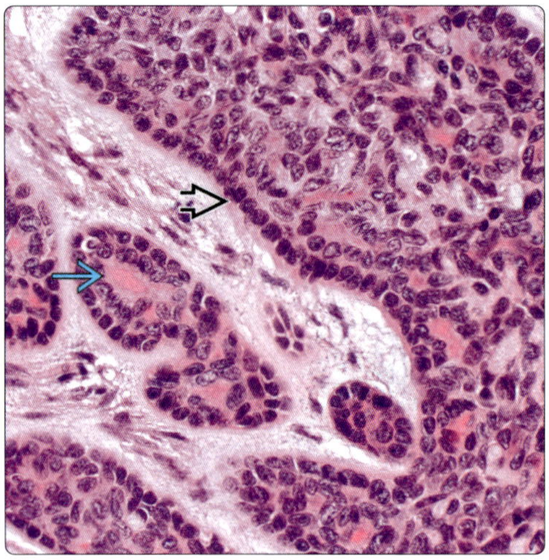

Basal Cell Adenocarcinoma

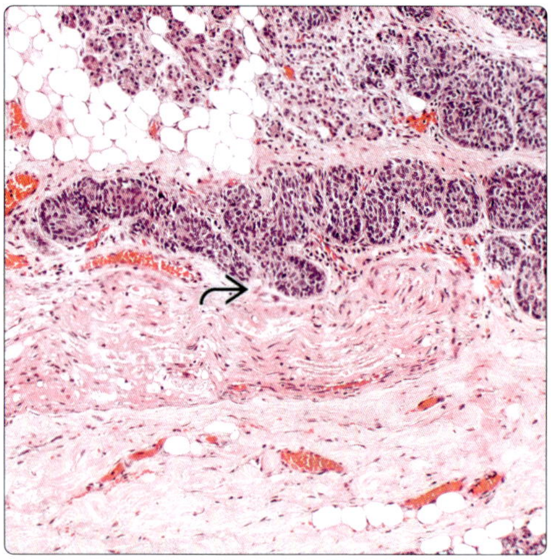

(Left) *In this margin reexcision, residual adenoid cystic carcinoma is present as scattered, deceptively bland, tubular glands* →*. This challenging diagnosis may be suspected due to the lack of circumscription. Nerves at margins should be carefully examined for perineural invasion.* **(Right)** *Adenoid cystic carcinoma can be difficult to recognize at the periphery, as tubules may be scant. Cribriform glands with hyperchromatic nuclei and scattered mitoses* → *confirm the malignant nature of these cells.*

Adenoid Cystic Carcinoma

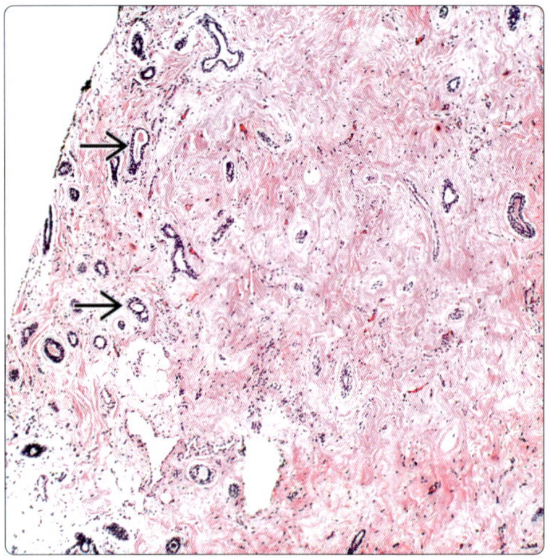

Adenoid Cystic Carcinoma

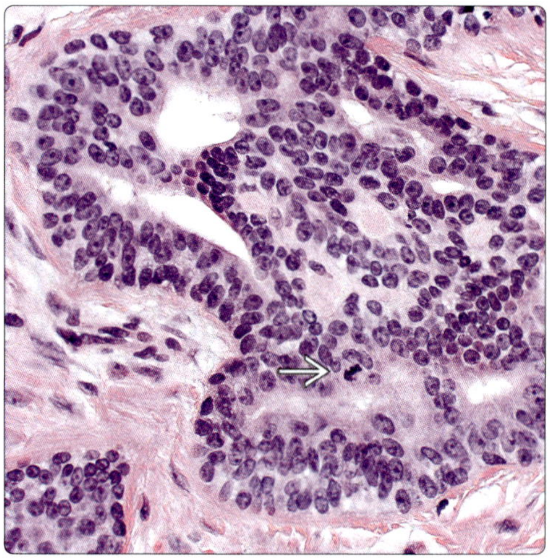

(Left) *The solid variant of adenoid cystic carcinoma may or may not have overt cytologic features of malignancy. Here, perineural invasion is present* →*. Distinction from other basaloid carcinomas is only possible when the more recognizable tubular or cribriform patterns* → *are also present.* **(Right)** *Primary high-grade neuroendocrine carcinoma cannot be distinguished from metastatic small cell carcinoma and Merkel cell carcinoma on frozen section. Clinical history and immunostains are needed.*

Adenoid Cystic Carcinoma: Solid Type

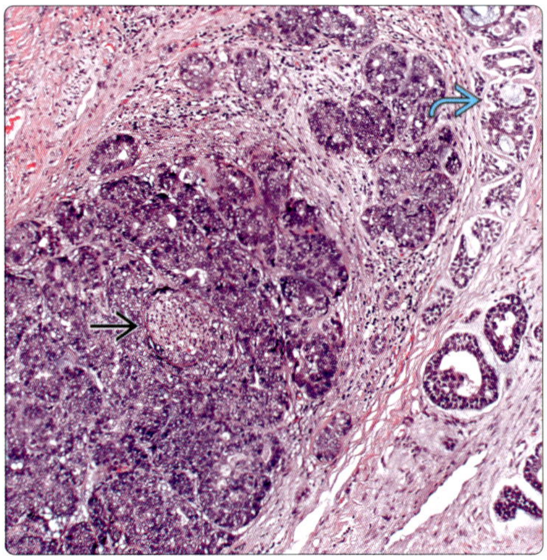

Neuroendocrine Carcinoma

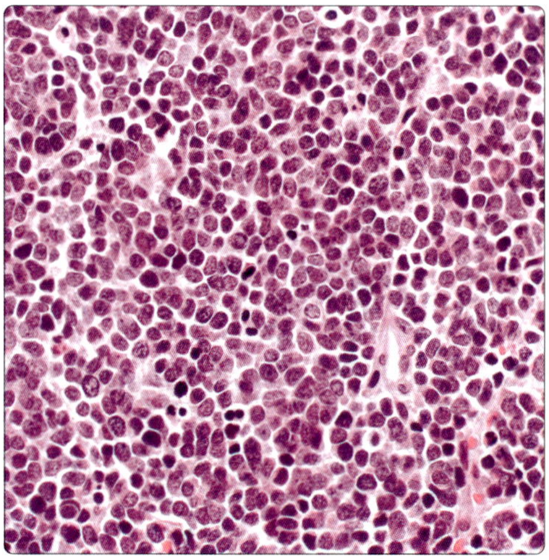

Polymorphous Adenocarcinoma

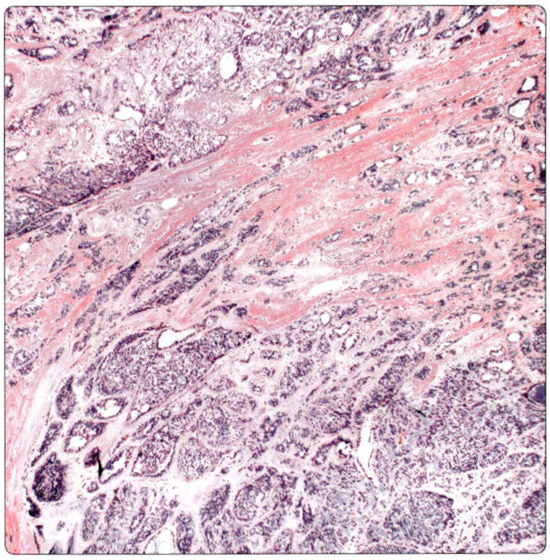

Polymorphous Adenocarcinoma

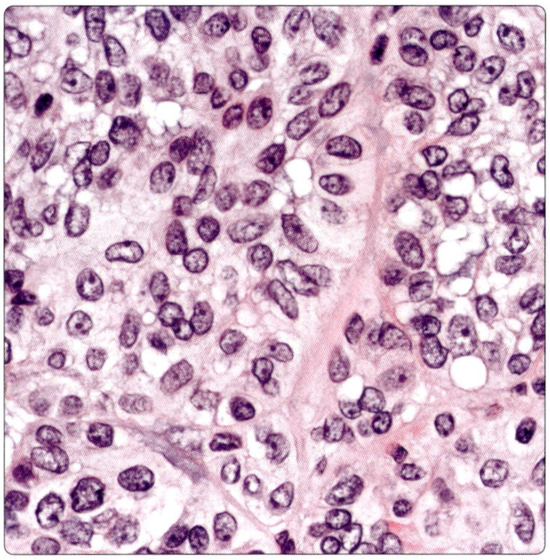

(Left) *Polymorphous adenocarcinoma is a malignancy of minor salivary glands that is architecturally diverse with solid, tubular, and cribriform growth. In small biopsy specimens, distinction from pleomorphic adenoma may be impossible. In such cases, a diagnosis of a low-grade salivary gland neoplasm is appropriate.* **(Right)** *Nuclei in polymorphous adenocarcinoma are uniform with fine chromatin and rare mitoses. In contrast, adenoid cystic carcinoma has angulated, hyperchromatic nuclei.*

Acinic Cell Carcinoma

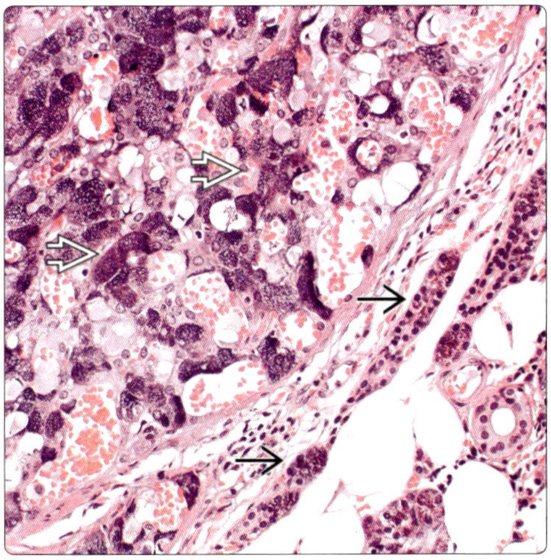

Acinic Cell Carcinoma

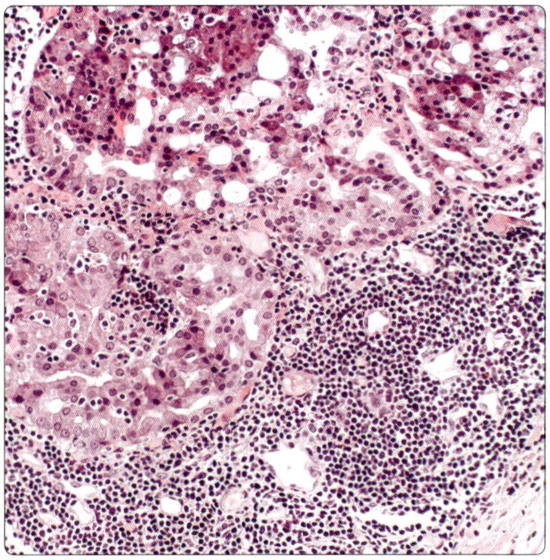

(Left) *Acinic cell carcinoma is recognized by the presence of serous acinar differentiation. The granular amphophilic cytoplasm in the tumor cells ➡ is similar to that of the adjacent benign serous acinar cells ⇒. If not evident on H&E, PAS with diastase will highlight cytoplasmic zymogen granules.* **(Right)** *Acinic cell carcinoma (shown here) and mucoepidermoid carcinoma frequently have an associated reactive lymphoid infiltrate that can mimic tumor metastatic to a lymph node.*

Epithelial-Myoepithelial Carcinoma

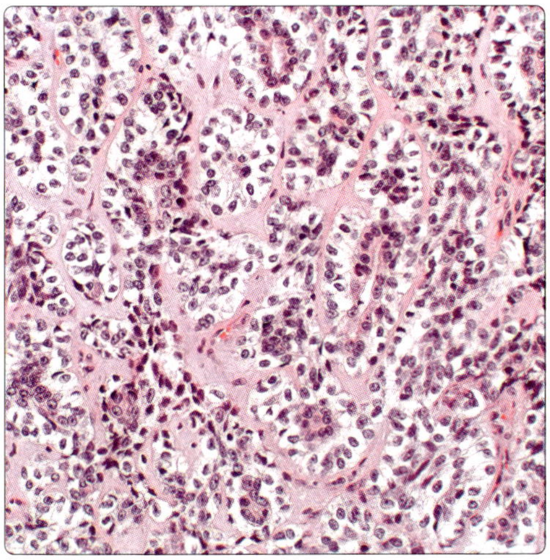

Clear Cell Carcinoma

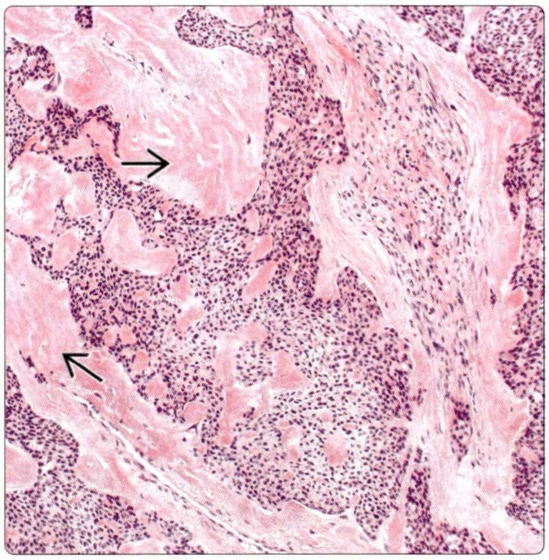

(Left) *Clear cell change is seen in many salivary tumors. In epithelial-myoepithelial carcinoma, the biphasic proliferation has prominent clear myoepithelial cells surrounding ductal cells.* **(Right)** *Clear cell carcinoma is an indolent malignancy of minor salivary glands characterized by sheets and cords of clear cells with infiltrative growth. The clear cells have a squamoid rather than myoepithelial phenotype. Hyalinized collagenous stroma is a common feature ⇒.*

(Left) *Low-grade cytologic features of this mucoepidermoid carcinoma make recognition of this isolated gland as tumor present at margin quite difficult.* (Right) *In this high-grade mucoepidermoid carcinoma, the cells are largely squamoid with pronounced atypia. Scattered cells bearing mucin vacuoles ⇒ are present. Extensive keratinization typifies squamous cell carcinoma, likely metastatic, rather than mucoepidermoid carcinoma.*

Low-Grade Mucoepidermoid Carcinoma

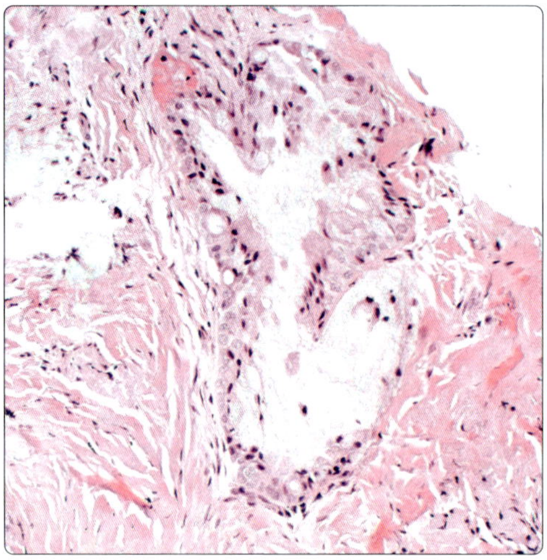

High-Grade Mucoepidermoid Carcinoma

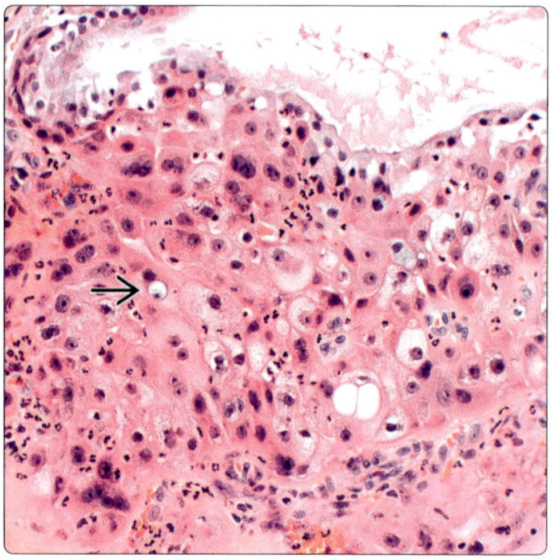

(Left) *Mucoepidermoid carcinoma may exhibit prominent oncocytic features. For low-grade tumors, the differential diagnosis is mainly of oncocytoma, whereas high-grade tumors overlap with rare oncocytic carcinomas. Intracellular mucin vacuoles ⇒ are present.* (Right) *Nonspecific clear cell morphology may be prominent in mucoepidermoid carcinoma, especially within the population of epidermoid cells as seen here. Intracytoplasmic mucin vacuoles ⇒ and squamoid features enable proper diagnosis.*

Oncocytic Mucoepidermoid Carcinoma

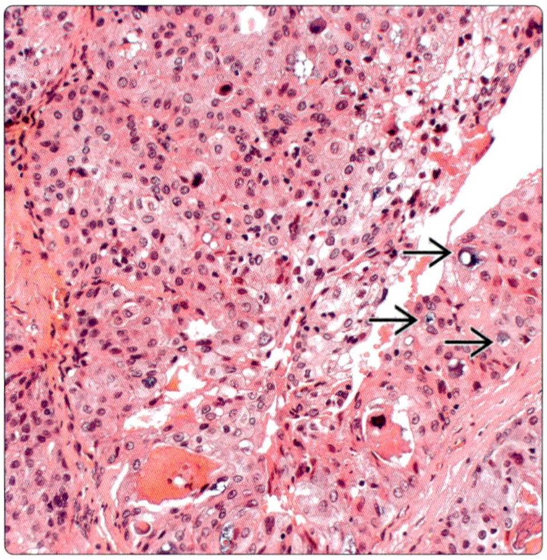

Clear Cell Mucoepidermoid Carcinoma

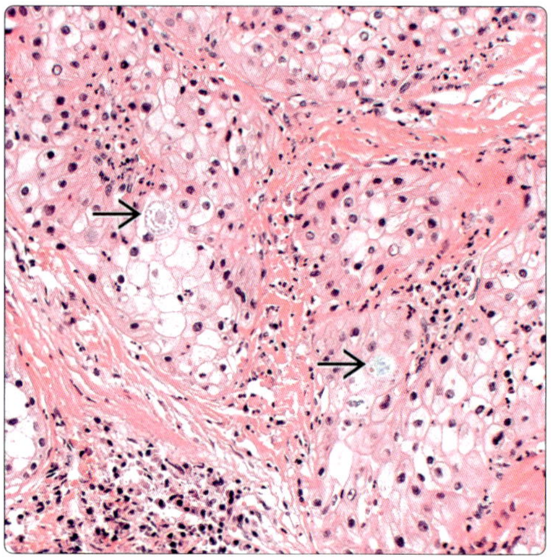

(Left) *Salivary duct carcinoma bears a striking resemblance to comedo-type breast cancer. This high-grade malignancy exhibits intraductal growth with comedonecrosis ⇒. An invasive component ⇒ is almost always present.* (Right) *Secretory carcinoma resembles secretory breast carcinoma morphologically and shares the same translocation. Note the back-to-back tubules lined by eosinophilic tumor cells filled with luminal, colloid-like secretory material.*

Salivary Duct Carcinoma

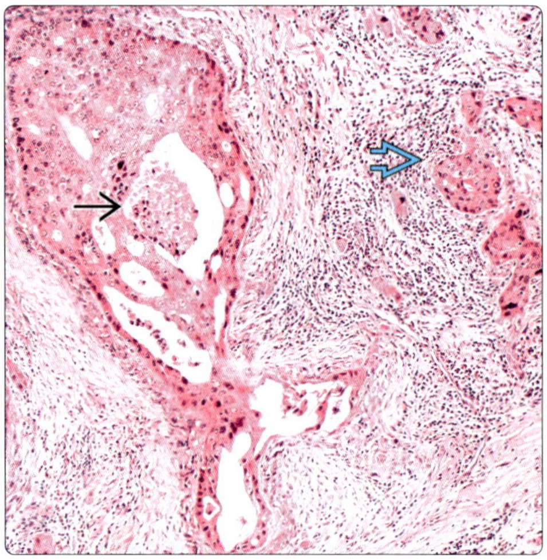

Secretory Carcinoma

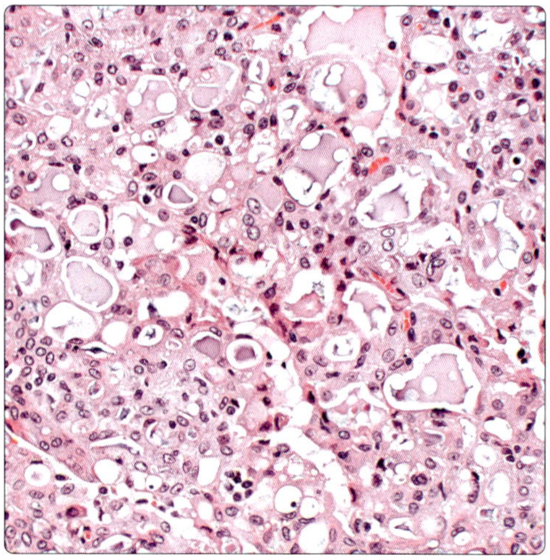

Contents

Warthin Tumor

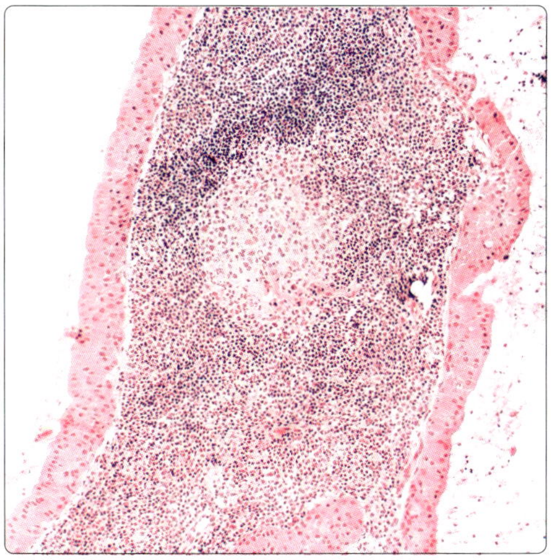

Oncocytoma

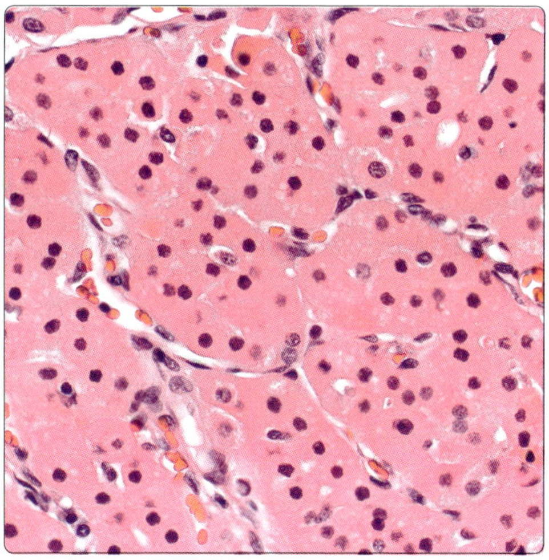

(Left) *A number of salivary gland tumors exhibit oncocytic differentiation. Warthin tumor characteristically has a bilayered oncocytic epithelium lining a core with reactive lymphoid cells. Squamous metaplasia may raise concern for malignancy, but true squamous cell carcinoma in Warthin tumor is rare.* **(Right)** *Oncocytoma is comprised of nests and cords of cells with abundant uniform granular eosinophilic cytoplasm. Clear cell change can also be seen. If multifocal, nodular oncocytic hyperplasia should be considered.*

Mucocele

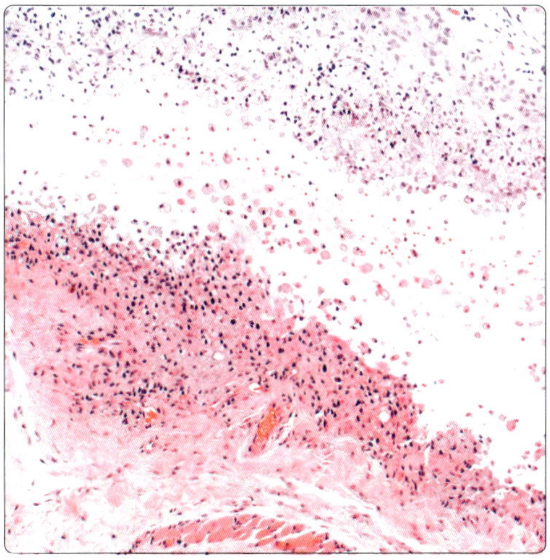

Radiation Atypia

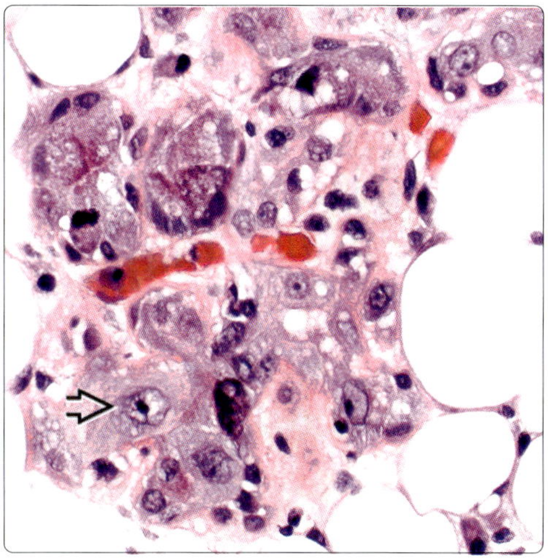

(Left) *Cystic salivary lesions require careful attention to the cyst-lining cells for appropriate classification, a task made more difficult by limited frozen section sampling. Sheets of muciphages line the wall of this mucocele and may be mistaken for tumor cells from a mucoepidermoid carcinoma or a cystic acinic cell carcinoma.* **(Right)** *Following radiation, salivary glands undergo acinar atrophy with ductal metaplasia. Isolated atypical nuclei ⇨ may also be seen consistent with treatment effect.*

Epithelial Inclusions

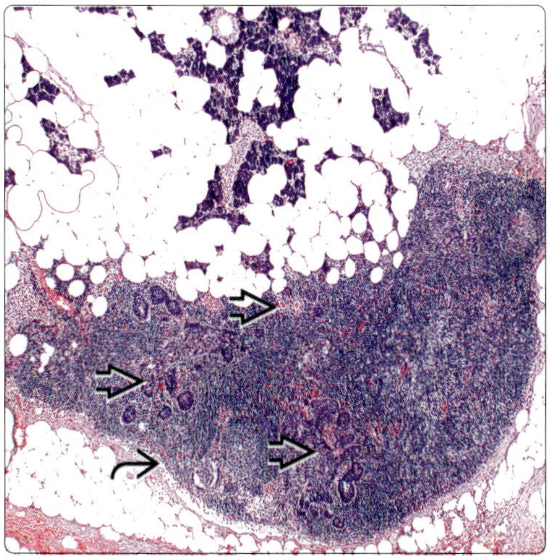

Necrotizing Sialometaplasia

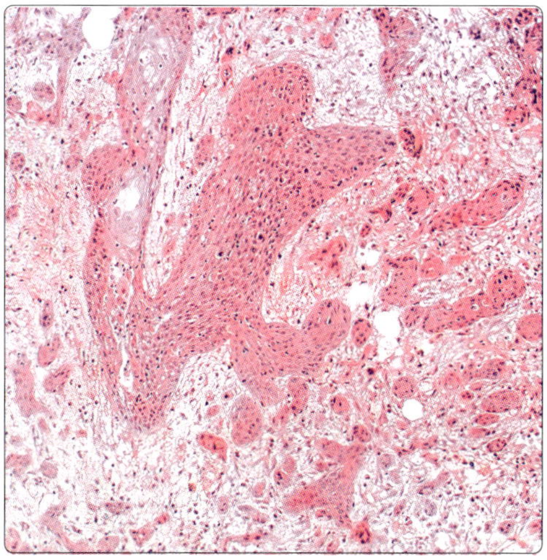

(Left) *Epithelial inclusions in intraparotid lymph nodes may be mistaken for metastatic carcinoma. This lymph node is only partially encapsulated ↪ and contains epithelial islands within the nodal parenchyma ⇨.* **(Right)** *Necrotizing sialometaplasia exhibits a pseudoinfiltrative appearance with islands of benign or reactive-appearing squamous epithelium. The relatively uniform distribution of these islands can be seen as they branch off of salivary ducts undergoing squamous metaplasia.*

SURGICAL/CLINICAL CONSIDERATIONS

Goal of Consultation

- Most common intraoperative consultation (IOC) is to ensure that malignant skin tumor has been completely excised
- IOC is rarely used to establish primary diagnosis of tumor

Change in Patient Management

- Additional skin will be taken around tumor to achieve clear margins if initially positive

Clinical Setting

- Skin tumors are usually diagnosed with shave, punch, or small excisional biopsy
  - Most carcinomas submitted for IOC are basal cell carcinoma (BCC) or squamous cell carcinoma (SCC)
  - Rarely, FS's may be performed on Merkel cell carcinoma or adnexal carcinomas
  - Completely freezing small lesions for primary diagnosis is not recommended
- Minimal margins may be taken to optimize cosmetic results (typically by Mohs surgery)
- In general, FS should **not** be performed on **melanocytic lesions**
  - FS artifacts and sampling errors compromise evaluation of these lesions
    - FS diagnosis of melanoma suffers from low sensitivity and specificity
    - Often difficult to distinguish melanoma in situ from melanocytic hyperplasia in sun-damaged skin
  - Diagnosis should be based on well-fixed and oriented permanent sections

SPECIMEN EVALUATION

Gross

- Specimen is usually oriented skin ellipse
  - Punch biopsies and shave biopsies may rarely be submitted for FS
- Specimen is described
  - Size of specimen, depth of excision, color of skin
  - Size, color, and borders (circumscribed or irregular) of all lesions
    - Type of lesion (papular, macular, nodular, etc.)
    - Distance of lesion(s) from margins
    - Site of original lesion may be difficult to see due to prior biopsy
  - Diagram showing orienting sutures, ink colors, and site of FS is helpful
- Specimen is serially sectioned

Frozen Section

- Section of skin with closest perpendicular margin(s) and deep margin is frozen
  - Orientation should be perpendicular to skin surface to measure distance
  - Sections should be deep enough through block to clearly show all margins
- En face margins may be useful to evaluate entire margin (used in Mohs)

MOST COMMON DIAGNOSES

Squamous Cell Carcinoma

- Grossly forms nodular mass &/or indurated area with central ulcer
- Invasion of dermis by enlarged, atypical epithelioid cells with eosinophilic cytoplasm
- Squamous eddies often present, especially in well- and moderately differentiated tumors
- Poorly differentiated and spindle cell variants may be difficult to diagnose without immunohistochemistry
- Overlying SCC in situ (Bowen disease) or actinic keratosis (AK) typically present

Basal Cell Carcinoma

- Grossly well-circumscribed erythematous papules to nodules
- Proliferation of atypical basaloid cells with peripheral palisading and mucinous stroma

Basal Cell Carcinoma: Clinical Appearance

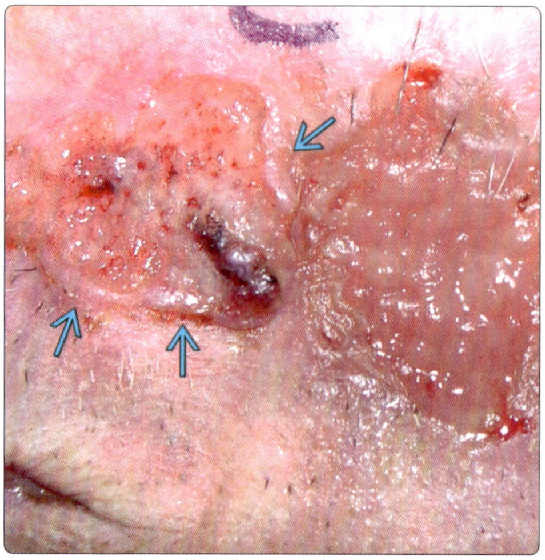

Basal Cell Carcinoma: Architectural Features

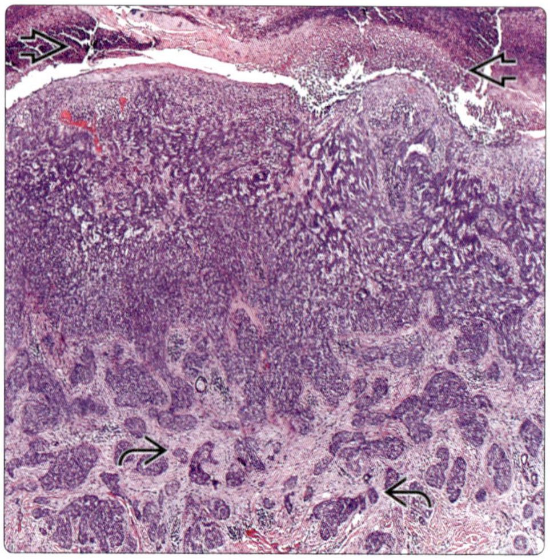

(Left) *This large nodular and infiltrative basal cell carcinoma arose on the cheek of this patient. The tumor forms an eroded plaque with characteristic rolled borders* ⮕. **(Right)** *This large basal cell carcinoma has nodular and micronodular* ⮕ *features and is associated with diffuse overlying ulceration of the epidermis with dense serum crust and degenerating neutrophils* ⮕.

- Stromal retraction artifact typically seen on permanent sections may not be present on FS
- Cells are uniform in appearance and mitoses can be abundant
- Superficial-multicentric, nodular, and micronodular types most common

Merkel Cell Carcinoma

- Much less common than SCC and BCC but far more aggressive tumor
- Proliferation of markedly atypical basaloid cells in dense nodular and sheet-like collections
- Mitoses and apoptotic bodies are numerous; necrosis often seen

Adnexal Carcinomas

- Microcystic adnexal carcinoma: Low-grade tumor with superficial follicular differentiation, deeper infiltrative ductal structures
  - Perineural invasion common but need deep biopsy/excision to identify
- Eccrine and apocrine carcinomas: Infiltrative ductal structures lined by small, dark cells (eccrine) or larger cells with abundant eosinophilic cytoplasm (apocrine)
- Sebaceous carcinoma: Lobules, nodules, and sheet-like collections of enlarged, atypical clear cells with abundant, multivacuolated cytoplasm

REPORTING

Frozen Section

- Presence or absence of tumor
- Confirmation/identification of tumor type
  - May not be able to give definitive type on FS (i.e., poorly differentiated and sarcomatoid carcinomas)
- Margin status
  - Positive or negative margin(s)
- Perineural invasion, if present
  - Surgeon may choose to remove additional tissue for wider margin

PITFALLS

Hair Follicles vs. BCC

- Tangential sections of hair follicles can mimic BCC
  - Oriented perpendicular to epidermis (BCC usually has parallel orientation)
  - Round to oval shape rather than irregular borders of BCC
    - Both hair follicles and BCC have peripheral palisading
  - Follicles have associated structures, including sebaceous glands and arrector pili muscles
    - Hair shafts and lumina helpful if present
  - Typically surrounded by fibrous tissue, not myxoid stroma
    - Clefting between epithelium and stroma not present, as in BCC
      - This feature may not be seen on frozen section
  - Hair follicles usually lack mitoses and apoptosis

Eccrine Ducts vs. Infiltrative or Morpheaform-Type BCC

- Eccrine ducts usually oriented perpendicular to epidermis
  - Present in normal dermis; sclerotic stroma is absent
  - Round in shape
  - May be in small groups
  - Usually 2 cell layers; cells lack cytologic atypia, cells show more cytoplasm
  - No retraction artifact
- Crushed eccrine ducts can resemble BCC on FS

Pseudoepitheliomatous Hyperplasia vs. SCC

- Pseudoepitheliomatous hyperplasia is a common reaction pattern, which may be associated with
  - Chronic irritation or trauma (i.e., lichen simplex chronicus and prurigo nodularis)
  - Deep fungal infections
  - Dermal/subcutaneous lesions: Dermatofibroma, granular cell tumor, anaplastic large cell lymphoma
  - Previous biopsy/surgery sites
- Cells may be enlarged and show reactive changes but lack high-grade cytologic atypia, increased mitoses, or infiltrative features
  - Inflammatory infiltrate is usually present

SCC vs. BCC

- Basosquamous carcinoma (BCC variant with squamous differentiation) and basaloid SCC can be difficult to distinguish, even on permanent sections
  - Look for areas of more conventional BCC or SCC, palisading and mucinous stroma for BCC, overlying AK or SCC in situ for SCC

Actinic Keratosis vs. SCC

- Superficial and tangentially embedded biopsies can make it difficult to distinguish SCC from AK
- AK may show proliferative features in some cases, with elongated rete ridges
  - No detached or infiltrative areas, although tangential sectioning makes it difficult to distinguish from invasive SCC

Multifocal Carcinoma

- Multiple foci may be present with
  - BCC: Superficial-multicentric type (often shows skip areas of several rete), infiltrative and morpheaform types, micronodular type
  - Recurrent carcinoma: Intervening scar may separate areas of tumor
    - If scar involves margins, cannot exclude residual underlying/adjacent tumor

Adnexal Carcinoma vs. Metastasis

- May be impossible to distinguish without complete clinical history &/or immunohistochemical studies
  - Should defer to permanents (and immunohistochemistry) in most cases

SELECTED REFERENCES

1. Moncrieff MD et al: False-negative rate of intraoperative frozen section margin analysis for complex head and neck nonmelanoma skin cancer excisions. Clin Exp Dermatol. 40(8):834-8, 2015
2. Onajin O et al: Frozen section diagnosis for non-melanoma skin cancers: correlation with permanent section diagnosis. J Cutan Pathol. 42(7):459-64, 2015
3. Gayre GS et al: Outcomes of excision of 1750 eyelid and periocular skin basal cell and squamous cell carcinomas by modified en face frozen section margin-controlled technique. Int Ophthalmol Clin. 49(4):97-110, 2009

Contents

(**Left**) *Skin ellipses are generally oriented with a suture at one tip and the margins labeled as a clock face. The specimen is sectioned along the short axis. The closest approach of the lesion to the margin should be chosen for intraoperative margin evaluation.* (**Right**) *Large skin ellipses can have the nonepidermal (deep and peripheral) surfaces, inked in 4 colors in order to identify the margin quadrants.*

Skin Ellipse: Orientation and Sectioning

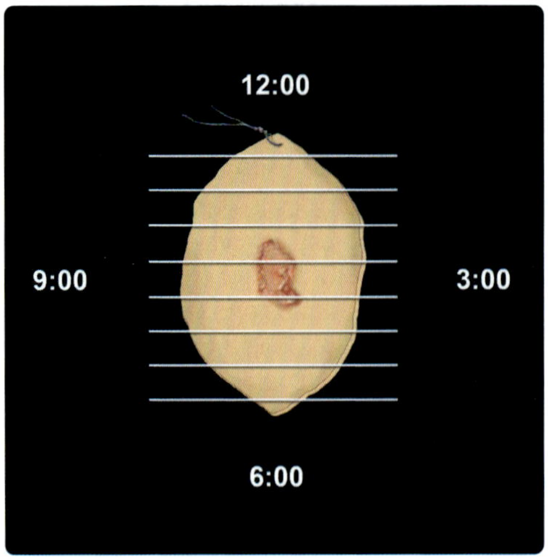

Large Skin Ellipse: Inking of Margins

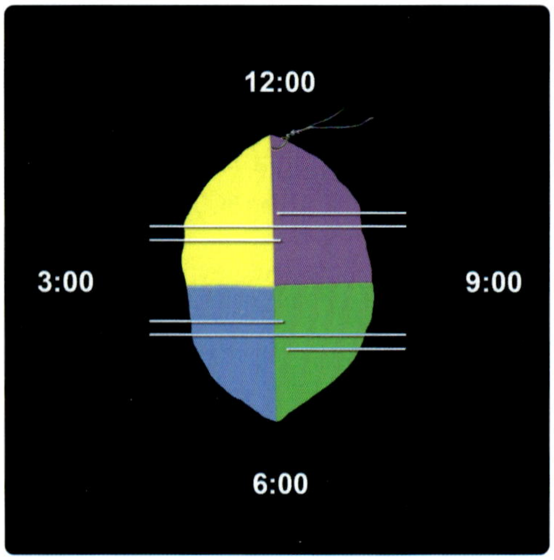

(**Left**) *The tip margins of a skin ellipse are generally evaluated as en face sections. These margins are usually negative, as they should be far from the lesion. However, any lesion in the frozen section is considered to be at the margin* ➔*.* (**Right**) *An entire cross section of a large skin ellipse may be too large for a single frozen section. Multiple tissue sections can be used to evaluate the margins. The color of the ink identifies the location of the cutaneous and deep margins.*

Skin Ellipse: En Face Tip Margin

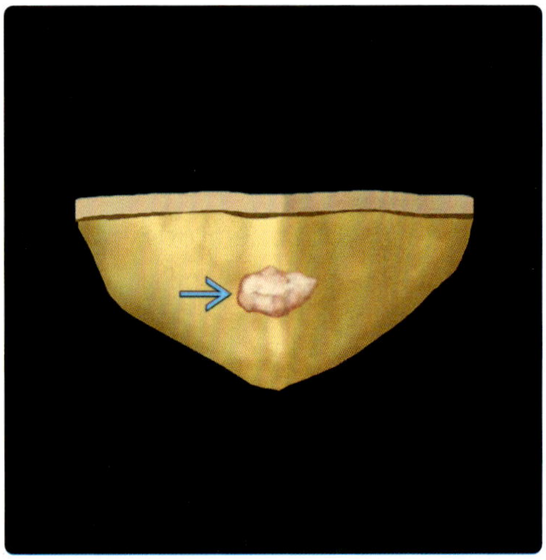

Skin Ellipse: Margins

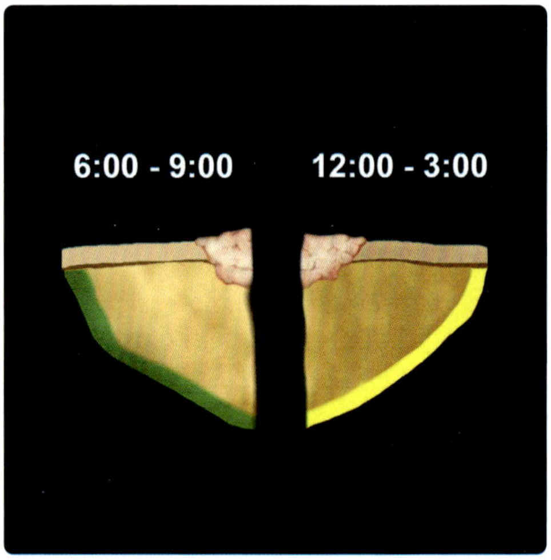

(**Left**) *Small skin ellipses are generally inked in 2 colors on the nonepidermal surface. The section taken for frozen section should be the complete cross section with the closest approach of the tumor to the margin.* (**Right**) *Small skin ellipses can generally be examined as a complete cross section such that margins on both side of the ellipse can be evaluated. The color of the ink identifies the locations of the margins.*

Small Skin Ellipse: Inking Margins

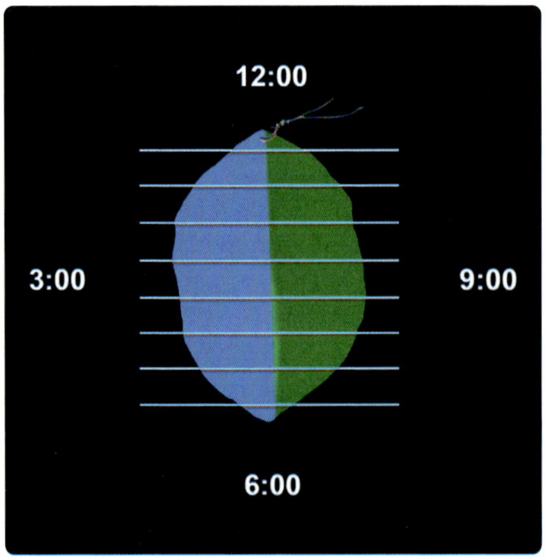

Small Skin Ellipse: Complete Cross Section

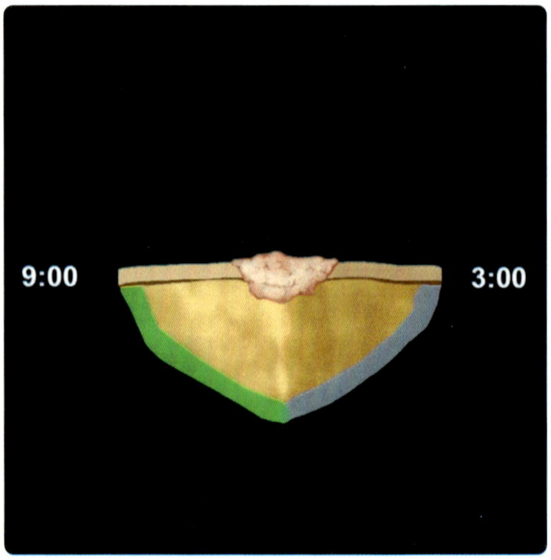

Superficial Basal Cell Carcinoma

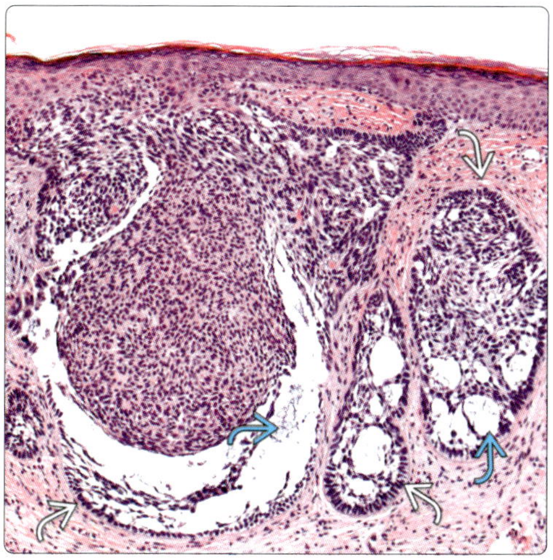

Basal Cell Carcinoma: Frozen Section

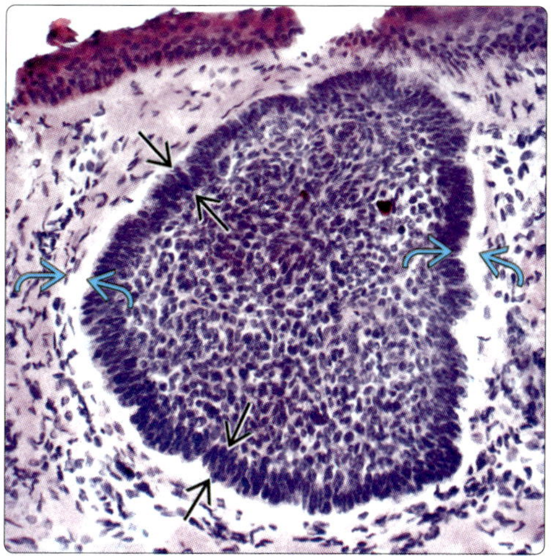

(Left) *This basal cell carcinoma on frozen section extends downward from the overlying epidermis. There are several superficial dermal nodules of crowded hyperchromatic-staining basaloid cells with areas of peripheral palisading . Collections of mucin are easily identified.* **(Right)** *This superficial dermal nodule of a basal cell carcinoma is composed of atypical, hyperchromatic basaloid cells with areas of peripheral palisading . Retraction artifact is easily identified. However, this feature may not be seen in frozen sections.*

Basal Cell Carcinoma With Numerous Apoptotic and Mitotic Figures

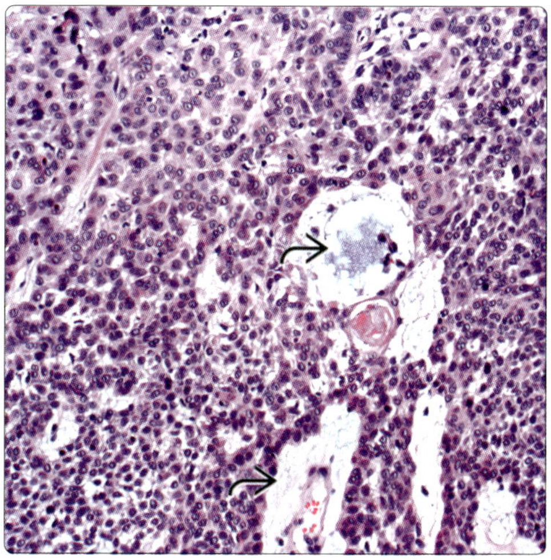

Nodular Basal Cell Carcinoma: Cytologic Features

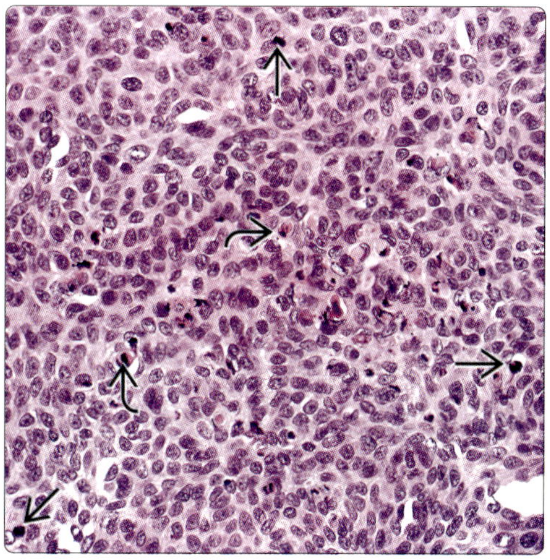

(Left) *This basal cell carcinoma shows a relatively uniform population of crowded cells. Multiple apoptotic and mitotic figures are present. Collections of mucin are often seen in basal cell carcinoma.* **(Right)** *This nodular basal cell carcinoma shows a dense, sheet-like proliferation of atypical basaloid cells with high nuclear:cytoplasmic ratios and numerous apoptotic and mitotic figures .*

Basal Cell Carcinoma: Cytologic Features on Frozen Section

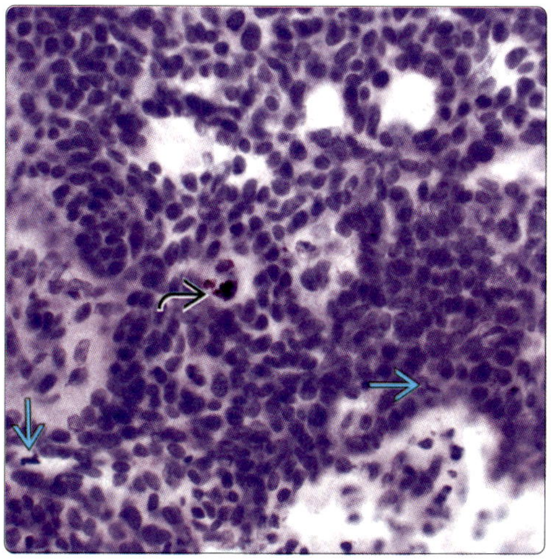

Basal Cell Carcinoma With Perineural Invasion

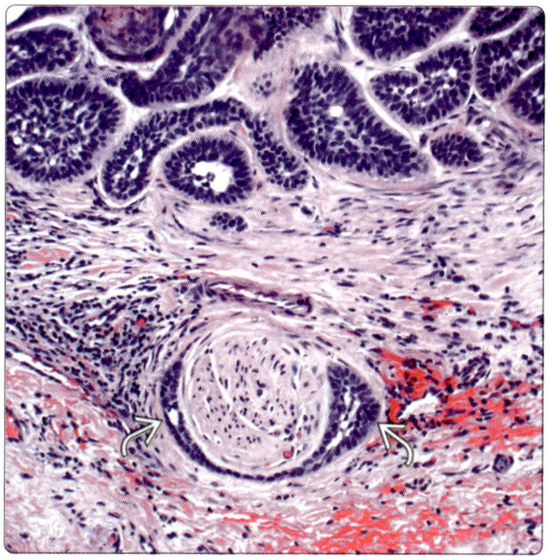

(Left) *This basal cell carcinoma consists of crowded hyperchromatic-staining nuclei. Several mitotic figures are present . Note the focal cytoplasmic pigmentation , which is commonly seen in basal cell carcinoma.* **(Right)** *Although relatively uncommon, perineural invasion can be seen in basal cell carcinoma, especially larger, deeply invasive tumors such as this micronodular basal cell carcinoma.*

(Left) *This elderly woman has developed a small squamous cell carcinoma (SCC) → in an area of sun damaged skin on her forehead. The tumor has been marked for surgical removal.* (Right) *This SCC in situ on frozen section is identified by the presence of full thickness squamous nuclear atypia →, pleomorphism, and mitotic figures →.*

Squamous Cell Carcinoma: Clinical Photograph

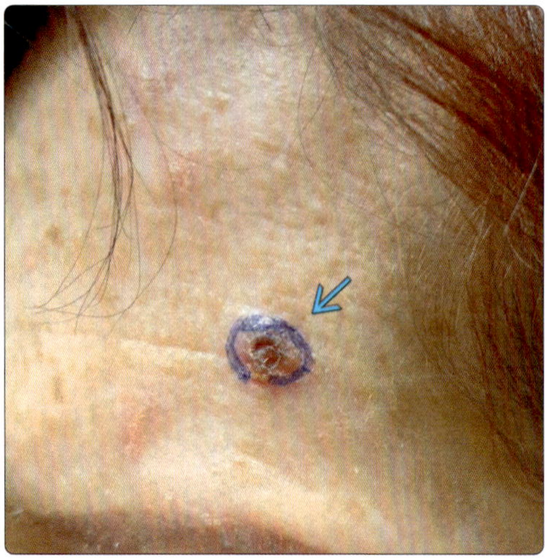

Squamous Cell Carcinoma in Situ: Frozen Section

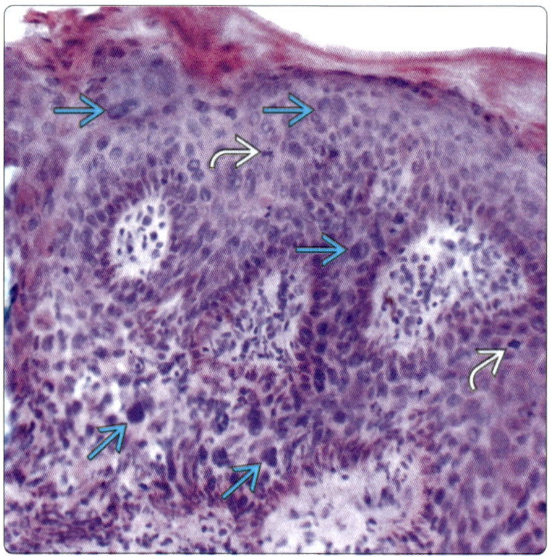

(Left) *SCC in situ typically arises in actinic keratoses in sun-damaged skin but may also occur rarely in a seborrheic keratosis or a verruca vulgaris (as in this case). Note prominent epidermal papillomatosis → and overlying hyperkeratosis and parakeratosis.* (Right) *This well- to moderately differentiated invasive SCC has prominent keratin pearls → and is associated with a sclerotic stroma with scattered inflammatory cells. It can sometimes be difficult to distinguish reactive stromal cells from spindled tumor cells.*

Squamous Cell Carcinoma In Situ Arising in Verruca Vulgaris

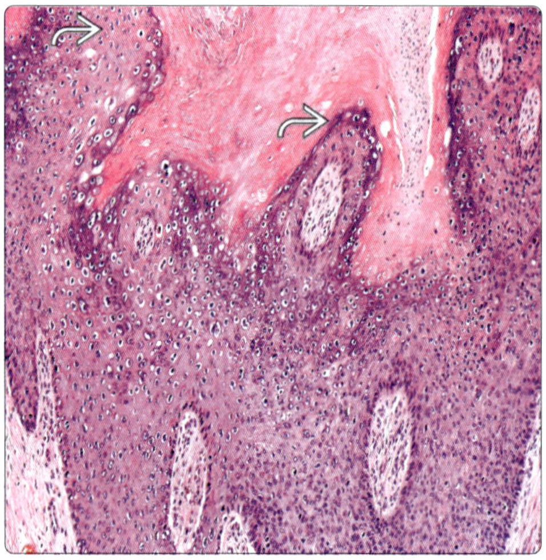

Invasive Squamous Cell Carcinoma, Well- to Moderately Differentiated

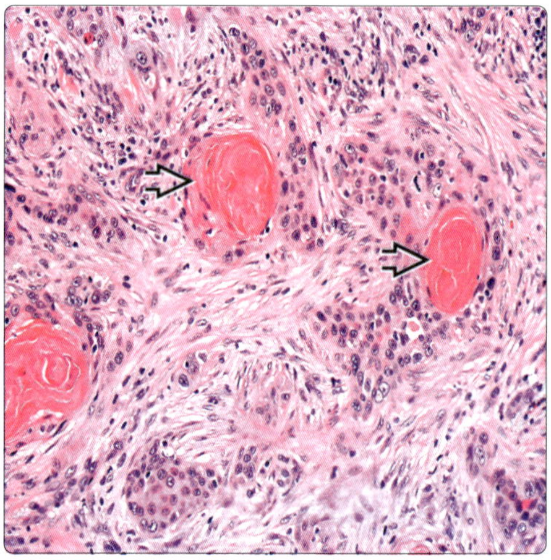

(Left) *Acantholytic invasive SCC shows scattered cystic spaces containing dyscohesive squamous cells →. This variant of SCC may mimic an adenocarcinoma (pseudoglandular SCC) or even an angiosarcoma (pseudovascular SCC).* (Right) *High-grade/poorly differentiated invasive SCC shows a sheet-like proliferation of atypical and pleomorphic epithelioid and multinucleated tumor cells with hyperchromatic nuclei, prominent nucleoli →, and abundant glassy-appearing eosinophilic cytoplasm →.*

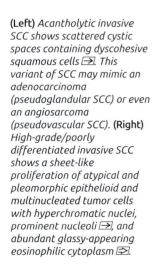

Acantholytic (Adenoid) Squamous Cell Carcinoma

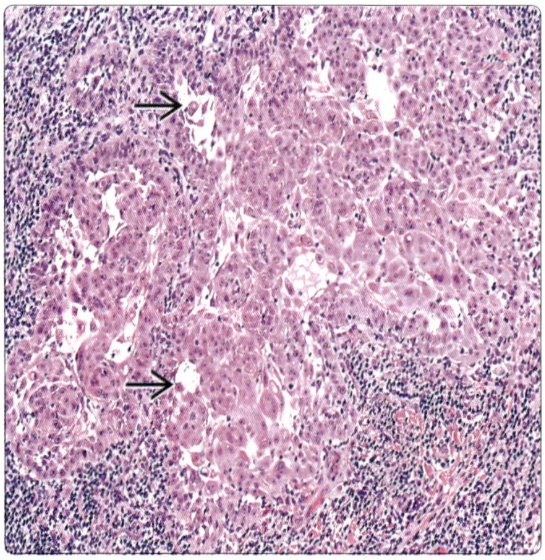

Invasive Squamous Cell Carcinoma, Poorly Differentiated

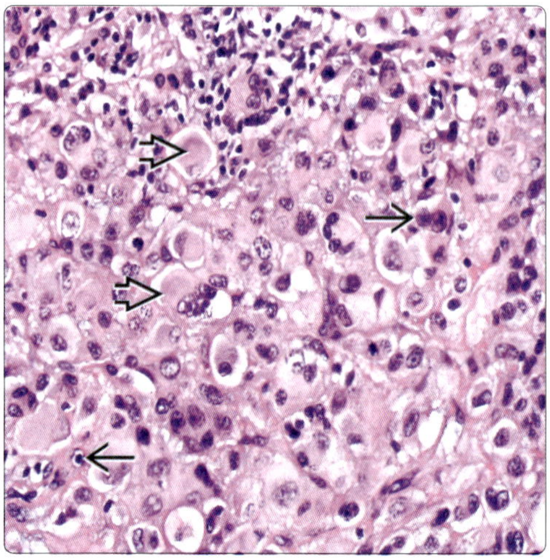

Invasive Well-Differentiated Squamous Cell Carcinoma

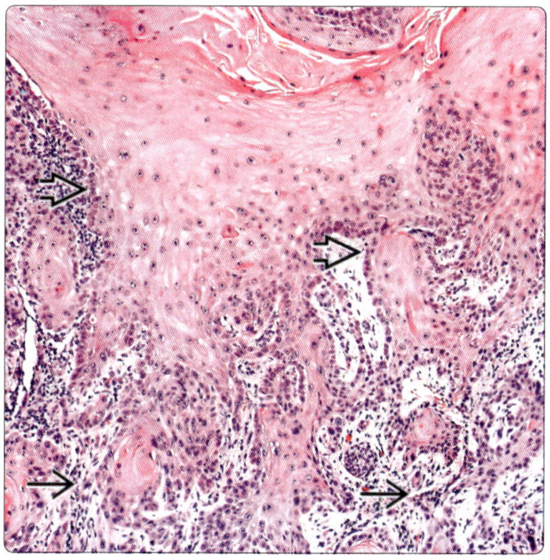

Invasive Squamous Cell Carcinoma With Desmoplastic Features

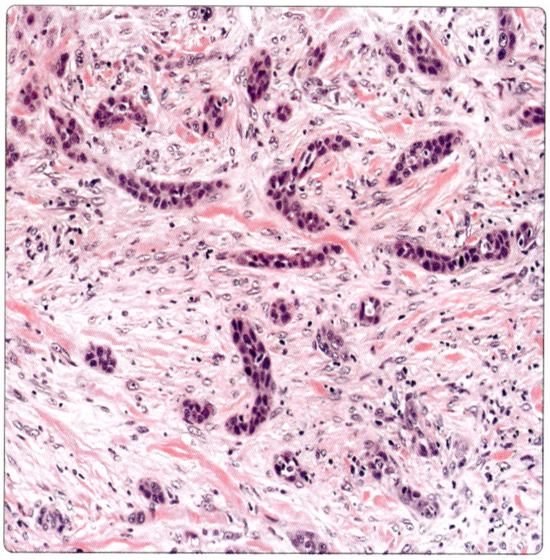

(Left) *This invasive well-differentiated SCC arose in association with an overlying actinic keratosis ⇒. The invasive front of the carcinoma forms irregular nests in the stroma →.* **(Right)** *This invasive SCC shows infiltrative cords in a sclerotic stoma, characteristic of the desmoplastic variant of this cancer. These are clinically more aggressive variants of SCC.*

Microcystic Adnexal Carcinoma

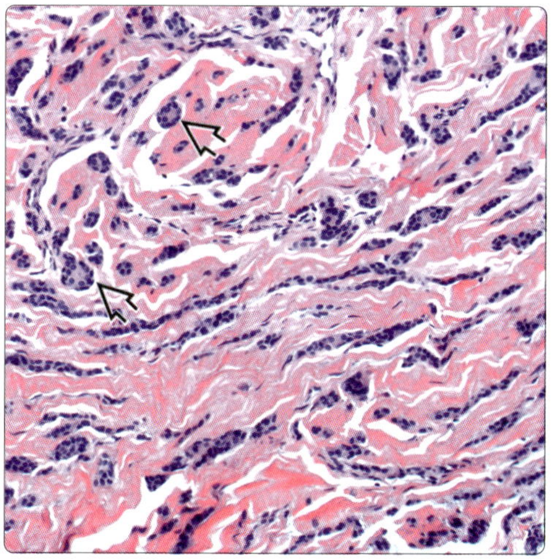

Invasive Adnexal Carcinoma

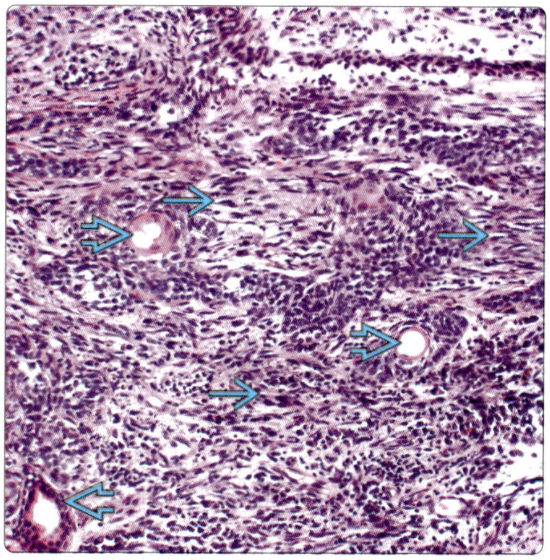

(Left) *This is a deeply invasive adnexal carcinoma (microcystic adnexal carcinoma). Note the infiltrative cords and scattered ductal-like structures ⇒. Despite the low-grade cytologic appearance, these are typically deeply invasive tumors with perineural invasion.* **(Right)** *This is a rare adnexal sarcomatoid carcinoma (porocarcinoma with sarcomatoid features). Note the scattered, well-differentiated ductal structures ⇒, which are surrounded by infiltrative atypical spindle cells →.*

Merkel Cell Carcinoma

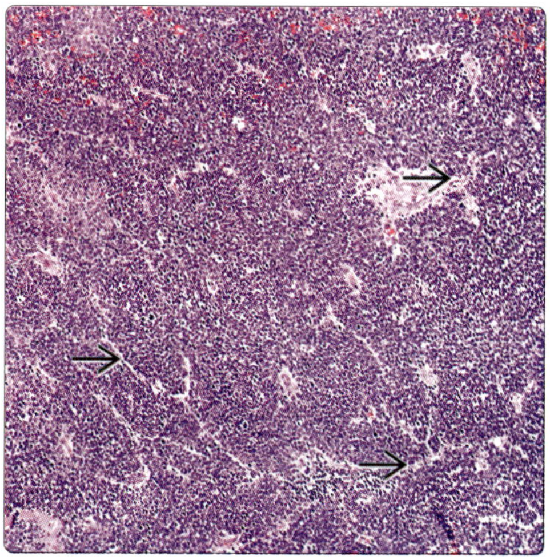

Merkel Cell Carcinoma: Cellular Detail

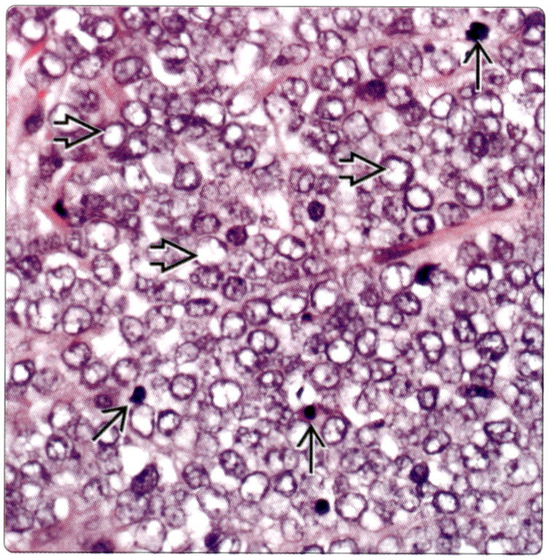

(Left) *Merkel cell carcinoma is an aggressive neuroendocrine carcinoma that consists of broad cords, nodules, and sheet-like collections of highly atypical basaloid cells. There is only very scant intervening stroma → between the neoplastic cells, and no palisading or mucinous material is present.* **(Right)** *Nuclear clearing ⇒ is often seen in Merkel cell carcinoma, a feature not identified in basal cell carcinoma or SCC. Note the numerous apoptotic and mitotic figures → present.*

Skin: Evaluation for Toxic Epidermal Necrolysis vs. Staphylococcal Scalded Skin Syndrome

SURGICAL/CLINICAL CONSIDERATIONS

Goal of Consultation

- To distinguish between toxic epidermal necrolysis (TEN)/Stevens-Johnson syndrome (SJS) and staphylococcal scalded skin syndrome (SSSS)

Change in Patient Management

- Appropriate treatment will be initiated depending on diagnosis

Clinical Setting

- TEN/SJS and SSSS can present with diffuse areas of exfoliated skin and can be difficult to distinguish
  - Erythema multiforme (EM) is generally more limited in extent than TEN/SJS and involves < 10% of body surface area
    - Typically associated with Herpes infection
  - TEN/SJS can rapidly progress to blistering and loss of skin and mucous membranes over wide areas
    - Occurs in adults more often than children
      - Mortality can be as high as 50%
    - May require withdrawal of causative medications and treatment with steroids or intravenous immunoglobulin
      - Thought to be due to cell-mediated hypersensitivity reaction to medications (more commonly) or infectious organisms (less commonly and usually less severe)
- SSSS presents with skin tenderness and large bullae
  - More common in pediatric patients than adults
  - Treated with antibiotics

SPECIMEN EVALUATION

Gross

- Specimen is typically fragment of exfoliated skin
  - Skin is rolled as tightly as possible using forceps
  - Roll is cross sectioned
- Shave or punch biopsies may be submitted for evaluation
  - Sectioned vertically to include full epidermal thickness

Frozen Section

- Cross sections of coils are embedded such that sections will be perpendicular to skin surface
- Shave or punch biopsies should be completely embedded with sections perpendicular to skin surface

MOST COMMON DIAGNOSES

Toxic Epidermal Necrolysis

- TEN, SJS, and EM major are on a spectrum and show essentially identical histologic features
- Cleavage plane occurs along dermal-epidermal junction
- Mild inflammation with exocytosis of scattered lymphocytes is typically present
- Dyskeratosis of keratinocytes present and often full-thickness necrosis (especially in more severe cases)

Staphylococcal Scalded Skin Syndrome

- Cleavage plane occurs near granular cell layer
- Only most superficial aspect of epidermis (stratum corneum layer) is seen on membrane rolls
- No or minimal inflammation should be present
  - Necrotic keratinocytes should not be present

REPORTING

Frozen Section

- Location of cleavage plane and presence or absence of inflammation and epidermal dyskeratosis/necrosis

PITFALLS

Poor Tissue Sections

- Specimens may be very friable, making it difficult to embed and obtain good sections

SELECTED REFERENCES

1. Mishra AK et al: A systemic review on staphylococcal scalded skin syndrome (SSSS): a rare and critical disease of neonates. Open Microbiol J. 10:150-9, 2016
2. Hosaka H et al: Erythema multiforme, Stevens-Johnson syndrome and toxic epidermal necrolysis: frozen-section diagnosis. J Dermatol. 37(5):407-12, 2010

Toxic Epidermal Necrolysis: Clinical Appearance

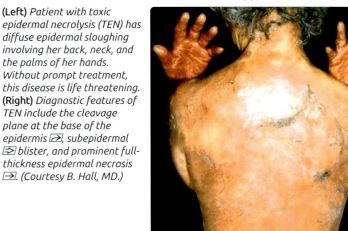

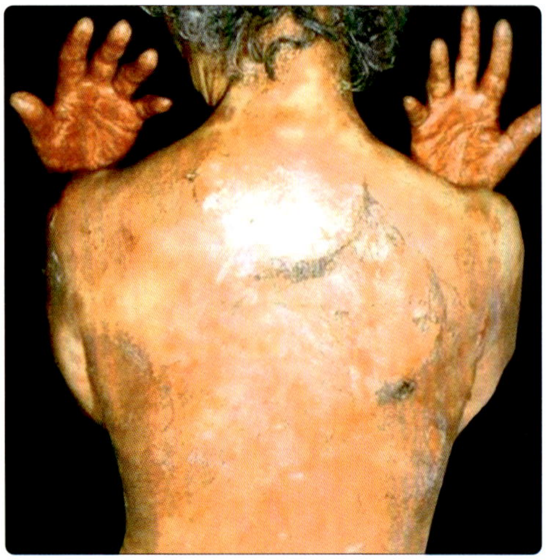

Toxic Epidermal Necrolysis: Histologic Appearance

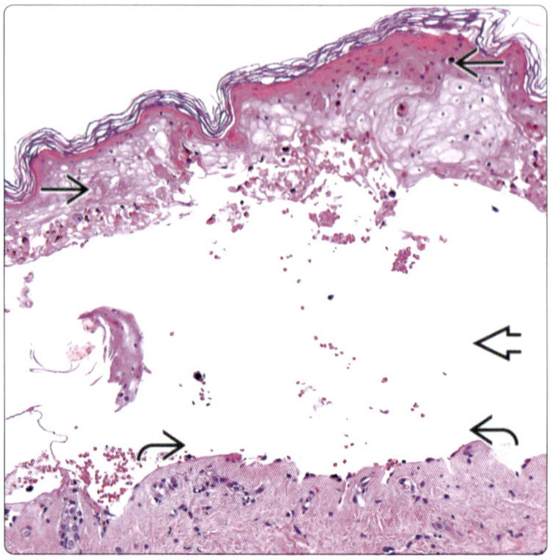

(Left) *Patient with toxic epidermal necrolysis (TEN) has diffuse epidermal sloughing involving her back, neck, and the palms of her hands. Without prompt treatment, this disease is life threatening.* **(Right)** *Diagnostic features of TEN include the cleavage plane at the base of the epidermis ➙, subepidermal ⇨ blister, and prominent full-thickness epidermal necrosis ➙. (Courtesy B. Hall, MD.)*

Toxic Epidermal Necrolysis: Clinical Appearance

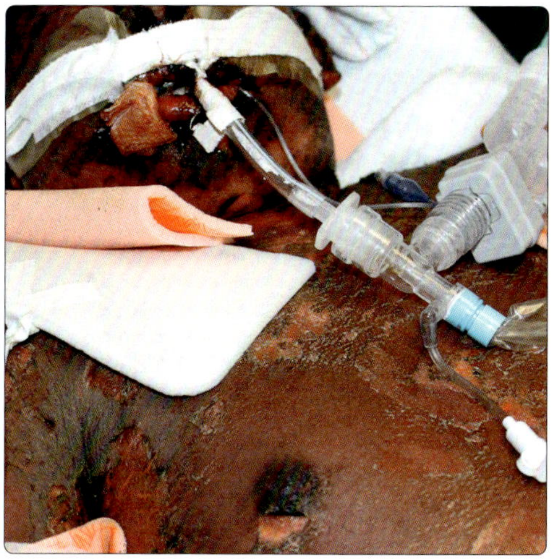

Toxic Epidermal Necrolysis: Inflammation

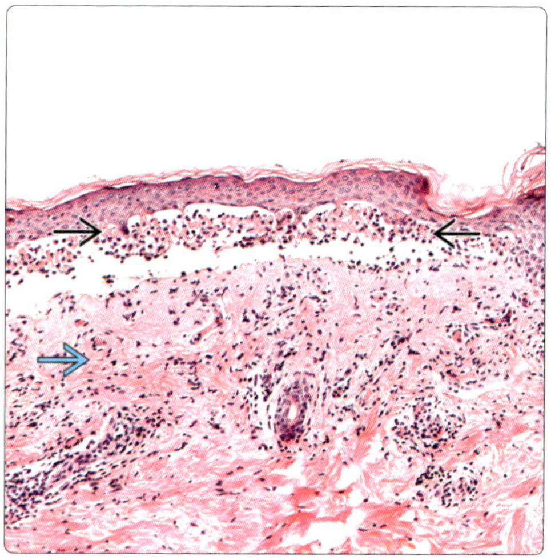

(Left) *TEN presents clinically as diffuse epidermal sloughing and shows involvement of the mucous membranes, which may result in a requirement for intubation. (Courtesy H. R. Jalian, MD.)* **(Right)** *TEN (bullous erythema multiforme) is characterized by a subepidermal bullous cavity filled with degenerating inflammatory cells and necrotic keratinocytes →. Only a mild inflammatory infiltrate is present in the dermis →. (Courtesy J. Jackson, MD.)*

Toxic Epidermal Necrolysis: Subepidermal Bulla

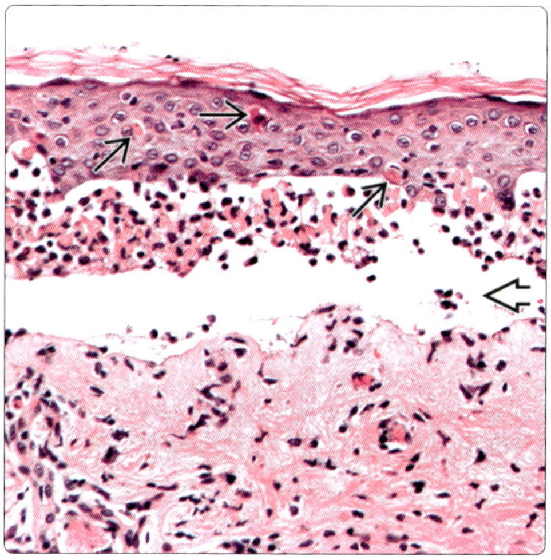

Toxic Epidermal Necrolysis: Edge of Bulla

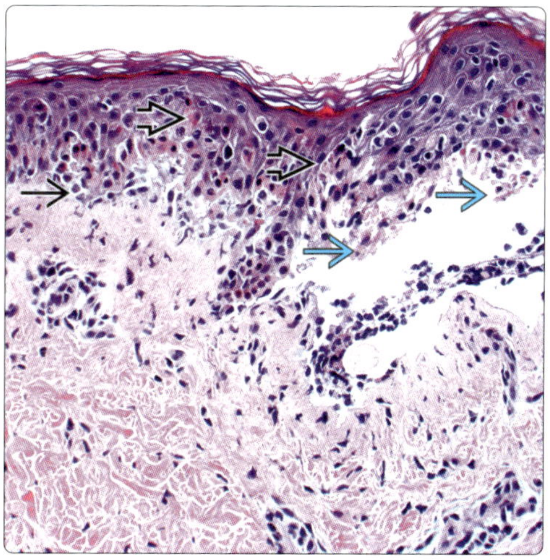

(Left) *This case of TEN (bullous EM) demonstrates subepidermal bulla formation ⇨ with necrotic keratinocytes and inflammatory cells, the majority lymphocytes. Scattered necrotic keratinocytes → are seen in the epidermis. (Courtesy J. Jackson, MD.)* **(Right)** *TEN at the edge of a bulla demonstrates interface changes along the dermal-epidermal junction with clear spaces around keratinocytes →. Many necrotic/apoptotic keratinocytes are in the epidermis ⇨ and within the bullous space →.*

Staphylococcal Scalded Skin Syndrome

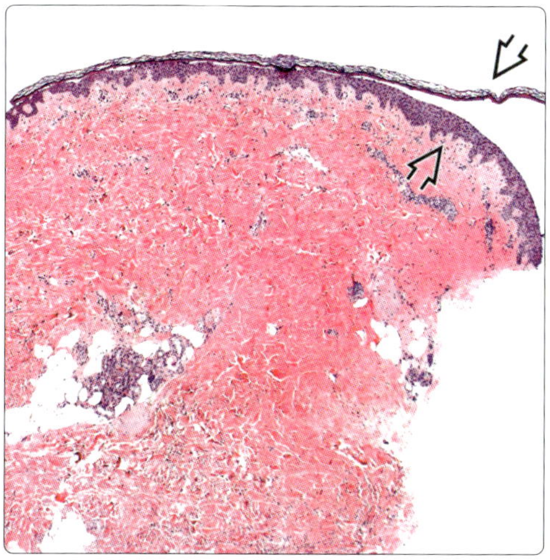

Staphylococcal Scalded Skin Syndrome: Sterile Subcorneal Blister

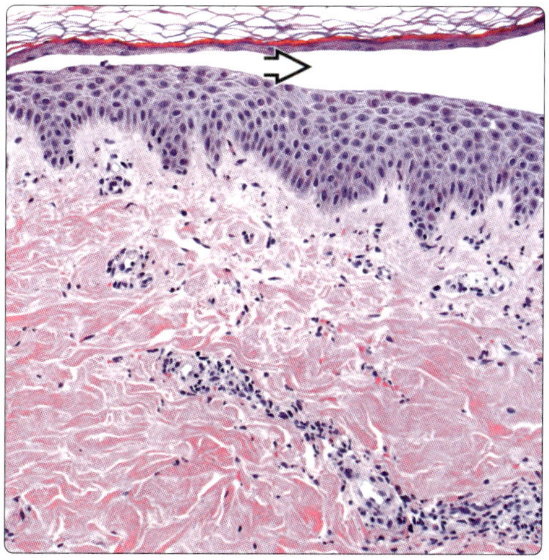

(Left) *The clinical differential diagnosis for TEN often includes SSSS. However, the pathologic appearances are very different. A biopsy of SSSS demonstrates a sterile subcorneal blister ➱ lacking significant inflammation or epidermal necrosis.* **(Right)** *SSSS shows a sterile subcorneal blister ⇨ space lacking intrabullous inflammatory cells. The cleavage plane is in the granular cell layer, leaving the remaining layers of the epidermis intact. Note the lack of interface inflammation and necrotic/dyskeratotic cells.*

Contents

SURGICAL/CLINICAL CONSIDERATIONS

Goal of Consultation

- Determine if lesional tissue is present at margin of skin excision by examining en face sections
- In theory, entire margin is examined on frozen sections (FS)

Change in Patient Management

- Additional tissue, embedded with en face margins, is excised if tumor is present at initial margin
- Process repeated until margins are free of lesional tissue

Mohs Technique

- Mohs micrographic surgery (MMS, also Mohs surgery, chemosurgery, or Mohs chemosurgery) is specialized technique
- Skin lesion is generally excised with 45° beveled edge through surrounding subdermal tissue
- Tissue is inked, and map is created
- Entire cut edge (peripheral margins and deep margin) is flattened into single plane
  - Beveled edge aids in being able to flatten entire surgical margin
- Specimen is embedded with en face margin (deep) side up
- Areas of residual carcinoma (positive areas) are correlated to map to identify location
- Additional tissue in positive areas is removed with beveled edge, and process is repeated

Clinical Setting

- Method for removal of skin cancer that examines 100% of microscopic tissue margins at time of surgery
- Pioneered by Frederic Mohs (general surgeon)
- Currently uses FS to examine margins
- Benefits
  - Very high cure rates for skin cancer: 99% for basal cell carcinoma (BCC), 94% for squamous cell carcinoma (SCC)
  - Tissue preservation: Minimum amount of noncancerous tissue is removed
  - Immediate identification of positive margins
  - Immediate tissue reconstruction and repair
- Indications for MMS
  - Recurrent skin cancers
    - Extent of involvement may be difficult to appreciate clinically after prior surgery
  - High-risk locations
    - Periorbital, perinasal, periauricular, perioral, scalp, digital, anogenital
  - Perineural invasion
    - This occurs in more aggressive tumors, and extent of involvement cannot be determined clinically
  - Large size (> 2 cm)
  - Higher risk histologic subtypes
    - BCC: Morpheaform, infiltrating, micronodular
    - SCC: Poorly differentiated, deeply invasive, spindle cell type, desmoplastic

SPECIMEN EVALUATION

Gross

- Specimen is oriented and inked by surgeon
- Specimen is described
  - Size of skin excision, depth of excision, color of normal skin
  - Size, type, color, and borders of lesion
  - Distance of lesion from peripheral margins on skin surface
- Central portion of lesion may be curetted away in order to facilitate pliability and flattening of specimen
- Edges of specimen are pressed down such that entire peripheral margin is in same plane as deep margin
  - This can be done with tissue pressed flat onto glass slide
    - This helps in making sure entire margin is in same plane
    - Ability to see margin through slide aids in making sure tissue is adequately flattened and that no air bubbles are present

Frozen Section

- Small excisions are embedded in 1 block
  - Large excisions can be sectioned into 4 blocks and each embedded separately

Clinical Photograph of Mohs Surgery Patient

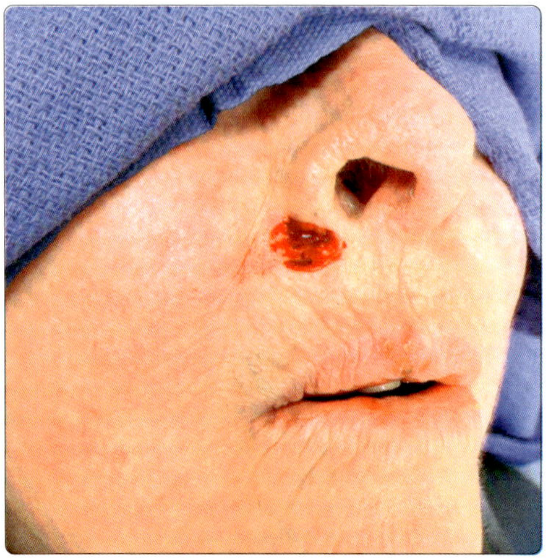

Gross Image of Mohs Surgery Specimen

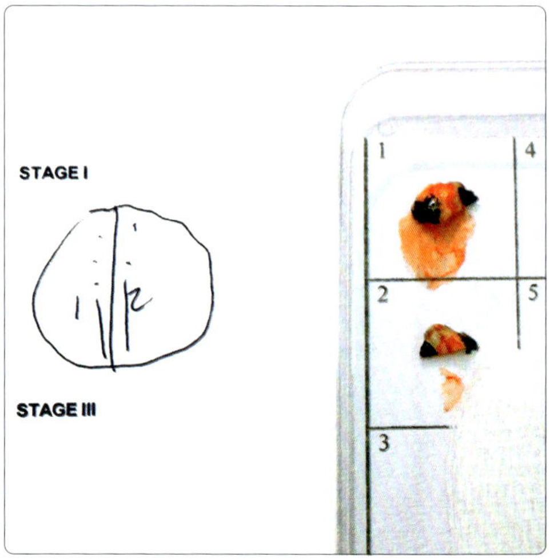

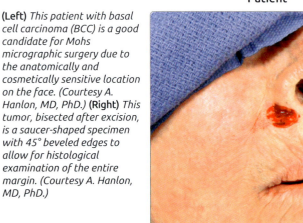

(Left) *This patient with basal cell carcinoma (BCC) is a good candidate for Mohs micrographic surgery due to the anatomically and cosmetically sensitive location on the face. (Courtesy A. Hanlon, MD, PhD.)* **(Right)** *This tumor, bisected after excision, is a saucer-shaped specimen with 45° beveled edges to allow for histological examination of the entire margin. (Courtesy A. Hanlon, MD, PhD.)*

- Tissue is embedded with true margin (inked) at the upper surface of the block
  - 1st tissue section is true margin
    - Facing of block should be discouraged (can lead to false-positive margins)
  - Deeper sections are farther away from margin
- H&E &/or toluidine blue can be used to stain slides

MOST COMMON DIAGNOSES

Basal Cell Carcinoma

- Nodular type
  - Basaloid cells in circumscribed nests with peripheral palisading
  - Mucinous stroma
  - Characteristic tumor-stromal retraction is helpful but may not be seen in FS
- Superficial-multicentric type
  - Multiple nests of tumor cells attached to epidermis
  - False-negative margins can occur as tumor has discontinuous growth pattern
- Morpheaform type
  - Tumor infiltrates as thin bands of tumor cells
  - Cells have bland nuclei and can be difficult to distinguish from normal cells
  - Chronic inflammatory cells and desmoplasia can make tumor difficult to detect on FS
- Micronodular type
  - Growth pattern as multiple separate round nests of cells in dermis and subcutaneous tissue
  - Stromal reaction may not be present

Squamous Cell Carcinoma

- Proliferation of atypical cells with abundant, eosinophilic-staining cytoplasm
- Foci of keratinization often present (especially in well- and moderately differentiated cases)
  - Poorly differentiated carcinomas with spindle cell pattern may be more difficult to detect and differentiate from scar
- Overlying actinic keratosis (AK) or SCC in situ typically present
- Perineural invasion can occur
  - Potential source of positive margins and recurrence if not recognized
  - Sometimes associated with perineural lymphocytic infiltrate

Squamous Cell Carcinoma In Situ

- Synonyms include Bowen disease and erythroplasia of Queyrat (penile)
- Full-thickness atypia and disorder of epidermis
- Often scattered mitoses throughout entire thickness of epidermis
- False-negative margins can occur, as tumor sometimes has discontinuous growth pattern or may be multicentric
  - Recurrence can also occur due to involvement of skin appendages

Melanoma In Situ

- Controversial whether these lesions should be excised using MMS
  - Some Mohs surgeons prefer "slow Mohs"
    - Tissue is fixed and processed for permanent sections
    - Slides are interpreted the following day
    - Advantages: Tissue conservation and better processing of fixed tissue vs. frozen tissue
    - Disadvantage: Delayed margin assessment and closure
- Proliferation of confluent to near-confluent atypical melanocytes, in single units and irregular nests
- Upward scatter of melanocytes into stratum spinosum
- During/after MMS
  - Immunohistochemical staining may be used to highlight melanocytes

Atypical Fibroxanthoma

- Spindle cells and bizarre, atypical giant cells
- During MMS, immunohistochemistry for CD10 may be used to help define tumor extent

Dermatofibrosarcoma Protuberans

- Grows in very irregular, infiltrative fashion
- Relatively monomorphous, bland spindle cells, often in storiform pattern
- Highly infiltrative into fat, often in honeycomb pattern
- During MMS, CD34 immunohistochemistry may be used to help define tumor extent

Merkel Cell Carcinoma

- Blue cells in nodules, sheets, or trabecular pattern
- High mitotic rate
- Molding of nuclei is often present

Microcystic Adnexal Carcinoma

- May resemble desmoplastic trichoepithelioma superficially
- Deeply infiltrative
- Often with perineural invasion

Sebaceous Carcinoma

- Nodular basophilic to clear cell tumor with variable number of sebocytes
- During MMS, Oil Red O may be used to highlight sebocytes

Extramammary Paget Disease

- Large cells with abundant cytoplasm scattered through epidermis
- During MMS, PAS stain or immunohistochemistry for cytokeratin 7 may be used to highlight atypical cells

Other Adnexal Tumors

- Examples include trichoepithelioma and trichoblastoma (especially with atypical features on face), primary mucinous carcinoma, hidradenocarcinoma

REPORTING

Frozen Section

- Confirmation/identification of tumor type
  - Identification of perineural invasion, if present
- Positive or negative margins
- Dense lymphocytic infiltrates or fibrosis at margin may be indication for reexcision for some surgeons
- If epidermis is not present at margin, this should be noted
  - Tissue may not be representative of true margin

PITFALLS

False-Negative Results Due to Improper Specimen Processing

- Tissue may be too thick, folded, or fractured
  - Can prevent complete visualization of margins
  - May be secondary to poor processing or tissue characteristics (e.g., presence of bone)
- Bubbles, nicks, or wrinkles may be present
  - Can prevent complete visualization of margins
  - May be secondary to poor processing or tissue characteristics (e.g., presence of bone)
  - Pressing tissue onto glass slide while freezing minimizes these artifacts
- Artifactual change (freezing, electrodessication) can destroy epidermal morphology
- Staining may be poor quality

Lymphocytes vs. Carcinoma

- Dense infiltrates of lymphocytes or other inflammatory cells can be associated with carcinomas
  - Can sometimes obscure tumor
  - Lymphocytes at margins should raise suspicion that there may also be tumor present

False-Negative Margin Due to Discontinuous Growth Pattern

- Some carcinomas, particularly BCC, either grow as multiple foci or appear to do so
- Although normal tissue is at margin, entire tumor may not be removed
- Some tumor types may require wider margins to ensure complete removal
  - Morpheaform, superficial-multicentric, and multinodular BCC

Basal Cell Carcinoma vs. Normal Hair Follicles

- Normal hair follicles (or portions of hair follicles) may be difficult to distinguish from BCC
  - Tangential sectioning can make normal hair follicles more difficult to recognize
- Normal hair follicles
  - Round to oval overall shape (not irregular)
  - Hair shafts (lumina), if present, very helpful
  - No clefting between follicle and stroma
  - Fibrous sheath may be present
  - Papillary mesenchymal bodies invaginate into follicle at base

Basal Cell Carcinoma vs. Basaloid/Follicular Hyperplasia

- Basaloid follicular proliferations may be extensive in some patients
- May be present in epidermis overlying another benign lesion
- Basaloid follicular proliferations
  - Oriented vertically around hair follicle
    - May see central hair shaft
    - May show areas of follicular differentiation
  - No clefting between proliferation and stroma
  - Few to absent necrotic keratinocytes

Actinic Keratosis (AK) vs. Squamous Cell Carcinoma In Situ

- Not full-thickness atypia or disorder
- Generally has alternating pattern of parakeratosis and orthokeratosis
- Typically spares adnexal structures
- Presence of AK can confound margin assessment
  - Comparison of FS findings with original biopsy may be helpful

Tumor vs. Scar

- Bland spindle cell tumors (dermatofibrosarcoma protuberans, spindle cell SCC) can be difficult to distinguish from scar
- BCC stroma may be difficult to distinguish from scar; toluidine blue staining may be helpful in this differential
- Scar
  - Blood vessels often prominent, verticalized
  - Thickened collagen bundles may be present between fibroblasts

Melanoma In Situ vs. Solar Damage

- Patients may have extensive solar damage (field effect) with tumor-free skin having increase in melanocytes
  - Comparing marginal tissue with normal tissue from another sun-exposed site on patient may help
- Melanocytes can be difficult to see on FS
- In general, melanocytic lesions should not be frozen

Multiple Tumors or Other Lesions

- Patients with extensive solar damage may have additional (undiagnosed) skin lesions
- Incidental tumors/findings can confuse evaluation for primary lesion
  - Incidental tumors
    - Intradermal or compound melanocytic nevi, neurofibroma, epidermal inclusion cyst or milium, seborrheic keratosis, solar lentigo, AK
  - Incidental findings (salivary glands on face, lymph nodes, calcification/ossification)

Eccrine Sweat Glands vs. Carcinoma

- Eccrine glands
  - Round overall shape; may see grouping
  - May see pink cuticle lining lumen
  - Islands generally small and lined by 2-cell layers
- Crushed eccrine glands may be difficult to distinguish from BCC

SELECTED REFERENCES

1. Zabielinski M et al: Laboratory errors leading to nonmelanoma skin cancer recurrence after Mohs micrographic surgery. Dermatol Surg. 41(8):913-6, 2015
2. Taylor BR et al: Facing the block and false positives in Mohs surgery: a retrospective study of 2,198 cases. Dermatol Surg. 39(11):1662-70, 2013
3. Tehrani H et al: Does the dual use of toluidine blue and hematoxylin and eosin staining improve basal cell carcinoma detection by Mohs surgery trainees? Dermatol Surg. 39(7):995-1000, 2013
4. Trimble JS et al: Rapid immunostaining in Mohs: current applications and attitudes. Dermatol Surg. 39(1 Pt 1):56-63, 2013
5. Green JS et al: Mohs frozen tissue sections in comparison to similar paraffin-embedded tissue sections in identifying perineural tumor invasion in cutaneous squamous cell carcinoma. J Am Acad Dermatol. 67(1):113-21, 2012

Mohs Section of Basal Cell Carcinoma

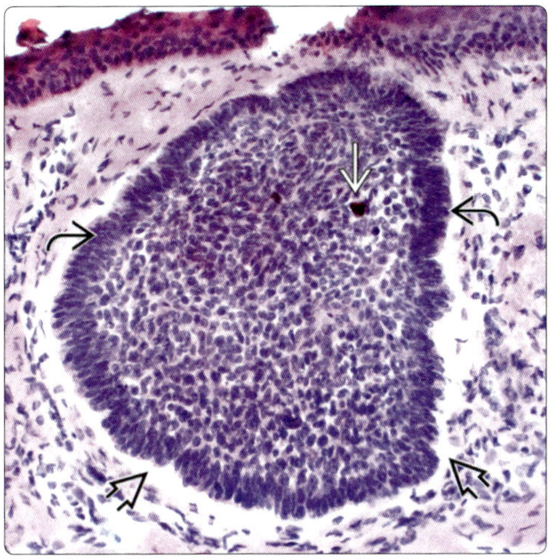

Mohs Section of Basal Cell Carcinoma: Cellular Detail

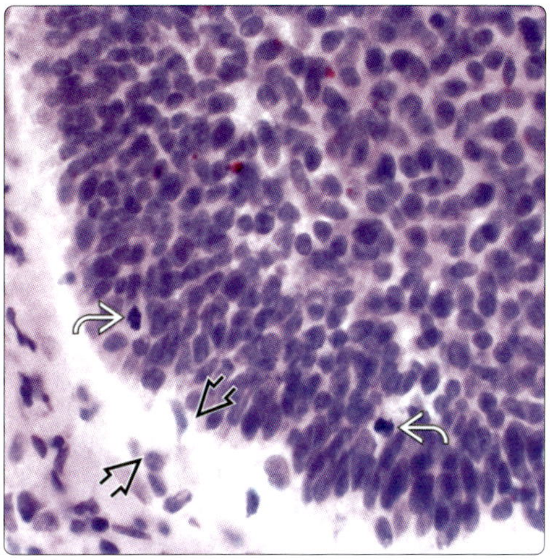

(Left) *Mohs section shows involvement by BCC at the en face margin. Note the prominent peripheral palisading* ↪ *and tumor-stromal retraction artifact* ⇨*. Focal melanin pigmentation is also identified* ➡*.* **(Right)** *BCC is characterized by monomorphic tumor cells with nuclear hyperchromasia but without prominent nucleoli. Cytoplasm is scant, giving a crowded appearance. Mitotic figures* ↪ *can be frequent but are scattered in this case. Stromal retraction* ⇨ *is characteristic.*

Frozen Section of Squamous Cell Carcinoma In Situ

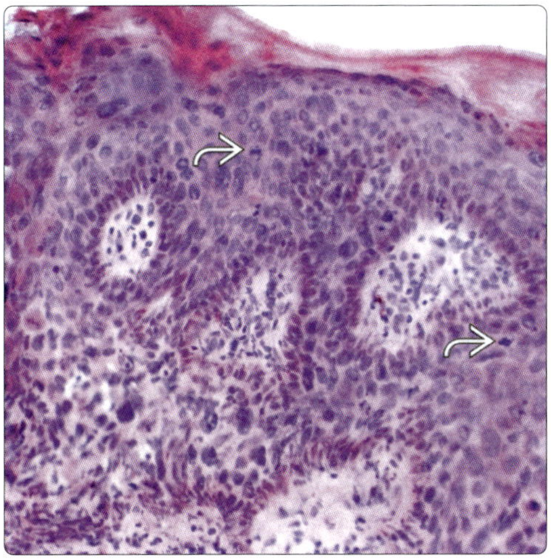

Mohs Section of Squamous Cell Carcinoma

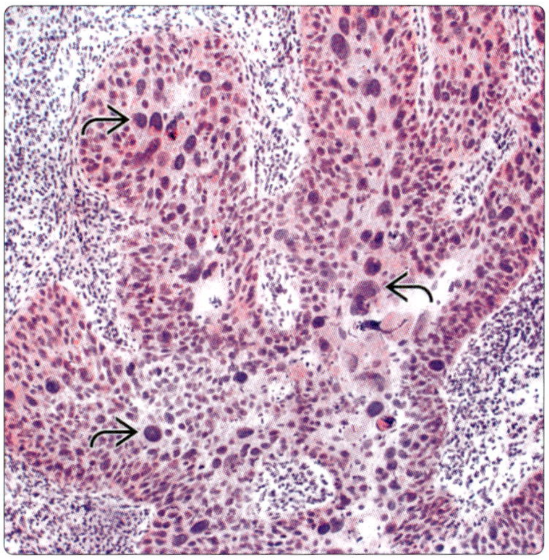

(Left) *Squamous cell carcinoma in situ (SCCis) is characterized by disordered keratinocytes throughout the entire epidermis with multiple mitoses at all levels of the epidermis* ↪*.* **(Right)** *After BCC, squamous cell carcinoma (SCC) is the most common tumor typically excised by Mohs surgery. The tumor is composed of large, atypical cells with irregular nuclei* ↪ *and abundant eosinophilic-staining cytoplasm.*

Slow Mohs Section of Melanoma In Situ (Lentigo Maligna Type)

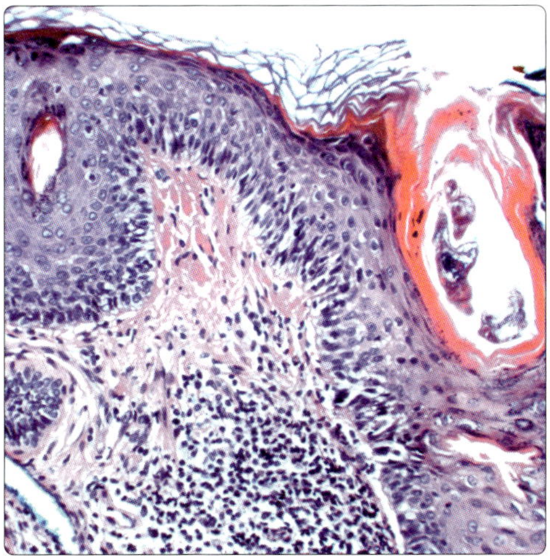

Mohs Section of Tangentially Embedded Hair Follicles

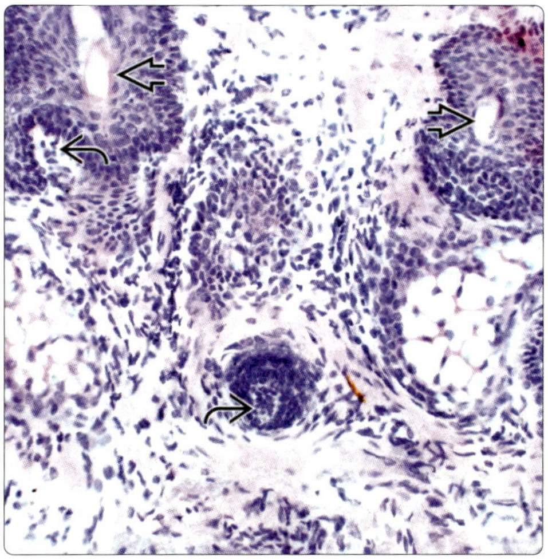

(Left) *This is a so-called slow Mohs section (rapidly processed paraffin-embedded histologic section) of melanoma in situ, lentigo maligna type. Due to the significant artifacts associated with frozen sections of melanoma, this is the preferred method for excising melanoma in situ in sensitive sites.* **(Right)** *Tangentially sectioned hair bulbs/peribulbar regions can be difficult to distinguish from nests of BCC. Note, however, the presence of papillary mesenchymal bodies* ↪ *and focal lumina* ⇨*.*

Mohs Micrographic Surgery: Skin Lesion

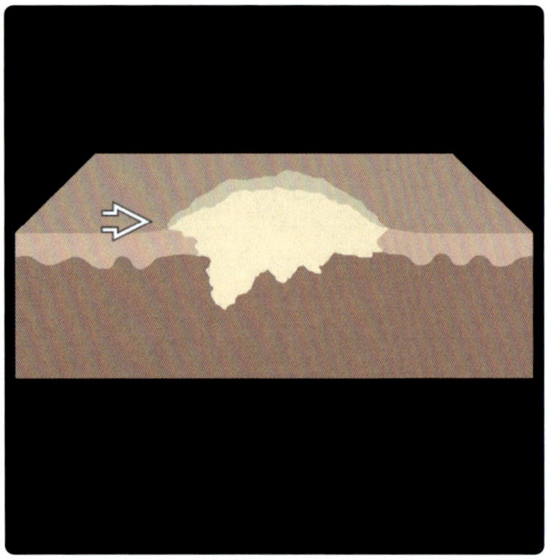

Mohs Micrographic Surgery: Curetting of Skin Cancer

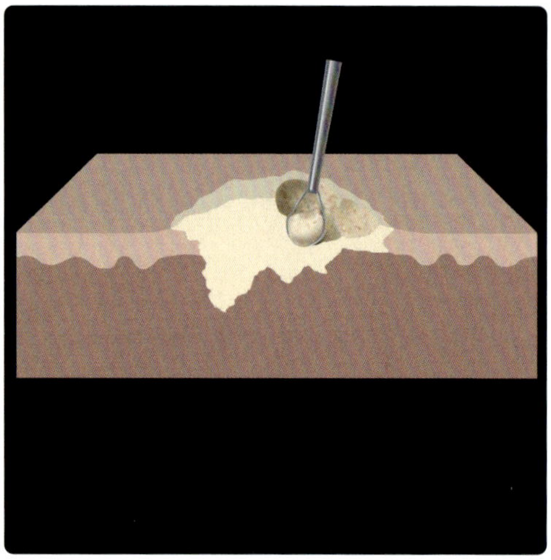

(Left) *Mohs micrographic surgery is designed to remove a minimal amount of tissue when excising squamous cell and basal cell skin cancers ➡. It is primarily used for diffusely infiltrative cancers (including those with perineural invasion); cancers in cosmetically and functionally important areas, such as the head and neck; recurrent tumors; and large (> 1 cm) tumors.* **(Right)** *The 1st step in the surgical procedure is curettage or excision to debulk the center of the carcinoma.*

Mohs Micrographic Surgery: Tumor Bed After Curetting

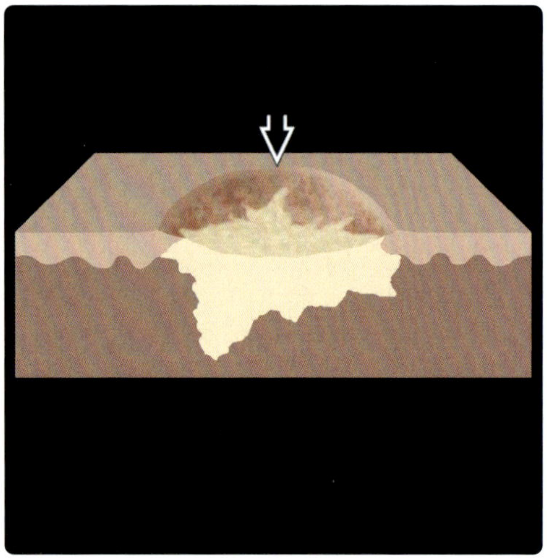

Mohs Micrographic Surgery: Excision of Cancer

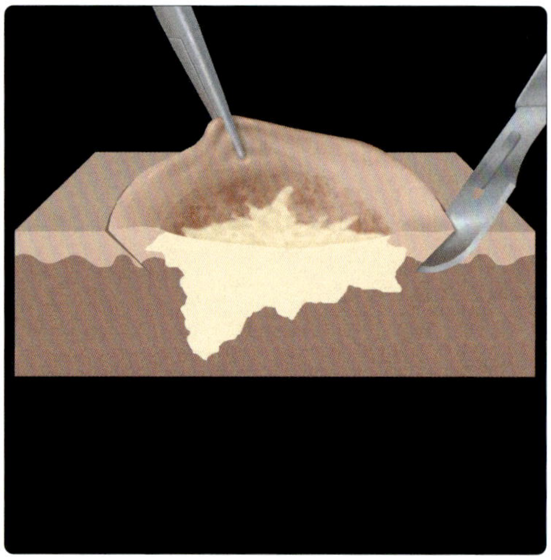

(Left) *The removal of the bulk of the cancer ➡ creates more pliability in the subsequent excisional specimen. Pliability is important in order to later bring all of the margins into the same plane of section.* **(Right)** *The surgeon removes the cancer using an excisional plane at ~ 45° to the edge of the cancer. The goal is to obtain tumor-free margins while excising the minimal amount of normal tissue.*

Mohs Micrographic Surgery: Excisional Specimen

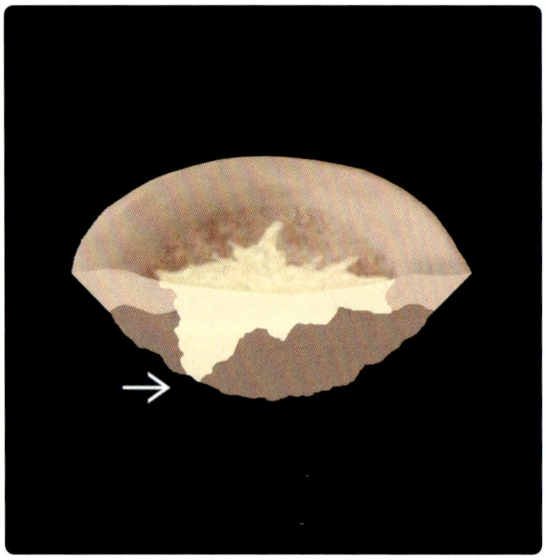

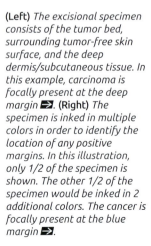

Mohs Micrographic Surgery: Inking Excisional Specimen

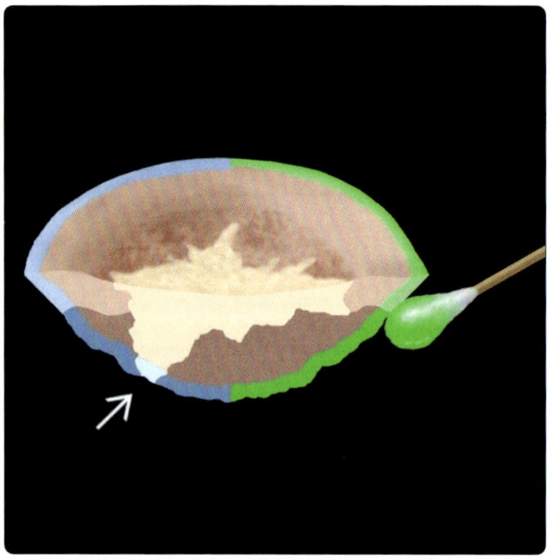

(Left) *The excisional specimen consists of the tumor bed, surrounding tumor-free skin surface, and the deep dermis/subcutaneous tissue. In this example, carcinoma is focally present at the deep margin ➡.* **(Right)** *The specimen is inked in multiple colors in order to identify the location of any positive margins. In this illustration, only 1/2 of the specimen is shown. The other 1/2 of the specimen would be inked in 2 additional colors. The cancer is focally present at the blue margin ➡.*

Mohs Micrographic Surgery: Manipulating Margin Into Single Plane

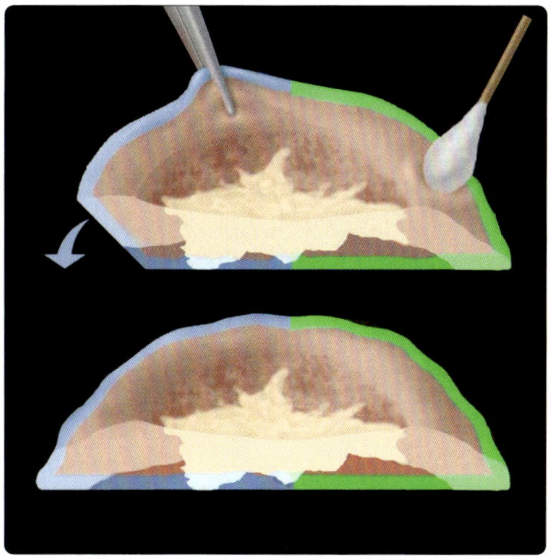

Mohs Micrographic Surgery: Adding Embedding Medium

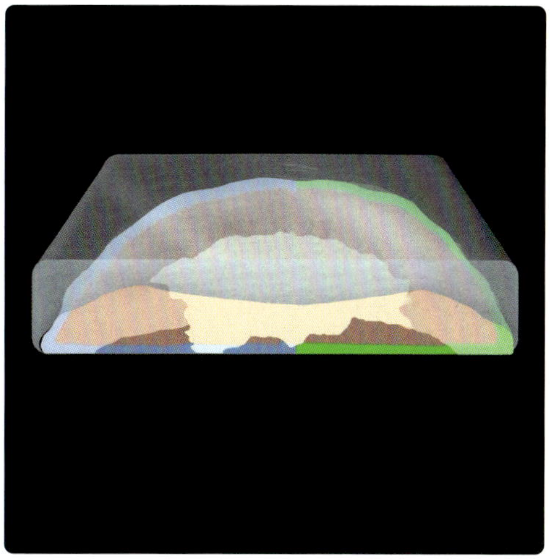

(Left) *The edges of the specimen are pressed down to form a single flat surface on a glass slide. The epidermal margin is in the same plane with the deep and peripheral margins. Large specimens may be cut in 1/2 or 1/4 if too large to fit on a glass slide.* **(Right)** *After the specimen is in the proper orientation, the specimen is covered with embedding medium and completely frozen.*

Mohs Micrographic Surgery: Inverting Specimen

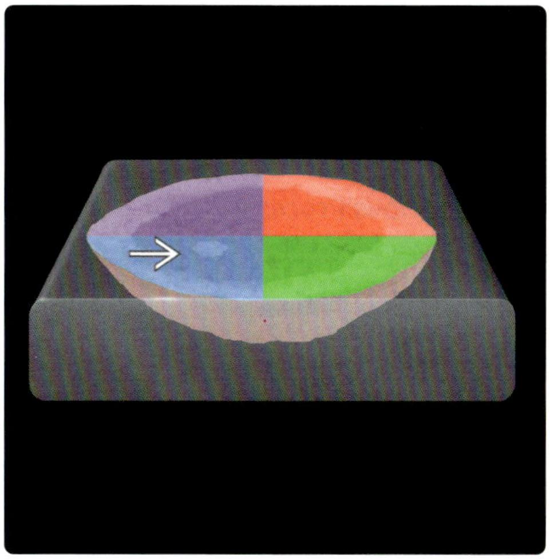

Mohs Micrographic Surgery: Tissue Sections

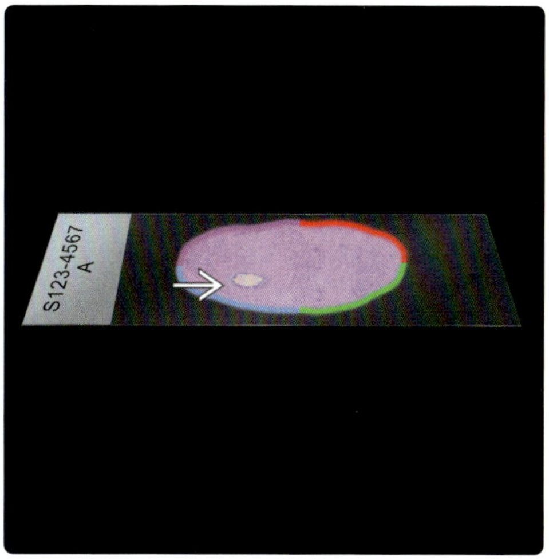

(Left) *The specimen, frozen in the embedding medium, is inverted such that the margin is face up. The block is mounted on a metal chuck in preparation for sectioning on the cryostat. The area of the positive margin* ➡ *is present in the portion of the margin inked in blue.* **(Right)** *The 1st frozen section is the true margin. The tissue sections show 100% of the en face margin of the specimen. Any cancer present on the slide* ➡ *is present at the margin. The portion of the tumor bed with residual cancer is identified according to the ink color.*

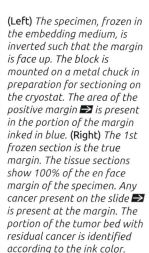

Mohs Micrographic Surgery: Reexcision

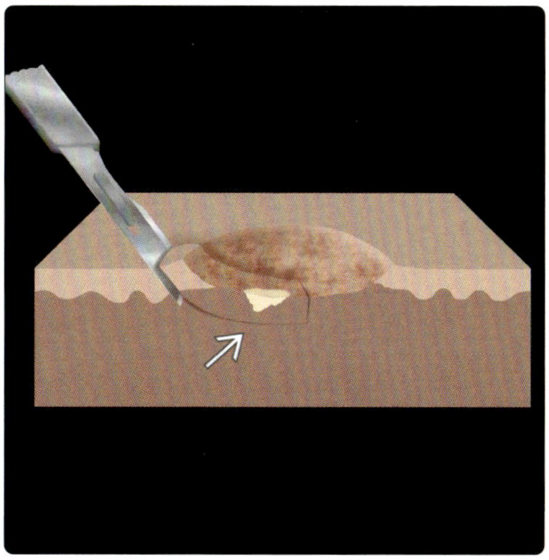

Mohs Micrographic Surgery: Evaluation of Reexcision Specimen

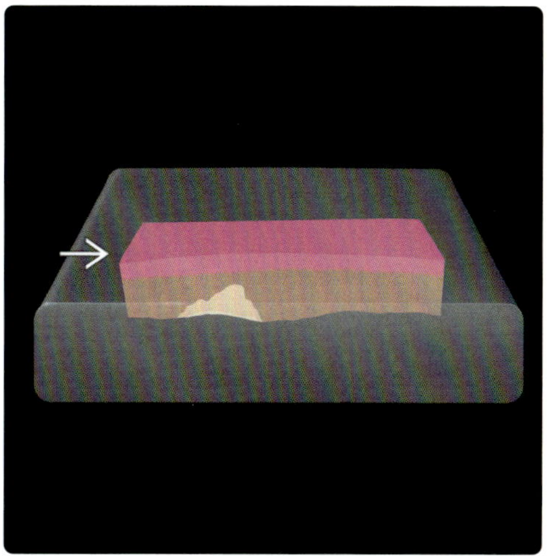

(Left) *Areas of cancer at the margin are identified by frozen section examination. The location of residual cancer is determined by the orientation and the ink colors. The specific area of involvement* ➡ *is reexcised.* **(Right)** *The side of the specimen representing the new margin can be marked with ink* ➡*. The new margin is embedded such that the new margin is sectioned first. This procedure can be repeated until the final margin is free of carcinoma.*

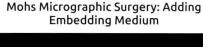

SURGICAL/CLINICAL CONSIDERATIONS

Goal of Consultation

- Establish diagnosis of necrotizing fasciitis (NF)
- Identify viable tissue beyond area of infection

Change in Patient Management

- Diagnosis may prompt immediate wide surgical debridement &/or amputation

Clinical Setting

- Rapidly progressive infection that causes death in up to 33% of patients
- 1/3 of cases are caused by *Streptococcus*, but polymicrobial infections are also common
  - Other pathogens include: *Staphylococcus, Enterococcus, Bacteroides, Clostridium, Escherichia coli, Acinetobacter, Klebsiella*
- Initial spread is horizontal with small bullae
  - In later stages, larger hemorrhagic bullae and necrosis of skin and deep tissues occur
- Initial symptoms are difficult to distinguish from cellulitis or abscess
  - Fever, swelling, and exquisite pain out of proportion to clinical findings are characteristic of NF

SPECIMEN EVALUATION

Gross

- Incisional biopsy, including skin, subcutaneous tissue, and underlying fascia
- Tissue may be taken for culture if not already obtained in operating room

Frozen Section

- Entire specimen is usually embedded
- Orientation of frozen section should be perpendicular to skin surface

Cytology

- Cytologic preparations are not usually made, as they are insufficient for specific diagnosis

MOST COMMON DIAGNOSES

Necrotizing Fasciitis

- Definite features of NF, which distinguish it from other entities in differential, are best appreciated when biopsy occurs within 4 days of onset of symptoms
  - Liquefactive necrosis of epidermis, dermis, and superficial fascia
  - Neutrophilic infiltration of deep dermis and fascia
  - Fibrinous thrombi and inflammation/destruction of arteries and veins
  - Microorganisms within necrotic fascia, subcutis, and dermis
    - Organisms often can be seen on H&E sections
    - Can be confirmed on Gram stains (permanent sections)

Cellulitis

- Neutrophilic infiltration of dermis and superficial subcutis
  - Involvement of deep subcutaneous tissue not seen
- Bacterial organisms identified on H&E &/or Gram stains

Erysipelas

- Rapidly spreading variant of cellulitis with vesiculobullous features

PITFALLS

Infection vs. Noninfectious Process

- Only rare neutrophils may be seen in some cases
- Numerous organisms can be present in absence of inflammatory infiltrate

SELECTED REFERENCES

1. Marchesi A et al: Necrotizing fasciitis in aesthetic surgery: a review of the literature. Aesthetic Plast Surg. 41(2):352-358, 2017
2. Faraklas I et al: A multi-center review of care patterns and outcomes in necrotizing soft tissue infections. Surg Infect (Larchmt). 17(6):773-778, 2016
3. Stegeman SA et al: The value of frozen section biopsy in diagnosing necrotizing fasciitis: proposal of a new grading system. J Tissue Viability. 21(1):13-6, 2012

Necrotizing Fasciitis: Clinical Appearance

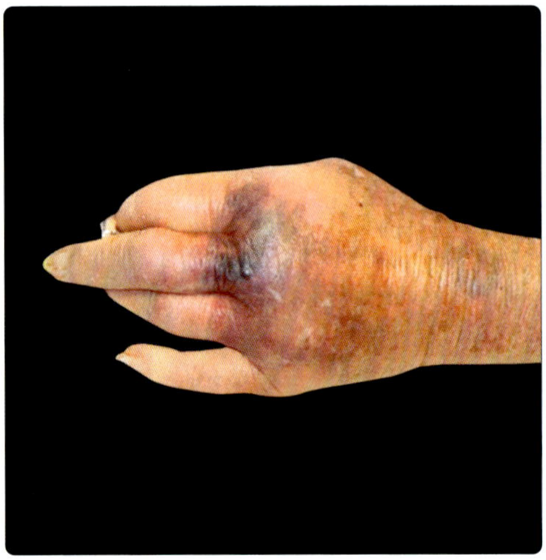

Necrotizing Fasciitis: Histologic Appearance

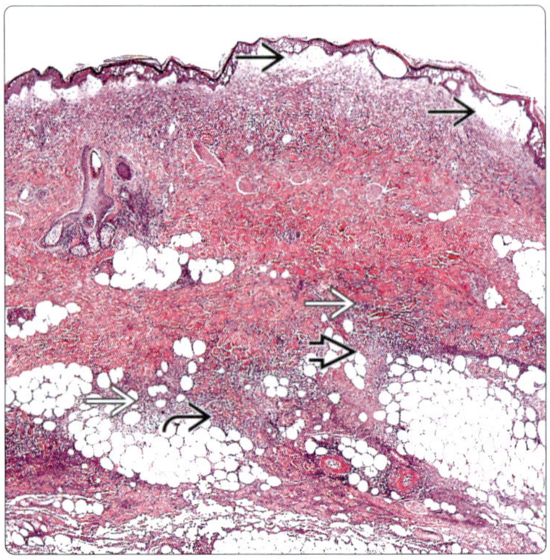

(Left) *A swollen, tender, and erythematous hand with exquisite pain is typical of necrotizing fasciitis. Aggressive debridement and sometimes amputation may be necessary to prevent the infection from spreading. (Courtesy C. Rhodes, MD.)* **(Right)** *Necrotizing fasciitis often shows areas of marked subepidermal edema ➔ with superficial, deep dermal ➔ and subcutaneous tissue ➔ necrosis. Scattered foci of inflammation are seen ➔. (Courtesy L. Layfield, MD.)*

Necrotizing Fasciitis Involving Limb

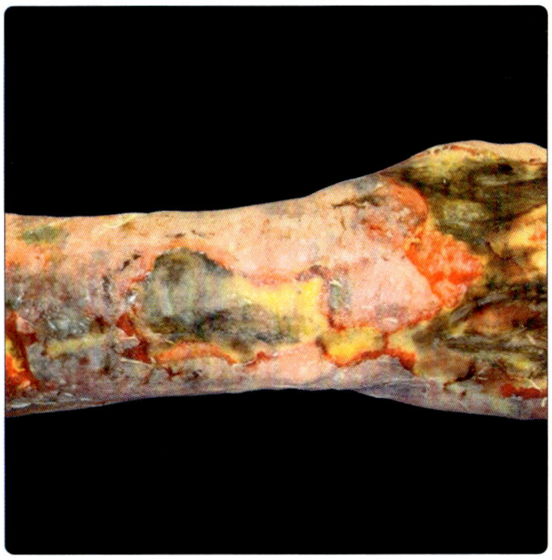

Necrotizing Fasciitis

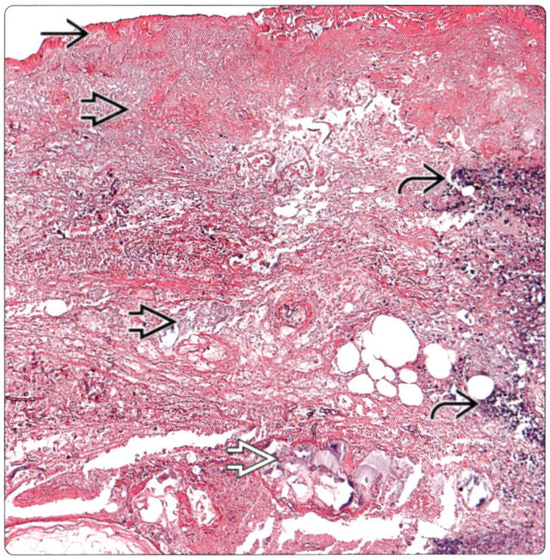

(Left) *Necrotizing fasciitis has caused extensive skin and subcutaneous necrosis of this distal extremity. This was a very aggressive case that required amputation.* **(Right)** *Necrotizing fasciitis often shows areas of necrosis involving the epidermis ➙, superficial and deep dermis ⇨, and deep subcutaneous tissue ➡. Inflammation ➚ is typically seen at the interface between viable areas and necrotic tissue. In contrast, cellulitis is usually restricted to the dermis and superficial subcutaneous tissue.*

Necrotizing Fasciitis: Vascular Involvement

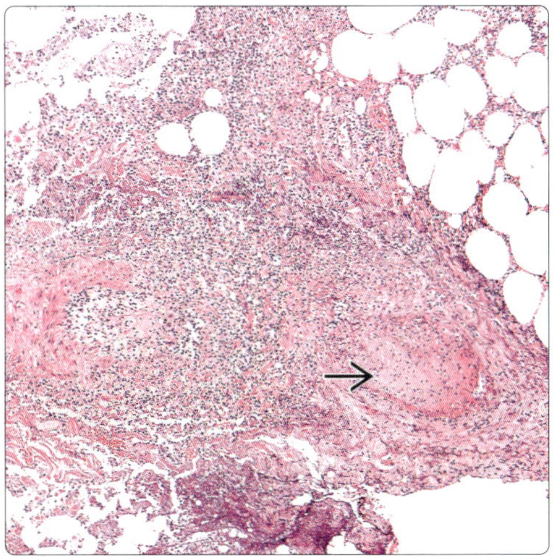

Necrotizing Fasciitis: Bacteria

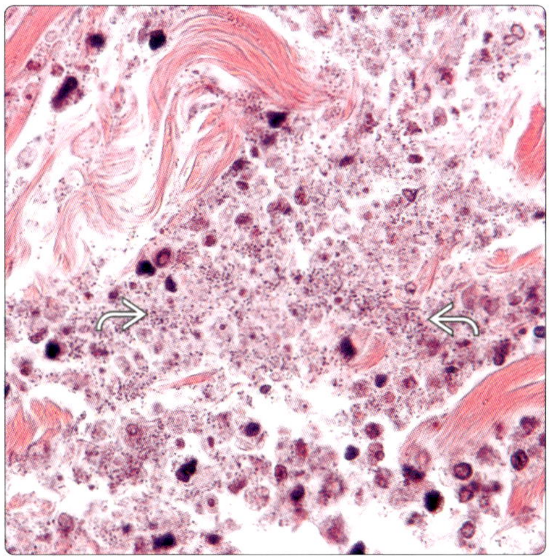

(Left) *Fibrinoid necrosis of vessels ➙ is commonly seen in necrotizing fasciitis, along with an intense neutrophilic infiltrate often containing numerous bacteria. Blood vessels may also be occluded by fibrin thrombi. (Courtesy L. Layfield, MD.)* **(Right)** *Large numbers of bacteria can often be seen on H&E stains in cases of necrotizing fasciitis. In this case, degenerating inflammatory cells are associated with numerous small, cocci-like bacterial organisms ➚. (Courtesy L. Layfield, MD.)*

Necrotizing Fasciitis: Clostridium

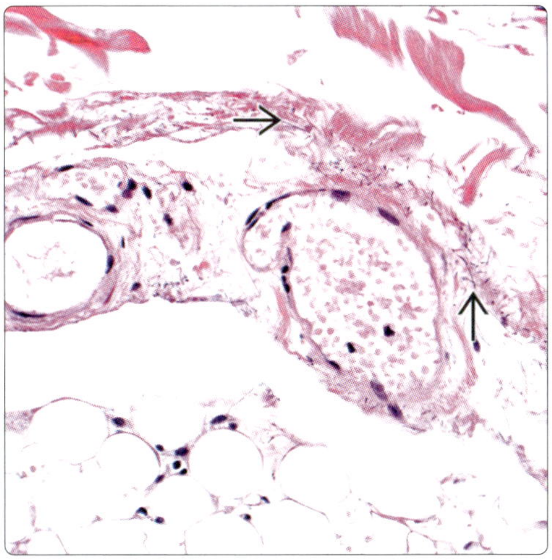

Necrotizing Fasciitis: Gram Stain

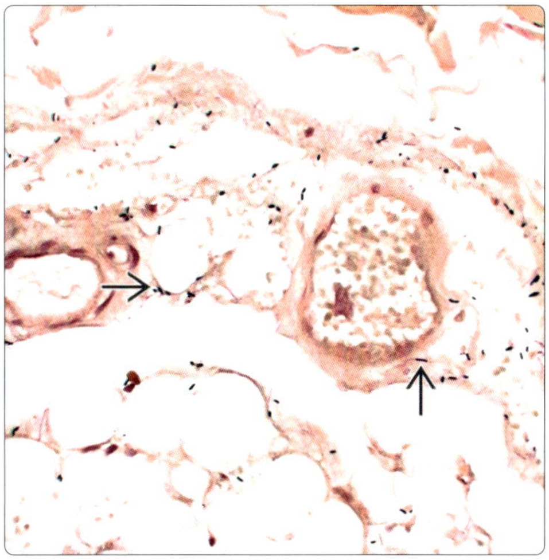

(Left) *Numerous rod-shaped bacteria ➙ are present adjacent to blood vessels on an H&E stain of this rare case of clostridial necrotizing fasciitis. Inflammation was deceptively minimal in this case. In other cases, Gram stains are necessary to identify bacteria.* **(Right)** *Special stains for organisms are generally not performed during an intraoperative consultation for necrotizing fasciitis. In this case, a Gram stain performed on a permanent section highlights multiple variably gram-positive rods of Clostridium ➙.*

SURGICAL/CLINICAL CONSIDERATIONS

Goal of Consultation

- Ensure sufficient tissue is available for eventual diagnosis
- Allocate tissue for special studies
- If specimen is definitive resection, margins may be evaluated grossly

Change in Patient Management

- Additional tissue may be taken until diagnostic tissue has been acquired
- For definitive resections, additional tissue may be taken to achieve tumor-free margins

Clinical Setting

- Patients typically present with large soft tissue mass, which may or may not be symptomatic
- Biopsy for diagnosis is necessary to determine best course of treatment
  - Some patients may be treated with presurgical radiation &/or chemotherapy
  - Surgery for malignant lesions is generally more extensive with greater morbidity than that for benign lesions
    - Definitive surgical treatment should not be based solely on frozen section diagnosis

SPECIMEN EVALUATION

Gross: Biopsies

- Representative portion may be frozen to guide apportionment of tissue for special studies
- Entire specimen should not be frozen
  - If small, surgeon may be queried as to whether additional tissue will be available
- Tissue is allocated for special studies according to likely diagnosis and amount of tissue
  - Formalin
    - Thin (0.2-0.3 cm) slices of tumor should be placed in formalin as soon as possible
    - Slices should be thin enough such that they can easily fit into cassette without additional slicing
  - Frozen
    - Small sections of tumor are frozen in embedding medium
    - This tissue can be used for DNA and mRNA studies
    - Frozen section remnant can be used for this purpose if amount of tissue is limited
  - Electron microscopy (EM)
    - Tumor is cut into small cubes (< 0.1 cm per side) using sharp blade and placed in fixative for EM (i.e., glutaraldehyde)
  - Cytogenetics
    - Tumor must be sterile and viable
  - Hematopathology fixatives
    - If lymphoma is in differential diagnosis, tissue may be saved in fixatives, such as B-Plus

Gross: Resections

- All structures in specimen are identified
- Orientation should be provided by surgeon
  - If orientation is unclear, surgeon should be consulted before proceeding
- Inspect outer surface for areas suspicious for tumor involvement
- Selectively ink areas of true margins
  - Multiple colors of ink can help to identify different margins
- Serially section specimen
- Identify all lesions
  - Tissue can be allocated for ancillary studies as appropriate
- Distance from each margin should be recorded
  - In general, minimal 2-cm margin should be achieved &/or excision to tissue plane

Frozen Section

- Small portion of tumor may be frozen to document lesional tissue and to help guide apportionment of tissue
- Margins are generally not frozen for evaluation

Nodular Fasciitis

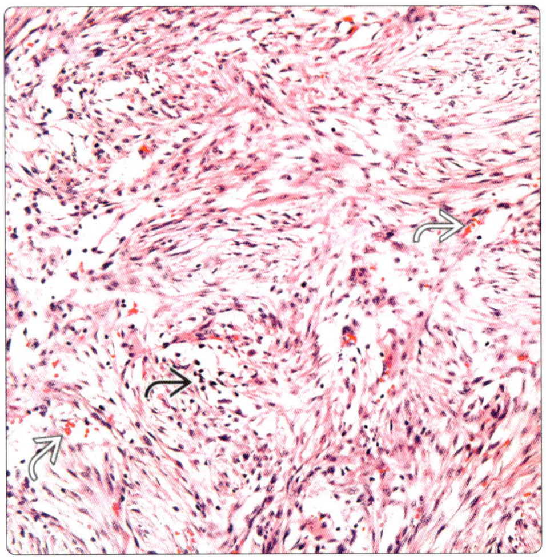

Leiomyosarcoma

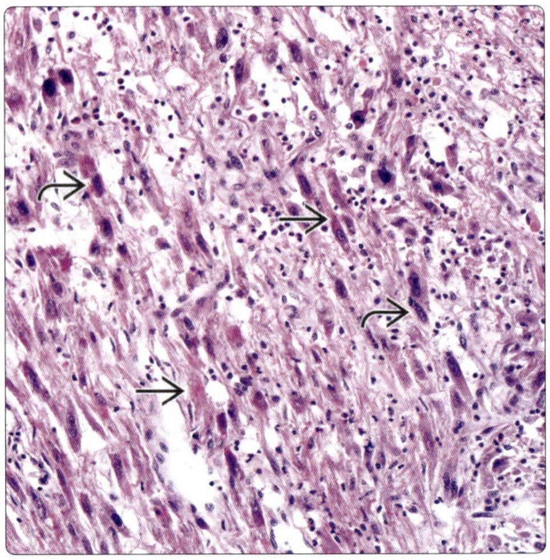

(Left) *Nodular fasciitis is a relatively common spindle cell proliferation with a storiform pattern, mitoses, lymphocytes ⮫, and extravasated erythrocytes ⮫. This lesion can be easily mistaken for a sarcoma.* **(Right)** *Leiomyosarcoma is a sarcoma composed of fascicles of highly atypical, spindle-shaped cells with oval to elongated, cigar-shaped nuclei ⮫ and abundant eosinophilic-staining cytoplasm →.*

Cytology

- Smears of tumor may be performed for evaluation in conjunction with frozen sections

MOST COMMON DIAGNOSES

Dermatofibroma/Fibrous Histiocytoma

- Proliferation of spindled and histiocytoid-appearing cells with collagen entrapment in dermis
- Cellular variants show dense collections of spindle cells with less conspicuous collagen trapping, especially in center of lesion

Dermatofibrosarcoma Protuberans

- Monotonous proliferation of spindle cells in storiform arrays in deep dermis and subcutis
- Collagen entrapment not present but can also be lacking in center of cellular dermatofibroma

Neurofibroma

- Small, bland spindled cells with wavy nuclei in myxoid to collagenous stroma
- Degenerative (ancient) changes with large, hyperchromatic, and pleomorphic-appearing nuclei can be seen

Schwannoma

- Encapsulated spindle cell tumor with alternating cellular (Antoni A) and hypocellular (Antoni B) areas
- Often deeper-seated and encapsulated tumors, in contrast to neurofibromas
- Also can show ancient changes with cells showing large, hyperchromatic-, and pleomorphic-appearing nuclei

Nodular Fasciitis and Other Pseudosarcomas

- Benign spindle cell proliferation with storiform pattern
- Can be easily mistaken for sarcoma, especially on frozen sections, if not considered in differential diagnosis
- Mitoses are frequent but not atypical

Leiomyoma

- Fascicles of spindle cells with blunt-ended (cigar-shaped) nuclei
- Lack significant atypia or mitotic activity in most cases

Leiomyosarcoma

- Presents in older adults, deep soft tissues of extremities and retroperitoneum
- Fascicles of eosinophilic-staining spindle cells with cigar-shaped nuclei and perinuclear vacuoles

Atypical Fibroxanthoma

- Presents in heavily sun-damaged skin of older adults
- Atypical and pleomorphic spindle cells with numerous mitotic figures

Pleomorphic Sarcoma

- Deep soft tissues
- Proliferation of markedly atypical and pleomorphic-appearing large cells with abundant cytoplasm

Liposarcoma

- Deep soft tissues of extremities and retroperitoneum
- Often difficult to obtain interpretable frozen sections, given abundance of fat in most tumors
- Dedifferentiated liposarcoma shows solid areas of undifferentiated spindle cells or heterologous elements, including malignant osteoid or cartilage

Rhabdomyosarcoma

- Usually in children, embryonal subtype most common
- Alveolar rhabdomyosarcoma shows proliferation of round cells with dyscohesion pattern

REPORTING

Gross: Margin Evaluation

- Distance of tumor from margins can be provided

Frozen Section: Specimen Adequacy

- Specific diagnosis is rarely necessary and usually not possible, unless it is recurrence or metastasis of previously diagnosed tumor
    - Report "spindle cell tumor, classification deferred to permanent sections" in most cases

Cytology

- Description of cytologic findings may be given (i.e., spindled, epithelioid, or rhabdoid cells)

PITFALLS

Benign Spindle Cell Tumors vs. Sarcoma

- Definitive characterization of spindle cell tumors may be impossible on frozen sections
- Nuclei appear more atypical on frozen section, and it can be difficult to distinguish myxoid stroma from edema
- Greater sampling and immunohistochemical studies on permanent sections often necessary for definitive diagnosis
    - Therefore, deferring classification to permanent is usually appropriate for intraoperative reporting

Reactive Peritumoral Tissue

- There is often a rim of reactive fibrosis and inflammation at periphery of tumor
- Surgeon may not sample actual lesional tissue
- Tissue reaction can be mistaken for spindle cell proliferation
- Pathologist should request additional tissue if definitive lesional tissue is not seen

Treated Tumors

- Sarcomas may be treated with chemotherapy &/or radiation prior to excision
- It can be very difficult to distinguish treatment-related changes from residual tumor
- Ideally, margins will consist of normal tissue and not tumor bed or surgical site changes

SELECTED REFERENCES

1. Kurtulan O et al: Diagnostic power and pitfalls of intraoperative consultation (frozen section) in rhabdomyosarcoma. Turk Patoloji Derg. 31(1):16-23, 2015
2. Ashford RU et al: The role of intra-operative pathological evaluation in the management of musculoskeletal tumours. Recent Results Cancer Res. 179:11-24, 2009
3. Bui MM et al: Practical issues of intraoperative frozen section diagnosis of bone and soft tissue lesions. Cancer Control. 15(1):7-12, 2008
4. Ashford RU et al: Surgical biopsy with intra-operative frozen section. An accurate and cost-effective method for diagnosis of musculoskeletal sarcomas. J Bone Joint Surg Br. 88(9):1207-11, 2006

(Left) *Cutaneous neurofibromas are fairly well-circumscribed, but unencapsulated, tumors arising in the dermis. Although they may occur in neurofibromatosis type 1, the majority of localized cutaneous tumors are sporadic in nature.* (Right) *Schwannomas are nerve sheath tumors composed of spindle cells. Some have characteristic alternating Antoni A and B areas. Areas of nuclear palisading (Verocay bodies) are part of the Antoni A areas. Antoni B areas are hypocellular.*

Neurofibroma

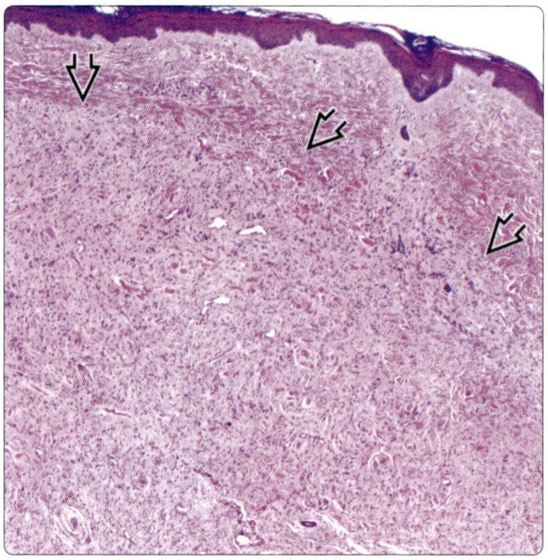

Schwannoma

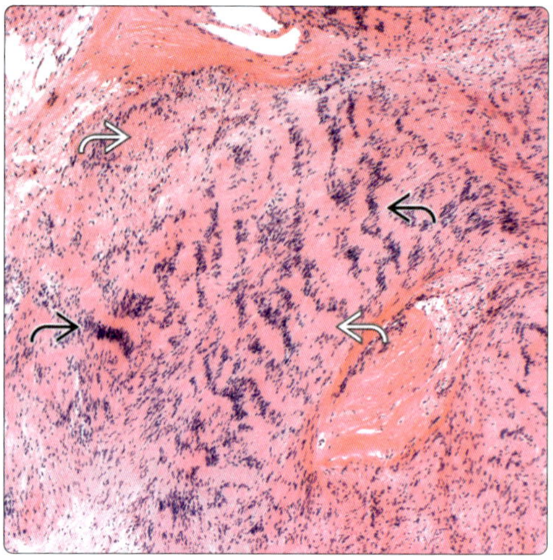

(Left) *Cellular fibrous histiocytoma/dermatofibroma (DF) shows epidermal acanthosis and a thin grenz zone separating the tumor from the epidermis. The lesion contains many spindled fibroblastic cells, a few foamy histiocytes, and often lacks the prominent collagen trapping typical of most DFs.* (Right) *This DFSP is a cellular spindle cell tumor involving the deep dermal and subcutaneous tissue with honeycombing fat entrapment. The epidermis and superficial dermis are spared.*

Cellular Fibrous Histiocytoma/Dermatofibroma

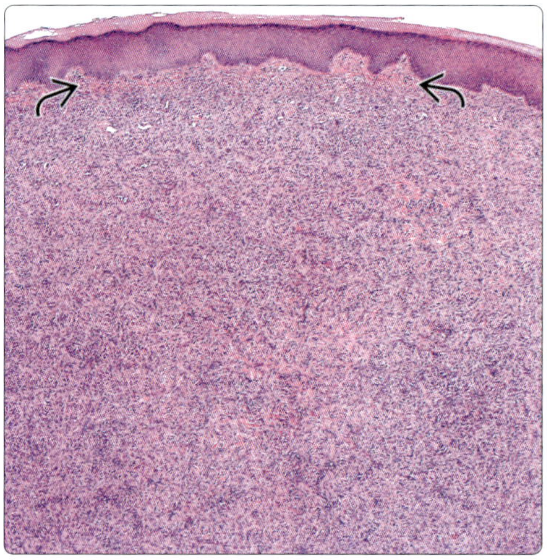

Dermatofibrosarcoma Protuberans

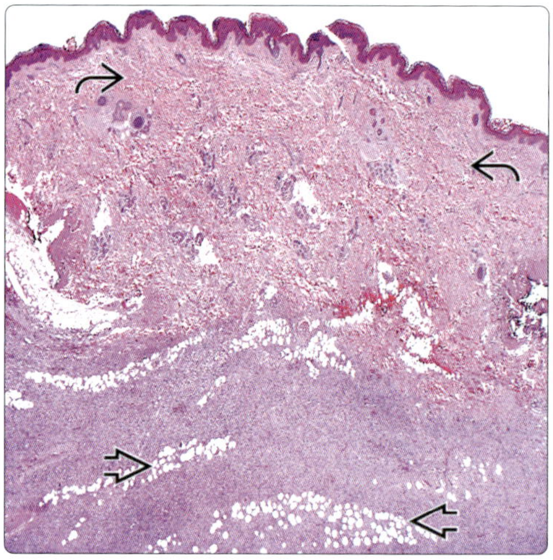

(Left) *Fibrosarcoma (arising in a DFSP) displays dense cellularity, prominent cytologic atypia, and multiple mitotic figures. The tumor is arranged in a fascicular or herringbone architecture, which is not seen in most other sarcomas.* (Right) *High-grade myxofibrosarcoma shows spindle cells with cytologic atypia and several large, multinucleated cells. Multiple small, branching blood vessels are typically present. A diagnosis of "malignant spindle cell neoplasm" would be adequate on frozen section.*

Fibrosarcoma

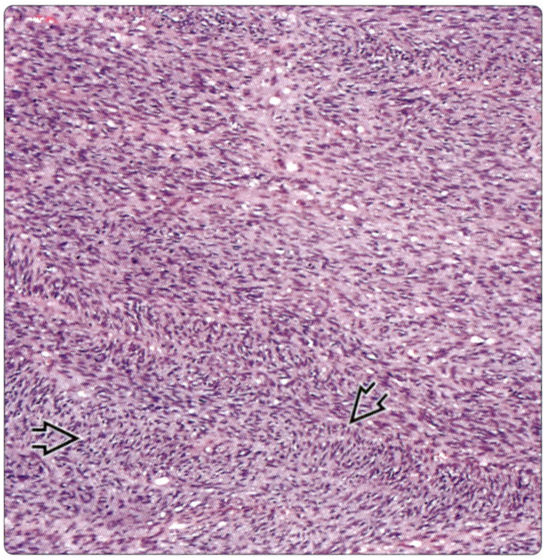

Myxofibrosarcoma

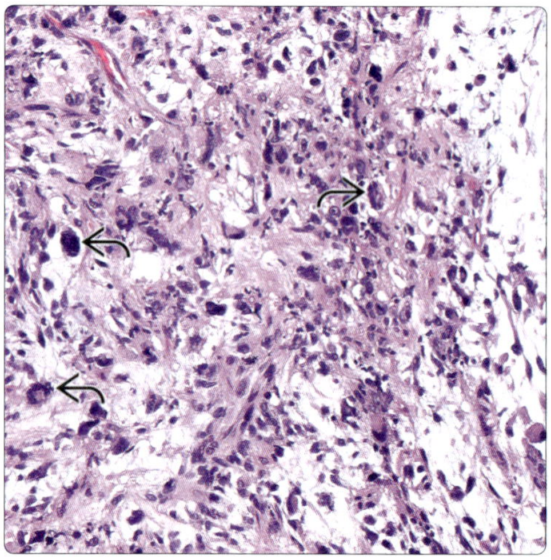

Atypical Fibroxanthoma

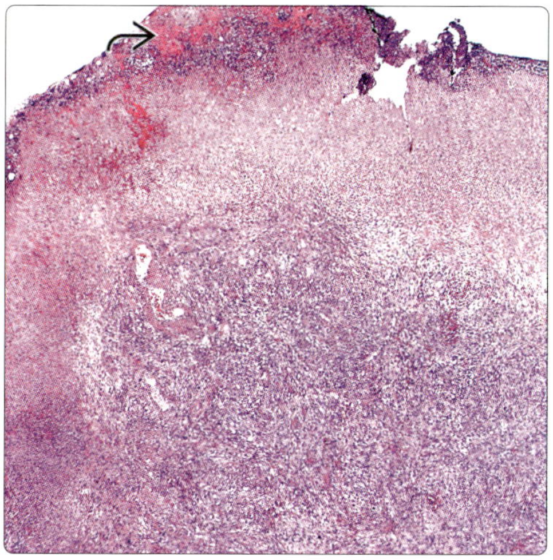

Atypical Fibroxanthoma: High Power

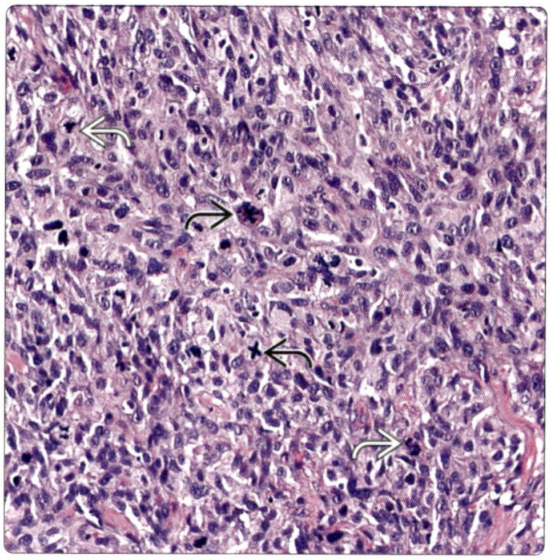

(Left) *This atypical fibroxanthoma (AFX) consists of a large, dermal-based atypical nodular to sheet-like collection of spindled and epithelioid tumor cells with overlying ulceration and serum crust.* **(Right)** *This AFX is characterized by a cellular proliferation of large, highly atypical, and pleomorphic spindled- to epithelioid-appearing cells with numerous mitoses, including several frankly atypical forms. Deeply invasive tumors are typically considered a type of pleomorphic sarcoma.*

Cutaneous Rhabdomyosarcoma

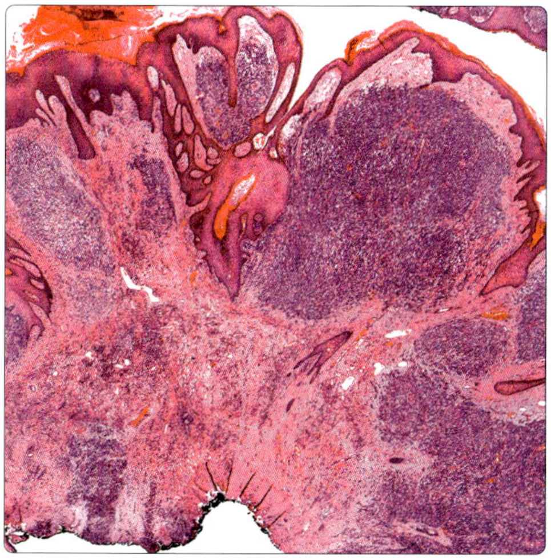

Alveolar Rhabdomyosarcoma

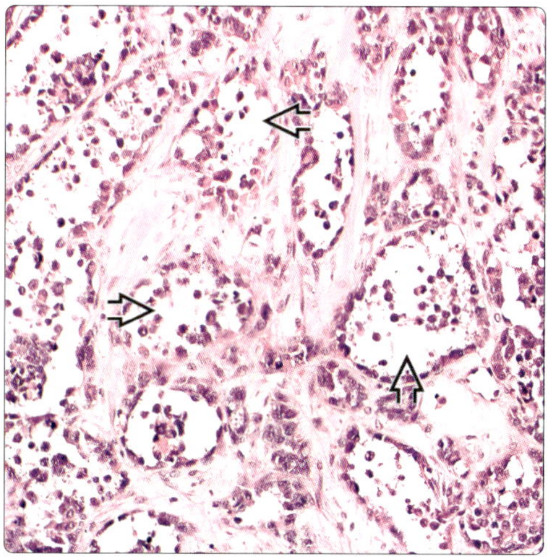

(Left) *This cutaneous rhabdomyosarcoma from the ear is a polypoidal tumor with extensive infiltration of the dermis by hypercellular sheets of fairly uniform, small blue (hyperchromatic-staining) round to ovoid cells. (Courtesy S. Billings, MD.)* **(Right)** *This example of alveolar rhabdomyosarcoma shows nests of round cells separated by fibrous septa. There is central dyscohesion and tumor cell necrosis forming clear spaces, somewhat resembling the appearance of pulmonary alveoli. (Courtesy S. Billings, MD.)*

Dedifferentiated Liposarcoma

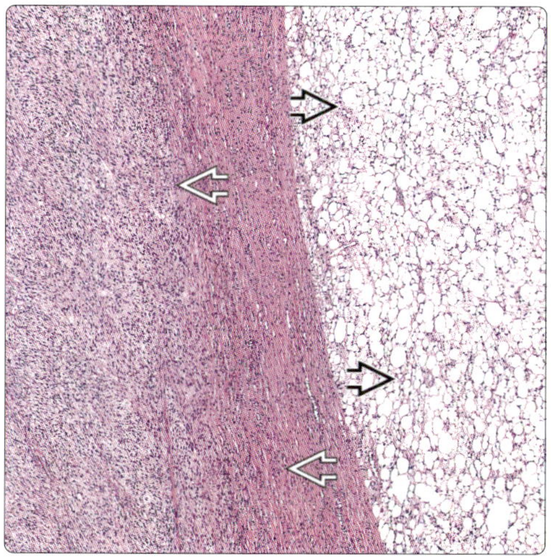

Metastatic Melanoma

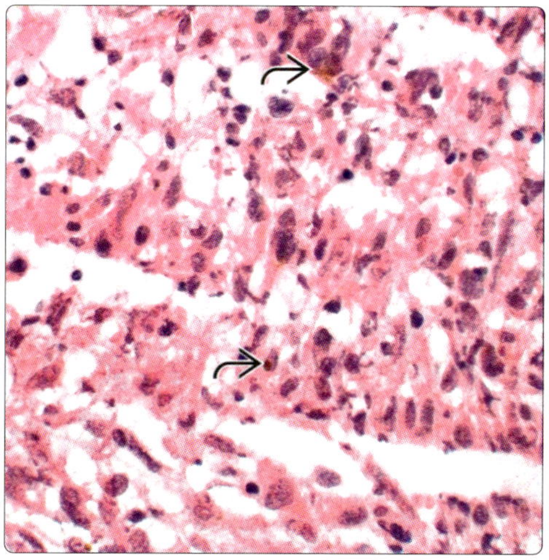

(Left) *This dedifferentiated liposarcoma shows an undifferentiated spindle cell component on the left with an abrupt transition to an atypical lipomatous tumor (well-differentiated liposarcoma) on the right.* **(Right)** *This melanoma that has metastasized to soft tissue, consisting of atypical, spindle-shaped to epithelioid-appearing cells, could be mistaken for a soft tissue tumor without the appropriate clinical history and ancillary studies on permanent sections.*

Contents

SURGICAL/CLINICAL CONSIDERATIONS

Goal of Consultation

- Provide diagnosis to guide further intraoperative management
- Allow for proper handling of tissue for ancillary studies

Change in Patient Management

- Some tumors, such as myxopapillary ependymoma and meningioma will undergo complete resection
- Other tumors, such as astrocytoma, require biopsy for diagnosis but usually cannot undergo complete resection
- Some lesions require only provisional diagnosis to guide tissue allocation for special studies
  - Molecular studies and flow cytometry (lymphoma)
  - Electron microscopy (differential diagnosis of meningioma, identification of metastatic tumors)
  - Microbiologic culture (inflammatory lesions)

Clinical Setting

- There are 3 main settings in which patients with spinal cord lesions require tissue biopsy
- **New onset of localizing signs** (e.g., paraparesis, nerve root symptoms)
- **Systemic illnesses with risk of impending cord compression, requiring emergency therapy**
  - Metastatic carcinoma, sarcoma
  - Lymphoma or plasmacytoma
  - Suspected infection (e.g., epidural abscess)
- **Patients with germline mutations**
  - Neurofibromatosis, type 1
    - Optic pathway gliomas (usually pilocytic)
    - Cerebral, cerebellar, and spinal cord diffuse astrocytomas
    - Spinal nerve root neurofibromas (nodular and plexiform)
    - Spinal nerve root plexiform schwannomas
  - Neurofibromatosis, type 2
    - Bilateral vestibular schwannomas
    - Multiple meningiomas (may affect cord)
    - Ependymomas of spinal cord parenchyma, always benign
    - Meningioangiomatosis (cortex)
  - von Hippel-Lindau disease
    - Single or multiple hemangioblastomas (may affect cord)

NEUROIMAGING

Presurgical Imaging

- Location and appearance of lesion on MR is essential for developing most likely differential diagnosis
  - This information should be available to pathologist at time of intraoperative consultation
    - Pathologist should review imaging prior to consultation
- Helps provide safety net to ensure final diagnosis incorporates both microscopic and macroscopic features of lesion

Neuroanatomic Location

- Para- or extraspinal, bony spine, and epidural
  - Metastasis
  - Sarcoma
  - Lymphoma or plasmacytoma
  - Infection
  - Nerve sheath tumors
- Intradural, extramedullary
  - Meningioma
  - Metastasis
  - Nerve sheath tumors
  - Cysts
  - Vascular malformations
- Distal (filum terminale, cauda equina)
  - Paraganglioma
  - Myxopapillary ependymoma
  - Metastasis
- Intramedullary
  - Astrocytoma
  - Ependymoma

Ependymoma

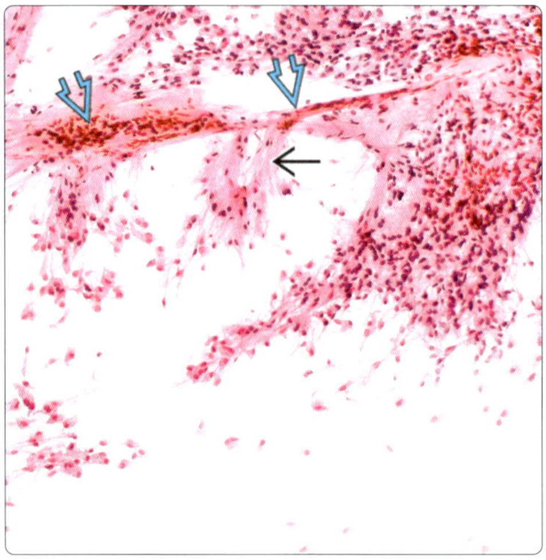

Ependymoma

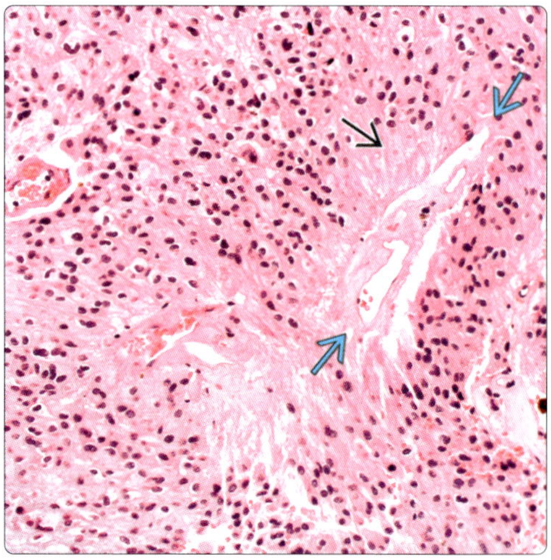

(Left) *A smear from an ependymoma shows uniform cell nuclei and fibrillary cytoplasm ➔ that extend to blood vessels ⇨. This pattern forms perivascular pseudorosettes in tissue sections.* **(Right)** *A blood vessel ⇨ shows a surrounding radial array of low-grade ependymoma tumor cells. The fibrillary tumor cell processes ➔ form a nucleus-free zone (perivascular pseudorosette). Anaplastic ependymomas have much more cellularity, pleomorphism, brisk mitotic activity, and microvascular proliferation.*

  - Cysts
  - Syrinx

Signal Characteristics

- Contrast enhancement
  - Vascularity
- Hypodensity
  - Necrosis
  - Cystic change

SPECIMEN EVALUATION

Gross

- Usually very few distinctive macroscopic characteristics
  - Gliomas: Soft, gray-translucent, gelatinous texture
  - Metastatic carcinoma: Red or tan, gritty consistency, can be necrotic
  - Nerve sheath tumors: Rubbery, fibrous tissue
  - Abscess: Purulent material

Frozen Section

- Important not to use entire specimen (may be only specimen received)
- A minute fragment is set aside for cytologic preparation
- Frozen section method
  - Perch tissue to be frozen on small bead of embedding medium, but do not cover with medium
  - Freeze quickly with light touch of metal heat extractor or cryospray to avoid ice crystals in tissue
  - Step section carefully into block on cryostat when making slides
- Some specimens are best evaluated using only cytologic preparations without frozen section
  - Very small specimens
  - Suspected infectious disease
  - Specimens with dense calcification

Cytologic Preparations

- Smear method
  - Place 1-3 pinhead-sized fragments 1/3 of way down glass slide
  - Use 2nd slide to gently smear tissue
- Touch preparation method
  - Use for firm/calcified/fibrous lesions
  - Gently and rapidly touch tissue (held gently in forceps) to slide surface
    - Make only 1 touch imprint
    - If > 1 is made, some will have drying artifact
- Place immediately in fixative to avoid drying artifact
- Entire slide must be scanned, as lesions may be heterogeneous

MOST COMMON DIAGNOSES

Ependymoma (WHO Grade II)

- Frozen section
  - Variably cellular, with perivascular pseudorosettes, ependymal tubules or canals, and small intracytoplasmic vacuoles (lumina)
  - Microvascular proliferation and infarct-like necrosis are of no prognostic significance
- Smear
  - Glial tumor cells with uniform oval nuclei, often with small nucleoli
  - Cytoplasmic processes, radially arranged around blood vessels, ± vascular cell proliferation
  - Occasional intracytoplasmic lumina as well as cilia and terminal bars (blepharoplasts) in tubules
- Difficulties
  - Must distinguish from astrocytoma, as ependymoma requires resection

Astrocytoma (WHO Grade II)

- Frozen section
  - Cellularity slightly greater than normal cord parenchyma
  - Cytologic atypia may be mild
  - Elongated nuclei in infiltrating cells in white matter
  - No mitoses, microvascular proliferation, or necrosis
- Smear
  - Fibrillary background clearer than in frozen
  - Individual cytologically atypical nuclei (hyperchromatic, irregularly shaped, enlarged compared to normal glia)
- Difficulties
  - Findings must correlate with neuroimaging
    - Diffuse astrocytoma is not contrast enhancing
    - Enhancement implies higher grade
  - Distinction from reactive processes, such as myelitis or demyelination, may require special studies
    - Diagnosis may need to be deferred to permanent sections

Anaplastic Ependymoma (WHO Grade III)

- Frozen section and smear
  - Higher cellularity, pleomorphism, and mitoses than in grade II ependymoma
  - Necrosis prominent
  - Ependymal tubules or perivascular pseudorosettes may not be present
- Difficulties
  - Evidence of ependymal differentiation may be scarce, making distinction from anaplastic astrocytoma or glioblastoma multiforme challenging

Anaplastic Astrocytoma (WHO Grade III) and Glioblastoma (WHO Grade IV)

- Frozen section
  - Dense cellularity, pleomorphism, brisk mitotic activity
  - Microvascular proliferation with glomeruloid profiles
  - In glioblastoma, necrosis, sometimes pseudopalisading
- Smear
  - Cytologically malignant cells (hyperchromasia, high nuclear:cytoplasmic ratio, irregular nuclear outline, mitoses)
  - Coarse fibrillary background
  - Knotted and blind-ending glomeruloid vessels
  - In glioblastoma, necrosis, sometimes with apoptotic debris
- Difficulties
  - If small sample, grading may need to be deferred
  - It can be difficult to distinguish from metastatic carcinoma or lymphoma

Meningioma

- Identical to tumors in cranial meninges

  - Grading usually does not need to be established on frozen section
    - However, presence of atypical or anaplastic features should be communicated to neurosurgeon.
- **Meningioma, WHO grade I**
  - Fibrous, meningothelial, transitional, psammomatous, secretory, angiomatous, microcystic subtypes
    - Often of psammomatous type in spinal cord
  - Meningothelial whorls with psammoma bodies may be seen on touch prep
  - Syncytial groupings of cells with broad, flat eosinophilic cytoplasm, nuclei with fine dusty chromatin and smooth nuclear borders
- **Atypical meningioma, WHO grade II**
  - Frozen section or smear
    - Prominent mitotic activity
    - Sheet-like growth (disordered architecture), small cell change, prominent nucleoli, hypercellularity, necrosis (in absence of embolization)
    - **Or** chordoid or clear cell morphology
- **Anaplastic meningioma, WHO grade III**
  - Frozen section or smear
    - ≥ 20 mitoses/10 HPF
    - **Or** atypia in excess of that seen in grade II (resembling carcinoma, melanoma, or sarcoma)
    - **Or** rhabdoid or papillary features in majority of tumor
- If uncertain, grading can be deferred while commenting on atypical features

Metastatic Carcinoma

- May affect any spinal compartment (bony spine, disc, paravertebral soft tissues, dura, cord parenchyma)
- Most frequently from prostatic, breast, or gastrointestinal primaries

Lympho- or Myeloproliferative Disorders

- May affect any spinal compartment (bony spine, disc, paravertebral soft tissues, dura, cord parenchyma)
  - Plasmacytoma and chloroma are solid masses
  - Leptomeningeal involvement by systemic lymphoma is usually segmental &/or multifocal

Sarcoma

- Can arise from bone, cartilage, or soft tissues
- Identical to those in other sites
  - Chordoma and chondrosarcoma
  - Malignant peripheral nerve sheath tumor

Paraganglioma

- Usually seen in cauda equina region
- Identical to those in other sites
  - Tumor cells grow in zellballen (cohesive nests of tumor cells) surrounded by sustentacular cells
  - Nuclei are uniform, round to oval, and have neuroendocrine appearance (salt and pepper chromatin)
  - Cytoplasm is eosinophilic and finally granular
  - Delicate blood vessels surround tumor cell nests

Nerve Root Lesions

- Schwannoma, neurofibroma
- Single or multiple (in setting of tumor syndromes)
- Histologic appearance identical to those seen elsewhere in body
  - Plexiform variants suggest tumor syndrome (e.g., neurofibromatosis)

Infections

- Epidural abscess
  - Potentially fatal
  - Neutrophils and necrosis in epidural tissue
- Meningitis, myelitis: Rarely biopsied
- Tissue should be saved for microbiologic culture

Vascular Lesions

- Dural venous anomaly (Foix-Alajouanine syndrome)
  - Ischemic changes with calcifications, iron deposition, macrophages
  - Rarely biopsied

Cysts

- Distinguishable by their lining cells &/or contents
  - Arachnoid cyst
    - Flattened to cuboidal epithelium, clear cerebrospinal fluid contents, ± psammoma bodies
  - Neurenteric/bronchogenic cyst
    - Columnar epithelium, may be intestinal type
  - Syringomyelia (pseudocyst)
    - Glial lining with Rosenthal fibers
- Rarely sent for intraoperative consultation

REPORTING

Frozen Section and Cytology

- Confirmation that lesional tissue has been obtained (i.e., biopsy only)
  - Exception is ependymoma, which should be diagnosed if possible
    - Can be resected if recognized
- Allocation for microbiology or molecular studies
- Important to document potential limitations to diagnosis (e.g., small specimen size)

PITFALLS

Undersampling of Glial Neoplasms

- Small biopsies may not sample areas of anaplasia
  - Final diagnosis may undergrade tumor
  - Correlation with imaging is crucial to judge whether biopsy is representative
- Tumors can be surrounded by piloid gliosis giving impression of pilocytic astrocytoma
- Additional biopsies should be requested if appearance seems inconsistent with imaging features

Recognition of Inflammatory Processes

- Cytologic preparations may help in recognition of inflammatory cells

SELECTED REFERENCES

1. Lee HS et al: The basics of intraoperative diagnosis in neuropathology. Surg Pathol Clin. 8(1):27-47, 2015
2. Kresak JL et al: CNS intraoperative consultation: a survival guide for non-neuropathologists. Methods Mol Biol. 1180:369-76, 2014
3. Folkerth RD: Smears and frozen sections in the intraoperative diagnosis of central nervous system lesions. Neurosurg Clin N Am. 5(1):1-18, 1994

High-Grade Glioma

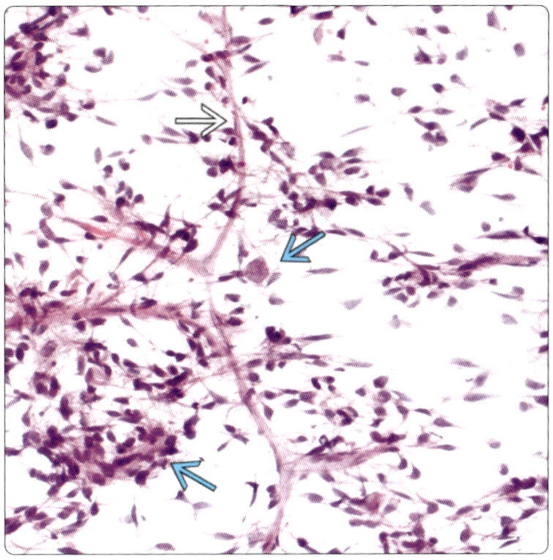

High-Grade Glioma and Reactive Gliosis

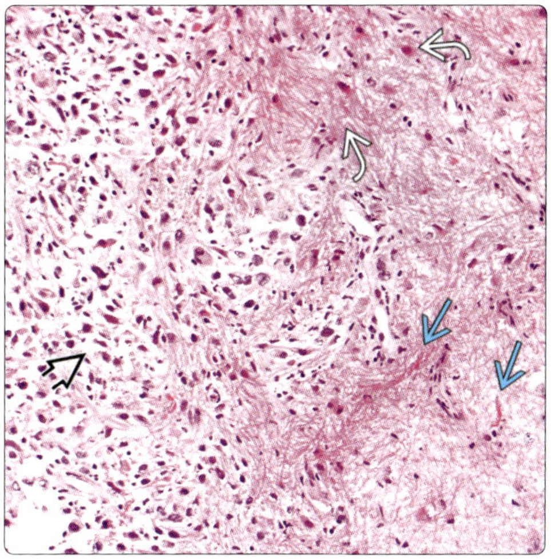

(Left) *A smear of a spinal tumor shows numerous elongated atypical glial cells. Differential diagnosis includes ependymoma and high-grade glioma. Nuclear pleomorphism and the lack of a perivascular arrangement around the blood vessel support a diagnosis of high-grade glioma.* **(Right)** *Spinal cord high-grade glioma can be surrounded by reactive gliosis. In a case of a small biopsy from the reactive edge, the presence of Rosenthal fibers can be misleading for a pilocytic astrocytoma.*

Myxopapillary Ependymoma

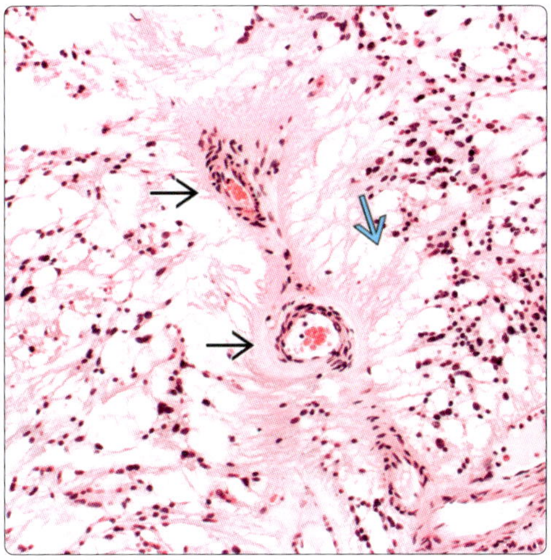

Myxopapillary Ependymoma

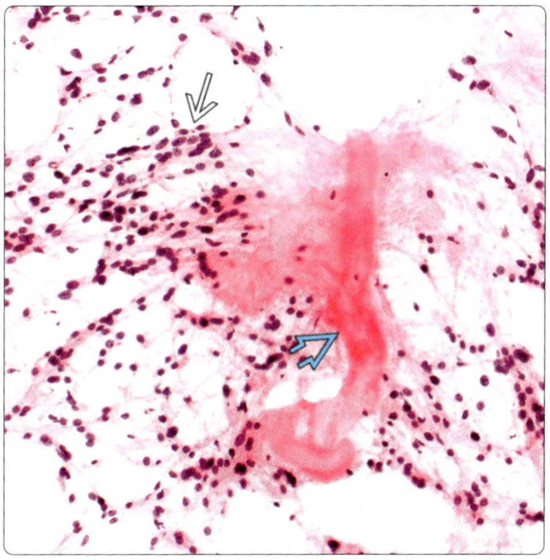

(Left) *A myxopapillary ependymoma shows vaguely papillary arrangements of tumor cells surrounding thickened blood vessels. Myxoid material is present between cell processes. Necrosis, if present, does not have prognostic significance.* **(Right)** *A smear preparation of a myxopapillary ependymoma shows a typical myxoid background and uniform, bland, slightly fibrillary tumor cells around blood vessels. The blood vessels are often hyalinized. Mitotic activity is rare.*

Chordoma

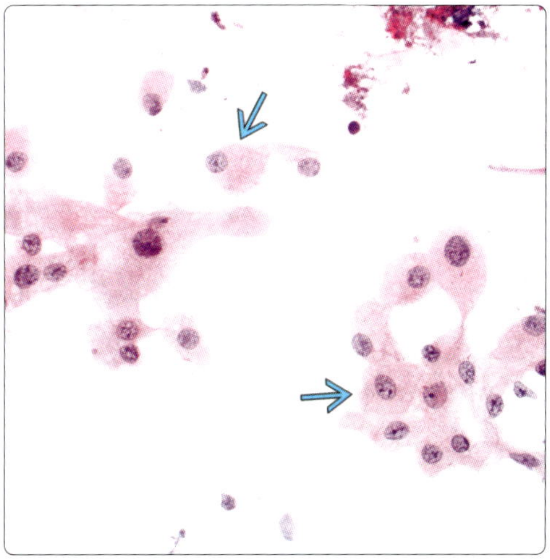

Chordoma

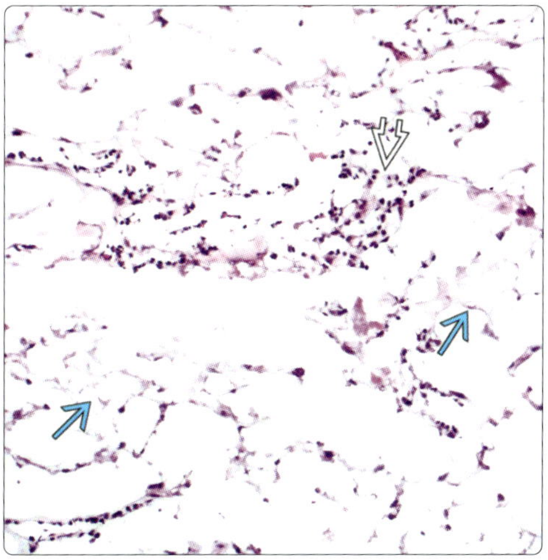

(Left) *A smear of a chordoma shows small epithelioid uniform cells with bland cytology. Lack of mitotic activity, nucleoli, and necrosis is typical. However, anaplastic chordoma can show marked pleomorphism and necrosis.* **(Right)** *Frozen section diagnosis of chordoma can be challenging due to freezing artifact. Variable amounts of chondroid matrix is present and cells are small and bland. Lack of primitive cartilage distinguishes it from chondrosarcoma.*

Paraganglioma

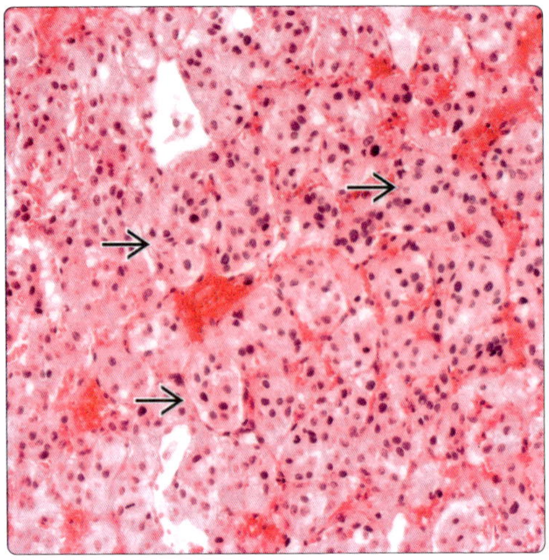

Metastatic Adenocarcinoma

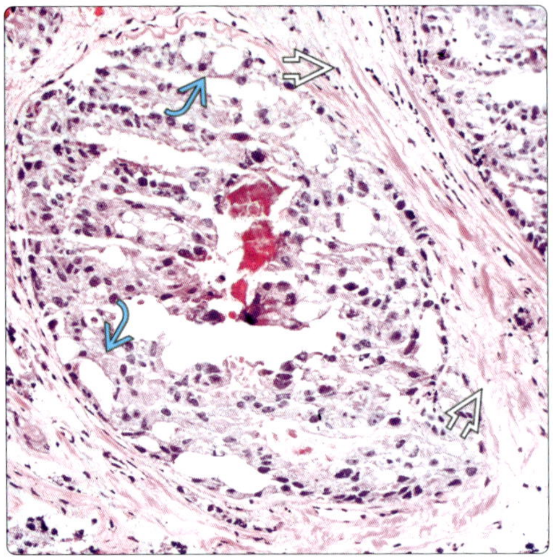

(Left) *Paragangliomas occur most frequently in the cauda equina region. They tend to be circumscribed, vascular tumors with histologic features identical to paragangliomas arising in other sites, including Zellballen arrangements → with fine intervening capillaries.* **(Right)** *Metastatic tumors are the most common malignancies of the spine. Metastatic prostate adenocarcinoma shows glandular nodules → separated by thick fibrous bands →. Vertebral lesions are often osteolytic.*

Metastatic Squamous Carcinoma

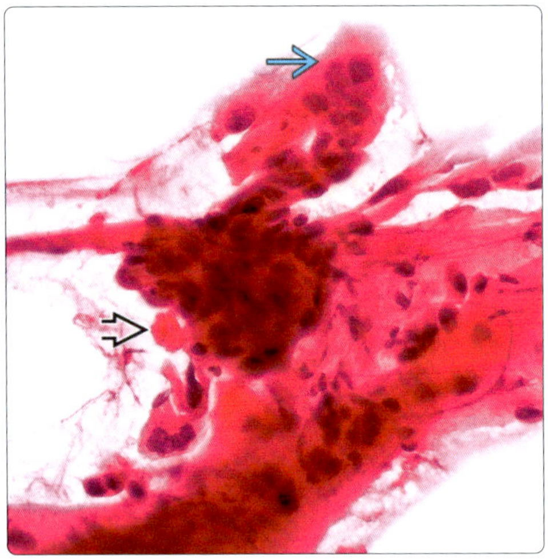

Metastatic Squamous Carcinoma

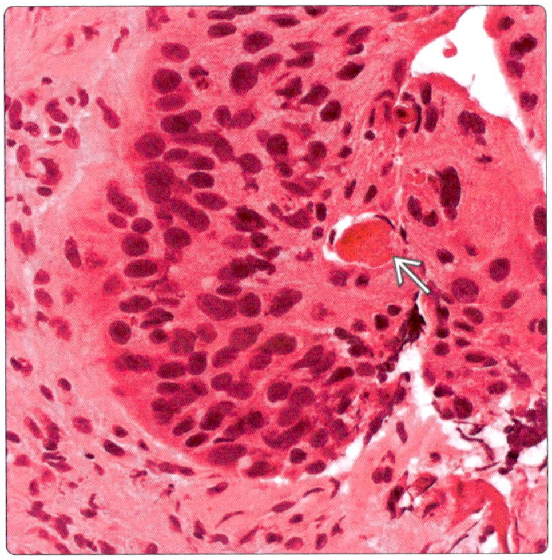

(Left) *This smear shows metastatic squamous cell carcinoma to the spine. Vaguely whorled groups of cells, some with enlarged nuclei and nucleoli →, are noted, as well as dyskeratotic bodies → in connective tissue.* **(Right)** *This frozen section shows fibrous tissue with nests of epithelioid cells. A dyskeratotic body → supports a diagnosis of metastatic squamous cell carcinoma. A history of prior carcinoma of this histologic type is important to make this diagnosis with confidence.*

Vertebral Plasmacytoma

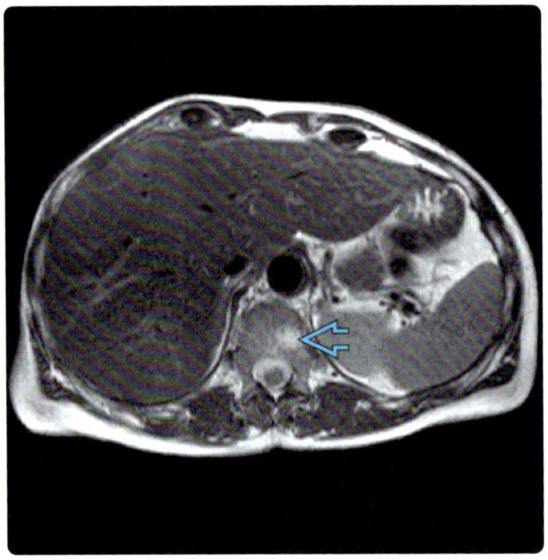

Vertebral Plasmacytoma

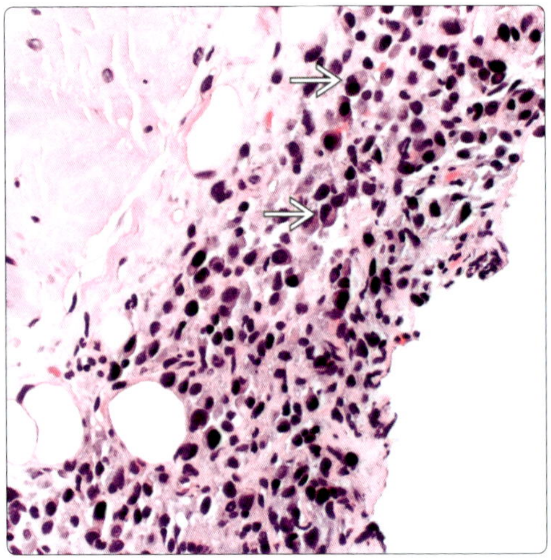

(Left) *Axial MR shows abnormal signal characteristics involving a lateral vertebral body and paravertebral soft tissues → corresponding to a plasmacytoma in a patient with plasma cell dyscrasia.* **(Right)** *Atypical plasmacytoid cells, with perinuclear hof (clearing) →, infiltrate fibroadipose tissue in a biopsy from the paravertebral soft tissue. It may be quite difficult to recognize the plasmacytoid features of these cells on frozen section or on intraoperative cytologic preparations.*

Schwannoma: Gross Appearance

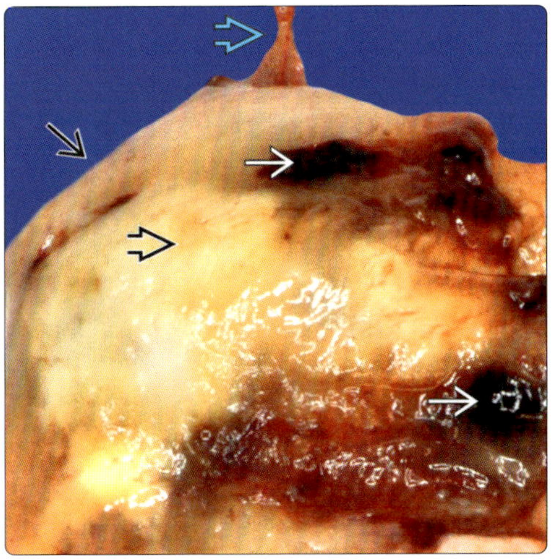

Schwannoma

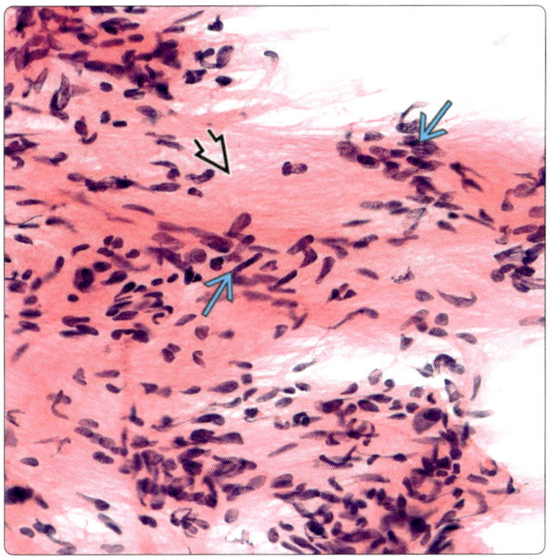

(Left) *This schwannoma arises from a peripheral nerve. The tumor has a thick tan capsule and a heterogeneous yellow appearance with foci of hemorrhage. Necrosis is usually not seen in these tumors.* **(Right)** *The cytologic appearance of schwannoma includes syncytial groupings of tumor cells with blunt-ended or tapering nuclei. A characteristic anuclear zone surrounded by cigar-shaped nuclei (Verocay body) can be noted on the smear.*

Malignant Peripheral Nerve Sheath Tumor

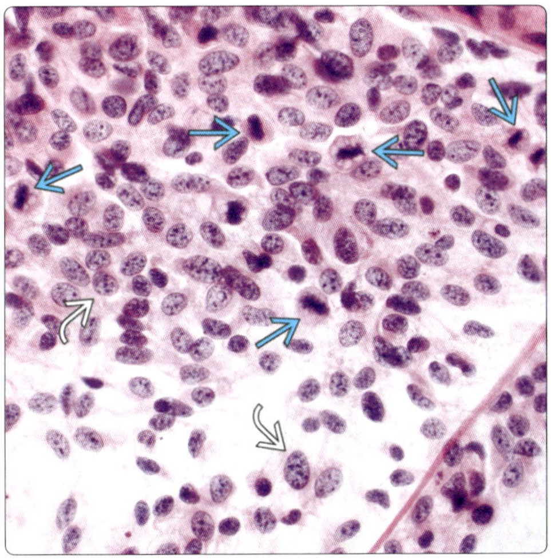

Malignant Peripheral Nerve Sheath Tumor

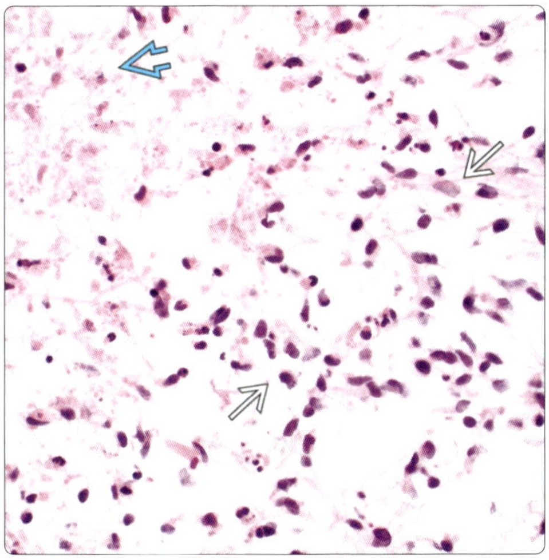

(Left) *In striking contrast with a benign nerve sheath tumor, a malignant peripheral nerve sheath tumor is hypercellular. Cells become epithelioid or pleomorphic and the tumor shows numerous mitotic figures.* **(Right)** *Frozen section of a malignant peripheral nerve sheath tumor shows pleomorphic spindle cells and necrosis. Compared to a cytologic preparation, mitotic activity might be difficult to appreciate due to freezing artifact.*

Osteoblastoma

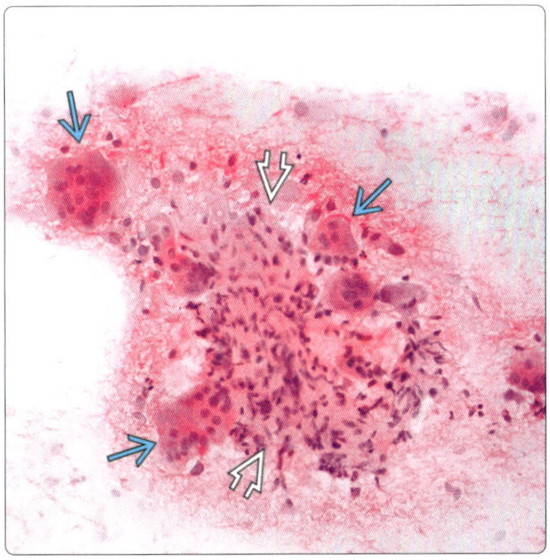

Osteoblastoma

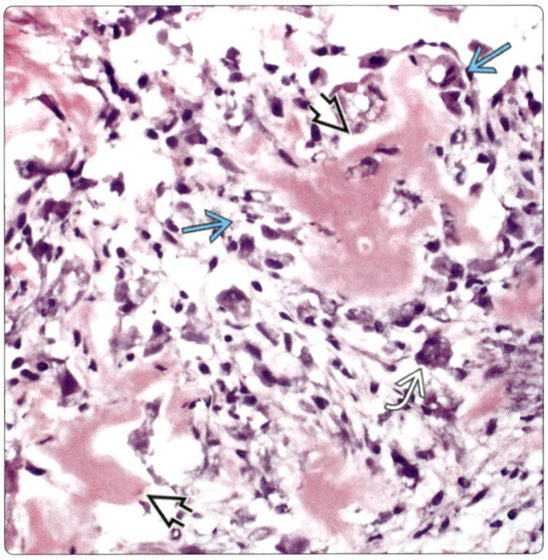

(Left) *Bone tumors can be challenging on frozen section and correlation with radiologic appearance is critical. A smear of an osteoblastoma shows a mixed population of bland mono- and multinuclear cells. Differential diagnosis includes giant cell tumor of bone.* **(Right)** *Osteoid arranged in anastomosing trabeculae and rimmed by osteoblasts is seen in osteoblastoma. Mitotic figures are rare. Some tumors show cartilaginous matrix. Multinucleated cells can be difficult to identify on frozen section.*

SURGICAL/CLINICAL CONSIDERATIONS

Goal of Consultation

- Diagnosis to guide intraoperative management and to take tissue for ancillary studies when appropriate
- Evaluation of proximal and distal margins

Change in Patient Management

- If carcinoma is identified, additional lymph nodes may be sampled
- If tumor is present at margin, additional tissue may be resected

Clinical Setting

- Diagnosis will usually have been made by endoscopic biopsy
  - In unusual cases, such biopsies are inconclusive, and goal of intraoperative consultation is to ensure diagnostic tissue is obtained
- Carcinomas may be excised with goal of cure
- In advanced-stage disease, stomach may be resected for palliation

SPECIMEN EVALUATION

Gross

- Anatomic structures present are identified
  - Esophagus: May be present at proximal margin
  - Stomach: May be complete or partial gastrectomy
  - Proximal duodenum: May be present at distal margin
- Outer aspect of specimen is examined to identify
  - Serosal penetration or tumor present at radial margin
  - Grossly positive lymph nodes
- Proximal, distal, and radial margins are identified
  - If stomach has been transected (i.e., partial gastrectomy), margin can be difficult to identify after stomach is opened
  - Radial margin is rarely involved and not typically evaluated intraoperatively
- Locations of any lesions are identified by palpation or by inserting finger into lumen
  - Stomach is opened in such a way as to not transect lesion
  - Margins should be inked or otherwise identified in order to distinguish true margin from cut edges
- After opening, all lesions are identified and gross distance to margins documented
  - Size, shape, color, consistency, and depth of infiltration
  - Location
    - Cardia, fundus, antrum, greater or lesser curvature, anterior or posterior wall
    - Muscularis propria
  - Distance from margins
    - Measure as soon as possible, as muscularis contracts
- If prior diagnosis has not been established by biopsy, frozen section evaluation may be helpful to determine need for ancillary studies

Frozen Section

- Gross evaluation of mucosal margins for intestinal-type carcinoma or muscularis margins for gastrointestinal stromal tumor (GIST) is generally very reliable to determine margin involvement
- Gross evaluation of margins is not reliable for tumors that involve muscularis propria
  - Infiltration of intestinal-type carcinomas within muscularis propria
  - Signet ring cell carcinomas within muscularis propria
- Frozen sections, including muscularis propria, must be evaluated
- If grossly evident tumor is close to margin, perpendicular section at closest approach can be evaluated
- If tumor is difficult to identify grossly, en face sections evaluate greater area of margin

MOST COMMON DIAGNOSES

Carcinoma: Intestinal Type

- Most commonly arise in antrum
- Usually grossly evident as raised mucosal lesion with central ulceration
  - Mucosal folds generally do not radiate from ulcerated center

Gastric Signet Ring Cell Carcinoma: Gross Appearance

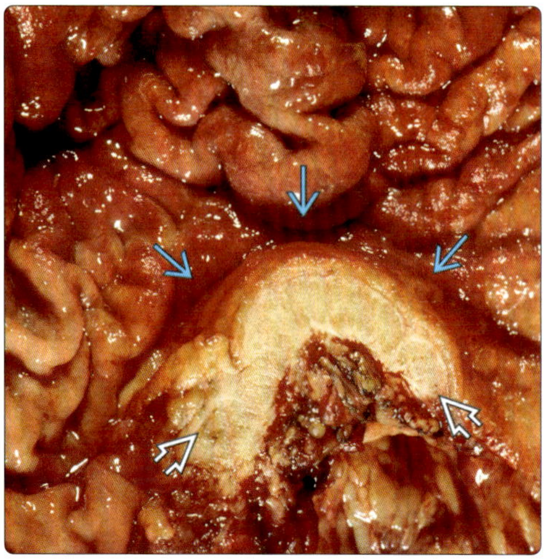

Gastric Signet Ring Cell Carcinoma

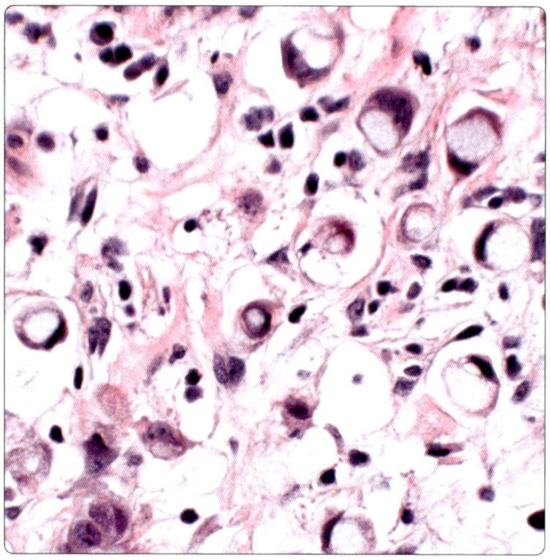

(Left) *Signet ring cell carcinomas diffusely invade the wall of the stomach, causing marked thickening of the muscularis propria* ➔ *called "linitis plastica." The overlying mucosa* ⇨ *is normal in appearance.* **(Right)** *Gastric signet ring cells have abundant foamy cytoplasm and bland nuclei and can be very difficult to detect. It is very helpful to know the histologic type of primary carcinoma before evaluating a frozen section.*

Carcinoma: Signet Ring Cell Type

- Most common in prepyloric region or body of stomach
- Typically has diffuse infiltrative pattern in mucosa and muscularis
  - Mucosal involvement may be subtle area of erosion or not be present
  - Tumor usually involves much larger area than grossly evident lesion
- On cross section, muscularis is thickened and firm (linitis plastica)
- Margins cannot be reliably evaluated by gross inspection
  - Frozen sections may be difficult to interpret due to subtle appearance of these carcinomas
  - Tissue section must be full thickness with both muscularis and mucosa
- Tumor diffusely infiltrates as single cells
  - Can resemble histiocytes, plasma cells, or other types of lymphocytes
  - Nuclei should be larger than those of normal gastric cells

Ulcer

- Occurs in distal stomach
  - Mucosal folds may radiate from center of ulcer
- Edges are usually flat or only slightly heaped up
- ~ 2% of ulcers thought to be benign clinically prove to be malignant
  - More likely for ulcers > 2 cm in size

Gastrointestinal Stromal Tumor (GIST)

- Stomach is most common site for GIST (60-70% of cases)
  - Arise from interstitial cells of Cajal present in muscularis propria
  - Majority are benign
  - Lymph node metastases are rare (< 2%)
- Cut surface is tan and homogeneous
  - Lack whorled gross appearance of smooth muscle tumors
- Overlying mucosa is generally intact
- Small tumors may be removed by small partial gastrectomies
- Spindle cell pattern is most common (70%)
  - Arranged in fascicles with uniform nuclei
  - Hyalinization and myxoid change common
  - Nuclei may be indented by vacuole at one pole
- Epithelioid pattern is less common (30%)
  - Round epithelioid cells, clear cytoplasm
- Other spindle cell lesions also occur in stomach but are less common
  - Leiomyoma, leiomyosarcoma, peripheral nerve sheath tumor
  - Diagnosis often requires extensive sampling and immunohistochemical studies
  - If spindle cell lesion has unusual appearance, report as "spindle cell lesion, final classification deferred to permanent sections"
  - Specific diagnosis is not necessary intraoperatively

Lymphoma

- 1/2 of gastrointestinal lymphomas arise in stomach
  - Most common in distal stomach
    - Rarely involve pyloric region
- Infiltrate wall of stomach
  - Gastric folds may appear hypertrophied
  - Mass or shallow ulcer without raised margins may be present
  - May closely resemble gross appearance of signet ring cell carcinoma

Neuroendocrine Lesions

- Range from neuroendocrine cell hyperplasia to grossly evident tumors
  - Tumors form circumscribed submucosal masses
- Clinical setting varied
  - Longstanding hypergastrinemia due to gastric body atrophic gastritis and achlorhydria
    - Multiple small lesions confined to mucosa
  - Multiple endocrine neoplasia/Zollinger-Ellison syndrome with hypertrophic gastropathy
    - Multiple tumors present
  - Sporadic (gastric mucosa normal)
    - Tumors are usually larger and present at higher stage
- Small neoplasms are limited to mucosa and superficial submucosa

REPORTING

Frozen Section

- Diagnosis: Can be provided when appropriate
  - Primary diagnosis has generally been made by prior endoscopic biopsy
- Report "spindle cell tumor, final classification deferred to permanent sections" for probable GIST
  - Classification as benign or malignant should be made on permanent sections
- Margins
  - Proximal and distal margins are reported as positive or negative for tumor

PITFALLS

Signet Ring Cell Carcinoma

- Tissue can look grossly normal but be involved by carcinoma
- Metastatic lobular carcinoma of breast can have very similar appearance
  - Targetoid mucin vacuoles are more characteristic of signet ring cells in breast cancer
    - Gastric signet ring cells more commonly have numerous small vacuoles
    - However, both types of signet ring cells can be seen in both types of cancer
  - Lobular carcinoma of breast can have subtle clinical and imaging appearance and can present with distant metastases with occult primary

SELECTED REFERENCES

1. Jones GE et al: Breast cancer metastasis to the stomach may mimic primary gastric cancer: report of two cases and review of literature. World J Surg Oncol. 5:75, 2007
2. Shen JG et al: Influence of a microscopic positive proximal margin in the treatment of gastric adenocarcinoma of the cardia. World J Gastroenterol. 12(24):3883-6, 2006
3. Shen JG et al: Intraoperative frozen section margin evaluation in gastric cancer of the cardia surgery. Hepatogastroenterology. 53(72):976-8, 2006

(Left) *The most common type of gastric carcinoma resembles colon carcinoma (intestinal type). The tumor forms a mass arising from the mucosa with heaped-up borders* ➡ *and central ulceration* ⇨*. The extent of the carcinoma can usually be predicted by gross examination.* (Right) *Benign ulcers* ➡ *of the distal stomach may require resection due to hemorrhage. Unlike gastric cancers, the edges around the ulcer are not heaped up. Radiating gastric folds converge at the center of the ulcer.*

Gastric Carcinoma With Central Ulceration: Gross Appearance

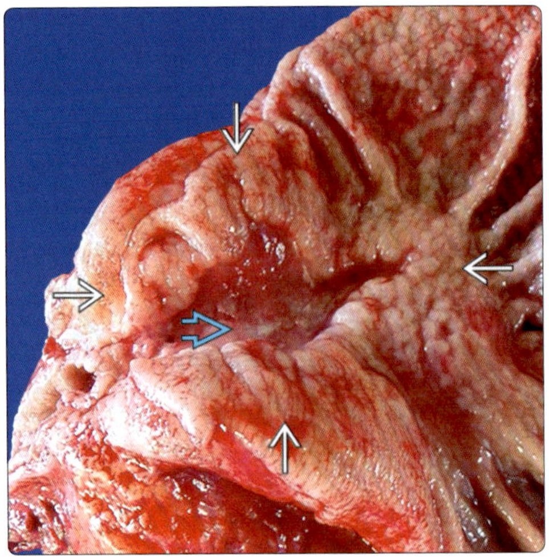

Benign Gastric Ulcer: Gross Appearance

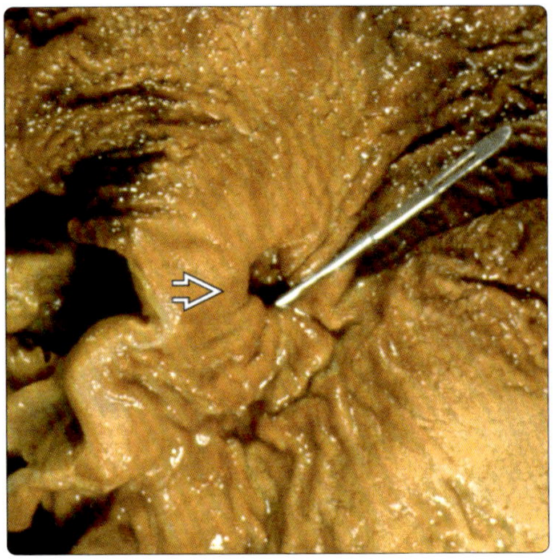

(Left) *In addition to documenting the absence of tumor, frozen sections in distal/total gastrectomy should also confirm that the margin actually represents duodenum and not the stomach. Presence of villi and submucosal mucus glands* ⇨ *help in this distinction.* (Right) *Poorly differentiated gastric carcinomas can be diffusely invasive and not apparent grossly. This gastric margin shows invasive carcinoma in the muscularis propria* ⇨*. The overlying mucosa* → *is free of carcinoma.*

Duodenal Margin

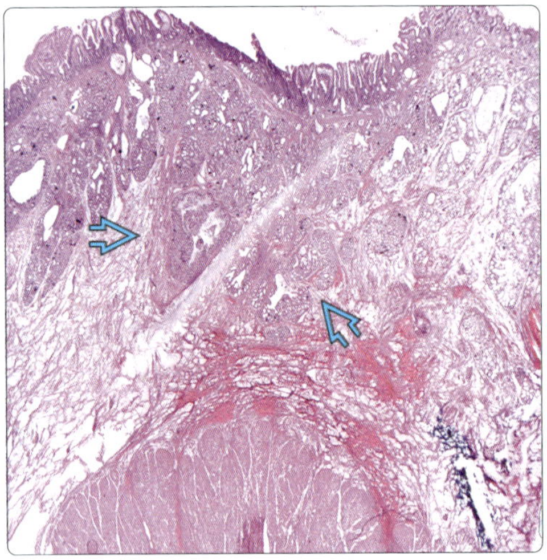

Stomach: Positive Margin

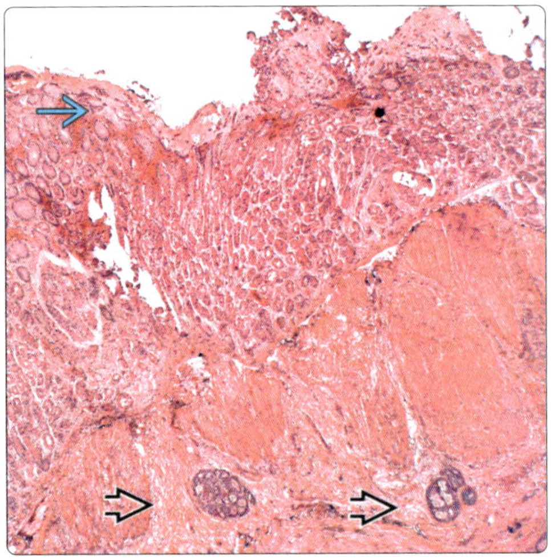

(Left) *Gastric neuroendocrine tumors arise from cells in the mucosa and grow as circumscribed submucosal masses. This carcinoid* ⇨ *has formed a submucosal mass. Note the intact overlying gastric mucosa* ➡*.* (Right) *Neuroendocrine tumors range from well-differentiated tumors, as seen here, to poorly differentiated high-grade tumors. Grading is not important for intraoperative consultation. However, knowing the type of tumor helps in the evaluation of margins.*

Gastric Carcinoid: Gross Appearance

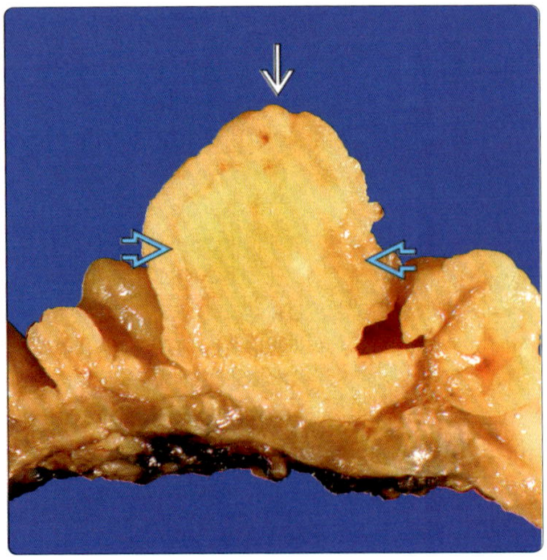

Gastric Neuroendocrine Neoplasm

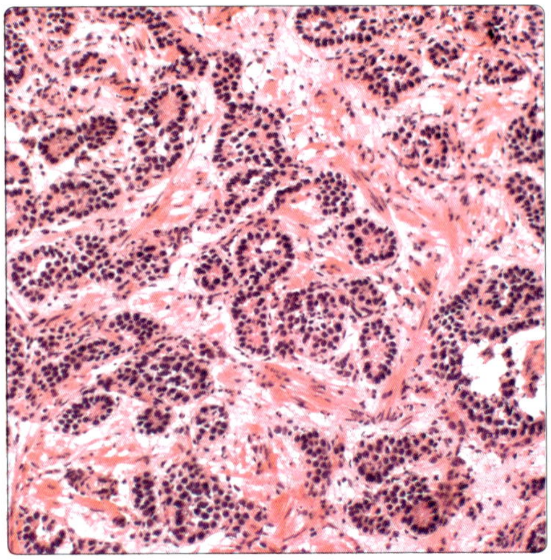

Gastrointestinal Stromal Tumor

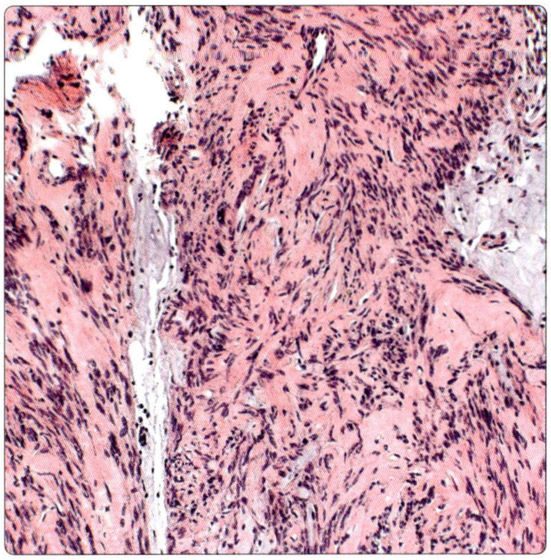

Gastrointestinal Stromal Tumor

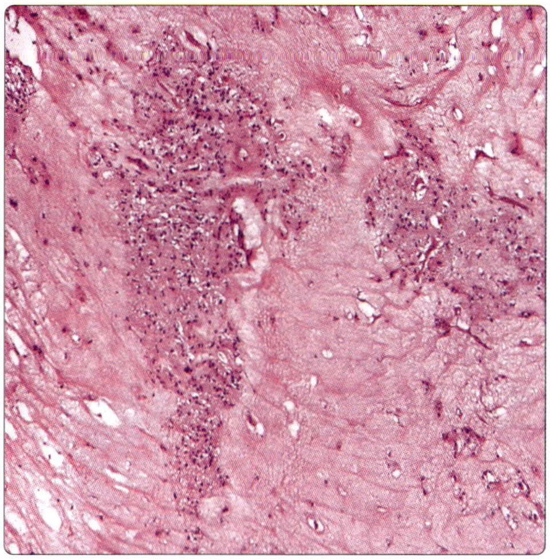

(Left) *A nodule in the muscularis propria of the stomach is most likely a gastrointestinal stromal tumor (GIST). The most common type (70% of tumors) is composed of spindle cells, as seen here. Less commonly (30% of tumors), epithelioid cells are seen.* **(Right)** *GISTs can be solitary but may also occur as multinodular tumors in a myxoid stroma as shown in this example of an succinate dehydrogenase (SDH)-deficient GIST.*

Gastrointestinal Stromal Tumor

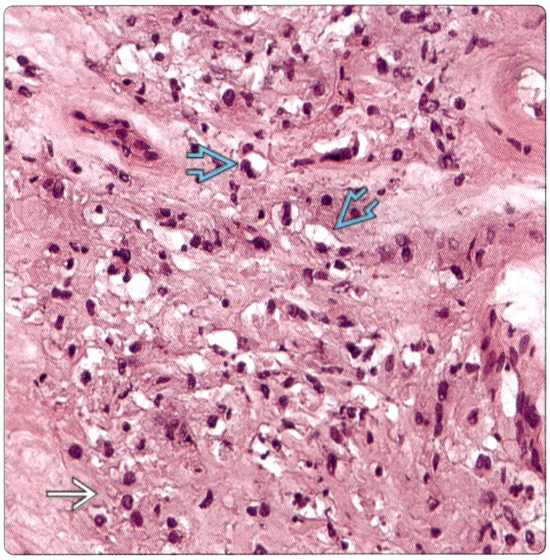

Metastatic Renal Cell Carcinoma to Stomach: Gross Appearance

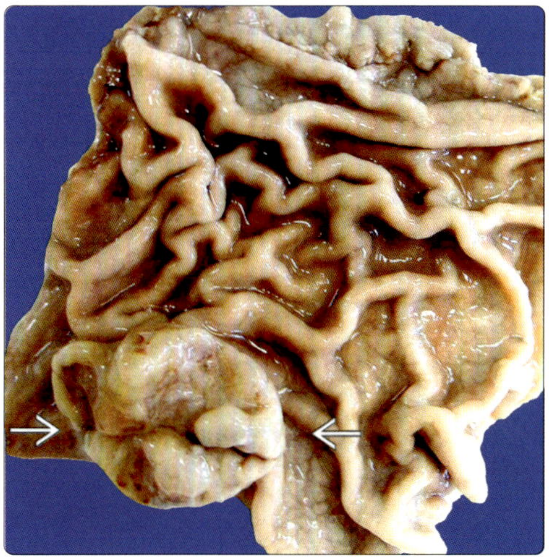

(Left) *SDH-deficient GISTs typically show an epithelioid morphology* ➡ *with prominent paranuclear vacuoles* ⇨. **(Right)** *Melanoma and carcinomas of lung, breast, and esophagus are the most common tumors to metastasize to the stomach. The majority (65%) are solitary lesions and present as a submucosal tumor* ➡. *Although most can be diagnosed by endoscopic biopsy, resection may be undertaken in some cases if a diagnosis cannot be obtained or a primary tumor cannot be excluded.*

Metastatic Renal Cell Carcinoma to Stomach

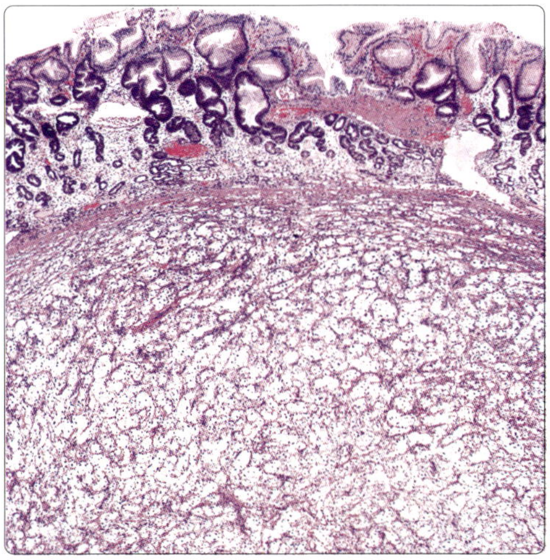

Metastatic Lobular Carcinoma to Stomach

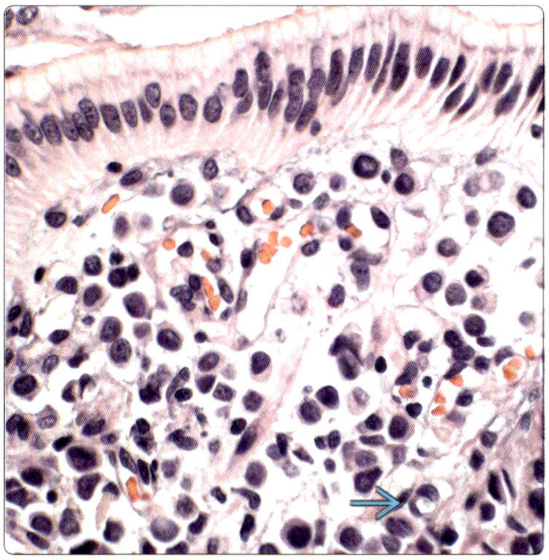

(Left) *Metastatic tumors to the stomach can usually be recognized by a histologic appearance different than those typical for gastric tumors, such as this clear cell renal cell carcinoma.* **(Right)** *Gastric signet ring cell carcinomas and lobular breast carcinomas can be identical in appearance. A clue to identifying this as a metastasis is a cell with a prominent central mucin vacuole* ⇨. *This appearance is more commonly seen in breast signet ring cells but can also be seen in gastric signet ring cells.*

Contents

SURGICAL/CLINICAL CONSIDERATIONS

Goal of Intraoperative Consultation

- Evaluate thyroid nodule or mass for malignancy
  - Intraoperative consultation (IOC) is rarely needed if preoperative fine-needle aspiration (FNA) was definitive for papillary carcinoma or benign process
  - IOC can be helpful if preoperative FNA was suspicious for papillary carcinoma, inconclusive, or not performed
- There is rarely need to evaluate margins
  - Papillary and follicular carcinomas usually do not invade into surrounding tissue, and systemic therapy with radioactive iodine is very effective in eliminating microscopic residual disease
  - Anaplastic thyroid carcinomas are diffusely invasive and can rarely be resected with negative margins

Change in Patient Management

- Additional surgery may be performed if carcinoma is present
  - Papillary thyroid carcinoma
    - Complete thyroidectomy
    - Lymph node evaluation and possible dissection
  - Follicular thyroid carcinoma
    - Complete thyroidectomy
  - Medullary thyroid carcinoma
    - Complete thyroidectomy
    - Lymph node evaluation and possible dissection
    - Evaluation of parathyroid glands for adenomas
    - Surgeon should be aware 10-15% of patients will also have pheochromocytoma

SPECIMEN EVALUATION

Gross

- Thyroid is weighed and measured
- Outer surface is examined
  - Normal thyroid has smooth outer surface
  - Attached soft tissue &/or muscle may be indicative of tumor invasion
  - Parathyroid glands are not usually present
- Thyroid is oriented according to shape of lobes and concave posterior surface
  - Isthmus joins 2 lobes at inferior aspect of thyroid
- Outer surface is inked
- Gland is serially sectioned from superior to inferior
  - Normal thyroid has uniform beefy red surface
  - All nodules are identified and measured
    - Single nodule is likely to be adenoma or carcinoma
    - Multiple nodules are more likely to be hyperplasia or adenomatous nodules
  - Nodules previously sampled by FNA should be identified
    - Site of prior FNA may be evident as area of fibrosis and hemorrhage
  - Irregular or ill-defined firm masses are possibly malignant
  - Well-circumscribed masses usually benign (> 80%)
  - Cystic masses are usually benign
    - Infrequent papillary carcinomas are cystic

Frozen Section

- If irregular or ill-defined, firm mass is present and prior diagnosis has not been made by FNA, frozen section (FS) can be useful
  - Tissue chosen should include edge of mass and surrounding tissue
- If well-circumscribed encapsulated mass is present, FS is rarely helpful
  - > 80% are benign
  - Entire capsule must be examined microscopically before benign diagnosis can be established
  - Capsular and vascular invasion can be very focal
  - Artifacts and tissue loss introduced during preparation of FS can preclude optimal diagnosis on permanent section
  - In general, this type of lesion should be examined only by permanent sections

Cytology

- Cytologic preparations can be made by touch or scrape preparations
  - Cytologic preparations are very useful to diagnose papillary carcinomas, as nuclear features are more clearly observed

(Left) *Papillary thyroid carcinoma is the most common thyroid malignancy (> 80%). The majority are diagnosed by preoperative FNA, but intraoperative diagnosis based on a classic gross appearance and cytologic features is also highly accurate.* **(Right)** *Encapsulated solitary masses are most commonly adenomas but can also be carcinomas (~ 20%). The final diagnosis is best determined by extensive sampling of the capsule on permanent sections. Frozen section is generally not helpful.*

Papillary Carcinoma: Gross Appearance

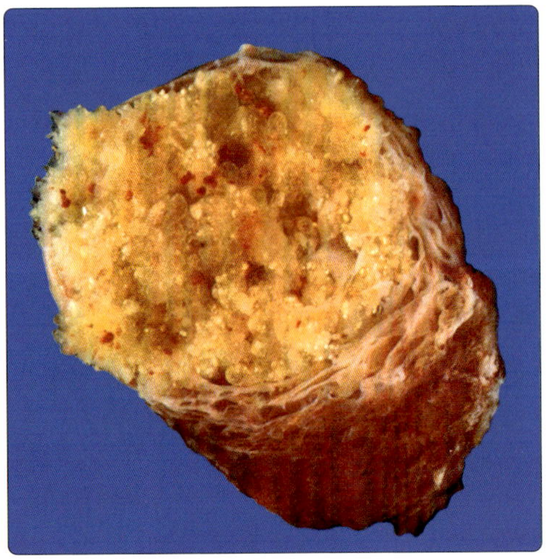

Encapsulated Thyroid Nodule: Gross Appearance

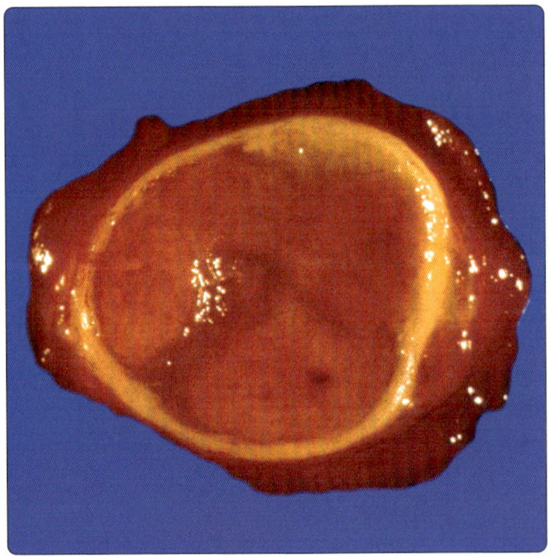

Contents

- Diagnosis of papillary carcinoma can be made on nuclear features alone
- FS artifact can mimic papillary carcinoma
  - Nuclear enlargement, nuclear clearing, nuclear change resembling pseudoinclusions
  - These changes are absent on cytologic preparations
- Cytologic preparations and FS provide complementary information

Reliability

- Preoperative FNA and FS can be used together to accurately diagnose thyroid lesions
- FNA positive for papillary carcinoma (Bethesda VI)
  - FNA is > 97% accurate for this diagnosis
  - In majority of cases, FS would only confirm this diagnosis
  - In minority of cases in which diagnosis is not confirmed by FS, FNA is more likely correct diagnosis
    - Therefore, there is little to no benefit to performing FS in this setting
- FNA suspicious for papillary thyroid carcinoma (Bethesda V)
  - 60-75% of these lesions will prove to be papillary carcinoma
  - FS &/or cytologic examination can be helpful to establish diagnosis at surgery
- FNA suggestive of follicular neoplasm (Bethesda IV)
  - 15-30% of these lesions will prove to be carcinoma; however, diagnosis is difficult to accomplish intraoperatively as it requires evaluation of entire capsule
  - Definite diagnosis of carcinoma is only possible in rare cases (< 5%)
  - These lesions are best evaluated on permanent sections
- FNA showing atypical cells of undetermined significance (Bethesda III)
  - 5-10% of these lesions will prove to be papillary carcinoma
  - FS &/or cytologic examination can be helpful in some cases
- FNA interpreted as benign (Bethesda II)
  - < 1% of these lesions will prove to be malignant
  - IOC may detect 1/3 of cases of malignancy but can also result in false-positive diagnoses
  - These lesions are best evaluated on permanent sections
- FNA insufficient for diagnosis or not performed (Bethesda I)
  - IOC is very accurate if follicular lesions are not included
  - For papillary carcinomas, sensitivity is > 95% and specificity approaches 100%

MOST COMMON DIAGNOSES

Papillary Thyroid Carcinoma

- Most common thyroid malignancy (75-85% of total)
- 90% have irregular or ill-defined margin
  - Often firm but may be soft
  - White or tan; may have finely granular or nodular texture due to papillae
  - Average size: 2-3 cm (ranges from < 0.5 cm to > 4 cm)
  - Calcifications (psammoma bodies) are common (gritty texture when sectioned)
    - Present in fibrovascular cores of papillae
    - Very specific for papillary carcinoma
  - Small carcinomas can look like pale gray, depressed scar
  - ~ 15% are cystic
- 10% are circumscribed with thick capsule
  - Grossly resemble follicular adenomas and carcinomas
  - Cytologic preparation may be helpful to look for nuclear features
  - If definitive diagnosis cannot be made cytologically, lesion is best evaluated on permanent sections
- 20-60% are multicentric
- Preoperative FNA is diagnostic for ~ 90% of papillary carcinomas
  - IOC is not required in this situation
- Preoperative FNA is suspicious for papillary carcinoma in ~ 10% of cases
  - In many cases, definitive diagnosis of papillary carcinoma can be made by IOC
  - Cytologic preparations are helpful to identify diagnostic nuclear features
- Nuclear features are diagnostic
  - Intranuclear inclusions (cytoplasmic invaginations)
    - Very specific; only seen in papillary carcinomas and hyalinizing trabecular adenomas
    - Only present in ~ 30% of papillary carcinomas and may be infrequent
    - Inclusions have well-defined borders and are same color as cytoplasm
    - Frozen crystallization artifact does not have well-defined borders and usually creates central nuclear clearing
  - Nuclear clefts or grooves
    - Not completely specific for papillary carcinoma; can also be seen in benign lesions
    - Common finding; present in > 80% of carcinomas
  - Enlarged overlapping nuclei with irregular nuclear borders
    - Has appearance of nest of eggs
  - Optically clear (ground-glass) nuclei
    - This feature is not present in FS
      - Chromatin clearing is artifact of formalin fixation
    - This appearance can be mimicked by bubbly chromatin due to FS artifact
- Papillary growth pattern is present in majority of cases
  - Diagnostic of papillary carcinoma in majority of cases
    - Psammoma bodies often present in papillae
    - Can be mimicked by cystic degeneration in benign lesions and papillary ingrowth or pseudopapillae in Graves disease
- Minority of papillary carcinomas have follicular growth pattern
  - Classification of encapsulated lesions with follicular pattern has changed
    - Thyroid tumors previously diagnosed as noninvasive encapsulated follicular variant of papillary thyroid carcinoma (EFVPTC) are now termed noninvasive follicular neoplasm with papillary-like nuclei (NIFTP)
    - Carcinomas with vascular &/or tumor capsule invasion are classified as invasive EFVPTC
  - If nonencapsulated, classified as follicular variant of papillary carcinoma

- Rare diffuse sclerosing variant of papillary carcinoma may be difficult to identify on FS
  - Dense lymphocytic infiltrate may obscure tumor cells
  - Tumor cells may be scant in sclerotic stroma
  - Numerous psammoma bodies are important clue, but it may difficult to obtain good quality sections

Noninvasive Follicular Neoplasm With Papillary-Like Nuclei

- Encapsulated neoplasms with papillary nuclear features without invasion are called NIFTP
- Diagnostic criteria
  - Encapsulation or clear demarcation
  - Nuclear features of papillary thyroid carcinoma
  - Follicular growth pattern
  - < 1% papillae
  - No psammoma bodies
  - < 30% solid/trabecular/insular growth
  - Nuclear score 2-3
  - No capsular or vascular invasion
- As with all follicular-patterned neoplasms, diagnosis is made
  - Only after complete evaluation of capsule
  - Not during IOC

Follicular Carcinoma

- 2nd most common thyroid malignancy (10-20% of cases)
- Solitary mass that may be circumscribed or irregular
  - Majority are minimally invasive
    - Circumscribed cancers usually have thick capsules (> 1 mm)
    - Gross appearance can be identical to adenoma
  - Widely invasive follicular carcinomas are rare in USA
- IOC is of no value for circumscribed lesions diagnosed on FNA as follicular neoplasm or Hürthle cell neoplasm
  - FNA cannot distinguish follicular carcinoma from adenoma
  - Follicular carcinoma is distinguished from follicular adenoma by examining entire capsule microscopically
    - Invasion may be very focal in minimally invasive carcinomas
    - FS artifact &/or tissue loss during preparation of FS can preclude eventual definitive diagnosis
    - It is not practical to examine entire capsule by FS
- Preferable to defer diagnosis of follicular lesions to permanent sections

Follicular Adenoma

- Well-circumscribed mass that may have thin or thick capsule
  - Entire capsule must be examined microscopically to confirm lesion is benign
  - Preferable to defer diagnosis of follicular lesions to permanent sections
- Cells have round and regular nuclei lacking nuclear features diagnostic of papillary thyroid carcinoma
  - Cytologic features cannot distinguish benign from malignant follicular lesions
- Hürthle cell adenoma (oncocytoma) has characteristic brown color
  - Central scar may be present
  - Cells have abundant eosinophilic granular cytoplasm
  - Colloid with concentric laminations can mimic psammoma bodies
- Some adenomas are cystic
  - Papillary projections of residual parenchyma into cystic space should not be mistaken for true papillae
  - Papillae of papillary carcinoma will have fibrovascular cores and will not contain follicles

Medullary Thyroid Carcinoma

- Only 5-8% of thyroid malignancies
- Grossly circumscribed masses with soft and fleshy or firm and gritty consistency
  - Not encapsulated
  - Color ranges from gray/white to yellow/brown
  - Necrosis and hemorrhage may be present
  - Size can range from < 1 cm to replacement of entire gland
  - Often multicentric
- Usually have typical neuroendocrine appearance
  - Round or spindle-shaped cells
  - Uniform nuclei with dispersed chromatin and inconspicuous nuclei
  - Lack colloid formation
  - Amyloid (due to extracellular calcitonin deposition) is often difficult to see on FS
  - Variants with clear cells, pigment, giant cells, pseudopapillae as well as other types occur
- IOC is not needed if preoperative FNA was definitive for medullary thyroid carcinoma
- If diagnosis is 1st made on FS, surgeon must be aware that 10-15% of patients will also have pheochromocytoma
  - Release of catecholamines from tumor during surgery without adequate α-adrenergic blockade can result in significant morbidity and mortality
- ~ 25% of medullary carcinomas are associated with germline mutations
  - Patients with multiple endocrine neoplasia type 2 are also at risk for pheochromocytoma and parathyroid neoplasms

Anaplastic Thyroid Carcinoma

- Rare thyroid malignancy (< 5%)
- Carcinomas are pale gray and firm to hard
- Tumors have solid growth pattern with marked nuclear pleomorphism
- Rarely seen as IOC as many patients are not surgical candidates due to diffuse infiltrative pattern
- Incisional biopsy with FS is performed usually to ensure adequacy of specimen for diagnosis
  - Specimen may consist of fragments of tumor along with fragments of strap muscles
  - Very unlikely to be diagnosed in intact thyroid gland

Multinodular Hyperplasia

- Gland is replaced by multiple nodules of varying sizes
  - Nodules are circumscribed and usually poorly encapsulated
  - Irregular scarring, hemorrhage, calcification, and cysts can be present
  - Colloid-rich appearance
- Nodules with central degeneration may be lined by residual parenchyma that resemble papillae

Contents

- Papillae-like structures point toward center of cyst rather than have infiltrative pattern, as is seen in carcinoma
- FS is not needed on intrathyroidal nodules unless mass suspicious for invasive carcinoma is present
  - Carcinomas in this setting are rare in USA (< 5%)

Lymphocytic Thyroiditis

- Gland is usually diffusely enlarged with homogeneous texture
  - Inflammation and fibrosis can cause nodularity
- Dense lymphocytic infiltrate, including germinal centers, admixed with oncocytic follicular cells involves entire gland

Lymphoma

- Incisional biopsy may be performed to submit tissue for lymphoma work-up
  - Diagnosis is usually made by FNA
- Majority are diffuse large B-cell lymphomas in older patients

Post-FNA Site Changes

- Be aware of post-FNA site changes that can mimic malignancy
- **Acute changes: Within 3 weeks from FNA to surgical removal**
  - Hemorrhage with hemosiderin-laden macrophages
  - Granulation tissue
  - Localized follicular destruction
  - Capsular alterations
  - Atypical cytological features with nuclear atypia, nuclear enlargement with clearing occurring near needle tract
  - Necrosis
  - Mitosis
- **Chronic changes: > 3 weeks from FNA to surgical removal**
  - Squamous metaplasia and oncocytic cell changes
  - Cytological atypia
  - Capsular pseudoinvasion
    - Linear hemorrhagic tract
    - Within needle tract there is chronic inflammatory infiltrate and hemorrhage
    - Follicular epithelium does not violate capsule
  - Vascular alterations
    - Dilated vascular spaces with papillary endothelial hyperplasia, thrombosis, and organization
    - Endothelial cell atypia
    - Artifactual implantation of tumor cells
    - Tumor cells float within vascular lumen and are not adherent to vessel wall
  - Infarction
  - Fibrosis
  - Calcification
  - Cholesterol clefts and foreign body giant cell granulomas
  - Cystic changes

Metastatic Carcinoma

- Rare diagnosis but should be considered in patients with history of malignancy
- Most common primary sites are kidney and breast, followed by colon and lung
- May become evident many years after original diagnosis
- Areas of necrosis are more common in metastases than primary carcinomas
  - Metastatic renal cell carcinoma often associated with blood lakes

Hyalinizing Trabecular Tumor

- Form circumscribed masses with abundant sclerotic stoma
- Tumor cells are elongated or spindle-shaped
  - Nuclei can have grooves and pseudoinclusions
  - Can be rare cause of false-positive result for papillary carcinoma on FNA
- Stroma is hyalinized and sclerotic
  - Psammoma bodies can be present

Paraganglioma

- Form circumscribed encapsulated masses
  - Typical nested pattern of neuroendocrine-type cells surrounded by sustentacular cells

Intrathyroidal Parathyroid Gland

- In rare circumstances, parathyroid gland can be located within thyroid
- Gland will have smooth border and paler appearance than surrounding thyroid tissue

REPORTING

Frozen Section

- Definitive diagnosis of carcinoma is reported when diagnostic features are present
  - No need to make definitive classification of tumor type or report histologic variants
- Report "follicular neoplasm, final classification deferred to permanent sections" for circumscribed masses without identified features of malignancy

Cytology

- Reported as positive for papillary thyroid carcinoma or not diagnostic of malignancy
- Diagnosis is deferred to permanent sections for follicular lesions

PITFALLS

Follicular Carcinoma vs. Adenoma

- Diagnosis of follicular carcinoma usually requires evaluation of entire capsule
- Distinction between carcinoma and adenoma is not one that should be attempted intraoperatively
- Report of "follicular neoplasm, final diagnosis deferred to permanent sections" is sufficient

Follicular-Patterned Thyroid Lesions vs. Pseudofollicular Parathyroid Lesions

- Differentiating parathyroid with pseudofollicular architecture from thyroid tissue can be challenging on intraoperative FSs
- Refractile and polarizable calcium oxalate crystals are frequently present in colloid of normal thyroid follicles
  - Crystals are flat and rhomboid or needle-shaped
    - Clear to light yellow in color
  - Crystals are rare in parathyroid tissue
- Crystal identification using polarization can aid in distinguishing thyroid from parathyroid tissue on FSs

Major Patterns and Diagnostic Categories

Pathological Features	Diagnostic Considerations
Follicular lesion	Adenomatous nodules
	Follicular neoplasm (defer)
	Follicular adenoma (defer)
	Follicular carcinoma (defer)
	Papillary thyroid carcinoma, follicular variant (defer)
	Nodular hyperplasia
Encapsulated follicular-patterned lesion	Follicular neoplasm (defer)
	Papillary thyroid carcinoma (defer)
	Noninvasive follicular neoplasm with papillary-like nuclear features (defer)
	Parathyroid lesion with follicular architecture
Papillary thyroid carcinoma with invasive features	Papillary thyroid carcinoma, including all variants
	Papillary thyroid carcinoma, follicular variant with invasion
Papillary thyroid carcinoma with papillae	Papillary thyroid carcinoma, classic type
	Papillary thyroid carcinoma, hobnail variant
Other	Confirm diagnosis
	Medullary thyroid carcinoma
	Lymphoma
	Anaplastic thyroid carcinoma
	Thyroiditis
	Parathyroid

Follicular Variant of Papillary Carcinoma vs. Adenoma

- If lesion is encapsulated, "follicular neoplasm, final diagnosis deferred to permanent sections" is sufficient
  - Nuclear features of papillary thyroid carcinoma may be focal and difficult to identify on FS during IOC

Post-FNA Changes vs. Carcinoma

- History of prior FNA should be provided
- Changes associated with FNA should not be mistaken for malignancy
  - Epithelial displacement into stroma
  - Nuclear atypia, enlargement, and clearing near needle track
  - Pseudovascular invasion due to artifactual displacement
  - Squamous metaplasia
  - Necrosis &/or hemorrhage

Lymphoma vs. Lymphocytic Thyroiditis

- May not be possible to distinguish on FS
- If lymphoma is possibility, tissue can be reserved for possible special studies for lymphoma

Lymphocytic Thyroiditis vs. Metastatic Carcinoma to Lymph Node

- Small peripheral nodules in nodular hyperplastic thyroid can appear to be perithyroidal lymph nodes to surgeon
  - Specimen may be sent for FS labeled as "lymph node"
- Dense lymphocytic infiltrate surrounding normal thyroid acini can be mistaken for metastatic carcinoma to lymph node
  - Thyroid nuclei will be normal without cytologic features of papillary carcinoma
  - Normal lymph node architecture will not be present
    - It is also possible for ectopic thyroid tissue to be present in normal lymph node
- Pathologist should inquire as to whether mass was present immediately adjacent to gland or if it was at separate site

Mimics of Papillary Carcinoma

- Nuclear clearing characteristic of papillary carcinomas can be mimicked by FS artifact
- Nuclear grooves and intranuclear inclusions can be present in hyalinizing trabecular adenomas
- Papillary ingrowths into cystic spaces can mimic true papillae

SELECTED REFERENCES

1. Haugen BR Md et al: The ATA guidelines on management of thyroid nodules and differentiated thyroid cancer task force review and recommendation on the proposed renaming of eFVPTC without invasion to NIFTP. Thyroid. 27(4):481-483, 2017
2. Kennedy JM et al: Thyroid frozen sections in patients with preoperative FNAs: review of surgeons' preoperative rationale, intraoperative decisions, and final outcome. Am J Clin Pathol. 145(5):660-5, 2016
3. Wong KS et al: Utility of birefringent crystal identification by polarized light microscopy in distinguishing thyroid from parathyroid tissue on intraoperative frozen sections. Am J Surg Pathol. 38(9):1212-9, 2014
4. Antic T et al: Thyroid frozen section: supplementary or unnecessary? Am J Surg Pathol. 37(2):282-6, 2013

Encapsulated Thyroid Neoplasm: Gross Appearance

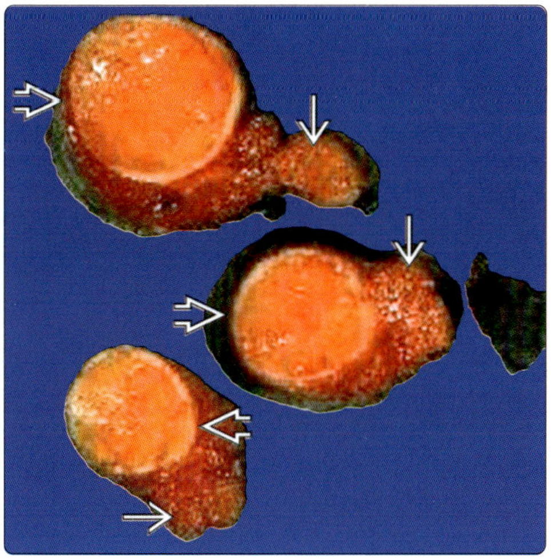

Follicular Neoplasm: Uniform Appearance

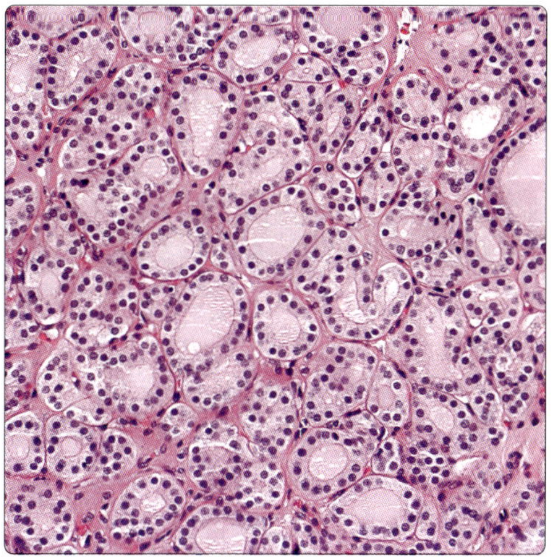

(Left) *Solitary circumscribed masses ➡ can be benign or malignant. Carcinomas tend to have thicker capsules (> 1 mm) and to be paler in color compared to the adjacent beefy red thyroid ➡. These lesions are best evaluated on permanent sections.* **(Right)** *Follicular neoplasms are typically composed of small uniform follicles lined by cells with round regular nuclei with dense chromatin without nucleoli. Unlike papillary carcinomas, cytologic features are not helpful to distinguish benign from malignant neoplasms.*

Follicular Carcinoma: Capsular Invasion

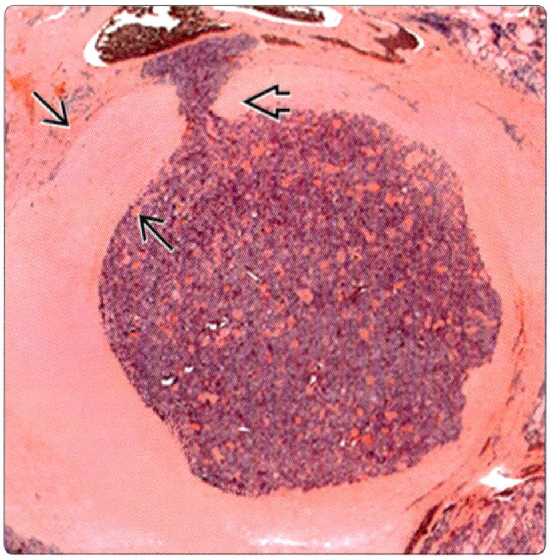

Follicular Neoplasm: Thick Fibrous Capsule

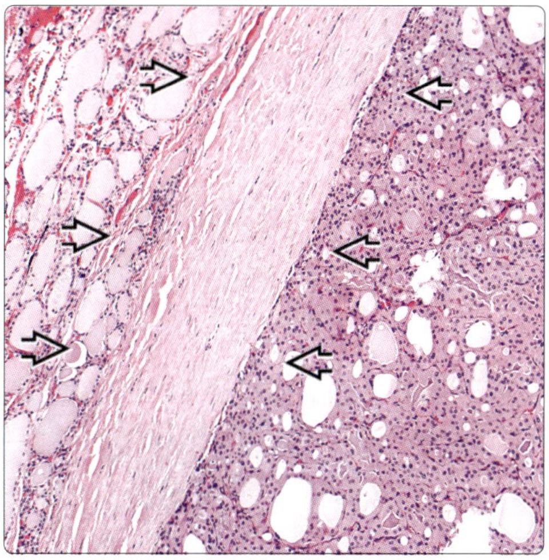

(Left) *Follicular carcinoma tends to have a thick capsule ➡. The entire capsule must be examined microscopically as diagnostic areas of capsular ➡ &/or vascular invasion can be quite focal. Frozen section artifact can make the evaluation of these features difficult.* **(Right)** *In this section, no capsular or vascular invasion is present ➡. However, this finding does not exclude carcinoma because the entire capsule must be examined microscopically. This examination is best made on permanent sections.*

Follicular Carcinoma: Lymph-Vascular Invasion

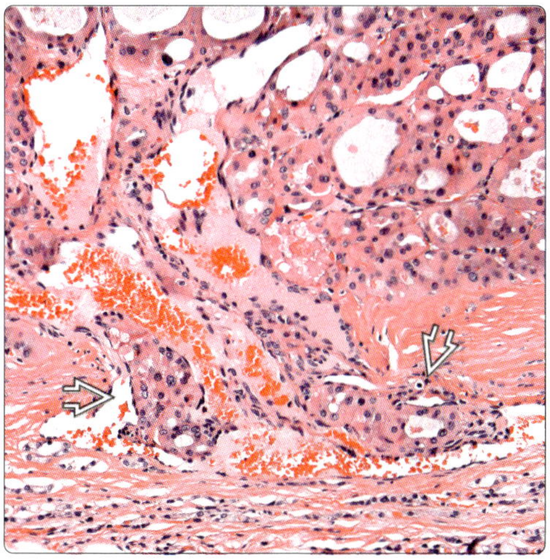

Follicular Carcinoma: Capsular and Vascular Invasion

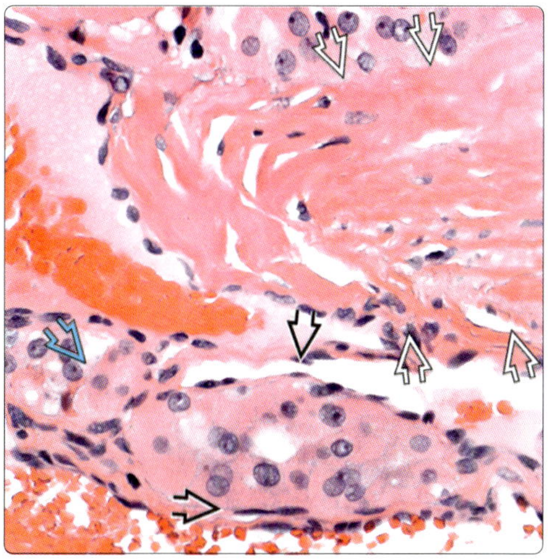

(Left) *Invasion through the capsule into a vascular space ➡ is diagnostic of follicular carcinoma and is best assessed on permanent sections. Possible artifacts due to freezing or prior needle track alterations would need to be considered in frozen sections.* **(Right)** *Vascular invasion ➡ must be identified within or outside of the tumor capsule ➡. The tumor cells must be within a vascular space and must be covered by endothelium ➡ or be attached to the wall and associated with a thrombus.*

Contents

(Left) This papillary thyroid carcinoma has the classic papillary growth pattern and typical nuclear features with hobnail cells. These carcinomas are usually reliably diagnosed by FNA. Confirmation by frozen section is not generally necessary. **(Right)** *Intranuclear pseudoinclusions ➔ are cytoplasmic invaginations (the same color as cytoplasm) that have a well-defined border. They are very specific for papillary carcinoma but can also be seen in rare trabecular hyalinizing adenomas.*

Papillary Thyroid Carcinoma: Papillary Architecture

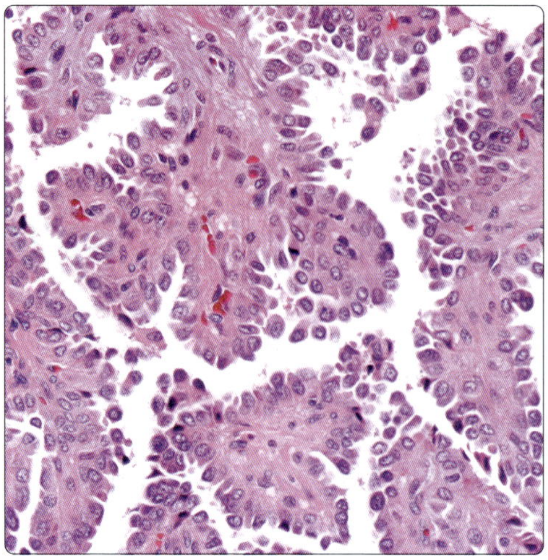

Papillary Carcinoma: Intranuclear Pseudoinclusions

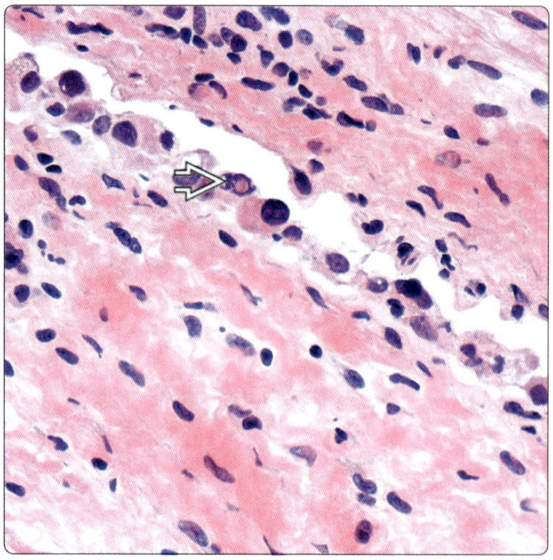

(Left) *Nuclear enlargement ➔ and overlapping nuclei are very characteristic of papillary carcinoma. Nuclear grooves ➔ are also present in the majority. Chromatin clearing is an artifact of formalin fixation and only seen in permanent sections.* **(Right)** *Nuclear features are more easily appreciated on cytologic preparations as there are no freezing artifacts. Intranuclear grooves ⮫ in the majority of tumor cells favor a diagnosis of papillary carcinoma.*

Papillary Carcinoma: Enlarged Nuclei

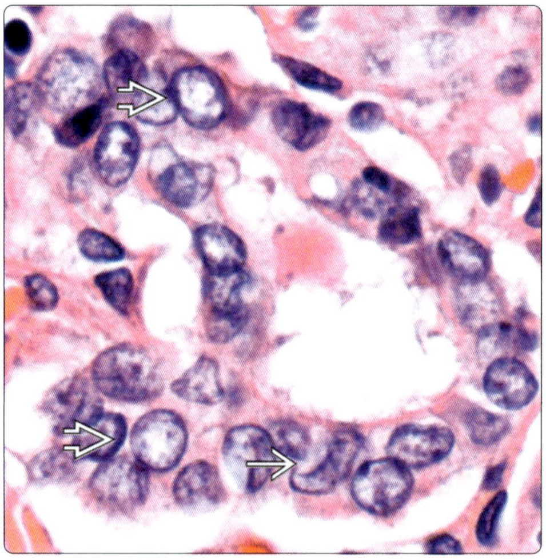

Papillary Carcinoma: Cytologic Preparation, Nuclear Grooves

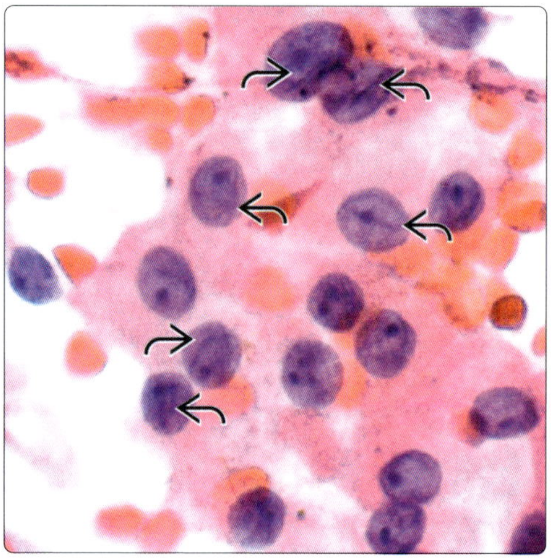

(Left) *The diagnosis of the follicular variant of papillary carcinoma is based on nuclear features. In this permanent section of a frozen section remnant, ice crystal artifact precludes optimal evaluation.* **(Right)** *Diagnostic optically clear nuclei are only present after formalin fixation and are not seen in tissue that has been frozen. The clearer chromatin in nuclei seen in this permanent section of a frozen section remnant is due to ice crystal artifact and can be seen in benign and malignant lesions.*

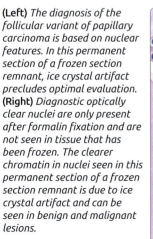

Papillary Carcinoma: Clearing Artifact

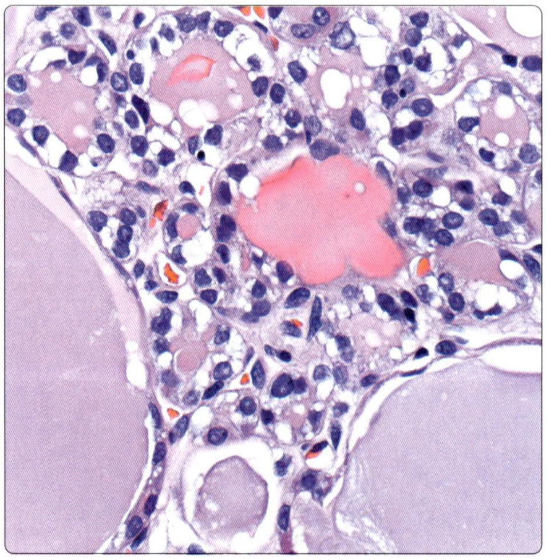

Papillary Carcinoma: Clearing Artifact

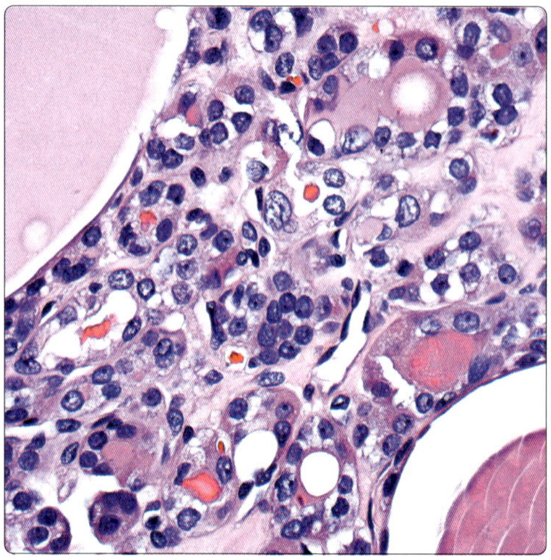

Calcium Oxalate Crystals

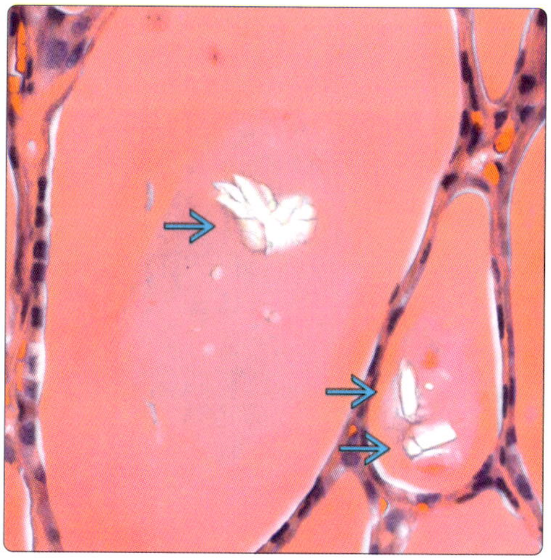

Calcium Oxalate Crystals: Polarization

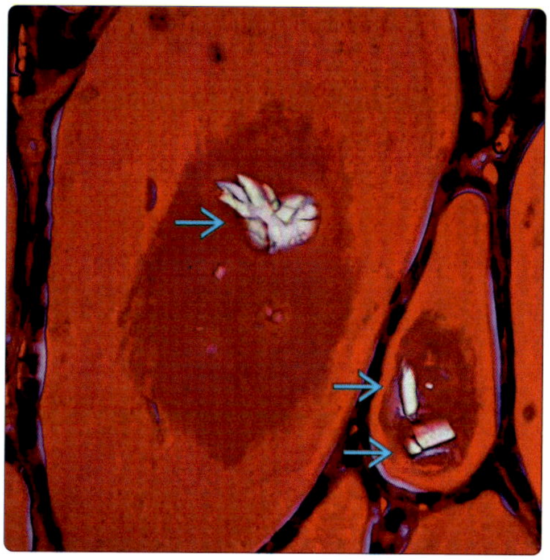

(Left) *Calcium oxalate crystals* → *are frequently identified within colloid of normal, hyperplastic, or neoplastic thyroid follicles. Crystals are rare or absent within parathyroid tissue. The crystals are rhomboid to needle-shaped and clear to pale yellow in color.* **(Right)** *Calcium oxalate crystals are present in colloid of normal and neoplastic thyroid follicles. They are more easily seen using polarized light* →. *Their presence can aid in distinguishing the thyroid from parathyroid tissue on frozen sections.*

Parathyroid Tissue

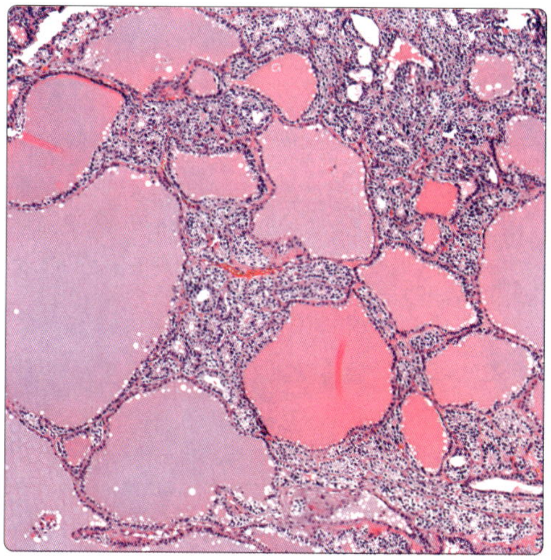

Solid Cell Nest Mimicking Papillary Thyroid Carcinoma

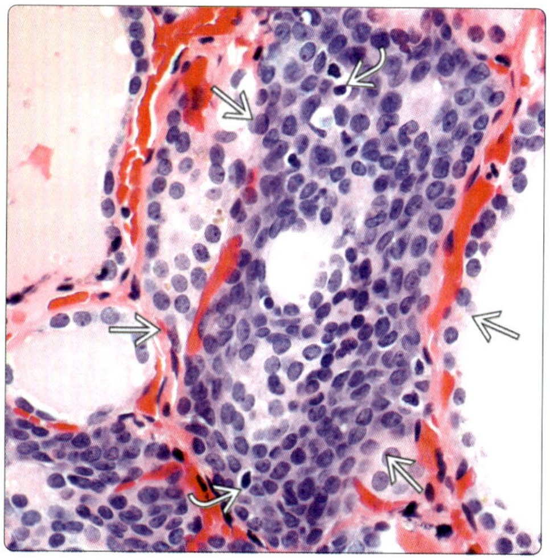

(Left) *Parathyroid tissue can closely resemble thyroid tissue when pseudofollicular areas are filled with colloid-like material. The absence of calcium oxalate crystals in the parathyroid, or their presence in thyroid, can sometimes be a helpful clue to the type of tissue.* **(Right)** *The presence of a large solid cell nest* → *on frozen section may be diagnostically challenging, as it may mimic papillary thyroid carcinoma. This solid cell nest obscures the follicular architecture. Note the presence of the characteristic epithelial lymphocytes* →.

Hyalinizing Trabecular Tumor

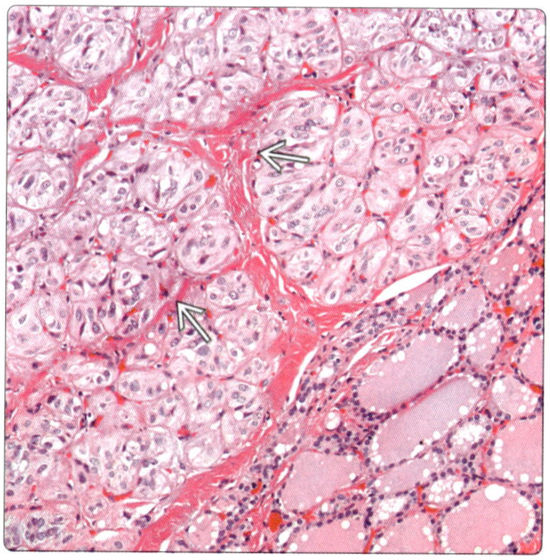

Hyalinizing Trabecular Tumor: Intranuclear Inclusions

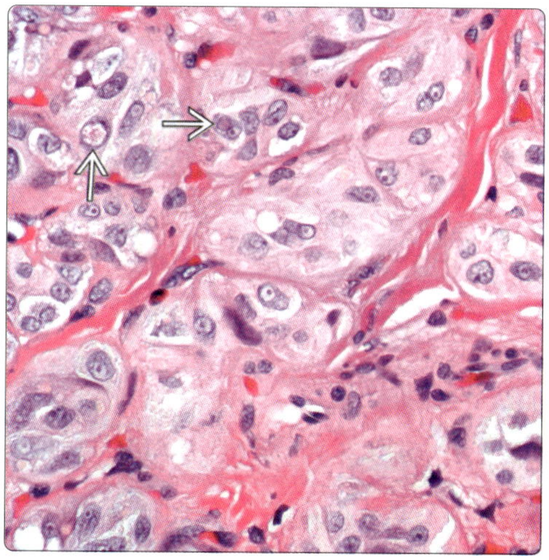

(Left) *Hyalinizing trabecular tumors are rare, benign neoplasms. The intratrabecular and extratrabecular fibrosis* → *associated with elongated spindle cells are clues to the diagnosis. Psammoma bodies may be present.* **(Right)** *Hyalinizing trabecular tumors can have intranuclear inclusions* → *as well as nuclear grooves. Thus a prior FNA may have been interpreted as "suspicious" for papillary carcinoma. Frozen section may be helpful to arrive at the correct diagnosis.*

Anaplastic Thyroid Carcinoma: Gross Appearance

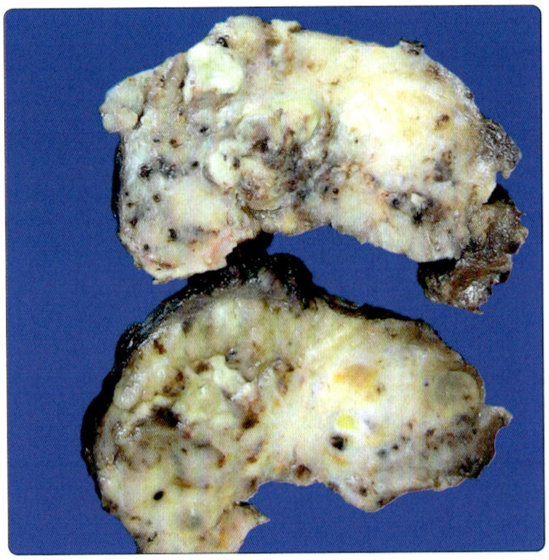

Anaplastic Carcinoma: Nuclear Pleomorphism

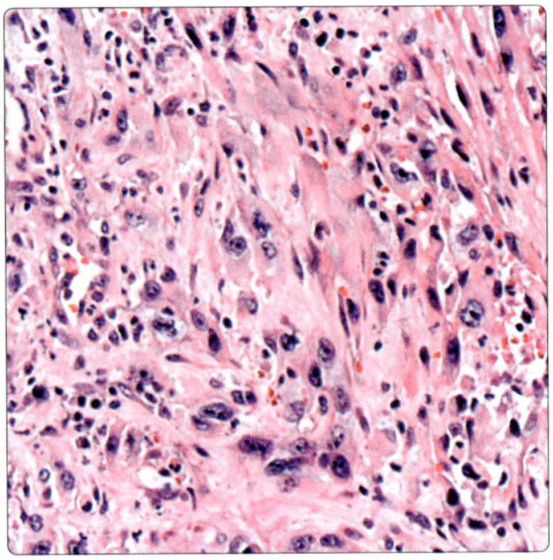

(Left) *Anaplastic thyroid carcinomas have a white-yellow variegated appearance with areas of hemorrhage and necrosis. An incisional biopsy may be performed with an intraoperative consultation to ensure adequacy of tissue for diagnosis. Due to extensive invasion into adjacent tissue, complete resection with negative margins is rarely possible.* **(Right)** *Anaplastic thyroid carcinomas consist of sheets of pleomorphic, highly atypical cells that are easily recognized as malignant on frozen section. Tumor necrosis may be present.*

Medullary Carcinoma: Gross Appearance

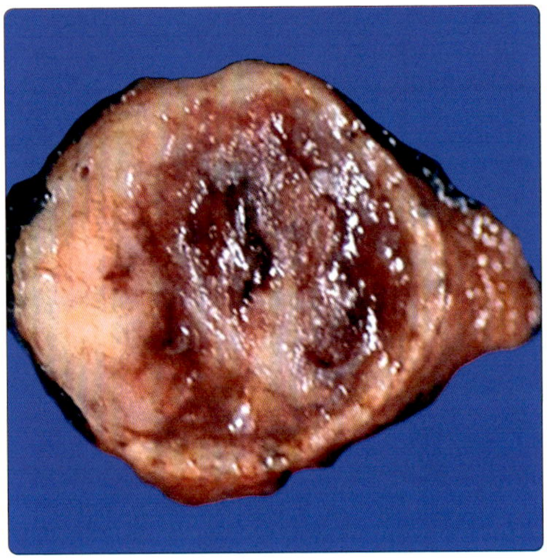

Medullary Carcinoma: Cytologic Preparation

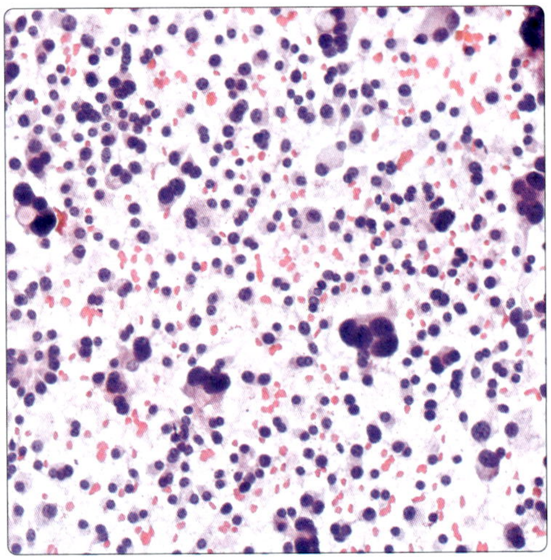

(Left) *This medullary thyroid carcinoma is well circumscribed, but not encapsulated, and replaces the majority of the thyroid lobe. The surface is gray-white and fleshy with focal areas of hemorrhage. These tumors are frequently multifocal.* **(Right)** *The cells of medullary thyroid carcinoma have a neuroendocrine appearance with regular round nuclei, dispersed chromatin (salt and pepper pattern), and inconspicuous nucleoli. Many cells have a plasmacytoid appearance with eccentric nuclei.*

Poorly Differentiated Thyroid Carcinoma: Gross Appearance

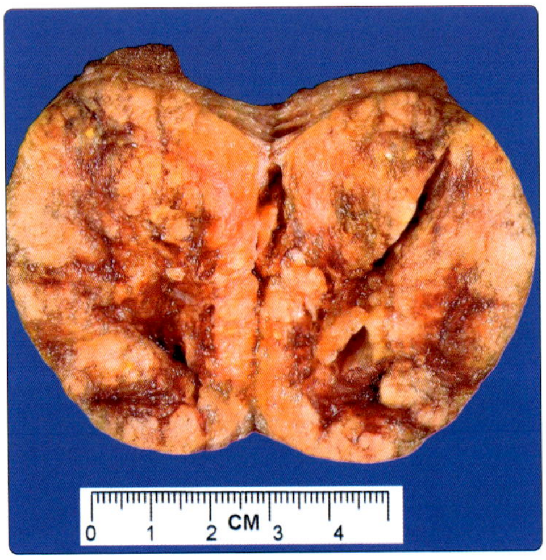

Poorly Differentiated Thyroid Carcinoma

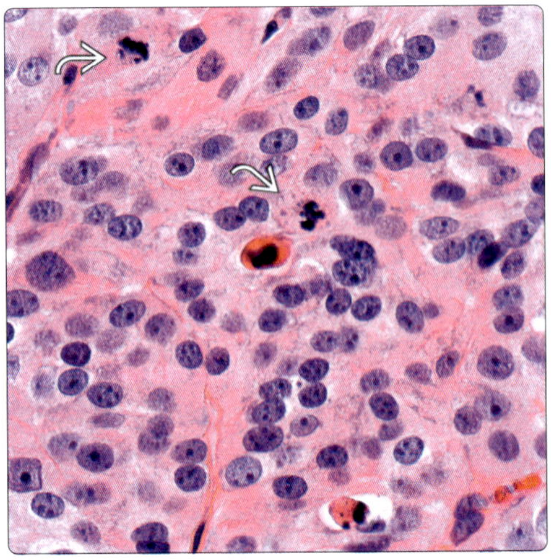

(Left) *Poorly differentiated thyroid carcinoma has a soft irregular cut surface, that shows areas of hemorrhage and necrosis. The tumor occupies most of the thyroid lobe with a minimal amount of uninvolved thyroid.* **(Right)** *Poorly differentiated thyroid carcinoma shows small- to medium-sized cells with round to oval nuclei and homogeneous chromatin, apoptotic bodies, and mitoses ➔. Extensive necrosis may be present. These carcinomas can have papillary and follicular patterns.*

Thyroid Paraganglioma

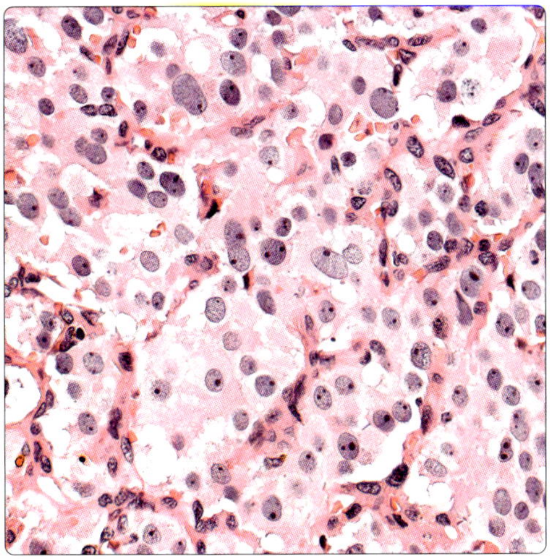

Metastatic Carcinoma to Thyroid: Gross Appearance

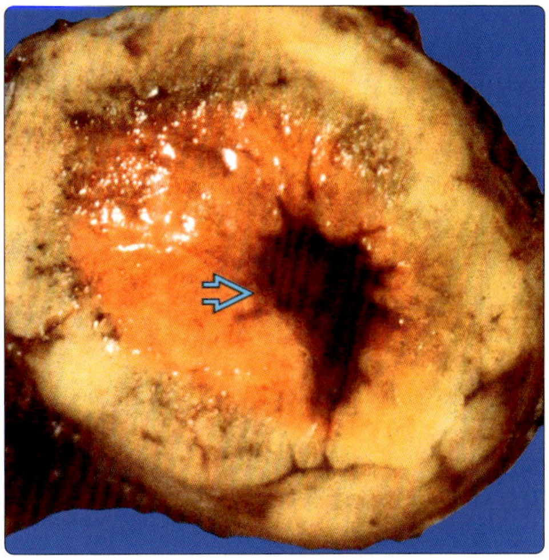

(Left) *Thyroid paraganglioma shows the characteristic alveolar nesting pattern of tumor cells (zellballen). The variably sized nests of tumor cells are surrounded by thin-walled vessels and sustentacular cells.* **(Right)** *The most common metastatic carcinomas to the thyroid are from the kidney and breast. This large thyroid nodule, considered to be a primary thyroid nodule, proved to be metastatic renal cell carcinoma. The prominent blood lake is typical of this tumor due to the delicate vasculature.*

Metastatic Breast Carcinoma to Thyroid

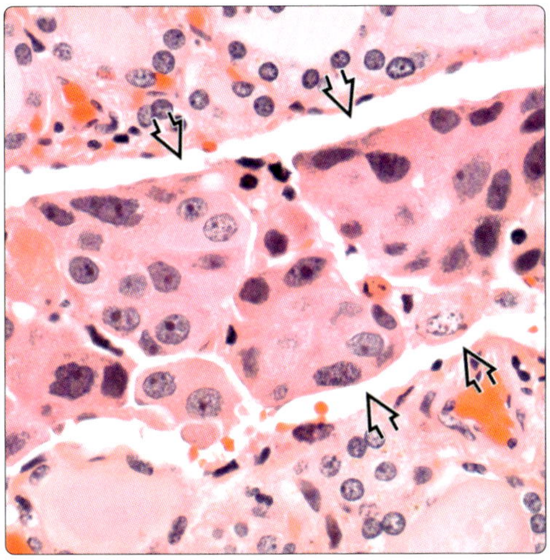

Metastatic Renal Cell Carcinoma to Thyroid

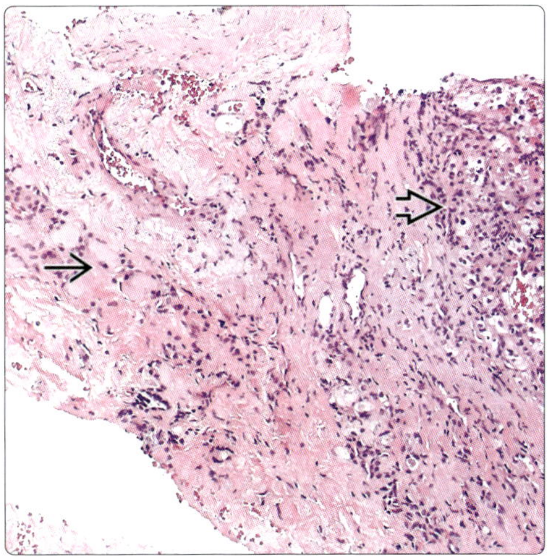

(Left) *This area of lymph-vascular invasion did not resemble the papillary thyroid carcinoma present elsewhere in the thyroid gland. The tumor in lymphatics proved to be metastatic disease of breast origin.* **(Right)** *This frozen section of a needle biopsy of a thyroid nodule shows metastatic clear cell renal cell carcinoma surrounded by fibrosis with rare residual thyroid follicles.*

Metastatic Papillary and Medullary Carcinomas to Lymph Node

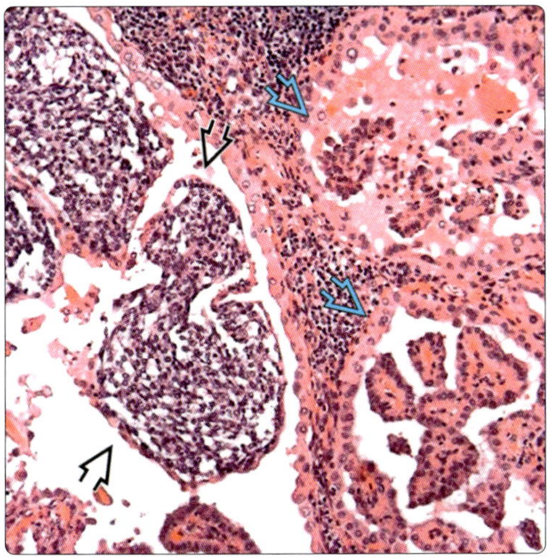

Lymphocytic Thyroiditis

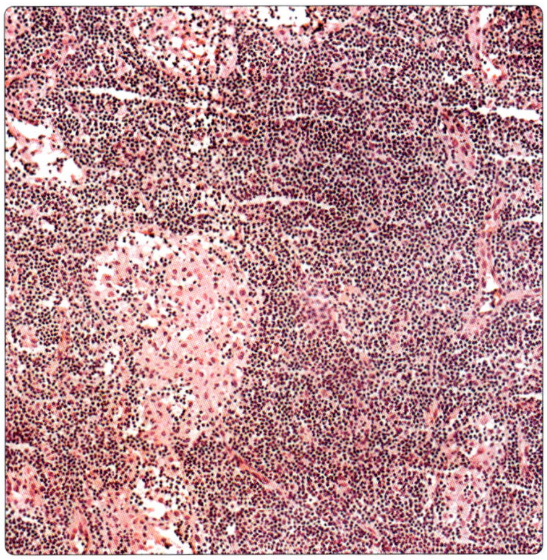

(Left) *Lymph node involvement is an important prognostic factor for papillary and medullary carcinoma. This is an unusual case with 2 primaries and metastases from both. Thyroid showed a large medullary carcinoma and a 0.2-cm papillary microcarcinoma.* **(Right)** *Lymphocytic infiltrates with germinal centers can diffusely involve the thyroid. If present in a peripheral nodule submitted as a lymph node, the presence of normal thyroid follicles within a lymphocytic infiltrate can be mistaken for metastatic carcinoma.*

SURGICAL/CLINICAL CONSIDERATIONS

Goal of Consultation

- Determine if ureteral margins on cystectomy specimen are free of urothelial carcinoma in situ & invasive carcinoma

Change in Patient Management

- Additional ureter may be resected to achieve tumor-free margins

Clinical Setting

- Cystectomies are usually performed for muscle invasive urothelial carcinomas (pT2) & therapy refractory urothelial carcinoma in situ
- Patients with positive margins may be at higher risk for recurrence within remaining upper urinary tract

SPECIMEN EVALUATION

Gross

- Small length of ureter is usually provided
- True margin should be identified if specimen is too long to be entirely frozen en face
  - Often identified by presence of stitch or clip at 1 end of ureter segment

Frozen Section

- Cross section of margin is embedded with true margin face up in order that 1st frozen section will be true margin
- If complete cross section of urothelium is not seen on initial sections, deeper levels should be obtained
- If extensive denudation of urothelium is present, additional levels may be obtained

MOST COMMON DIAGNOSIS

Urothelial Carcinoma In Situ

- Urothelium appears crowded & disorganized with loss of polarity & nuclear overlapping
- Full-thickness atypia is not required
- Due to loss of cell cohesion, prominent denudation may be present
- Underlying connective tissue may have associated vascular congestion & inflammation

REPORTING

Frozen Section

- Positive for carcinoma in situ &/or invasive carcinoma or negative for malignancy
- Atypical cells present
  - Surgeon may choose to send additional margins
    - Features are worrisome, but not diagnostic, for carcinoma

PITFALLS

Umbrella Cells

- Can be mistaken for tumor cells

Reactive Epithelial Changes

- Nuclei are enlarged but appear more uniform than carcinoma in situ & have vesicular nuclei with single small nucleolus
- Occasional mitotic figures may be present but should not be atypical
- Acute or chronic inflammation is often present within urothelium

Frozen Section Artifact

- Urothelial cells artifactually appear larger & more hyperchromatic on frozen section than on permanent sections

Subepithelial Involvement

- In rare instances, soft tissue & muscle layers of ureter may contain invasive urothelial carcinoma, whereas urothelial mucosa is uninvolved

SELECTED REFERENCES

1. Satkunasivam R et al: Utility and significance of ureteric frozen section analysis during radical cystectomy. BJU Int. 117(3):463-8, 2016
2. Gordetsky J et al: Ureteral and urethral frozen sections during radical cystectomy or cystoprostatectomy: an analysis of denudation and atypia. Urology. 84(3):619-23, 2014

Ureter Margin: Gross Appearance

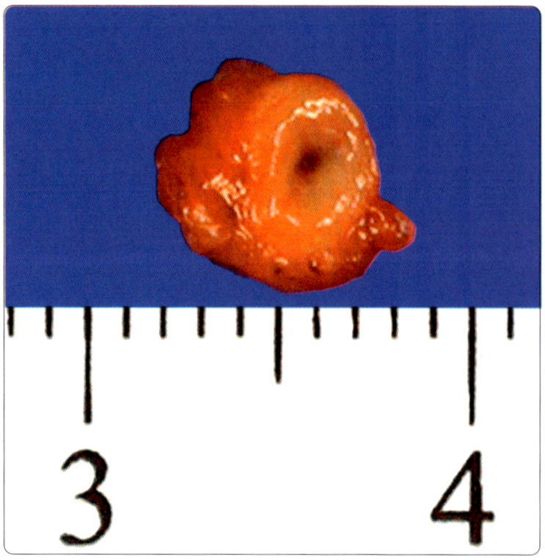

Ureter Margin: Frozen Section

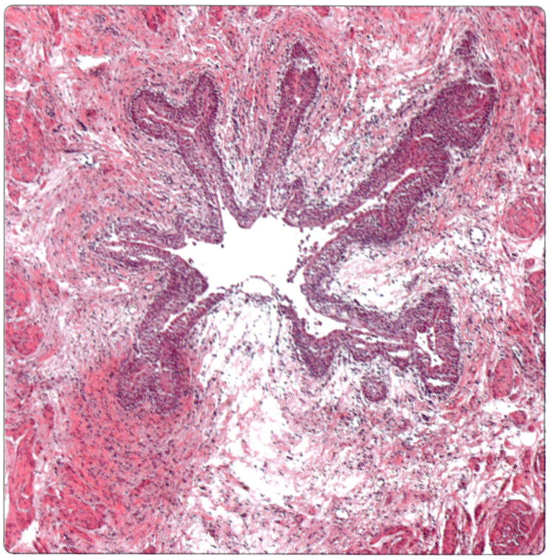

(Left) *A small length of ureter received for frozen section should be oriented & embedded in such a way that a complete cross section of the lumen is obtained for microscopic evaluation. (Courtesy A. Joiner, MD.)* **(Right)** *A complete cross section of the ureter is necessary to adequately evaluate the entire urothelium for the presence of carcinoma in situ. The lumen often has a star-shaped morphology on cross section.*

Normal Urothelium

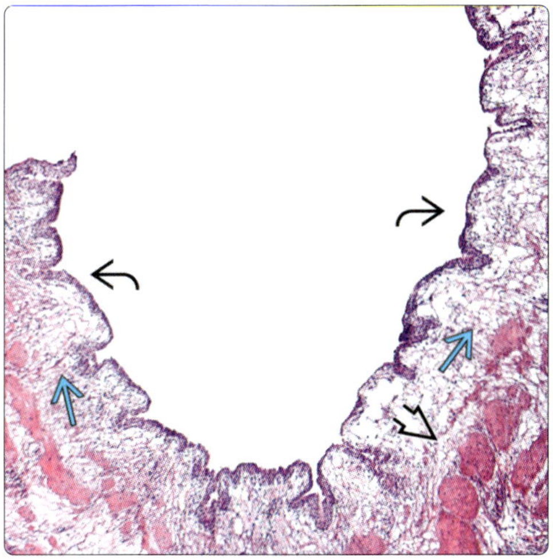

Normal Urothelium: Cytologic Features

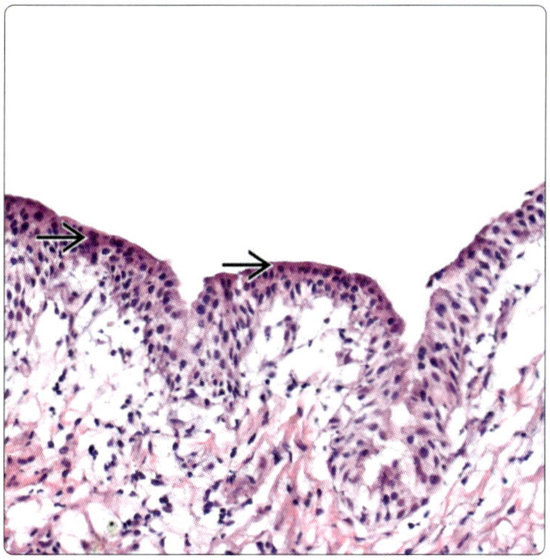

(Left) *The normal urothelial surface* ⇗ *has an undulating contour. The underlying loose connective tissue* ➔ *may appear edematous, inflamed, or fibrotic, especially if previous treatments or procedures have been performed. Bundles of smooth muscle make up the muscularis layer* ⇨. **(Right)** *Normal urothelium has cells with small, uniform nuclei. The cells have round to ovoid nuclei & lightly eosinophilic cytoplasm. A superficial layer of larger umbrella cells* ➔ *is present.*

Normal Urothelium: Umbrella Cells

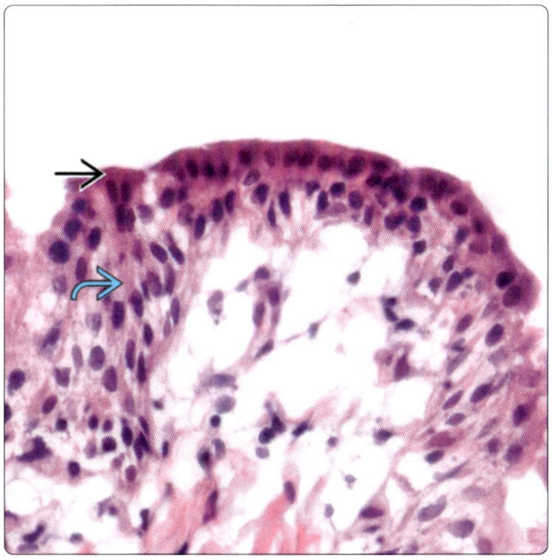

Normal Urothelium: Umbrella Cells

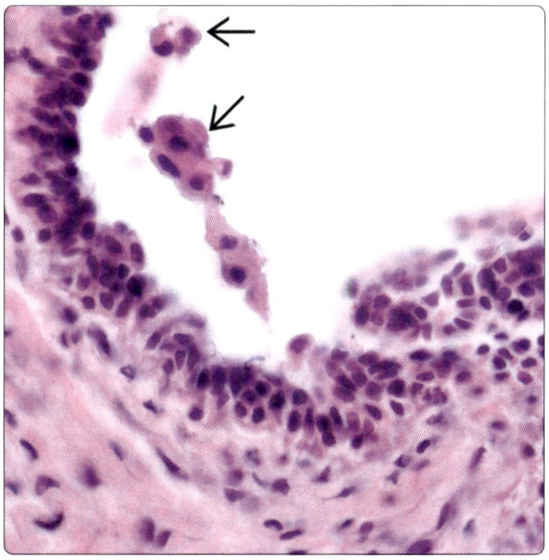

(Left) *The nuclei within the intermediate layer* ⇗ *of the urothelium are arranged longitudinally, perpendicular to the basement membrane. A single overlying layer of larger umbrella cells* ➔ *lines the luminal surface.* **(Right)** *Detached clusters of umbrella cells* ➔ *are present within the lumen of a normal ureter. This finding should not be confused with dyscohesive tumor cells. Umbrella cells are characterized by their abundant eosinophilic cytoplasm & may be binucleated.*

Normal Urothelium: Tangential Sectioning

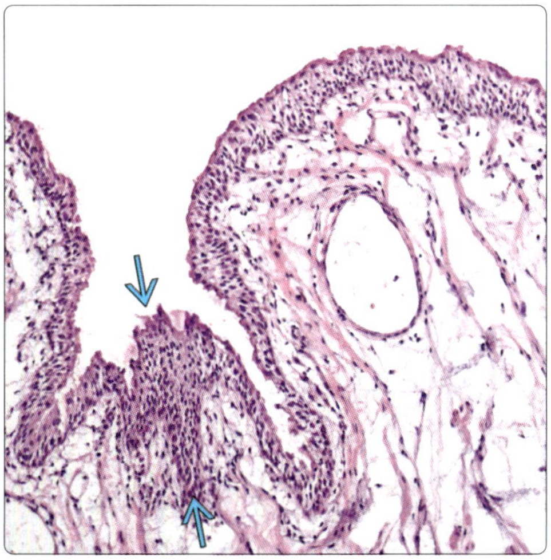

Normal Urothelium: Tangential Sectioning

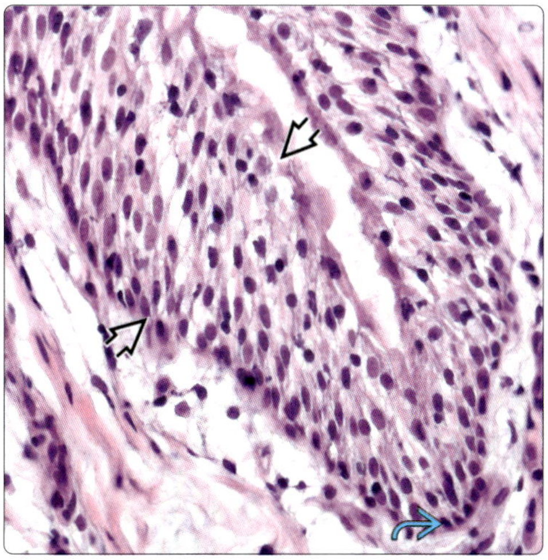

(Left) *This normal urothelium appears thickened in areas due to tangential sectioning* ➔. *However, the cells have small, uniform nuclei & normal polarity. The lamina propria is edematous & contains inflammatory cells.* **(Right)** *Although urothelium is normally 3-7 cell layers in thickness, tangential sectioning can artificially give an appearance of a thickened urothelium* ⇨. *The cells are uniform in size & shape with normal polarity. Small basal cells* ⇗ *are present adjacent to the basement membrane.*

(Left) *A permanent section of a ureter margin shows the typical star-shaped appearance of the lumen on cross section. The urothelium has an overall orderly appearance on low power with no nuclear enlargement or loss of normal polarity.* **(Right)** *The cells of normal urothelium have lightly eosinophilic cytoplasm & uniform, round to ovoid nuclei. A single umbrella cell layer ⮫ is present at the luminal surface. The subepithelial connective tissue contains scattered lymphocytes.*

Normal Ureter: Cross Section

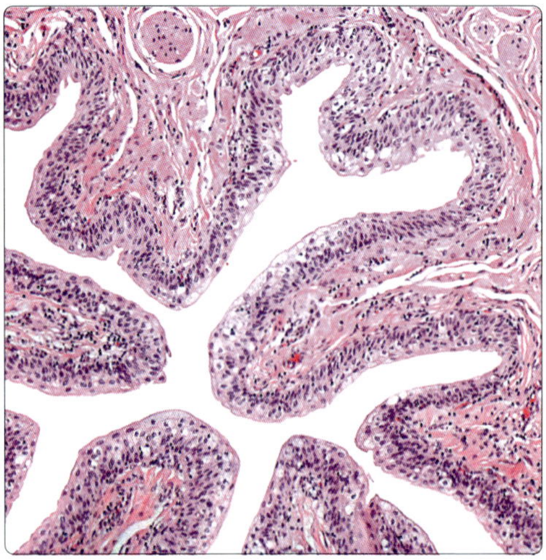

Ureter: Cytologic Features

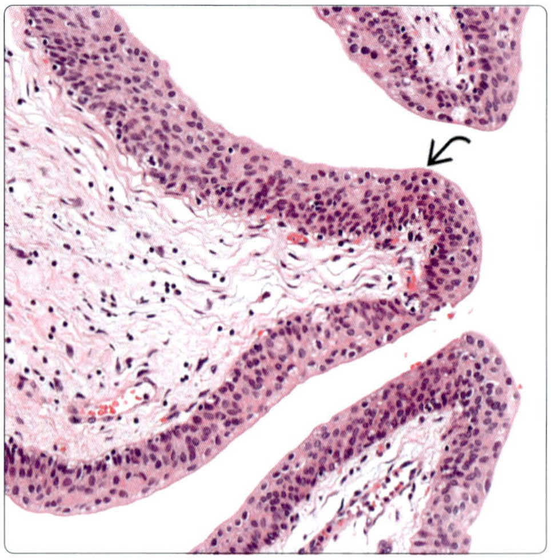

(Left) *Normal urothelium has uniform, orderly nuclei arranged perpendicular to the cell membrane. Occasional small, indistinct nucleoli may be present.* **(Right)** *This frozen section of the ureter margin is a complete cross section but is suboptimal because areas of the urothelium are missing ➙. Malignant cells are dyscohesive & are easily detached from the surface. Deeper levels through the tissue should be obtained to visualize the entire circumference of the margin.*

Normal Urothelium: Cytologic Features

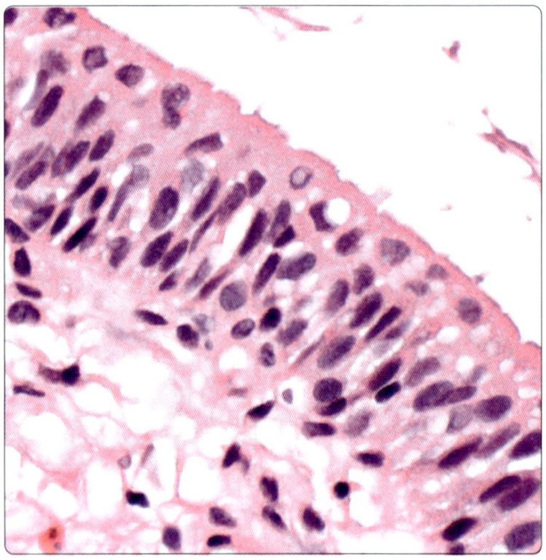

Ureter Margin: Denuded Epithelium

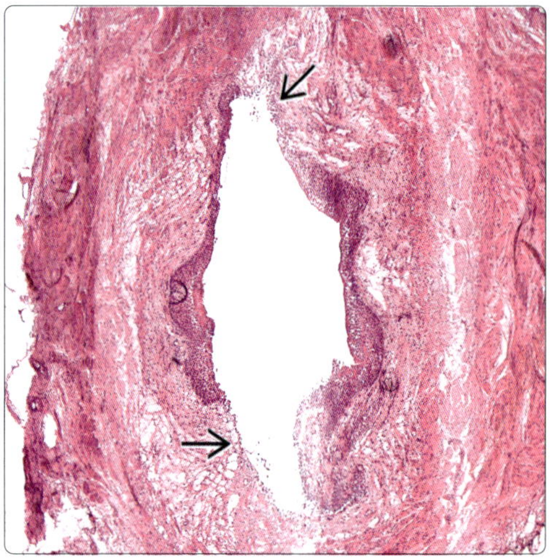

(Left) *von Brunn nests can be present within the ureter. The small nests have smooth, regular contours & are arranged in an orderly fashion. The interface with the underlying subepithelial connective tissue should be well-delineated without evidence of infiltration.* **(Right)** *von Brunn nests represent invaginations of urothelium into the underlying stroma. The nuclei of the cells within the von Brunn nests ⇨ share the bland cytologic features of the overlying normal urothelium ➙.*

von Brunn Nests

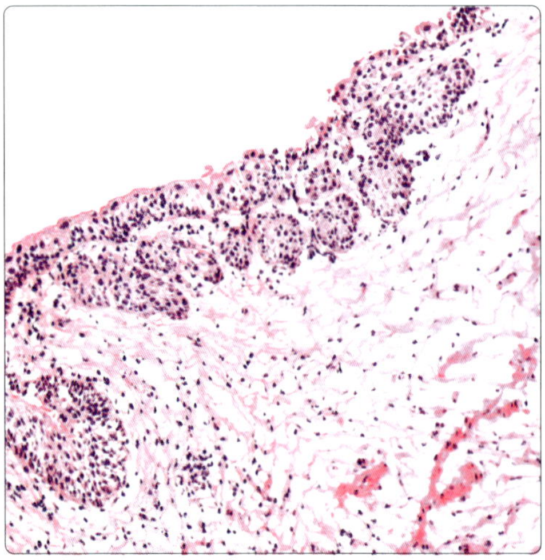

von Brunn Nests: Cytologic Features

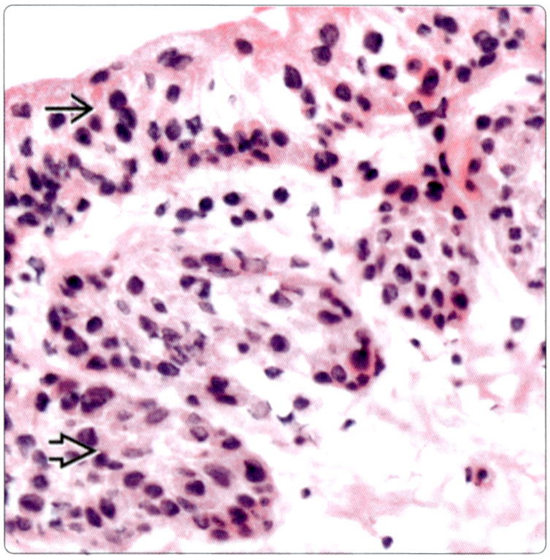

von Brunn Nests: Lobular Architecture

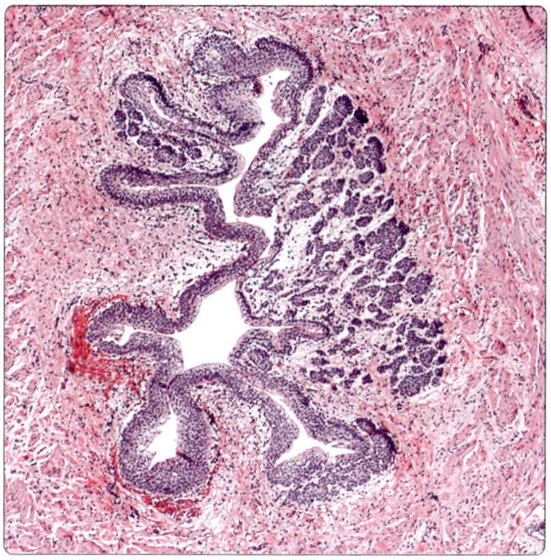

von Brunn Nests: Cytologic Features

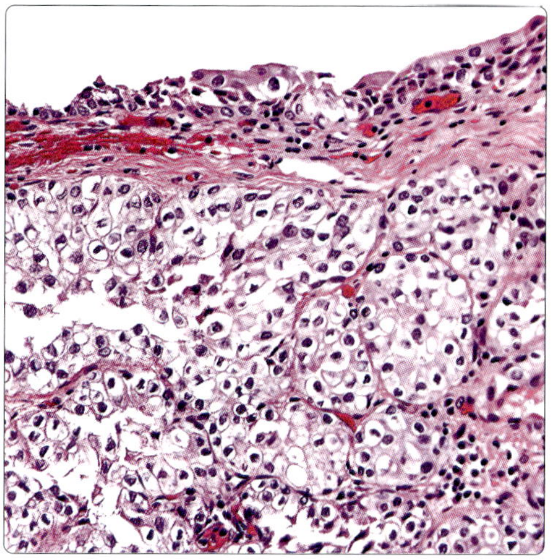

(Left) *At low power, the overall lobular architecture of von Brunn nests can be appreciated. The interface between the epithelial nests & the underlying stroma is linear, & no stromal reaction is present. (Courtesy J. McKenney, MD.)* **(Right)** *The urothelial cells in the von Brunn nests lack pleomorphism or hyperchromasia & share similar cytologic features to the normal surface urothelium, although mild nuclear enlargement can be present within the nests. (Courtesy J. McKenney, MD.)*

Reactive Urothelium

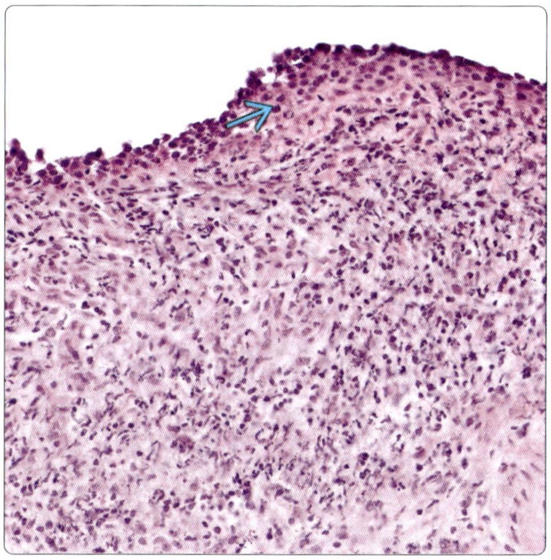

Reactive Urothelium: Cytologic Features

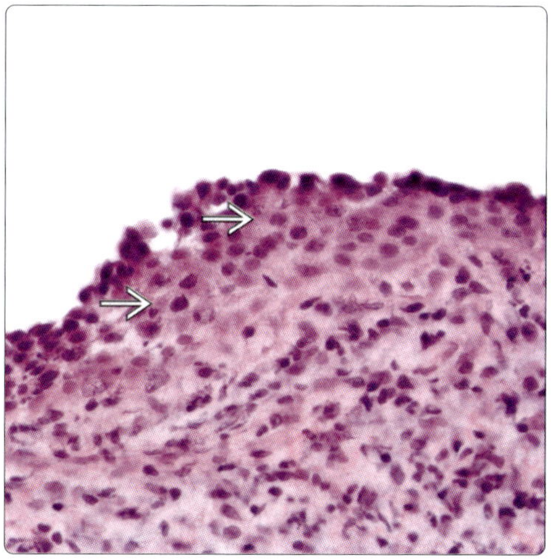

(Left) *An inflammatory infiltrate in the wall of the ureter or urothelium can cause reactive changes in the urothelial cells. Although the nuclei in reactive urothelium appear enlarged, they lack the pleomorphism & hyperchromasia of urothelial carcinoma in situ.* **(Right)** *The cells in reactive urothelium are enlarged but they appear uniform. The nuclei are round with a vesicular chromatin pattern & single nucleolus. Acute &/or chronic inflammatory cells are often present within the urothelium.*

Reactive Urothelium: Inflammatory Cells

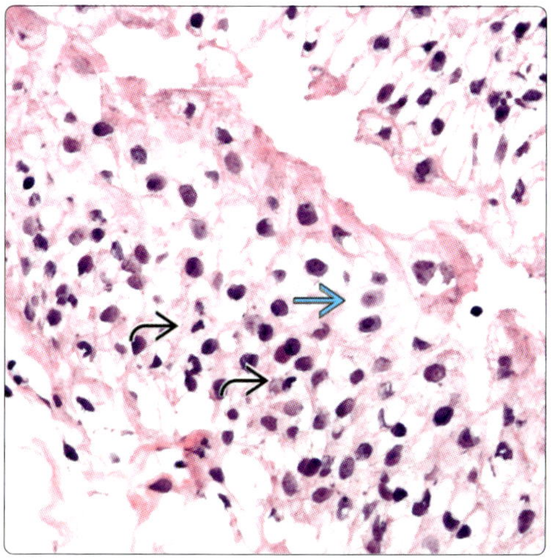

Reactive Urothelium: Inflammatory Infiltrate

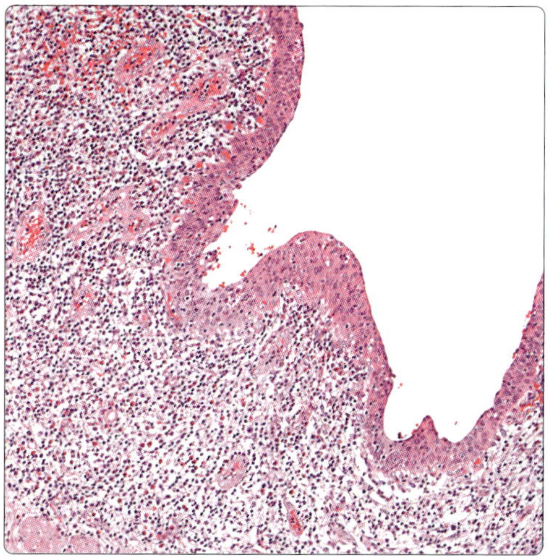

(Left) *In reactive urothelium, acute & chronic inflammatory cells are often identified within the urothelium. Although some loss of polarity may be present, the urothelium lacks the disorganized appearance of carcinoma in situ. The nuclei are often vesicular with a single nucleolus.* **(Right)** *An intense inflammatory infiltrate is present in this ureter. The cytoplasm in reactive urothelial cells may appear more brightly eosinophilic than that typically seen in normal urothelium.*

(Left) *Mitotic figures* ⇒ *may be identified within reactive urothelium, but atypical mitoses are absent. The nuclei lack pleomorphism & are vesicular with single nucleoli.* **(Right)** *Reactive urothelium* ⇒ *is characterized by enlarged cells with vesicular nuclei & occasional nucleoli. In contrast, the cells in the normal urothelium have smaller nuclei & lack nucleoli* ⇒.

Reactive Urothelium: Mitotic Figures

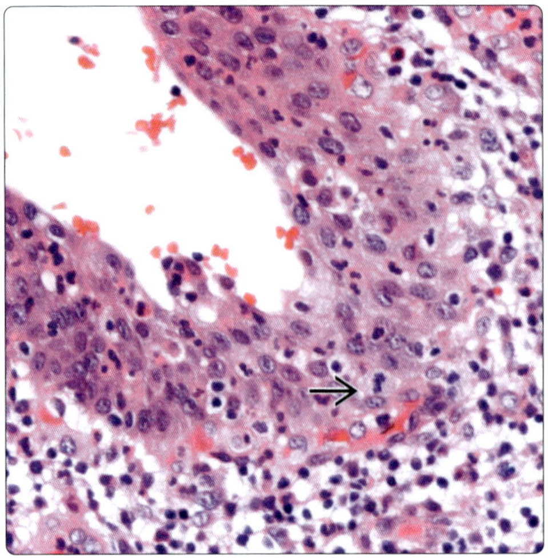

Reactive Urothelium: Cytologic Features

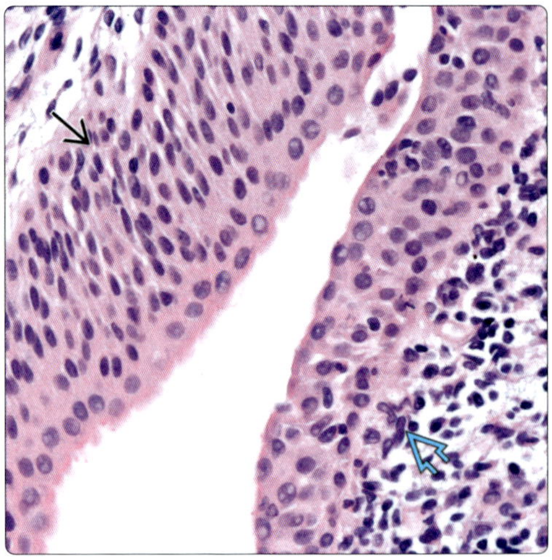

(Left) *Atypia can be identified at low power in carcinoma in situ. The cells appear hyperchromatic & enlarged. Dyscohesion of the cells is present with some of the cells having been sloughed off into the lumen* ⇒. **(Right)** *Urothelial carcinoma in situ is characterized by crowded overlapping cells. Prominent nucleoli* ⇒ *are present within some of the enlarged nuclei. These nuclei are more pronounced than the small indistinct nuclei of benign, reactive urothelium.*

Urothelial Carcinoma In Situ

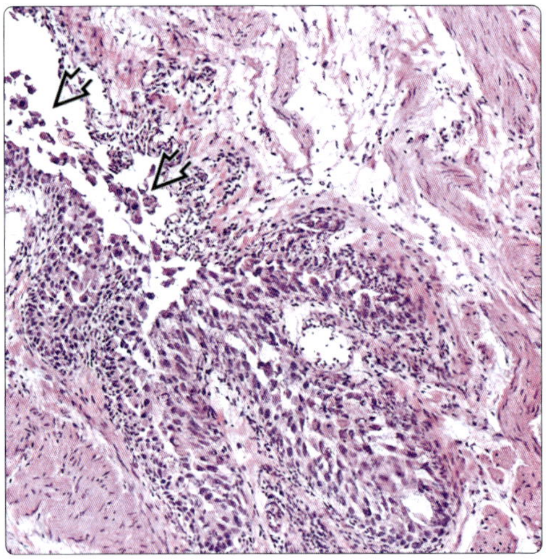

Urothelial Carcinoma In Situ: Cytologic Features

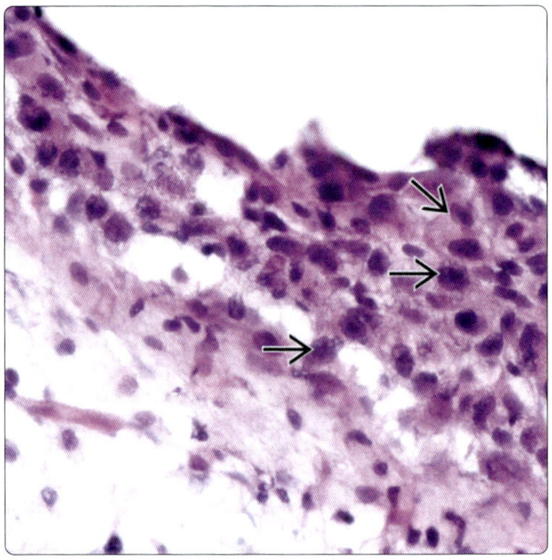

(Left) *The cells of carcinoma in situ appear enlarged & hyperchromatic at low power. Nuclear crowding & cellular dyscohesion are also evident. The subepithelial connective tissue may have increased inflammation & vascularity. It is important to distinguish neoplastic changes from reactive changes.* **(Right)** *The cells of urothelial carcinoma in situ have enlarged hyperchromatic nuclei & vary in size & shape. The cells have lost all polarity & appear crowded & disorganized. Mitotic figures are often present.*

Urothelial Carcinoma In Situ: Low-Power Appearance

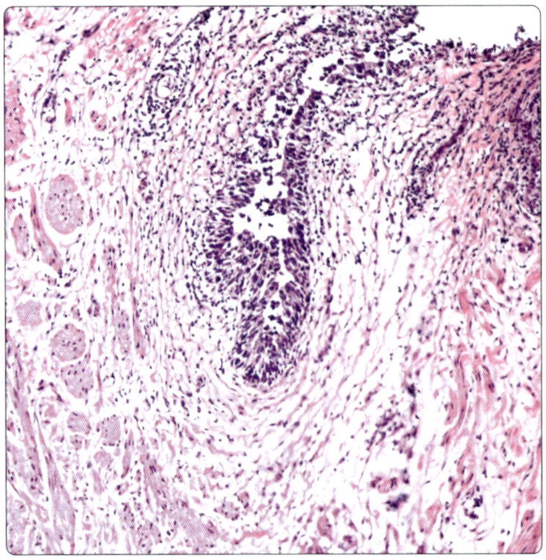

Urothelial Carcinoma In Situ: Cytologic Features

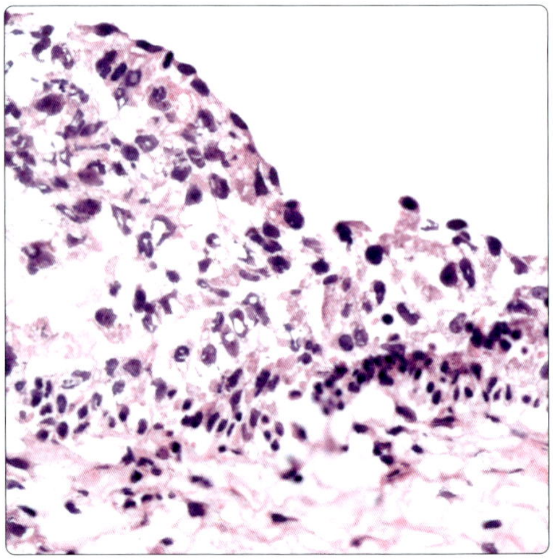

Urothelial Carcinoma In Situ: Mitotic Figures

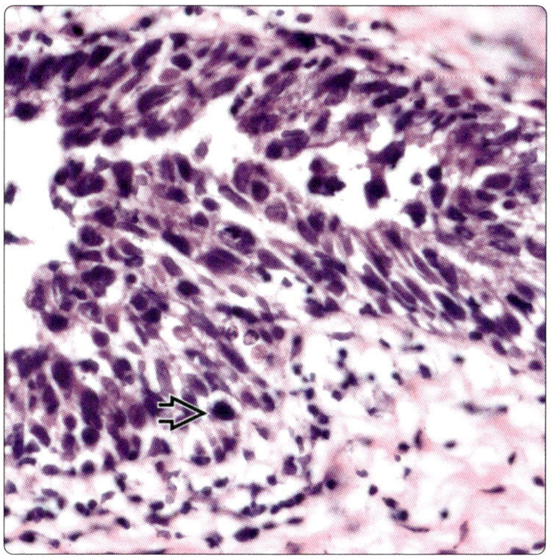

Urothelial Carcinoma In Situ: Denuded Epithelium

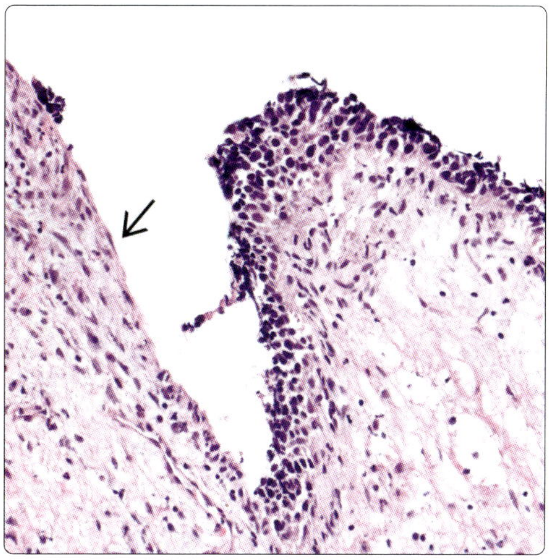

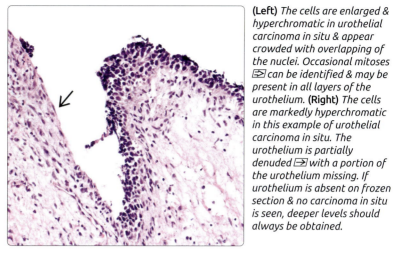

(Left) *The cells are enlarged & hyperchromatic in urothelial carcinoma in situ & appear crowded with overlapping of the nuclei. Occasional mitoses* ➡ *can be identified & may be present in all layers of the urothelium.* **(Right)** *The cells are markedly hyperchromatic in this example of urothelial carcinoma in situ. The urothelium is partially denuded* ➡ *with a portion of the urothelium missing. If urothelium is absent on frozen section & no carcinoma in situ is seen, deeper levels should always be obtained.*

Urothelial Carcinoma In Situ: Sloughed Tumor Cells

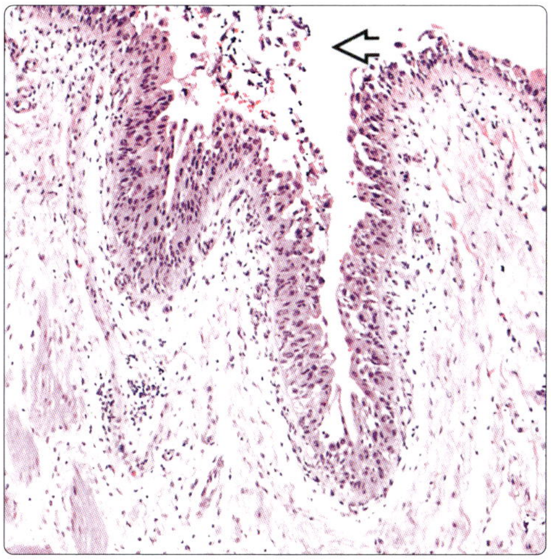

Urothelial Carcinoma In Situ: Cytologic Features

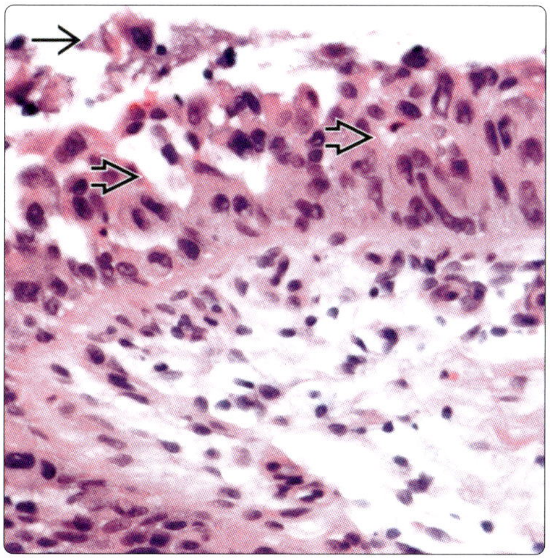

(Left) *This permanent section shows the overall hyperchromatic, disorganized appearance of the urothelium in carcinoma in situ at low power. The cells are dyscohesive, & sloughed urothelial cells are present within the lumen of the ureter* ➡*.* **(Right)** *Urothelial carcinoma in situ with nuclear crowding & disorganization as well as hyperchromasia & pleomorphism is clearly seen in this permanent section. The dyscohesion of the cells can be seen* ➡*. Sloughed carcinoma in situ cells are identified within the lumen* ➡*.*

Urothelial Carcinoma In Situ: Denuded Epithelium

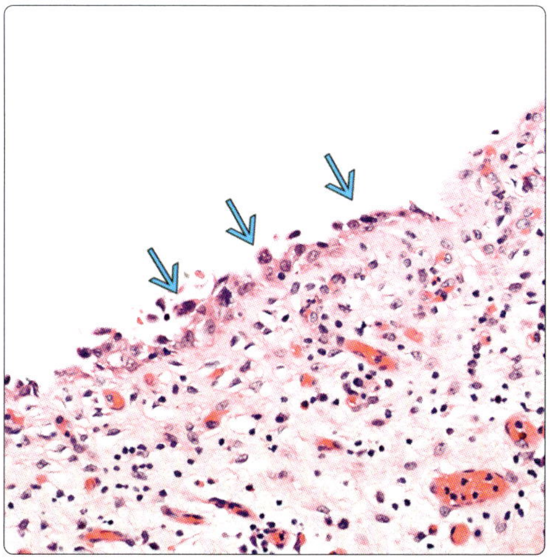

Pagetoid Urothelial Carcinoma In Situ

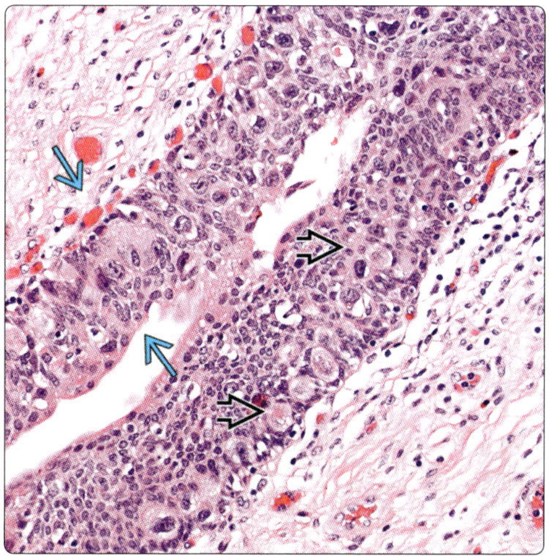

(Left) *Extensive denudation of urothelial carcinoma in situ may be present, leading to only a single layer of "clinging" atypical cells* ➡ *with nucleomegaly, hyperchromasia, & pleomorphism.* **(Right)** *Full-thickness atypia is not required for the diagnosis of urothelial carcinoma in situ. In some cases, pagetoid spread of cells is present with single cells or nests of cells* ➡ *undermining the benign urothelium. In this section, full-thickness atypia is present within the adjacent urothelium* ➡*.*

(Left) *Low-grade papillary urothelial carcinoma can occur within the ureter, & in some cases, multiple lesions are present. This frozen section shows fibrovascular cores → lined by atypical urothelium with enlarged nuclei & hyperchromasia. Overall, the nuclei appear uniform in size.* **(Right)** *This low-grade papillary urothelial carcinoma has hyperchromatic, uniform nuclei. The nuclei appear disordered & have lost their normal polarity.*

Low-Grade Papillary Urothelial Carcinoma

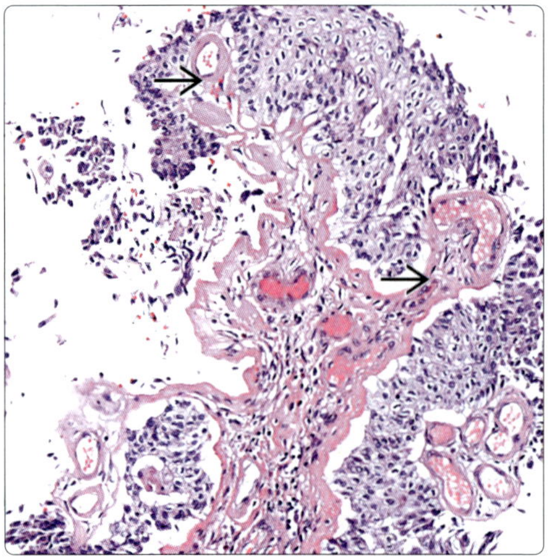

Low-Grade Papillary Urothelial Carcinoma: Cytologic Features

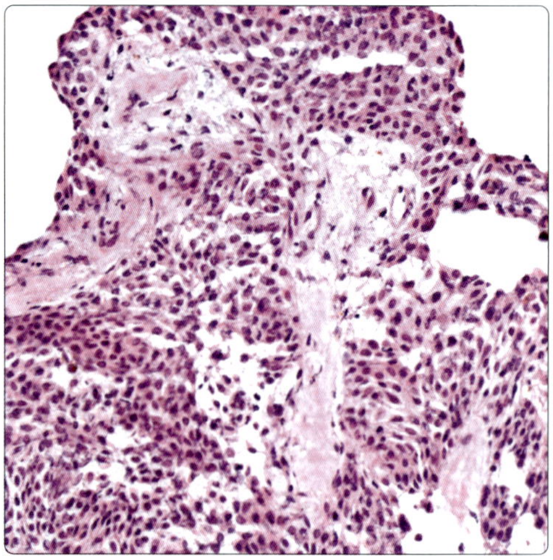

(Left) *The cells in this permanent section of low-grade papillary urothelial carcinoma appear uniformly enlarged with an overall disordered appearance. The pleomorphism & frequent mitotic figures that characterize high-grade papillary urothelial carcinoma are lacking.* **(Right)** *High-grade papillary urothelial carcinoma is identified by a central fibrovascular core → lined by hyperchromatic & pleomorphic cells. Prominent crowding & loss of polarity is present.*

Low-Grade Papillary Urothelial Carcinoma: Cytologic Features

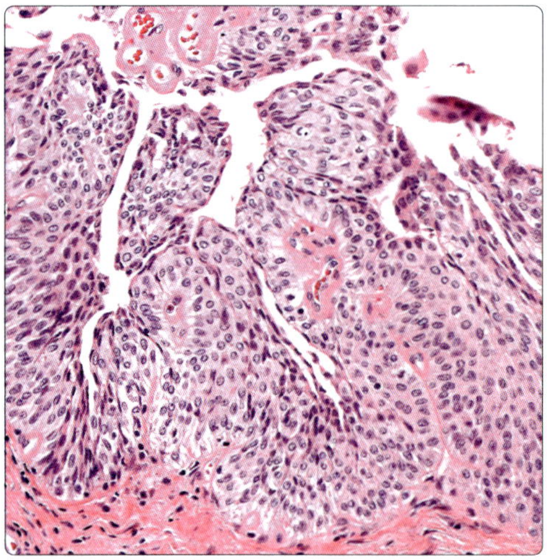

High-Grade Papillary Urothelial Carcinoma

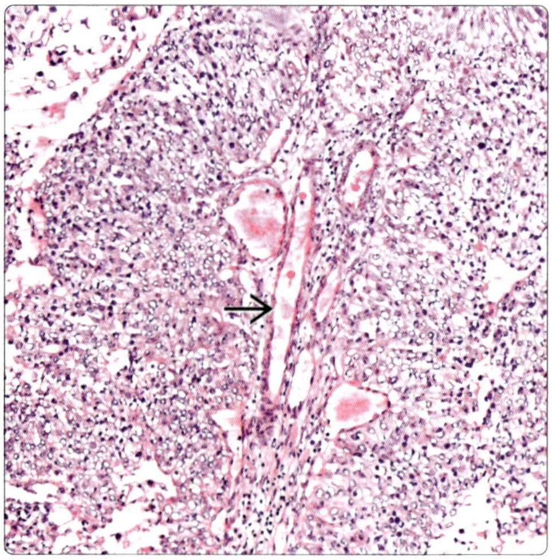

(Left) *High-grade papillary urothelial carcinoma is distinguished from low-grade urothelial carcinoma by higher grade enlarged nuclei with prominent nucleoli ↗ & numerous mitotic figures. The cells may be dyscohesive, resulting in denuded fibrovascular cores.* **(Right)** *Marked hyperchromasia & pleomorphism is evident in this high-grade papillary urothelial carcinoma. The cells appear more crowded when compared to low-grade papillary urothelial carcinoma, & mitoses are more frequent.*

High-Grade Papillary Urothelial Carcinoma: Cytologic Features

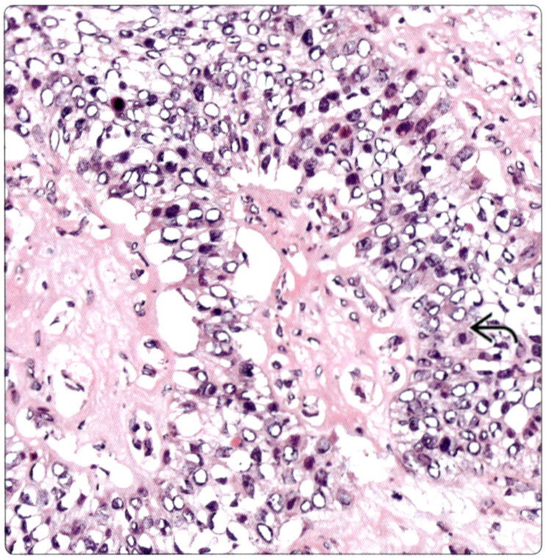

High-Grade Papillary Urothelial Carcinoma

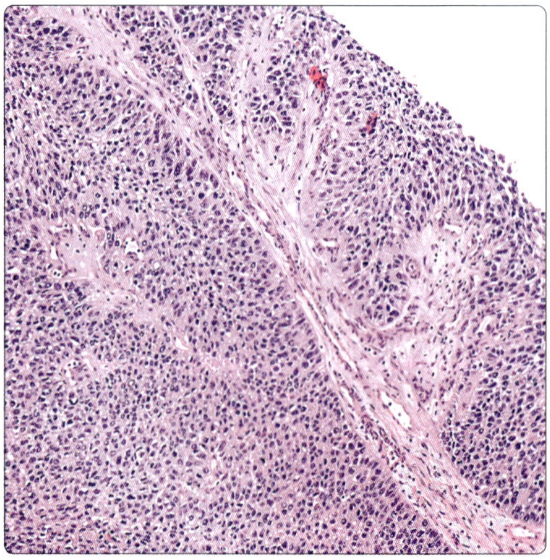

Invasive Urothelial Carcinoma

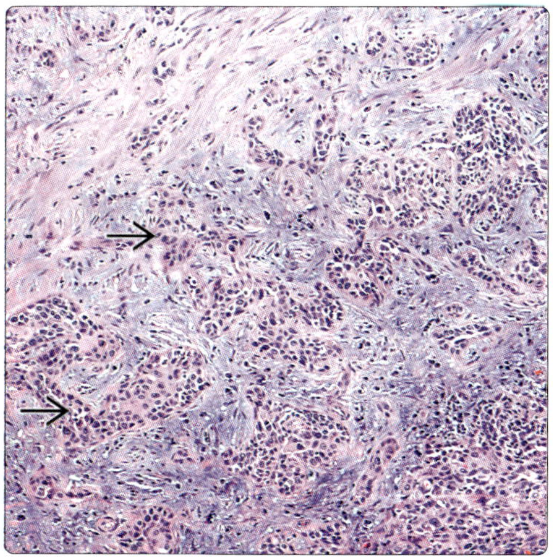

Invasive Urothelial Carcinoma: Cytologic Features

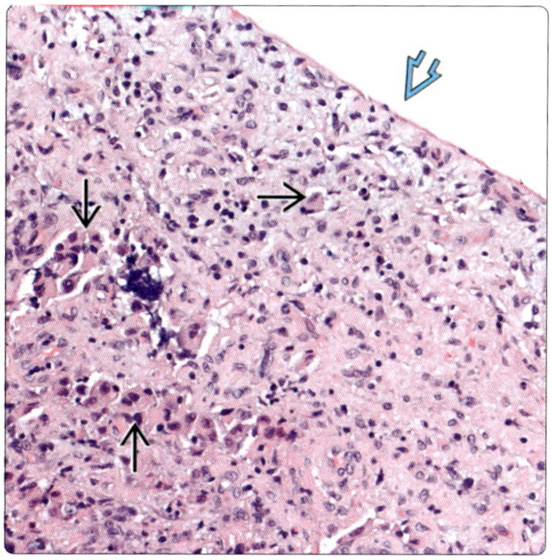

(Left) *It is unusual to find clinically undetected invasive urothelial carcinoma in a ureter margin. The infiltrative irregular tumor nests have incited a reactive desmoplastic stromal response in the subepithelial connective tissue. Chronic inflammation is present in the background.* **(Right)** *Single cells & nests of cells infiltrate the subepithelial connective tissue in this focus of invasive urothelial carcinoma. The overlying mucosa of the ureter is completely denuded.*

Invasive Urothelial Carcinoma: Cytologic Features

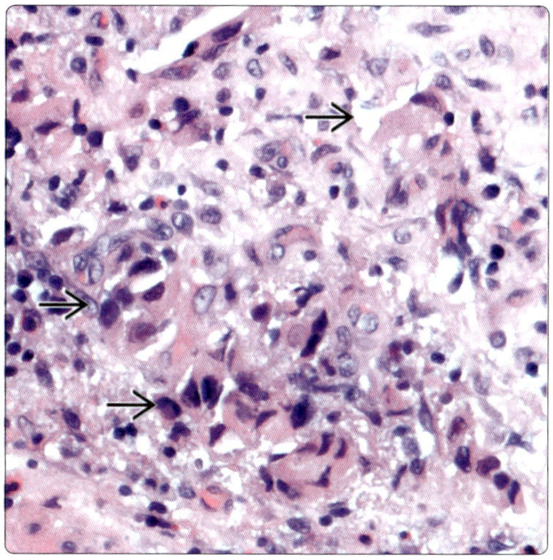

Invasive Urothelial Carcinoma: Invasion in Periureteral Adipose Tissue

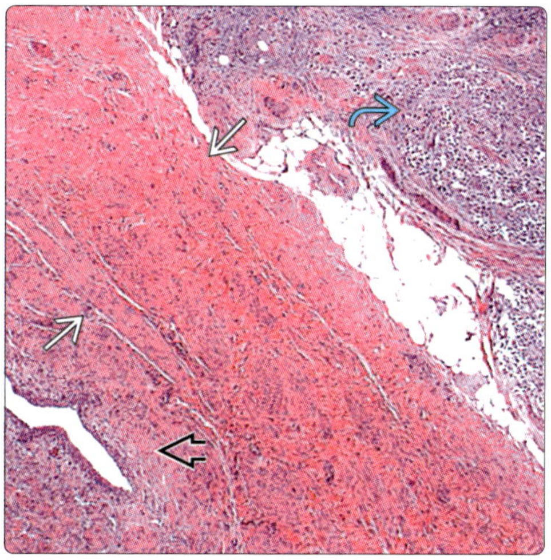

(Left) *This invasive urothelial carcinoma infiltrates in the subepithelial connective tissue as single cells & small nests with abundant eosinophilic cytoplasm.* **(Right)** *While the urothelium & muscular wall of this ureter appear unremarkable, the periureteral adipose tissue is involved with urothelial carcinoma. The muscular wall & surrounding adipose tissue can be positive for carcinoma, even though the surface urothelium is benign. (Courtesy J. McKenney, MD.)*

Plasmacytoid Urothelial Carcinoma

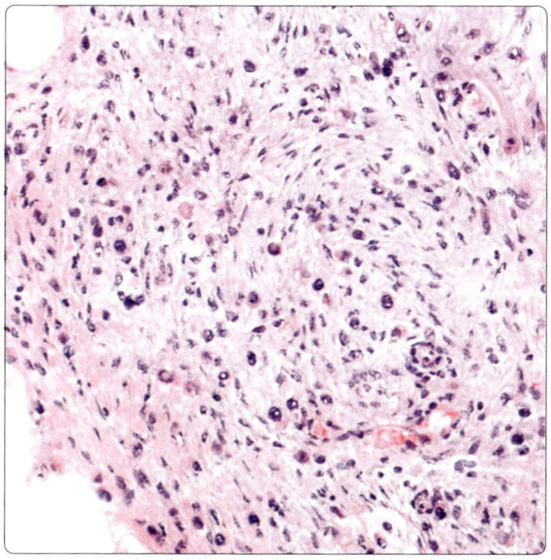

Plasmacytoid Urothelial Carcinoma: Cytologic Features

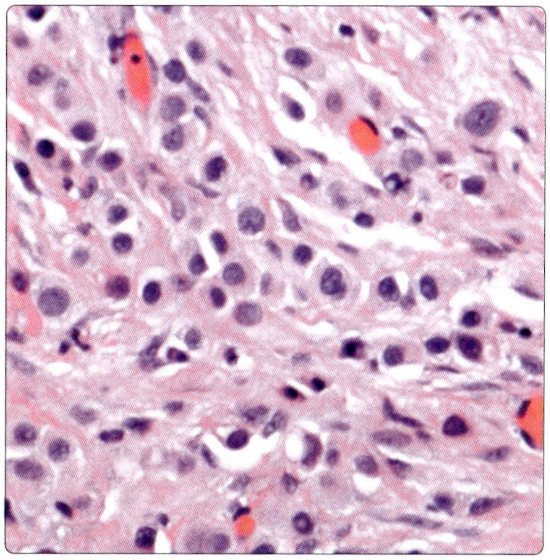

(Left) *Single, highly atypical cells with a plasmacytoid appearance infiltrate through the fibroadipose tissue surrounding the ureter. The presence of urothelial carcinomas, including the more aggressive variants, such as plasmacytoid & micropapillary, can be overlooked in ureter margins, as the surface urothelium may appear unremarkable.* **(Right)** *This urothelial carcinoma consists of dyscohesive cells with a plasmacytoid appearance arranged in linear arrays & as single cells in the ureteral wall.*

Contents

SURGICAL/CLINICAL CONSIDERATIONS

Goal of Consultation

- Determine if carcinoma is present with features indicating need for further staging

Change in Patient Management

- Surgeon may perform pelvic &/or paraaortic lymph node dissections if endometrial carcinoma with following features are present
  - Grade II or III
  - Invasion beyond 50% of myometrial thickness
  - Cervical involvement
  - Extensive lymph-vascular space invasion

Clinical Setting

- Diagnosis of carcinoma or endometrial intraepithelial neoplasia (EIN) will usually have been made with prior biopsy
  - Patients with serous or clear cell carcinoma will undergo hysterectomy and staging
  - Women with endometrioid carcinoma will undergo hysterectomy
    - Staging will be performed based on intraoperative evaluation of carcinoma
- Intraoperative consultation also may be requested during routine hysterectomy in absence of prior diagnosis of carcinoma if atypical findings are observed during surgery

SPECIMEN EVALUATION

Gross

- Orient uterus according to anterior and posterior aspects
  - Peritoneal reflection is lower on posterior surface and often comes to point
  - Peritoneal reflection is higher and blunter on anterior surface where bladder has been dissected away
  - If orientation is not possible, designate 2 aspects, "A" and "B"
- Outer surface of uterus is inspected for areas suspicious for direct tumor invasion or serosal implants
  - Any suspicious areas should be differentially inked
- Open uterus along lateral edges using scissors
  - In uteri with abnormally thick walls or laterally placed leiomyoma, probe may be inserted into cervical os and a long sectioning knife used to bivalve uterus
    - Using knife should be avoided if possible
      - More difficult to maintain section perpendicular to uterine wall: Depth of invasion is more difficult to determine in tangential section
- Inspect (but do not touch) endometrial lining for gross evidence of carcinoma
  - Pale yellow-tan, heaped-up, and firm areas
- Make serial transverse incisions at 5-mm intervals from mucosal surface to, but not through, serosa
  - Specimen should be kept intact to maintain orientation
- Myometrial invasion grossly appears as effacement of normal myometrial texture
  - Carcinoma often presents as tan-yellow-white homogeneous mass replacing normal myometrium
  - Depth of invasion can sometimes be determined grossly
- Surfaces of ovaries and fallopian tubes are carefully inspected
  - Ovaries are serially sectioned and inspected for any mass lesions

Frozen Section

- Section of area of suspected deepest invasion is frozen
- Areas of suspected cervical, fallopian tube, or ovarian involvement may be evaluated by frozen section as well

MOST COMMON DIAGNOSES

Endometrial Carcinoma

- ~ 50% of cases
- Endometrial lining may appear heaped-up
  - Carcinomas are typically pale yellow to tan and friable
- Histologic types
  - **Endometrioid**: Most common type, composed of glands lined by columnar epithelium
  - **Clear cell**: High-grade carcinoma with variable cytoplasmic clearing, tubulocystic glands with hobnail cells, and stromal hyalinization
  - **Serous**: High-grade carcinoma composed of slit-like glandular spaces lined by highly atypical cells with prominent nucleoli
  - **Carcinosarcoma**: Endometrioid, clear cell, or serous carcinomas with malignant mesenchymal (stromal) component
- Grade
  - Grade II or III is indication for staging biopsies
- Depth of invasion
  - Uterine wall is serially sectioned to identify greatest depth of invasion that can be seen grossly
  - Myometrial invasion is detected by effacement of normal myometrial texture
  - Invasion can be difficult to assess when carcinomas involve adenomyosis

Endometrial Stromal Sarcoma

- Usually diffusely infiltrative
- Lymph-vascular invasion can be seen as worm-like masses in myometrium
- Hemorrhage and necrosis may be present
- Irregular nests or tongues of malignant stromal cells or solid growth pattern

Endometrial Polyp

- ~ 10-15% of cases
- Usually, broad-based finger-like projection from endometrial wall
- Central portion consists of fibrous stroma, and surface is covered by endometrium
- Polyp should be assessed for atypical epithelium indicative of serous neoplasia

Adenomyosis

- ~ 10% of cases
- Normal endometrium is deeply embedded within myometrium
  - Can mimic invasion when involved by carcinoma
- Grossly consists of thick, trabeculated muscle fibers with small, pinpoint hemorrhages

FIGO Grading of Endometrial Carcinoma

Grade	Architectural Criteria	Nuclear Criteria
Well differentiated (GI)	≤ 5% solid growth	No notable nuclear atypia
Moderately differentiated (G2)	≤ 5% solid growth	Notable nuclear atypia (G3 nuclear atypia)
Moderately differentiated (G2)	6-50% solid growth	No notable nuclear atypia (G3 nuclear atypia)
Poorly differentiated (G3)	6-50% solid growth	Notable nuclear atypia (G3 nuclear atypia)
Poorly differentiated (G3)	> 50% solid growth	Not required

Endometrial Intraepithelial Neoplasia (EIN)

- Generally not grossly evident
- Closely packed glands with intervening stroma

REPORTING

Frozen Section

- In cases of EIN or atypical hyperplasia, frozen section diagnosis of "at least EIN in 1 examined section" is appropriate with note deferring further classification to more extensive sampling of endometrium
- If carcinoma is present, following features are reported
  - Type (endometrioid, clear cell, serous, or carcinosarcoma)
  - Grade
  - Depth of invasion
  - Cervical involvement
  - Serosal, ovarian, or fallopian tube involvement
- Attempt at diagnosis of type of carcinoma and depth of invasion should be made for each case
- If cervix and adnexa are grossly negative, this should be reported

Reliability of Intraoperative Assessment

- Grade is accurate in 67-96% of cases
- Depth of invasion is accurate in 85-95% of cases
- Cervical involvement is accurate in 65-96% of cases
- False-positive diagnoses
  - In ~ 9% of cases, > 50% myometrial invasion is reported but not confirmed on permanent sections
    - Carcinoma involving adenomyosis
    - Lymph-vascular invasion mistaken for invasion
- False-negative results
  - In ~ 10% of cases, myometrial invasion is not reported but is found on permanent sections
    - Diffusely invasive carcinoma with widely spaced glands may be missed

PITFALLS

Carcinomatous Involvement of Adenomyosis

- Depth of invasion can be difficult to determine when adenomyosis is present

Lymph-Vascular Invasion vs. Myometrial Invasion

- Tumor in deep lymphatics can be mistaken for myometrial invasion

Difficult Patterns of Invasion

- Adenoma malignum pattern of invasion
  - Some carcinomas are diffusely invasive with widely spaced glands and minimal desmoplastic response (adenoma malignum pattern)
  - Invasive glands may mimic adenomyosis or involvement of adenomyosis
    - Adenomyosis-like invasion may be identified by its irregular (yet smooth) borders
      - Adenomyosis typically displays smooth, rounded borders
    - Focal desmoplasia may be present
- **M**icrocystic, **el**ongated, and **f**ragmented (MELF) pattern of invasion
  - Patterns of myometrial invasion may be difficult to identify, especially MELF pattern
    - MELF may be identified at low power as myxoid areas or pockets of inflammation deep in myometrium
    - Malignant glands are often fragmented and composed of eosinophilic epithelium admixed with acute inflammatory cells
    - MELF frequently represents deepest extent of tumor invasion and is associated with higher rate of lymph node metastasis

Overestimating Histologic Grade

- Squamous morules, denoted by their whorling growth pattern, are solid and are not considered solid tumor growth that would lead to increase in grade
- Frozen section artifact must be considered when evaluating nuclear morphology for atypia

Tangential Sectioning of Uterine Wall

- Tangential section of uterine wall can make wall appear wider than it actually is
  - This could make it difficult to determine depth of invasion of carcinoma
- Opening uterus with scissors is less likely to lead to tangential sections than opening uterus with knife blade

SELECTED REFERENCES

1. Kisu I et al: Preoperative and intraoperative assessment of myometrial invasion in endometrial cancer: comparison of magnetic resonance imaging and frozen sections. Acta Obstet Gynecol Scand. 92(5):525-35, 2013
2. Turan T et al: Accuracy of frozen-section examination for myometrial invasion and grade in endometrial cancer. Eur J Obstet Gynecol Reprod Biol. 167(1):90-5, 2013
3. Akbayir O et al: Combined use of preoperative transvaginal ultrasonography and intraoperative gross examination in the assessment of myometrial invasion in endometrial carcinoma. Eur J Obstet Gynecol Reprod Biol. 165(2):284-8, 2012
4. Kumar S et al: A prospective assessment of the reliability of frozen section to direct intraoperative decision making in endometrial cancer. Gynecol Oncol. 127(3):525-31, 2012

Uterus: Orientation

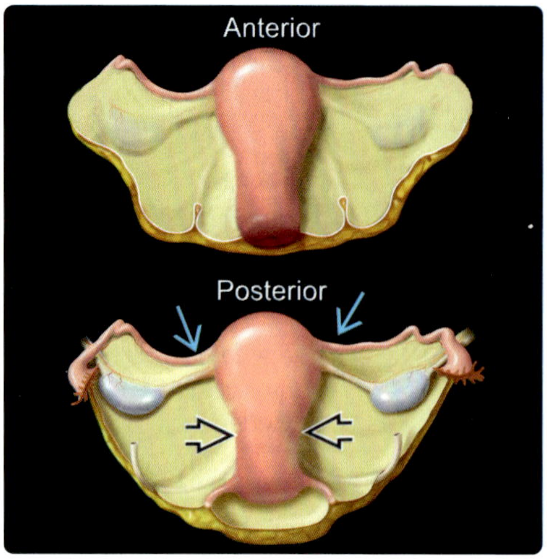

Uterus: Orientation

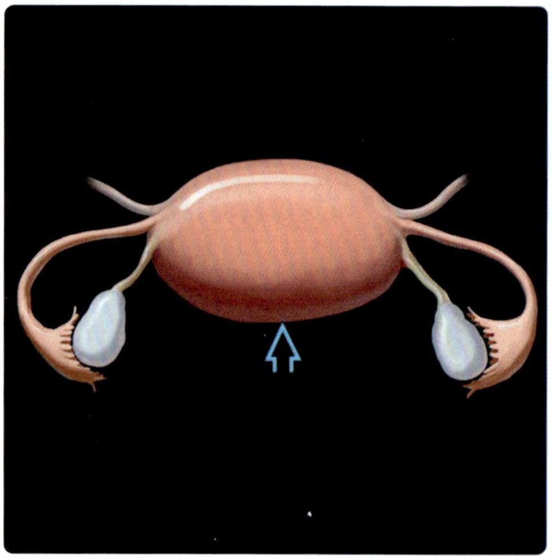

(Left) *Several landmarks may be used to orient a uterus as anterior/posterior. The adnexal structures* ➡ *project toward the posterior surface; the peritoneal reflection tracks deeper on the posterior aspect and will often be cauterized near the lower uterine segment* ➡. **(Right)** *When viewed from the top, the natural orientation of the adnexa will project to the posterior aspect* ➡.

Radical Hysterectomy

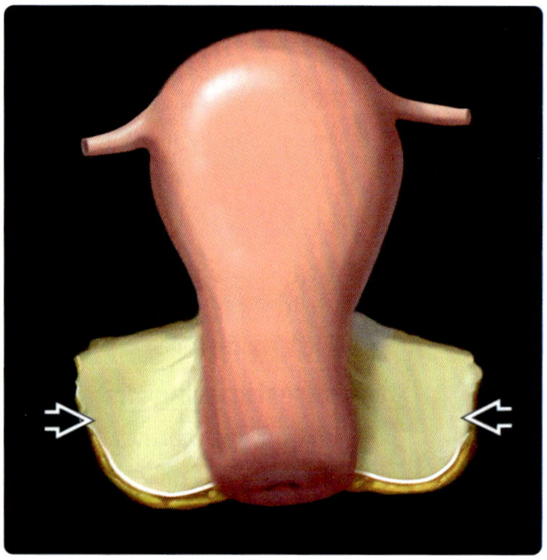

Uterus: Proper Opening Technique

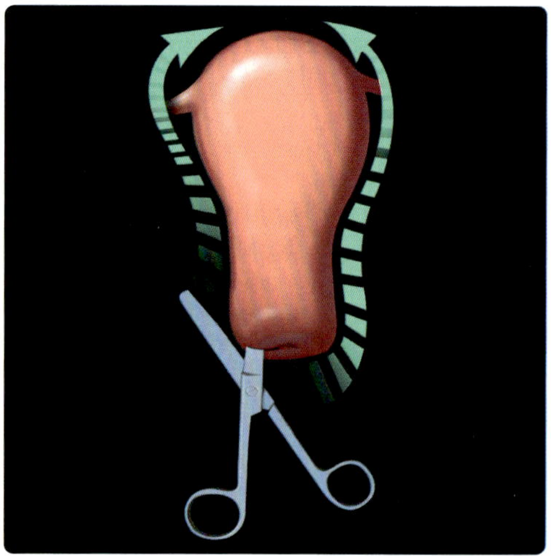

(Left) *Radical hysterectomies contain parametrial tissue* ➡, *which is inked, amputated, sectioned, and submitted before opening the uterus to prevent contamination with tumor fragments. In general, frozen section of cervical cancers is contraindicated.* **(Right)** *In most cases, the uterus should be opened laterally, starting through the cervix, with scissors. In cases of an abnormally thick wall or leiomyomata, a probe may be inserted into the cervical os, and a long knife may be used (this should be avoided if possible).*

Uterus: Tumor Sectioning

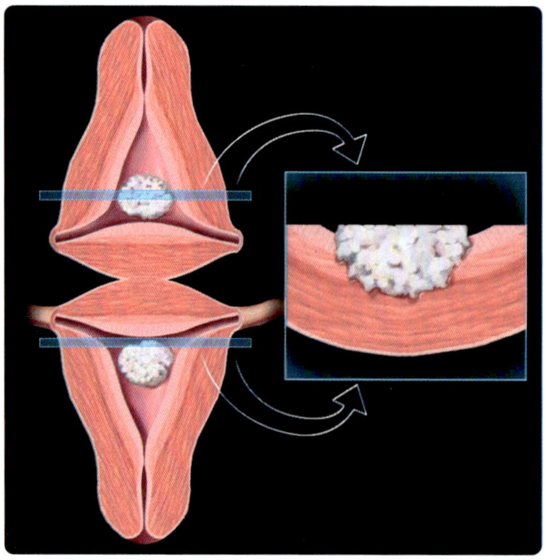

Endometrial Carcinoma: Depth of Invasion

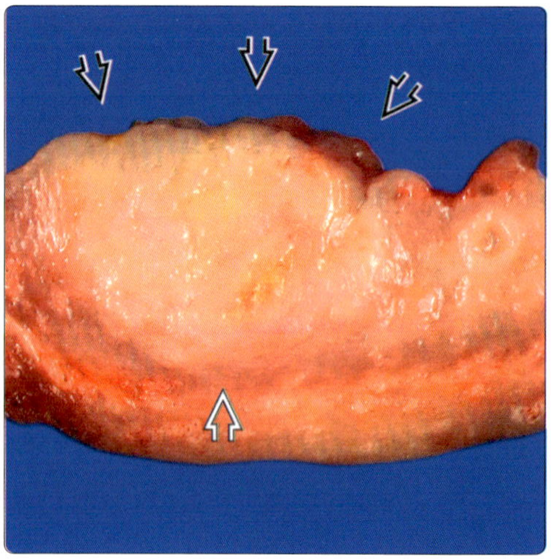

(Left) *The uterus should be sectioned at 5- to 10-mm intervals from the cervix to the superior aspect of the endometrial cavity. The deepest area of gross tumor invasion is submitted for frozen section: Full-thickness is preferable if possible.* **(Right)** *The depth of invasion of endometrial carcinoma* ➡ *into the myometrium is an important predictor of the likelihood of metastasis. The deepest extent of invasion* ➡ *is confirmed by frozen section.*

Endometrial Intraepithelial Neoplasia (Atypical Hyperplasia)

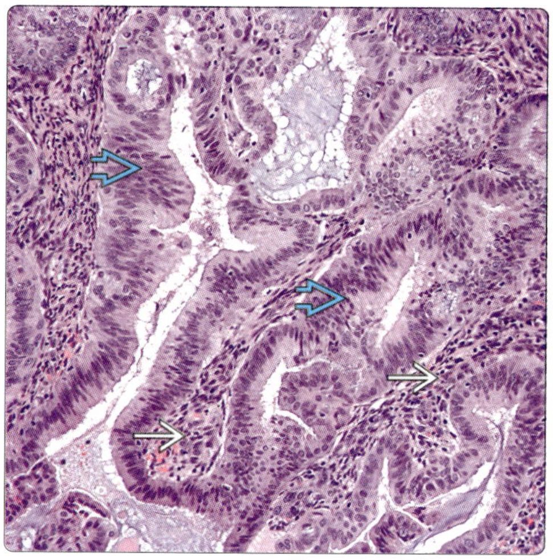

Low-Grade Endometrioid Carcinoma

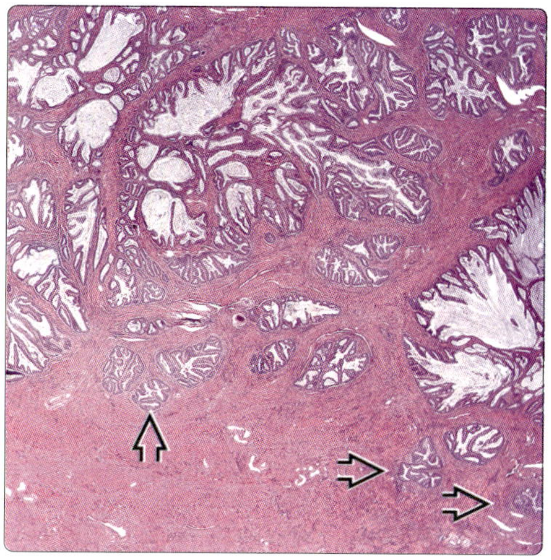

(Left) *Endometrial intraepithelial neoplasia, or atypical hyperplasia, is characterized by closely packed glands with some intervening stroma. In contrast, areas of cribriforming and back-to-back glands with thread-like stroma support a diagnosis of low-grade adenocarcinoma.* **(Right)** *Low-grade (FIGO grade I) adenocarcinoma is predominately gland forming with < 5% solid tumor growth and a low to intermediate nuclear grade. Small invasive nests of tumor are easily identifiable.*

High-Grade Endometrioid Carcinoma

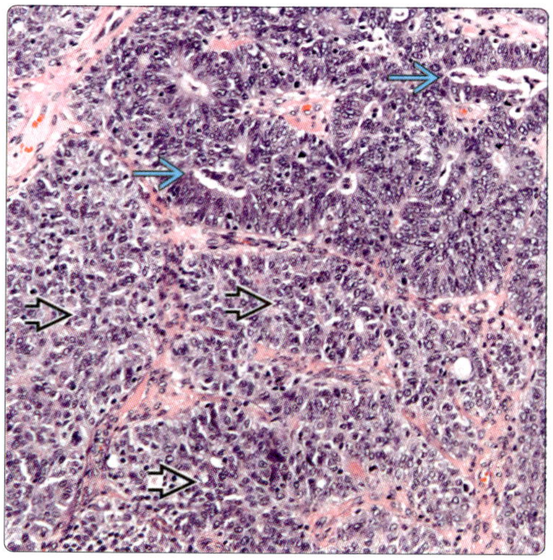

Endometrial Carcinoma: Squamous Morules

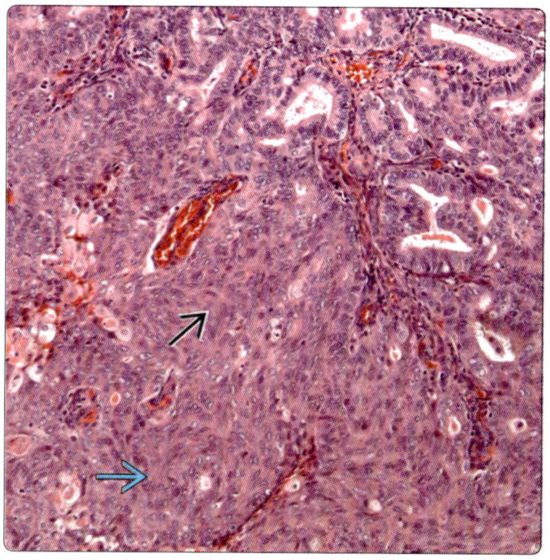

(Left) *High-grade adenocarcinoma consists of sheets of malignant cells as opposed to gland formation. Care should be taken not to misinterpret morular metaplasia, identified by its swirling growth pattern, as solid tumor growth.* **(Right)** *Squamous morular metaplasia may lead to overestimation of FIGO grade due to its appearance of solid growth. It can be recognized by its streaming or whorled growth pattern.*

Endometrioid Carcinoma: Adenoma Malignum

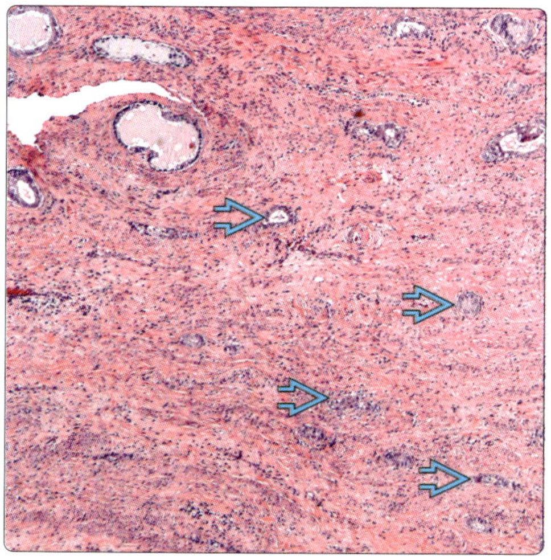

Endometrioid Carcinoma: Myometrial Invasion

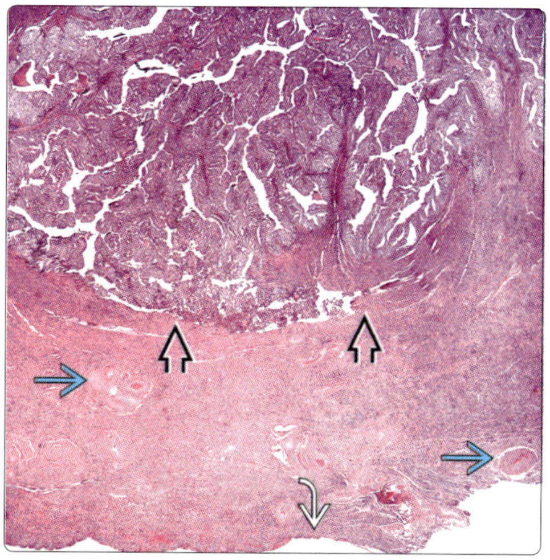

(Left) *Adenoma malignum-type invasion is the least common pattern of invasion in endometrioid adenocarcinoma. It is composed of scattered, benign-appearing glands that largely lack surrounding desmoplasia. These tumors may be impossible to identify grossly.* **(Right)** *A low-grade gland-forming carcinoma has a pushing growth pattern into the deep myometrium. Large caliber vessels are a helpful feature to identify deep myometrium in diffusely invasive cases. In this case, the serosal surface is present.*

Contents

(Left) *Low-power examination of microcystic, elongated, and fragmented glands (MELF) typically reveals small pockets of inflammation, myxoid change, or cystic change within the myometrium. The malignant epithelium is typically fragmented and cystic and is best identified at higher magnification.* **(Right)** *MELF myoinvasion is characterized by fragmented, eosinophilic epithelial cells, myxoid stroma, and an acute inflammatory response. It may often be seen deep to traditional forms of invasion.*

Microcystic, Elongated, and Fragmented Glands

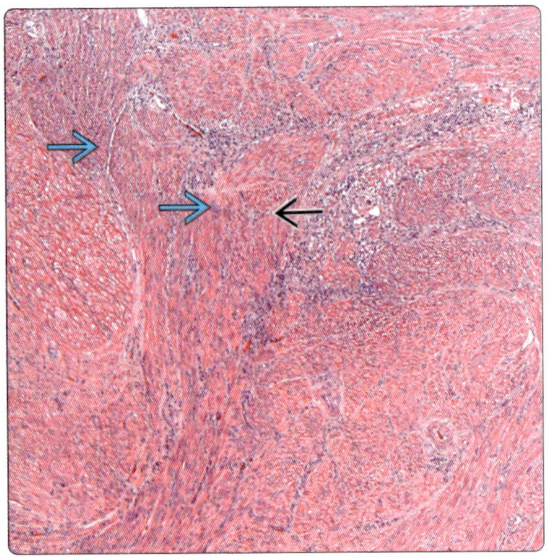

Microcystic, Elongated, and Fragmented Glands

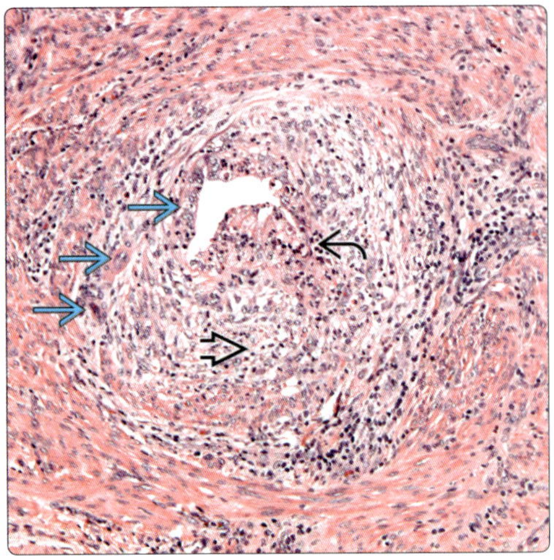

(Left) *Adenomyosis is identified by its smooth contour and occasionally by the condensation of endometrial stroma or benign glands at its periphery. In this example, adjacent invasive glands are bordered by a cuff of desmoplastic stroma, which may not always be present.* **(Right)** *Areas of adenomyosis-like invasion have smooth but irregular outer borders. Identification of focal desmoplasia, or singly dispersed glands, with no endometrial stroma are indicative of invasion.*

Invasion and Adenomyosis

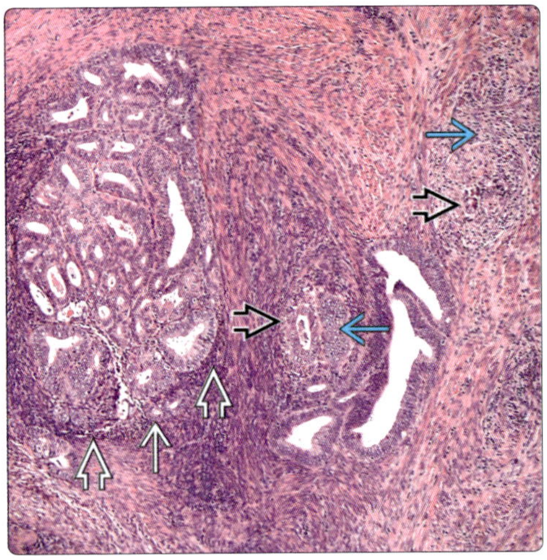

Adenomyosis-Like Invasion

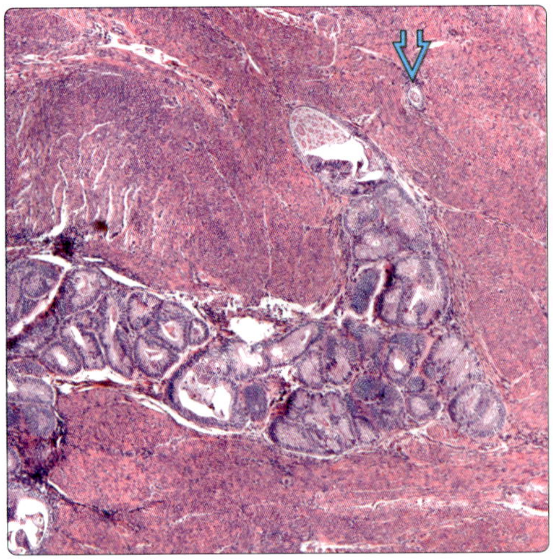

(Left) *One of the most common growth patterns of clear cell carcinoma is the tubulocystic pattern composed of dilated tubular spaces. The cells often have markedly pleomorphic nuclei with prominent nucleoli and areas of cytoplasmic clearing.* **(Right)** *A common growth pattern of clear cell carcinoma consists of papillae with hyalinized stromal cores. Note how the clear cells grow in a hobnail pattern from the papillae. Nuclear pleomorphism is present.*

Clear Cell Carcinoma: Tubulocystic Growth

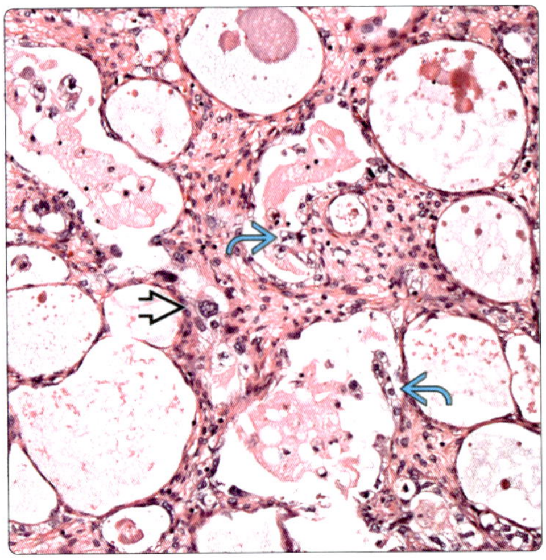

Clear Cell Carcinoma: Papillary Growth

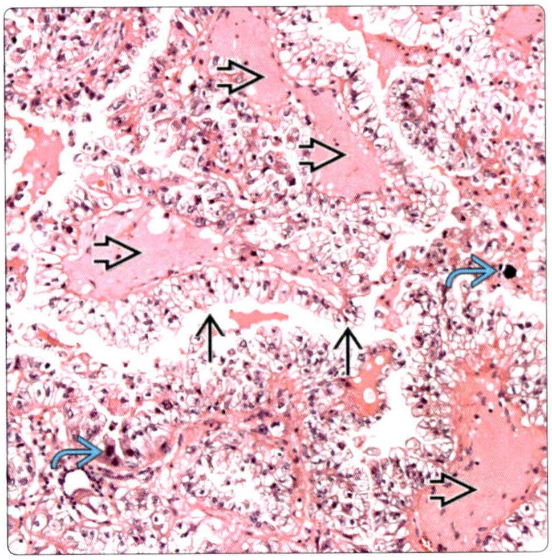

Serous Carcinoma: Cellular Features

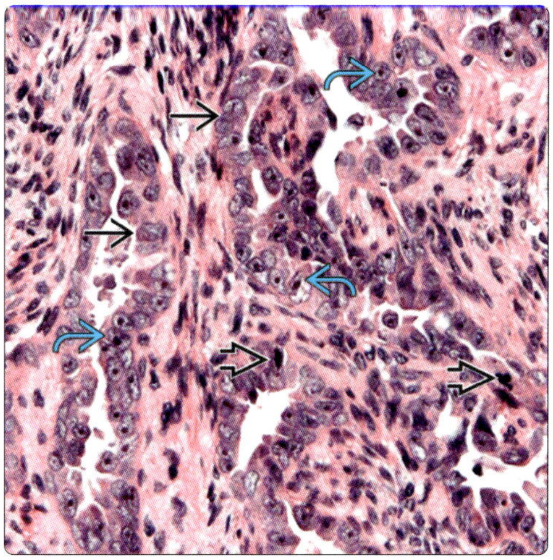

Serous Carcinoma: Architectural Pattern

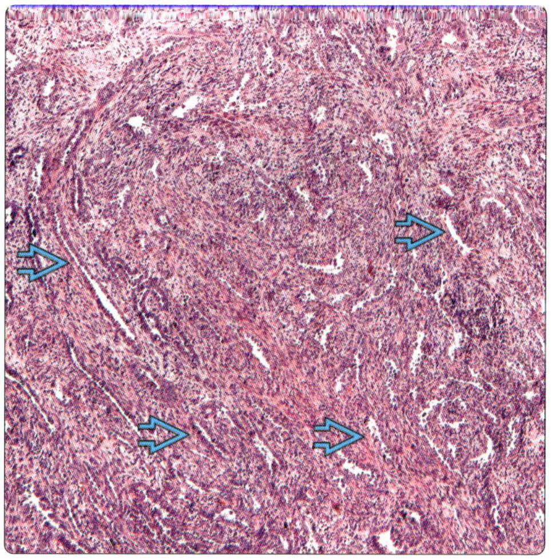

(Left) *Slit-like glands of serous carcinoma are often lined by a single layer of polygonal, eosinophilic tumor cells →. The nuclei are often enlarged, vesicular, and pleomorphic with prominent nucleoli →. Mitotic figures are typically abundant →.* **(Right)** *Serous carcinoma is remarkable for its slit-like glandular growth pattern → at low power. In contrast, endometrioid carcinoma forms round glands and the usual pattern of clear cell carcinoma consists of cysts and tubules.*

Endometrial Stromal Sarcoma

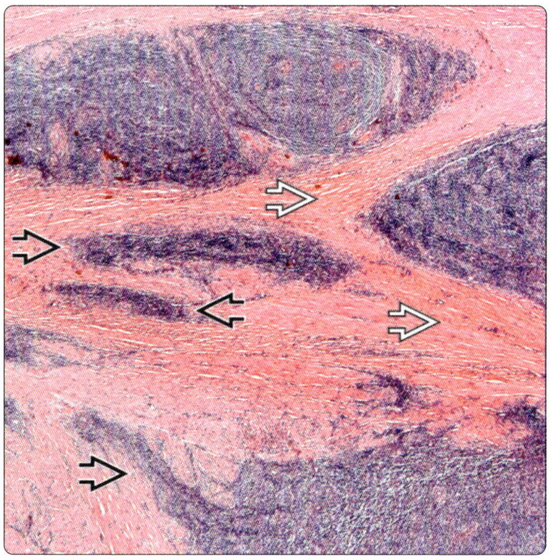

Endometrial Stromal Sarcoma

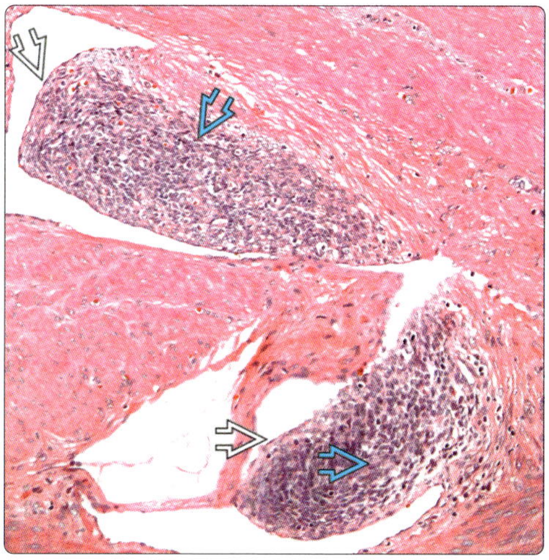

(Left) *Endometrial stromal sarcoma is best recognized at low power by its tongue-like growth pattern → that often extends deep into the myometrium →. However, high-grade solid carcinoma often lacks the tongue-like growth.* **(Right)** *Vascular invasion → is very common in low-grade endometrial stromal sarcoma. The tumor pushes into large vascular spaces, and the surface of the tumor is superficially lined by endothelium → that will be contiguous with the vessel wall.*

Carcinosarcoma

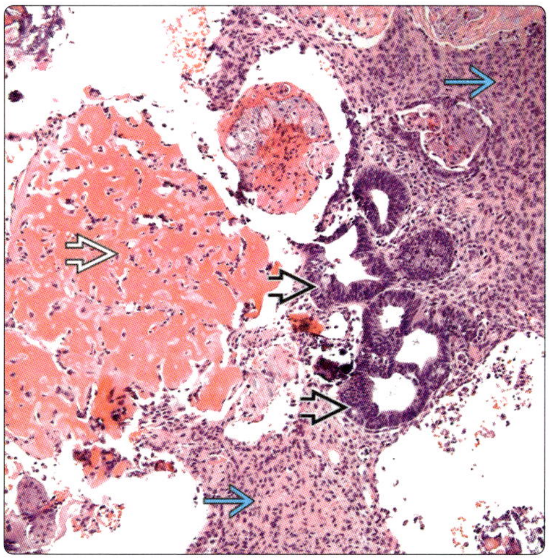

Endometrial Carcinoma: Extension to Cervix

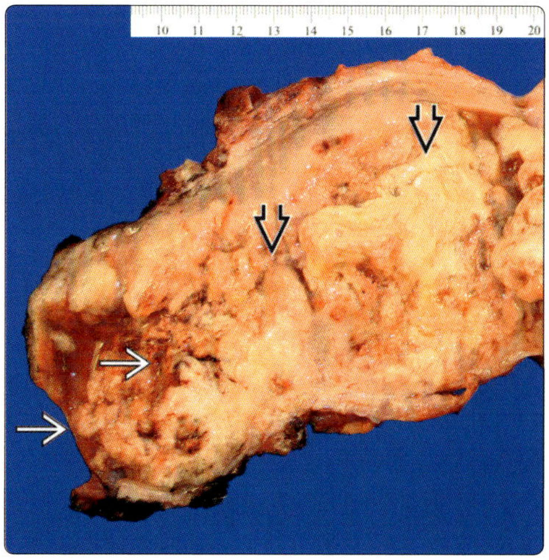

(Left) *Carcinosarcoma consists of a biphasic admixture of malignant epithelium → and malignant stromal components. The stromal component may be undifferentiated sarcoma → or may have cartilaginous, osseus →, skeletal muscle, or lipomatous differentiation.* **(Right)** *This extensive endometrial carcinoma fills the uterine cavity → and extends into the cervix →. Frozen section evaluation of the cervix to confirm involvement is important for staging.*

SURGICAL/CLINICAL CONSIDERATIONS

Goal of Consultation

- Document intrauterine pregnancy by detecting placental villi &/or recent implantation site

Change in Patient Management

- If intrauterine pregnancy is confirmed, patient can be managed conservatively
- If intrauterine pregnancy cannot be confirmed, patient should be closely monitored and surgery may be performed

Clinical Setting

- Pregnant women (elevated hCG) with vaginal bleeding or pelvic pain may have ectopic pregnancy
  - Ectopic pregnancy can result in fatal hemorrhage
- Transvaginal ultrasound and rapid hCG levels can be used to detect majority of ectopic pregnancies
  - In some cases, intrauterine pregnancy or tubal pregnancy is not evident by imaging techniques

SPECIMEN EVALUATION

Gross

- 3 different types of specimens
  - Endometrial curetting
  - Endometrial biopsy (Karmen biopsy)
  - Tissue from vaginal vault
- Rinse tissue free of blood with saline
- Float tissue in saline in Petri dish
- Examine tissue grossly or under dissecting microscope
  - Villi are white and spongy
    - Form complex architectural patterns with acute angle branching

Frozen Section

- Tissue most likely to contain villi is frozen
  - Confirmation of grossly evident villi by histologic examination is recommended
- Additional tissue should be frozen until villi are identified or until all tissue is examined
- If dissecting microscope is not available, areas of clotted blood should be frozen 1st as they are more likely to contain villi

MOST COMMON DIAGNOSES

Placental Villi

- Lined by circumferential cytotrophoblasts and outer layer of small syncytiotrophoblasts
  - Extravillous trophoblasts may be present
  - In 1st trimester, villi have irregular borders and are larger than more mature 2nd or 3rd trimester villi
- Stroma is hypocellular and small blood vessels may be present
  - Stroma becomes more cellular and number of vessels increases as pregnancy progresses
- In some cases of true intrauterine pregnancy, villi are not seen
  - Trophoblasts (of placental site or isolated) are necessary to confirm intrauterine pregnancy

Implantation Site

- Mononuclear intermediate trophoblasts
- Syncytiotrophoblasts
- Nitabuch fibrin (amorphous bright eosinophilic material)

Decidualized Endometrium

- Often develops in presence of ectopic pregnancy
  - Decidualized endometrium alone is not diagnostic of intrauterine pregnancy
- Stromal cells with abundant amphophilic cytoplasm and sheet-like architecture
  - Nuclei are often enlarged
  - Usually lacks Nitabuch fibrin

Placental Villi: Gross Appearance

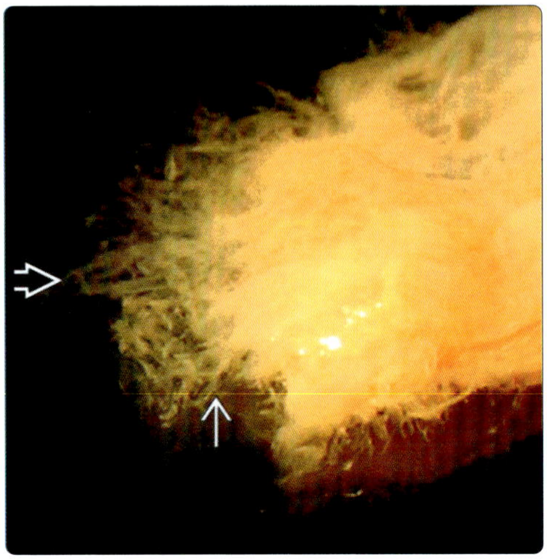

Placental Villi: Microscopic Appearance

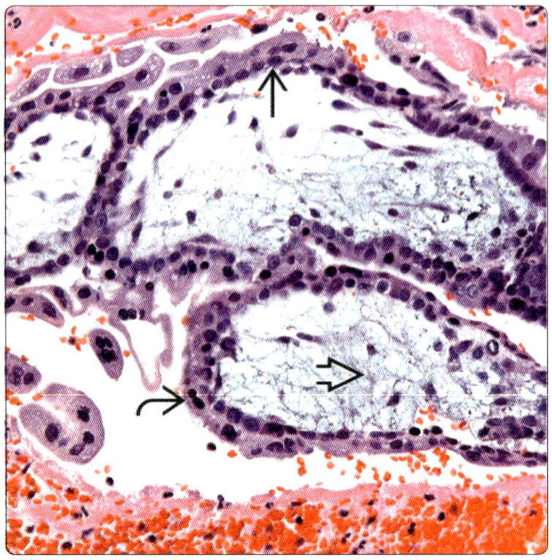

(Left) *Placental villi in saline can be identified using a dissecting microscope. The villi form small hair-like or tree-like structures* ➡ *with acute angle branching* ➡. *(Courtesy K. Sirois, BA.)* **(Right)** *Early villi from an intrauterine pregnancy display circumferential cytotrophoblasts* ⇨ *and small syncytiotrophoblasts* ⇨. *The stroma* ⇨ *is usually hypocellular and may have small blood vessels.*

Criteria for Diagnosis of Villi vs. Decidualized Endometrium

Type of Tissue	Color	Structure	Type of Branching	Consistency
Villi	White or pink	Complex 3D architecture (similar to shrub or sea anemone)	Acute angle branching	Springy, rapidly reexpands after being gently squeezed
Decidualized endometrium	Usually pink but may be white; more opaque than villi	Glandular and vascular structures; may mimic villi	Structures run in parallel and are not branched	Not springy

REPORTING

Frozen Section

- In presence of early, viable placental villi (± fresh implantation site), diagnosis of intrauterine pregnancy may be made
- Fresh implantation site, without placental villi, is highly suggestive of intrauterine pregnancy
  - Note should state that implantation site contamination from tubal pregnancy cannot be ruled out
- Rare scattered villi may represent contamination from ectopic site and should be communicated to consulting physician

Reliability

- In study in which all tissue was frozen, correct diagnosis was made in 93% of cases
  - Sensitivity: ~ 76%
  - Specificity: ~ 98%
  - Positive predictive value: ~ 95%
  - Negative predictive value: ~ 88%
- False-positive diagnosis of pregnancy
  - Rare (1-5%)
- False-negative diagnosis
  - 6-12% of cases
  - Diagnostic tissue is present in deeper levels of blocks used for frozen section
    - Frozen sections should be cut deep enough to have representative sections of all fragments

PITFALLS

Diagnosis Based Only on Gross Appearance

- Diagnosis of intrauterine pregnancy cannot be made by gross examination alone
- Microscopic examination by frozen section is mandatory

False-Positive Diagnosis of Intrauterine Pregnancy

- Contamination from ectopic pregnancy
  - Rare villi or scant implantation site may be present in endometrial curettings
- Changes due to previous pregnancy
  - Sclerotic villi can be mistaken for current, viable pregnancy
    - May be embedded in fibrin
    - Associated with chronic active inflammation
    - May be calcified
  - Remote (old) implantation site nodules can mimic fresh implantation site
    - Fewer extravillous trophoblasts are present
    - Fibrotic and hyalinized
- Decidualized endometrium
  - Reactive or degenerating decidua can mimic implantation site trophoblasts
- Endocervix
  - Fragments of edematous endocervix can simulate placental villi
  - Superficial lining cells are columnar and mucinous
  - Stroma has dense lymphoplasmacytic infiltrate

False Diagnosis of Inflammation

- Small fragments of embryonic mesenchyme resemble sheets of inflammation when viewed at low power

False Diagnosis of Malignancy

- Choriocarcinoma
  - Women may have markedly elevated hCG compared with normal gestations
    - Mitoses are typically frequent and may be atypical
    - Necrosis is often present
  - Early, proliferating, admixed intermediate trophoblasts, syncytiotrophoblasts, and cytotrophoblasts can mimic choriocarcinoma
    - Presence of villi excludes diagnosis of choriocarcinoma
- Clear cell adenocarcinoma or serous carcinoma
  - Arias-Stella effect: Normal but exaggerated change in endometrial tissue during pregnancy
    - Includes marked nuclear changes (increase in size, pleomorphism) and abundant cytoplasm with secretory changes (clear or eosinophilic)
    - May be mistaken for malignancy

False-Positive Diagnosis of Ectopic Pregnancy

- Making diagnosis of ectopic pregnancy based on lack of villi or implantation site
- Intrauterine pregnancy is not completely excluded even if diagnostic findings are not seen in endometrial curettings

SELECTED REFERENCES

1. Dhingra N et al: Arias-Stella reaction in upper genital tract in pregnant and non-pregnant women: a study of 120 randomly selected cases. Arch Gynecol Obstet. 276(1):47-52, 2007
2. Al-Ramahi M et al: The value of frozen section Pipelle endometrial biopsy as an outpatient procedure in the diagnosis of ectopic pregnancy. J Obstet Gynaecol. 26(1):63-5, 2006
3. Barak S et al: Frozen section examination of endometrial curettings in the diagnosis of ectopic pregnancy. Acta Obstet Gynecol Scand. 84(1):43-7, 2005
4. Heller DS et al: Reliability of frozen section of uterine curettings in evaluation of possible ectopic pregnancy. J Am Assoc Gynecol Laparosc. 7(4):519-22, 2000
5. Spandorfer SD et al: Efficacy of frozen-section evaluation of uterine curettings in the diagnosis of ectopic pregnancy. Am J Obstet Gynecol. 175(3 Pt 1):603-5, 1996

Contents

(Left) *Early placental villi are admixed with proliferating extravillous cytotrophoblasts and multinucleated syncytiotrophoblasts. The intermingling of the 2 types of extravillous trophoblasts can resemble choriocarcinoma. However, the presence of villi excludes this diagnosis.* **(Right)** *As the 1st trimester progresses, the villous stroma becomes more hypercellular, and the villi decrease in size. First trimester villi display irregular villous contours.*

Early Villi and Trophoblasts

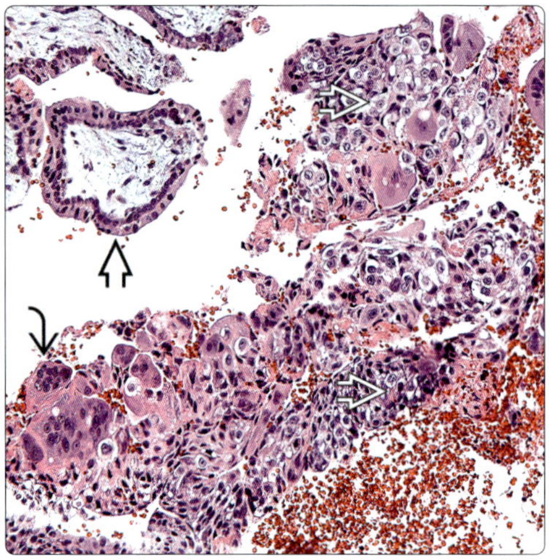

1st Trimester Villi

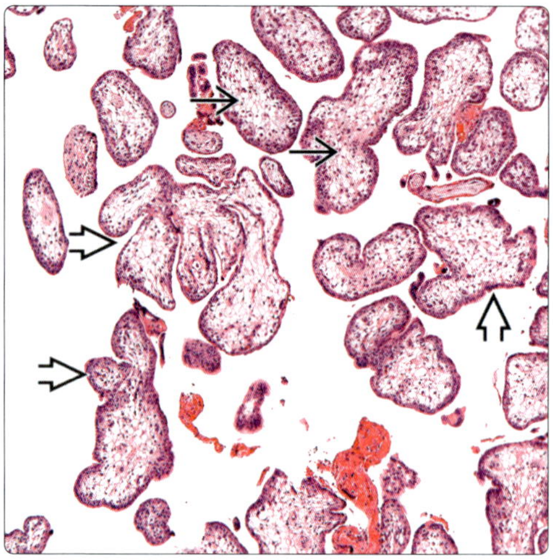

(Left) *Sclerotic villi encased in fibrin and acute and chronic inflammation may be seen in the setting of a recent prior pregnancy. By themselves, they are not diagnostic of a current, viable, intrauterine pregnancy. Note the associated calcifications.* **(Right)** *The endocervix, especially if edematous, may mimic placental villi. The presence of surface columnar, mucin-rich lining cells and a dense lymphoplasmacytic stromal infiltrate are features of villiform endocervical tissue.*

Sclerotic Villi

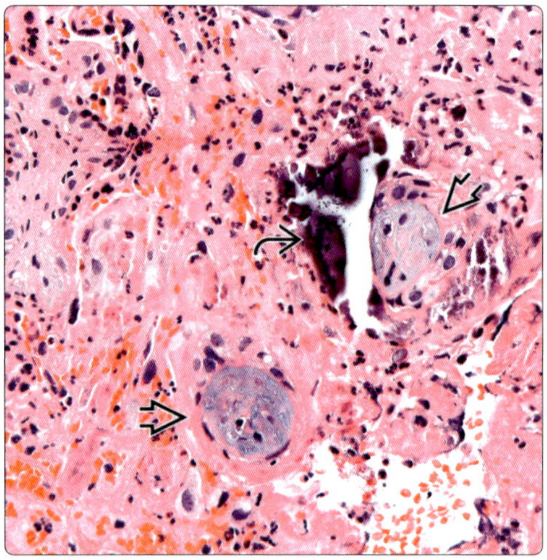

Endocervix

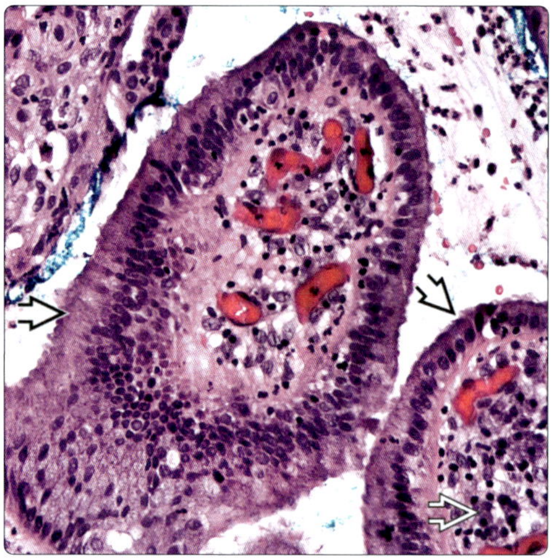

(Left) *Identification of a fresh implantation site is highly suggestive of an intrauterine pregnancy. The site should contain mononuclear intermediate trophoblasts, syncytiotrophoblasts, and Nitabuch fibrin, which is an amorphous, brightly eosinophilic material.* **(Right)** *A remote implantation site from a previous pregnancy must not be mistaken for fresh implantation. Old implantation sites contain fewer extravillous trophoblastic cells and are much more fibrotic and hyalinized.*

Fresh Implantation Site

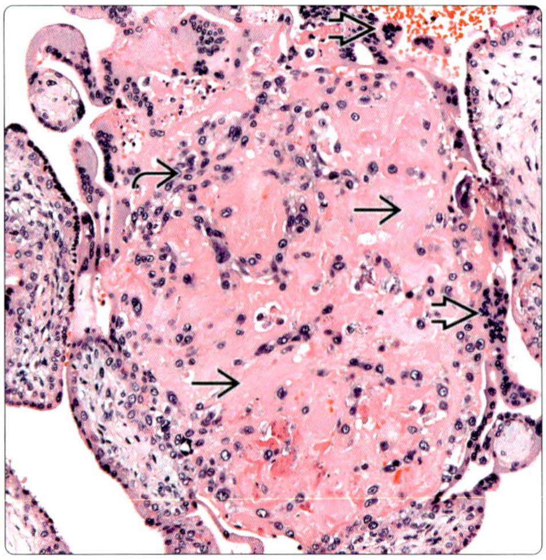

Remote Implantation Site

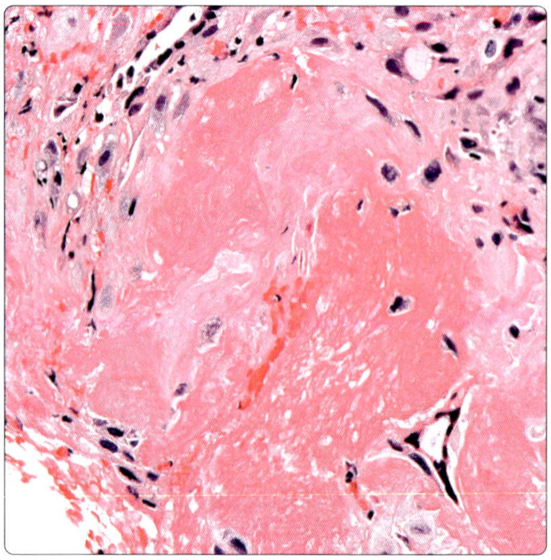

Contents

Decidualized Endometrium

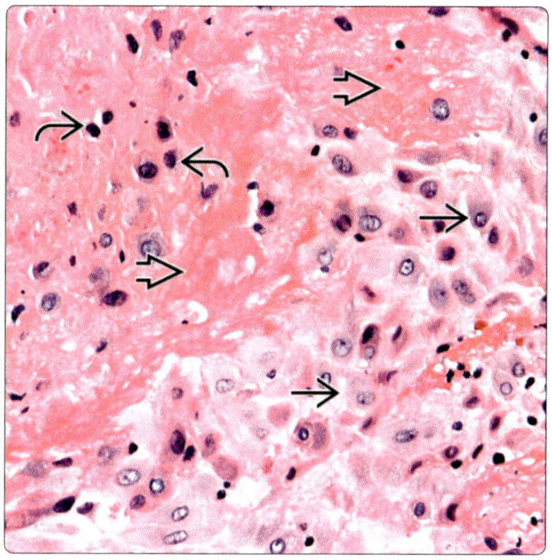

Reactive Decidua

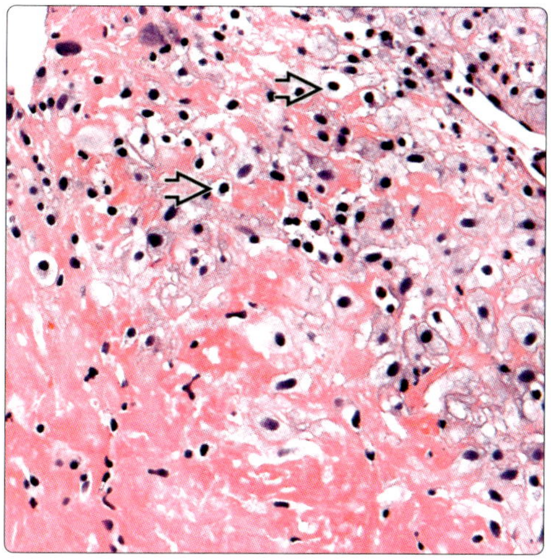

(Left) *Potential mimics of implantation site trophoblasts are decidualized endometrial stromal cells. Decidualized endometrial stroma is usually sheet-like and lacks the intervening Nitabuch fibrin (although it may be adjacent).* **(Right)** *Degenerating decidua is a mimic of extravillous trophoblasts. The degenerating cells may become pyknotic; however, they will maintain round, regular nuclear contours, helping to discriminate them from trophoblasts.*

Decidualized Endometrium

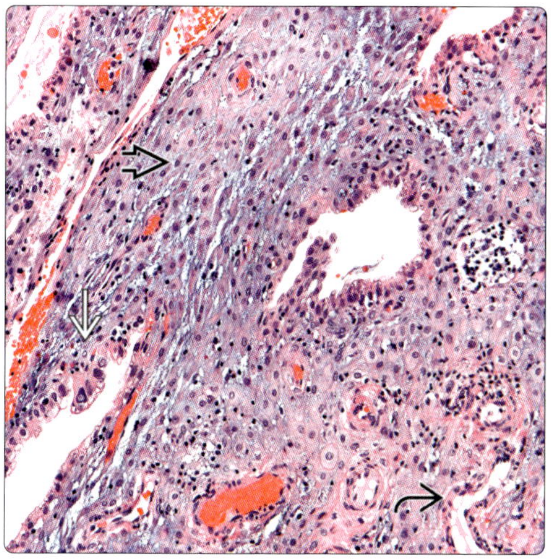

Arias-Stella Effect

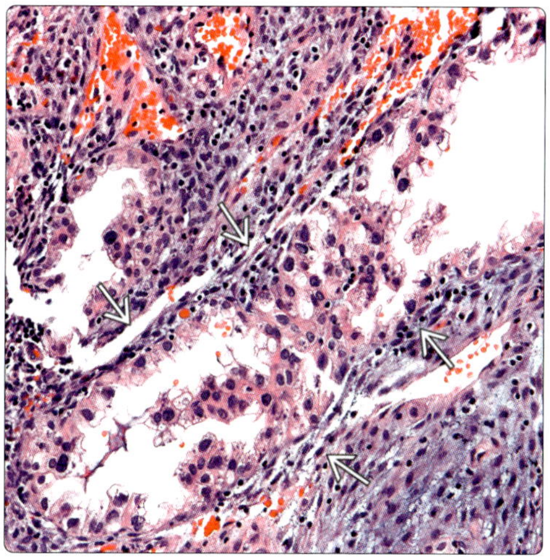

(Left) *Decidualized endometrium is composed of sheets of large, polygonal, eosinophilic stromal cells as well as endometrial glands. Arias-Stella effect may be present and should not be confused with malignancy.* **(Right)** *Arias-Stella effect includes hypersecretory change within endometrial glands. Nuclear enlargement, atypia, and hyperchromasia are usually present. The cytoplasm is frequently vacuolated and eosinophilic. These changes are not diagnostic of intrauterine pregnancy.*

Embryonic Tissue

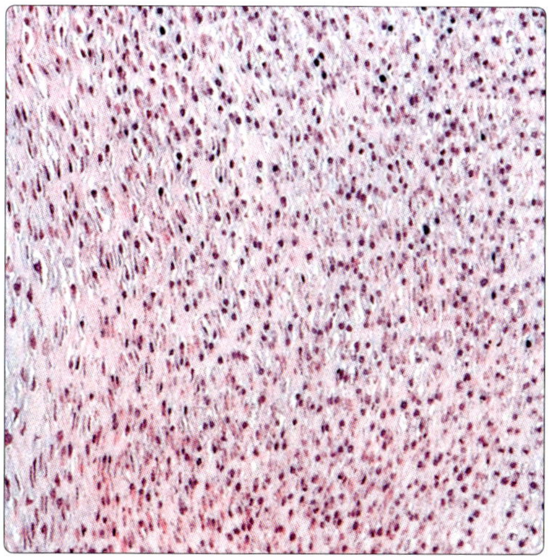

Embryonic Tissue

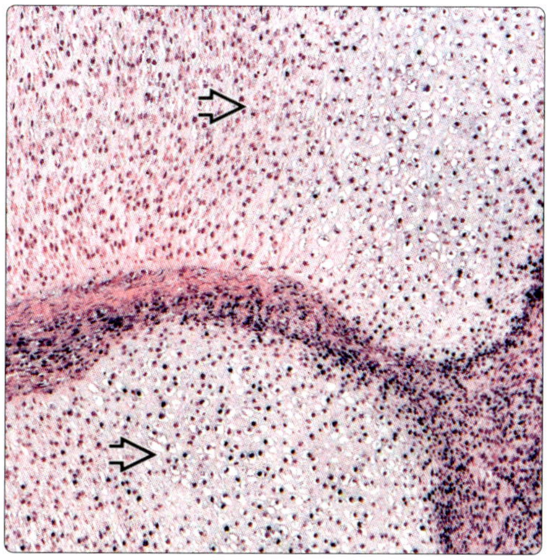

(Left) *Sheets of primitive-appearing mesenchymal tissue may represent an inadvertently sampled embryo. This tissue may be confused for inflammatory cells admixed with mucin.* **(Right)** *Embryonic mesenchyma may form "islands" or be arranged in a geographic pattern. An organized pattern of development can be helpful in differentiating primitive tissue from inflammation or other potential mimics.*

Contents

SURGICAL/CLINICAL CONSIDERATIONS

Goal of Consultation

- Evaluate presumed leiomyoma for malignancy

Change in Patient Management

- If malignancy is present, hysterectomy may be performed instead of myomectomy
- Additional biopsies of any suspicious peritoneal lesions may be performed

Clinical Setting

- Myomectomy may be performed for leiomyomas
  - Usually premenopausal women who wish to maintain their fertility
  - Diagnosis of malignancy will result in hysterectomy and should only be made when findings are definitive
- Morcellation of suspected leiomyomas has been used in past
  - ~ 1 of 352 women have unsuspected sarcoma
  - FDA recommended against this procedure for peri- or postmenopausal women in 2014
- Clinical features suspicious for malignancy include
  - Ultrasound showing irregular border or cystic areas
  - Large size and soft consistency
  - Rapid growth
    - However, leiomyomas can also exhibit rapid growth
  - Difficulty in removing lesion from uterine wall
    - This finding is more commonly associated with adenomyosis than malignancy

SPECIMEN EVALUATION

Gross

- Specimen usually consists of leiomyoma without surrounding tissue
- Specimen is serially sectioned at ~ 1-cm intervals
- Features suggestive of malignancy
  - Soft consistency
  - Necrosis or hemorrhage
  - Irregular or infiltrative borders
- Morcellated specimen may rarely be sent in laparoscopy bag
  - Fragments are carefully inspected for necrosis

Frozen Section

- Representative sections are selected from grossly suspicious lesions
- Areas suspicious for necrosis should be sampled along with adjacent viable tissue
  - Avoid sections that are entirely hemorrhagic or necrotic

MOST COMMON DIAGNOSES

Leiomyoma

- Grossly white, whorled, firm masses without necrosis or hemorrhage
  - Degenerative changes include carneous appearance (beefy red to brown discoloration) or cystic and mucoid areas
- Typically composed of intersecting fascicles of bland spindle cells with oval or cigar-shaped nuclei
- Conspicuous mitotic activity should be absent
  - Proliferation is stimulated by progesterone and mitoses may be increased during menstrual secretory phase
    - Postmenopausal hormone therapy or tamoxifen could also potentially increase mitotic rate
  - Proliferation can also be stimulated by recent surgical manipulation (i.e., curettage)
  - Atypical mitotic figures are indicative of at least atypical smooth muscle neoplasm
- Tumor cell necrosis should be absent
  - Hyaline or infarct-type necrosis may be present
  - Some drugs can cause necrosis &/or hemorrhage
    - Oral contraceptives, progestogens, tranexamic acid, gonadotropin-releasing hormone
  - Recent surgical manipulation can cause necrosis
- Nuclear atypia should be absent
  - Leiomyomas may have bizarre nuclei (also termed symplastic or pleomorphic leiomyomas)
    - Large cells with bizarrely shaped multilobated nuclei or polynucleation

Leiomyoma, Hysterectomy: Gross Appearance

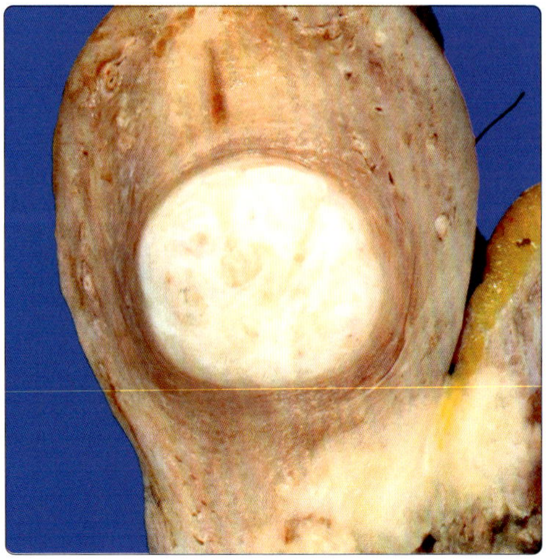

Leiomyomas, Myomectomy: Gross Appearance

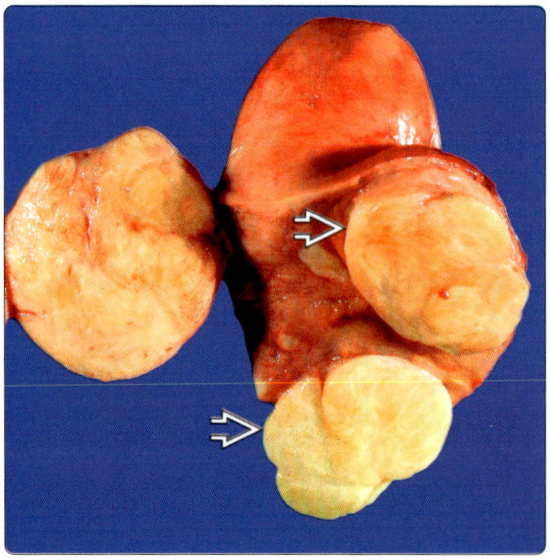

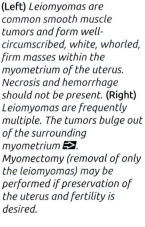

(Left) *Leiomyomas are common smooth muscle tumors and form well-circumscribed, white, whorled, firm masses within the myometrium of the uterus. Necrosis and hemorrhage should not be present.* **(Right)** *Leiomyomas are frequently multiple. The tumors bulge out of the surrounding myometrium* ➡*. Myomectomy (removal of only the leiomyomas) may be performed if preservation of the uterus and fertility is desired.*

- Some degenerating nuclei can mimic mitotic figures
- Usually scattered among cells without atypical nuclei
  - Nuclear atypia associated with carcinoma is usually present throughout tumor

Leiomyosarcoma

- Rare; only 1-3 women per 1,000 initially thought to have leiomyoma are diagnosed with sarcoma
  - Majority are > 40 years of age
  - More likely if mass has been increasing in size
- Gross features can identify lesions more likely to be malignant
  - Large size (> 10 cm)
  - Gray to yellow color
  - Soft consistency
  - Infiltrative borders
  - Necrosis (may be green in color) or hemorrhage
  - Vascular involvement
- Usually solitary or dominant lesion if there are other leiomyomas
- Majority are composed of spindle cells with nuclear pleomorphism
  - Epithelioid variants have rounded cells with moderate amounts of cytoplasm and may resemble carcinomas
  - Myxoid types have abundant myxoid stroma
  - However, leiomyomas can also have epithelioid or myxoid appearances
- 3 features are evaluated to determine malignancy
  - Coagulative necrosis
    - Presence of coagulative tumor cell necrosis in isolation is highly suggestive of leiomyosarcoma
  - Increased mitotic activity
    - Spindle cell: > 10 mitoses per 10 HPF
    - Myxoid: ≥ 2 per 10 HPF
    - Epithelioid: > 5 per 10 HPF (if moderate to severe atypia)
  - Nuclear atypia
    - Assessed at low power (10x)
    - Usually present throughout malignant tumors rather than focal
- Leiomyosarcoma can be diagnosed if following features are present
  - Necrosis and increased mitotic rate (± nuclear atypia)
  - Increased mitotic rate combined with severe, diffuse nuclear atypia (± necrosis)
- Report as "atypical smooth muscle neoplasm, final classification deferred to permanent sections" if atypical features are present but are insufficient for diagnosis of leiomyosarcoma

Adenomatoid Tumor

- Benign tumor of mesothelial cells
  - Often incidental finding
- Poorly circumscribed soft mass within myometrium
  - Usually located near serosal surface
- Solid, cystic, and angiomatoid patterns
  - Nuclear atypia and mitoses should be absent

Adenomyosis/Adenomyoma

- Benign endometrial glands are embedded within myometrium
- Smooth muscle appears thickened with coarse trabeculations, may be mass-forming (adenomyoma)
- Small punctate hemorrhage can be present

Endometrial Stromal Sarcoma

- Tumor can be diffusely infiltrative
- Lymphovascular invasion may appear as worm-like masses within myometrium
- Adjacent abdominal and pelvic tissues may be invaded

Intravenous Leiomyomatosis

- Surgeon may find pelvic veins are filled with worm-like plugs of tumor
- Microscopically have same benign appearance as leiomyomas

Diffuse Leiomyomatosis

- Very rare (< 20 cases)
- Entire uterus is replaced by confluent nodules of smooth muscle

REPORTING

Frozen Section

- Report "leiomyoma" if there are no atypical nuclei, necrosis, or increased mitotic activity
- Report "smooth muscle neoplasm, favor leiomyosarcoma, final diagnosis deferred to permanent sections" if sufficient features are present for diagnosis of malignancy
  - Atypical features present are stated
- Report "atypical smooth muscle neoplasm, final diagnosis deferred to permanent sections" if atypical features are present but insufficient for malignancy
  - Additional frozen sections may be helpful
  - Atypical features present are stated
- Report "poorly differentiated spindle cell neoplasm, final diagnosis deferred to permanent sections" if lesion is poorly differentiated and does not resemble leiomyosarcoma

PITFALLS

Nonneoplastic Atypical Features

- Benign alterations in leiomyomas due to surgery or drug use can raise concern for malignancy
  - Can cause increased mitoses and necrosis
- Previous uterine artery embolization procedures may cause ischemic degeneration, necrosis, and nuclear atypia

Fragmented Specimen

- Fragmented and morcellated specimens should be thoroughly evaluated grossly for necrosis
  - Definite diagnosis should be avoided unless gross and microscopic features are definitive

SELECTED REFERENCES

1. Taylan E et al: Contained morcellation: review of current methods and future directions. Front Surg. 4:15, 2017
2. Cui RR et al: Risk of occult uterine sarcoma in presumed uterine fibroids. Clin Obstet Gynecol. 59(1):103-18, 2016
3. Ip PP et al: Uterine smooth muscle tumors other than the ordinary leiomyomas and leiomyosarcomas: a review of selected variants with emphasis on recent advances and unusual morphology that may cause concern for malignancy. Adv Anat Pathol. 17(2):91-112, 2010

(**Left**) *This leiomyoma shows hydropic degeneration that can occur in large lesions. The soft, cystic changes ➡, edema, and mottled color should not be mistaken for malignancy. Normal smooth muscle ➡ is usually present.* (**Right**) *Conventional leiomyomas are composed of varying amounts of bland, spindled cells that are arranged in intersecting fascicles. Obvious nuclear atypia should be absent at low power.*

Leiomyoma With Cystic Degeneration: Gross Appearance

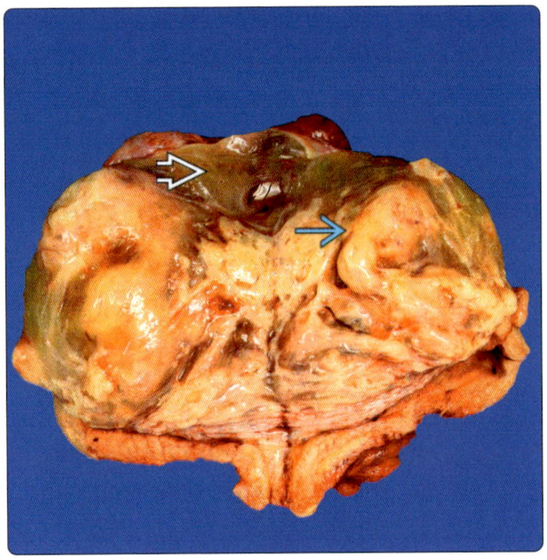

Leiomyoma

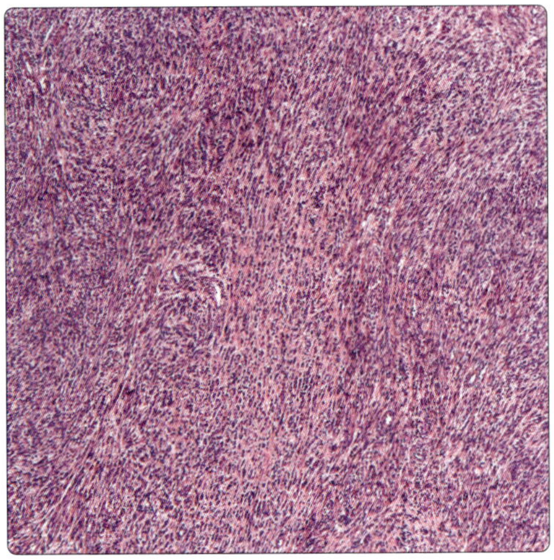

(**Left**) *Hemorrhagic infarction has produced a beefy appearance (so-called red degeneration) in this leiomyoma. This is typically seen in pregnant women. (From DP: Gynecological.)* (**Right**) *Occasionally, the nuclei in a cellular leiomyoma may palisade ➡ resembling the pattern seen in neural tumors. Adjacent areas usually show the conventional appearance of leiomyoma.*

Leiomyoma, Hemorrhagic Infarction: Gross Appearance

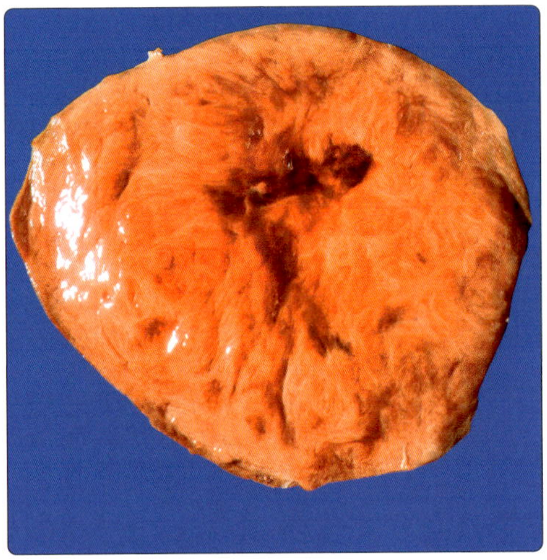

Neurilemmoma-Like Leiomyoma

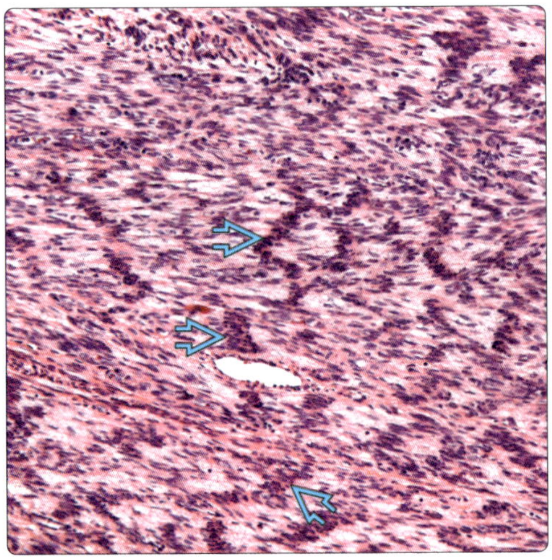

(**Left**) *Some leiomyomas undergo extensive infarction with secondary hemorrhage and necrosis, which may cause concern for sarcoma on gross inspection. (From DP: Gynecological.)* (**Right**) *In medically embolized leiomyomas, degenerative changes and infarction may be extensive ➡. Embolization material may be identified in vascular spaces ➡.*

Leiomyoma, Massive Infarction: Gross Appearance

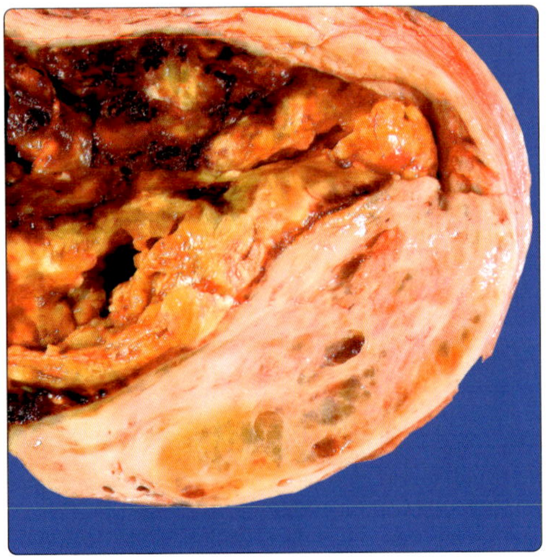

Leiomyoma: Embolization Material

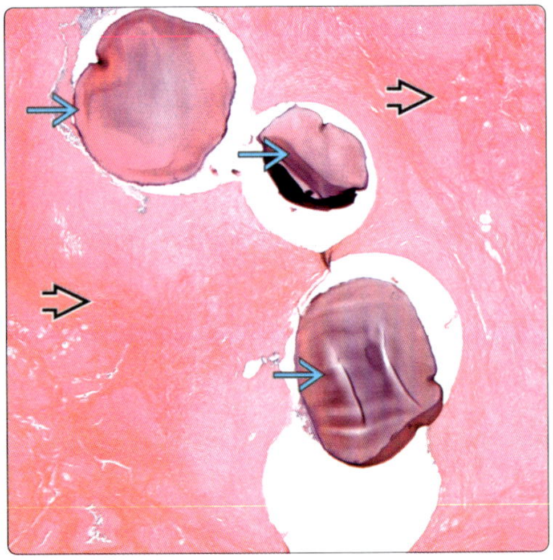

Highly Cellular Leiomyoma: Gross Appearance

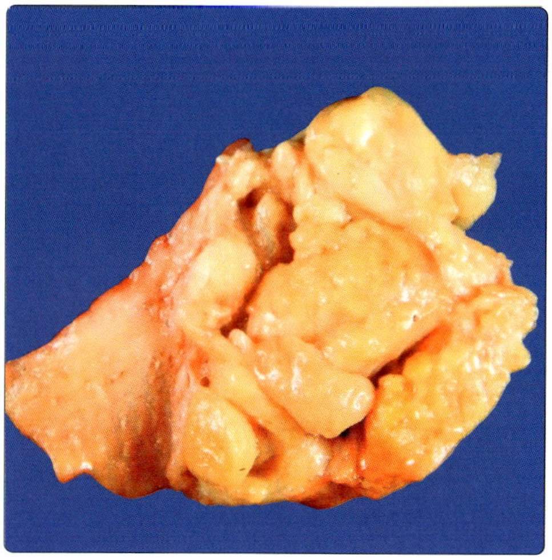

Highly Cellular Leiomyoma

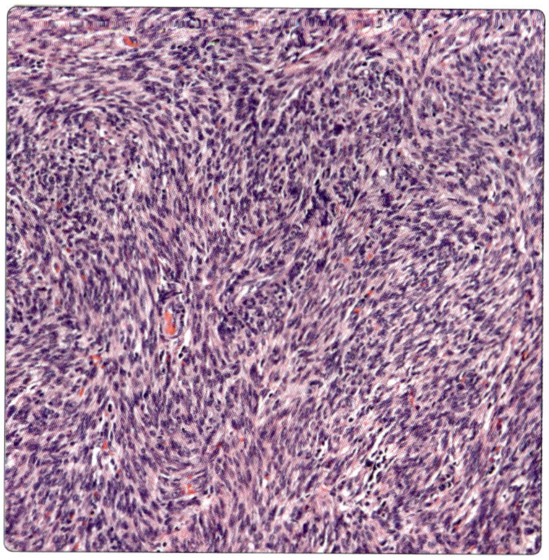

(Left) *A highly cellular leiomyoma often has a soft and tan to yellow cut surface when compared to conventional leiomyomas, which have a firm white whorled appearance. (From DP: Gynecological.)* **(Right)** *Markedly increased cellularity may be seen in some leiomyomas. The nuclei lack significant atypia and necrosis should be absent, as in this example. The mitotic count per HPF may be elevated, which can occur due to the increase in nuclear density.*

Hydropic Leiomyoma: Gross Appearance

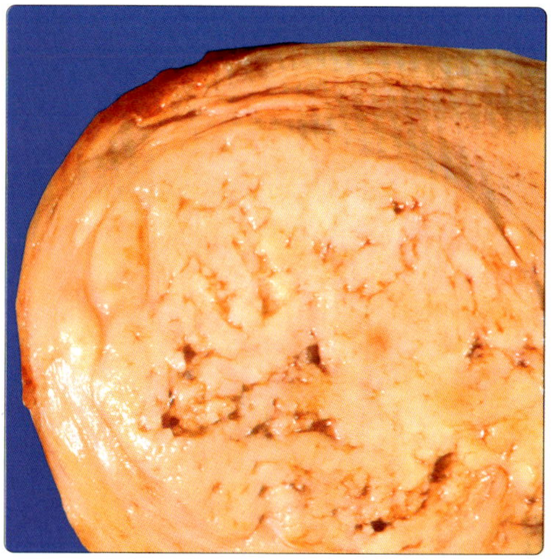

Leiomyoma: Hydropic Degeneration

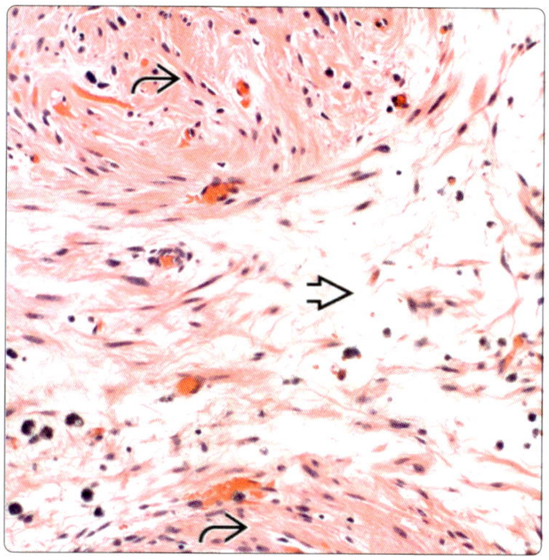

(Left) *A leiomyoma with hydropic change often shows a perinodular growth of the tumor on gross and microscopic examination due to abundant edema. Edema can be distinguished from myxoid change by "squeezing" the tumor. This extrudes abundant watery fluid. (From DP: Gynecological.)* **(Right)** *The edema fluid in hydropic degeneration in a leiomyoma is clear and appears to separate bundles of smooth muscle fibers. These changes must not be mistaken for myxoid change or necrosis.*

Leiomyoma: Hydropic Degeneration

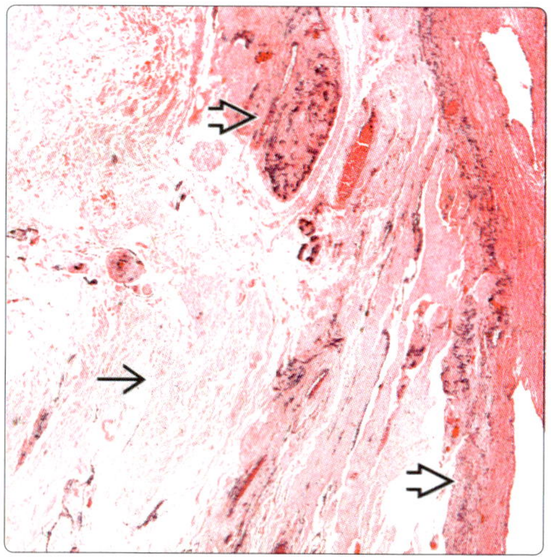

Leiomyosarcoma: Myxoid Change

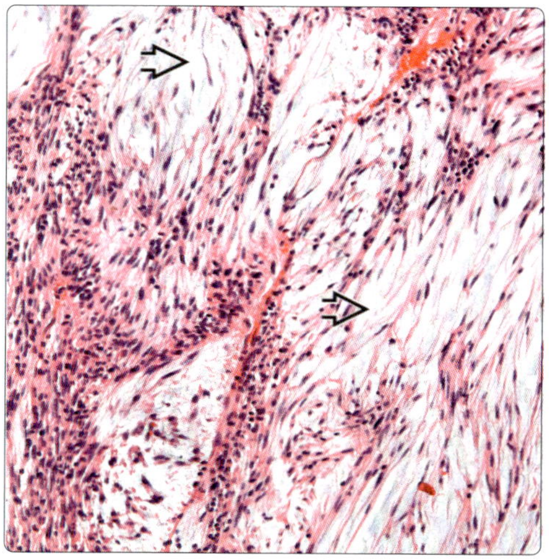

(Left) *Hydropic degeneration within a leiomyoma may mimic necrosis. Fascicles of normal smooth muscle alternate with edema fluid. Edema fluid is often clear to pink as opposed to myxoid change, which appears basophilic. No nuclear debris is present.* **(Right)** *Myxoid change is characteristic of a myxoid leiomyosarcoma. Myxoid extracellular matrix appears basophilic as opposed to edema fluid. In myxoid lesions, a much lower threshold of mitotic activity (≥ 2 mitoses per 10 HPF) and nuclear atypia are required.*

(Left) *Myxoid leiomyosarcoma often shows a gelatinous and shiny cut surface and may be deceptively well circumscribed from the surrounding myometrium ➡. (From DP: Gynecological.)* **(Right)** *A leiomyosarcoma may have a fleshy consistency ➡ with areas of necrosis ➡ and hemorrhage ➡. Additionally, an irregular infiltrative border ➡ is present. These gross features are highly suggestive of leiomyosarcoma.*

Myxoid Leiomyosarcoma: Gross Appearance

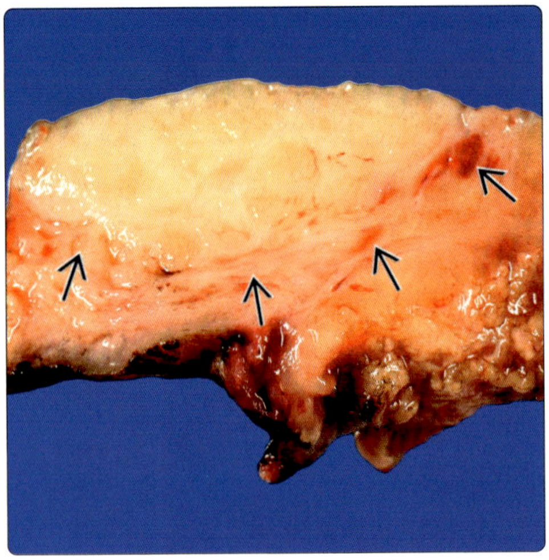

Leiomyosarcoma: Gross Appearance

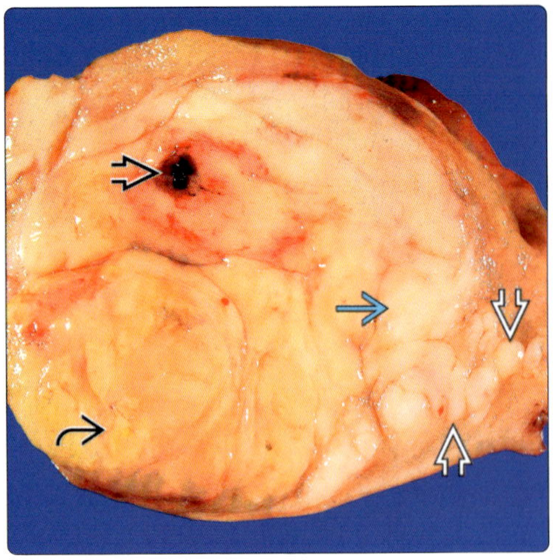

(Left) *A highly cellular histologic appearance should prompt the search for atypia (using a 10x objective, so-called low-power atypia) as well as mitotic activity to help classify this lesion as a leiomyosarcoma.* **(Right)** *True tumor cell necrosis has an abrupt interface ➡ with the adjacent viable atypical tumor cells ➡ and is highly suggestive of malignancy. Atypical degenerating cells and nuclear fragments ➡ are often present in the zones of necrosis and are a helpful diagnostic clue.*

Leiomyosarcoma: Increased Cellularity

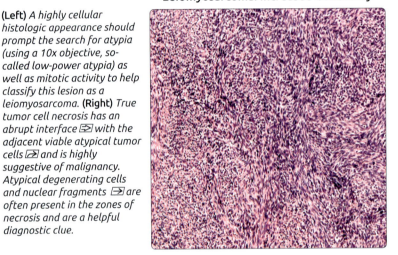

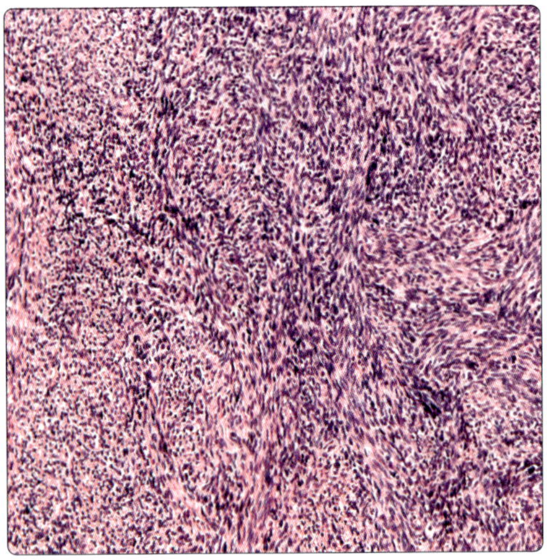

Leiomyosarcoma: Tumor Cell Necrosis

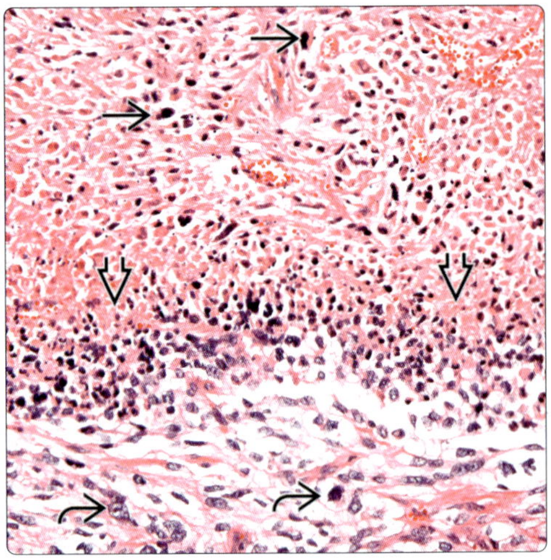

(Left) *Within zones of coagulative tumor cell necrosis, large, atypical, "ghost" cells ➡ may be identified. The finding of pleomorphic and necrotic cells can be helpful in distinguishing true coagulative necrosis in a leiomyosarcoma from degenerative necrosis in a leiomyoma.* **(Right)** *Occasional leiomyosarcomas have an epithelioid appearance instead of the traditional spindle cell morphology. They are composed of rounded cells ➡ with ample, eosinophilic cytoplasm, findings that may mimic a carcinoma.*

Leiomyosarcoma: Tumor Cell Necrosis

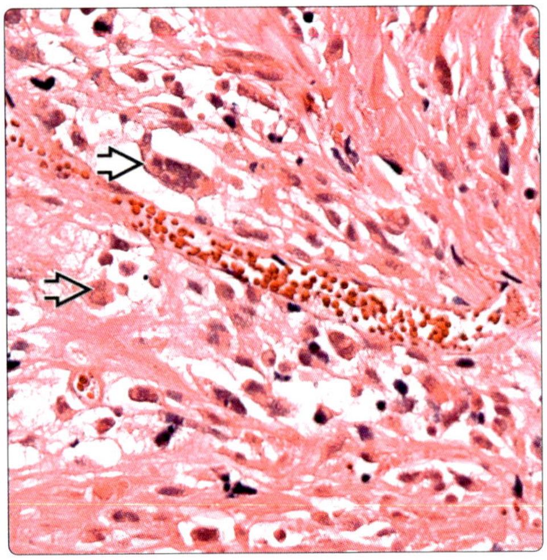

Epithelioid Leiomyosarcoma

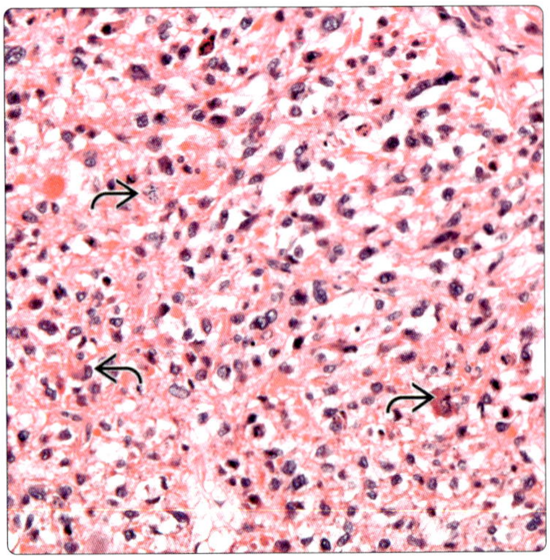

Leiomyosarcoma: Low-Power Atypia

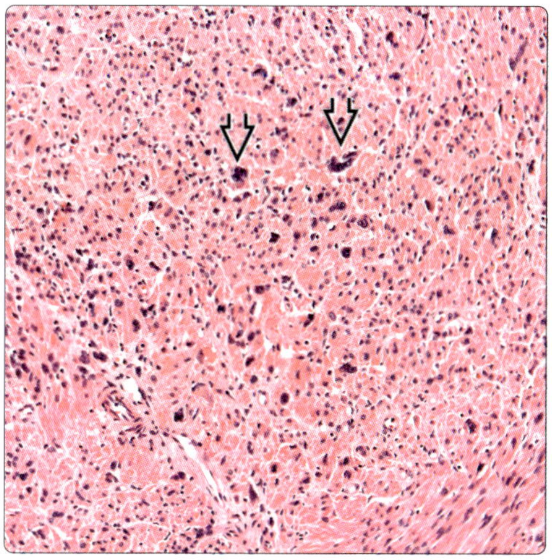

Leiomyosarcoma: Increased Mitotic Activity

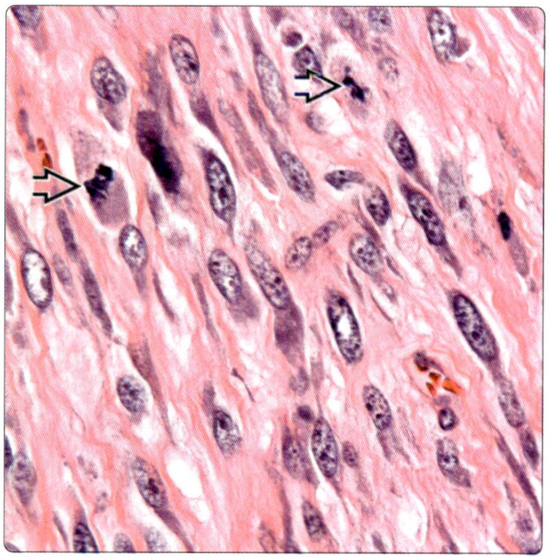

(Left) *Nuclear atypia ⇨, identifiable at low power (10x), is 1 of the 3 criteria used to diagnose leiomyosarcoma. Atypical smooth muscle tumors (not leiomyosarcoma) may display focal atypia, whereas diffuse atypia is suggestive of a malignant tumor.* **(Right)** *Mitotic figures ⇨ may be identified in any smooth muscle tumor. In the absence of nuclear atypia and necrosis, a diagnosis of "mitotically active leiomyoma" may be considered. Mitotic counts > 15 may indicate a potentially malignant tumor.*

Leiomyosarcoma: Atypical Mitotic Figure

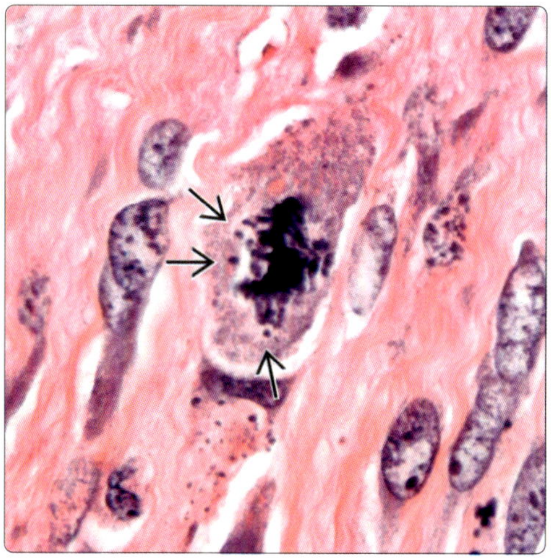

Endometrial Stromal Sarcoma: Gross Appearance

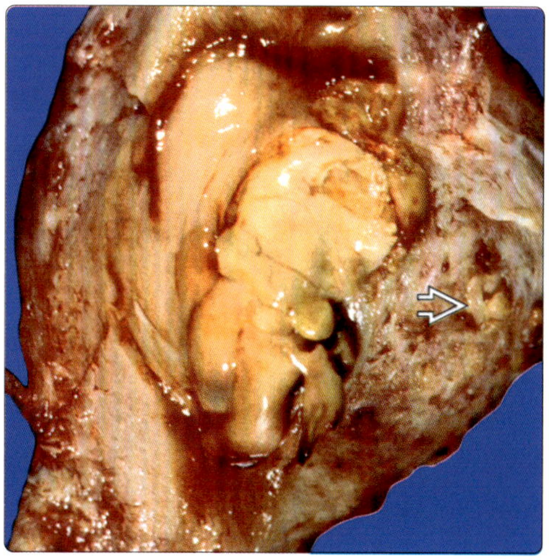

(Left) *The presence of atypical mitotic figures is indicative of genomic instability and may be a sign of malignancy. In this cell, lagging chromosomes ➔ are present around the periphery of the mitotic figure.* **(Right)** *Endometrial stromal sarcoma forms a multinodular, poorly defined mass with a tan-yellow and soft cut surface. Notice the presence of scattered worm-like plugs of tumor within myometrial vessels ➡. (From DP: Gynecological.)*

Intravenous Leiomyomatosis: Gross Appearance

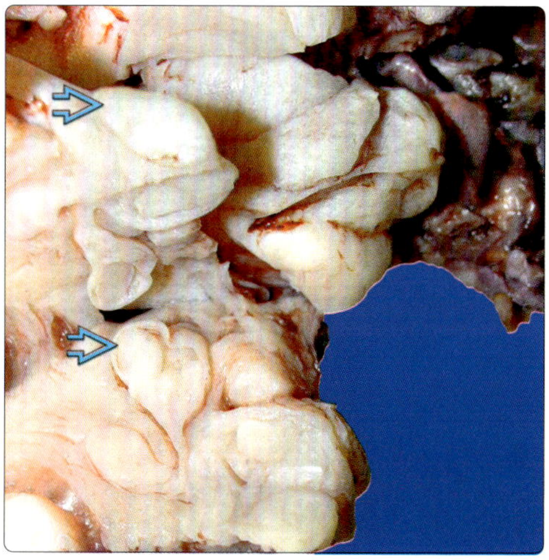

Adenomatoid Tumor

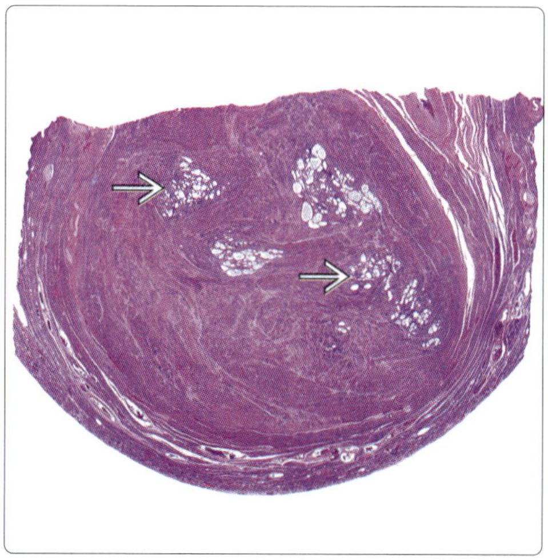

(Left) *Intravenous leiomyomatosis characteristically shows multiple worm-like plugs of tumor distending vascular spaces outside of leiomyomas ⇨. The proliferations have a white and bulging cut surface. (From DP: Gynecological.)* **(Right)** *This adenomatoid tumor is in its characteristic subserosal localization and consists of a neoplastic proliferation with small cystic spaces ➡ associated with prominent muscle hypertrophy mimicking a smooth muscle tumor. (From DP: Gynecological.)*

SURGICAL/CLINICAL CONSIDERATIONS

Goal of Consultation

- Determine if margins are involved by neoplastic or dysplastic process

Change in Patient Management

- Additional tissue will be taken to achieve tumor-free margins
- Narrow margins may be necessary for large lesions or lesions located near urethra, clitoris, or anus to avoid disfiguring surgery

Clinical Setting

- Margin evaluation is usually performed for squamous cell carcinoma (SCC) and rare cases of mesenchymal neoplasms with close margins
- Evaluation for other lesions is generally contraindicated
  - Paget disease and vulvar intraepithelial neoplasia
    - Often multifocal with irregular borders
  - Melanoma
    - Wide margins are preferable, making frozen section evaluation unnecessary

SPECIMEN EVALUATION

Gross

- Specimen orientation is identified and margins inked to maintain orientation
  - Diagrams are helpful to record features of complicated specimens
- All gross lesions are identified and distance to each margin recorded
  - If no gross lesion is present, surgeon may be able to identify closest margin of concern

Frozen Section

- A section to evaluate a close margin is taken perpendicular to gross lesion
- Tissue is oriented on chuck such that inked margin is clearly seen

MOST COMMON DIAGNOSES

Squamous Cell Carcinoma (SCC)

- Raised white mass, often with ulcerated center
  - Also papillary and endophytic growth patterns
- Consists of irregularly shaped nests of squamous epithelium in stroma below epithelial basal layer
  - Inverse maturation, presenting as increased eosinophilia, is a common feature

Vulvar Intraepithelial Neoplasia (VIN)

- Maculopapular red, brown, or white lesion(s)
- Dysplasia is classified as 2 types
  - Classic type
    - Low-grade dysplasia (condyloma): Mild increase in thickness of basal layer and cytopathic effect (e.g., binucleation, nuclear enlargement, and perinuclear halo formation)
    - High-grade dysplasia: Full-thickness loss of maturation with small cells and scant cytoplasm
  - Differentiated type: Severe basal atypia, abnormal keratinization, and maturation (differentiation) of upper layers of epidermis

REPORTING

Frozen Section

- Presence of SCC &/or dysplasia at margin, or distance from margin, is reported
- Severity of dysplasia (low grade or high grade)

PITFALL

Cautery Artifact

- Cautery can mimic high-grade dysplasia

SELECTED REFERENCES

1. Horn LC et al: Frozen section analysis of vulvectomy specimens: results of a 5-year study period. Int J Gynecol Pathol. 29(2):165-72, 2010
2. Baker P et al: A practical approach to intraoperative consultation in gynecological pathology. Int J Gynecol Pathol. 27(3):353-65, 2008

(Left) *The typical appearance of squamous cell carcinoma (SCC) is that of hypereosinophilic nests with irregular borders ➡ invading the dermis. Intense inflammation ➡ and desmoplasia may be present.* **(Right)** *Early invasive SCC can be identified by irregularly shaped nests surrounded by a desmoplastic response ➡. The cytoplasm is often hypereosinophilic ➡ (inverse maturation).*

Invasive Squamous Cell Carcinoma

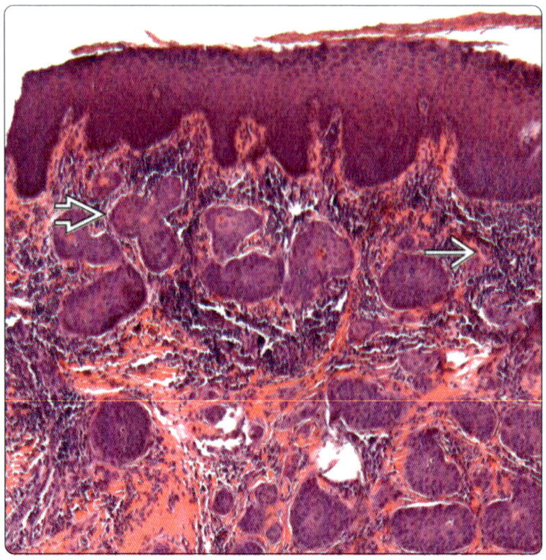

Invasive Squamous Cell Carcinoma

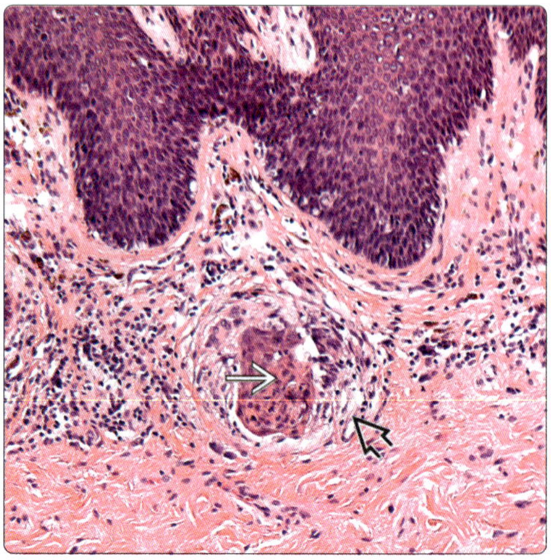

Low-Grade Squamous Intraepithelial Lesion

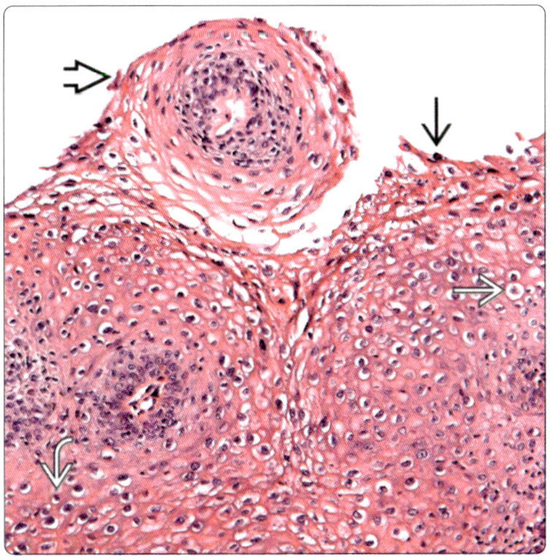

High-Grade Squamous Intraepithelial Lesion: Classic VIN

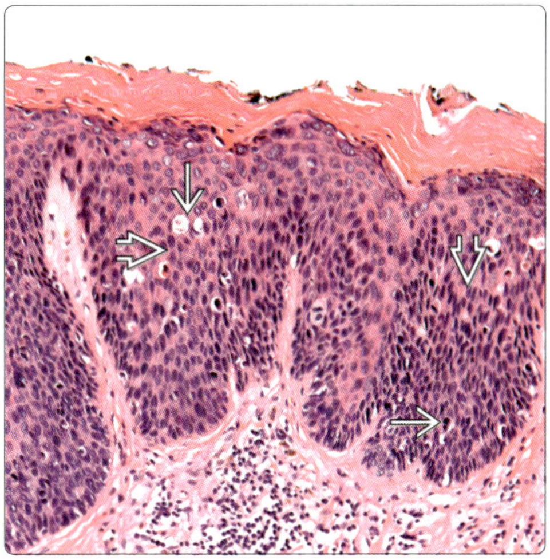

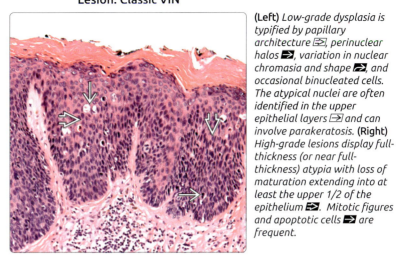

(Left) *Low-grade dysplasia is typified by papillary architecture, perinuclear halos, variation in nuclear chromasia and shape, and occasional binucleated cells. The atypical nuclei are often identified in the upper epithelial layers and can involve parakeratosis.* **(Right)** *High-grade lesions display full-thickness (or near full-thickness) atypia with loss of maturation extending into at least the upper 1/2 of the epithelium. Mitotic figures and apoptotic cells are frequent.*

High-Grade Dysplasia: Margin Involvement

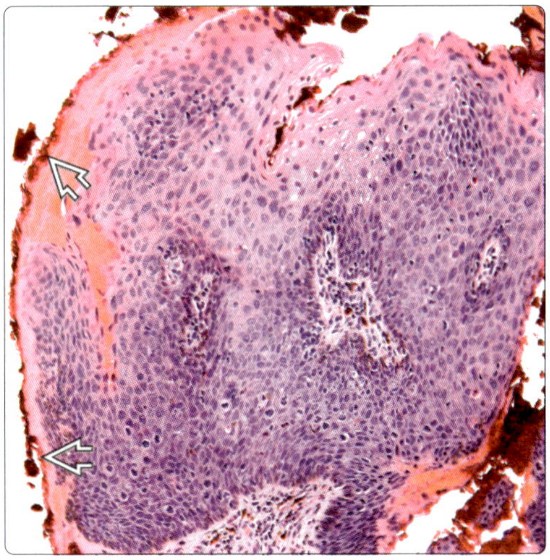

Differentiated Vulvar Intraepithelial Neoplasia

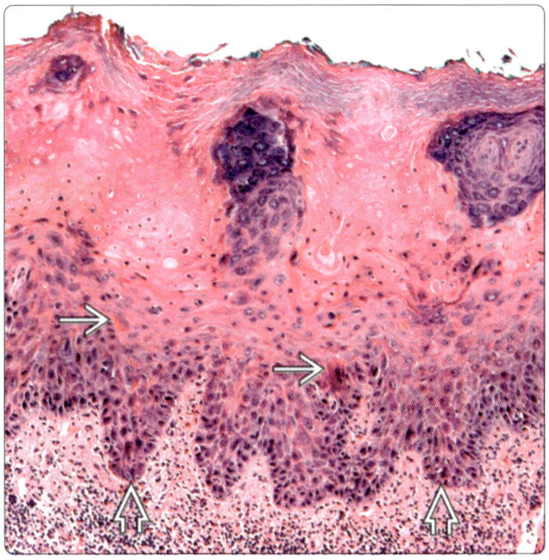

(Left) *The presence of low- or high-grade dysplasia at the margin is reported. Careful inking is helpful in identifying the true specimen edge. In this example, high-grade dysplasia is transected at the inked margin.* **(Right)** *Differentiated vulvar intraepithelial neoplasia is another form of high-grade dysplasia. It can be identified by severe basal atypia, abnormal keratinization with dyskeratotic cells, and superficial maturation. It is often associated with inflammatory dermatologic conditions.*

Paget Disease

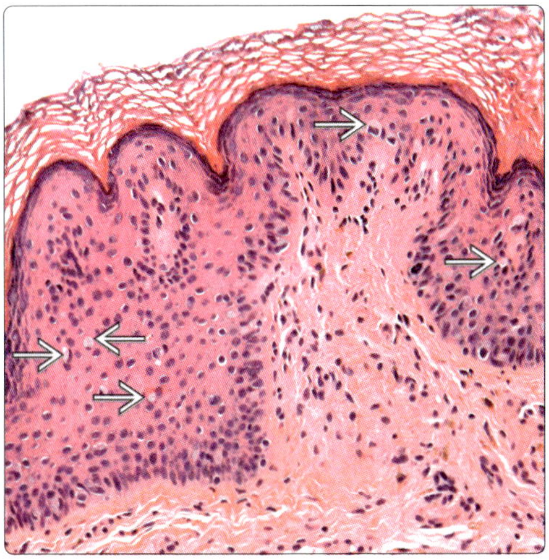

Melanoma In Situ

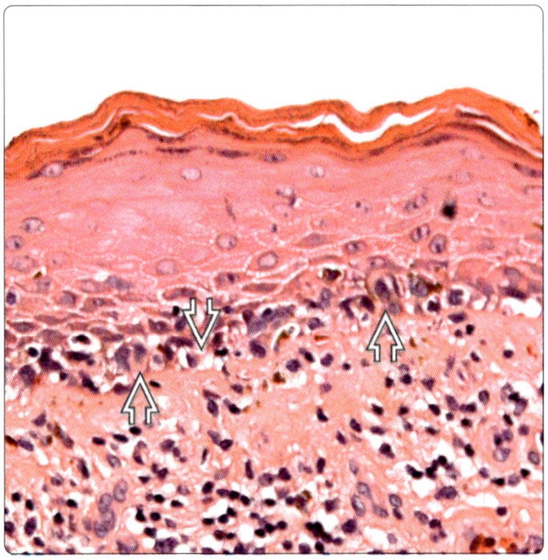

(Left) *Although it is generally contraindicated, frozen section evaluation of Paget disease may be requested. Pale gray, mucin-containing cells "floating upward" in an otherwise normal epidermis may be the only histologic feature. Margin involvement is often very subtle.* **(Right)** *In general, frozen section should not be used to evaluate margins on melanomas but may be requested when wide margins cannot be obtained. The presence of atypical melanocytes may be difficult to detect.*

INDEX

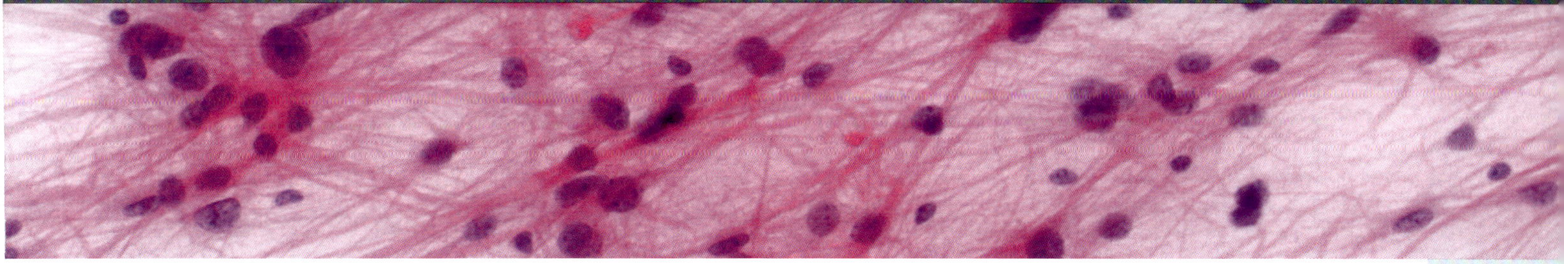

A

B

C

INDEX

INDEX

D

E

F

G

H

I

INDEX

J

K

L

N

O

P

INDEX

INDEX

Q

R

INDEX

S

T

U

V

W

X

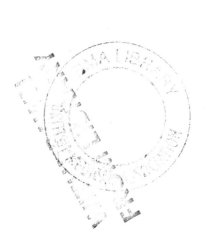